PRINCIPLES AND PRACTICE OF DIALYSIS

THIRD EDITION

PRINCIPLES AND PRACTICE OF DIALYSIS

THIRD EDITION

Editor

WILLIAM L. HENRICH, M.D.

Theodore E. Woodward Professor and Chairman
Department of Medicine
University of Maryland School of Medicine
Physician-in-Chief
University of Maryland Medical Center
Baltimore, Maryland

LIPPINCOTT WILLIAMS & WILKINS
A **Wolters Kluwer** Company

Philadelphia • Baltimore • New York • London
Buenos Aires • Hong Kong • Sydney • Tokyo

Acquisitions Editor: Timothy Y. Hiscock
Developmental Editor: Nicole Wagner
Production Editor: Thomas Boyce
Manufacturing Manager: Colin Warnock
Cover Designer: Christine Jenny
Compositor: Lippincott Williams & Wilkins Desktop Division
Printer: Maple Press

Library of Congress Cataloging-in-Publication Data

Principles and practice of dialysis / editor, William L. Henrich.— 3rd ed.
    p. ; cm.
    Includes bibliographical references and index.
    ISBN 0-7817-3881-4
    1. Hemodialysis. I. Henrich, William L.
    [DNLM: 1. Renal Dialysis. 2. Kidney Failure, Chronic—complications. 3. Kidney Failure, Chronic—therapy. WJ 378 P957 2003]
    RC901.7.H45P75 2003
    617.4′61059—dc21
                                                                2003047693

Care has been taken to confirm the accuracy of the information presented and to describe generally accepted practices. However, the authors, editor, and publisher are not responsible for errors or omissions or for any consequences from application of the information in this book and make no warranty, expressed or implied, with respect to the currency, completeness, or accuracy of the contents of the publication. Application of this information in a particular situation remains the professional responsibility of the practitioner.

The authors, editor, and publisher have exerted every effort to ensure that drug selection and dosage set forth in this text are in accordance with current recommendations and practice at the time of publication. However, in view of ongoing research, changes in government regulations, and the constant flow of information relating to drug therapy and drug reactions, the reader is urged to check the package insert for each drug for any change in indications and dosage and for added warnings and precautions. This is particularly important when the recommended agent is a new or infrequently employed drug.

Some drugs and medical devices presented in this publication have Food and Drug Administration (FDA) clearance for limited use in restricted research settings. It is the responsibility of the health care provider to ascertain the FDA status of each drug or device planned for use in their clinical practice.

10 9 8 7 6 5 4 3 2 1

For our housestaff, fellows and students, past, present and future: you are the inspiration for our work and our hope for brighter tomorrows

CONTENTS

CONTRIBUTING AUTHORS

Jorge Luis Ajuria, M.D. Department of Medicine, Senior Fellow, Division of Renal Diseases and Hypertension, George Washington University Medical Center, Washington, D.C.

Imran I. Ali, M.D. Director, Comprehensive Epilepsy Program, Department of Neurology, Medical College of Ohio, Toledo, Ohio

George R. Aronoff, M.D., F.A.C.P. Chief, Division of Nephrology, University of Louisville; Professor, Departments of Medicine and Pharmacology, University of Louisville, Louisville, Kentucky

Michael J. Berkoben, M.D. Associate Professor of Medicine, Duke University Medical Center, Durham, North Carolina

Anatole Besarab, M.D. Director of Clinical Research, Division of Nephrology and Hypertension, Henry Ford Hospital, Detroit, Michigan

Paola Boccardo, Biol.Sci.D Clinical Research Center for Rare Diseases 'Aldo e Cele Dacco', Villa Camozzi, Ranica; Negri Bergamo Laboratories, Mario Negri Institute for Pharmacological Research, Bergamo, Italy

Michael E. Brier, Ph.D. Kidney Disease Program, Division of Nephrology, University of Louisville School of Medicine, Louisville, Kentucky

Andrew E. Briglia, D.O. Department of Medicine, Nephrology Division, University of Maryland School of Medicine, Baltimore, Maryland

Wendy Weinstock Brown, M.D., M.P.H. Director, Clinical Nephrology, St. Louis Department of Veterans Affairs Medical Center; Professor, Internal Medicine, St. Louis University School of Medicine, St. Louis, Missouri

John M. Burkart, M.D. Nephrology Division, Bowman Gray School of Medicine; Professor of Medicine and Nephrology, Director of Outpatient Dialysis Services, Department of Nephrology, Wake Forest University Medical Center, Winston-Salem, North Carolina

Vito M. Campese, M.D. Department of Medicine, Nephrology Division, LAC/USC Medical Center; Professor of Medicine, Chief, Division of Nephrology, Keck School of Medicine, University of Southern California, Los Angeles, California

Charles B. Cangro, M.D. Assistant Professor, Department of Medicine-Nephrology, University of Maryland Hospital, Baltimore, Maryland

Thawee Chanchairujira, M.D. Department of Medicine, Siriraj Hospital, Mahidol University, Bangkok, Thailand

Srivasa B. Chebrolu, M.D. Research Associate, Nephrology Division of Medicine, VA Hospital, Hines, Illinois

Allan J. Collins, M.D., F.A.C.P. Director, Nephrology Analytical Services, Minneapolis Medical Research Foundation; Professor, School of Medicine, University of Minnesota, Minneapolis, Minnesota

Rochelle Cunningham, M.D. Assistant Professor, Department of Medicine, Division of Nephrology, University of Maryland School of Medicine, Baltimore, Maryland

Thomas A. Depner, M.D. Professor of Medicine, Nephrology Division, University of California, Davis, Medical Center, Sacramento, California

Béatrice Descamps-Latscha, M.D. Director of Research, INSERM U507, Necker Hospital, Paris, France

George T. Fantry, M.D. Director, Clinical Gastroenterology, Associate Professor, Department of Medicine, University of Maryland Medical Center, Baltimore, Maryland

Jeffrey C. Fink, M.D. Staff Physician, Department of Medicine, Associate Professor, Division of Nephrology, University of Maryland School of Medicine, Baltimore, Maryland

Lucy Fox, M.D., F.A.C.P. Renal Medicine Associates, Albuquerque, New Mexico

Eli A. Friedman, M.D. Distinguished Teaching Professor, Chief, Renal Disease Division, SUNY Downstate Medical Center, University Hospital, Brooklyn, New York

Miriam Galbusera, Biol.Sci.D   Head, Unit of Platelet Endothelial Cell Interaction, Negri Bergamo Laboratories, Mario Negri Institute for Pharmacological Research, Bergamo, Italy

Serafino Garella, M.D.   Chairman, Department of Medicine, Lutheran General Hospital, Park Ridge; Professor of Medicine, Department of Medicine, Chicago Medical School, North Chicago, Illinois

F. John Gennari, M.D.   Attending Physician, Department of Medicine, Fletcher Allen Health Care; Patrick Professor of Medicine, Department of Medicine, University of Vermont College of Medicine, Burlington, Vermont

Stuart L. Goldstein, M.D.   Medical Director, Renal Dialysis Unit, Texas Children's Hospital; Assistant Professor, Pediatrics, Baylor College of Medicine, Houston, Texas

Thomas A. Golper, M.D.   Professor of Medicine, Department of Medicine, Division of Nephrology, Vanderbilt University Medical Center, Nashville, Tennessee

Donna S. Hanes, M.D.   Clerkship Director, Department of Internal Medicine; Assistant Professor, Department of Medicine, University of Maryland, Baltimore, Maryland

William L. Henrich, M.D.   Physician-in-Chief, Department of Medicine, University of Maryland School of Medicine, Baltimore, Maryland

L. David Hillis, M.D.   Vice Chair, Department of Medicine, University of Texas Southwestern Medical Center, Dallas, Texas

Todd S. Ing, M.D., F.A.C.P.   Attending Physician, Department of Medicine, Veterans Affairs Hospital, Hines; Professor of Medicine, Department of Medicine, Stritch School of Medicine, Loyola University, Maywood, Illinois

Kathy L. Jabs, M.D.   Director, Pediatric Nephrology, Vanderbilt University Medical Center; Associate Professor, Department of Pediatrics, Vanderbilt University School of Medicine, Nashville, Tennessee

Paul Jungers, M.D.   Emeritus Professor of Nephrology, Faculty of Medicine, Necker-Enfants Malades, Paris, France

Toros Kapoian, M.D.   Medical Director, Dialysis, Robert Wood Johnson University Hospital; Associate Professor of Medicine, Department of Medicine, Division of Nephrology, University of Medicine and Dentistry of New Jersey–Robert Wood Johnson Medical School, New Brunswick, New Jersey

Paul L. Kimmel, M.D.   Attending Physician, Department of Medicine, George Washington University Hospital; Professor of Medicine, Division of Renal Diseases and Hypertension, George Washington University Medical Center, Washington, D.C.

David K. Klassen, M.D.   Medical Director, Kidney and Pancreas Transplantation, Department of Medicine, University of Maryland Hospital; Professor of Medicine, Department of Medicine, University of Maryland School of Medicine, Baltimore, Maryland

Stephen M. Korbet, M.D.   Associate Director, Nephrology, Department of Internal Medicine, Rush Presbyterian–St. Luke's Medical Center; Professor of Medicine, Department of Internal Medicine, Rush Medical College, Chicago, Illinois

Victoria A. Kumar, M.D.   Department of Nephrology, University of California, Davis, Medical Center, Davis, California

Richard A. Lafayette, M.D.   Associate Chair, Department of Medicine; Associate Professor, Department of Medicine, Stanford University Medical Center, Stanford, California

George Lai, M.D.   Associate Physician, The Permanente Medical Group, Kaiser Hayward, Hayward, California

Paul D. Light, M.D.   Associate Professor, Division of Nephrology, Department of Medicine, University of Maryland School of Medicine, Baltimore, Maryland

Ravindra L. Mehta, M.D.   Professor of Clinical Medicine, Department of Medicine, Division of Nephrology and Hypertension, University of California, San Diego, San Diego, California

Susan R. Mendley, M.D.   Director of Nephrology, Department of Pediatrics, University of Maryland Medical Center; Assistant Professor, Departments of Pediatrics and Medicine, University of Maryland School of Medicine, Baltimore, Maryland

Ayesa N. Mian, M.D.   Assistant Professor, Pediatric Nephrology, University of Maryland, Baltimore, Maryland

Anne Marie V. Miles, M.D., F.A.C.P.   Attending Physician in Nephrology, Northshore Medical Center, Miami, Florida

R. Tyler Miller, M.D.   Chief, Nephrology, Department of Medicine, Louis Stokes VAMC; Professor of Medicine and Physiology, Departments of Medicine and Physiology, Case Western Reserve University, Cleveland, Ohio

Sean W. Murphy, M.D.   Patient Research Center, The Health Sciences Center Memorial University of Newfoundland, St. John's, Newfoundland, Canada

B.V.R. Murthy, M.D.   Assistant Professor of Medicine, Division of Renal Diseases and Hypertension, University of Texas Houston Medical School, Houston, Texas

Svetlozar N. Natov, M.D.   Chief Medical Officer, Medical Director, Department of Medicine, Northeast Specialty Hospital, Braintree; Assistant Professor of Medicine, Division of Nephrology, Tufts New England Medical Center, Tufts University School of Medicine, Boston, Massachusetts

Andrew S. O'Connor, D.O.   Clinical Research Fellow, Department of Nephrology, MetroHealth Medical Center; Clinical Research Fellow, Division of Nephrology, Case Western Reserve University, Cleveland, Ohio

Biff F. Palmer, M.D.   Professor of Internal Medicine, Department of Internal Medicine, University of Texas Southwestern Medical School, Dallas, Texas

Patrick S. Parfrey, M.D., F.R.C.P.C., F.A.C.P.   Staff Nephrologist, Department of Medicine, Health Sciences Centre; University Research Professor, Department of Medicine, Memorial University, St. John's, Newfoundland, Canada

Brian J.G. Pereira, M.D.   President and Chief Executive Officer, New England Health Care Foundation, New England Medical Center; Louisa C. Endicott Professor of Medicine, Department of Medicine, Tufts University School of Medicine, Boston, Massachusetts

Andreas Pierratos, M.D., F.R.C.P.C.   Staff Nephrologist, Department of Medicine, Humber River Regional Hospital; Associate Professor, Department of Medicine, University of Toronto, Toronto, Ontario, Canada

Noor A. Pirzada, M.D.   Associate Professor, Department of Neurology, Medical College of Ohio Hospital, Toledo, Ohio

Giuseppe Remuzzi, M.D.   Director, Division of Nephrology and Dialysis, Azienda Ospedaliera, Ospedali Riuniti di Bergamo; Director, Negri Bergamo Laboratories, Mario Negri Institute for Pharmacological Research, Bergamo, Italy

Roger A. Rodby, M.D.   Associate Attending Physician, Department of Internal Medicine, Rush Presbyterian–St. Luke's Medical Center; Associate Professor of Medicine, Department of Internal Medicine, Rush Medical College, Chicago, Illinois

Daniel J. Salzberg, M.D.   Division of Nephrology, University of Maryland Medical System; Assistant Professor of Medicine, Department of Medicine, University of Maryland, Baltimore, Maryland

Steve J. Schwab, M.D.   Professor and Chair, Department of Medicine, Duke University Medical Center, Durham, North Carolina

Richard A. Sherman, M.D.   Professor of Medicine, University of Medicine and Dentistry of New Jersey, Robert Wood Johnson Medical School, New Brunswick, New Jersey

Donald J. Sherrard, M.D.   Chief, Nephrology and Specialty Primary Care, Puget Sound Health Care Systems; Professor, Department of Medicine, University of Washington, Seattle, Washington

Edith M. Simmons, M.D.   Clinical Fellow in Nephrology, Department of Nephrology, Vanderbilt University, Nashville, Tennessee

William J. Stone, M.D.   Chief of Nephrology, Medical Service, Veterans Administration Medical Center; Professor, Department of Medicine, Vanderbilt University, Nashville, Tennessee

Adina Tanasescu, M.D.   Division of Nephrology, Keck School of Medicine, University of Southern California, Los Angeles, California

Robert D. Toto, M.D.   Medical Director, Acute Dialysis Unit, Parkland Memorial Hospital; Professor of Medicine, Department of Internal Medicine, University of Texas Southwestern Medical Center of Dallas, Dallas, Texas

Antonios H. Tzamaloukas, M.D.   Chief, Renal Section, New Mexico Veterans Administration Health Care System; Professor, Department of Medicine, University of New Mexico, Albuquerque, New Mexico

Ravinder K. Wali, M.D.   Attending Physician, University Hospital; Assistant Professor, Department of Nephrology, University of Maryland School of Medicine, Baltimore, Maryland

Bradley A. Warady, M.D.   Chief, Section of Pediatric Nephrology, Director, Dialysis and Transplantation, Section of Pediatric Nephrology, The Children's Mercy Hospital; Professor of Pediatrics, Department of Pediatric Nephrology, University of Missouri-Kansas City School of Medicine, Kansas City, Missouri

Richard A. Ward, Ph.D.   Professor, Department of Medicine, University of Louisville, Louisville, Kentucky

B. Blake Weathersby, M.D.   Clinical Fellow, Division of Nephrology, Vanderbilt University School of Medicine, Nashville, Tennessee

Matthew R. Weir, M.D.   Director, Division of Nephrology, Department of Medicine, University of Maryland Hospital; Professor of Medicine, Department of Medicine, University of Maryland School of Medicine, Baltimore, Maryland

Jay Barry Wish, M.D.   Medical Director, Hemodialysis Services, University Hospitals of Cleveland; Professor, Department of Medicine, Case Western Reserve University, Cleveland, Ohio

Véronique Witko-Sarsat, Ph.D.   Director of Research, Department of Nephrology, Necker Hospital, Paris, France

Marsha Wolfson, M.D.   Senior Medical Director, Nephrology, U.S. Medical Affairs, Amgen, Inc., Thousand Oaks, California; Clinical Professor, Department of Medicine, Oregon Health Sciences University, Portland, Oregon

PREFACE

The practice of dialysis, like many practices in medicine, is a balance between science, clinical judgment and practicality. In recent years this practice has been improved by the publication of an increasing number of well-performed, rigorously conducted clinical trials complimented by a growing portfolio of well-executed translational science studies on the physiology of uremia. As is always the case, these new studies have altered practice while inevitably raising new questions that will require further investigation. In the aggregate, there is a sense that the field is moving, and practitioners are constantly being challenged to keep pace.

The third edition of *Principles and Practice of Dialysis* has been written in response to the ongoing need for current, but practically focused, information grounded on the latest and best evidence. Entirely new subjects discussed in this edition include Choosing the Best Dialysis Option in the Patient with Chronic Renal Failure, Nocturnal Dialysis, Oxidant Stress in ESRD, GI Complications in ESRD, Quality of Life and Rehabilitation in Dialysis Patients, Preparing Dialysis Patients for Renal Transplantation, and Current Outcomes for Dialysis Patients. Other topics have been re-approached and rewritten with the overall goal of always providing detailed information in an organized, accessible format.

It is the collective hope of everyone associated with *Principles and Practice of Dialysis* that this book will serve as a useful platform from which to guide therapy today while, at the same time, it points the way to tomorrow's discoveries that will improve the health of patients requiring dialytic therapy.

ACKNOWLEDGMENTS

I want to express my gratitude to the many authors whose excellent work is provided in the text. Their contributions will determine the ultimate success of this project. I also owe thanks to my administrative assistant, Ms. Phyllis Farrell, for her professional and cheerful assistance in the process of editing and organizing the final manuscript. Ms. Nicole Wagner and Mr. Tim Hiscock of Lippincott Williams & Wilkins also deserve thanks for their help and encouragement with all aspects of this project.

PRINCIPLES AND PRACTICE OF DIALYSIS

THIRD EDITION

CHOICE OF THE HEMODIALYSIS MEMBRANE

JORGE LUIS AJURIA AND PAUL L. KIMMEL

Since Congress passed the Medicare Act in 1972 that allocated federal funding for the end-stage renal disease (ESRD) program in the United States, the numbers of new patients initiated yearly on chronic renal replacement therapy has steadily grown. Most new patients receiving chronic renal replacement therapy in the United States are treated with hemodialysis (HD) rather than peritoneal dialysis (PD). Patients treated with HD today live longer in part because of better medical care, including but not limited to higher prescribed doses of therapy, improved dialyzer membrane design, the introduction of recombinant erythropoietin, and advances in calcium/phosphate management to prevent debilitating renal osteodystrophy (1–3).

Recognition of transient intradialytic leukopenia associated with cellulose-based membranes by Kaplow and Goffinet (4) began a new era of research on membrane biocompatibility that stimulated the development of new membrane materials. Advances in dialyzer design and membrane materials were supported by funding from the U.S. Artificial Kidney/Uremia Program of the National Institute of Arthritis, Metabolism, and Digestive Diseases. The development of chronic dialysis programs, vascular access technology, the hollow-fiber dialyzer, and formulation of the middle molecule hypothesis contributed significantly to advancements in membrane transport properties (5).

Despite medical and technologic advances over the past two decades, mortality among chronic ESRD patients remains high, and the choices facing the nephrology community in management decisions remain complex and often unresolved. This chapter focuses on dialyzer properties, types of dialyzer membrane materials available, what is known about the inflammatory response to bioincompatible membranes, and clinical sequelae in ESRD patients who are treated with chronic HD.

EPIDEMIOLOGY

The United States Renal Data System 2001 Annual Report showed that in 1999, more than 330,000 people in the United States with chronic ESRD required renal replacement therapy (6). Of these ESRD patients, approximately 64% received HD, 7% received PD, and the remaining 29% had a functioning

renal transplant. In the same year, 80,000 new ESRD patients were started on either HD or PD in the United States.

Comorbid medical conditions are commonly seen in patients requiring renal replacement therapy (7). The large burden of comorbidity in HD patients has an important effect on mortality, frequency of hospitalizations, and overall perception of quality of life. Sixty-seven thousand chronic ESRD patients, approximately 20% of the total number receiving renal replacement therapy in 1999, died with either a functioning renal transplant or while receiving dialysis (6). In the first year of renal replacement therapy, patients receiving HD had the highest mortality when compared with patients receiving PD or treated with a functioning transplant. This statistic was determined after adjustment for known predictors of mortality in ESRD patients: age, gender, race, and primary diagnosis of diabetes (8). Two-year mortality rates among all patients receiving renal replacement therapy remain about 20%. Cause-specific death rates from 1997 to 1999 in prevalent ESRD patients (ESRD patients treated with dialysis more than 1 year) age 20 and older were slightly higher among nondiabetic patients treated with HD when compared with PD. Prevalent ESRD patients with diabetes mellitus treated with PD had the highest mortality during this period of time. Of patients with ESRD who lived 10 or more years, approximately 69% had a functioning renal transplant, 29% received HD, and 3% received PD. Most patients with ESRD who die, will do so from cardiovascular or infectious causes while receiving chronic HD (6,9).

HEMODIALYSIS

The goals of HD are treatment of uremic symptoms, correction of acidemia, prevention of hyperkalemia and life-threatening electrolyte disorders, restoration of solute balance, and maintenance of volume status. For patients with ESRD treated with chronic HD, long-term goals are to ensure quality of life, maintain nutritional stability, and decrease morbidity and mortality. The introduction of recombinant human erythropoietin in the late 1980s alleviated the need for treatment of anemia in ESRD patients with multiple blood transfusions or administration of androgens (10–12).

Hemodialysis Operations

When HD is performed, two major circuits are involved: the blood circuit and the dialysate circuit (Fig. 1.1) (13). The blood circuit is composed of the patient, the vascular access, the tubing that transports blood to the HD machine, a dialyzer or artificial kidney, a HD machine, and tubing that returns blood to the patient. Extracorporeal circulation begins either at the "arterial" needle inserted into an arteriovenous anastomotic site or from a catheter port inserted in a large central vein (typically femoral, jugular, or subclavian). Blood flows from the patient at a rate of 200 to 400 mL/min. Blood is carried through the tubing from the vascular access site to the dialyzer under negative pressure produced by a blood pump in the HD machine. Blood is then typically transported through thousands of narrow hollow-fiber capillary tubes composed of a semipermeable membrane. Blood returns to the patient from the dialyzer through the "venous" blood tubing under positive pressure. The extracorporeal circulation terminates at either a venous needle at the arteriovenous anastomotic site or at a second venous catheter port. The dialysate circuit consists of concentrated dialysate that is mixed with treated water within the dialysis machine. The dialysate flows at a rate usually set between 500 to 800 mL/min countercurrent to blood in the compartment that immediately surrounds the hollow-fiber capillaries within the dialyzer. The dialysate flows into a drain after flowing through the dialyzer and is discarded.

Purity of water, in part to limit contamination, is maintained by treatment before mixing with concentrated dialysate in the dialysis machine. These functions are covered in guidelines issued by the Association for the Advancement of Medical Instruments (AAMI). In a typical water treatment design, municipal water is first routed through softeners and charcoal for the removal of chlorine. This is followed by flow through sediment filters, reverse osmosis systems, and ultraviolet lighting to control for microbial growth. Deionizing systems are used in the removal of aluminum and other metals. Treated water is pressurized and circulated for use with the dialysis machines and during reuse sterilization (14).

Diffusion and Ultrafiltration

Conventional HD involves two primary events: (a) correction of solute and electrolyte abnormalities and (b) volume removal by formation of a plasma ultrafiltrate. Thomas Graham (1805–1869), Chair of Chemistry at University College in London, first coined the term *dialysis* to describe the movement of

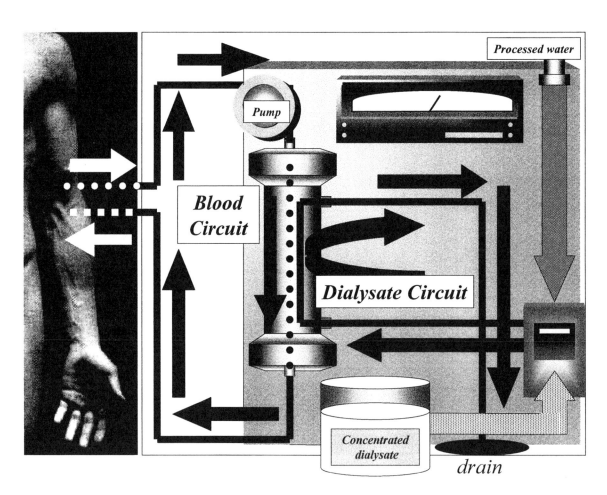

FIG. 1.1. Schematic representation of the hemodialysis operation. The blood circuit and the dialysate circuit interact at the dialyzer membrane.

colloids suspended in fluid through albumin-coated vegetable parchment into water. Graham's experiments demonstrated that solutes could be removed from fluids containing colloids and crystalloids (15). Nearly 150 years later, restoration of solute balance and correction of electrolyte abnormalities in HD patients is attained by the same diffusive transport. The hollow-fiber dialyzer is the most commonly used dialyzer in practice today in the United States. The parallel-plate dialyzer developed in the late 1960s is less commonly used. Both types of dialyzer contain four ports: two communicate with the blood circuit and two communicate with the dialysate circuit. In the hollow-fiber dialyzer, blood flows through thousands of hollow fibers surrounded by dialysate solution. The total membrane surface area available for solute transport in a hollow-fiber dialyzer is dependent on the number, length, and diameter of individual fibers (16). The individual fibers function as a semipermeable membrane between blood and dialysate. At the blood-dialysate capillary membrane interface, solutes and electrolytes diffuse down a concentration gradient from either the blood or dialysate compartment. Volume is removed from the patient when blood circulates through hollow fiber capillaries under negative pressure and a plasma ultrafiltrate is formed. The ultrafiltrate is formed in the dialysate compartment and then discarded through the drain. During ultrafiltration, solute and electrolytes are cleared from plasma by convective transport. Convective transport alone does not significantly alter plasma solute concentration. Plasma solute concentration is altered primarily by diffusive transport.

Urea Kinetic Modeling: *Kt/V*

Determination of adequacy of HD is a complicated and controversial topic that is discussed elsewhere. Candidates for unique toxins responsible for the uremic syndrome are many and are truly not known. Because uremic toxins are presumed to be both small and large solutes, urea removal has been used as one surrogate marker to measure the adequacy of prescribed HD. The use of urea clearance for dialysis adequacy is based on results from the National Cooperative Dialysis Study (NCDS) that used urea as a surrogate marker to determine parameters for prescribing adequate HD (17,18).

The urea reduction ratio (URR) and *Kt/V* are the most commonly used methods for estimating adequacy of prescribed dialysis (see Chapters 7 and 9 for a complete discussion). The amount of plasma cleared of urea during one dialysis session R can be estimated by the ratio of the postdialysis to the predialysis urea nitrogen serum concentration.

$$R = \frac{\text{Postdialysis serum urea nitrogen concentration}}{\text{Predialysis serum urea nitrogen concentration}}$$

The lower the ratio, the greater the amount of urea cleared. The URR is calculated by subtracting R from 1. For example, an R = 0.35 would be equivalent to a URR of 65.

The *Kt/V* was developed after the NCDS in an independent analysis by Gotch and Sargent (18) as an index for dialysis delivery. K represents the amount of urea cleared from total body water, measured in milliliters per minute. The value of K is dependent on patient height, weight, residual renal function, interdialytic weight gain, and the dialyzer's expected urea clearance as

determined by the manufacturer; t is the duration of dialysis in minutes; V is the volume of the patient's urea pool, measured in milliliters. Because urea is presumed to be freely distributed in all body compartments, the volume of urea distribution is assumed to approximate the volume of total body water. V is commonly taken to be 60% of total body weight in males and 50% total body weight in females. *Kt/V* correlates with the URR. Higher values of *Kt/V* and URR have been associated with decreased morbidity and mortality in chronic ESRD patients on maintenance dialysis in observational studies (9,14,17,19–22).

Urea kinetic modeling using *Kt/V* is plagued with many inaccuracies (13). The manufacturer's urea clearance data for a particular dialyzer can overestimate K by 15% to 20%. Dialyzer reuse and fiber clotting can decrease dialyzer urea clearance. The volume of distribution for urea, V, is less than the volume of total body water. Recirculation, improper collection of preserum and postserum blood urea nitrogen (BUN) samples as well as urea rebound can further contribute to inaccuracies in calculated *Kt/V*.

DIALYZER STRUCTURE

Membrane KoA

Diffusion of a solute across the membrane surface is dependent on solute size, molecular weight, and the blood-dialysate concentration gradient. Movement of a solute through a pore by diffusive transport is reduced as molecular size increases and approaches that of the pore. The rate of diffusion is inversely proportional to the molecular weight of the solute (23). An unstirred layer of fluid on either the blood or dialysate side of the membrane surface can decrease the effective concentration gradient across a membrane. Dialyzer design and blood flow rates affect the thickness of unstirred fluid layers (24,25).

Solute transport is dependent on the overall resistance (R_o) opposing transport from the center of the bloodstream to the center of the dialysate stream (Fig. 1.2) (26). The sum of all

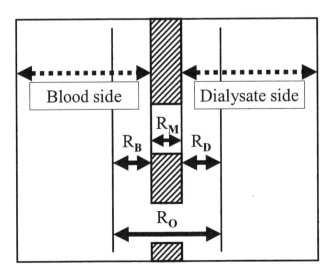

FIG. 1.2. Schematic representation of overall resistance (R_O) opposing transport from the center of the blood stream to the center of the dialysate stream. Blood side resistance (R_B) and dialysate side resistance (R_D) are dependent on blood and dialysate flow rates. Membrane resistance (R_M) depends on the thickness of the dialyzer membrane.

resistance encountered, referred to as mass transfer resistance, is expressed as

$$R_o = R_B + R_M + R_D$$

where R_o equals mass transfer resistance, R_B equals blood side resistance, R_M equals membrane resistance, and R_D equals dialysate side resistance. Blood flow rate, membrane structure, and dialysate flow rate determine mass transfer resistance (25). Increasing the blood flow rate will decrease R_B by decreasing unstirred layers on the blood side of the membrane. Likewise, dialysate side resistance can be decreased by increasing the rate of the dialysate flow and decreasing the extent of the unstirred layers on the dialysate side of the membrane (25).

The capacity of a dialyzer for maximal clearance of urea and solutes of similar molecular weight is described by the solute flux constant KoA, measured in milliliters per minute. KoA is a theoretical value determined by the manufacturer for a particular dialyzer, representing maximum urea clearance at infinite blood and dialysate flow rates (24). KoA is proportional to membrane surface area.

$$Ko = \frac{J/A}{\text{concentration gradient}}$$

$$KoA = \frac{J}{\text{concentration gradient}} \quad (23)$$

where Ko is the transport coefficient, A is the membrane area, and J is flux.

KoA is independent of membrane pore size, such that membranes with high KoA values can have small or large pores. Membranes with KoA values less than 500 mL/min are potentially less efficient at urea clearance, whereas membranes with a KoA greater than 700 mL/min have the potential for highly efficient urea clearance. The ultimate urea clearance achieved is dependent on blood flow rates, although other factors may affect the final result. If a low efficiency dialyzer is used with a KoA of 300 mL/min, doubling the blood flow rate from 200 to 400 mL/min would increase the urea clearance by approximately 25%. Comparably, doubling the blood flow rate of a high-KoA dialyzer (KoA = 800 mL/min) will increase urea clearance by 40% (24).

High-Flux Dialyzers and β₂-Microglobulin

The term *high-efficiency* refers to dialyzers with the capacity for high urea clearance (see Chapter 10 for details). The term *high-flux* refers to dialyzers with membranes that have large pore size and are able to clear solutes of larger molecular weight. High-flux dialyzers have higher ultrafiltration coefficients because of their larger pore size. Thin membranes with large pores have greater transport capacity. Not only do large pores allow diffusion of larger molecules with higher molecular weight but also smaller particles can more easily be transported through larger pores. This is of special significance with clearance of middle molecules such as β₂-microglobulin (27).

The Hemodialysis (HEMO) Study Group is a multicenter, randomized clinical trial with approximately 1,800 chronic ESRD patients, sponsored by the National Institute of Diabetes,

Digestive and Kidney Diseases (NIDDK), of the National Institutes of Health (NIH). The HEMO study was designed to assess the effect of HD dose and membrane flux on mortality and hospitalizations of ESRD patients treated with HD. The HEMO study proposed that the β₂-microglobulin clearance be used to define membrane permeability characteristics. A dialyzer with a β₂-microglobulin clearance less than 10 mL/min is described as a low-flux or low-permeability dialyzer, whereas a membrane with a β₂-microglobulin clearance greater than 20 mL/min is classified as a high-flux or high-permeability dialyzer (28). β₂-microglobulin is a low molecular weight protein (11,800 daltons) found on the surface of nucleated cells, where it functions as a light chain of the class I major histocompatibility complex [human leukocyte antigen (HLA)]. β₂-microglobulin is dissociated from the HLA complex and released into the extracellular fluid as a result of metabolism and cellular degradation. Daily production in a normal human averages 150 to 200 mg/day (29). In humans with normal renal function approximately 340 mg are filtered daily, 99.9% is reabsorbed in the proximal tubule, and maximal urinary excretion is approximately 370 µg/24 hours (30,31). Normal serum concentrations range from 1 to 3 mg/L. In patients treated with chronic HD, serum levels as high as 40 to 60 mg/L have been reported (32). Low-flux membranes do not remove significant amounts of β₂-microglobulin. Small amounts (100 to 200 mg/treatment) of β₂-microglobulin (33) can be removed by high-flux membranes through convective transport and adsorption to the membrane surface (34). Over time, accumulation of β₂-microglobulin can lead to the development of dialysis-related amyloidosis (35).

Preliminary results of the HEMO study announced at the National Kidney Foundation (NKF) meeting in April 2002 suggest that patients who received a prescribed HD dose (*Kt/V* > 1.05) or were dialyzed with low-flux membranes neither lived longer nor had fewer hospitalizations than patients who received an equilibrated *Kt/V* greater than 1.45 or were treated with high-flux dialyzers. Specific subgroup analyses may generate hypotheses regarding gender or duration of time on chronic HD; however, those hypotheses need further study (36).

DIALYZER MEMBRANES
Membrane Material

One property by which hemodialyzers can be categorized is by the chemical composition of the semipermeable membrane. The fibers may be composed of either cellulose monomers, modified cellulose monomers with addition of acetyl groups, synthetic polymers, or a combination of cellulose-based and synthetic polymers (Table 1.1) (24). Generally, cellulose based membranes are referred to as "bioincompatible" membranes, because of their ability to activate complement. In comparison to cellulose membranes, modified cellulose membranes and newer synthetic membranes are generally considered "biocompatible."

Evolution of the Dialyzer Membrane

In 1913, Abel, Roundtree, and Turner at Johns Hopkins Medical School in Baltimore were first to successfully remove solutes

TABLE 1.1. MEMBRANES AVAILABLE AND MATERIAL COMPOSITION

Membrane Type	Material
Cellulose	Regenerated cellulose
	Cuprammonium cellulose (Cuprophan)
	Cuprammonium rayon
	Cuprammonium saponified ester
Coated cellulose	Cuprammonium rayon coated with polyethylene glycol (PEG)
	Regenerated cellulose coated with vitamin E (Excebrane)
Substituted cellulose	Cellulose acetate (Cellulate)
	Cellulose diacetate
	Cellulose triacetate
Cellulo-synthetic	Cellosyn
	Hemophan
Synthetic	Polyacrylonitrile (PAN)
	Polyacrylonitrile co-polymerized with methalyl sulfonate (AN69)
	Polyamide
	Polycarbonate
	Polyethylene polyvinyl alcohol (EVAL)
	Polymethylmethacrylate (PMMA)
	Polysulfone

Modified from Hoenich NA, et al. Haemodialysis membranes: a matter of fact or taste? *Contrib Nephrol* 2001;133:81–104.

from the blood of nephrectomized animals by extracorporeal circulation through semipermeable celloidin tubes of 8 mm diameter and 40 cm length bathed in dialysis fluid (15). Georg Haas (1886–1971) is credited with the first human dialysis in 1924 using celloidin tubes of longer length (1.2 m), which provided greater membrane surface area for solute diffusion. Chicken intestine and animal peritoneum were investigated by Love in Chicago (1920) and Necheles in Hamburg (1925) as alternative animal-based membrane materials (15). Willem Johan Kolff used cellophane tubing made from regenerated cellulose originally manufactured for sausage casings as membrane material in the 1940s.

Cellulose-based membranes are derived from cotton or wood. Repetitive polysaccharide units on the cellulose membrane, similar to a bacterial cell wall structure, contain hydroxyl groups that provide a surface for activation of the complement pathway (37). Cellulose-based membranes in use throughout the 1960s were manufactured in the form of either continuous sheets or coiled tubing. Their small pore size, relatively large membrane thickness, and hydrophilic properties resulted in inefficient small solute removal with pronounced complement activation and leukopenia (4). Introduction of the modified flat plate dialyzers in the late 1960s improved the efficiency of small solute removal (38). Cuprophan, developed from regenerated cellulose by a different manufacture technique called the cuprammonium process, allowed manufacturers to develop thin, mechanically strong membranes with better diffusive transport of small solutes (5). Regenerated cellulose, cuprammonium cellulose (Cuprophan), and cuprammonium rayon are all cellulosic membranes made of unmodified cellulose monomers.

Modified cellulose and synthetic membranes with increased solute clearance were manufactured in an effort to minimize complement activation and increase clearance of uremic solutes and larger molecular-weight proteins (5). Developed in the 1960s, the first hollow-fiber dialyzer using cellulose acetate became available in the 1970s. Cellulose acetate membranes, composed of cellulose diacetate polymers, were the first modified cellulosic membranes in clinical use in which surface free hydroxyl groups were substituted with acetyl residues. Compared with regenerated cellulose membranes manufactured by the cuprammonium process, cellulose acetate membranes were characterized by increased permeability to water and larger solutes.

Cellulo-synthetic membranes (Hemophan), are cellulose-based membranes wherein the hydroxyl groups have been substituted with tertiary amino groups (39). Newer modified cellulosic membranes made from cellulose triacetate polymers have more complete acetylation of their hydroxyl moieties than those made of cellulose acetate polymers. Synthetic membranes developed during the late 1970s and early 1980s were more hydrophobic than regenerated cellulosic or cellulose-based membranes modified with acetyl residues. Porosity is a fixed and inherent quality of the synthetic material used and is determined by the manufacturing process. The porosity of the synthetic membrane determines the extent of solute flux (KoA) across its surface. Cellulose triacetate membranes have been shown to be comparable to synthetic membranes in relation to complement activation and cytokine production in a small number of studies (40,41). Use of synthetic membranes in the United States and worldwide has increased since their introduction and has exceeded 50% (2,33).

Endotoxins, Bacterial Contaminants, and Membrane Structure

Despite water treatment efforts, dialysate fluid contains bacteria and endotoxins with cytokine-inducing activity. Lipopolysaccharides (LPS) on the outer membrane of gram-negative bacteria consist of a toxic moiety referred to as lipid A, a core polysaccharide, and an O antigen polysaccharide side chain. LPS, also known as endotoxin, can produce fever and septic shock (42). Dialysis membranes may act as barriers to the transport of intact bacteria into the circulation (43). Endotoxins should not cross a typical dialyzer membrane because of their large molecular weight. However, LPS has been shown to cross membranes and retain their cytokine-inducing activity after traversing the membrane and entering the blood (44,45). This may be explained by transport of LPS fragments or other cytokine-activating substances through high-flux membranes (44,46,47).

Transport is mostly by diffusion and is influenced by membrane thickness as well as the physical and chemical composition of the membrane. LPS has been shown to adsorb to both cellulose-based and synthetic membrane surfaces (45). Synthetic membranes contain hydrophobic moieties that are able to bind hydrophobic pyrogens by hydrophobic interaction. Difference in charge between the membrane and bacterial products may also contribute to adsorption. Thicker membranes have a greater capacity to adsorb lipids of hydrophobic peptide-containing bacterial products (48). The large pore size of high-flux membranes can facilitate backfiltration of endotoxin from dialysate, and into the blood, resulting in complement activation (49,50). The backfiltration of dialysate contaminants has been proposed as a possible stimulant of C-reactive protein production by monocytes and macrophages in stable chronic dialysis patients (51).

BIOCOMPATIBILITY

Inflammatory Response

When blood circulates through a dialyzer, the host inflammatory response is variably stimulated by exposure to the HD membrane. Activation of the inflammatory response is probably dependent on the chemical composition of the membrane and the immune and genetic status of the patient, as well as contact of blood with the inert surface of the extracorporeal tubing.

Kaplow and Goffinet (4) were first to describe transient HD-related neutropenia observed in patients while undergoing extracorporeal circulation with cellulose membranes. Concomitant activation of the alternative complement pathway during dialysis with cellulose-based membranes was later described by Craddock and others (52–54). Elevation in serum cytokine levels correlate with elevation in serum complement levels and may be useful as markers of biocompatibility (55–58).

During HD, other humoral pathways such as the contact cascade (59) and cellular mechanisms such as expression of cell surface adhesion proteins by leukocytes (60,61) can be stimulated. In vivo and in vitro studies have demonstrated that exposure of blood to membranes results in variable activation of proteins of the coagulation cascade (52,62), platelets (62), and monocytes (63), as well as degranulation (64) and sequestration (52) of neutrophils. Cytokine production by macrophages and lymphocytes has been proposed as an explanation for acute fever and chronic amyloidosis in HD patients (65). The degree of host inflammatory response and activation of cellular mechanisms is variable and probably dependent at least in part on the chemical composition of the membrane used. The variability in the inflammatory response of blood when it comes into contact with a particular type of dialyzer membrane has been defined by Hakim (66) as the inherent biocompatibility of a membrane.

Adsorption and Clearance of Inflammatory Products by Membranes

Products of the inflammatory response may have one of three potential fates during HD: adsorption to the membrane surface (67–69), clearance from the blood to the dialysate (25,68), or circulation back to the patient. The degree of inflammatory response and serum levels of inflammatory mediators returning to the patient may depend on the type of membrane material, a membrane's protein adsorbing potential, and the magnitude of solute flux (67–69). Cheung et al. (68) demonstrated that activated complement products bind more readily to synthetic membranes than cellulose-based membranes. Measurement of activated complement serum levels drawn from the venous port detect nonadsorbed activated complement products and can underestimate the degree of complement activation by a synthetic membrane.

Because products of the inflammatory response such as complement and cytokines released from monocytes are relatively small molecules, newer high-flux membranes might clear more activated products from the blood during HD (25).

BIOLOGIC EVENTS AT THE MEMBRANE SURFACE

Protein Binding

Plasma protein adsorption onto the membrane surface is an initial event following blood-membrane contact. Adsorption is a result of electrostatic forces, hydrophobic forces, and hydrogen binding between protein and protein and between protein and membrane (33,70). Different membrane types can bind protein to varying degrees, as well as bind different types of protein. Plasma protein adsorption is often followed by platelet and leukocyte binding to the protein-coated membrane surface. Activation of biologic pathways by bound protein can result in thrombogenesis and activation of platelets, contact proteins, and complement.

Thrombogenesis and Platelet Activation

Negatively charged surfaces favor the binding of Hageman factor (factor XII), which can lead to activation of the intrinsic coagulation cascade and conversion of prothrombin to thrombin (33). Thrombin formation and protein deposition result in platelet activation, adherence, and morphologic change. Activated platelets release intracellular stores of thromboxane A_2, adenosine diphosphate (ADP), platelet factor 4 (PF4), and β-thromboglobulin (62,71). Further platelet aggregation and degranulation is induced by thromboxane A_2 and ADP (72). Thrombogenesis and clot formation result in decreased membrane surface area available for solute transport.

Dialysis membranes have been shown to variably activate factor XII (73). HD is associated with formation of platelet-leukocyte aggregates. All membrane types have been shown to form platelet-leukocyte aggregates with variable activation of platelets (62,74). Data suggest that Cuprophan membranes activate platelets more readily when compared with Hemophan or polysulfone membranes (74). Patients chronically dialyzed with polyacrylonitrile (PAN) membranes, when compared with patients chronically dialyzed with Cuprophan membranes, have been also chronically shown to have fewer episodes of arteriovenous fistula thrombosis, lower extremity thrombosis, and fatal pulmonary emboli (75).

Activation of the Contact Pathway

Binding of factor XII with circulating high-molecular-weight-kininogen (HMWK) complexed with prekallikrein leads to formation of activated kallikrein. Once activated, kallikrein is responsible for the release of bradykinin, a potent vasodilator that can decrease arterial resistance and mediate the inflammatory response. Inhibition of angiotensin-converting enzyme (ACE) breakdown of bradykinin has been implicated in the pathogenesis of anaphylactic reactions reported with the use of the AN69 membrane in patients treated with ACE inhibitors (76,77). Because ACE catalyzes breakdown of bradykinin, bradykinin accumulates in the presence of ACE inhibition. In vitro studies with human plasma incubated with AN69 membranes have shown bradykinin generation. Because of their more negatively charged surface, AN69 membranes are believed to activate the contact pathway to a greater degree (77), resulting in increased bradykinin-generating potential (59,76). The AN69 membrane reaction is pH dependent and enhanced in an acidic environment (78).

THE COMPLEMENT SYSTEM

Anaphylatoxins

The complement system functions as a major component of the inflammatory response against microbial agents and foreign particles. It is composed of 20 plasma proteins that can be activated in two different ways, through either the classical or the alternative pathway. The classical pathway is activated by antibody, whereas the alternative pathway is activated independent of antibody. Both pathways culminate with the formation of the membrane attack complex (MAC), C5b-9. Complement activation by dialyzer membranes is associated with the alternative pathway (52,79–81). The anaphylatoxins C3a and C5a are the major complement products generated via the alternative complement cascade. Anaphylatoxins are vasoactive peptides that increase vascular permeability by release of histamine from mast cells (82), stimulate the release of tumor necrosis factor (TNF) and cytokines from monocytes (83,84), and induce neutrophil degranulation (85). In addition, the potent chemotactic factor, complement C5a, causes neutrophil aggregation (85–87), release of free oxygen radicals (88), and altered expression of cell surface receptors that lead to neutrophil sequestration in the pulmonary microvasculature (60). Complement C5a has been shown to enhance release of β_2-microglobulin from peripheral blood monocytes (89).

Alternative Complement Pathway

Activation of the alternative complement pathway requires proteolytic cleavage of C3 into the anaphylatoxin C3a and the activated protein fragment C3b by a C3-cleaving enzyme complex (C3bBb) known as C3 convertase (Fig. 1.3). Complement C3b functions as a cofactor in the generation of new C3 convertase, thereby amplifying its own production as well as that of additional C3a. C3b expresses a binding site for factor B, a proenzyme of both C3 and C5 convertase. Once bound to C3b, factor B is subject to proteolytic cleavage into a 30-kd fragment (Ba) and a larger 80-kd fragment (Bb) by factor D, a plasma serine protease. The larger factor B fragment (Bb) attaches to C3b forming C3bBb, the C3 convertase. The newly generated C3 convertase cleaves another C3 into C3a and C3b, further amplifying the cascade reaction. Similarly, two activated C3b fragments combine with one factor B fragment (Bb) to form the C5 convertase. C5 convertase generates complement C5a and C5b. Complement C5b initiates formation of the MAC (C5b-9), the terminal pathway of the alternative complement system. Hydrophobic binding of the cylindrically shaped MAC to the lipid bilayer of target cells results in membrane disintegration in the vicinity of the integrated complex in addition to formation of transmembrane channels that lead to hypotonic lysis (90).

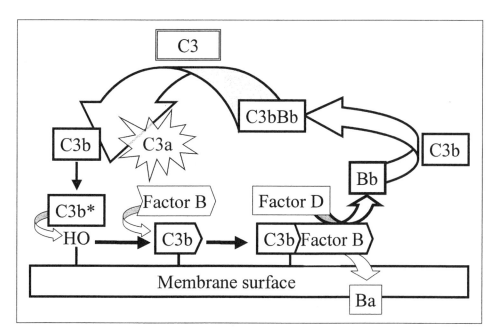

FIG. 1.3. Proposed mechanism for activation of the alternative complement pathway and formation of anaphylatoxin C3a at the dialyzer membrane surface. A free hydroxyl group on the dialyzer membrane surface hydrolyzes the thiolester bond of the activated C3b* fragment. Factor B binds to membrane-bound C3b and is cleaved by Factor D to form Bb. The Bb fragment binds to a free C3b to form the C3 convertase (C3bBb). C3 convertase splits C3 into free C3b and the anaphylatoxin C3a.

Whereas factor B activates the alternative complement cascade by interacting with complement C3b, factor H inactivates the C3b fragment by competitively inhibiting factor B from binding to C3b. Binding of factor H to the C3 convertase will also displace Bb from the protein-cleaving complex, rendering it inactive. When bound to complement C3, factor H functions as a cofactor for the enzymatic degradation of C3b to iC3b. Complement protein iC3b has neutrophil-modulating properties.

Complement Activation and the Membrane Surface

Early experiments demonstrated that levels of C3a and C5a measured from venous ports during HD were greater when cellulose-based membranes were used compared with the effect noted with noncellulosic membranes (54,67). Because cellulose is a polysaccharide composed of hydroxylated glucosan rings, it was suggested that the hydrophilic property of the membrane surface was associated with the degree of complement activation (37). Specifically, hydrolysis of the thiolester bond contained within the activated C3b fragment by free hydroxyl groups on the membrane surface might result in binding of C3b to the membrane surface where it could activate complement (91). When complement C3a and C5a levels were measured in patients dialyzed with either Cuprophan, an unsubstituted cellulosic membrane, or cellulose acetate dialyzers, where 70% of the hydroxyl groups are modified by acetyl residues, complement levels drawn from the venous port were significantly lower in patients dialyzed with cellulose acetate membranes (92,93). The lower levels of activated complement products measured in the venous ports of the patients dialyzed with the cellulose acetate membranes were attributed to the dialyzers' greater hydrophobic properties, resulting from the acetyl moieties on the membrane surface. Subsequent experiments by Cheung et al. (81) analyzing complement proteins eluted from Cuprophan and cellulose acetate membranes demonstrated that binding of factor B and factor H played pivotal roles in complement activation during dialysis. Interestingly, the total amount of complement proteins bound to the cellulose acetate membrane was approximately 20 times that bound to the Cuprophan membrane. However, Cuprophan adsorbed more factor B in proportion to factor H, resulting in more activated C3b membrane-bound and available for complement activation. In contrast, cellulose acetate had proportionally more factor H bound, resulting in accelerated inactivation of C3b.

Membranes are also known to adsorb significant quantities of activated complement products to their surface (94). Cheung et al. (68) demonstrated with in vitro studies that total C3a generation was significantly greater using a high-flux PAN membrane compared with Cuprophan membranes. Total C3a generation was determined by summation of measured concentration of complement C3a in the supernatant and the amount adsorbed to the membrane. Less complement C3a was generated by contact with the cellulosic membrane, and more complement C3a was generated during contact with the synthetic membranes. Because less complement was adsorbed to the membrane surface of the regenerated cellulosic membrane, more remained in the fluid phase. Surprisingly, the synthetic membrane stimulated greater amounts of complement; however, because of its ability to adsorb protein, less was available in the fluid phase that could reenter the patient's circulation. Other investigators have demonstrated that adsorption is also a factor in the removal of factor D, an important cofactor in the formation of C3a convertase (95), as well as cytokines (96) and β_2-microglobulin (34).

Serum levels of activated complement measured from the venous port are greatest approximately 15 to 20 minutes after initiation of dialysis, with gradual return to predialysis levels by the end of dialysis (67). Recent investigations of complement activity after dialysis with different types of membranes demonstrated variable suppression of the classical and alternative complement pathways despite normalization of serum complement concentration to predialysis levels. There was less suppression of the complement pathways in patients dialyzed with PAN and polyethylene glycol (PEG) coated cellulose membranes when compared with cellulose membranes. Factor H levels were shown to be higher in serum from patients dialyzed with cellulose membranes compared with levels measured in patients dialyzed with PAN membranes (97). Eosinophilia can occur during HD and has been associated with allergy to dialyzers with exaggerated activation of complement during HD (98,99). Eosinophil counts were linked to levels of circulating cytokines (99).

Neutrophils

Craddock et al. and others (52,79,100) demonstrated that activation of the alternative complement pathway is associated with transient neutropenia. Upregulation of cell surface integrin receptors on neutrophils causes their margination and sequestration in the pulmonary vasculature (60,61). Entrapment of neutrophils in the pulmonary vasculature results in the fall of arterial oxygen levels (PaO_2) and alterations in the carbon monoxide diffusing capacity of the lung (D_{LCO}) (79,101). Neutropenia begins to resolve within 15 minutes after initiation of dialysis (4,53). Simultaneous downregulation of selectin cell adhesion molecules has been suggested as a possible mechanism for resolution of neutropenia (102).

Numerous studies have demonstrated neutrophil degranulation and release of reactive oxygen species, including superoxide anion, hydrogen peroxide, hydroxyl radicals, and hypochlorous acid, in patients treated with chronic HD (103–105). Advanced oxidation protein products have been shown to be highest in patients treated with HD when compared with patients treated with PD or nondialyzed uremic patients with advanced chronic renal failure (106). Advanced glycation end products are associated with the pathogenesis of aging, as well as accelerated atherosclerosis and β_2-microglobulin amyloid arthropathy (107,108).

Monocytes and Cytokine Production

Patients undergoing HD using cellulose derived membranes show evidence of elevated levels of circulating interleukin-1 (IL-1) (109–112) and TNF before dialysis with further increase after dialysis (57,63). IL-1 produced by macrophages and monocytes affects immune cells, fibroblast proliferation, acute phase reaction mediator synthesis by hepatocytes, and bone resorption (113). IL-1 augments antigen-specific activity by release of interleukin-2 (IL-2) (114) and B-cell mitogenesis (115). Release of IL-2 stimulates T-cell proliferation and clonal expansion of antigen-specific T cells (116), as well as stimulation of phagocytosis and antibody production (117,118).

Complement C3a and C5a can induce IL-1 and TNF-α transcription in mononuclear cells, which can prime inflammatory cells for the translation of cytokines (119). This may result from endotoxin entering the bloodstream from the dialysis fluid (120) or by direct contact with certain membranes (83). IL-1 release and arachidonic acid metabolism in human mononuclear leukocytes has also been demonstrated after exposure to cuprammonium membranes independent of complement activation (121). In an in vitro study by Betz et al. (121), brief contact of human monocytes, platelets, or glomerular epithelial cells with a cellulose based membrane resulted in increased intracellular concentration of calcium, followed by release of prostaglandin E_2 (PGE_2), thromboxane B_2 (TXB_2), and IL-1 independent of complement activation. Monocyte production of interleukin-12 (IL-12), interleukin-6 (IL-6), and interleukin-10 (IL-10) has also been demonstrated in patients undergoing regular dialysis with Hemophan or polyamide dialyzers (122).

We compared plasma concentrations of complement-activated factors C3a and C5a simultaneously with plasma levels of IL-1 and the T-cell growth factor IL-2 in patients treated with Cuprophan, cuprammonium rayon modified cellulose, and Hemophan membranes (57). Circulating levels of IL-1 and IL-2 increased significantly during HD treatments using all three membranes. Patients treated with Cuprophan and Hemophan dialyzers had significantly higher levels of IL-1 compared with patients treated with a modified cellulose dialyzer at 30 and 60 minutes and after HD. In contrast to IL-1, there were no differences in mean circulating IL-2 levels in patients treated with different dialyzer membranes.

IL-6 is a multifunctional cytokine that regulates immune reactions and is principally responsible for acute-phase protein synthesis. IL-6 induces synthesis of serum amyloid A (SAA), C-reactive protein, and α_1-acid glycoprotein, while suppressing synthesis of negative acute-phase proteins, including albumin and transferrin. IL-6 stimulates muscle catabolism (123,124) and serum levels correlate with markers of malnutrition, such as weight loss and serum albumin level (125). Serum IL-6 levels predict degree of hypoalbuminemia, hypocholesterolemia, and mortality in ambulatory HD patients (111,126). C-reactive protein and SAA serum levels have prognostic value in predicting cardiovascular events (127). Uremic patients dialyzed with Cuprophan membranes and uremic patients not treated with renal replacement therapy have higher serum IL-6 levels compared with normal healthy controls and uremic patients dialyzed with polymethylmethacrylate membranes (111,128). The overproduction of proinflammatory cytokines IL-1 and IL-6 may impair immune function (129) or enhance development of amyloidosis (130).

Imbalance between production of reactive oxygen species and antioxidant defense mechanisms results in oxidative stress (see Chapter 20 for a discussion). It is speculated that oxidative stress in HD patients could be involved in accelerated atherosclerosis, amyloidosis, and anemia (131). A dialyzer membrane coated with vitamin E has been recently developed (132). The membrane is composed of a cellulose base chemically fixed to a hydrophilic polymer and fluorocarbon resin. The fluorocarbon resin binds an aliphatic alcohol that is hydrophobically bound to vitamin E (132). Vitamin E has been shown to reduce LPS-induced production of TNFα (133), IL-1 (134), and IL-6 (135). Early in vitro and in vivo studies in chronic HD patients treated with the vitamin-E coated membrane have demonstrated reduced production of IL-6 and reduction in markers of oxidative stress (132,136–139).

We demonstrated that ESRD patients treated with either HD or PD had increased capacity for cellular cytokine production compared with normal controls (116). Elevated cellular cytokine production in both HD and PD patients suggests that cytokine production is not solely a biocompatibility effect. We concluded that patients with renal disease have increased IL-2 production per level of IL-1, unaffected by type or presence of renal replacement therapy. Elevated serum levels of preactivated T-cells with abnormal mitogen-induced IL-2 activity have been demonstrated in patients treated with HD and uremic patients with chronic renal failure not yet treated with renal replacement therapy (140).

DIALYZER MEMBRANE AND CLINICAL SEQUELAE

Survival

In observational studies, chronic ESRD patients treated with synthetic membranes have lower rates of cause-specific mortality and hospitalization when compared with chronic patients treated with cellulosic membranes (141,142). The United States Renal Data System (USRDS) Case-Mix Adequacy Study provided survival data on a sample of approximately 6,000 patients receiving chronic HD treatment in 1990. Data abstracted included patient comorbidities, delivered dose of dialysis, and type of membrane used. Results suggested that dose of dialysis delivered as defined by the urea Kt/V was associated with lower mortality (2,19,143,144).

In the USRDS Case-Mix Adequacy Study, type of dialyzer membrane used was associated with patient survival, when stratified by membrane composition and adjusted for Kt/V and patient comorbidities. Membranes were grouped into three main categories by chemical composition: unsubstituted cellulose, modified cellulose, and synthetic. After adjusting for the presence of comorbid factors such as patient demographics, presence or absence of coronary artery disease, diabetes, pulmonary disease, serum albumin concentration, and dose of delivered dialysis, the relative risk of mortality in patients dialyzed with modified cellulose or synthetic membranes was 25% less ($p < 0.001$) than that of patients treated with unsubstituted cellulose membranes (142). We were able to show similar findings in a small group of patients with ESRD receiving chronic HD in Washington, DC (111). Hakim et al. (142) suggested that differences in patient survival observed with the use of various dialyzer membranes could be attributed to membrane biocompatibility, as well as difference in membrane flux (145), because modified cellulose and synthetic membranes often have higher ultrafiltration coefficients than membranes made from unsubstituted cellulose (146). Other explanations for observed differences in patient survival may be related to clearance of middle molecules (147), better achievement of dry weight with the use of ultrafiltration control machines, and the potential for better medical care at HD centers committing greater financial resources to patients and prescribing more expensive modified cellulose or synthetic membranes (148).

Improved serum albumin levels in stable ESRD patients switched from cuprammonium to polysulfone membranes has been demonstrated (149). However, the impact of membrane biocompatibility on serum albumin levels remains controversial. Not all studies have demonstrated a beneficial effect on serum albumin levels (150). In a recent cross-over study, IL-6 production by peripheral blood mononuclear cells (PBMCs) from HD patients treated with Cuprophan, cellulose diacetate, and synthetically modified cellulose membranes correlated with serum albumin and C-reactive protein levels (151). Patients treated with the synthetically modified membrane were found to have significantly reduced spontaneous release of IL-6 by cultured PBMC, and reduced serum levels of C-reactive protein.

The significance of elevated serum C-reactive protein levels in HD patients is a topic of current investigations (152–157). Early observational studies suggest that the presence of a chronic microinflammatory state in patients treated with chronic HD may predict cardiovascular risk and mortality. Hypoxemia, silent ischemia, and cardiac arrhythmias are known intradialytic complications (52,79,158–160). A correlation between membrane selection and cardiovascular events has not been clearly demonstrated. However, the combination of acetate dialysate buffer and cuprammonium membranes has been associated with adverse cardiac and pulmonary events (161). A trend toward normalization of lipoprotein profiles in patients treated with high-flux dialyzers independent of dietary or other interventions has also been shown in several studies (162–164).

For patients undergoing HD three times a week, chronic complement activation and cytokine production induced by membranes may be associated with increased susceptibility to infection (54,111), increased protein catabolism (123–125), and development of β_2-myoglobulin amyloidosis (89). We were able to show in a predominately African-American, urban, HD population that higher levels of circulating proinflammatory cytokines were associated with mortality, whereas immune parameters reflecting improved T-cell function were associated with survival, independent of other medical risk factors (111).

β_2-Microglobulin and Amyloidosis (see Chapter 23)

There may be a higher incidence of amyloid bone disease in patients undergoing dialysis with cellulose-based membranes (165–167). In a prospective, cross-over study by Zaoui et al. (89), in vitro studies using PBMC obtained from chronic HD patients first treated with Cuprophan membranes then treated with polymethylmethacrylate membranes, a significant increase in cellular expression of β_2-microglobulin was observed in the group treated with Cuprophan that later reversed with the use of

polymethylmethacrylate membranes. Accumulation of β_2-microglobulin in chronic HD patients has also been associated with endotoxin contamination of the dialysate (168,169) and chronic systemic inflammation associated with enhanced cytokine production (170). Proteases and reactive oxygen species are involved in the polymerization of β_2-microglobulin into amyloid (170,171). These findings would suggest that use of biocompatible membranes could slow the development of amyloid deposition or formation in patients treated with long-term HD.

Recent studies by Leypoldt et al. (172) compared β_2-microglobulin plasma concentrations before, during, and after the use of low-flux and high-flux dialyzers. Patients treated with low-flux dialyzers had increased β_2-microglobulin concentrations during dialysis, with decreased β_2-microglobulin concentrations measured after dialysis. The increase in β_2-microglobulin plasma concentration during dialysis with the low-flux membrane was attributed to decreased circulating blood volume and decreased clearance resulting from smaller pore size. Patients treated with high-flux dialyzers had 27% lower β_2-microglobulin plasma concentrations during dialysis; however, plasma concentrations 1 hour after dialysis were only reduced 14%. The rebound in plasma concentration may be attributed to unequal distribution of β_2-microglobulin in the extracellular compartment or shedding of β_2-microglobulin by cell surfaces (172).

DIALYZER REUSE

Dialyzer reuse has been practiced for several decades, and the trend to use reprocessed dialyzers has increased steadily in U.S. dialysis centers (see Chapter 2) (2,173). In addition to lowering the cost of dialysis, reuse of dialyzers has been shown to decrease complement activation (53), as well as the incidence of the "first use" syndrome (174,175). Chenoweth et al. (53) demonstrated that serum levels of complement C3a, in patients undergoing dialysis with reused Cuprophan hollow-fiber dialyzers sterilized with formalin, were approximately 20% to 30% of those observed with "first use" dialyzers. Neutropenia, associated with complement activation, also decreased with subsequent reuse of the same dialyzer. The findings suggested that C3b or C3b-derived fragments deposited during first use, or other circulating proteins, remained bound to the membrane, blocking subsequent complement activation during reuse.

Early studies had shown increased survival among patients dialyzed with reprocessed dialyzers (174,176,177). Later studies reported an increase in risk of death among patients treated with reprocessed dialyzers (178,179). The reasons, however, for any potential increased mortality are not fully understood. It has been speculated that decreased clearance of uremic toxins, decreased dialyzer membrane surface area, change in membrane permeability, and loss of structural integrity of reused dialyzers may lead to a decrease in the delivered dose of dialysis (173,180,181). Data regarding the effect of dialyzer reuse on urea and β_2-microglobulin clearance extracted from the HEMO study were recently evaluated. β_2-microglobulin clearance decreased, remained unchanged, or increased with reuse depending on the type of membrane used. Urea clearance decreased only slightly (1% to 2% per ten reuses) regardless of porosity of the membrane or reprocessing method (182).

In vivo cross-over studies comparing clearance of small (urea and creatinine) and middle molecular weight (β_2-microglobulin) molecules in patients dialyzed with low-flux, high-efficiency cellulose, and high-flux polysulfone dialyzers reused 20 times demonstrated significant decrease in urea and creatinine clearance with the high-flux polysulfone dialyzer. In contrast, urea and creatinine clearance increased with reuse of the cellulosic membrane. β_2-microglobulin clearance remained the same during reuse of the cellulose membrane, whereas β_2-microglobulin clearance increased in the polysulfone dialyzer with subsequent reuse (183).

Decrease in small molecular weight solute clearance with reused synthetic membranes had also been demonstrated with PAN dialyzers compared with Cuprophan dialyzers with seven reuses (184). Preservation of urea and creatinine clearance with reprocessed cellulosic dialyzers after reuse has also been observed in other studies (31,185). The type of processing may also have an impact on differential clearance (173). The impact of dialyzer reuse on mortality remains unanswered in the absence of carefully designed and executed randomized controlled trials (173).

Choice of Membrane in Acute Renal Failure

Mortality in acute renal failure (ARF) can be as high as 50% (186–188), with increased risk in patients requiring renal replacement therapy (189). In the management of ARF, indications for initiation of renal replacement therapy, choice of dialysis mode, intensity of prescribed dialysis, and choice of membrane biocompatibility remain controversial decisions that may affect patient recovery and survival (190,191).

It has been speculated that membrane biocompatibility may have an impact on patient survival and renal recovery rates. It had been observed that infiltration of the injured kidney with activated leukocytes may delay recovery from ARF (192–195). Although there have been extensive studies on blood-dialyzer membrane interactions in patients with chronic renal failure, there are few data regarding the effect of different dialyzer membranes on the stimulation of inflammatory mediators during HD for ARF (196–198). Early observational and randomized controlled studies found improved survival and renal recovery in patients with ARF treated with biocompatible membranes (197,199–201). Recent studies have not demonstrated a benefit (202–205). There is considerable variability within all the studies regarding the membrane selection, composition, and flux properties. In addition, patient characteristics, follow-up time, dialysis adequacy, and sample size were not consistent between the studies (195). A recent metaanalysis of ten previously published prospective trials comparing the use of cellulose-based membranes and synthetic membranes in ARF found a significant survival advantage in patients treated with synthetic membranes when compared with those treated with unmodified cellulose (206). There was no association between membrane type and recovery of renal function. The impact of membrane biocompatibility on clinical outcome in the setting of ARF remains a subject of ongoing debate.

CONCLUSION

A nephrologist must balance a number of variables when choosing between a variety of different dialyzer membranes. The wide range of different dialyzers to choose from may have different short-term and long-term patient outcomes. The membrane biocompatibility profile, KoA, and flux must be tailored to the individual patient comorbidities, size, vascular access, and nutritional status. The shift toward treatment of chronic renal failure patients with high-flux synthetic membranes has steadily grown in the past decade. Whether the differential effects of dialyzers on biocompatibility markers, volume, and solute clearance mediate changes in clinically meaningful long-term outcomes remains to be seen.

Although ESRD patients treated with HD have shown increased survival, morbidity and mortality remain high. With increasing numbers of patients developing ESRD and starting HD, the financial cost and economic constraints on outpatient dialysis centers and management of individual patients have increased. At the same time, reimbursement rates for chronic HD patients are decreasing. This economic reality limits the choice of dialyzers and encourages reuse. Reuse of dialyzer membranes has served to limit expense; however, the clinical impact of dialyzer reuse on patient health remains to be seen. The nephrologist must use his or her best judgment to match the characteristics of the dialyzers available to the patient's specific needs, given a literature that provides few discrete answers.

REFERENCES

1. Parker TF, et al. Survival of hemodialysis patients in the United States is improved with a greater quantity of dialysis. *Am J Kidney Dis* 1994;23:670–680.
2. Port FK, et al. Trends in treatment and survival for hemodialysis patients in the United States. *Am J Kidney Dis* 1998;32(S4):S34–S38.
3. Ritz E, et al. Osteodystrophy in the millennium. *Kidney Int* 1999; [Suppl 73]:S94–S98.
4. Kaplow L, et al. Profound neutropenia during the early phase of hemodialysis. *JAMA* 1968;203:133–135.
5. Cheung AK, et al. The hemodialysis membranes: a historical perspective, current state and future prospect. *Semin Nephrol* 1997;17: 196–213.
6. United States Renal Data System (USRDS). 2001 annual data report: atlas of end-stage renal disease in the United States. Bethesda, MD: National Institutes of Health, National Institute of Diabetes and Digestive and Kidney Diseases, 2001.
7. Keane WF, et al. Influence of comorbidity on mortality and morbidity in patients treated with hemodialysis. *Am J Kidney Dis* 1994;24: 1010–1018.
8. Port FK. Morbidity and mortality in dialysis patients. *Kidney Int* 1994;46:1728–1737.
9. Bloembergen WE, et al. Relationship of dose of hemodialysis and cause-specific mortality. *Kidney Int* 1996;50:557–565.
10. Eschbach JW, et al. Improvement in the anemia of chronic renal failure with fluoxymesterone. *Ann Intern Med* 1973;78:527–532.
11. Neff MS, et al. A comparison of androgens for anemia in patients on hemodialysis. *N Engl J Med* 1981;304:871–875.
12. Eschbach JW, et al. Correction of anemia of end-stage renal disease with recombinant human erythropoietin. *N Engl J Med* 1987;316: 73–78.
13. Miles AM, et al. Center and home chronic hemodialysis: outcome

and complications. In: Schrier RW, ed. *Diseases of the kidney and urinary tract*. Philadelphia: Lippincott Williams & Wilkins, 2001: 2979–3005.

14. Collins AJ. High-flux, high-efficiency procedures. In: Henrich WL, ed. *Principles and practice of dialysis*. Baltimore: Williams & Wilkins, 1994:76–88.

15. Drukker W. Haemodialysis: a historical review. In: Maher JF, ed. *Replacement of renal function by dialysis*. Dordrecht, the Netherlands: Kluwer Academic, 1989:20–86.

16. Gohl H, et al. Membranes and filters for hemofiltration. In: Henderson LW, et al., eds. *Hemofiltration*. Berlin: Springer-Verlag, 1986: 63–64.

17. Lowrie EG, et al. Effect of the hemodialysis prescription on patient morbidity: report from the National Cooperative Dialysis Study. *N Engl J Med* 1981;305:1176–1181.

18. Gotch FA, et al. A mechanistic analysis of the National Cooperative Dialysis Study (NCDS). *Kidney Int* 1985;28:526–534.

19. Hakim RM, et al. Effects of dose of dialysis on morbidity and mortality. *Am J Kidney Dis* 1994;23:661–669.

20. Collins AJ, et al. Urea index and other predictors of hemodialysis patient survival. *Am J Kidney Dis* 1994;23:272–282.

21. Held PJ, et al. The dose of hemodialysis and patient mortality. *Kidney Int* 1996;50:550–556.

22. Port FK, et al. Dialysis dose and body mass index are strongly associated with survival in hemodialysis patients. *J Am Soc Nephrol* 2002;13:1061–1066.

23. Winchester JF, et al. Theory of dialysis. In: Briggs JD, et al., eds. *Renal dialysis*. London: Chapman & Hall Medical, 1994:1–8.

24. Van Stone JC. Hemodialysis apparatus. In: Daugirdas JT, et al., eds. *Handbook of dialysis*. Boston: Little, Brown, 1994:30–52.

25. Clark WR, et al. Effect of membrane composition and structure on solute removal and biocompatibility in hemodialysis. *Kidney Int* 1999;56:2005–2015.

26. Sargent JA, et al. Principles and biophysics of dialysis. In: Maher JF, ed. *Replacement of renal function by dialysis: a textbook of dialysis*. Dordrecht, the Netherlands: Kluwer Academic, 1989:87–143.

27. Leypoldt JK. Solute fluxes in different treatment modalities. *Nephrol Dial Transplant* 2000;15[Suppl]:3–9.

28. Greene T, et al. Design and statistical issues of the hemodialysis (HEMO) study. *Con Clin Trials* 2000;21:502–525.

29. Karlsson FA, et al. Turnover in humans of β2-microglobulin: the constant chain of HLA-antigens. *Eur J Clin Invest* 1980;10:293–300.

30. Schardijn G, et al. Urinary β2-microglobulin in upper and lower urinary tract infections. *Lancet* 1979;1:805–807.

31. Churchill DN, et al. Dialyzer re-use: a multiple crossover study with random allocation to order of treatment. *Nephron* 1988;50:325–331.

32. Schardijn GHC, et al. β2-microglobulin: its significance in the evaluation of renal function. *Kidney Int* 1987;32:635–641.

33. Hoenich NA, et al. Haemodialysis membranes: a matter of fact or taste? *Contrib Nephrol* 2001;133:81–104.

34. Goldman M, et al. Removal of β2-microglobulin by adsorption on dialysis membranes. *Nephrol Dial Transplant* 1987;2:576–577.

35. Gorevic PD, et al. Beta-2 microglobulin is an amyloidogenic protein in man. *J Clin Invest* 1985;76:2425–2429.

36. Eknoyan G, et al. For the HEMO Study Group. Effect of dialysis dose and membrane flux in maintenance hemodialysis. *N Engl J Med* 2002;347:2010–2019.

37. Chenoweth DE. Complement activation during hemodialysis: clinical observations, proposed mechanisms, and theoretical implications. *Artif Organs* 1984;8:281–290.

38. Lysaght MJ. Evolution of hemodialysis membranes. *Contrib Nephrol* 1995;113:1–10.

39. Cheung AK. Biocompatibility of hemodialysis membranes. *J Am Soc Nephrol* 1990;1:150–161.

40. Hoenich NA, et al. Clinical comparison of high-flux cellulose acetate and synthetic membranes. *Nephrol Dial Transplant* 1994;9:60–66.

41. Grooteman M, et al. Cytokine profiles during clinical high-flux dialysis: no evidence for cytokine generation by circulating monocytes. *J Am Soc Nephrol* 1997;8:1745–1754.

42. Neidhardt FC. Bacterial structures. In: Ryan KJ, ed. *Sherris medical microbiology: an introduction to infectious diseases*. Norwalk, CT: Appleton & Lange, 1994:11–24.

43. Lonnemann G. Chronic inflammation in hemodialysis: the role of contaminated dialysate. *Blood Purif* 2000;18:214–223.

44. Lonnemann G, et al. Detection of endotoxin-like interleukin-1 inducing activity during in vitro dialysis. *Kidney Int* 1988;33:29–35.

45. Laude-Sharpe M, et al. Induction of IL-1 during hemodialysis: transmembrane passage of intact endotoxins (LPS). *Kidney Int* 1990;38: 1089–1094.

46. Bingel M, et al. Human interleukin-1 production during dialysis. *Nephron* 1986;43:161–163.

47. Lonnemann G, et al. Permeability of dialyzer membranes to TNFα-inducing substances derived from water bacteria. *Kidney Int* 1992;42: 61–68.

48. Lonnemann G. Should ultrapure dialysate be mandatory? *Nephrol Dial Transplant* 2000;15[Suppl]:55–59.

49. Baurmeister U, et al. Dialysate contamination and back filtration may limit the use of high-flux dialysis membranes. *ASAIO Trans* 1989;35: 519–522.

50. Bigazzi R, et al. High-permeable membranes and hypersensitivity-like reactions: role of dialysis fluid contamination. *Blood Purif* 1990;8: 190–198.

51. Panichi V, et al. C-reactive protein as a marker of chronic inflammation in uremic patients. *Blood Purif* 2000;18:183–190.

52. Craddock PR, et al. Hemodialysis leukopenia. pulmonary vascular leukostasis resulting from complement activation by dialyzer cellophane membranes. *J Clin Invest* 1977;59:879–888.

53. Chenoweth DE, et al. Anaphylatoxin formation during hemodialysis: comparison of new and re-used dialyzers. *Kidney Int* 1983;24: 770–774.

54. Hakim RM, et al. Biocompatibility of dialysis membranes: effects of chronic complement activation. *Kidney Int* 1984;26:194–210.

55. Luger A, et al. Blood-membrane interaction in hemodialysis leads to increased cytokine production. *Kidney Int* 1987;32:84–88.

56. Schindler R, et al. Gene expression of interleukin-1 beta during hemodialysis. *Kidney Int* 1993;43:712–721.

57. Varela MP, et al. Biocompatibility of hemodialysis membranes: interrelations between plasma complement and cytokine levels. *Blood Purif* 2001;19:370–379.

58. Horl WH. Hemodialysis membranes: interleukins, biocompatibility, and middle molecules. *J Am Soc Nephrol* 2002;15[Suppl 1]:29–35.

59. Krieter DH, et al. Anaphylactoid reactions during hemodialysis in sheep are ACE inhibitor dose-dependent and mediated by bradykinin. *Kidney Int* 1998;53:1026–1035.

60. Arnaout MA, et al. Increased expression of an adhesion promoting surface glycoprotein in the granulocytopenia of hemodialysis. *N Engl J Med* 1985;312:457–462.

61. Alvarez V, et al. Differentially regulated cell surface expression of leukocyte adhesion receptors on neutrophils. *Kidney Int* 1991;40: 899–905.

62. Hakim RM, et al. Hemodialysis associated platelet activation and thrombocytopenia. *Am J Med* 1985;78:575–580.

63. Luger A, et al. Blood-membrane interaction in hemodialysis leads to increased cytokine production. *Kidney Int* 1987;32:84–88.

64. Kaupke CJ, et al. Effect of hemodialysis on leukocyte adhesion receptor expression. *Am J Kidney Dis* 1996;27:244–252.

65. Henderson LW, et al. Hemodialysis hypotension: the interleukin hypothesis. *Blood Purif* 1983;1:3–8.

66. Hakim RM. Clinical Implications of hemodialysis biocompatibility. *Kidney Int* 1993;44:484–494.

67. Chenoweth DE, et al. Anaphylatoxin formation during hemodialysis: effects of different dialyzer membranes. *Kidney Int* 1983;24: 764–769.

68. Cheung AK, et al. Activation of complement by hemodialysis membranes: polyacrylonitrile binds more C3a than cuprophan. *Kidney Int* 1990;37:1055–1059.

69. Pascual M, et al. Is adsorption an important characteristic of dialysis membranes? *Kidney Int* 1996;49:309–313.

70. Marshall JW, et al. Adherence of blood components to dialyzer membranes: morphological studies. *Nephron* 1974;12:157–170.

71. Green D, et al. Elevated β-thromboglobulin in patients with chronic renal failure: effect of hemodialysis. *J Lab Clin Med* 1980;95: 679–685.

72. Vazari ND, et al. Effect of hemodialysis on contact group of coagulation factors, platelets, and leukocytes. *Am J Med* 1984;77:437–441.

73. Schulman G, et al. Bradykinin generation by dialysis membranes: possible role in anaphylactic reaction. *J Am Soc Nephrol* 1993;3: 1563–1569.

74. Gawez MP, et al. Platelet-leukocyte aggregates during hemodialysis: effect of membrane type. *Artif Organs* 1999;23:29–36.

75. Simon P, et al. Enhanced platelet aggregation and membrane biocompatibility: possible influence on thrombosis and embolism in hemodialysis patients. *Nephron* 1987;45:172–173.

76. Tielemans C, et al. Anaphylactoid reactions during hemodialysis on AN69 membranes in patients receiving ACE inhibitors. *Kidney Int* 1990;38:982–984.

77. Verresen L, et al. Bradykinin is a mediator of anaphylactoid reactions during hemodialysis with AN69 membranes. *Kidney Int* 1994;45: 1497–1503.

78. Brophy P, et al. AN-69 membrane reactions are pH-dependent and preventable. *Am J Kidney Dis* 2001;38:173–178.

79. Craddock PR, et al. Complement and leukocyte-mediated pulmonary dysfunction in hemodialysis. *N Engl J Med* 1977;296: 769–774.

80. Hakim RM, et al. Complement activation and hypersensitivity reactions to dialysis membranes. *N Engl J Med* 1984;311:878–882.

81. Cheung AK, et al. Activation of the alternative pathway of complement by cellulosic hemodialysis membranes. *Kidney Int* 1989;36: 257–265.

82. Johnson AR, et al. Release of histamine from mast cells by the complement peptides C3a and C5a. *Immunology* 1975;28:1067–1080.

83. Haeffner-Cavaillon N, et al. C3a (C3a$_{desArg}$) induces production and release of interleukin-1 by cultured human monocytes. *J Immunol* 1987;139:794–799.

84. Schindler R, et al. Recombinant C5a stimulates transcription rather than translation of IL-1 and TNF: priming of mononuclear cells with recombinant C5a enhances cytokine synthesis induced by LPS, IL-1 or PMA. *Blood* 1990;76:1631–1635.

85. Hammerschmidt DE, et al. Complement-induced granulocyte aggregation in vivo. *Am J Pathol* 1981;102:146–150.

86. Craddock PR, et al. Complement (C5a)-induced granulocyte aggregation in vitro: a possible mechanism of complement-mediated leukostasis and leukopenia. *J Clin Invest* 1977;60:260–264.

87. Yancey KB, et al. Studies of human C5a as a mediator of inflammation in normal human skin. *J Clin Invest* 1985;75:486–495.

88. Sacks T, et al. Oxygen radicals mediate endothelial cell damage by complement-stimulated granulocytes: an in vitro model of immune vascular damage. *J Clin Invest* 1978;61:1161–1167.

89. Zaoui P, et al. Effect of dialysis membrane on β$_2$-microglobulin production and cellular expression. *Kidney Int* 1990;38:962–967.

90. Parker CJ, et al. Mechanisms of immune destruction of erythrocytes. In: Lee GR, et al., eds. *Wintrobe's clinical hematology.* Philadelphia: Lippincott Williams & Wilkins, 1999:1191–1209.

91. Law SA, et al. Binding reaction between the third human complement protein and small molecules. *Biochemistry* 1981;20:7457–7463.

92. Ivanovich P, et al. Symptoms and activation of granulocytes and complement with two dialysis membranes. *Kidney Int* 1983;24:758–763.

93. Cheung AK, et al. Compartmental distribution of complement activation products in artificial kidneys. *Kidney Int* 1986;30:74–80.

94. Pascual M, et al. Is adsorption an important characteristic of dialysis membranes? *Kidney Int* 1996;49:309–313.

95. Schaefer RM, et al. Enhanced biocompatibility with a new cellulosic membrane: cuprophan vs. hemophan. *Blood Purif* 1987;5:262–267.

96. Goldfarb S, et al. Proinflammatory cytokines and hemofiltration membranes. *J Am Soc Nephrol* 1994;5:228–232.

97. Ohi H, et al. Cellulose membranes suppress complement activation in patients after hemodialysis. *Am J Kidney Dis* 2001;38:384–389.

98. Bodner G, et al. Dialysis-induced eosinophilia. *Nephron* 1982;32: 63–66.

99. Hertel J, et al. Eosinophilia and cellular responsiveness in hemodialysis patients. *J Am Soc Nephrol* 1992;3:1244–1252.

100. Amadori A, et al. Hemodialysis leukopenia and complement function with different dialyzers. *Kidney Int* 1983;24:775–781.

101. Fawcett S, et al. Haemodialysis-induced respiratory changes. *Nephrol Dial Transplant* 1987;2:161–168.

102. Himmelfarb J, et al. Modulation of granulocytes LAM-1 and MAC-1 during dialysis—a prospective, randomized controlled trial. *Kidney Int* 1992;41:388–395.

103. Nguyen AT, et al. Hemodialysis membrane-induced activation of phagocyte oxidative metabolism detected in vivo and in vitro within microamounts of whole blood. *Kidney Int* 1985;28:158–167.

104. Himmelfarb J, et al. Reactive oxygen species production by monocytes and polymorphonuclear leukocytes during dialysis. *Am J Kidney Dis* 1991;17:271–276.

105. Descamps-Latscha B, et al. Establishing the relationship between complement activation and stimulation of phagocyte oxidative metabolism in hemodialyzed patients: a randomized prospective study. *Nephron* 1991;59:279–285.

106. Witko-Sarat V, et al. Advanced oxidation protein products as a novel marker of oxidative stress in uremia. *Kidney Int* 1996;49:1304–1313.

107. Miyata T, et al. Implication of an increased oxidative stress in the formation of advanced glycation end products in patients with end-stage renal failure. *Kidney Int* 1997;51:1170–1181.

108. Descamps-Latscha B, et al. Immune system dysregulation in uremia: role of oxidative stress. *Blood Purif* 2002;20:481–484.

109. Port FK, et al. The role of dialysate in the stimulation of interleukin-1 production during clinical hemodialysis. *Am J Kidney Dis* 1987;10: 118–122.

110. Lonnemann G, et al. Detection of endotoxin-like interleukin-1 inducing activity during in vitro hemodialysis. *Kidney Int* 1988;33: 29–35.

111. Kimmel PL, et al. Immunologic function and survival in hemodialysis patients. *Kidney Int* 1998;54:236–244.

112. Linnenweber S, et al. Effects of dialyzer membrane in interleukin-1β (IL-1β) and IL-1β-converting enzyme in mononuclear cells. *Kidney Int* 2001;59[Suppl 78]:S282–S285.

113. Dinarello CA. Interleukin-1 and the pathogenesis of the acute-phase response. *N Engl J Med* 1984;311:1413–1418.

114. Smith KA, et al. The functional relationship of the interleukins. *J Exp Med* 1980;151:1551–1556.

115. Freedman AS, et al. Pre-exposure of human B cells to recombinant IL-1 enhances subsequent proliferation. *J Immunol* 1988;141: 3398–3404.

116. Kimmel PL, et al. Effect of renal replacement therapy on cellular cytokine production in patients with renal disease. *Kidney Int* 1990; 38:129–135.

117. Smith KA, et al. Interleukin-2 regulates its own receptors. *Proc Natl Academy Sci U S A* 1985;82:864–868.

118. Kishi H, et al. Induction of IgG secretion in a human B cell clone with recombinant IL-2. *J Immunol* 1985;134:3104–3107.

119. Schindler R, et al. Transcription, not synthesis of interleukin-1 and tumor necrosis factor by complement. *Kidney Int* 1990;37:85–93.

120. Okusawa S, et al. C5a induction of human interleukin-1: synergistic effect with endotoxin or interferon-gamma. *J Immunol* 1987;139: 2635–2640.

121. Betz M, et al. Cuprammonium membranes stimulate interleukin-1 release and arachidonic acid metabolism in monocytes in the absence of complement. *Kidney Int* 1988;34:67–73.

122. Girndt M, et al. Influence of dialysis with polyamide vs. hemophan hemodialyzers on monokines and complement activation during a 4-month long-term study. *Nephrol Dial Transplant* 1999;14:676–682.

123. Goodman MN. Interleukin-6 induces skeletal muscle protein breakdown in rats. *Proc Soc Exp Biol Med* 1994;205:182–185.

124. Tsujinaka T, et al. Interleukin-6 receptor antibody inhibits muscle atrophy and modulates proteolytic systems in interleukin-6 transgenic mice. *J Clin Invest* 1996;97:244–249

125. Kaizu Y, et al. Interleukin-6 may mediate malnutrition in chronic hemodialysis patients. *Am J Kidney Dis* 1998;31:93–100.

126. Bologa RM, et al. Interleukin-6 predicts hypoalbuminemia, hypocholesterolemia, and mortality in hemodialysis patients. *Am J Kidney Dis* 1998;32:107–114.

127. Liuzzo G, et al. The prognostic value of C-reactive protein and serum amyloid A protein in severe unstable angina. *N Engl J Med* 1994;331: 417–424.

128. Memoli B, et al. Role of different dialysis membranes in the release of interleukin-6-soluble receptor in uremic patients. *Kidney Int* 2000;58: 417–424.

129. Girndt M, et al. Production of interleukin-6, tumor necrosis factor alpha and interleukin-10 in vitro correlates with the immune defect in chronic hemodialysis patients. *Kidney Int* 1995;47:559–565.

130. Van Ypersele de Strihou C, et al. Effect of dialysis membrane and patient's age on signs of dialysis-related amyloidosis. The Working Party on Dialysis Amyloidosis. *Kidney Int* 1991;39:1012–1019.

131. Morena M, et al. Why hemodialysis patients are in a prooxidant state? What could be done to correct the pro/antioxidant imbalance. *Blood Purif* 2000;18:191–199.

132. Galli F, et al. Bioreactivity and biocompatibility of a vitamin E-modified multi-layer hemodialysis filter. *Kidney Int* 1998;54:580–589.

133. Bulger EM, et al. Enteral vitamin E supplementation inhibits the cytokine response to endotoxin. *Arch Surg* 1997;132:1337–1341.

134. Devaraj S, et al. The effects of alpha tocopherol supplementation on monocyte function. decreased lipid oxidation, interleukin-1 beta secretion, and monocyte adhesion to endothelium. *J Clin Invest* 1996; 98:756–763.

135. Cannon JG, et al. Acute phase response in exercise. II. Associations between vitamin E, cytokines, and muscle proteolysis. *Am J Physiol* 1991;260:R1235–R1240.

136. Buoncristiani U, et al. Oxidative damage during hemodialysis using a vitamin-E-modified dialysis membrane: a preliminary characterization. *Nephron* 1997;77:57–61.

137. Girndt M, et al. Prospective crossover trial of the influence of vitamin E-coated dialyzer membranes on T-cell activation and cytokine induction. *Am J Kidney Dis* 2000;35:95–104.

138. Satoh M, et al. Oxidative stress is reduced by the long-term use of vitamin E-coated dialysis filters. *Kidney Int* 2001;59:1943–1950.

139. Shimazu T, et al. Effects of a vitamin E-modified dialysis membrane on neutrophil superoxide anion radical production. *Kidney Int* 2001; 59[Suppl 78]:S137–S143.

140. Beaurain G, et al. In vivo T-cell preactivation in chronic uremic hemodialyzed and non-hemodialyzed patients. *Kidney Int* 1989;36: 636–644.

141. Himmelfarb J, et al. Biocompatibility and risk of infection in hemodialysis patients. *Nephrol Dial Transplant* 1994;9[Suppl 2]: 138–144.

142. Hakim RM, et al. Effect of the dialysis membrane on mortality of chronic hemodialysis patients. *Kidney Int* 1996;50:566–570.

143. Collins AJ, et al. Urea index and other predictors of hemodialysis patient survival. *Am J Kidney Dis* 1994;23:272–282.

144. Held PJ, et al. The dose of hemodialysis and patient mortality. *Kidney Int* 1996;50:550–556.

145. Koda Y, et al. Switch from conventional to high-flux membrane reduces the risk of carpal tunnel syndrome and mortality of hemodialysis patients. *Kidney Int* 1997;52:1096–1101.

146. Hoenich NA, et al. Comparison of membranes used in the treatment of end-stage renal failure. *Kidney Int* 1988;33[Suppl 24]:S44–S48.

147. Leypoldt JK, et al. Effect of dialysis membranes and middle molecule removal on chronic hemodialysis patient survival. *Am J Kidney Dis* 1999;33:349–355.

148. Hirth RA, et al. Extent and sources of geographic variation in Medicare end-stage renal disease expenditures. *Am J Kidney Dis* 2001; 38:824–831.

149. Tayeb JS, et al. Effect of biocompatibility on hemodialysis membranes on serum albumin levels. *Am J Kidney Dis* 2000;35: 606–610.

150. Locatelli F, et al. Effects of different membranes and dialysis technologies on patient treatment tolerance and nutritional parameters. *Kidney Int* 1996;50:1293–1302.

151. Memoli B, et al. Changes of serum albumin and C-reactive protein are related to changes of interleukin-6 release by peripheral blood mononuclear cells in hemodialysis patients treated with different membranes. *Am J Kidney Dis* 2002;39:266–2273.

152. Owen WF, et al. C-reactive protein as an outcome predictor for maintenance hemodialysis patients. *Kidney Int* 1998;54:627–636.

153. Lederer SR, et al. Ultrapure dialysis fluid lowers the cardiovascular morbidity in patients on maintenance hemodialysis by reducing continuous microinflammation. *Nephron* 2002;91:452–455.

154. Van Tellingen A, et al. Intercurrent clinical events are predictive of plasma C-reactive protein levels in hemodialysis patients. *Kidney Int* 2002;62:632–638.

155. Schwedler SB, et al. Advanced glycation end products and mortality in hemodialysis patients. *Kidney Int* 2002;62:301–310.

156. Wanner C, et al. Inflammation and cardiovascular risk in dialysis patients. *Kidney Int* 2002;61[Suppl 80]:99–102.

157. Qureshi AR, et al. Inflammation, malnutrition, and cardiac disease as predictors of mortality in hemodialysis patients. *J Am Soc Nephrol* 2002;13[Suppl 1]:S28–S36.

158. Morrison G, et al. Mechanism and prevention of cardiac arrhythmias in chronic hemodialysis patients. *Kidney Int* 1980;17:600–611.

159. Cardoso M, et al. Hypoxemia during hemodialysis: a critical review of the facts. *Am J Kidney Dis* 1988;11:281–297.

160. Kimura K, et al. Cardiac arrhythmias in hemodialysis patients: a study of incidence and contributory factors. *Nephron* 1989;53: 201–207.

161. Munger MA, et al. Cardiopulmonary events during hemodialysis: effects of dialysis membranes and dialysate buffers. *Am J Kidney Dis* 2000;36:130–139.

162. Josephson MA, et al. Improved lipid profiles in patients undergoing high-flux dialysis. *Am J Kidney Dis* 1992;20:361–366.

163. Seres DS, et al. Improvement of plasma lipoprotein profiles during high-flux dialysis. *J Am Soc Nephrol* 1993;3:1409–1415.

164. Blankestijn PJ. Hemodialysis using high-flux membranes improves lipid profiles. *Clin Nephrol* 1994;42[Suppl 1]:48–51.

165. Stone WJ, et al. Beta-2-microglobulin amyloidosis in long-term dialysis patients. *Am J Nephrol* 1989;9:177–183.

166. Bommer J, et al. Determinants of plasma β2 microglobulin concentration: possible relation to membrane biocompatibility. *Nephrol Dial Transplant* 1987;2:22–25.

167. Zingraff J, et al. Influence of haemodialysis membranes on β2-microglobulin kinetics: in vivo and in vitro studies. *Nephrol Dial Transplant* 1988;3:284–290.

168. Schindler R, et al. Plasma levels of bactericidal/permeability-increasing protein (BPI) and lipo-polysaccharide-binding protein (LBP) during hemodialysis. *Clin Nephrol* 1993;40:346–351.

169. Friedlander MA, et al. Role of dialysis modality in responses of blood monocytes and peritoneal macrophages to endotoxin stimulation. *Am J Kidney Dis* 1993;22:11–23.

170. Miyata T, et al. Involvement of beta 2-microglobulin modified with advanced glycation end products in the pathogenesis of hemodialysis-associated amyloidosis. Induction of human monocyte chemotaxis and macrophage secretion of tumor necrosis factor-alpha and interleukin-1. *J Clin Invest* 1994;93:521–528.

171. Hou FF, et al. Beta(2)-microglobulin modified with advanced glycation end products delays monocyte apoptosis. *Kidney Int* 2001;59: 990–1002.

172. Leypoldt JK, et al. β2-microglobulin after hemodialysis. *Kidney Int* 1999;56:1571–1577.

173. Kimmel PL, et al. Dialyzer reuse and the treatment of patients with end-stage renal disease by hemodialysis. *J Am Soc Nephrol* 1998;9: 2153–2156.

174. Kant KS, et al. Multiple use of dialyzers: safety and efficacy. *Kidney Int* 1981;19:728–738.

175. Daugirdas JT, et al. First-use reactions during hemodialysis: a definition of subtypes. *Kidney Int* 1988;33[Suppl 24]:S37–S43.

176. Wing AJ, et al. Mortality and morbidity of reusing dialyzers: a report

by the registration committee of the European Dialysis and Transplant Association. *Br Med J* 1978;2:853–855.

177. Held PJ, et al. Survival analysis of patients undergoing dialysis. *JAMA* 1987;257:645–650.

178. Held PJ, et al. Analysis of the association of dialyzer reuse practices and patient outcomes. *Am J Kidney Dis* 1994;23:692–708.

179. Feldman HI, et al. Effect of dialyzer reuse on survival of patients treated with hemodialysis. *JAMA* 1996;276:620–625.

180. Sherman RA, et al. The effect of dialyzer reuse on dialysis delivery. *Am J Kidney Dis* 1994;24:924–926.

181. Matos JPS, et al. Effects of dialyzer reuse on the permeability of low-flux membranes. *Am J Kidney Dis* 2000;35:839–844.

182. Cheung AK, et al. Effects of hemodialysis reuse on clearances of urea and β2-microglobulin. The Hemodialysis (HEMO) study group. *J Am Soc Nephrology* 1999;10:117–127.

183. Murthy BVR, et al. Effect of formaldehyde/bleach reprocessing on in vivo performances of high-efficiency cellulose and high-flux polysulfone dialyzers. *J Am Soc Nephrol* 1998;9:464–472.

184. Vanholder RC, et al. Performance of cuprophane and polyacrylonitrile dialyzers during multiple use. *Kidney Int* 1988;24[Suppl 24]:S55–S56.

185. Pereira BJG, et al. Impact of single use versus re-use of cellulose dialyzers on clinical parameters and indices of biocompatibility. *J Am Soc Nephrol* 1996;7:861–870.

186. Chertow GM, et al. Prognostic stratification in critically ill patients with acute renal failure requiring dialysis. *Arch Intern Med* 1995;155:1505–1511.

187. Douma CE, et al. Predicting mortality in intensive care patients with acute renal failure treated with dialysis. *J Am Soc Nephrol* 1997;8:111–117.

188. Nolan CR, et al. Hospital-acquired acute renal failure. *J Am Soc Nephrol* 1998;9:710–718.

189. Lien J, et al. Risk factors influencing survival in acute renal failure treated by hemodialysis. *Arch Intern Med* 1985;145:2067–2069.

190. Vanholder R, et al. Does biocompatibility of dialysis membranes affect recovery of renal function and survival? *Lancet* 1999;354:1316–1318.

191. Karsou SA, et al. Impact of intermittent hemodialysis variables on clinical outcomes in acute renal failure. *Am J Kidney Dis* 2000;35:980–991.

192. Badr KF, et al. Preservation of the glomerular capillary ultrafiltration coefficient during rat nephrotoxic serum nephritis by a specific leukotriene D4 receptor antagonist. *J Clin Invest* 1988;81:1702–1709.

193. Harris KP, et al. Effect of leukocyte depletion on the function of the post-obstructed kidney in the rat. *Kidney Int* 1989;36:210–215.

194. Yoshioka T, et al. Glomerular dysfunction induced by polymorphonuclear leukocyte-derived oxygen species. *Am J Physiol* 1989;257:F53–F59.

195. Schulman G, et al. Complement activation retards resolution of acute ischemic renal failure in the rat. *Kidney Int* 1991;40:1069–1074.

196. Horl WH, et al. Neutrophil activation in acute renal failure and sepsis. *Arch Surg* 1990;125:651–654.

197. Schiffl H, et al. Biocompatible membranes in acute renal failure: a prospective case-controlled study. *Lancet* 1994;344:570–572.

198. Jaber BL, et al. Impact of dialyzer membrane selection on cellular response in acute renal failure: a crossover study. *Kidney Int* 2000;57:2107–2116.

199. Hakim RM, et al. Effect of the dialysis membrane in the treatment of patients with acute renal failure. *N Engl J Med* 1994;331:1338–1342.

200. Schiffl H, et al. Biocompatible membranes place patients with acute renal failure at increased risk of infection. *ASAIO J* 1995;41:M709–M712.

201. Himmelfarb J, et al. A multicenter comparison of dialysis membranes in the treatment of acute renal failure requiring dialysis. *J Am Soc Nephrol* 1998;9:257–266.

202. Kurtal H, et al. Is the choice of membrane important for patients with acute renal failure requiring hemodialysis? *Artif Organs* 1995;19:391–394.

203. Jorres A, et al. Hemodialysis-membrane biocompatibility and mortality of patients with dialysis-dependent acute renal failure: a prospective randomized multicenter trial. *Lancet* 1999;354:1337–1340.

204. Gastaldello K, et al. Comparison of cellulose diacetate and polysulfone membranes in the outcome of acute renal failure: a prospective randomized study. *Nephrol Dial Transplant* 2000;15:224–230.

205. Albright RC, et al. Patient survival and renal recovery in acute renal failure: randomized comparison of cellulose acetate and polysulfone membrane dialyzers. *Mayo Clin Proc* 2000;75:1141–1147.

206. Subramanian S, et al. Influence of dialysis membranes on outcomes in acute renal failure: a meta-analysis. *Kidney Int* 2002;62:1819–1823.

REUSE OF HEMODIALYSIS MEMBRANES IN CHRONIC DIALYSIS THERAPY

PAUL D. LIGHT

HISTORICAL INTRODUCTION

Reprocessing and reuse of dialyzers has been practiced since the original Kill dialyzers were handmade at the advent of hemodialysis (1964) (1,2). The practice of disinfection of a dialyzer for additional treatments for the same patient increased in the mid-1970s after the introduction of hollow-fiber dialyzers (3). The high cost of synthetic membranes, which became available in the 1970s, accelerated the reuse practice. The steady increase in reuse was stimulated by clinical and economic influences and opposed by concerns for the safety of the patients and staff (4). Areas of concern included infectious risks resulting from inadequate sterilization, ineffective dialysis delivery, and long-term exposure to germicide agents. Clinical benefits of reuse initially centered on reduction of complement activation via the alternate pathway by cellulosic membrane interactions with blood. In short-term studies, reuse was shown to improve the biocompatibility of cellulosic membranes after reprocessing (5,6). Reduction in complement activation by reprocessing improved dialysis-associated leukopenia and leukocyte sequestration in the pulmonary capillaries, associated with dyspnea and hypoxemia (7–11).

Any beneficial effect on complement activation is less substantial for substituted cellulosic and synthetic membranes for which activation of complement is significantly less without reprocessing (12). Reuse of these more biocompatible-type membranes is associated with a reduction in cytokine stimulation, which may significantly contribute to long-term benefits, such as improved malnutrition and reduced susceptibility to infection (13,14). Whether these beneficial outcomes are demonstrated for the newest biocompatible membranes is controversial and awaits scientific study.

Early reports suggested that dialyzer reprocessing reduced the incidence of first-use syndrome (FUS) as well as many intradialytic symptoms (11,15–21). FUS is an anaphylactoid IgE-mediated reaction, which occurs during the first use of a dialyzer. The very earliest reports suggested FUS was more frequent in centers reprocessing dialyzers (22). There is no clear documented relationship between FUS and complement activation (10,23). Sensitization to ethylene oxide used as a factory sterilant is now thought to cause FUS (24–29). Reduction in the incidence of FUS can no longer be considered a valid benefit of reuse, unless ethylene oxide cannot be adequately rinsed by conventional techniques in sensitized individuals. Studies in the 1980s did not show a beneficial reduction of intradialytic symptoms, particularly hypotension and hypoxemia with reuse (11,30).

Single-center studies from the 1980s suggested that reuse practices were safe, based on similar mortality for reuse and non-reused populations (4,17,31–33). Congressional concern was raised over the safety of reuse practices when the incidence of leukopenia was shown to be higher in centers performing reprocessing with bleach (34). In response to congressional concerns, a prospective cohort study for incident patients (1989–90) was initiated. A differential relative risk for patient mortality associated with reuse was reported in 1994 (35). This study demonstrated a 13% increased mortality for non-hospital-based units using peracetic acid/hydrogen peroxide (PAM) (Renalin) and 17% increased mortality when the germicide glutaraldehyde was used. However, for hospital-based units using the same germicides, mortality was equivalent. These observations have been confirmed by subsequent studies, using successive prevalent patient groups (36,37), but over this time period the type of dialyzers employed changed. Low-flux dialyzers were the predominate dialyzer used in the earliest observational periods, but high-flux dialyzers were increasingly used in the later observational periods. Any increased mortality risk associated with the use of these germicides in a specific type of facility has decreased with each more recent time interval studied. Mortality now shows similar results, but the trends persist (36).

These studies had many methodologic constraints that make inferences on mechanisms difficult (38). The problems include the identification of the entire reuse process with the germicide employed; inability to ensure random assignment; lack of a control for patient comorbidities, which have previously been shown to influence mortality; and limited control for center-effects (36,38–42).

During the time period of these observational studies, techniques and disinfection practices have evolved. Chemical disinfectant has been the predominant type of disinfection employed during the entire history of reuse; heat disinfection, first described in 1991, is currently employed in only 5% of facilities (7,43). Formaldehyde was the most prevalent disinfectant until the late 1980s (44), when toxicity concerns lead to an increasing use of the germicide PAM. A small number of facilities use glutaraldehyde, but its toxicity has limited its use to 5% of facilities.

Dialyzer reprocessing was initially performed manually. Patient safety concerns centered on the delivery of the proper concentrations of sterilants and complete filling of the dialyzer with sterilant. Exposure to toxic chemicals was a major risk for both patients and staff. Automated equipment, available in the 1980s, offered improved safety by decreasing the risk of human error. By the 1990s, 60% of facilities used automated reuse.

Critics of reuse have sited loss of dialyzer performance with repeated processing as a threat to the delivery of adequate dialysis with reprocessed dialyzers (45). Irrespective of germicide or the reprocessing technique employed, losses of small molecule clearance and ultrafiltration for low-flux, low-urea clearance membranes have been predictable (46). Concern for the continued delivery of adequate dialysis based on the reduction in surface area with reprocessing is effectively managed by monitoring the delivered dialysis dose as recommended by the Dialysis Outcomes Quality Initiative (DOQI) adequacy guidelines (47). Several double-blinded, randomized clinical trials have not shown an increased risk of pyrogenic reactions with dialyzer reuse (10,16, 20,48). Early episodes of reprocessing-related infections resulting from inadequate sterilization were related to ineffective germicide dose (49,50), time of exposure, or inactivation of germicide (51–54). No recent reports have occurred since the Centers for Disease Control and Prevention (CDC) promulgated new reprocessing guidelines in association with Association for the Advancement of Medical Instrumentation (AAMI) standards (55).

Reduced mortality in association with the use of high-flux membranes has recently been reported (36,56). Potential causal explanations have centered on increased middle- and large-molecule clearance with high-flux dialyzers and/or improved biocompatibility of these membranes, which has been shown to be associated with cause-specific reduction of infectious and cardiovascular mortality (13). Additional investigations in this area are certainly warranted.

PREVALENCE

By 1982 approximately 20% of dialysis centers practiced reuse (44). Beginning with the availability of hollow-fiber dialyzers, both economic and medical benefits promoted the steady increase in dialyzer reuse in the United States (44). With the change in reimbursement from a reasonable charge basis to a fixed composite rate, reuse participation increased rapidly to more than 80% of all patients and dialysis facilities (Fig. 2.1) (43). Although the medical benefits reportedly favoring reuse have changed over the decades, economic influences have increasingly forced cost containment to afford technology that offers health benefits to the end-stage renal disease (ESRD) population.

The markedly increased use of reprocessed dialyzers has been stimulated by economic factors. When dialyzers that were both high-flux and more biocompatible became available, they were so expensive that reuse became an economic necessity. In the 1980s, the development of automated systems for processing dialyzers contributed to the attractiveness of reuse. The 1996 United States Renal Data System (USRDS) annual report documented that 60% of reuse facilities employed automated techniques. When facilities that perform both manual and auto-

Year	No. of centers	No. (%) reusing dialyzers
1976	750	135 (18)
1980	956	179 (19)
1982	1015	435 (43)
1983	1120	579 (52)
1984	1201	693 (58)
1985	1250	764 (61)
1986	1350	855 (63)
1987	1486	948 (64)
1988	1586	1058 (67)
1989	1726	1172 (68)
1990	1882	1310 (70)
1991	2046	1453 (71)
1992	2170	1569 (72)
1993	2304	1688 (73)
1994	2449	1835 (75)
1995	2647	2048 (77)
1996	2808	2261 (81)
1997	3077	2523 (82)
1999	3478	2788 (80)
2000	3669	2935 (80)

FIG. 2.1. Hemodialysis centers having dialyzer reuse programs, 1976–2000, United States. (From Tokars JI, et al. National surveillance of dialysis-associated diseases in the United States, 2000. *Semin Dial* 2002;15[3]:165, with permission.)

mated reprocessing are included, this increases to nearly 75% (57). Automated techniques are generally more reliable and predictable with better computer-generated quality assurance monitoring capabilities.

The purported risks and benefits of reuse have varied since the 1980s. The first cited benefit of a decreased incidence of FUS (5,6,20,58) has been discredited. An article by Held (59) showed a higher mortality rate for hemodialysis units using PAM, when combined with manual reprocessing techniques. However, a follow-up study, using a very large number of patients, did not demonstrate a survival disadvantage associated with the automated reprocessing of dialyzers (35). Recent evidence shows substantially lower morbidity for patients treated with the more expensive high-flux compared with low-flux dialyzers (36,56). Medical benefits still recommend dialyzer reuse in the fixed rate reimbursement system available in the United States.

Reuse is considerably less prevalent in other parts of the world with less than 10% of European dialysis patients using reused dialyzers (60). The higher reimbursement available in these locales provides more incentive for longer dialysis with more expensive dialyzers. In Japan, reimbursement is significantly higher than the

United States, but reuse is prohibited by law (35). However, in developing countries, limited resources and the considerable cost of high-flux membrane dialyzers have stimulated reuse.

The National Kidney Foundation recommends that every patient be allowed to decline reuse, and most centers document patient understanding of the risks and benefits by signing informed consents (61). Eight percent of patients at facilities providing reuse do not use reprocessed dialyzers. These patients have a lower prescribed dialysis prescription and are more likely to be treated with low-flux dialyzers (62).

TYPES OF REUSE

Automated reuse systems offer safety advantages by decreasing the risk of human error, ensuring the correct concentration of germicide and adequate filling of the dialyzer with the germicide, and verifying that a dialyzer has been treated with sterilant. Some newer machines provide the ability to process multiple dialyzers simultaneously. Manual techniques, although requiring less capital outlay, are associated with relatively higher labor costs, which favors use of automated systems.

Both automated and manual reprocessing techniques employ the same process steps. The major steps in this process are rinsing, cleaning, measurement of dialyzer performance, disinfection, and germicide removal. Automated systems deliver highly reproducible cleaning cycles and a variety of quality control tests, including measurements of fiber-bundle volume (FBV), ultrafil-tration coefficient, and pressure-leak test with accurate assignment of results to the proper dialyzer. Labels produced by computerized automated systems facilitate correct dialyzer assignment.

Almost all reuse procedures employ a chemical means of disinfection; heat processing is performed in only 4% of dialysis facilities. Using heat as a sterilizing method for reprocessing dialyzers offers the potential advantage of eliminating staff and patient exposure to germicides (7). However, the high temperatures (100° to 105°C) originally involved in this procedure produced significant thermal stress on the structure of the membrane reducing the number of reuses, particularly for polysulfone dialyzers (7,63). Consequently, heat sterilization at lower temperatures ranging from 95° to 100°C has been combined with a low concentration of a disinfectant, such as 0.7% to 1.0% formaldehyde. Sterilization was possible for the combined process with lower temperatures. Recently, Levine et al. (64) have demonstrated excellent germicide effectiveness using 1.5% citric acid with relatively low temperatures (95° to 100°C), associated with a mean of 13 reuses, when using polysulfone membranes. Demonstration of the effectiveness of this technique for other membrane types may lead to increased use of this process in the future.

Initially, formaldehyde was the most commonly used germicide for reuse (44). By the 1990s, 40% of reuse facilities used either PAM or formaldehyde and less than 10% used glutaraldehyde as the germicide (44). As of 2000, 59% of dialysis facilities used PAM germicide, 36% used formalin, and approximately an equal percentage (4%) used either heat or glutaraldehyde (Fig. 2.2) (43).

| Year | Percent of centers using method | | | |
	Formaldehyde	Peracetic acid	Glutaraldehyde	Heat
1983	94	5	<1	—
1984	86	12	3	—
1985	80	17	3	—
1986	69	28	3	—
1987	62	34	4	—
1988	54	40	6	—
1989	47	46	7	—
1990	43	49	8	—
1991	42	50	9	—
1992	40	52	8	<1
1993	40	51	8	1
1994	40	52	7	1
1995	38	54	7	1
1996	36	54	7	3
1997	34	56	7	3
1999	33	58	6	3
2000	31	59	5	4

FIG. 2.2. Methods for reprocessing dialyzers in hemodialysis centers, 1983–2000, United States. (From Tokars JI, et al. National surveillance of dialysis-associated diseases in the United States, 2000. *Semin Dial* 2002; 15[3]:165, with permission.)

THE RATE OF REUSE

The potential for decreased solute transport resulting from either alterations in membrane integrity or loss of fiber bundles from occlusion and/or thrombosis are major limiting factors to the number of times that a dialyzer can be reprocessed (46,65). The CDC reported that the median number of reuses nationally was 14, although the maximum number of reuses varies widely among centers (44). The greater the number of reuses, the lower the cost of the dialyzer component for the cost of treatment. A cost advantage is apparent for up to 30 reuses.

BLOOD CELLULOSIC INTERACTIONS

Reported clinical benefits have been a major stimulus for dialyzer reuse. However, the clinical benefit purported to favor reuse has changed. Early in the history of reuse, evidence supporting reduction in the FUS (5,6,20,58) and reduced activation of the complement system induced by blood-cellulose membrane interactions (5,65–67) were the purported clinical benefits supporting dialyzer reprocessing. In recent years, evidence in support of improved survival characteristics for patients receiving dialysis with more biocompatible membranes has been mounting (36,56,68). These very expensive membranes favor reusing the dialyzers on the basis of economic necessity.

The FUS describes the range of clinical symptoms experienced by some patients when exposed to new dialyzers. The syndrome ranged in intensity from mild symptoms of chest and back pain to bronchospastic reactions and occasionally anaphylactic shock (58). Hakim et al. (69) showed that this syndrome was associated with exaggerated complement activation resulting in the highest peak levels of anaphylactins, C3a and C5a, in symptomatic patients. However, there is no clear relationship between complement activation and FUS (10,63). Curiously, there were more FUS reactions in centers practicing reuse (22). The currently favored hypothesis holds that this syndrome is an anaphylactoid IgE-mediated allergic reaction from sensitization to ethylene oxide used by many manufacturers to maintain sterility in packaged dialyzers (24–26,70). However, the incidence of FUS is now extremely low (44) and the current biocompatible dialyzers are still packaged with ethylene oxide. More studies are needed to define the cause of the condition.

Craddock et al. (71) first showed that the complement cascade was activated early during dialysis when cellulosic membranes are exposed to blood. Cellulosic membranes are highly polar with numerous free hydroxy groups, which can activate the complement cascade (72). Resulting activation of the alternate pathway leads to a reduction in total hemolytic complement activity and increased levels of anaphylactins, C3a and C5a (5), and levels decreased after dialyzers were reprocessed (5). Vasodilatation, bronchospasm, and increased vascular permeability are responsible, in part, for clinical symptoms (5,58).

In addition, other pathways including the kinin and interleukin systems are activated with increased levels of bradykinin (73) contributing to the likelihood of hypotension (74). After several hours delay, interleukin-1 (IL-1) production is stimulated in monocytes under the influence of C3a and C5a (74,75). Hakim et al. (76,77) have shown that recurrent stimulation and activation of neutrophils by both compliment and interleukin activation leads to impaired phagocytic function that may contribute to immune deficiency state of uremia (see Chapter 21). Chronic stimulation of the interleukin system is thought to contribute to long-term hemodialysis complication of dialysis amyloid and possibly malnutrition (68,78). For unclear reasons cytokine levels, particularly interleukin-1 (IL-1) levels, are variable when measured in the dialyzed population. Studies rely on high levels of IL-1 receptor antagonist to confirm chronic cytokine activation. Biocompatible membranes may also improve dialysis morbidity, that is, dialysis-induced amyloidosis (68), malnutrition (78), and infection, by reducing cytokine activation that has been shown to stimulate β_2-microglobulin production (79).

Adequate reprocessing of cellulosic membranes was convincingly demonstrated to reduce complement activation. Studies from Chenoweth et al. (5) show that levels of C3a and C5a and leukopenia are significantly reduced compared with non-reused dialyzers after reprocessing (Figs. 2.3 and 2.4). Ultrastructural studies demonstrated that membranes reprocessed with formaldehyde are coated with a thin layer of protein. Subsequent studies have shown that C3b is firmly bound to the membrane after reprocessing and adherent C3a renders the dialyzer incapable of further complement activation (5). However, the type of germicide use can effect the biocompatibility of the reprocessed cellulosic dialyzer. Sodium hypochlorite can reverse the beneficial effects of reprocessing with formaldehyde by scrubbing clean this protective protein layer when used in high concentrations for prolonged periods. This observation stimulated congressional concern for safety evaluation of patients receiving reprocessed dialyzers (34).

Reduction in complement activation results in a significant improvement in the neutropenia, usually seen with the first use of cellulosic membranes (44). As a result of complement activation, white blood cells with complement attached are sequestered in the pulmonary capillary bed. Limiting complement attachment also improves dialysis-related hypoxemia (80).

The newer, more biocompatible membranes, especially the synthetic membranes, are distinguished by little or no activation of the complement system (12). Therefore, any purported benefit for reuse in reducing complement activation with these membranes is not a legitimate claim. Cellulosic membranes reprocessed with bleach maintained the membrane's ability to activate the complement system. When bleach was used in conjunction with formaldehyde, β_2-microglobulin clearance by F80B dialyzer was enhanced substantially, whereas reprocessing without bleach substantially decreased the β_2-microglobulin clearance (81). Results from the USRDS Dialysis Morbidity and Mortality Study (DMMS) showed reprocessing of synthetic membranes was associated with lower mortality when bleach was used in the process (37). It is unclear whether the benefit is derived from the ability of the reprocessing technique to allow continued adsorption or by altering membrane characteristics to permit better middle-molecule clearance. These data underscore the importance of

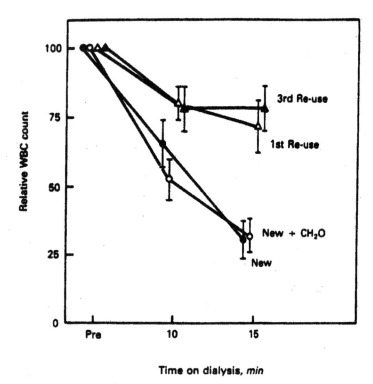

FIG. 2.3. Hemodialysis-associated leukopenia observed with different types of cuprophan dialyzers. Patients were dialyzed with new (N-11, ●), formalin-fixed new (N = 8, O), or reused dialyzers (first re-use, N = 11, △; third re-use, N = 10, ▲) and their peripheral blood leukocyte counts determined during the initial phases of hemodialysis. Each *data point* represents the mean ± standard error of the mean (SEM) of duplicate determinations in each patient. (From Chenoweth DE, et al. Anaphylatoxin formation during hemodialysis: comparison of new and re-used dialyzers. *Kidney Int* 1983;24:772, with permission.)

the recommendation made in the Hemodialysis (HEMO) Study Group, that middle-molecule clearance with biocompatible membranes must be evaluated within the context of the entire reuse procedure (56). This and other data are lending new support to middle-molecule clearance as an important factor for reducing dialysis-related mortality (37,81,82). Bio-

compatible membranes may also improve dialysis morbidity, that is, dialysis-induced amyloidosis, by reducing cytokine and compliment activation that stimulates β_2-microglobulin production (66,68). Reprocessing of biocompatible membranes offers the clinical benefit of improved mortality made economically feasible by the reuse practice (68,82,83).

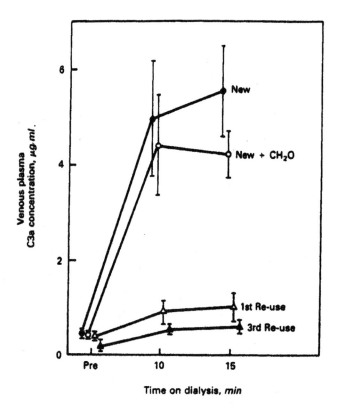

FIG. 2.4. Generation of C3a antigen during the initial phases of hemodialysis. Patients dialyzed with either new (N = 11, ●) or formalin-fixed new (N = 8, O) cuprophan dialyzers exhibit significant levels of C3a antigen in their venous plasma. Dialyzer reuse, either one time (N = 11, △) or three times (N = 10, ▲), produces significantly less complement activation. Each *data point* represents the mean ± standard error of the mean (SEM) of duplicate determinations performed on plasma samples from each individual. (From Chenoweth DE, et al. Anaphylatoxin formation during hemodialysis: comparison of new and re-used dialyzers. *Kidney Int* 1983;24:772, with permission.)

SAFETY

In the 1980s, Gotch (45,46) extensively evaluated low-flux dialyzers for concerns that reprocessing dialyzers may compromise the delivery of prescribed dialysis dose because of the predictable reduction of effective membrane surface area resulting from thrombosis/clotting of the fiber bundles. Gotch demonstrated that loss of small molecules solute clearance could be predicted by the change in the aggregate volume of patent hollow fibers contained within the blood compartment of a hollow-fiber dialyzer, FBV. Urea clearance fell by only 10% if the FBV was greater than 80% of the original volume. To a certain extent this small molecular weight solute removal was compensated by increased flow in the remaining fiber bundles (45). However, meaningful tests of FBV cannot be performed with plate dialyzers because their blood compartment volume changes with the amount of transmembrane pressure applied. Only hollow-fiber dialyzers are used in the reuse process.

AAMI standards (84) prohibit reprocessing dialyzers with inadequate small molecule solute clearance, for which a FBV of less than 80% of its baseline value is an indirect indicator. Caution is recommended in assuming an orderly relationship between FBV and delivered Kt/V, because dialyzer clearances may vary independent of the blood compartment volume (85). At least one study has shown that an unexpectedly significant drop in delivered Kt/V was observed after just four reuses (85,86). A possible explanation includes a loss of FBV during the intradialytic process by clotting that is cleared by the rinsing step of the reuse process before measurement of FBV. The use of the FBV is inadequate to evaluate a loss of ultrafiltration and larger molecule clearance, which is increasingly linked to better patient survival for high-flux membranes (16,56,68).

Loss of dialyzer ultrafiltration has little clinical impact because these types of membranes require pairing with machines using sophisticated ultrafiltration controls. The dialyzer ultrafiltration coefficient (K_uf), an indirect measure of membrane mass transfer properties, has been shown to fall slightly after reuse with PAM but increases after reuse with formaldehyde and bleach (87). Whether a change in the ultrafiltration coefficient is the result of changes in membrane resistance or surface area is not known, but at present these alterations do not limit ultrafiltration for machines with ultrafiltration controls (88).

Change in middle-molecule clearance after reprocessing dialyzers with bleach, formaldehyde, or PAM has produced widely variable results depending on the membrane type and the germicide process used (56,89,90). Bleach and formaldehyde reprocessing of a F80B dialyzer markedly increased β_2-microglobulin clearance with little increase observed when the same dialyzer was reprocessed with bleach and PAM (81). In addition, final results from the DMMS showed increased β_2-microglobulin clearance for synthetic membranes after reuse with bleach, particularly for high-flux polysulfone membranes, whereas use of PAM as the disinfectant appeared to have the opposite effect (37). Because of the variations in dialyzer design among manufacturers, the effects of a specific reuse process on one dialyzer cannot be generalized to dialyzers with similar membranes from other companies (81). Most importantly, these studies found substantially lower mortality in addition to improved clearances associated with better middle-molecule clearances (56,68,81,82).

Increased protein loss has been reported when bleach is used as a cleaning agent in conjunction with formaldehyde disinfection of polysulfone membranes (91); the amount of protein loss decreased after bleach was removed from the process (92). Considerably smaller protein losses have been reported for polysulfone dialyzers exposed to repeated bleach and formaldehyde reprocessing (93); insignificant protein loss was observed with peracetic acid or heat (94). Significant albumin loss, the result of protein sieving, could potentiate protein malnutrition and predisposes to hypoalbuminemia, an independent risk factor of mortality (14). Leypoldt and others have highlighted the importance of specific knowledge of the effect on both small- and middle-molecule clearance (37,56,82) and albumin loss (81,91) for each combination of dialyzer and germicide/bleach combination to ensure delivery of optimal dialysis therapy.

POTENTIAL HAZARDS OF DIALYZER REUSE

Since the advent of reuse processes, a number of concerns have been raised regarding potential long-term hazards. These hazards include ineffective dialysis because of poorly functioning dialyzers, infections resulting from inadequate sterilization, and deleterious effects from long-term exposure to germicide agents.

Potentially Ineffective Dialysis

That reprocessed dialyzers may jeopardize the delivery of effective dialysis is a legitimate concern based on the progressive loss of the membrane surface area with each successive reprocessing (46,58). Loss of small molecule clearance is objectively predictable as a function of the residual FBV for low-flux, low-urea clearance dialyzers (40,45). Exceptions to this relationship could occur, if the surface area was reduced during dialysis by occluded fibers, which were opened by the rinsing process before the measurement of FBV. A recent study has shown that optimizing the heparin loading dose and infusion rate with achievement of whole blood intradialytic clotting time of 150% of the predialysis value will significantly increase dialyzer reuse rates (95). In addition, prevention of fiber-bundle occlusion by air with careful preparation of the dialyzer for reprocessing at the dialysis station is necessary to maximize the number of reuses and preserves the predictability of solute clearance by measurement of FBV.

Studies have shown that cellulosic membranes have predictable losses of urea, creatinine, or phosphorus clearances, irrespective of the processing technique employed (46,58,87); however, patient-specific monitoring of the delivered dialysis dose must verify delivery of adequate dialysis (47). The monitoring of FBV may not reliably predict small-molecule and does not predict middle-molecule clearance for high-performance membranes (96). The clearance of β_2-microglobulin can be increased, decreased, or unchanged depending on the combination of dialyzer and cleaning agents used (56,89,90). These studies mandate that both small- and possibly middle-molecule clearances of reprocessed dialyzers must be tested under clinical conditions (37,56,82).

INFECTION RISK

The risks of microbiologic infections, resulting from inadequate sterilization or improper storage of the dialyzer, and an increase in pyrogenic reactions have been considered potential hazards facing the reuse program. Several outbreaks of infections in dialysis patients have been well documented. Non-tuberculous mycobacteria (NTM) are frequently found in tap water and are more resistant than *Pseudomonas aeruginosa* and other gram-negative bacteria to disinfection (97,50). Disinfection with at least 4% formaldehyde is necessary to eradicate NTM without use of ancillary procedures such as heat sterilization. An outbreak in 1985 resulted from improper preparation of formaldehyde by the staff of the dialysis unit (51). Fourteen of 27 infected patients died of various medical complications over the ensuing year. In 1990, an outbreak of gram-negative bacteremia was reported initially from centers in California and subsequently in other centers (52,53,98,99). The germicide concentration (PAM) was found to have varied markedly in these manually reprocessed dialyzers, suggesting that an ineffective concentration of germicide was used to reprocess the dialyzers (98). Another center experienced an outbreak of bacteremia related to inadequate sterilization of the dialyzer O-rings (100). The dialyzer headers were removed to clear clots but the O-rings were not replaced before reprocessing the dialyzer. Responding to the outbreaks, the CDC heightened surveillance of reuse processes at dialysis facilities and AAMI guidelines have been modified to specify the proper germicide concentrations (101). Since implementation of these modifications, there have been few reports of bacteremic outbreaks resulting from improper dialyzer processing techniques (102).

Reports from the CDC and others suggest that there was an increased risk of pyrogenic reactions associated with dialyzer reprocessing (103,104). Pyrogenic reactions are manifested as fever, chills, myalgia, nausea, and hypotension. Early in the history of reuse, disruption in the integrity of the dialysis membrane as a result of germicides was thought to be responsible for these reactions (105). Investigation of outbreaks of pyrogenic reactions, evaluated by the CDC between 1985 to 1993, revealed microbiologic contamination of the water for reuse exceeded the AAMI guidelines level in each instance (106). Several comparative and double-blinded, randomized trials have not shown an increase of pyrogenic reactions with dialyzer reuse (8,10,20,48).

Backfiltration of contaminants present in the dialysate water or failure to use dialysate quality water for all reuse steps is thought to expose patients to chronic, low-level endotoxin stimulation, especially with high-flux dialyzers (see Chapter 10) (107–109). The virtually ubiquitous elevation of C-reactive protein in ESRD patients is explained, in part, by chronic stimulation of interleukin-6 (IL-6) production by monocytes on the basis of the backfiltration of endotoxins from dialysate water (110,111). Studies have shown that the use of ultrapure water or point of delivery filtration of dialysate has resulted in decrease in IL-6 production (112). The 1997 National Kidney Foundation position paper on reuse recommends that AAMI standards set the lowest acceptable water bacterial counts and endotoxin levels at 200 cfu/mL and 2 EU/mL, respectively (61).

There is no evidence that dialyzer reuse is associated with viral transmission to patients or dialysis personnel if CDC and AAMI guidelines are followed (113,84). The CDC advises against reuse of dialyzers for patients who are hepatitis B surface antigen positive. However, there are no recommendations against dialyzer reuse for patients with hepatitis C or human immunodeficiency virus (HIV) infections. We exclude the HIV-positive population from participation in the reuse program to avoid inadvertent exposure of noninfected patients to mislabeled dialyzers.

TOXICITY OF LONG-TERM ACCUMULATIVE EXPOSURE TO DIALYZER REUSE

Chronic exposure to formaldehyde has been associated with the formation of antibodies to the erythrocyte N-antigen (102,114–117). In NN and MM phenotypic individuals, the interaction of formaldehyde with a terminal sialic acid of the N-antigen results in an immunologically active altered N-antigen. The anti N-like antibodies were first seen 12 to 18 months after first exposure but disappeared if formaldehyde exposure was eliminated. The early assays for residual formaldehyde were insensitive, leading to exposure. Clinical hemolysis is uncommon, although ongoing low-grade hemolysis has been reported (21). In addition, early transplant failure in some cases has been reported (114,118). This complication is largely attributable to the insensitivity of the early tests for residual formaldehyde. It is mandatory to monitor for removal of most germicides before dialyzer reuse. Rinsing of the dialyzer against dialysate should not be interrupted before use to remove any germicide that may have leached out of the packing or header material, which can act as sinks for the germicide (117,119).

Some patients on angiotensin-converting enzyme (ACE) inhibitors have experienced an anaphylactoid symptom complex associated with reprocessed dialyzers sterilized with PAM (120–122). Discontinuation of reprocessed dialyzer use lead to resolution of this symptom, despite continuation of the ACE inhibitor (120). Although the cause of this symptom complex is unclear, one hypothesis suggests that for some patients an interaction between the reuse sterilant and the ACE inhibitor acts to inhibit degradation of kinin. Anaphylactoid symptoms have also occurred if dialyzers packed with ethylene oxide are not used promptly after rinsing (123).

Germicide handling has potential risk for staff members. Reuse staff, who are chronically exposed to formaldehyde, have developed allergic reactions (124–126). Glutaraldehyde contact exposure can produce a chronic dermatitis. Spills of germicides, particularly formaldehyde, are associated with eye irritation, whereas the combination of formaldehyde and bleach produces chlorine gas and formic acid, which leads to nausea, vomiting, and airway irritation if exposure is sufficient. Interaction of PAM and bleach can produce hydrochloric acid, and skin contact to PAM can cause burning (127).

MORTALITY

Single-center studies in the late 1980s generally found similar mortality for patients that reused dialyzers compared with patients that did not reuse dialyzers (8,10,31,33,128,129). At this time dialyzers employed predominately cellulosic membranes. High-dose bleach used in automated reuse systems was associated with profound leukopenia; lower concentrations of bleach commonly used for manual reprocessing did not cause these symptoms. Consequently, additional population-based studies were initiated to further examine the safety of reuse practices: the Case Mix Severity Study (34) and a USRDS-sponsored study performed by Held et al. (35).

The Case Mix Severity Study evaluated 3,163 of 5,281 patients, who started on dialysis between 1986 to 1987. This preliminary study was not able to document a significant mortality risk in patients treated with reuse (34). There was, however, a trend toward increased mortality for reprocessing using PAM with manual, but not automated, processing (34). Subsequently, Held et al. (35) analyzed facility-specific data, combining the USRDS and CDC databases for 1989 to 1990, a time period when low-flux dialyzers were reprocessed with formalin. This study observed a trend toward increased mortality in patients treated with manually reprocessed dialyzers using the sterilant PAM. This conclusion, a matter of concern, was not consistent with the findings among patients treated in hospital-based dialysis facilities who experienced no apparent toxic effect from PAM or glutaraldehyde. The conclusions were flawed by an oversimplified condensation of all factors involved in the reuse process into a single indicator, germicide use.

Feldman et al. (36) initiated a point prevalence study of 66,097 ESRD patients developing two cohorts of patients, which were prospectively studied: a group using reprocessed dialyzers was compared with a group not using reprocessed dialyzers. This study, as opposed to the Held et al. study (35), included patients surviving less than 90 days, adjusted for a few comorbidity factors associated with survival and added more reuse process-related factors, including frequency of water testing and number of reuses, but included no important treatment factors such as Kt/V or hematocrit. This unit level analysis showed some conflicting results in this intention to treat analysis. For low-flux dialyzers, overall mortality was increased 13% for PAM and 10% for glutaraldehyde in freestanding units; however, for hospital-based units, mortality was lower for PAM and unchanged for the glutaraldehyde reuse compared with non-reuse. Results of an analysis from a smaller subset of units employing high-flux dialyzers provided conflicting findings when compared with facilities using low-flux dialysis: mortality was modestly lower in the units using PAM germicide (RR = 0.79) but similar for formaldehyde compared with units using non-reprocessed low-flux dialyzers. The authors cautioned that the different survival characteristics could be explained by lack of adjustment for patient-specific comorbidities, such as quality of dialysis, nutrition, and anemia (36).

In response to these conflicting results, two initiatives were fostered by the National Institute of Diabetes, Digestive and Kidney Diseases (NIDDK): the prospective randomized controlled trial of morbidity and mortality influences in hemodialysis including dialyzer reuse (HEMO) trial (56) and the USRDS special study, the DMMS (38).

As reported by Ebben et al. (38), the DMMS study used point prevalence Medicare patients using conventional treatment (no high-flux dialyzers) and adjusted for facility and for-profit status and patient-specific and unit demographics but continued to use only patient comorbidities available in the HCFA (CMS) data-base. The results of this study generally supported the findings of Held et al. (35) and Feldman et al. (36), but the mortality risk trend had lost significance, so that mortality for patients treated in facilities that reused dialyzers was now similar to that for patients treated at facilities that did not reuse dialyzers. The increased use of larger synthetic membranes, now associated with reduced mortality, may have obscured continued higher risk from certain reprocessing techniques, so the authors still advised monitoring for a potential increased relative mortality risk when PAM and glutaraldehyde are employed as the germicide (38).

Collins et al. (41) restudied the association between germicide reuse and mortality but included additional patient-specific comorbidities and unit-specific practices to reduce potential heterogeneity in the reuse and non-reuse cohorts. Controlling for these additional factors, the analysis demonstrated greater mortality risk only for patients in freestanding for-profit units using manual reprocessing techniques. Data were not available for adjustment for center effects. However, reanalysis using comorbidity factors, known to be independently linked with mortality, such as hematocrits, suggested that factors including severity of disease, comorbidity, hematocrit, and presumably adequacy might have a greater influence on mortality than the reuse practices themselves. The lack of random assignment of patient survival-related factors across study cohorts may have influenced the apparent association between germicide use and mortality observed in all these studies (35,36,38,41).

Substantially lower mortality associated with the use of synthetic dialyzers treated with bleach compared with no bleach during reuse procedures was a significant finding of the DMMS study (37). This study supports the hypothesis that clearance of substances beyond the small molecule range may be important in predicting mortality. Results from the Hemodialysis (HEMO) Study Group demonstrated variable responses on β_2-microglobulin clearances for different combinations of dialyzer and reprocessing reagents employed but a lower mortality risk was associated with higher vitamin B_{12} clearance, even at the same Kt/V (56). Recently, clearance of molecules of this size has become more important because of the lower mortality observed with greater vitamin B_{12} clearances (16,56,68). In the future, the choice of reuse dialyzers must be based on sustained in vivo performance of small- and middle-molecule clearance with acceptable albumin loss under facility-specific reuse practices, including the use of bleach, dialyzer, and germicide.

Without the benefit of a randomized control trial, the possibility remains that other significant survival-related aspects of care and not simply the germicide employed were responsible for any observed differences in mortality risk demonstrated by these studies (35–38,41,56). With this caveat, it appears that there is no detectable difference in mortality using high-flux dialyzers treated with germicide. In all cases, the reuse processes must conform to the National Kidney Foundation (NKF) guidelines and AAMI standards (61,84).

REPROCESSING TECHNIQUE

The major steps in dialysis reprocessing are identification, rinsing, cleaning, measurement of dialysis performance, disinfec-

TABLE 2.1. MAJOR REPROCESSING STEPS

1. Rinsing
2. Cleaning
3. Test of dialyzer performance
4. Disinfection
5. Germicide removal

tion, sterilization, and germicide removal (Table 2.1). With the availability of automated equipment in the 1980s, both manual and automated methods have been employed to reprocess dialyzers. Automated systems improve safety by decreasing the risk of human error, by ensuring adequate exposure to the proper concentrations of germicide and adequate filling of the dialyzer with germicide, and by accurate assigning of testing results.

IDENTIFICATION

Dialyzer identification is an essential step in the reprocessing procedure ensuring that individual patients receive treatment with only their assigned dialyzer. Tracking of dialysis performance across its reuse history must be accurately matched with the properly identified dialyzer to ensure that a dialyzer with unacceptable characteristics is discarded. Number of reuses, residual FBV, results of the various tests, and the technician who reprocessed the dialyzer are the important characteristics monitored for quality control. Multiple checks must employ both staff and patient to ensure that, once reprocessed, the same patient exclusively uses a dialyzer.

RINSING

The water quality for this and every subsequent step must meet the AAMI standard for water used to produce dialysate. Residual blood must be rinsed from the dialyzer to preserve fiber-bundle patency and reduce the aggregation of organic matter that may potentiate bacterial growth. The blood prime should be returned to the patient by flushing with heparinized saline. Removal of residual blood is accomplished by reverse osmosis with dialysate while the dialyzer is still at the dialysis station. The dialyzer should receive a pressurized rinse of both the blood and the dialysate compartment as soon as possible. Headers, if removable, are cleared of clots and must be reapplied before cleaning. If pressurized rinsing must be delayed, the dialyzer should be refrigerated. Water used for rinsing must meet the same AAMI standards as water use to prepare the dialysate (84). When manual techniques are used water purity, pressure, flow rate and type of flow (continuous or pulsatile), and use of reverse ultrafiltration must be specified to ensure uniformity of practice.

CLEANING

After rinsing, any residual blood is removed from the dialyzer by chemical cleaning agents. Sodium hypochlorite diluted to 1% or

less dissolves clots and organic deposits that occlude fibers. Hydrogen peroxide, 3% or less, and PAM are also commonly used. When combinations of chemicals are used in the cleaning process, it is mandatory that each chemical is completely removed before use of the next agent to protect against degradation of the germicide or production of noxious fumes. Cleaning of the dialyzer is facilitated by reverse ultrafiltration from the dialysate to the blood compartment at 15 to 20 psi. Reverse ultrafiltration continues until the effluent from the blood compartment is clear. Automated systems ensure that the exposure time and sterilant concentration meet the manufacturer's recommendations. Manual reprocessing must verify these parameters regularly, preferably daily. The manufacturer's recommended test must document removal of the sterilant after a standardized rinse time.

TEST OF DIALYZER PERFORMANCE

Pressure tests ensure the integrity of the membrane, its clearance, and ultrafiltration properties. A reprocessed dialyzer must withstand a pressure load without membrane rupture. The blood path integrity test works by generating a transmembrane pressure across the membrane and observing for a pressure fall in either the blood or the dialysate compartment. The pressure gradient, at least 20% above the highest operating pressure, is produced by installation of either pressurized air or nitrogen into the blood side of the membrane or by production of a vacuum on the dialysate side. The dialyzer is discarded if there is a pressure drop exceeding 10% during exposure to this transmembrane pressure.

TEST OF FIBER-BUNDLE VOLUME (FBV)

Both automated and manual techniques measure the FBV, defined as the volume of liquid in the blood compartment after displacement of any liquid by air, with the initial reprocessing and after each cleaning. When the residual FBV falls to 80% of the initial volume, AAMI standards require discarding of the dialyzer. An indicator of ultrafiltration (K_uf) can be measured by determining the volume of water passing through the membrane at a given pressure and temperature. Failure to achieve the target ultrafiltration goal with a properly functioning volumetric control mechanism should prompt reevaluation of the reprocessing method.

DISINFECTANT AND STERILIZATION

High-level disinfection is accomplished by installation of a germicide in both the blood and dialysate compartments of the dialyzer. The germicide must remain in the dialyzer for a specific amount of time, depending on the product used. Most centers allow exposure for 24 hours. PAM, formaldehyde, and glutaraldehyde are the most common germicides used (43). PAM offers the advantage of qualifying as a sterilant able to kill bacterial spores, but the dialyzer must be completely filled, because it does not develop a vapor pressure. If formaldehyde alone is used at room temperature, a 4% solution is the minimal concentration recommended by the CDC (55). Water used for preparation of the germicide solution must meet the same AAMI standards as water used to prepare the dialysate (84). Heat disinfection is a nonnoxious alternative, which offer the advantage of limiting patient and staff exposure to chemicals (7). The combination of bleach with the heat process reduced the number of reuses from damage to the dialyzer casing (64). The combination of heat and citric acid allows disinfection with lower temperatures (95° to 100°C) and a higher number of reuses (64). This promising technique is costly but deserves further study.

For manual reprocessing the presence of the germicide in the process is either documented by the use of an indicator substance in the stock solution or each dialyzer should be checked individually. Daily verification that batch solution has the proper concentration of the germicide, as well as spot checks of the germicide and its concentration in individual dialyzers, is required. Complete mixing of the germicide is necessary to avoid outbreaks of pyrogenic reactions or infections, which were caused by incomplete mixing of germicide in the early history of reuse. The dialyzer cap and O ring (if employed) must be processed by the germicide along with the dialyzer or separately, using ethylene oxide gas or steam, because failure to include these items in the disinfection process have caused an outbreak of infections (100).

Germicide removal is initiated by flushing of the blood compartment, followed by a saline flushing of the dialysate compartment, taking care to remove any trapped air to allow complete germicide removal.

INSPECTION

Before use, the blood circuit must be checked for residual germicide by the dialysis technician and rechecked by another technician or the patient, using manufacturer recommended reagent test kits designed specifically for the germicide employed. Dialyzers then receive a final inspection for subjective fiber discoloration or the presence of clots in the header. A failure at any step should result in the dialyzer being discarded.

SUMMARY

Dialyzer reuse has been employed in dialysis therapy for more than 30 years; any significant survival disadvantage for patients using reprocessed low-flux dialyzers has decreased over time when reprocessing adheres to AAMI standards (84) and follows KDP recommendations (61). Mounting evidence supports a survival benefit associated with higher middle- and large-molecule clearance offered by the more biocompatible, high-flux dialyzers, but the high cost of these dialyzers continues to provide an economic incentive favoring reuse. Reprocessing high-flux dialyzers is safe and extends their availability to more patients. Use of heat disinfection with citric acid, which is associated with little protein loss and patient exposure to noxious chemicals, will require

continued study with a variety of dialyzers of different membrane types (64). In the future, the selection of the components of the reuse process (e.g., bleach, dialyzer, membrane type, as well as germicide) must be based on the preservation of in vivo small- and middle-molecule clearance with minimal protein loss under facility-specific clinical reuse practice.

REFERENCES

1. Pollard TI, et al. A technique for storage and multiple re-use of the Kiil dialyzer and blood tubing. *ASAIO J* 1967;13:24–28.
2. Gotch FA, et al. Chronic hemodialysis with the hollow fiber artificial kidney (HFAK). *Trans Am Soc Artif Int Organs* 1969;5:87–96.
3. Lazarus JM, et al. Hollow fiber kidney reuse. *Dial Transplant* 1973; 2:14–16.
4. Shusterman NH, et al. Reprocessing of hemodialyzers: a critical appraisal. *Am J Kidney Dis* 1989;14:81–91.
5. Chenoweth DE, et al. Anaphylatoxin formation during hemodialysis: comparison of new and re-used dialyzers. *Kidney Int* 1983;24:770–774.
6. Cheung AK, et al. Activation of the alternative pathway of complement activation by cellulosic hemodialysis membranes. *Kidney Int* 1989;36:257–265.
7. Schoenfeld P, et al. Heat disinfection of polysulfone hemodialyzers. *Kidney Int* 1995;47:638–642.
8. Kant KS, et al. Multiple use of dialyzers: safety and efficacy. *Kidney Int* 1981;19:728–738.
9. Stroncek DF, et al. Effect of dialyzer reuse on complement activation and neutropenia in hemodialysis. *J Lab Clin Med* 1984;104:304–311.
10. Churchill DN, et al. Dialyzer reuse—a multiple crossover study with random allocation in order of treatment. *Nephron* 1988;50:325–331.
11. Cheung AK, et al. A prospective study on intradialytic symptoms associated with reuse of hemodialyzers. *Am J Nephrol* 1991;11:397–401.
12. Cheung AK, et al. Compartmental distribution of complement activation products in artificial kidneys. *Kidney Int* 1986;30:74–80.
13. Bloembergen WE, et al. Relationship of dialysis membrane and cause-specific mortality. *Am J Kidney Dis* 1999;33:1–10.
14. Stenvinkel P, et al. Strong association between malnutrition, inflammation, and atherosclerosis in chronic renal failure. *Kidney Int* 1999; 55:1899–1911.
15. Dumler F, et al. Effect of dialyzer reprocessing methods on complement activation and hemodialyzers restarted symptoms. *Artif Organs* 1987;11:128–131.
16. Ouseph R, et al. Maintaining blood compartment volume in dialyzers reprocessed with peracetic acid maintains KT/V but not β_2 microglobulin removal. *Am J Kidney Dis* 1997;30:501–506.
17. Robson M, et al. Effect of first and subsequent use of hemodialyzers on patient well-being. *Am J Nephrol* 1986;6:101–107.
18. Vanholder R, et al. Influence of reuse and reuse sterilants on the first-use syndrome. *Artif Organs* 1987;11:137–139.
19. Charoenpanich R, et al. Effect of first and subsequent use of hemodialyzers on patient well-being: the rise and fall of a syndrome associated with new dialyzer use. *Artif Organs* 1987;11:123–127.
20. Bok DV, et al. Effect of multiple use of dialyzers on intradialytic symptoms. *Proc Clin Dial Transplant Forum* 1980;10:92–99.
21. Lemke HD. Hypersensitivity reactions during hemodialysis: the choice of methods and assays. *Nephrol Dial Transplant* 1994;9[Suppl 2]:120–125.
22. Center for Infectious Diseases. National surveillance of dialysis-associated diseases in U.S., 1989. Atlanta, GA: Centers for Disease Control, Public Health Service, Department of Health and Human Service, 1992.
23. Kaufman AM, et al. Clinical experience with heat sterilization for reprocessing dialyzers. *ASAIO* 1992;38:M338.
24. Bommer J, et al. Ethylene oxide (ETO) as a major cause of anaphylactoid reactions in dialysis (review). *Artif Organs* 1987;11:111–117.
25. Poothullil J, et al. Anaphylaxis from the products of ethylene oxide gas. *Ann Intern Med* 1975;82:58–60.

26. Grammer LC, et al. IgE against ethylene oxide-altered human serum albumin in patients with anaphylactic reactions to dialysis. *J Allergy Clin Immunol* 1985;76:511–514.

27. Foret M, et al. Hypersensitivity reactions during hemodialysis in France. *Proc Eur Dial Transplant Assoc* 1985;22:181–191.

28. Nicholls AJ, et al. Anaphylactoid reactions due to hemodialysis, hemofiltration, or membrane plasma separation. *BMJ* 1982;285: 1607–1609.

29. Popli S, et al. Severe reactions with cuprophane capillary dialyzers. *Artif Organs* 1982;6:312–315.

30. Pereira BJG, et al. Impact of single use versus reuse of cellulose dialyzers on clinical parameters and indices of biocompatibility. *J Am Soc Nephrol* 1996;7:861–870.

31. Pollak V, et al. Repeated use of dialyzers is safe: long-term observations on morbidity and mortality in patients with end stage renal disease. *Nephron* 1986;42:217–223.

32. Jacobs C, et al. Combined reports on regular dialysis and transplantation in Europe. *Proc Eur Dial Transplant Assoc* 1977;14:3–67.

33. Held PJ, et al. Survival analysis of patients undergoing dialysis. *JAMA* 1987;257:645–650.

34. Dialyzers. Food and Drug Administration Talk Paper. Washington, DC: U.S. Department of Health and Human Services, Oct. 13, 1992:792–846.

35. Held PJ, et al. Analysis of the association of dialyzer reuse practices and patient outcomes. *Am J Kidney Dis* 1994;23:692–708.

36. Feldman HI, et al. Effect of dialyzer reuse on survival of patients treated with hemodialysis. *JAMA* 1993;276:620–625.

37. Port FK, et al. Mortality risk by hemodialyzer reuse practice and dialyzer membrane characteristics: results from the USRDS dialysis morbidity and mortality study. *Am J Kidney Dis* 2001;37:276–286.

38. Ebben JP, et al. Impact of disease severity and hematocrit level on reuse-associated mortality. *Am J Kidney Dis* 2000;35:244–249.

39. Fink JC, et al. Effect of center- versus patient-specific factors on variations in dialysis adequacy. *J Am Soc Nephrol* 1991;12:164–169, 2001.

40. Agodoa LYC, et al. Reuse of dialyzers and clinical outcomes: fact or fiction. *Am J Kidney Dis* 1998;32[Suppl 4]:S88–S92.

41. Collins AJ, et al. Dialysis unit and patient characteristics associated with reuse practices and mortality: 1989–1993. *J Am Soc Nephrol* 1998;9:2108–2117.

42. Kimmel PL, et al. Dialyzer reuse and the treatment of patients with end-stage renal disease by hemodialysis. *J Am Soc Nephrol* 1998;9: 2153–2156.

43. Tokars JI, et al. National surveillance of dialysis-associated diseases in the United States, 2000. *Semin Dial* 2002;15(3):162–171.

44. Tokars JI, et al. National surveillance of dialysis associated diseases in the United States. *ASAIO J* 1994;40:1020–1031.

45. Gotch FA. Solute and water transport and sterilant removal in reused dialyzers. In: Deane N, et al., eds. *Guide to reprocessing of hemodialyzers*. Dordrecht, the Netherlands: Martinus Nijhoff, 1986:39–63.

46. Gotch FA. The effects of dialyzer reprocessing techniques on dialyzer solute transport. In: *AAMI standards and recommended practices: dialysis*. Arlington, VA: 1996:3.

47. *NKF-DOQI clinical practice guidelines for hemodialysis adequacy*. New York: National Kidney Foundation, 1997:24.

48. Fleming SJ, et al. Dialyzer reprocessing with Renalin. *Am J Nephrol* 1991;11:27.

49. Favero MS, et al. Dialysis-associated infections and their control. In: Bennett JV, et al., eds. *Hospital infections,* 3rd ed. Boston: Little Brown, 1992:375–403.

50. Favero MS. Nontubercular mycobacterial infections in hemodialysis patients—Louisiana. *Morbid Mortal Wkly Rep* 1983;32:244–245.

51. Carson LA, et al. Prevalence of nontuberculous mycobacteria in water supplies of hemodialysis centers. *Appl Environ Microbiol* 1988;54: 3122–3125.

52. Centers for Disease Control and Prevention. Bacteremia associated with reuse of disposable hollow-fiber hemodialyzers. *Morb Mortal Wkly Rep* 1986;35:417–418.

53. Vanholder R, et al. Waterbone *Pseudomonas* septicemia due to deficient disinfectant mixing during reuse. *Int J Artif Organs* 1992;15:19–24.

54. Flaherty JP, et al. An outbreak of gram-negative bacteremia traced to contaminated O-rings in reprocessed dialyzers. *Ann Intern Med* 1993; 119:1072–1078.

55. Association for the Advancement of Medical Instrumentation (AAMI). *Standards and recommended practices: dialysis*. Arlington, VA: 1996:3.

56. Cheung AK, et al. Effects of hemodialyzer reuse on clearances of urea and β_2-microglobulin. *J Am Soc Nephrol* 1999;10:117–127.

57. USRDS 1996 annual data report. The USRDS dialysis morbidity and mortality study (wave I). *Am J Kidney Dis* 1996;28[Suppl 2]:S58–S78.

58. Daugirdas JT, et al. First-use reactions during hemodialysis: a definition of subtypes. *Kidney Int* 1988;33[Suppl 24]:S37–S43.

59. National Institutes of Diabetes and Digestive and Kidney Diseases. The USRDS case mix study, preliminary results on dialyzer reuse. Presented to an open meeting of the Food and Drug Administration, Oct. 8, 1992.

60. Fassbender W, et al. Combined report on regular dialysis and transplantation in Europe. *Nephrol Dial Transplant* 1991;6[Suppl 1]:5–35.

61. National Kidney Foundation report on dialyzer reuse. Task force on reuse of dialyzers, council on dialysis, National Kidney Foundation. *Am J Kidney Dis* 1997;30:859–871.

62. Okechukwu CN, et al. Characteristics and treatment of patients not reusing dialyzers in reuse units. *Am J Kidney Dis* 2000;36:991–999.

63. Dolovich J, et al. Allergy to ethylene oxide in chronic dialysis patients. *Artif Organs* 1984;8:334–337.

64. Levin NW, et al. The use of heated citric acid for dialyzer reprocessing. *J Am Soc Nephrol* 1995;6:1578–1585.

65. Laude-Sharp M, et al. Induction of IL-1 during hemodialysis: transmembrane passage of intact endotoxins (LPS). *Kidney Int* 1991;38: 1089–1094.

66. Urena P, et al. Permeability of cellulosic and non-cellulosic membranes to endotoxin subunits and cytokine production during in vitro hemodialysis. *Nephrol Dial Transplant* 1992;7:16–28.

67. Hakim RM, et al. Effect of dialyzer reuse on leukopenia, hypoxemia and total hemolytic complement system. *ASAIO Trans* 1980;26:159–164.

68. Koda Y, et al. Switch from conventional to high-flux membrane reduces the risk of carpal tunnel syndrome and mortality of hemodialysis patients. *Kidney Int* 1997;52:1096–1101.

69. Hakim RM, et al. Complement activation and hypersensitivity reactions to dialysis membranes. *N Engl J Med* 1984;311:878–882.

70. Rockel A, et al. Ethylene oxide and hypersensitivity reactions in patients on hemodialysis. *Kidney Int* 1988;33[Suppl 24]:S62–S67.

71. Craddock PR, et al. Complement and leukocyte-mediated pulmonary dysfunction in hemodialysis. *N Engl J Med* 1977;296:769–774.

72. Lysaght MJ. Evolution of the hemodialysis membranes. *Contrib Nephrol* 1995;113:1–10.

73. Verresen L, et al. Bradykinin is a mediator of anaphylactoid reactions during hemodialysis with AN69 membranes. *Kidney Int* 1994;45: 1497–1503.

74. Herbelin A, et al. Influence of uremia and hemodialysis on circulating interleukin-1 and tumor necrosis factor. *Kidney Int* 1990;37:116–125.

75. Bingel M, et al. Plasma interleukin-1 activity during hemodialysis: the influence of dialysis membranes. *Nephron* 1988;50:273–276.

76. Hakim RM, et al. Biocompatibility of dialysis membranes: effect of chronic complement activation. *Kidney Int* 1984;26:194–200.

77. Vanholder R, et al. Phagocytosis in uremia and hemodialysis patients: a prospective and cross over sectional study. *Kidney Int* 1991;39: 320–327.

78. Parker TF III, et al. Effect of the hemodialysis membrane biocompatibility on nutritional parameters in chronic hemodialysis patients. *Kidney Int* 1996;49:551–556.

79. Cheung AK. Biocompatibility of hemodialysis membranes. *J Am Soc Nephrol* 1990;1:150–161.

80. Davenport A, et al. The effect of dialyzer reuse on peak expiratory flow rate. *Respir Med* 1990;84:17–21.

81. Murthy BVR, et al. Effect of formaldehyde/bleach reprocessing on in vivo performances of high-efficiency cellulose and high-flux polysulfone dialyzers. *J Am Soc Nephrol* 1998;9:464–472.

82. Leypoldt JK, et al. Effect of dialysis membranes and middle molecule removal on chronic hemodialysis patient survival. *Am J Kidney Dis* 1999;33:349–355.

83. Hakim RM, et al. The effect of membrane biocompatibility on plasma β$_2$-microglobulin levels in chronic hemodialysis patients. *J Am Soc Nephrol* 1996;7:472–478.
84. Keen M. Formaldehyde and glutaraldehyde. In: *AAMI standards and recommended practices: dialysis.* Arlington, VA: 1996;3:335–343.
85. Delmez J, et al. Severe dialyzer dysfunction undetectable by standard reprocessing validation tests. *Kidney Int* 1989;36:478–484.
86. Sherman RA, et al. The effect of dialyzer reuse on dialysis delivery. *Am J Kidney Dis* 1994;24:924–926.
87. Fleming SJ, et al. Dialyzer reprocessing with Renalin. *Am J Nephrol* 1991;11:27–30.
88. Krivitski NM, et al. In vivo measurement of hemodialyzer fiber bundle volume: theory and validation. *Kidney Int* 1998;54:1751–1758.
89. Peterson J, et al. The effects of reprocessing cuprophane and polysulfone dialyzers on β$_2$-microglobulin removal from hemodialysis patients. *Am J Kidney Dis* 1991;17:174–178.
90. Westhuyzen JW, et al. Effect of dialyzer reprocessing with Renalin on serum beta-2 microglobulin and complement activation in hemodialysis patients. *Am J Nephrol* 1992;12:29–36.
91. Kaplan AA, et al. Dialysis protein losses with bleach processed polysulphone dialyzers. *Kidney Int* 1995;47:573–578.
92. Ikizler TA, et al. Amino acid and albumin losses during hemodialysis. *Kidney Int* 1994;46:830–837.
93. Kaysen GA, et al. Mechanism of hypoalbuminemia in hemodialysis patients. *Kidney Int* 1995;48:510–516.
94. Gotch FA, et al. Effects of reuse with peracetic acid, heat, and bleach on polysulfone dialyzers. *J Am Soc Nephrol* 1995;415(abst).
95. Ouseph R, et al. Improved dialyzer reuse after population pharmacodynamic model to determine heparin doses. *Am J Kidney Dis* 2000;35:89–94.
96. Vanholder RC, et al. Performance of cuprophane and polyacrylonitrile dialyzer during multiple use. *Kidney Int* 1988;33:S55–S56.
97. Bolan G, et al. Infections with mycobacterium chelonei patients receiving dialysis and using processed dialyzers. *J Infect Dis* 1985;152:1013–1019.
98. Lowry PW, et al. Mycobacterium chelonae infection among patients receiving high-flux dialysis in a hemodialysis clinic in California. *J Infect Dis* 1990;161:85–90.
99. Beck-Sague CM, et al. Outbreak of gram-negative bacteremia and pyrogenic reactions in a hemodialysis center. *Am J Nephrol* 1990;10:397–403.
100. Bland LA, et al. Recovery of bacteria from reprocessed high-flux dialyzers after bacterial contamination of the header spaces and O-rings. *ASAIO Trans* 1989;35:315–316.
101. Gordon SM, et al. Pyrogenic reactions in patients receiving conventional, high-efficiency, or high-flux hemodialysis treatments with bicarbonate dialysate containing high concentrations of bacteria and endotoxin. *J Am Soc Nephrol* 1992;2:1436–1444.
102. Welbel SF, et al. An outbreak of gram-negative bloodstream infections in chronic hemodialysis patients. *Am J Nephrol* 1995;15:1–4.
103. Gordon SM, et al. Pyrogenic reactions associated with the reuse of disposable hollow-fiber hemodialyzers. *JAMA* 1988;260:2077–2081.
104. Tokars JI, et al. National surveillance of dialysis associated diseases in the United States. *ASAIO J* 1993;42:219–229.
105. Bland LA, et al. Effect of chemical germicides on the integrity of hemodialyzers membranes. *ASAIO J* 1988;34:172–175.
106. Arduino MJ, et al. Pyrogenic reactions associated with the reuse of disposable hollow-fiber hemodialyzers. *JAMA* 1988;260:2077–2081.
107. Pegues DA, et al. A prospective study of pyrogen reactions in hemodialysis patients using bicarbonate dialysis fluids filtered to remove bacteria and endotoxin. *J Am Soc Nephrol* 1992;3:1002–1007.
108. Clark WR. Quantitative characteristics of hemodialyzer solute and water clearance. *Semin Dial* 2001;14:32–36.
109. Alter MJ, et al. Reuse of hemodialyzers: results of nationwide surveillance for adverse effects. *JAMA* 1988;260:2073–2076.
110. Panichi V, et al. Plasma C-reactive protein is linked to back-filtration associated interleukin-6 production. *ASAIO J* 1998;44:M415–M417.
111. Arici M, et al. End-stage renal disease, atherosclerosis, and cardiovascular mortality: is C-reactive protein the missing link? *Kidney Int* 2001;59:407–414.
112. Tielemans C, et al. Effects of ultrapure and non-sterile dialysate on the inflammatory response during in vitro hemodialysis. *Kidney Int* 1996;49:236–243.
113. Center for Disease Control and Prevention (CDC). Recommendations for preventing transmission of infections among hemodialysis patients. *MMWR* 2001;RR5:50.
114. Shaldon S, et al. Dialysis associated autoantibodies. *Proc EDTA* 1976;13:339–347.
115. Lewis K, et al. Formation of anti-N-like antibodies in dialysis patients: effects of different methods of dialyzer rinsing to remove formaldehyde. *Clin Nephrol* 1981;15:39–43.
116. Kaehny WD, et al. Relationship between dialyzer reuse and the presence of anti-N-like antibodies in chronic hemodialysis patients. *Kidney Int* 1977;12:59.
117. Ng YY, et al. Anti-N form antibody in hemodialysis patients. *Am J Nephrol* 1995;15:374–378.
118. Belzer FO, et al. Red cell cold agglutinins as a cause of failure of renal allotransplantation. *Transplantation* 1971;11:422–424.
119. Stragier A, et al. Rinsing time and disinfectant release of reused dialyzers: comparison of formaldehyde, hypochlorite, warexin, and Renalin. *Am J Kidney Dis* 1995;26:549–553.
120. Pegues DA, et al. Anaphylactoid reactions associated with reuse of hollow-fiber hemodialyzers and ACE inhibitors. *Kidney Int* 1992;43:1232–1237.
121. Schmitter L, et al. Anaphylactic reactions with the addition of hypochlorite to reuse in patients maintained on reprocessed polysulfone hemodialyzers and ACE inhibitors. *ASAIO Trans* 1993;39:75(abst).
122. Salem M, et al. Adverse effects of dialyzers manifesting during the dialysis session. *Nephrol Dial Transplant* 1994;9[Suppl 2]:127–137.
123. Hakim RM, et al. Formaldehyde kinetics and bacteriology in dialyzers. *Kidney Int* 1985;28:936–943.
124. Bousquet J, et al. Allergy to formaldehyde and ethylene oxide. *Clin Rev Allergy* 1991;9:357–370.
125. Kramps JA, et al. Measurement of specific IgE antibodies in individuals exposed to formaldehyde. *Clin Exp Allergy* 1989;19:509–514.
126. Bousquet J, et al. Allergy in long-term hemodialysis. *J Allergy Clin Immunol* 1988;81:605–610.
127. Fischbach LJ. Renalin: qualification as a dialyzer sterilant. In: *AAMI standards and recommended practices: dialysis.* Arlington, VA: 1996;3:195–199.
128. Kerr PG, et al. The effects of reprocessing high-flux polysulfone dialyzers with peroxyacetic acid on beta-2 microglobulin removal in hemodiafiltration. *Am J Kidney Dis* 1992;19:433–438.
129. National Kidney Foundation Executive Committee Meeting. National Kidney Foundation Report on dialyzer reuse. *Am J Kidney Dis* 1988;11:1–6.

3

DIALYSATE COMPOSITION IN HEMODIALYSIS AND PERITONEAL DIALYSIS

BIFF F. PALMER

Patients with end-stage renal disease (ESRD) depend on dialysis to maintain fluid and electrolyte balance. In both hemodialysis and peritoneal dialysis, solutes diffuse between blood and dialysate such that, over the course of the procedure, plasma composition is restored toward normal values. The makeup of the dialysate is of paramount importance in accomplishing this goal. This chapter reviews recent developments on how the dialysate can be manipulated to improve patient tolerance. Individualizing the dialysate composition is likely to gain increasing importance given the advancing age and increasing number of comorbid conditions found in ESRD patients.

DIALYSATE COMPOSITION IN HEMODIALYSIS

In most outpatient settings, patients receive hemodialysis using dialysate prepared in bulk and delivered via a central delivery system so that the composition of the dialysate is the same for all patients. Although most patients tolerate the procedure when administered in this fashion, many patients suffer from hemodynamic instability or symptoms of dialysis disequilibrium. One strategy to improve the clinical tolerance to dialysis is to adjust the dialysate composition according to the individual characteristics of the patient.

Dialysate Sodium

As dialysis has evolved there has been continued interest in adjusting the dialysate sodium (Na) concentration in an attempt to improve the tolerability of the procedure. In the early days of dialysis a low Na dialysate was typically used to reduce the complications of chronic volume overload such as hypertension and congestive heart failure. With reduced dialysis treatment times it, however, became apparent that such therapy contributed to hemodynamic instability by exacerbating the decline in plasma osmolality (particularly early in the dialysis procedure) and intravascular volume. Subsequent studies demonstrated that raising dialysate Na to between 139 and 144 mEq/L was associated with improved hemodynamic stability and general tolerance to the procedure (1–4).

There was concern that an increased dialysate Na concentration would produce a dipsogenic effect resulting in increased weight gain and poor blood pressure control. Studies addressing this issue confirmed that a higher dialysate Na modestly increased interdialytic weight gain. However, this excess weight was found to be readily removed with improved tolerance to ultrafiltration (3).

More recently, there has been interest in varying the concentration of Na in the dialysate during the procedure so as to minimize the potential complications of a high Na solution while retaining the beneficial hemodynamic effects. A high dialysate Na concentration is used initially with a progressive reduction toward isotonic or hypotonic levels by the end of the procedure. This method allows for a diffusive Na influx early in the session to prevent the rapid decline in plasma osmolality resulting from the efflux of urea and other small molecular weight solutes. During the remainder of the procedure, when the reduction in osmolality accompanying urea removal is less abrupt, the lower dialysate Na level minimizes the development of hypertonicity and any resultant excessive thirst, fluid gain, and hypertension in the interdialytic period.

As shown in Table 3.1, several studies have compared the hemodynamic and symptomatic effects of a dialysate in which the Na concentration is varied during the procedure to that in which the Na concentration is fixed. Dumler et al. (5) used a dialysate Na of 150 mEq/L during the initial 3 hours of dialysis at the time of ultrafiltration; the dialysate Na was decreased to 130 mEq/L for the last hour. The control group was dialyzed against Na concentration fixed at 140 mEq/L. Use of the high/low Na hemodialysis was associated with a smaller decline in systolic pressure as well as fewer symptomatic hypotensive episodes.

Other investigators have varied dialysate Na according to a Na-gradient protocol in which the Na is set to decrease from a high to a low level over the course of a dialysis session. The mixed results from these experiences are shown in Table 3.1. Raja et al. (6) and Daugirdas et al. (7) found no measurable benefit. Acchiardo et al. (8) found a reduction in hypotensive episodes, and Sadowski et al. (9) had similar results in young patients. The linear and step Na modeling programs have been

TABLE 3.1. SUMMARY OF RECENT STUDIES EXAMINING THE EFFECTS OF NA GRADIENT PROTOCOLS

Study	Design	Intervention[a]	Results
Dumler et al., 1979 (5)	10 patients, cross-over design	Fixed 140 vs. high (150)/low (130), Uf only with 150	50% decrease in cramping episodes (no statistical comparison possible)
Raja et al., 1983 (6)	10 patients, cross-over design	Fixed (135 and 140) vs. high (145)/low (135) vs. low (135)/ high (145)	No difference in hypotensive episodes between high/low and 140 but both better than 135 and low/high protocols
Daugirdas et al., 1985 (7)	7 patients, cross-over design	Fixed (143, 135) vs. gradient (160 to 133)	No difference in hypotensive episodes or cramps between 3 groups
Acchiardo et al., 1991 (8)	39 patients, cross-over design	Fixed 140 vs. gradient (149 to 140 linear, exponential, step)	50% reduction in hypotensive episodes and cramps with gradient protocol
Sadowski et al., 1993 (9)	16 patients (16–32 years of age), cross-over design	Fixed (138) vs. gradient (149 to 138, linear, exponential, step)	Decrease in intradialytic and interdialytic morbidity with gradient, no differences in symptomatic hypotension
Levin et al., 1996 (10)	11 symptomatic patients and 5 asymptomatic patients, cross-over design	Fixed (140) vs. ramped Na (155–160 to 140) and Uf, each individually tailored	Significant decrease in dialysis morbidity with ramped protocol
Sang et al., 1997 (11)	23 patients, cross-over design	Fixed (140) vs. gradient (155 to 140, linear or step)	Decrease in cramps and hypotension with gradient but only 22% of patients with significant benefit

[a]Units for Na values are mEq/L.

found to be better in lowering the risk of intradialytic headache as compared with the exponential program. The linear program was the only individual program that alleviated interdialytic cramps; the most striking reduction in the risk for posttreatment hypotension occurred with the step program.

Differences in the incidence of symptomatic hypotension during dialysis or in the degree of interdialytic weight gain between the fixed or variable Na protocols have been difficult to demonstrate. Levin et al. (10) studied a group of patients who were specifically selected because of the frequent occurrence of symptoms on dialysis such as headaches, cramps, and lightheadedness. In a cross-over trial, these patients were assigned either to a fixed Na dialysate and a constant rate of ultrafiltration or to a gradient protocol in which the initial Na concentration and ramping pattern were individually adjusted to minimize thirst. Use of the patient-specific Na gradient profiles was associated with improvement in all patients with headache and in 70% of patients with lightheadedness. Most patients reported an increase in thirst, but there were no differences in interdialytic weight gain or in predialysis and postdialysis mean arterial pressure. Using a more general dialysis population, Sang et al. (11) compared a linear or step Na gradient (155 to 140 mEq/L) protocol with a fixed Na dialysate (140 mEq/L). In this study, Na modeling was associated with a significant reduction in cramps and symptomatic hypotension. However, these benefits were followed by increasing thirst, fatigue, and weight gain between dialysis sessions, as well as a higher predialysis blood pressure. The authors concluded that only 22% of patients had a significant benefit from the modeling programs. Finally, a study by Movilli et al. (12) found improved blood volume preservation by using a pattern of high to low Na change (160 to 133 mEq/L); the changes in blood pressure were similar between this high to low variation and conventional dialysis.

In summary, the available data suggest that in most chronic dialysis patients, changing the dialysate Na during the course of the treatment offers little advantage over a constant dialysate Na

of between 140 to 145 mEq/L. The inability to clearly demonstrate a superiority of Na modeling may be due to the fact that the time-averaged concentration of Na was similar in many of the comparative studies. For example, a linear decline in dialysate Na from 150 to 140 mEq/L will produce approximately the same postdialysis serum Na as occurs when a dialysate Na of 145 mEq/L is used throughout the procedure. In addition the optimal time-averaged Na concentration whether administered in a modeling protocol or with a fixed dialysate concentration is likely to vary from patient to patient as well as in the same patient during different treatment times (13). This variability is supported by studies demonstrating wide differences in the month to month predialysis Na concentration in otherwise stable dialysis patients (14).

Nevertheless, in selected patients Na modeling may be of benefit (Table 3.2). Patients initiating dialysis with marked azotemia are often deliberately dialyzed so as to decrease the urea concentration slowly over the course of several days to avoid the development of the dialysis disequilibrium syndrome. The use of a high/low-Na dialysate in these patients may minimize fluid shifts into the intracellular compartment and decrease the tendency for neurologic complications. In this regard, Heineken et

TABLE 3.2. INDICATIONS AND CONTRAINDICATIONS FOR USE OF NA MODELING (HIGH/LOW PROGRAMS)

Indications
    Intradialytic hypotension
    Cramping
    Initiation of hemodialysis in setting of severe azotemia
    Hemodynamically unstable patient (as in intensive care unit setting)
Contraindications
    Intradialytic development of hypertension
    Large interdialytic weight gain induced by high Na dialysate
    Hypernatremia

al. (15), using hypertonic dialysate Na, reported reductions (without complications) in the urea concentration by 60% to 70% over 3 to 4 hours in patients with initial urea levels in excess of 200 mg/mL. Na modeling may also be beneficial in patients suffering frequent intradialytic hypotension, cramping, nausea, vomiting, fatigue, or headache. In such patients the modeling protocol can be individually tailored to minimize increased thirst, weight gain, and hypertension. Combining dialysate Na profiling with a varying rate of ultrafiltration may provide additional benefit in particularly symptomatic patients. Use of this combined approach may be of particular benefit in ensuring hemodynamic stability in patients with acute renal failure in the intensive care unit (16).

When prescribing a Na gradient protocol it is important to monitor the patient for evidence of a progressive increase in total body Na. In some patients a high/low Na protocol can lead to large interdialytic weight gain or cause intradialytic hypertension (Table 3.2). Such adverse effects are more likely to occur when the time-averaged Na concentration is greater than the patient's predialysis serum Na concentration (17). In this setting, use of a low dialysate Na during the terminal phase of the procedure does not guarantee negative Na balance. As a result, individualizing the protocol to ensure neutral Na balance is important (18).

A Na gradient protocol can be administered in such a way that the amount of Na exchanged is the same as with a fixed Na dialysate while better preserving blood volume during ultrafiltration (12). Similar findings have been reported by Coli et al. (19–22), using a technique termed profiled hemodialysis. This technique is based on a mathematical model in which baseline patient characteristics are used to construct a patient specific Na profile dialysate before each treatment. Initial experience with this procedure has shown improved cardiovascular hemodynamics when compared with a fixed dialysate Na concentration despite the same total mass of Na being removed (21,22).

In hypertensive patients, adjusting the protocol to achieve negative Na balance may be of therapeutic benefit in the long-term control of blood pressure. In this regard, Flanigan et al. (23) recently compared a fixed dialysate Na of 140 mEq/L to a gradient protocol in which the dialysate Na was lowered in an exponential fashion from 155 to 135 mEq/L and then held constant at 135 mEq/L for the final half hour of the procedure. Ultrafiltration was discontinued during the final half hour of the session. Use of the variable Na dialysate permitted a 50% reduction in the dose of antihypertensive medications without significant changes in predialysis blood pressure or interdialytic weight gain. Although not specifically measured, use of the terminal low Na period may have caused a decrease in the total body exchangeable Na thus accounting for improved blood pressure control in Na-sensitive patients.

In dialysis patients interdialytic Na and water loads vary from one patient to another and from treatment to treatment. Water balance can be achieved by making total ultrafiltrate volume equal to interdialytic weight gain. Current research is focusing on ways in which the dialysate Na concentration can be adjusted to more accurately match intradialytic Na removal with interdialytic Na intake. In this manner, management of Na balance would be made similar to management of fluid intake.

The ability of dialysis to accurately regulate fluid balance has become highly refined over the years (although choosing the target dry weight and reaching it are more problematic). A similar accuracy in the maintenance of Na balance requires that the dialysate Na concentration be individualized such that with each treatment a constant end-session plasma Na concentration is reached. If over time end-dialysis weight and plasma Na concentration are kept constant, (assuming no change in Na distribution volume) one can assume that the patient will be in Na balance. As currently practiced the dialysate Na concentrations whether fixed or varied are not chosen with the primary aim of achieving Na balance. This approach risks a pathologic excess in the total Na mass, which over time can lead to clinical manifestations of volume overload such as hypertension or congestive heart failure.

To properly calculate the dialysate Na concentration required to maintain Na balance, measurement of the patient's plasma water Na concentration at the beginning of the treatment is required. Conductivity measurements can be used as a surrogate of Na concentration because there is a linear correlation between these parameters. Locatelli et al. (24,25) have recently described the use of a biofeedback system that allows for the automatic determination of plasma water and dialysate conductivity such that blood sampling can be avoided. With these measurements along with session time, desired weight loss, and expected end-treatment plasma water conductivity, the dialysate conductivity is automatically adjusted to achieve the prescribed final plasma water conductivity. Application of this conductivity kinetic model to patients treated with a variant of hemodiafiltration achieves near zero hydro-sodium balance and improves intradialytic cardiovascular stability (24). Newer technology will allow for plasma water and dialysate conductivity to be measured repetitively during the procedure allowing automatic adjustment of the dialysate Na on-line throughout the procedure (26,27).

With increased ability to individualize the dialysate Na concentration one can envision a scenario in which a patient initiated on hemodialysis is initially treated with a dialysate Na concentration designed to achieve negative Na balance. Once the patient becomes normotensive or requires minimal amounts of antihypertensive medications, the dialysate Na can be adjusted on a continual basis to ensure that Na balance is maintained. Achieving the optimal total body Na content will likely become just as important as determining an accurate dry weight.

Dialysate Potassium

In most chronic outpatient dialysis centers there is little individualization of the dialysate potassium concentration. Rather, most patients are dialyzed with a potassium bath that is prepared centrally and delivered with a concentration fixed at 1 or 2 mEq/L. When using a fixed dialysate potassium it is difficult to predict the exact amount of potassium that will be removed in a given dialysis session. Typically, one should not expect more than about 80 to 100 mEq of potassium removal even with the use of a potassium-free dialysate. In addition, there will be marked variability in the amount of potassium removed from patient to patient despite similar predialysis potassium levels and dialysis regimens. This variability can be explained by the fact that potassium movement from the intracellular to the extracellular space and ultimately into the dialysate is influenced by several patient-specific factors.

The removal of excess potassium by dialysis is achieved by the use of a dialysate with a potassium concentration lower than that of plasma creating a gradient favoring potassium removal; its rate is largely a function of this gradient (28). Plasma potassium concentration falls rapidly in the early stages of dialysis, but as the plasma concentration falls, potassium removal becomes less efficient. Because potassium is freely permeable across the dialysis membrane, movement of potassium from the intracellular space to the extracellular space appears to be the limiting factor in potassium removal. Factors that importantly dictate the distribution of potassium between these two spaces include changes in acid-base status, tonicity, glucose and insulin concentration, and catecholamine activity (Table 3.3).

The movement of potassium between the intracellular and extracellular space is influenced by changes in acid-base balance that occur during the dialysis procedure (29,30). Extracellular alkalosis causes a shift of potassium into cells, whereas acidosis results in potassium efflux from cells. During a typical dialysis there is net addition of base to the extracellular space, which promotes cellular uptake of potassium and therefore attenuates the removal of potassium during dialysis. With routine dialysis the change in blood pH is of small magnitude and the effect on potassium removal is not profound. By contrast, dialysis in patients who are acidotic will result in less potassium removal because potassium is shifted into cells as the serum bicarbonate rises. Weigand et al. (31) described five patients in whom the serum potassium concentration decreased during dialysis even though the dialysate potassium concentration was higher than the original serum potassium concentration. The decline in potassium concentration occurred in association with a marked rise in the pH. In one patient the decline in potassium concentration was of such a magnitude that she became quadriplegic and developed respiratory failure. There appears to be no difference in potassium removal whether acetate or bicarbonate is chosen as the dialysate buffer.

Conversely, the serum potassium concentration can influence the net addition of base. Redaelli et al. (32) found that a potassium-free dialysate was associated with less bicarbonate uptake as compared with a dialysate that contained a potassium concentration of 2 mEq/L. It was postulated that a lower potas-

sium dialysate that results in a high plasma-to-dialysate potassium concentration gradient causes less hydrogen ion movement from the intracellular space to the extracellular space and hence less downward titration of the extracellular bicarbonate concentration. As a result, the concentration gradient favoring diffusion of bicarbonate from the dialysate to the extracellular space is reduced. This relationship should be considered when dialyzing an acidotic patient.

Insulin is known to stimulate the cellular uptake of potassium and can therefore influence the amount of potassium removal during dialysis. This effect of insulin was demonstrated in studies comparing potassium removal using glucose-containing and glucose-free dialysates (33,34). The use of a glucose-free dialysate was found to result in greater amounts of potassium removal when compared with the use of a glucose-containing bath. The use of a glucose-free dialysate would be expected to result in lower levels of insulin. As a result, there is increased movement of potassium to the extracellular space where it becomes available for dialytic removal.

Changes in plasma tonicity can affect the distribution of potassium between the intracellular and extracellular space (29). Administration of hypertonic saline or mannitol is sometimes used in the treatment of hypotension during dialysis. These agents would be expected to favor potassium removal during dialysis because the resultant increased tonicity would favor potassium movement into the extracellular space. There are no studies addressing whether there is any significant clinical benefit with this approach.

Beta-adrenergic stimulation is known to shift potassium into cells and lower the extracellular concentration. Inhaled beta stimulants have been reported to be effective in the acute treatment of hyperkalemia, so such therapy before dialysis may lower the total amount of potassium removed during the dialytic procedure. Allon et al. (35) found that the cumulative dialytic potassium removal was significantly lower in patients who were treated with nebulized albuterol 30 minutes before the procedure as compared with patients in whom the albuterol treatment was omitted.

Alterations in serum potassium concentration during dialysis can conceivably have important effects on systemic hemodynamics. A decrease in serum potassium concentration during hemodialysis would be predicted to increase systemic vascular resistance. Hypokalemia has been shown to increase resistance in skeletal muscle, skin, and coronary vascular beds, possibly through effects on the electrogenic Na-K pump in the sarcolemmal membranes of vascular smooth muscle cells (36). In addition, decreased serum potassium concentration may enhance the sensitivity of the vasculature to endogenous pressor hormones (37).

Despite the potential for hypokalemia to increase systemic vascular resistance, Pogglitsch et al. (38) found the incidence of hypotensive episodes were, in fact, reduced when supplemental potassium was administered during the final 30 minutes of dialysis. One explanation for this seemingly paradoxical finding rests on the known interaction between hypokalemia and the autonomic nervous system. For example, hypokalemia has been found to be associated with dysautonomia in patients with hyperaldosteronism (39). It is reasonable to speculate that in patients with advanced renal failure, who already have a propen-

TABLE 3.3. FACTORS AFFECTING POTASSIUM (K) REMOVAL DURING HEMODIALYSIS

Shifts K into cell thereby ↓ dialytic K removal
  Exogenous insulin
  Glucose containing dialysate vs. glucose free dialysate
  Beta agonists
  Correction of metabolic acidosis during dialysis
Shifts K to extracellular space or impairs cell K uptake thereby ↑
Dialytic K removal
  Beta blockers
  Alpha-adrenergic receptor stimulation
  Hypertonicity

sity for autonomic insufficiency, a fall in plasma potassium may uncover or cause impairment in sympathetic responses (40).

In support of this suggestion, Henrich et al. (41) found that hypokalemic dialysis was accompanied by a fall in plasma catecholamine concentration as compared with dialysis in which serum potassium concentration was held constant. Moreover, despite similar reductions in blood pressure, the isokalemic dialysis group had a significant increase in heart rate after dialysis, whereas the hypokalemic group demonstrated no significant change. Further studies are needed to investigate the effects of fluctuations in serum potassium concentration during dialysis on the autonomic nervous system.

Changes in serum potassium concentration during dialysis may also influence systemic hemodynamics through effects on myocardial performance. Dialysis is associated with an increase in contractility, which can be attributed to an increase in ionized serum calcium. Increased ionized calcium is most closely related to improved ventricular contractility, but modifying effects of concomitant decreases in potassium may also be important. Haddy et al. (42) have demonstrated that the inotropic effect of increased serum calcium concentration is enhanced by simultaneous decreases in plasma potassium concentration. In this regard, Wizemann et al. (43) found that improvement in myocardial contractility during a series of isovolemic dialysis maneuvers was related to a simultaneous increase in plasma calcium and decrease in plasma potassium concentration. In the presence of an elevated plasma potassium concentration, a high plasma calcium concentration failed to exert a significant inotropic effect.

An increase in peripheral vascular resistance secondary to the development of hypokalemia could have potential detrimental effects on dialysis efficiency. This decrease in efficiency would result from decreased blood flow to urea-rich tissues such as skeletal muscle and in effect increase the amount of body wide recirculation. In support of this possibility, Dolson et al. (44) found that a dialysate potassium concentration of 1.0 mmol/L as compared with 3.0 mmol/L resulted in lower values for both the urea reduction ratio and *Kt/V* in 14 patients with ESRD. By contrast, Zehnder et al. (45) found no effect of dialysate potassium on dialysis adequacy. Although more studies are needed in this area, it is likely that any effect of a low dialysate potassium concentration to decrease dialysis adequacy is small in magnitude. In addition, increasing the dialysate potassium concentration to improve dialysis adequacy will increase the risk of hyperkalemia during the interdialytic period.

Most patients dialyzed with a fixed potassium dialysate tolerate the procedure well and do not suffer from complications of hypokalemia or hyperkalemia. Nevertheless, there are clinical conditions in which an individualized dialysate potassium concentration may be useful. Patients with underlying heart disease, particularly in the setting of digoxin therapy, are prone to arrhythmias as hypokalemia develops toward the end of a typical treatment. The risk of arrhythmias is also increased in the early stages of a dialysis session when the plasma potassium concentration may still be normal but rapidly declining (46). The sudden reduction in the plasma potassium concentration during the initial portions of the dialysis procedure has recently been shown to unfavorably alter the QTc (a marker of risk of ventricular arrhythmias) even in dialysis patients without obvious heart disease (47,48).

With these considerations in mind, Redaelli et al. (49) have studied the effects of modeling the dialysate potassium concentration in such a way as to minimize the initial rapid decline in the plasma potassium concentration. Patients with frequent intradialytic premature ventricular complexes were dialyzed using a dialysate with a fixed (2.5 mEq/L) potassium or one with an exponentially declining potassium (from 3.9 to 2.5 mEq/L), which maintained a constant blood to dialysate potassium gradient of 1.5 mEq/L throughout the procedure. In the fixed dialysate group, the blood to dialysate potassium gradient decreased over the treatment from 3.0 mEq/L to 1.4 mEq/L. The variable potassium dialysate decreased premature ventricular complexes, a finding most evident during the first hour of the procedure. The total drop in the serum potassium concentration was no different between the fixed and variable potassium dialysates.

In addition to decreasing arrhythmias, maintenance of a constant blood to dialysate potassium concentration may prove useful in patients who tend to develop worsening hypertension during the course of the dialysis procedure. Hypokalemia increases resistance in skeletal muscle, skin, and coronary vascular beds possibly through effects on the electrogenic Na-K pump in the sarcolemmal membranes of vascular smooth muscle cells (50). In addition, decreased serum potassium concentration may enhance the sensitivity of the vasculature to endogenous presser hormones (51). In chronic dialysis patients, postdialysis rebound hypertension is greater with a 1.0 mEq/L than with a 3.0 mEq/L potassium dialysate (52). Although not yet studied, preventing the initial rapid decline in the plasma potassium concentration with a ramped dialysate potassium may help attenuate the hypertensive response that some patients exhibit toward the end of a dialysis treatment.

In summary, because of kinetics of potassium movement from the intracellular to the extracellular space one can expect only up to 70 to 90 mEq of potassium to be removed during a typical dialysis session. As a result, one should not overestimate the effectiveness of the dialytic procedure in the treatment of severe hyperkalemia. The total amount removed will exhibit considerable variability and will be influenced by changes in acid-base status, changes in tonicity, changes in glucose and insulin concentration, and catecholamine activity. Given the tendency for the plasma potassium to rise in the immediate postdialysis time period, the most efficient way to remove excess potassium stores would be to prescribe 2- to 3-hour periods of dialysis separated by several hours (53). Studies examining the hemodynamic effect of potassium fluxes during hemodialysis are limited. More importantly, deliberate alterations in dialysate potassium concentration to effect hemodynamic stability would not be without risk. Use of low potassium dialysate concentration may contribute to arrhythmias, especially in those patients with underlying coronary artery disease or those taking digoxin. On the other hand, use of dialysate with high potassium concentration may predispose patients to predialysis hyperkalemia. In patients who are at high risk for arrhythmias on dialysis, modeling the dialysate potassium concentration so as to maintain a constant blood to dialysate potassium gradient throughout the procedure may be of clinical benefit (Table 3.4).

TABLE 3.4. CONSIDERATIONS WHEN INDIVIDUALIZING COMPONENTS OF THE DIALYSATE

Dialysate Component	Advantage	Disadvantage
Na Increased	More hemodynamic stability, less cramping	Dipsogenic effect, increased interdialytic weight gain, ? chronic hypertension
Decreased (rarely used)	Less interdialytic weight gain	Intradialytic hypotension and cramping more common
Ca Increased	Suppression of PTH, promotes hemodynamic stability	Hypercalcemia with vitamin D and Ca-containing phosphate binders
Decreased	Permits greater use of vitamin D and calcium-containing phosphate binders	Potential for negative calcium balance, stimulation of PTH, slight decrease in hemodynamic stability
K Increased	Less arrhythmias in setting of digoxin or coronary heart disease, less rebound hypertension	Limited by hyperkalemia
Decreased (ramped dialysate K ideal, prevents rapid initial decline in plasma K)	Greater dietary intake of K with less hyperkalemia, ? improvement in myocardial contractility	Increased arrhythmias, may exacerbate autonomic insufficiency
HCO₃ Increased	Corrects chronic acidosis thereby benefits nutrition and bone metabolism	Postdialysis metabolic alkalosis
Decreased	Less metabolic alkalosis	Potential for chronic acidosis
Mg Increased	? Less arrhythmias, ? hemodynamic benefit	Hypermagnesemia
Decreased	Permits use of Mg-containing phosphate binders	Hypomagnesemia
PO₄ (rarely added to dialysate)	Treats or prevents hypophosphatemia in malnourished, chronic disease state, overdose setting, daily dialysis	Hyperphosphatemia

PTH, parathyroid hormone.

Dialysate Buffer

Acetate Buffer

The early use of bicarbonate as the base in dialysis solutions required a cumbersome system in which CO_2 was continuously bubbled through the dialysate to lower pH to prevent the precipitation of calcium and magnesium salts. As a result, in the early 1960s acetate became the standard dialysate buffer used to correct uremic acidosis and to offset the diffusive losses of bicarbonate during hemodialysis. Over the next several years, reports began to accumulate linking routine use of acetate with cardiovascular instability and hypotension during dialysis. In particular, critically ill patients undergoing acute hemodialysis, especially with the use of large surface area dialyzers, were found to exhibit vascular instability when exposed to acetate in dialysis fluid. Given these observations, bicarbonate-containing dialysate began to reemerge as the principal dialysate buffer especially as advances in biotechnology made the use of bicarbonate dialysate less expensive and less cumbersome to use. Because acetate is still used as the principal dialysate buffer in some centers, the following paragraphs compare the clinical effects of acetate and bicarbonate dialysate.

During a routine dialysis in which acetate is used as the buffer there are large fluxes of both acetate and bicarbonate across the dialyzer with little overall net gain in base (54). Because the acetate dialysate lacks bicarbonate there is diffusion of actual bicarbonate from the blood into the dialysate. In addition, potential bicarbonate is lost from the blood in the form of organic anions such as citrate, lactate, pyruvate, beta-hydroxybutyrate, and acetoacetate because these anions diffuse across the dialyzer and into the dialysate (55). The pH of blood exiting the dialysis cartridge does not fall because CO_2 diffuses from the blood as well. Despite this large efflux of potential and actual bicarbonate from the body, there is a net gain of alkali because of the greater influx of acetate as it diffuses from the dialysate into the blood. Acetate is normally metabolized in muscle to acetyl CoA. Acetyl CoA is then metabolized in the Krebs cycle to CO_2 and water with formation of one bicarbonate molecule for each molecule of acetate metabolized. The metabolism of acetate to carbon dioxide can contribute up to 40% of the total energy expenditure during dialysis (56). In addition, acetate-containing dialysate is associated with significant increases in the plasma concentration of ketone bodies (57). The accelerated ketogenesis and the extra caloric burden seen with acetate dialysate does not appear to be associated with an impairment in glucose utilization or change in plasma insulin during the procedure.

Chronic hemodialysis patients metabolize acetate at a reduced rate as compared with control patients (58). Decreased rates of metabolism of acetate to bicarbonate can potentially result in accumulation of acetate. This accumulation of acetate is magnified with use of dialyzers with large surface areas that allow for transfer of acetate to the plasma compartment at rates greater than a patient's ability to metabolize it. The consequent increase in blood concentration of acetate has been associated with nausea, vomiting, fatigue, and, more importantly, hemodynamic instability.

There are a number of mechanisms by which acetate might predispose to vascular instability (Table 3.5). Acetate, possibly by its conversion to adenosine, has vasodilatory properties that can directly decrease peripheral vascular resistance. In addition, acetate might increase venous capacity leading to a decrease in cardiac filling (59). These vasodilatory effects of acetate are further augmented through the release of interleukin-1. Interleukin-1 has vasodilatory properties and its activity is increased

TABLE 3.5. MECHANISMS BY WHICH ACETATE BUFFER CONTRIBUTES TO HEMODYNAMIC INSTABILITY

Directly decreases peripheral vascular resistance (in approximately 10% of patients)
Stimulates release of the vasodilator compound, interleukin-1
Induction of metabolic acidosis via bicarbonate loss through the dialyzer
Associated with arterial hypoxemia and increases in oxygen consumption
? Myocardial effects of acetate

from 8 to 12 times normal by standard acetate hemodialysis (60).

In addition to direct vasodilatory properties, incomplete acetate oxidation can lead to acid-base changes that can adversely affect hemodynamics. Metabolism of acetate to bicarbonate in an amount less than the diffusive losses of bicarbonate through the dialyzer will result in a decreased concentration of serum bicarbonate. A decrease in serum bicarbonate concentration can result in mild metabolic acidosis that may take 2 to 3 hours after dialysis to correct (61). Such loss of bicarbonate through the dialyzer contributes to vascular instability in addition to any direct vascular effects of acetate (62).

Arterial hypoxemia occurs with the use of acetate dialysate and may also contribute to vascular instability. During acetate dialysis there is diffusive loss of soluble carbon dioxide from blood to dialysate. In an attempt to maintain normal blood carbon dioxide concentration, pulmonary hypoventilation occurs resulting in hypoxemia. In addition, metabolism of acetate leads to an increase in oxygen consumption further exacerbating any decrease in oxygenation. In susceptible individuals, acetate may provoke subendocardial schemia by deleteriously affecting myocardial oxygen balance (63).

Despite the association of acetate with a higher frequency of symptoms in some studies, there is a poor correlation between symptoms and signs and blood acetate concentration (64–66). In an attempt to reconcile this discrepancy, Vinay et al. (67) studied a large population of dialysis patients and concluded that true acetate intolerance only occurred in about 10% of the dialysis population. The patients found intolerant were unable to metabolize acetate optimally and were predominately female. Because muscle is the primary site of metabolism of acetate, a reduced muscle mass often found in females might account for the reduced metabolism of acetate. Similarly, malnourished and elderly patients may be more predisposed to acetate intolerance by such a mechanism.

During conventional hemodialysis with acetate the vasoconstrictive response to hypovolemia is masked by the vasodilatory tendency induced by the diffusive nature of the therapy. It is unclear, however, whether inability to vasoconstrict during conventional hemodialysis is related to use of acetate or rather a fall in serum osmolality. In this regard, several studies have found that vascular instability with acetate dialysis is generally improved with use of a higher Na dialysate concentration. In addition, substitution of bicarbonate for acetate as the base constituent in the dialysate has been purported to markedly improve symptoms on dialysis. It has been difficult to prove,

however, whether bicarbonate dialysate can independently further improve hemodynamic and symptomatic tolerance to hemodialysis especially when a higher dialysate osmolality is used. Wehle et al. (68) found no added benefit of bicarbonate over acetate particularly if dialysate Na was increased to 145 mEq/L. Henrich et al. (69) in a comparative study of acetate and bicarbonate dialysis using a dialysate Na concentration of 140 mEq/L demonstrated strikingly similar hemodynamic responses. In a later study, Velez et al. (70) noted that with high-Na dialysates (141 mEq/L) no detectable differences between bicarbonate and acetate were found with respect to cardiac output, mean blood pressure, or orthostatic tolerance to standing after dialysis. With use of a dialysate Na of 130 mEq/L, however, bicarbonate dialysate was associated with greater stability of blood pressure on standing after dialysis.

Controversy exists as to the overall effects of acetate and bicarbonate buffers on ventricular performance. Administration of sodium acetate as a bolus injection in dogs results in marked decreases in myocardial contractile force and blood pressure (71). If given, however, as a continuous infusion no definite depression of myocardial function is observed (72). Aizawa et al. (73) compared the effects of acetate and bicarbonate hemodialysis on cardiac function using phonocardiography. Left ventricular function was depressed to a greater extent with acetate than after bicarbonate dialysis.

The negative inotropic effect attributed to acetate has been contested by other reports in which sodium acetate was found to increase ventricular performance. Nitenberg et al. (74) using angiographic techniques studied left ventricular function in seven patients with plasma acetate concentrations comparable to that found during sodium acetate hemodialysis. An increase in cardiac index, ejection fraction, and maximum velocity of circumferential fiber shortening (VCF) not attributable to alterations in heart rate, preload, or afterload was demonstrated after sodium acetate infusion. Mansell et al. (75) noted that patients who developed hyperacetatemia during regular dialysis were still able to maintain an increased cardiac output. Schick et al. (76) studied nine patients in a double-blind cross-over manner and demonstrated improvement of left ventricular mean VCF of equal magnitude with both acetate and bicarbonate hemodialysis. Ruder et al. (77) performed a double-blind, cross-over study of 36 patients comparing acetate and bicarbonate hemodialysis with respect to baseline left ventricular function. In patients with depressed VCF, hemodialysis with either buffer resulted in improvement of ventricular function with mean VCF significantly higher after bicarbonate dialysis as compared with acetate. In patients with normal VCF only bicarbonate dialysis produced significantly better ventricular function. In contrast, Leunissen et al. (78,79) found increases in VCF in patients with normal left ventricular function with either acetate or bicarbonate dialysis. In patients with compromised left ventricular function, only bicarbonate dialysis resulted in significant increase in VCF.

The disparity of results in studies of effects of dialysate composition on cardiac function may in part result from failure to distinguish effects of volume removal. In this regard, Nixon et al. (80) demonstrated that dialysis with acetate with or without volume removal produced an increase in contractility. Mehta et al. (81) performed isovolemic dialysis and found that mean VCF improved to the same extent with both acetate and bicarbonate dialysis. Anderson et al. (82) studied left ventricular performance with two-dimensional echocardiography in five patients under three different cardiac filling volumes before and after a standard isovolemic hemodialysis. Cardiac performance as assessed by VCF improved comparably with acetate or bicarbonate under conditions of increased or decreased preloads.

In summary, many years of experience with acetate as the principal buffer in dialysate has not borne out concerns that acetate would be associated with long-term adverse consequences. In most chronic stable dialysis patients, cardiac function is improved with acetate or bicarbonate-containing dialysate. Under conditions in which a dialysate Na of more than 140 mEq/L is used, bicarbonate offers no apparent hemodynamic advantage over acetate. By contrast, use of a bicarbonate bath may provide more hemodynamic stability than acetate under conditions of a low Na dialysate concentration (less than 135 mEq/L) or in patients who are truly acetate intolerant. In addition, bicarbonate-containing dialysate improves platelet function to a greater extent than does acetate and may be less arrhythmogenic in susceptible patients (83,84). In either case, it should be pointed out that as high-efficiency and especially high-flux dialysis becomes more widely used, acetate-containing dialysate will become a thing of the past. The increased clearance seen with these procedures would allow the rate of influx of acetate to exceed the maximal rate of metabolism such that acid-base balance could not be maintained.

Bicarbonate Buffer

Bicarbonate is now the principal buffer used in dialysate. Producing bicarbonate dialysate requires a specifically designed system that mixes a bicarbonate concentrate and an acid concentrate with purified water. The acid concentrate contains a small amount of either lactic or acetic acid and all the calcium and magnesium. The exclusion of these cations from the bicarbonate concentrate prevents the precipitation of magnesium and calcium carbonate that would otherwise occur in the setting of a high bicarbonate concentration. During the mixing procedure the acid in the acid concentrate will react with an equimolar amount of bicarbonate to generate carbonic acid and carbon dioxide. The generation of carbon dioxide causes the pH of the final solution to fall to approximately 7.0 to 7.4. This more acidic pH as well as the lower concentrations of calcium and magnesium in the final mixture allows for these ions to remain in solution. The final concentration of bicarbonate in the dialysate is generally fixed in the range of 33 to 38 mmol/L (Fig. 3.1).

The use of a bicarbonate dialysate is associated with a number of potential complications (85,86). The liquid bicarbonate concentrate can be responsible for microbial contamination of the final dialysate largely because the bicarbonate concentrate is an excellent bacterial growth medium. This complication can be minimized by short storage time as well as filtration of the concentrate during the production procedure. Use of a bicarbonate cartridge can further minimize this complication. This device allows for the bicarbonate concentrate to be produced on-line by passing water through a column containing powdered bicarbon-

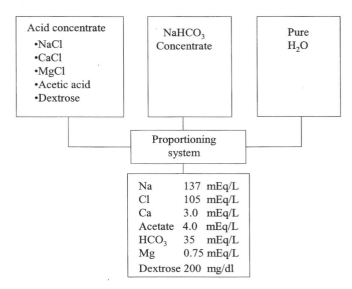

FIG. 3.1. Components of the dialysate circuit in which bicarbonate serves as the buffer source.

ate. The concentrate is produced and proportioned immediately before mixing with the acid concentrate. Hypoxemia may occur during bicarbonate dialysis when high concentrations of bicarbonate are used. This complication appears to be the result of suppressed ventilation secondary to the increase in pH and serum bicarbonate concentration. In addition, excessively high levels of bicarbonate in the dialysate may result in acute metabolic alkalosis causing mental confusion, lethargy, weakness, and cramps.

The factors that determine bicarbonate requirements in hemodialysis patients include acid production during the interdialytic period, the removal of organic anions during the hemodialysis procedure, and the buffer deficit of the body. Because these factors are likely to vary from patient to patient there is increasing interest in individualizing the dialysate bicarbonate concentration. The optimal level of dialysate bicarbonate would be a concentration low enough to prevent significant alkalosis in the postdialytic period and yet be high enough to prevent predialysis acidosis (87,88).

Maintaining a predialysis total CO_2 concentration of greater than 23 mmol/L can be achieved in most patients by individually adjusting the dialysate bicarbonate concentration. Oettinger et al. (89) found that 75% of patients exceeded this level with a dialysate bicarbonate concentration of 42 mmol/L (89). Use of this high bicarbonate dialysate did not result in progressive alkalemia, even in patients beginning the study with a normal predialysis total CO_2 using a standard bicarbonate dialysate concentration of 36 mmol/L. In addition, the high bicarbonate dialysate did not cause hypoxia or hypercarbia or alter the predialysis calcium, ionized calcium, or phosphorus.

Using high bicarbonate dialysate may improve nutrition and bone metabolism. Graham et al. (90) examined protein turnover in a group of chronic dialysis patients in whom dialysate bicarbonate concentration was increased from 35 to 40 mmol/L; supplemental oral bicarbonate therapy was given to two patients whose predialysis tCO_2 (total CO_2) concentration did not exceed 23 mmol/L. The mean tCO_2 concentration increased from 18.5 to 24.8 mmol/L during the high bicarbonate dialysate. Correction of the acidosis was associated with a significant decrease in protein degradation as suggested by leucine kinetic studies. In a similarly designed study, these investigators found an increase in the sensitivity of the parathyroid glands to calcium in patients using a dialysate bicarbonate concentration of 35 or 40 mmol/L (91).

Another strategy that may be effective in improving the acidosis of chronic dialysis patients is to use citric acid in place of acetic acid in the acid concentrate. In a recent study of 22 patients, use of citric acid decreased the number of patients with a predialysis bicarbonate concentration less than 23 mEq/L from 14 to 7 (92). Use of the citric acid dialysate was also associated with an increased delivered dose of dialysis, an effect postulated to be due to improved membrane permeability resulting from citrate's local anticoagulant effect. Improved membrane permeability with greater diffusive flux of bicarbonate from dialysate to blood or metabolism of citrate to bicarbonate in liver and muscle are the most likely explanations for the improvement in bicarbonate concentration.

The bicarbonate concentration used in most dialysis centers is set at 35 mmol/L and rarely adjusted. Given the increasing evidence that correction of chronic acidosis is of clinical benefit, increased consideration should be given to adjusting the bicarbonate concentration with the goal of maintaining the predialysis tCO_2 concentration at greater than 23 mmol/L. In some patients, supplemental oral bicarbonate therapy will be required to achieve this goal. Substitution of citric acid for acetic acid in the acid concentrate is a maneuver worthy of further investigation.

Dialysate Magnesium

The usual concentration of magnesium in the dialysate is 0.5 to 1.0 mEq/L and is only rarely manipulated. In an attempt to minimize the development of hypercalcemia associated with the use of calcium-containing phosphate binders and vitamin D, there has been interest in using magnesium-containing compounds as a phosphate binder. The use of oral magnesium requires the use of a low magnesium dialysate concentration so as to avoid the development of hypermagnesemia. Depending on which magnesium salt is used, this strategy has had variable success (93,94).

Use of oral $Mg(OH)_3$ in association with a magnesium-free dialysate had little or no effect on phosphate and increased mean serum magnesium to 4.3 mg/dL. In addition, diarrhea was a frequent side effect. More favorable results have been reported with oral $MgCO_3$. O'Donovan et al. (95) reported good control of the serum phosphorus level using oral $MgCO_3$ and a magnesium-free dialysate. On this regimen diarrhea was mild and transient and the serum concentration of magnesium did not change. More recently, Kelber et al. (96) examined the feasibility of using a magnesium-free dialysate in the setting of high-efficiency dialysis. Despite the use of oral $MgCO_3$, patients developed severe muscle cramping that was immediately relieved by adding magnesium back to the dialysate. It was determined that measured magnesium removal exceeded the estimated predialysis extracellular fluid magnesium pool. By contrast, a dialysate magnesium of 0.6 mg/dL in combination with oral $MgCO_3$ was well tolerated.

Use of this later regimen was then examined in a prospective randomized cross-over study (97). Patients were studied while taking $MgCO_3$ and one half the usual dose of $CaCO_3$ along with a dialysate magnesium of 0.6 mg/dL and again while ingesting $CaCO_3$ given in the usual dose with a dialysate magnesium of 1.8 mg/dL. There was no difference in the serum concentrations of phosphorus, calcium, or magnesium between the two phases of the study. In addition, the $MgCO_3$-low $CaCO_3$ regimen permitted a greater amount of intravenous calcitriol to be used without the development of hypercalcemia. It was concluded that use of oral $MgCO_3$ as a phosphate binder and a low dialysate magnesium concentration may be a useful strategy in patients who develop hypercalcemia during treatment with calcitriol and $CaCO_3$ (Table 3.4).

Dialysate Calcium

Until recently, dialysate calcium concentrations (typically 3.5 mEq/L) that result in a net flux of calcium into the patient were widely used. The substitution of calcium for aluminum phosphate binders and the wider use of high doses of intravenous 1,25 $(OH)_2$ vitamin D both may be complicated by the development of hypercalcemia. The use of a high dialysate calcium concentration can further contribute to this problem and can limit the use of calcium-containing phosphate binders and vitamin D.

Given these considerations, dialysate calcium concentrations have generally fallen. Using a dialysate calcium concentration of 2.5 mEq/L, Slatopolsky et al. (98) was able to control the serum phosphorus in 21 patients with calcium carbonate at an average daily dose of 10.5 g with no instances of hypercalcemia. In an earlier study using a dialysate calcium concentration of 3.5 mEq/L, large doses of calcium carbonate were also effective in controlling the serum phosphorus but only at the expense of several instances of hypercalcemia (99). The beneficial effect of combining high-dose calcium-containing phosphate binders with a low dialysate calcium concentration has been confirmed by other investigators as well (100,101). In a similar manner, Van der Merwe et al. (102) treated patients with secondary hyperparathyroidism with high-dose oral calcitriol combined with a low calcium dialysate concentration. During the course of the study there was a significant fall in the parathyroid hormone (PTH) level and alkaline phosphatase concentration without the development of hypercalcemia.

Despite the enthusiasm for use of low calcium dialysate some recent studies have emphasized that such an approach requires careful monitoring to ensure that the patient does not develop negative calcium balance or worsening secondary hyperparathyroidism. Argiles et al. (103) found that serum immunoreactive parathyroid hormone (iPTH) levels increased significantly in patients treated with a 2.5 mEq/L dialysate calcium bath compared with a control group of patients dialyzed with a dialysate calcium of 3.0 mEq/L. This increase in iPTH occurred despite 2.4-fold more oral $CaCO_3$ ingested in the low dialysate calcium group. Although the increase in oral calcium intake was not sufficient to prevent the stimulation in iPTH, subsequent treatment with 1,25 (OH)₂ vitamin D was effective in reversing the rise in iPTH levels.

Similar results were reported by Fernandez et al. (104) in a group of patients sequentially dialyzed against a 3.5 mEq/L and then 2.5 mEq/L calcium bath. While on the low calcium dialysate, there was a significant increase in both serum iPTH as well as serum alkaline phosphatase levels. These changes occurred despite the fact that oral calcium carbonate was administered at doses ranging from 3 to 6 g/day while on the low calcium dialysate. As determined by clearance studies, the authors suggested that the low calcium dialysate resulted in negative calcium balance that, in turn, contributed to the worsening hyperparathyroidism. Furthermore, the maintenance of a normal serum calcium concentration noted in the study occurred at the expense of PTH-induced calcium mobilization from bone. Using measurements of total and ionized calcium in serum as well as in spent dialysate, Argiles et al. (105) have confirmed that a 2.5 mEq/L calcium dialysate is associated with negative calcium balance. Based on the potential of a 2.5 mEq/L dialysate calcium to cause negative calcium balance and to worsen secondary hyperparathyroidism, these authors now use a dialysate calcium of at least 3.0 mEq/L in most chronic dialysis patients (106).

In addition to effects on metabolic bone disease varying the dialysate calcium concentration can affect hemodynamic stability during dialysis. Maynard et al. (107) studied 12 patients in a prospective cross-over trial and found that a high dialysate calcium concentration (3.75 mEq/L) was associated with significantly less fall in both systolic blood pressure and mean arterial pressure than a low calcium dialysate (2.75 mEq/L). In a double-blind prospective study, Sherman et al. (108) studied 20 patients who underwent alternate hemodialysis with dialysate calcium concentrations of 2.5 and 3.5 mEq/L. The use of a low dialysate calcium concentration was associated with a minor but statistically significant reduction in mean blood pressure during hemodialysis. This effect may become clinically important in patients with congestive heart failure. One study found that a 3.5 mEq/L calcium dialysate offered clear hemodynamic benefits over a 2.5 mEq/L dialysate in patients with an ejection fraction of less than 40% (109).

In patients prone to intradialytic hypotension who are at risk for hypercalcemia, dialysate calcium profiling can be used as a strategy to improve hemodynamic stability and yet minimize the potential for hypercalcemia (110). In one study patients were dialyzed for 4 hours in which the dialysate calcium concentration was set low (1.25 mmol/L) for the first 2 hours and then increased to 1.75 mmol/L for the last 2 hours (110). Use of the varying dialysate calcium concentration was associated with greater hemodynamic stability as compared with a fixed dialysate calcium concentration of either 1.25 or 1.5 mmol/L. This hemodynamic benefit was accomplished via an increase in cardiac output. At the end of 3 weeks there was no difference in the predialysis ionized calcium concentration between the three groups.

Changes in serum calcium concentration may influence blood pressure through alterations in either systemic vascular resistance or the determinants of cardiac output or both. In an attempt to determine the physiologic mechanisms for calcium-induced changes in systemic arterial pressure, Fellner et al. (111)

studied hemodynamic variables that determine arterial blood pressure as a function of changes in dialysate calcium concentration. Eight patients underwent hemodialysis three times within a single week with dialysate calcium concentrations of 1.0 mEq/L, 3.5 mEq/L, or 5.0 mEq/L. As in previous studies, changes in blood calcium concentration correlated directly with blood pressure. In addition, higher levels of calcium augmented left ventricular stroke volume and cardiac output while leaving total vascular resistance unchanged. It was concluded that alterations in blood calcium concentration affected blood pressure primarily through changes in left ventricular output rather than in peripheral vascular tone.

In addition to changes in ionized calcium concentration, hemodialysis leads to alterations in several factors that could conceivably be responsible for the observed changes in ventricular function. Henrich et al. (112) performed a series of dialysis maneuvers to determine the contribution of dialyzable toxins, ionized calcium, and acidemia to left ventricular performance during routine hemodialysis. The dialysate of each maneuver was adjusted to produce three effects: (a) isovolemic dialysis in which neither ionized calcium nor bicarbonate was allowed to increase (this procedure tested the effects of uremic toxin removal), (b) isovolemic dialysis during which ionized calcium increased but bicarbonate was held constant, and (c) isovolemic dialysis in which bicarbonate increased but ionized calcium was kept constant. Echocardiographic studies showed that left ventricular end-diastolic and end-systolic volumes decreased and ejection fraction and VCF increased only in the procedure in which plasma ionized calcium increased. This study suggested that the rise in ionized calcium is a major element in the observed improvement in myocardial contractility. Similar findings were recently reported by Lang et al. (113). Using dialysates differing only in calcium concentration, myocardial contractility was shown to correlate directly with plasma ionized calcium. The mechanism by which increases in ionized calcium seen during hemodialysis lead to enhanced ventricular function is not known.

In summary, the dialysate calcium concentration has implications with regards to metabolic bone disease and hemodynamic stability. As with the other dialysate constituents, the calcium concentration should be individually tailored to the patient. In patients who are prone to intradialytic hypotension avoidance of a low dialysate calcium concentration may be of benefit. On the other hand, the use of a lower calcium concentration in the dialysate will allow the use of increased doses of calcium-containing phosphate binders and lessen any dependence on aluminum-containing binders. In addition, use of 1,25 (OH)₂ vitamin D can be liberalized so as to reduce circulating levels of PTH with less fear of inducing hypercalcemia. However, when using low dialysate calcium concentrations (<3.0 mEq/L), one must monitor the patients closely to ensure that negative calcium balance does not develop (as might occur when substituting Renalgel for calcium phosphate binders) and that iPTH levels remain in an acceptable range (114).

Dialysate Phosphate

In patients with mild to moderate hyperphosphatemia, hemodialysis has been estimated to remove 250 to 325 mg/day of phosphorus when extrapolated to an average week (115,116). Because a diet that provides adequate protein may provide approximately 900 mg of phosphorus daily, it follows that dialysis cannot provide adequate control of phosphate by itself. Rather management of hyperphosphatemia requires a combination of dietary restriction, oral phosphate binders, and dialysis.

The limited ability of dialysis to remove phosphorus is primarily related to the kinetics of phosphorus distribution within the body and not inadequate clearance across the dialyzer. In a typical dialysis session the rate of phosphorus removal is greatest during the initial stages of the procedure and then progressively declines to a low constant level toward the end of the treatment. This decline is due to the decrease in plasma concentration and the slow efflux of phosphorus from the intracellular space and/or mobilization from bone stores. Although dialysis membranes differ with respect to plasma clearance of phosphate, it is the slow transfer of phosphorus to the extracellular space where it becomes accessible for dialytic removal that is the most important factor limiting phosphorus removal (117–119).

There are only a few situations in which one might consider adding phosphorus to the dialysate (Table 3.4). Hypophosphatemia can be an occasional finding in the chronic dialysis patient who is malnourished and suffering from some chronic disease state. In such patients adding phosphorus to the dialysate may be an effective means to treat hypophosphatemia without having to use a parenteral route of administration. The phosphate must be added to the bicarbonate component of a dual proportioning system to avoid the precipitation of calcium phosphate that would result from addition to the calcium-containing acid concentrate. Kaye et al. (120) described three hypophosphatemic dialysis patients who were treated by adding phosphorus to the dialysate in a single proportioning system. In these patients phosphate was added to a bicarbonate concentrate that contained no calcium. To avoid hypocalcemia, calcium was infused into the venous drip chamber as a 10% $CaCl_2$ solution. A final phosphate concentration of 1 to 2 mmol/L was found effective in correcting the hypophosphatemia by the end of a 4-hour session.

Another situation in which addition of phosphate to the dialysate may be useful is in the setting of an overdose. In a patient with normal renal function and a normal serum phosphate concentration, use of a phosphate-free dialysate will commonly result in hypophosphatemia. In most circumstances the hypophosphatemia is of short duration and is of little clinical consequence. However, some intoxications may increase the risk for complications of hypophosphatemia such that addition of phosphate to the dialysate may be warranted.

Finally, hypophosphatemia has been noted in patients treated with prolonged daily nocturnal hemodialysis (121). In this setting, adding phosphate to the dialysate may prove useful as a means to normalize the serum phosphate concentration.

In summary, most outpatient hemodialysis patients are currently treated with a dialysate that is prepared in bulk and delivered by way of a central delivery system (Table 3.4). As the age and number of comorbid diseases continue to increase in the dialysis population it is likely that individually tailored dialysates will play an important role in improving the tolerability of the dialysis procedure.

DIALYSATE COMPOSITION IN PERITONEAL DIALYSIS

Similar to the strategy in hemodialysis, the composition of the dialysis solution for peritoneal dialysis is designed to create favorable concentration gradients across the peritoneal membrane so as to achieve maximal removal of endogenous waste products, to maintain acid-base and electrolyte balance near normal, and to maintain the extracellular fluid volume constant (Table 3.6). As with hemodialysis, the composition of the dialysate can be individually modified for ultrafiltration and clearance needs (Table 3.6).

Osmotic Agents

The addition of a solute to render the dialysate hyperosmolar relative to plasma creates an osmotic gradient that results in the net movement of water into the peritoneal cavity. The degree of hypertonicity, the time that the fluid is allowed to dwell in the abdomen, and the hydraulic permeability of the peritoneal membrane determine the volume of fluid removed. Clinically, the magnitude of ultrafiltrate is determined by subtracting the volume of fluid instilled in the abdomen from the effluent volume.

In commercially available peritoneal dialysates glucose is the most commonly used osmotic agent used to enhance ultrafiltration. The concentrations available range from 1.36% glucose (1.5% dextrose) to 3.86% glucose (4.25% dextrose). Both the

TABLE 3.6. ADVANTAGES AND DISADVANTAGES OF NEW PERITONEAL DIALYSIS SOLUTIONS

Solution	Advantage	Disadvantage
Icodextran	Sustained ultrafiltration in overnight dwell in CAPD, long dwell in APD, and during peritonitis, avoids effects of glucose absorption, iso-osmotic	Skin reactions (<10%), maltose accumulation
Amino acids	Improves malnutrition	Azotemia and metabolic acidosis
Bicarbonate and bicarbonate/lactate buffer	Improved biocompatibility because of neutral pH, ↓ glucose degradation products	Two chamber bags to separate Ca and Mg from bicarbonate
Glucose sterilized separately at lower pH	Improved biocompatibility, ↓ glucose degradation products	Two chamber bags required

APD, automated peritoneal dialysis; CAPD, continuous ambulatory peritoneal dialysis.

ultrafiltration rate and the time until osmotic equilibrium is reached are directly related to the glucose concentration used. Using 2-L exchanges with cycle times up to 6 hours, solutions containing 1.5% dextrose will generate 100 to 200 mL of net ultrafiltrate (122). Solutions containing 4.25% under the same conditions will generate up to 800 mL of net ultrafiltrate. By increasing the frequency of exchanges this ultrafiltrate volume can be increased to as high as 1 L/hour using the 4.25% solution. Over time the osmolality of the dialysate declines as a result of water movement into the peritoneal cavity and absorption of dialysate glucose. By 4 hours of dwell using the 1.5% solution, the tonicity of the dialysate is essentially equal to that of plasma and the glucose concentration of the dialysate decreases to approximately one half the original value.

The use of glucose as an osmotic agent is well recognized to have several deficiencies. The absorption of glucose contributes substantially to the caloric intake of patients on continuous peritoneal dialysis (123,124). This carbohydrate load over time is thought to contribute to progressive obesity, hypertriglyceridemia, and decreased nutrition as a result of loss of appetite and decreased protein intake. In addition, an increasing body of literature suggests that the high glucose concentrations and high osmolality of the currently available solutions adversely affect the function of the peritoneal membrane importantly contributing to technique failure over time (125).

Ultrafiltration failure resulting from increased permeability of small molecular weight solutes is one of the most frequent reasons patients are transferred from peritoneal to hemodialysis. This increase in permeability can be traced to an increase in the number of blood vessels in the peritoneal membrane effectively enlarging the vascular peritoneal surface area (126). High glucose concentrations have been linked to this process of neoangiogenesis through a variety of mechanisms to include stimulation of vascular endothelial growth factor and toxic effects of advanced glycosylation end-products and glucose degradation products (127,128).

The bioincompatibility of glucose-containing solutions has prompted a search for alternative osmotic agents. Experimental and some clinical studies have been performed using substances such as fructose, sorbitol, xylitol, dextran, and gelatin (129–132). For one reason or another these agents have either been proven unsafe or ineffective as an osmotic agent. Glycerol has received some interest as an osmotic agent particularly in patients with diabetes. This agent is not dependent on insulin for metabolism and may allow for better and easier glucose control in the diabetic population (133).

One of the most promising new peritoneal dialysis solutions uses glucose polymers as the osmotic agent (134,135). These compounds can be administered as a solution that is iso-osmolar to plasma because they generate an ultrafiltrate through the process of colloid osmosis. This process is based on the principle that water is transported from capillaries in the direction of impermeable large solutes rather than down an osmotic gradient as occurs with glucose-containing solutions. The icodextran-based dialysis solution is a polymer of glucose that is now available in several countries. In a 6-hour dwell, the 7.5% icodextran solution generates an ultrafiltrate volume that is higher than that generated by 1.5% dextrose despite having a lower osmolality

(285 vs. 347 mOsm/kg). With prolonged dwell times of 8 to 12 hours, the icodextran solution provides equivalent or higher ultrafiltrate volumes than that generated by the 4.25% dextrose solution (486 mOsm/kg) (136). The ability to maintain a colloid osmotic pressure for prolonged periods of time makes this solution ideal for overnight dwells in patients on continuous ambulatory peritoneal dialysis (CAPD) as well as daytime dwells for those on automated peritoneal dialysis regimens.

In patients with ultrafiltration failure who would otherwise be transferred to hemodialysis, use of icodextran has been shown to extend the time that patients remain on peritoneal dialysis by many months (137). In addition use of icodextran is associated with less weight gain, improved lipid control, and less hyperinsulinemia as compared with dextrose-containing solutions (138). It is likely that icodextran will become the preferred agent for the long dwell in most peritoneal dialysis patients (136,139).

Because patients on peritoneal dialysis have a high incidence of protein-calorie malnutrition, in part, resulting from daily losses of protein and amino acids into the dialysate, studies have also examined the feasibility of using amino acids as a replacement for glucose as an osmotic agent (140,141). Use of amino acids should augment the amino acid intake and reduce the net amino acid losses of the patient potentially providing additional nutrition to the patient. The overall absorption of amino acids in various solutions ranges from 60% to 90% depending on the concentration used and the length of the dwell (142). One 2-L bag of 1.0% solution can provide at least 14 g of amino acids. Importantly, these solutions have no major impact on the transport characteristics of the peritoneal membrane and are as effective osmotic agents as glucose (142).

Initial studies using amino acid containing solutions were unimpressive with regards to showing an improvement in nutritional parameters. Moreover, use of these solutions was associated with significant increases in the blood urea nitrogen concentration and development of metabolic acidosis. More recent studies have used amino acid containing dialysates that have been altered to provide the optimal balance between essential and nonessential amino acids required for a chronic renal failure patient (143–145). Kopple et al. (144) studied the effectiveness of the 1.1% amino acid solution (Nutrineal; Baxter Healthcare) in a group of patients who were clinically malnourished. The patients were fed a constant diet and the number of amino acid exchanges per day was adjusted so that the total daily dietary protein plus dialysate amino acid intake would be 1.1 to 1.3 g/kg/day. Patients required one to two daily exchanges of the amino acid solution to achieve this goal. The amino acid dialysate was associated with positive nitrogen balance that remained significant throughout the study. In addition, there was net protein anabolism as directly demonstrated from radiolabeled N-glycine studies. Patients tolerated the treatment well; however, some patients developed mild metabolic acidemia.

This same solution has been examined in 15 stable CAPD patients in whom malnutrition was not an entry criterion (145). In this study one 2-L exchange of the 1.1% solution was performed at lunchtime to ensure the simultaneous uptake of sufficient carbohydrates. Previous experience with parenteral nutrition has shown that optimal utilization of amino acids occurs when there is combined uptake of nonprotein calories and amino acids. Over the 3 months of the study there was a significant increase in the serum albumin concentration whether baseline malnutrition was present or not. Use of the dialysate in this manner did not result in acidosis although the blood urea nitrogen increased by 20%. Other studies have also confirmed that this 1.1% amino acid is effective in providing a nutritional benefit particularly in patients who are malnourished (143).

In summary, glucose remains the standard osmotic agent used in peritoneal dialysis solutions. In an attempt to develop a more physiologic solution, various new osmotic agents are now under investigation. It is likely that icodextran will be used with greater frequency in peritoneal dialysis patients particularly as the osmotic agent for long dwell times. In patients with evidence of ultrafiltration failure, use of icodextran may extend the time certain patients can remain on peritoneal dialysis before having to switch to hemodialysis. Amino acid containing solutions also show promise for patients with evidence of malnutrition. To limit the development of azotemia and acidosis the use of these solutions will likely be confined to one exchange per day.

Dialysate Buffer

The buffer present in most commercially available peritoneal dialysate solutions is lactate. In patients with normal hepatic function, lactate is rapidly converted to bicarbonate such that 1 mM of lactate absorbed generates 1 mM of bicarbonate. Even with the most vigorous peritoneal dialysis, there is no appreciable accumulation of circulating lactate (146). The rapid metabolism of lactate to bicarbonate maintains the high dialysate-to-plasma lactate gradient necessary for continued absorption. This absorption may be somewhat less with use of dialysate that contains higher concentrations of dextrose. Under these conditions increased ultrafiltrate formation may dilute the concentration of lactate in the peritoneal cavity and therefore decrease the concentration gradient for diffusion. Lactate is normally provided as a racemic mixture of the dextro and levo isomers in approximately equal concentrations. There is some evidence that the natural isomer (L-lactate) is more rapidly absorbed than the D-isomer (D-lactate) (147).

The pH of commercially available peritoneal dialysis solutions is purposely made acidic by adding hydrochloric acid to prevent dextrose caramelization during the sterilization procedure. Once instilled into the abdomen the pH of the solution rises to values greater than 7.0. The acidic nature and buffer composition of currently available solutions further contributes to the bioincompatibility of peritoneal dialysate (125,148,149).

To address this issue, neutral pH solutions buffered with bicarbonate or with a mixture of bicarbonate and lactate have been introduced into clinical practice. Up until recently bicarbonate was not able to be used as the buffer in peritoneal dialysis solutions because calcium and magnesium would precipitate in the presence of bicarbonate in the setting of an alkaline pH. Omitting magnesium and calcium from the dialysate was not an option because patients undergoing chronic peritoneal dialysis would develop deficits of these divalent cations. These limitations have largely been overcome by the development of a two-chamber dialysate bag in which one chamber contains the bicarbonate or buffer and the other contains a solution with calcium

and magnesium. The system is designed so that the two solutions are mixed just before entering the patient and thus avoids the problem of precipitation. In addition to having a neutral pH, there are less glucose degradation products because the bicarbonate is sterilized separately from the other components of the solution.

In a recent randomized trial of 106 patients, a pH neutral bicarbonate/lactate-based peritoneal dialysis solution was compared with the conventional acidic lactate buffered solution in which markers of peritoneal membrane integrity and inflammation were examined (150). At the end of 6 months, patients treated with the pH neutral solution had a significantly greater increase in the dialysate CA 125 (a marker of viability and cell mass of the mesothelium). The same group also had a significantly greater decrease in dialysate hyaluronan (a marker of inflammation in the peritoneal cavity). The pH neutral solution is associated with less inflow pain, and no adverse effect has been demonstrated on peritoneal transport. Use of the pH neutral solution has also been shown to result in long term improvement in peritoneal macrophage function as compared with conventional solutions (151).

The dual-chamber bag has also been used to separate glucose from the other solution components. The advantage of this setup is that glucose can be sterilized at a much lower pH as compared with a single-chamber bag and as a result the formation of glucose degradation products is markedly reduced. Mixing of the two components at the time of abdominal installation effectively raises the pH. The application of this solution has been studied in a randomized trial of 80 patients (152). As compared with conventional treatment, patients treated with the study solution had significantly greater dialysate CA 125 and significantly lower dialysate hyaluronan. Over a 24-month follow-up there were no adverse effects on parameters of peritoneal transport.

In summary, a great deal of progress has been made to improve the biocompatibility of peritoneal dialysis solutions. Both experimental and clinical studies demonstrate that these solutions are much better at preserving peritoneal membrane function. Because no one solution is ideal it is likely that in the future each patient will be prescribed a combination of fluids to meet specific individual needs. One can envision a daily regimen in a patient on CAPD consisting of one exchange of amino acids, two exchanges of bicarbonate/glucose, and an overnight exchange of icodextran (153). Future studies will be required to determine the efficacy of various combinations.

Dialysate Sodium

The Na concentration in the ultrafiltrate during peritoneal dialysis is usually less than the extracellular fluid such that there is a tendency for water loss and the development of hypernatremia. Commercially available peritoneal dialysates have a Na concentration of 132 mEq/L to compensate for this tendency toward dehydration. This effect is most pronounced with increasing frequency of exchanges and with increasing dialysate glucose concentrations. Use of the more hypertonic solutions with frequent cycling can result in significant dehydration and hypernatremia. As a result of stimulated thirst, water intake and weight may increase resulting in a vicious cycle.

The use of a low Na dialysate does lead to net Na removal and can predispose to hypotension in patients with inadequate Na intake. In the occasional patient who is unable to increase dietary Na, the dialysate Na concentration can be raised to decrease the amount of Na removal so that extracellular fluid volume can be maintained.

Dialysate Potassium

Potassium is cleared by peritoneal dialysis at a rate similar to that of urea. With CAPD and 10 L of drainage per day, approximately 35 to 46 mEq of potassium is removed per day. Daily potassium intake is usually greater than this amount and yet significant hyperkalemia is uncommon in these patients (154). Presumably potassium balance is maintained by increased colonic secretion of potassium as well as some residual renal excretion. Given these considerations potassium is not routinely added to the dialysate.

Maximal removal of potassium with peritoneal dialysis is approximately 10 mEq/hour even in the setting of severe hyperkalemia (155). It should be noted that removal rates with Kayexalate enemas far exceed this value and may approach 30 mEq/hour. In patients undergoing frequent exchanges, hypokalemia may develop. In these instances potassium can be added to the dialysate to achieve a final concentration of 2 to 3 mEq/L. This is particularly important in patients receiving digoxin because the development of hypokalemia can precipitate arrhythmias.

Dialysate Magnesium

Initially the standard peritoneal dialysis solution contained 1.5 mEq/L magnesium. The concentration has since been lowered to 0.5 mEq/L to lessen the frequency of hypermagnesemia that was observed with the higher magnesium concentration. As discussed with hemodialysis, a lower dialysate magnesium concentration may allow use of magnesium salts as an additional calcium-free phosphate binder.

Dialysate Calcium

As discussed previously, patients with progressive chronic renal failure have a tendency to develop hypocalcemia. To avoid negative calcium balance as well as potentially suppressing circulating PTH, commercially available peritoneal dialysis solutions evolved to contain a calcium concentration of 3.5 mEq/L (1.75 mmol/L). This concentration is equal to or slightly greater than the ionized concentration in the serum of most patients. As a result, there is net calcium absorption in most patients when using a conventional dialysis regime such as $3 \times 1.5\%$ glucose and $1 \times 4.5\%$ glucose solutions (156). When ultrafiltration volume is high, as occurs with use of 4.25% dextrose concentration at high rates of exchange, net transfer of calcium can be reversed such that calcium balance becomes negative.

As the use of calcium-containing phosphate binders has increased, hypercalcemia has became a common problem when using the 3.5 mEq/L calcium dialysate. This complication has been particularly common in patients treated with peritoneal dialysis because these patients have a much greater incidence of adynamic bone disease as compared with hemodialysis patients (157). In fact, the continual positive calcium balance associated with the 3.5 mEq/L solution has been suggested as a contributing factor in the development of this lesion. The low bone turnover state typical of this disorder impairs the accrual of administered calcium contributing to the development of hypercalcemia. As a result there has been increased interest in using a similar strategy as has been employed in hemodialysis—namely, lower the calcium content of the dialysate. This strategy can allow for increased usage of calcium-containing phosphate binders as well as more liberal use of $1,25 (OH)_2$ vitamin D to effect decreases in the circulating level of PTH. In this manner, the development of hypercalcemia can be minimized.

Several studies have confirmed that a stable serum calcium concentration can be maintained when using low calcium dialysis solutions (158–160). In a large randomized controlled multicenter trial, Weinreich et al. (159) studied 103 stable CAPD patients comparing 1.0 mmol/L versus 1.75 mmol/L calcium solutions over 6 months (159). Aluminum-containing binders were given in place of $CaCO_3$ in cases of hypercalcemia. In the low calcium group, serum calcium levels were maintained within the normal range with a threefold reduction in the incidence of hypercalcemia and significant reduction in the need for $Al(OH)_3$ as compared with the conventional dialysate. One concern with use of a low calcium dialysate is that PTH levels might be stimulated. However, in this study, PTH levels remained within the desired range. In addition there was no radiologic sign of renal osteodystrophy or demineralization of bones. More recently, Johnson et al. (160) reported data from a randomized, prospective, double-blind trial in 45 CAPD patients comparing treatment with 1.25 mmol/L and 1.75 mmol/L dialysate calcium over 12 months. In this study the low calcium dialysate was associated with less hypercalcemia and at the same time permitted larger quantities of calcitriol and $CaCO_3$ to be prescribed. Increased use of these agents, however, may explain why use of $Al(OH)_3$ could not be reduced in the low calcium group. Increased doses of calcitriol can preserve the need for $Al(OH)_3$ by increasing intestinal calcium absorption thereby limiting the maximum dose of $CaCO_3$ that could be used and by increasing phosphate absorption thereby increasing the total dose of phosphate binders required for satisfactory phosphate control. In addition, PTH levels increased in the low calcium group but values returned toward baseline after the first 6 months of the study. Bone mineralization studies showed no differences between the two groups.

In summary, peritoneal dialysis solutions are widely available with a calcium concentration of either 1.25 or 1.75 mmol/L. The decision to use one concentration or the other should be made on an individual basis. Most patients can be treated with a dialysis solution that contains 1.75 mmol/L calcium. On the other hand, a low dialysate calcium solution offers a valuable therapeutic option to treat patients with increased doses of calcium-containing phosphate binders and calcitriol with a much lower incidence of hypercalcemia. Close monitoring of patients is required when using a low calcium solution so as to ensure that secondary hyperparathyroidism is not exacerbated. This is particularly so in patients who are questionably compliant with their calcium-containing phosphate binders. Monitoring of bone mineralization is also indicated with long-term use of low calcium dialysate.

REFERENCES

1. Odgen D. A double-blind crossover comparison of high and low-sodium dialysis. *Proc Clin Dial Transplant Forum* 1978;8:157–165.
2. Swartz RD, et al. Preservation of plasma volume during hemodialysis depends on dialysate osmolality. *Am J Nephrol* 1982;2:189–194.
3. Henrich WL, et al. The chronic efficacy and safety of high sodium dialysate: double-blind, crossover study. *Am J Kidney Dis* 1982;2:349–353.
4. Bihaphala S, et al. Comparison of high and low-sodium bicarbonate and acetate dialysis in stable chronic hemodialysis patients. *Clin Nephrol* 1985;23:179–183.
5. Dumler F, et al. Sequential high/low sodium hemodialysis: an alternative to ultrafiltration. *Trans Am Soc Artif Intern Organs* 1979;25:351–353.
6. Raja R, et al. Sequential changes in dialysate sodium (D_{Na}) during hemodialysis. *Trans Am Soc Artif Intern Organs* 1983;24:649–651.
7. Daugirdas JT, et al. A double-blind evaluation of sodium gradient hemodialysis. *Am J Nephrol* 1985;5:163–168.
8. Acchiardo SR, et al. Is Na modeling necessary in high flux dialysis. *Trans Am Soc Artif Organs* 1991;37:M135–M137.
9. Sadowski RH, et al. Sodium modelling ameliorates intradialytic and interdialytic symptoms in young hemodialysis patients. *J Am Soc Nephrol* 1993;4:1192–1198.
10. Levin A, et al. The benefits and side effects of ramped hypertonic sodium dialysis. *J Am Soc Nephrol* 1996;7:242–246.
11. Sang GLS, et al. Sodium ramping in hemodialysis: a study of beneficial and adverse effects. *Am J Kidney Dis* 1997;29:669–677.
12. Movilli E, et al. Blood volume changes during three different profiles of dialysate sodium variation with similar intradialytic sodium balances in chronic hemodialyzed patients. *Am J Kidney Dis* 1997;30:58–63.
13. Sherman RA. Intradialytic hypotension: an overview of recent, unresolved and overlooked issues. *Semin Dial* 2002;15:141–143.
14. Flanigan MJ. Role of sodium in hemodialysis. *Kidney Int* 2000;[Suppl 76];76:S72–S78.
15. Heineken FS, et al. Intercompartmental fluid shifts in hemodialysis patients. *Biotechnol Prog* 1987;3:69.
16. Paganini EP, et al. The effect of sodium and ultrafiltration modelling on plasma volume changes and haemodynamic stability in intensive care patients receiving haemodialysis for acute renal failure: a prospective, stratified, randomized, cross-over study. *Nephrol Dial Transplant* 1996;11:32–37.
17. Song J, et al. Time-averaged concentration of dialysate sodium relates with sodium load and interdialytic weight gain during sodium-profiling hemodialysis. *Am J Kidney Dis* 2002;40:291–301.
18. Petitclerc T, et al. Electrolyte modelling: is dialysate sodium profiling actually useful? *Nephrol Dial Transplant* 1996;11:35–38.
19. Coli L, et al. Clinical use of profiled hemodialysis. *Artif Organs* 1998;22:724–730.
20. Ursino M, et al. Mathematical modeling of solute kinetics and body fluid changes during profiled hemodialysis. *Int J Artif Organs* 1999;22:94–107.
21. Coli L, et al. Evidence of profiled hemodialysis efficacy in the treatment of intradialytic hypotension. *Int J Artif Organs* 1998;21:398–402.
22. Coli L, et al. A simple model applied to selection of the sodium profile during profiled hemodialysis. *Nephrol Dial Transplant* 1998;13:404–416.
23. Flanigan MJ, et al. Dialysate sodium delivery can alter chronic blood pressure management. *Am J Kidney Dis* 1997;29:383–391.
24. Locatelli F, et al. Effect of on-line conductivity plasma ultrafiltrate kinetic modeling on cardiovascular stability of hemodialysis patients. *Kidney Int* 1998;53:1052–1060.
25. Locatelli F, et al. On-line monitoring and convective treatment modalities: short-term advantages. *Nephrol Dial Transplant* 1999;14 [Suppl 3]:92–97.
26. Petitclerc T. Recent developments in conductivity monitoring of haemodialysis session. *Nephrol Dial Transplant* 1999;14:2607–2613.
27. Bosetto A, et al. Sodium management by dialysis conductivity. *Adv Ren Replace Ther* 1999;6:243–254.
28. Feig PV, et al. Effect of potassium removal during hemodialysis on the plasma potassium concentration. *Nephron* 1981;27:25.
29. Spital A, et al. Potassium homeostasis in dialysis patients. *Semin Dial* 1988;1:14–20.
30. Ketchersid TL, et al. Dialysate potassium. *Semin Dial* 1991;4:46–51.
31. Weigand C, et al. Life threatening hypokalemia during hemodialysis. *Trans Am Soc Artif Intern Organs* 1975;25:416.
32. Redaelli B, et al. Potassium removal as a factor limiting the correction of acidosis during dialysis. *Proc EDTA* 1982;19:366.
33. Ward RA, et al. Hemodialysate composition and intradialytic metabolic, acid base and potassium changes. *Kidney Int* 1987;32:129.
34. Sherman RA, et al. Variability in potassium removal by hemodialysis. *Am J Nephrol* 1986;6:284.
35. Allon M, et al. Effect of albuterol treatment on subsequent dialytic potassium removal. *Am J Kidney Dis* 1995;26:607–613.
36. Brace RA, et al. Local effects of hypokalemia on coronary resistance and myocardial contractile force. *Am J Physiol* 1974;227:590–597.
37. Linas SL. The role of potassium in the pathogenesis and treatment of hypertension. *Kidney Int* 1991;39:771–786.
38. Pogglitsch H, et al. The cause of inadequate haemodynamic reactions during ultradiffusion. *Proc Eur Dial Transplant Assoc* 1978;8:245–252.
39. Biglieri EG, et al. Abnormalities of renal function and circulatory reflexes in primary aldosteronism. *Circulation* 1966;33:78–86.
40. Henrich WL. Hemodynamic instability during hemodialysis. *Kidney Int* 1986;30:605–612.
41. Henrich WL, et al. Competitive effects of hypokalemia and volume depletion on plasma renin activity, aldosterone and catecholamine concentrations in hemodialysis patients. *Kidney Int* 1977;12:279–284.
42. Haddy FJ, et al. Effects of generalized changes in plasma electrolyte concentration and osmolarity on blood pressure in the anesthetized dog. *Circ Res* 1969;24:I59–I74.
43. Wizemann V, et al. Acute effects of dialysis on myocardial contractility: influence of cardiac status and calcium/potassium ratio. *Contrib Nephrol* 1986;52:60–68.
44. Dolson GM, et al. Low dialysate [K+] decreases efficiency of hemodialysis and increases urea rebound. *J Am Soc Nephrol* 1998;9:2124–2128.
45. Zehnder C, et al. Low-potassium and glucose-free dialysis maintains but enhances potassium removal. *Nephrol Dial Transplant* 2001;16:78–84.
46. Redaelli B. Electrolyte modelling in haemodialysis—potassium. *Nephrol Dial Transplant* 1996;11:39–41.
47. Cupisti A, et al. Potassium removal increases the QTc interval dispersion during hemodialysis. *Nephron* 1999;82:122–126.
48. Lorincz I, et al. QT dispersion in patients with end-stage renal failure and during hemodialysis. *J Am Soc Nephrol* 1999;10:1297–1302.
49. Redaelli B, et al. Effect of a new model of hemodialysis potassium removal on the control of ventricular arrhythmias. *Kidney Int* 1996;50:609–617.
50. Brace RA, et al. Local effects of hypokalemia on coronary resistance and myocardial contractile force. *Am J Physiol* 1974;227:590–597.
51. Linas SL. The role of potassium in the pathogenesis and treatment of hypertension. *Kidney Int* 1991;39:771–786.
52. Dolson G, et al. Acute decreases in serum potassium augment blood pressure. *Am J Kidney Dis* 1995;26:321–326.
53. Ketchersid TL, et al. Dialysate potassium. *Semin Dial* 1991;4:46–51.
54. Gotch FA, et al. Hydrogen ion balance in dialysis therapy. *Artif Organ* 1982;6:387.
55. Gennari FJ. Acid-base balance in dialysis patients. *Kidney Int* 1985;28:678–688.
56. Skutches CL, et al. Contributions of dialysate acetate to energy metabolism. *Kidney Int* 1983;23:57.
57. Akanji A, et al. Effect of acetate on blood metabolites and glucose tolerance during haemodialysis in uraemic non-diabetic and diabetic subjects. *Nephron* 1991;57:137–143.
58. Henrich WL. Hemodynamic instability during hemodialysis. *Kidney Int* 1986;30:605–612.

59. Daugirdas JT. Dialysis hypotension: a hemodynamic analysis. *Kidney Int* 1991;39:233–246.
60. Lonnemann G, et al. Plasma interleukin-1 activity in humans undergoing hemodialysis with regenerated cellulosic membranes. *Lymphokine Res* 1987;6:63–70.
61. Vinay P, et al. Acetate metabolism during hemodialysis: metabolic consideration. *Am J Nephrol* 1987;7:337.
62. Malberti F, et al. The influence of dialysis fluid composition on dialysis tolerance. *Nephrol Dial Transplant* 1987;2:93–98.
63. Wolff J, et al. Effects of acetate and bicarbonate dialysis on cardiac performance, transmural myocardial perfusion and acid-base balance. *Int J Artif Organs* 1986;9:105–110.
64. Pagel MD, et al. Acetate and bicarbonate fluctuations and acetate intolerance during dialysis. *Kidney Int* 1982;21:513–518.
65. Mansell MA, et al. Incidence and significance of rising blood acetate levels during hemodialysis. *Clin Nephrol* 1979;12:22–25.
66. Heneghan WF. Acetate, bicarbonate and hypotension during hemodialysis. *Am J Kidney Dis* 1982;2:302–304.
67. Vinay P, et al. Acetate metabolism and bicarbonate generation during hemodialysis: 10 years of observation. *Kidney Int* 1987;31:1194–1204.
68. Wehle B, et al. The influence of dialysis fluid composition on the blood pressure response during dialysis. *Clin Nephrol* 1978;10:62–66.
69. Henrich WL, et al. High sodium bicarbonate and acetate hemodialysis: double-blind crossover comparison of hemodynamic and ventilatory effects. *Kidney Int* 1983;24:240–245.
70. Velez RL, et al. Acetate and bicarbonate hemodialysis in patients with and without autonomic dysfunction. *Kidney Int* 1984;26:59–65.
71. Kirkdendol PL, et al. A comparison of the cardiovascular effects of sodium acetate, sodium bicarbonate and other potential sources of fixed base in hemodialysate solutions. *Trans Am Soc Artif Intern Organs* 1977;23:399–405.
72. Kirkendol PL, et al. Cardiac and vascular effects of infused sodium acetate in dogs. *Trans Am Soc Artif Intern Organs* 1978;24:714–717.
73. Aizawa Y, et al. Depressant action of acetate upon the human cardiovascular system. *Clin Nephrol* 1977;8:477–480.
74. Nitenberg A, et al. Analysis of increased myocardial contractility during sodium acetate infusion in humans. *Kidney Int* 1984;26:744–751.
75. Mansell MA, et al. The effect of hyperacetatemia on cardiac output during regular hemodialysis. *Clin Nephrol* 1982;18:130–134.
76. Schick EC, et al. Comparison of the hemodynamic response to hemodialysis with acetate or bicarbonate. *Trans Am Soc Artif Intern Organs* 1983;24:25–28.
77. Ruder MA, et al. Comparative effects of acetate and bicarbonate hemodialysis on left ventricular function. *Kidney Int* 1984;27:768–773.
78. Leunissen KML, et al. Influence of left ventricular function on changes in plasma volume during acetate and bicarbonate dialysis. *Nephrol Dial Transplant* 1987;2:99–103.
79. Leunissen KML, et al. Acetate or bicarbonate for haemodialysis. *Nephrol Dial Transplant* 1988;3:1–7.
80. Nixon JV, et al. Effect of hemodialysis on left ventricular function. *J Clin Invest* 1983;71:377–384.
81. Mehta BR, et al. Effects of acetate and bicarbonate hemodialysis on cardiac function in chronic dialysis patients. *Kidney Int* 1983;24:782–787.
82. Anderson LE, et al. Comparative effects of bicarbonate and acetate dialysis on left ventricular function. *Clin Res* 1984;32:874A.
83. Turi S, et al. The effects of bicarbonate and acetate haemodialysis on platelet cyclic AMP concentration, thromboxane B_2 release and aggregation. *Pediatr Nephrol* 1991;5:327–331.
84. Fantuzzi S, et al. Hemodialysis-associated cardiac arrhythmias: a lower risk with bicarbonate? *Nephron* 1991;58:196–200.
85. Van Stone JC. Bicarbonate dialysate: still more to learn. *Semin Dial* 1994;7:168–169.
86. Leunissen KML, et al. Bicarbonate dialysis: a review and future perspectives. *Semin Dial* 1994;7:186–191.
87. Alpern RJ, et al. The clinical spectrum of chronic metabolic acidosis: homeostatic mechanisms produce significant morbidity. *Am J Kidney Dis* 1997;29:291–302.
88. Bailey JL. Metabolic acidosis and protein catabolism: mechanisms and clinical implications. *Miner Electrolyte Metab* 1998;24:13–19.
89. Oettinger CW, et al. Normalization of uremic acidosis in hemodialysis patients with a high bicarbonate dialysate. *J Am Soc Nephrol* 1993; 3:1804–1807.
90. Graham KA, et al. Correction of acidosis in hemodialysis decreases whole-body protein degradation. *J Am Soc Nephrol* 1997;8:632–637.
91. Graham KA, et al. Correction of acidosis in hemodialysis patients increases the sensitivity of the parathyroid glands to calcium. *J Am Soc Nephrol* 1997;8:627–631.
92. Ahmad S, et al. Dialysate made from chemicals using citric acid increases dialysis dose. *Am J Kidney Dis* 2000;35:493–499.
93. Guillot AP, et al. The use of magnesium-containing phosphate binders in patients with end-stage renal disease on maintenance hemodialysis. *Nephron* 1982;30:114–117.
94. Oe PL, et al. Long-term use of magnesium hydroxide as a phosphate binder in patients on hemodialysis. *Clin Nephrol* 1987;28:180–185.
95. O'Donovan R, et al. Substitution of aluminum salts by magnesium salts in control of dialysis hyperphosphataemia. *Lancet* 1986;1: 880–882.
96. Kelber J, et al. Acute effects of different concentration of dialysate magnesium during high-efficiency dialysis. *Am J Kidney Dis* 1994; 24:453–460.
97. Delmez JA, et al. Magnesium carbonate as a phosphorus binder: a prospective, controlled, crossover study. *Kidney Int* 1996;49:163–167.
98. Slatopolsky E, et al. Long-term effects of calcium carbonate and 2.5 mEq/L calcium dialysate on mineral metabolism. *Kidney Int* 1989; 36:897.
99. Slatopolsky E, et al. Calcium carbonate as a phosphate binder in patients with chronic renal failure undergoing dialysis. *N Engl J Med* 1986;315:157.
100. Sawyer N, et al. High-dose calcium carbonate with stepwise reduction in dialysate calcium concentration: effective phosphate control and aluminum avoidance in haemodialysis patients. *Nephrol Dial Trans* 1989;4:105–109.
101. Teruel J, et al. Satisfactory control of secondary hyperparathyroidism with low-calcium dialysate in patients not receiving vitamin D. *Mineral Electrolyte Metab* 1997;23:19–24.
102. Van der Merwe WM, et al. Low calcium dialysate and high-dose oral calcitriol in the treatment of secondary hyperparathyroidism in haemodialysis patients. *Nephrol Dial Transplant* 1990;5:874–877.
103. Argiles A, et al. Calcium kinetics and the long-term effects of lowering dialysate calcium concentration. *Kidney Int* 1993;43:630–640.
104. Fernandez E, et al. Low-calcium dialysate stimulates parathormone secretion and its long-term use worsens secondary hyperparathyroidism. *J Am Soc Nephrol* 1995;6:132–135.
105. Argiles A, et al. Calcium balance and intact PTH variations during haemodiafiltration. *Nephrol Dial Transplant* 1995;10:2083–2089.
106. Argiles A, et al. Low-calcium dialysate worsens secondary hyperparathyroidism. *J Am Soc Nephrol* 1996;7:635–636.
107. Maynard JC, et al. Blood pressure response to changes in serum ionized calcium during hemodialysis. *Ann Intern Med* 1986;104: 358–361.
108. Sherman RA, et al. The effect of dialysate calcium levels on blood pressure during hemodialysis. *Am J Kidney Dis* 1986;8:244–247.
109. van der Sande FM, et al. Effect of dialysate calcium concentrations on intradialytic blood pressure course in cardiac-compromised patients. *Am J Kidney Dis* 1998;32:125–131.
110. Kyriazis J, et al. Dialysate calcium profiling during hemodialysis: use and clinical implications. *Kidney Int* 2002;61:276–287.
111. Fellner SK, et al. Physiological mechanisms for calcium-induced changes in systemic arterial pressure in stable dialysis patients. *Hypertension* 1989;13:213–218.
112. Henrich WL, et al. Increased ionized calcium and left ventricular contractility during hemodialysis. *N Engl J Med* 1984;310:19–23.
113. Lang RB, et al. Left ventricular contractility varies directly with blood ionized calcium. *Ann Intern Med* 1988;108:524–529.
114. Ritz E, et al. What is the appropriate dialysate calcium concentration for the dialysis patient? *Nephrol Dial Transplant* 1996;11:91–95.
115. DeSoi CA, et al. Does the dialysis prescription influence phosphate removal. *Semin Dial* 1995;8:201–203.
116. Hou S, et al. Calcium and phosphorus fluxes during hemodialysis with low calcium dialysate. *Am J Kid Dis* 1991;18:217–224.
117. Schuck O, et al. Kinetics of phosphorus during hemodialysis and the

calculation of its effective dialysis clearance. *Clin Nephrol* 1997;47: 379–383.

118. Shinaberger JH, et al. Phosphate removal by conventional dialysis, high efficiency dialysis, and high flux hemodiafiltration. *Kidney Int* 1987;31:245.

119. Delmez J, et al. Hyperphosphatemia: its consequences and treatment in patients with chronic renal disease. *Am J Kidney Dis* 1992;19:303–317.

120. Kaye M, et al. Correction of hypophosphatemia in patients on hemodialysis using a calcium-free dialysate with added phosphate. *Clin Nephrol* 1991;35:130–133.

121. Pierratos A, et al. Nocturnal hemodialysis: three-year experience. *J Am Soc Nephrol* 1998;9:859–868.

122. Nolph KD. Continuous ambulatory peritoneal dialysis (CAPD). *Am J Nephrol* 1981;1:1.

123. Grodstein GP, et al. Glucose absorption during continuous ambulatory peritoneal dialysis. *Kidney Int* 1981;19:564.

124. Nolph KD, et al. Equilibration of peritoneal dialysis solutions during long dwell exchanges. *J Lab Clin Med* 1979;93:246.

125. Jorres A, et al. Biocompatibility of peritoneal dialysis fluids. *Int J Artif Organs* 1992;15:79–83.

126. Mateijsen MA, et al. Vascular and interstitial changes in the peritoneum of CAPD patients with peritoneal sclerosis. *Perit Dial Int* 1999;19:517–525.

127. Zweers MM, et al. Vascular endothelial growth factor in peritoneal dialysis: a longitudinal follow-up. *J Lab Clin Med* 2001;137:125–132.

128. Davies SJ, et al. Peritoneal glucose exposure and changes in membrane solute transport with time on peritoneal dialysis. *J Am Soc Nephrol* 2001;12:1046–1051.

129. Raja RM, et al. Peritoneal dialysis with fructose dialysate. *Ann Intern Med* 1973;79:511.

130. Yen TS. Experimental study of peritoneal dialysis using xylitol containing solution. *J Formosan Med Assoc* 1970;69:292.

131. Bischel MD, et al. Peritoneal dialysis with sorbitol versus dextrose dialysate. *Nephron* 1974;12:449.

132. Gjessing J. The use of dextrose as a dialyzing fluid in peritoneal dialysis. *Acta Med Scand* 1969;185:237.

133. Matthys E, et al. Extended use of glycerol containing dialysate in diabetic CAPD patients. *Perit Dial Bull* 1987;7:10.

134. Vanholder R, et al. Osmotic agents in peritoneal dialysis. *Kidney Int* 1996;50:S86–S91.

135. Mistry C, et al. A randomized multicenter clinical trial comparing isosmolar Icodextrin with hyperosmolar glucose solutions in CAPD. *Kidney Int* 1994;46:496–503.

136. Pecoitis-filho R, et al. Future of icodextran as an osmotic agent in peritoneal dialysis. *Kidney Int* 2002;62[Suppl 81]:S80–S87.

137. Krediet R, et al. Use of icodextran in high transport ultrafiltration failure. *Kidney Int* 2002;62[Suppl 81]:S53–S61.

138. Gokal R, et al. Metabolic and laboratory effects of icodextran. *Kidney Int* 2002;62[Suppl 81]:S62–S71.

139. Plum J, et al. Efficacy and safety of a 7.5% icodextran peritoneal dialysis solution in patients treated with automated peritoneal dialysis. *Am J Kidney Dis* 2002;39:862–871.

140. Young GA, et al. The use of an amino acid based CAPD fluid over 12 weeks. *Nephrol Dial Transplant* 1989;4:285.

141. Bruno M, et al. CAPD with an amino acid dialysis solution: a long term, cross-over study. *Kidney Int* 1989;35:1189.

142. Faller B. Amino-acid based dialysis solutions. *Kidney Int* 1996;50: S81–S85.

143. Misra M, et al. Nutritional effects of amino acid dialysate (Nutrineal) in CAPD patients. *Adv Perit Dial* 1996;12:311–314.

144. Kopple J, et al. Treatment of malnourished CAPD patients with an amino acid based dialysate. *Kidney Int* 1995;47:1148–1157.

145. Faller B, et al. Clinical evaluation of an optimized amino-acid solution for peritoneal dialysis. *Nephrol Dial Transplant* 1995;10: 1432–1437.

146. Fine A. Metabolism of D-lactate in the dog and in man. *Perit Dial Int* 1989;9:99.

147. Rubin J, et al. Stereospecific lactate absorption during peritoneal dialysis. *Nephron* 1982;31:224.

148. Feriani M. Buffers: bicarbonate, lactate, and pyruvate. *Kidney Int* 1996;50:S75–S80.

149. Coles G. Towards a more physiologic solution for peritoneal dialysis. *Semin Dial* 1995;8:333–335.

150. Jones S, et al. Bicarbonate/lactate-based peritoneal dialysis solution increases cancer antigen 125 and decreases hyaluronic acid levels. *Kidney Int* 2001;59:1529–1538.

151. Jones S, et al. Continuous dialysis with bicarbonate/lactate-buffered peritoneal dialysis fluids results in a long-term improvement in ex vivo peritoneal macrophage function. *J Am Soc Nephrol* 2002;13 [Suppl 1]:S97–S103.

152. Rippe B, et al. Long-term clinical effects of a peritoneal dialysis fluid with less glucose degradation products. *Kidney Int* 2001;59: 348–357.

153. Gokal R. Peritoneal dialysis in the 21st century: an analysis of current problems and future developments. *J Am Soc Nephrol* 2002;13[Suppl 1]:S104–S116.

154. Nolph KD, et al. Autoregulation of sodium and potassium removal during continuous ambulatory peritoneal dialysis. *Trans Am Soc Artif Int Organs* 1980;26:334.

155. Brown ST, et al. Potassium removal with peritoneal dialysis. *Kidney Int* 1973;4:67.

156. Weinreich T. Low or high calcium dialysate solutions in peritoneal dialysis? *Kidney Int* 1996;50:S92–S96.

157. Sherrard D, et al. The spectrum of bone disease in end-stage renal failure—an evolving disorder. *Kidney Int* 1993;43:436–442.

158. Cunningham J, et al. Dialysate calcium reduction in CAPD patients treated with calcium carbonate and alfacalcidol. *Nephrol Dial Transplant* 1992;7:63–68.

159. Weinreich T, et al. Low dialysate calcium in continuous ambulatory peritoneal dialysis: a randomized controlled multicenter trial. *Am J Kidney Dis* 1995;25:452–460.

160. Johnson D, et al. A randomized trial comparing 1.25 mmol/L calcium dialysate to 1.75 mmol/L calcium dialysate in CAPD patients. *Nephrol Dial Transplant* 1996;11:88–93.

4

HEMODIALYSIS VASCULAR ACCESS

MICHAEL J. BERKOBEN AND STEVE J. SCHWAB

Hemodialysis sustains life in three general circumstances: acute renal failure, poisonings, and end-stage renal disease (ESRD). Successful hemodialysis in any of these circumstances requires access to large blood vessels capable of supporting rapid extracorporeal blood flow. Immediate and temporary access to the circulation in acute renal failure and in poisonings is easily achieved by the percutaneous insertion of dual-lumen dialysis catheters into the femoral, internal jugular, or (if necessary) subclavian veins.

The establishment and maintenance of vascular access in ESRD, however, provides a greater challenge. Adequate dialytic therapy requires reliable, long-term access to the circulation. Vascular access that is beset with complications exacts considerable morbidity and mortality. Reliable, long-term access to the circulation in ESRD is best achieved by the construction of an endogenous (nonsynthetic) arteriovenous fistula. Less desirable is the construction of a synthetic arteriovenous fistula.

When reading this chapter, one should not lose sight of the fact that careful preparation for endogenous arteriovenous fistula creation well before the need for hemodialysis is often the single most important step that the nephrologist can take to ensure long-term, complication-free access to the circulation.

ACUTE VASCULAR ACCESS

Scribner Shunt

The clinical application of acute and chronic hemodialysis received a boost in 1960 when Scribner and Quinton introduced the external arteriovenous fistula (1). Silastic tubes fitted with Teflon tips are inserted into the radial artery and cephalic vein at the wrist or into the posterior tibial artery and saphenous vein at the ankle. The artery and vein are ligated distal to the insertion site. During hemodialysis, the silastic tubes are connected directly to the blood tubing. When the Scribner shunt is not in use, the tubes are joined by a Teflon connector.

Scribner shunts have fallen out of favor for several reasons. Surgical insertion is necessary, and thrombosis rates are high. Inadvertent dislodgment may occur. In addition, ligation of the artery and vein sacrifices a potential permanent vascular access site. Scribner shunts are now rarely used for acute or chronic hemodialysis.

Double-lumen Hemodialysis Catheters

Double-lumen central venous catheters are the preferred form of vascular access for acute hemodialysis. Central venous catheters can be inserted at the bedside using the Seldinger technique and may support extracorporeal blood-flow rates greater than 300 mL/min. Separation of the arterial and venous ports minimizes recirculation of blood (Fig. 4.1). Central venous catheters may be used for conventional hemodialysis and for continuous venovenous hemodialysis.

Catheter Materials

Polyurethane, polyethylene, and polytetrafluoroethylene (PTFE) are the preferred polymers for catheters. Their rigidity at room temperature allows bedside insertion, and their softness at body temperature minimizes the risk of vein perforation during prolonged catheterization (2). Polyurethane has been reported to be the most flexible and least thrombogenic of the three materials (2).

Although silicone is the softest and least thrombogenic material, its softness necessitates the use of a peel-away sheath for percutaneous insertion (3). Insertion of silicone catheters via internal or external jugular venotomy is an alternative approach.

Catheter Insertion Sites

Dual-lumen hemodialysis catheters may be inserted into the femoral, internal jugular, or subclavian veins. Because subclavian vein catheter placement may lead to subclavian vein stenosis, subclavian vein catheters should not be placed in patients who will ultimately require fistula creation for chronic hemodialysis.

Femoral Vein

The femoral vein is cannulated immediately below the inguinal ligament. Cannulation of the femoral vein requires less skill, less experience, and less time than cannulation of other central veins. Femoral vein cannulation is an invaluable technique for patients with pulmonary edema because it may be performed with the patient in the semirecumbent position.

The incidence of life-threatening complications is lower for femoral vein cannulation than for internal jugular and subclavian vein cannulation. Complications of femoral vein cannula-

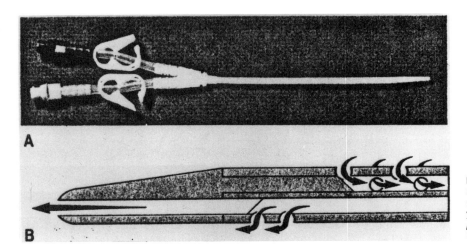

FIG. 4.1. A: Acute hemodialysis catheter. **B:** Separation of arterial and venous lumens minimizes recirculation of blood. (From Schwab SJ. Hemodialysis vascular access. In: Jacobson HR, et al., eds. *The principles and practice of nephrology.* Philadelphia: BC Decker, 1991:766–772, with permission.)

tion include ileofemoral vein thrombosis, arteriovenous fistula, retroperitoneal hemorrhage from vein perforation, and hemorrhage from accidental puncture of the femoral artery. Patients with femoral vein catheters must remain at bed rest in the hospital. To minimize the risk of infection, femoral vein catheters should not remain in place longer than 5 to 7 days.

The length of the femoral dialysis catheter is important. Kelber et al. (4) demonstrated that significant urea recirculation occurs when 15-cm catheters are used but not when 24-cm catheters are used. Increasing blood-flow rates through 15-cm catheters increases recirculation and does not increase dialysis efficiency. It is recommended that femoral catheters be at least 19-cm long so that the catheter tip resides in the inferior vena cava.

Subclavian Vein

The subclavian vein is cannulated by placing the introducer needle directly beneath the midpoint of the clavicle and aiming at the suprasternal notch. The needle is passed beneath the clavicle while remaining parallel to the sagittal plane. Subclavian vein catheters are comfortable and secure. They may be left in place for weeks and do not require that the patient remain in the hospital.

Subclavian vein cannulation requires more skill and may lead to more serious complications than femoral vein cannulation. Subclavian vein catheterization may lead to subclavian vein stenosis, precluding fistula placement in the ipsilateral arm. As mentioned previously, subclavian vein catheters should not be placed in patients for whom chronic hemodialysis is anticipated.

Internal Jugular Vein

In the anterior approach, the introducer needle enters the skin at a 20-degree angle to the sagittal plane, two fingerbreadths above the clavicle between the sternal and clavicular heads of the sternocleidomastoid muscle. The needle is aimed at the ipsilateral nipple. Internal jugular vein catheters may remain in place for weeks and do not require that the patient remain in hospital. In our experience, internal jugular catheters are less comfortable (despite the introduction of looped port extensions) and less secure than subclavian catheters. However, internal jugular

vein cannulation carries a lower risk of pneumothorax and central vein stenosis than does subclavian vein cannulation and is, in our opinion, the preferred technique.

Complications of Central Vein Cannulation

Insertion Complications

Insertion complications become less likely as the operator gains experience (5). The incidence of serious insertion complications is higher for subclavian vein and internal jugular vein cannulation than for femoral vein cannulation. Table 4.1 lists the most common insertion complications.

Atrial arrhythmias may result from endocardial irritation by the guidewire or catheter but are generally of no clinical significance (6). Ventricular arrhythmias occur in roughly 20% of patients but rarely require therapy (7).

Inadvertent arterial puncture is a common insertion complication. Manual pressure will prevent significant hematomata from femoral artery and carotid artery puncture, even in patients with bleeding diatheses (8). Although serious hemorrhage complicates less than 1% of subclavian vein catheterization attempts (9,10), we do not recommend attempts at subclavian vein catheterization in patients with coagulopathies or severe thrombocytopenia because of the difficulty of applying direct manual pressure to the subclavian artery.

Pneumothorax follows 1% to 5% of subclavian vein cannulations (5,9,10) but less than 0.1% of internal jugular vein cannulations (5,10). To minimize the chance of fatal pneumothorax, two rules must be followed:

TABLE 4.1. ACUTE HEMODIALYSIS CATHETER INSERTION COMPLICATIONS

Atrial and ventricular dysrhythmias
Arterial puncture
Hemothorax
Pneumothorax
Air embolism
Perforation of central vein or cardiac chamber
Pericardial tamponade

1. The operator should never attempt cannulation of the subclavian vein ipsilateral to the only healthy lung.
2. An unsuccessful attempt at subclavian cannulation may still lead to pneumothorax. A chest radiograph should be obtained before cannulation of the contralateral subclavian is attempted.

Perforations of the superior vena cava or cardiac chamber may lead to hemothorax, mediastinal hemorrhage, pericardial tamponade, and death (10). These complications are rare but are more likely following subclavian vein cannulation than following internal jugular vein cannulation, perhaps because of the curved path that a subclavian catheter must follow. To minimize the chance of perforation during insertion, the operator must never advance the catheter without protection by a J-tipped guidewire (11). A chest radiograph must be obtained following insertion to confirm that the catheter is within a central vein. If the catheter tip is in the right atrium, the catheter should be pulled back to prevent right atrial perforation. Prolonged catheterization may lead to erosion and perforation of the superior vena cava; pericardial tamponade should be considered in the hypotensive hemodialysis patient with a central venous dialysis catheter.

Air embolism rarely complicates central vein cannulation (10), but care should be taken to avoid accidental introduction of air through the introducer needle, dilator, or catheter.

Injuries to the brachial plexus (12), trachea (13), and recurrent laryngeal nerve (14) are rare complications of internal jugular vein cannulation.

At our institution, a handheld ultrasound device may be used in difficult cases. Ultrasonographic confirmation of target vein patency before cannulation prevents futile attempts at cannulation of thrombosed veins. In addition, the introducer needle may be inserted under direct ultrasonographic visualization. Fewer needle passes are required for successful cannulation when the ultrasound device is used (15).

Infection

Catheter-related infection, most commonly resulting from *Staphylococcus aureus* and *Staphylococcal epidermidis,* exacts considerable morbidity and even mortality. The mechanism of infection is migration of bacteria from the patient's skin through the catheter insertion site and down the outer surface of the catheter or contamination of the catheter lumen during hemodialysis (16). Rarely, infection is caused by infusion of infected solutions (16).

The risk of infection increases with the duration of catheterization (9,16–18). A recent study has defined the risk of bacteremia from temporary hemodialysis catheters (18). The risk of bacteremia from femoral catheters was 3.1% for up to 1 week of catheterization but increased to 10.7% by 2 weeks. Femoral catheters should, therefore, be removed after 1 week. Patients must be bed-bound during the period of catheterization. Prolonged catheterization of the subclavian and internal jugular veins carries less risk. For internal jugular catheters, the risk of bacteremia was 5.4% up to 3 weeks but increased to 10.3% by the fourth week. In individual patients, we believe that the risk

TABLE 4.2. PREVENTION OF ACUTE HEMODIALYSIS CATHETER INFECTION

Skin disinfection with 2% aqueous chlorhexidine at the time of insertion
Sound insertion technique
Skin disinfection with chlorhexidine or povidone-iodine solution at each hemodialysis treatment
Application of povidone-iodine ointment or mupirocin ointment to the catheter insertion site at each dressing change
Dry gauze dressings
Use of face shield or surgical mask by patients and nurses during connection and disconnection procedures
Limited duration of catheterization

of infection from prolonged catheterization should be weighed against the risk of repeated catheter insertion. Evidence of exit-site infection, even in the absence of systemic symptoms, should prompt catheter removal. Exit-site infection presages bacteremia, presumably because the absence of a cuff permits migration of bacteria along the tunnel and outer surface of the catheter.

Other preventive measures are listed in Table 4.2. Disinfection with 2% aqueous chlorhexidine at the time of insertion is preferred to disinfection with povidone-iodine or isopropyl alcohol (19). Hemodialysis catheters should not be used for infusions or blood sampling. After catheter placement and at the end of each hemodialysis treatment, the skin should be disinfected using chlorhexidine or povidone-iodine solution. Next, povidone-iodine ointment (20) or mupirocin ointment should be applied to the exit site. Lastly, a dry gauze dressing rather than an occlusive dressing should be applied (21).

A febrile hemodialysis patient with a central venous catheter should be presumed to have catheter-related bacteremia unless there is strong evidence to the contrary. Rigors are especially suggestive of bacteremia. Blood cultures should be obtained, the catheter removed, and antibiotics administered. A new catheter may be placed once the patient defervesces. Antibiotic therapy should be continued for 2 to 3 weeks. In the event of metastatic infection (e.g., vertebral osteomyelitis or endocarditis), a longer course of antibiotic therapy will be required. The management of *S. aureus* bacteremia is detailed later in the discussion of Permcath-related bacteremia.

Catheter Thrombosis

Intracatheter thrombus impedes extracorporeal blood flow. Treatment consists of instilling alteplase (recombinant human tissue plasminogen activator) reconstituted to a concentration of 1 mg/mL in volumes sufficient to fill the catheter lumens for 30 to 120 minutes (22). This procedure may be repeated if necessary. If catheter occlusion persists, catheter exchange may be performed using a J-tipped guidewire.

Extracatheter or mural thrombosis is a less frequent but more serious complication (23). Arm edema is the presenting sign of subclavian vein occlusion and warrants catheter removal. Systemic anticoagulation may be administered, but permanent occlusion is likely. Symptoms subside as collateral drainage develops, but placement of permanent vascular access in the involved arm is permanently precluded.

Central Vein Stenosis

Subclavian vein stenosis may occur after placement of subclavian dialysis catheters (24–26). Central vein stenosis occurs less commonly after placement of internal jugular catheters (27,28). Arm edema is the presenting complaint of subclavian vein stenosis, but it may develop only after placement of an ipsilateral arteriovenous fistula. It is not known whether fistulas uncover unrecognized stenoses or whether they are necessary for their development. It should be noted, however, that central vein stenosis has developed in the absence of antecedent catheterization. Also, central vein stenosis may become clinically evident months after ipsilateral fistula placement (29). It is possible, then, that ipsilateral fistulas may initiate or hasten the development of central vein stenoses. Regardless of the mechanism of stenosis formation, we do not recommend that subclavian catheters be placed in those patients in whom fistula placement is anticipated. The treatment of central vein stenoses is discussed later in this chapter.

PERMANENT VASCULAR ACCESS

Vascular access remains the Achilles' heel of chronic hemodialysis. Vascular access that is beset with complications is costly to both the patient and society; vascular access failure is the most frequent cause of hospitalization for patients with ESRD. The primary arteriovenous fistula is the form of vascular access most likely to provide long-term complication-free vascular access. The importance of careful preparation for primary arteriovenous fistula placement months before the need for hemodialysis cannot be overemphasized.

Types of Permanent Vascular Access

The types of permanent vascular access are listed in Table 4.3.

Primary Arteriovenous Fistulas

First described by Brescia et al. in 1961 (30), the primary arteriovenous fistula remains the best form of permanent vascular access. These endogenous fistulas are usually created by a side-to-side or end-to-side vein-to-artery anastomosis of the cephalic vein and radial artery at the wrist. Brachial-cephalic fistulas at the elbow and transposed brachial-basilic fistulas may also be created. Although 24% to 27% of primary arteriovenous fistulas thrombose within the first few postoperative weeks or fail to achieve sufficient caliber to permit cannulation (31,32), most mature within 2 to 6 months. Once mature, native fistulas have excellent long-term patency rates and rarely become infected. The authors have seen primary arteriovenous fistulas provide adequate vascular access for 20 years.

Unfortunately, a minority of patients in most hemodialysis centers have functional endogenous fistulas. Use of cephalic veins for phlebotomy or intravenous cannulation can prevent successful fistula construction. In addition, elderly and diabetic patients comprise an increasing proportion of patients entering chronic hemodialysis programs; the vascular anatomy of elderly and diabetic patients often precludes successful native fistula creation.

Synthetic Arteriovenous Grafts

Synthetic fistulas are composed of PTFE. PTFE grafts are typically placed in the forearm in either a loop (brachial artery to basilic vein) or straight (distal radial artery to basilic vein) configuration. Within 3 to 4 weeks, fibrous tissue secures the graft in its subdermal tunnel and helps achieve hemostasis at needle puncture sites. Although PTFE will withstand numerous thrombectomies and revisions, PTFE grafts are more prone to thrombosis and infection that are primary arteriovenous fistulas. By 3 years, most grafts have been lost to thrombosis or infection. On occasion, the material wears out after repeated needle puncture.

TABLE 4.3. TYPES OF PERMANENT VASCULAR ACCESS

Type of Access	Patency Rates	Advantages	Disadvantages
Primary arteriovenous fistula	60%–70% at 1 year 50%–65% at 2–4 years	Low thrombosis and infection rates May provide complication-free access for many years (few if any interventions required to maintain patency)	May require 6 months or more to mature 24%–27% fail to mature
PTFE grafts	62%–83% at 1 year 50%–77% at 2 years	Require only 3 weeks to mature	Thrombosis and infection rates higher than those for primary fistulas (many interventions required to maintain patency)
Tunneled cuffed catheters	30%–74% at 1 year	May be used immediately No risk of arterial steal Morbidity of insertion and removal low No needle puncture required for hemodialysis	Chronically low blood flow rates may lead to inadequate dialysis High rate of catheter-related bacteremia and metastatic infection
Subcutaneous ports attached to catheters	Device survival as high as 90% at 6 months (38)	May have longer survival rates and lower infection rates than do tunneled cuffed catheters May not need to be removed in cases of bacteremia	More difficult to remove than tunneled cuffed catheters

PTFE, polytetrafluoroethylene.

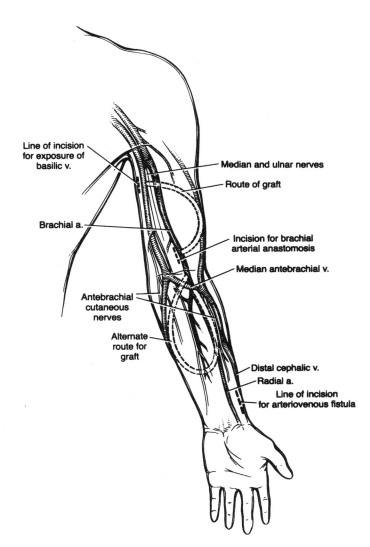

Line of incision
for exposure of
basilic v.

Median and ulnar nerves

Route of graft

Brachial a.

Incision for brachial
arterial anastomosis

Median antebrachial v.

Antebrachial
cutaneous
nerves

Alternate
route for
graft

Distal cephalic v.

Radial a.

Line of incision
for arteriovenous fistula

FIG. 4.2. Looped forearm graft and upper arm graft. (From Stickel DL. Renal dialysis access procedures. In: Sabiston DC Jr, ed. *Atlas of general surgery.* Philadelphia: WB Saunders, 1994:90–98, with permission.)

Fortunately, PTFE grafts can be placed in many sites. Following forearm graft loss, a new PTFE graft can be placed in the upper arm, chest wall (axillary artery to axillary vein and axillary artery to jugular vein), or thigh (femoral artery to femoral vein). Fig. 4.2 depicts a looped forearm graft and an upper arm graft.

Tunneled Cuffed Catheters

Double-lumen silastic or silicone catheters with felt cuffs (such as Permcath from Quinton Instrument Company, Seattle, Wash., and others) are inserted through a subcutaneous tunnel under fluoroscopic guidance into an internal jugular vein (Fig. 4.3), external jugular vein, subclavian vein, or, if necessary, femoral vein. The right internal jugular vein is the preferred insertion site. When compared with the left internal jugular vein approach, the right internal jugular vein approach offers a less curved route to the superior vena cava, a lower risk of complications (27,28,33), better catheter function, and a lower rate of central vein stenosis and thrombosis (33,34). The catheter tip should reside at the junction of the superior vena cava and right atrium or in the right atrium to ensure a high blood-flow rate.

Because of the risk of subclavian vein stenosis, subclavian vein catheterization should be performed only if jugular vein catheterization is not possible. Cuffed catheters may be used immediately after insertion.

Cuffed double-lumen catheters are the least desirable form of permanent vascular access. Intracatheter thrombosis and fibrin sheath formation on the external surface of the catheter often limit extracorporeal blood flow. Moss et al. (34) found that these catheters provided a mean blood-flow rate of only 243 mL/min when used as long-term vascular access. In a recent study from our institution, only 73% of catheters were able to consistently provide extracorporeal blood-flow rates of 400 mL/min, despite prompt lytic therapy for catheter thrombosis and prompt mechanical removal of fibrin sheaths (35). More importantly, catheter-related infection is common and may lead to metastatic infection and even death (see later). The use of cuffed double-lumen silastic catheters should be restricted to those patients whose endogenous or synthetic fistulas have not yet matured, to those who have exhausted all fistula sites, and to those who cannot tolerate the increase in cardiac output associated with fistula construction.

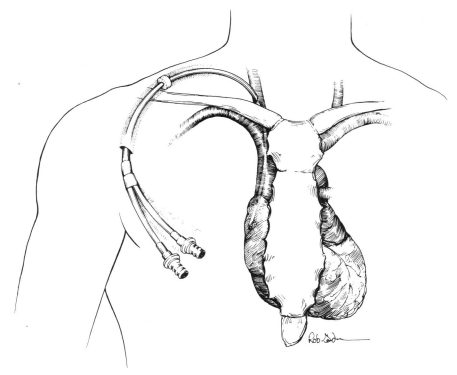

FIG. 4.3. Cuffed double-lumen silastic catheter inserted through a subcutaneous tunnel into the right internal jugular vein. (From Schwab SJ, et al. Prospective evaluation of a Dacron cuffed hemodialysis catheter for prolonged use. *Am J Kidney Dis* 1988;11:166–169, with permission.)

Subcutaneous Ports with Catheters

Recent studies have demonstrated the utility of subcutaneous ports attached to catheters. These devices consist of a subcutaneous port implanted beneath the clavicle to which is attached a catheter that is tunneled to the right internal jugular vein. Two such systems exist—the LifeSite Hemodialysis Access System (Vasca, Inc., Tewksbury, Mass.) and Dialock (Biolink Corp., Middleboro, Mass.). In the case of the LifeSite system (36), two ports, each attached to a single catheter, are implanted. Each port is accessed transcutaneously with a dialysis needle. In the case of Dialock (37), a single port is attached to two catheters, and the port is accessed transcutaneously with two needles. Compared with tunneled cuffed hemodialysis catheters, the LifeSite device, when used with 70% isopropyl alcohol as the disinfectant, provided higher blood flow rates, had a lower infections rate, and had a higher device survival rate (38). Use of the Dialock system may also result in a lower infection rate than that reported for tunneled cuffed catheters (37,39).

Preparation for Vascular Access Placement

The radial cephalic primary arteriovenous fistula at the wrist of the nondominant arm is the preferred form of vascular access for chronic hemodialysis. Careful planning is necessary to achieve successful fistula creation. The patient and primary care physician must be instructed that the patient's morbidity on chronic hemodialysis will largely be determined by the adequacy of his or her vascular access (40). Patients should be taught to protect the vasculature of the nondominant arm; they should not permit placement of radial artery catheters and cephalic vein catheters. If possible, venipuncture should be avoided altogether in the nondominant arm.

A history of subclavian vein catheter placement or current or previous transvenous pacemaker placement ipsilateral to the planned access site should prompt preoperative venography to exclude central vein stenosis or occlusion; the presence of an untreatable central vein lesion precludes ipsilateral access placement. The radial cephalic fistula should be created 6 to 8 months before the anticipated need for hemodialysis. If this fistula is slow to mature, ligation of major venous side branches may speed maturation. If radial-cephalic fistula construction is not possible, brachial-cephalic fistula construction at the elbow is the next best option (41).

In those patients in whom neither radial cephalic nor brachial cephalic primary fistula creation is possible, a synthetic graft or a transposed brachial-basilic primary fistula should be placed in the nondominant arm (41). The choice should be determined by the patient's vascular anatomy and by the preference of the vascular surgeon. The synthetic graft may be placed in either the forearm (looped graft from brachial artery to basilic vein preferred) or the upper arm (brachial artery to proximal basilic vein). Although an upper arm graft may be expected to have a higher blood-flow rate and longer patency, forearm graft placement will preserve potential access sites in the proximal limb. Again, the choice should be determined by the patient's vascular anatomy and by the preference of the surgeon. The transposed brachial-basilic fistula is created by making an incision from the forearm to the axilla along the course of the basilic vein, dividing the vein where it is too small to use, and mobilizing the vein toward the axilla where it is anastomosed to the brachial artery. In some hands, transposed brachial-basilic fistulas are less likely to thrombose than are upper arm grafts (42). Following vascular access loss in both arms, a PTFE graft may be placed in the chest wall or in the thigh.

The use of cuffed double-lumen catheters and subcutaneous ports attached to catheters should be restricted to patients whose native or synthetic fistulas have not yet matured and to patients in whom native or synthetic fistula placement is not possible.

Vascular Access Blood Flow and Patency

The chief determinant of vascular access adequacy and patency is access blood flow. As discussed later in this chapter, inadequate blood flow results in recirculation of blood within the access and decreases the efficiency of dialysis. Perhaps more importantly, low access blood-flow rates lead to access thrombosis and access loss.

Vascular access blood flow depends on the type, the location, and the age of the access. Initial blood-flow rates in primary arteriovenous fistulas are only 200 to 300 mL/min (43) but increase to greater than 800 mL/min as the venous drainage system dilates (44). Blood-flow rates in synthetic fistulas are high initially (45,46) but may fall with time because of progressive intimal and fibromuscular hyperplasia in the venous outflow system. Investigators have demonstrated that grafts with blood-flow rates less than 600 mL/min are more likely to clot than grafts with blood-flow rates greater than 600 mL/min (47–49). Grafts constructed using more proximal arteries have higher blood-flow rates (43,46) and may have higher patency rates.

The cumulative patency rate is defined as the percentage of accesses that remain patent at a given time regardless of the need for revision and thrombectomy. Cumulative patency rates for primary arteriovenous fistulas have been reported to be 60% to 70% at 1 year and 50% to 65% at 2 to 4 years (31,50). Cumulative patency rates for PTFE grafts have been reported to be 62% to 83% at 1 year and 50% to 77% at 2 years (31,32,50–54). Fifty percent or fewer of synthetic grafts are patent beyond 3 years. The lower cumulative patency rates for primary arteriovenous fistulas are due to early fistula failure; approximately one fourth of these fistulas fail to mature. After correction for early failure, cumulative patency rates are at least as high as patency rates for PTFE grafts (31,32,50). In addition, native fistulas require fewer interventions to maintain patency than do synthetic fistulas. At our institution, intractable thrombosis accounts for roughly 80% of access loss, infection for roughly 20%, and vascular steal for a small percentage of access loss.

Tunneled cuffed catheters and subcutaneous ports attached to catheters may be used for permanent vascular access or for temporary vascular access in those patients awaiting fistula maturation. When the tunneled cuffed catheter is used for permanent vascular access, the catheter survival rate is 30% to 74% at 1 year (34,35,55–57). Intracatheter clotting and extracatheter fibrin sheath formation are common but may be treated with

tissue plasminogen activator and catheter stripping, respectively (see later). Infection is the leading cause of catheter loss. When used for temporary vascular access, almost all tunneled cuffed catheters function satisfactorily until elective removal (35). We await long-term studies of subcutaneous ports attached to catheters.

Vascular Access Complications

Access Thrombosis

Fistula Thrombosis

Thrombosis is the leading cause of fistula loss. Thrombosis within 1 month of fistula construction is likely due to technical errors in fistula construction or to premature cannulation of the fistula. After the first month, the thrombosis rate is 0.5 to 0.8 episodes per patient-year (58). Synthetic fistulas thrombose much more frequently than do endogenous fistulas.

Nearly 90% of graft thromboses are associated with stenoses of the venous outflow tract (31,59–61). These lesions are characterized by intimal and fibromuscular hyperplasia (31,62). Most venous stenoses develop at or within 2 to 3 cm of the vein-graft anastomosis (63). The remainder develop in more proximal veins, in central veins, or in the graft itself. Subclavian vein stenoses are associated with previous subclavian vein catheterization and with transvenous pacemaker placement (24,29,64). Intragraft stenoses are reported to result from pseudointimal hyperplasia (62) and fibroblastic ingrowth through needle puncture sites (65).

A minority of graft thromboses occur in the absence of an identifiable anatomic lesion. Hypotension, intravascular volume depletion, and graft compression during sleep may decrease graft flow and lead to graft thrombosis. Excessive graft compression by patients or dialysis staff attempting to achieve hemostasis following dialysis may lead to graft thrombosis; complete and accurate treatment records may allow the identification and retraining of those individuals who apply excessive pressure. The prevention and treatment of fistula thrombosis is discussed later in this chapter.

Tunneled Cuffed Catheter Thrombosis

Malfunction of cuffed hemodialysis catheters is very common. A study from our institution described 163 consecutive episodes of catheter malfunction in 121 catheters (35). Intraluminal instillation of urokinase reestablished an extracorporeal blood-flow rate of at least 300 mL/min in 121 cases; these episodes were presumably due to intracatheter clotting. The remaining 42 cases were studied by contrast injection into the catheter and digital subtraction angiography. Fibrin sheath formation on the catheter tip was detected in 38 of these 42 cases. Two cases were due to malposition of the catheter tip, and two cases were due to technical errors made at the time of catheter insertion. The fibrin sheath was successfully stripped from the catheter in 36 of the 38 cases. In this procedure, a gooseneck snare is passed through a common femoral vein sheath into the right atrium. The snare encircles the catheter and strips away the fibrin sheath as it is retracted (Fig. 4.4).

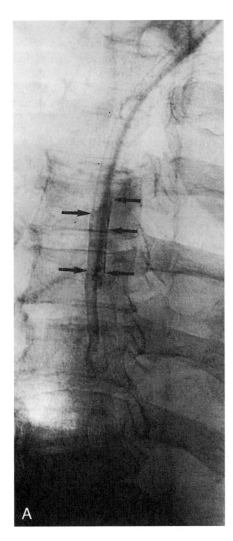
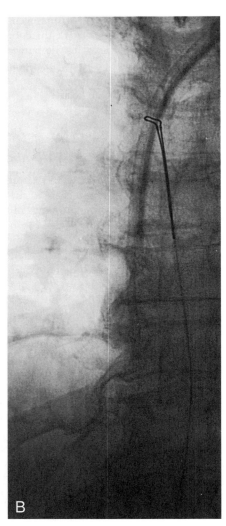

FIG. 4.4. A: Contrast injection into the lumen of a cuffed catheter demonstrates a fibrin sheath. **B:** A gooseneck snare encircles the cuffed catheter. (From Suhocki PV, et al. Silastic cuffed catheters for hemodialysis vascular access: thrombolytic and mechanical correction of malfunction. *Am J Kidney Dis* 1996;28:379–386, with permission.)

Intraluminal urokinase instillation at the hemodialysis unit has been the first step in the treatment of cuffed catheter malfunction. However, urokinase is not currently available in the American market. As of this writing, instillation of alteplase (recombinant human tissue plasminogen activator) is the first step (22). If this procedure does not restore catheter function, contrast injection and angiography should be performed to detect fibrin sheath formation or catheter malposition. Fibrin sheath formation may be treated by stripping or by replacement of the catheter over a guidewire. Infusion of urokinase through both ports at a rate of 20,000 U per port per hour for 6 hours is also an effective treatment for fibrin sheaths and refractory intraluminal clots (57). Again, however, urokinase is not currently available in the American market. A malpositioned catheter should be repositioned with a snare or may be replaced over a guidewire.

Infection

Vascular access infection is a serious and, in some cases, life-threatening problem.

Fistula and Synthetic Graft Infection

Native fistula infections are uncommon; they are usually localized and can usually be treated successfully with antibiotic therapy (31). However, because these are endovascular infections, it has been recommended that they be treated as subacute bacterial endocarditis—with 6 weeks of antibiotic therapy (66).

Synthetic fistula infections are not uncommon; they are the second most common cause of fistula loss (31,51,67) and the most common cause of bacteremia in hemodialysis patients (68–71). Gram-positive cocci—*S. aureus* and, less commonly, *S. epidermidis* and streptococcal species—are the culprits in most cases. Gram-negative bacteria account for roughly 15% of episodes of bacteremia in hemodialysis patients (68–71).

Some risk factors for graft infection are beyond the nephrologist's control. Intravenous drug use (31), dermatitis overlying the graft, and poor personal hygiene (71) predispose patients to graft infection. Femoral grafts have a high infection rate (72,73), most likely because of the proximity of the graft to the perineum. Nevertheless, preventive measures should be undertaken. We strongly believe that patients should wash the skin overlying their grafts with soap and water before each hemodialysis treatment. This practice may decrease the likelihood of inadvertent introduction of bacteria into the bloodstream during graft cannulation. Monitoring of graft cannulation and infection records may allow one to identify hemodialysis staff who employ poor needle insertion technique.

Fever, chills, and rigors are the typical presenting complaints of the bacteremic hemodialysis patient. Physical evidence of graft infection is often absent. The febrile hemodialysis patient with a synthetic fistula should be presumed to have graft-associated bacteremia unless the history, physical examination, and initial investigations provide strong evidence to the contrary. Blood cultures should be obtained. Initial antibiotic therapy should be effective against gram-positive organisms (including *Enterococcus*) and against gram-negative organisms. At our institution, we administer loading doses of vancomycin (20 mg/kg) and either gentamicin (2 mg/kg) or tobramycin (2 mg/kg). Because methicillin-resistant *S. aureus* (MRSA) and coagulase-negative staphylococci are common culprits, a β-lactam antibiotic should not be used as an empiric agent. The antibiotic regimen can be simplified if blood cultures yield a culprit. If staphylococci are isolated that are susceptible to β-lactam antibiotics, a β-lactam should be substituted for vancomycin unless the patient has a β-lactam allergy.

Patients with gram-positive bacteremia who defervesce promptly in response to antibiotic therapy and whose grafts have no associated pustule or abscess can often be successfully treated with intravenous antibiotics alone. However, extensive graft infection may be present even when the physical examination is unremarkable. If fever or bacteremia persists, strong consideration should be given to graft excision. Staphylococcal bacteremia has a propensity to lead to metastatic infection; endocarditis, osteomyelitis, septic pulmonary emboli, empyema, septic arthritis, and meningitis have been reported. Persistent fever or bacteremia should also prompt one to search for evidence of metastatic infection. In hemodialysis patients with *S. aureus* bacteremia, this search should include transesophageal echocardiography to exclude infective endocarditis. If fever and bacteremia promptly remit and if there is no evidence of metastatic infection, a 3-week course of antibiotic should suffice. Otherwise, a 6-week or longer course of antibiotic therapy is required. Regardless of the length of therapy, blood cultures should be obtained after completion of therapy to ensure that the infection has been eradicated. Gram-negative infections less commonly lead to metastatic infection, and a 2- to 3-week course of antibiotic therapy should suffice.

Evaluation by the vascular surgeon is mandatory if a pustule or abscess overlies the graft. Localized infection of the graft may be treated by simple incision and drainage or by partial graft excision and bypass grafting. Extensive infection necessitates total graft excision. Grafts placed within the past month must be completely excised even if the infection is thought to be localized; because these grafts are incompletely incorporated into surrounding tissue, the infection is unlikely to be localized (74). Finally, it should be noted that bleeding through an area of eroded skin overlying a synthetic graft may be the initial manifestation of graft infection. "Herald bleeding" mandates evaluation by the vascular surgeon.

Cuffed Catheter Infection

Cuffed catheter infection deserves special attention. At each hemodialysis treatment, the exit site should be examined, and, to reduce the risk of infection, povidone-iodine ointment (20) or mupirocin ointment and a dry gauze dressing (21) should be applied to the exit site. Occlusive dressings should be avoided; they trap any drainage and create a moist environment at the exit site. Exit-site and tunnel infections may be treated without catheter removal if systemic symptoms of infection are absent and if blood cultures yield no growth. Exit-site infections (erythema, crusting, scant drainage) may be treated with topical antibiotic therapy. Tunnel drainage should prompt parenteral antibiotic therapy; if there is no response to therapy, the catheter should be removed. In our experience, copious purulent tunnel drainage cannot be eradicated without catheter removal.

In recent years, much has been learned about bacteremia associated with cuffed catheters. Catheter-related bacteremia is very common. In a series from Duke, 41 of 102 patients with cuffed hemodialysis catheters experienced 62 episodes of bacteremia (75). Sixty-four percent of episodes were due to gram-positive cocci, 29% to gram-negative bacilli, and 5% to both gram-positive and gram-negative organisms. The most common pathogen was *S. aureus*. Antibiotic treatment without catheter removal was attempted in 38 instances but failed in 26; catheter removal was ultimately necessary in these 26 instances because of evidence of persistent infection. Nine of the 41 bacteremic patients developed complications: osteomyelitis in six, septic arthritis in one, infective endocarditis in four, and death in two. All patients with complications had gram-positive bacteremia. Attempted catheter salvage did not appear to increase the risk of complications. We have also described several cases of epidural abscess associated with catheter-related bacteremia (76). The only consistent initial complaint was severe back pain. All cases were due to staphylococci. Excruciating back pain in a hemodialysis patient with current or previous bacteremia should prompt magnetic resonance imaging of the spine (76,77).

Because of this experience, we do not recommend treatment of catheter-related bacteremia with the catheter in place. A standard practice has been to administer antibiotics, to remove the catheter, and to reinsert another at a new central venous site after eradication of bacteremia (negative blood cultures for at least 48 hours). Intravenous antibiotic therapy is continued for 3 weeks. A search for metastatic infection should be undertaken if fever persists or recurs, including transesophageal echocardiography in those with *S. aureus* bacteremia (78,79). This approach has several disadvantages, however. A several-day hospital stay is often required. At least one hemodialysis treatment via a temporary femoral vein catheter is usually required. Placement of a new tunneled cuffed catheter leads to use (and perhaps eventual loss) of another central venous access site. Because of these disadvantages, alternative approaches have been proposed.

Shaffer (80) has demonstrated that, in the absence of tunnel or exit-site infection, catheter-related bacteremia may be treated by antibiotic therapy and catheter exchange over a guidewire using the same venous insertion site with creation of a new tunnel and exit site. Beathard (81) has reported that, in patients with mild symptoms and without tunnel or exit-site infection, catheter exchange may be performed using the same venous insertion site, tunnel, and exit site. Antibiotic therapy is then administered for 3 weeks. This approach was successful in 87.8% of patients. We believe that antibiotic therapy combined with catheter exchange is a satisfactory approach to catheter-related bacteremia not associated with exit-site or tunnel infection. This approach preserves central venous access sites and limits hospital stays. Catheter removal is mandatory, however, in patients with catheter-related bacteremia associated with a tender or erythematous tunnel or with purulent exit-site drainage, in unstable patients, and in patients in whom symptoms of infection persist after 36 hours (82).

Another approach has been to leave the catheter in place and administer a 3-week course of parenteral antibiotic therapy along with antibiotic lock solution at the end of each hemodialysis treatment. The rationale for this approach is that biofilms coat the luminal surfaces of catheters within days of placement and may be a source of continued bacteremia if the catheter is left in place. Instillation of highly concentrated antibiotic solutions (roughly 100-fold higher than therapeutic plasma concentrations) into catheter lumens at the end of each hemodialysis treatment may eliminate these biofilms. In a recent series, this approach was successful in only 51% of patients (83). However, only two infections in the series were due to *S. aureus*. Because of these drawbacks, this approach cannot yet be recommended.

Antibiotic Dosing Strategies

As described previously, empiric antibiotic therapy for the hemodialysis patient with suspected bacteremia consists of vancomycin 20 mg/kg and gentamicin 2 mg/kg or tobramycin 2 mg/kg. Vancomycin therapy should be continued if blood cultures yield enterococci or MRSA. Subsequent vancomycin doses of 500 mg after each hemodialysis treatment maintain prehemodialysis serum vancomycin levels above 10 μg/mL in most cases (84).

If the aminoglycoside is to be continued, subsequent doses of 1 mg/kg should be administered. Prolonged administration of an aminoglycoside in combination with vancomycin is discouraged because of the risk of otovestibulotoxicity.

If the isolated organism is susceptible to cefazolin, we recommend that this antibiotic be used. Recommended regimens include 2 g administered after each hemodialysis treatment or 20 mg/kg (rounded to the nearest 500-mg increment) administered after each hemodialysis treatment (85). Use of cefazolin for susceptible strains of *S. aureus* should help limit the emergence of vancomycin resistance. In 1999, strains of *S. aureus* with intermediate resistance were reported in two chronic dialysis patients. One patient had a peritoneal catheter (86), and the other had a central venous catheter and synthetic graft (87). Both had MRSA infections and were treated with a prolonged course of vancomycin therapy. It was proposed that prolonged exposure to vancomycin and the continued presence of prosthetic material acted to produce vancomycin resistance.

Congestive Heart Failure

If fistula blood flow exceeds 20% of cardiac output, high-output congestive heart failure may develop in patients with ventricular dysfunction (88). Reduction of fistula blood flow by banding or interposition of a tapered synthetic segment may reduce symptoms (89–91). Fistula takedown should be performed in refractory cases.

Hand Ischemia

Hand ischemia following fistula placement may be due to arterial insufficiency or venous hypertension. Arterial insufficiency results from direct shunting of arterial blood through the low-resistance fistula and from vascular steal, in which blood flows retrograde from the palmar arch through the radial artery into the fistula (92). Symptoms of hand ischemia usually decrease in the weeks following fistula construction, but close observation is warranted. If symptoms are severe (coldness or loss of motor function), fistula blood flow may be reduced by banding or by interposition of a tapered synthetic graft (89–91). If symptoms persist or if hand viability is threatened, fistula takedown should be performed.

Venous hypertension may occur after side-to-side anastomosis of the radial artery and cephalic vein. In the presence of a proximal venous stenosis or occlusion, there may be retrograde blood flow through the fistula and arterialization of the distal venous system; the pressure in the venous system of the hand will approach arterial pressure (92,93). Treatment consists of ligation of the distal vein and correction of the venous stenosis.

Aneurysms and Pseudoaneurysms

True aneurysms occur very commonly in native fistulas and generally cause no problems. Surgical intervention is required only if the aneurysm compromises the arterial anastomosis (94).

Pseudoaneurysms of synthetic grafts appear as progressive damage to the graft material leads to inability to seal needle puncture sites. Pseudoaneurysms may rapidly expand or may threaten the viability of the overlying skin. Surgical intervention should be considered in these circumstances to prevent hemorrhage. Surgical treatment consists of excision of the involved graft segment and placement of an interposition graft.

Prospective Identification of Venous Stenoses

As venous stenoses evolve, intraaccess pressure increases and access blood flow decreases. Eventually, the access may fail; nearly 90% of access thromboses are associated with venous stenoses (31,59–61). The preferred methods for the prospective detection of venous stenoses are serial measurement of access blood flow and measurement of static venous dialysis pressure (95). For reasons given later, neither method is in widespread use. Fortunately, the nephrologist may use other methods for the prospective detection of venous stenoses (Table 4.4). Prospective detection of venous stenoses followed by either percutaneous transluminal angioplasty (PTA) or surgical revision decreases fistula thrombosis rates and prolongs access survival (60,63,96–100).

Physical Evidence

Arm edema is a common indicator of subclavian stenosis, and difficulty with needle placement is an indicator of intragraft

TABLE 4.4. METHODS FOR THE PROSPECTIVE IDENTIFICATION OF VENOUS STENOSES

Physical examination and clinical assessment (difficulty with needle placement, prolonged bleeding following hemodialysis)
Venous dialysis pressure
   Dynamic venous dialysis pressure
   Static venous dialysis pressure
Access recirculation
   Urea recirculation
   Direct measurements of access recirculation (blood temperature monitoring method, saline dilution method, ultrasound dilution method)
Access blood flow
   Doppler ultrasonography
   Magnetic resonance
   Ultrasound dilution
   Conductance dilution
   Thermal dilution

stenosis (64). Prolonged bleeding after hemodialysis may indicate venous stenosis. Physical examination may be used to estimate access blood flow (101). A thrill at the arterial, midgraft, and venous segments is associated with an access blood-flow rate greater than 450 mL/min. A pulse without thrill is associated with a lower access blood-flow rate.

Venous Dialysis Pressure

Either dynamic venous dialysis pressure (venous dialysis pressure in the presence of extracorporeal blood flow) or static venous dialysis pressure (venous dialysis pressure in the absence of extracorporeal blood flow) may be measured. Measurement of static venous dialysis pressure is preferred but requires either a special device or more dialysis staff time.

Measurement of dynamic venous dialysis pressure is the least expensive method for the prospective detection of venous stenoses. However, dynamic venous dialysis pressure is affected by factors other than venous stenosis, rendering it the least reliable method for detecting venous stenoses. Because needle gauge and extracorporeal blood-flow rate affect dynamic venous dialysis pressure, these factors must be held constant. It is recommended that dynamic venous dialysis pressure be measured through 15-gauge needles at an extracorporeal blood-flow rate of 200 mL/min. In addition, different hemodialysis machines have different pressure monitors and different types and lengths of tubing. Each hemodialysis unit, then, must establish its own threshold pressure. Threshold dynamic venous dialysis pressures range from 125 to 150 mm Hg (102). These variables have led to wide differences among hemodialysis units in their ability to use this technique. The measurement of dynamic venous dialysis pressure is less sensitive and specific than measurement of access blood flow and is very prone to operator error. Indeed, some hemodialysis units have been unable to use this technique. Measurement of access blood flow and measurement of static venous dialysis pressure are the preferred techniques for the prospective detection of venous stenoses.

Dynamic venous dialysis pressure should be measured during each hemodialysis treatment. If the dynamic pressure exceeds

the threshold during three consecutive treatments or if the dynamic pressure is steadily increasing, fistulography should be performed and any venous stenosis should be treated. The efficacy of this strategy for the prospective detection and treatment of venous stenoses has been demonstrated by numerous investigators (60,61,63,97,103).

Elevated static venous dialysis pressures are also highly predictive of the presence of venous stenoses. Besarab et al. (96) measured static venous dialysis pressure by inserting a stopcock-transducer system between the venous needle and the venous blood line. Static venous dialysis pressure was measured every 3 to 4 months. Fistulography was performed if static venous dialysis pressure/systolic blood pressure was equal to 0.4, and angioplasty was performed if stenoses resulted in a luminal diameter reduction greater than 50%. As this protocol evolved, the angioplasty rate at their institution increased 13-fold, the thrombosis rate decreased 70%, and the access replacement rate decreased 79%. The measurement of static venous dialysis pressure in this manner requires special equipment. Simplified techniques may allow widespread application of this approach. A new static intraaccess pressure surveillance protocol is detailed in the most recent *Clinical Practice Guidelines for Vascular Access* (104).

Urea Recirculation

Hemodialysis access recirculation occurs when dialyzed blood returning through the venous needle reenters the extracorporeal circuit through the arterial needle. It is important to measure access recirculation for two reasons. First, reentry of dialyzed blood into the extracorporeal circuit reduces solute concentration gradients across the dialysis membrane and thereby reduces the efficiency of dialysis. Second, high degrees of access recirculation indicate low access blood flow and herald access thrombosis.

Recirculation is usually caused by a venous stenosis that decreases access blood flow or by reversed needles (see Chapter 5 for a complete discussion). When the access blood-flow rate is lower than that demanded by the blood pump, reentry of dialyzed blood into the extracorporeal circuit is necessary to meet the demand of the blood pump (Fig. 4.5). Less commonly, recirculation results from arterial stenosis.

Access recirculation is calculated from the following formula.

$$\text{Percentage recirculation} = ((\text{Systemic [BUN]} - \text{Arterial blood line [BUN]})/(\text{Systemic [BUN]} - \text{Venous blood line [BUN]})) \times 100$$

where, ideally, the systemic blood urea nitrogen (BUN) concentration is equal to the BUN concentration in the blood entering the fistula. One can see that access recirculation exists whenever the concentration of urea in arterial line blood is lower than the concentration of urea in systemic blood, indicating reentry of dialyzed blood into the arterial line.

The chief source of error in the determination of access recirculation lies with the determination of the systemic urea concentration. The systemic urea concentration is assumed to be equal to the urea concentration in blood entering the access. Traditionally, systemic blood has been sampled from a peripheral vein in the contralateral arm ("three-needle method"). This

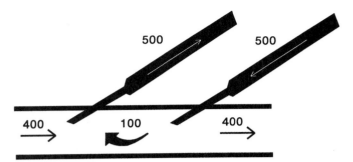

FIG. 4.5. Access recirculation is 20% because extracorporeal blood flow exceeds access blood flow. (From Depner TA. Techniques for prospective identification of venous stenosis. *Adv Ren Replace Ther* 1994;1:119–130, with permission.)

method has been found to be inadequate because of two phenomena: arteriovenous disequilibrium and venovenous disequilibrium.

The first phenomenon that renders the three-needle sampling method inadequate is arteriovenous disequilibrium (or cardiopulmonary recirculation) (105–108). Dialyzed blood (with a low urea concentration) returns to the central veins, dilutes blood returning from the systemic circulation (with a high urea concentration), and reduces the urea concentration in central venous blood (Fig. 4.6). The urea concentration in blood leaving the left heart and entering the hemodialysis access will be lower than the urea concentration in peripheral venous blood. Use of the peripheral vein BUN in the recirculation formula, then, will result in overestimation of access recirculation. The degree of arteriovenous disequilibrium increases with increasing extraction of urea by the dialyzer, with increasing extracorporeal blood-flow rate, and with decreasing cardiac output. With increasing extracorporeal blood-flow rate or with decreasing cardiac output, a greater proportion of the cardiac output courses through the dialyzer, increasing the dilution of peripheral venous blood by dialyzed blood.

The second phenomenon that accounts for the different urea concentrations in peripheral venous blood and in blood entering the access is venovenous disequilibrium (105–107,109). Perfusion of the arm contralateral to the hemodialysis access is low during hemodialysis; urea removal in that limb is diminished in comparison to well-perfused compartments. As a result, the urea concentration is higher in the veins of the contralateral arm than in central venous blood and in blood entering the access. This difference increases with time. Again, use of the peripheral vein BUN concentration in the recirculation formula will result in overestimation of access recirculation.

Fortunately, there is an alternative to the three-needle method. Sherman (110) has devised the method described in Table 4.5. In this two-needle method, the extracorporeal blood-flow rate is decreased to 120 mL/min for 10 seconds to clear the arterial line of recirculated blood. Systemic blood is then sampled from the arterial line after the blood pump is shut off. This technique reduces but does not eliminate the effect of arteriovenous disequilibrium; systemic blood obtained in this manner

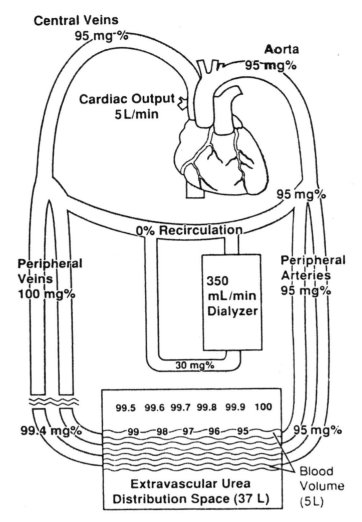

FIG. 4.6. Arteriovenous recirculation. Dialyzed blood bypasses the systemic circulation, dilutes blood returning from the body, and decreases the concentration of urea in central venous blood. Because the concentration of urea in blood leaving the left heart and entering the access will be lower than the concentration of urea in peripheral venous blood, use of the peripheral vein blood urea nitrogen (BUN) in the recirculation formula will lead to overestimation of access recirculation. In this case, access recirculation is absent, but the percentage of urea recirculation using the peripheral vein method is (100 − 95)/(100 − 30) × 100 or 7%. (From Sherman RA. Recirculation revisited. *Semin Dial* 1991;4:221–223, with permission.)

TABLE 4.5. PROTOCOL FOR THE MEASUREMENT OF UREA RECIRCULATION

Turn off ultrafiltration 30 minutes after the initiation of hemodialysis
Draw arterial (A) blood line and venous (V) blood line samples
Immediately decrease extracorporeal blood flow rate to 120 mL/min
Turn blood pump off exactly 10 seconds after decreasing blood flow rate
Clamp arterial line immediately above port
Draw systemic (S) sample from arterial line port
Measure blood urea nitrogen (BUN) in the three samples
Percentage recirculation = (S − A)/(S − V) × 100

Adapted from *NKF-K/DOQI Clinical practice guidelines for vascular access.* New York: National Kidney Foundation, 2001:48, with permission.

will more closely approximate blood entering the hemodialysis access.

The threshold urea recirculation value that should prompt one to request fistulography is not known. Because access recirculation should not occur unless the access blood-flow rate is less than the extracorporeal blood-flow rate demanded by the blood pump (111), any degree of access recirculation is abnormal. Indeed, the blood temperature monitoring method and the saline dilution method have demonstrated that recirculation is absent in well-functioning fistulas (112,113). These techniques directly measure access recirculation and do not require urea measurements; the effects of arteriovenous and venovenous disequilibrium are completely eliminated. These techniques require special equipment and are not yet in widespread use.

Unfortunately, threshold values of urea recirculation have been determined using the three-needle (peripheral vein) method, which overestimates access recirculation (114,115). When the recommended two-needle method is used, urea recirculation values greater than 10% should prompt further investigation (110). When values exceed 20%, the possibility of reversed needle placement should be considered before fistulography is requested (110). The blood temperature monitoring method and the saline dilution method provide more accurate measurements of recirculation but require special equipment and are not in widespread use. If recirculation exceeds 5% when measured by these techniques, fistulography should be requested (110).

Access Blood Flow

Because the chief determinant of vascular access patency is access blood flow, sequential measurement of access blood flow is the preferred method for the prospective monitoring of vascular accesses. Doppler evaluation, magnetic resonance, and ultrasound dilution are the techniques that have been most extensively studied. Unfortunately, these techniques require special equipment and are not in widespread use.

Doppler flow is predictive of access patency. Shackleton et al. (47) reported that, in synthetic grafts, Doppler flow less than 450 mL/min had a sensitivity of 83% and a specificity of 75% for the development of thrombosis within 2 to 6 weeks. Rittgers et al. (46) reported a mean blood flow of 307 mL/min in synthetic grafts that clotted within 2 weeks and a mean blood flow of 849 mL/min in synthetic grafts that remained patent. The expense and interobserver variability of Doppler blood-flow measurements have precluded its widespread use. In addition, Doppler measurements cannot be performed during the hemodialysis treatment because the needles prevent proper measurement. Magnetic resonance provides accurate measurements of access flow but is expensive (116).

Access blood flow may also be measured by ultrasound dilution, conductance dilution, or thermal dilution. A detailed description of the ultrasound dilution technique (117,118) is beyond the scope of this chapter. In brief, the hemodialysis blood lines are reversed. The blood pump is set at a rate of 300 mL/min and ultrafiltration is turned off. A bolus of isotonic saline is then injected into the venous port. Because the velocity of ultrasound in blood is determined primarily by the blood protein concentration, the isotonic saline will dilute blood protein and change the sound velocity in proportion to the concentration of injected saline in the blood. An ultrasound flow sensor on the arterial line measures blood flow in the tubing by a transit-time method and simultaneously detects saline dilution of the blood by measuring the velocity of an ultrasound beam. These measurements permit calculation of access blood flow. This technique yields accurate measurements and may be performed during the hemodialysis treatment.

A recent study from our institution demonstrated the utility of surveillance of access blood flow by the ultrasound dilution technique (119). Access blood flow measurements were performed monthly. If access blood flow was less than 600 mL/min or if access blood flow fell by 20% and was less than 1,000 mL/min, fistulography was performed. All patients who agreed to fistulography were found to have significant access stenoses. PTA increased access flow by 20% in 80% of the patients. The thrombosis rate for patients in this study was lower than that for historical controls. Of the 10 episodes of thrombosis that occurred during the study period, eight occurred in patients who did not keep appointments for fistulography or who refused surgical revision after unsuccessful PTA. We are hopeful that ultrasound dilution technology will be incorporated into hemodialysis machines and that serial measurements of access blood flow using the ultrasound dilution method will supplant other methods for the prospective detection of access stenoses.

Other Indicators

An unexplained decrease in the amount of hemodialysis delivered may signal the presence of venous stenosis. A very low arterial prepump pressure that prevents adequate extracorporeal blood flow should lead one to suspect arterial inflow stenosis.

Treatment of Venous Stenoses and Fistula Thrombosis

PTA is effective for the treatment of venous stenoses of both native and synthetic fistulas. Dilatation of *hemodynamically significant* venous stenoses (stenoses accompanied by elevated venous dialysis pressure, decreased access blood flow, elevated access recirculation, unexplained decline in delivered *Kt/V*, or physical evidence of stenosis) improves access function and prolongs access survival (60,63,96,97). The importance of prospective detection of venous stenosis cannot be overemphasized; patency rates are far higher for stenotic accesses angioplastied before thrombosis than for accesses angioplastied at the time of thrombolysis (60,120–122). Angioplasty is well tolerated by patients; hospitalization is not required, and hemodialysis may be performed immediately after the procedure. Venous stenoses may also be corrected by surgical revision. This approach, however, requires hospitalization and, by extending the fistula up the arm, sacrifices a segment of vein and eliminates a potential vas-

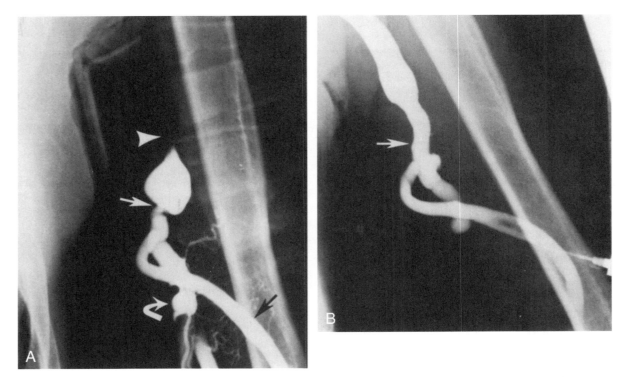

FIG. 4.7. Stenosis at vein-graft anastomosis **(A)** before and **(B)** after percutaneous transluminal angioplasty. (From Schwab SJ, et al. Transluminal angioplasty of venous stenoses in polytetrafluoroethylene vascular access grafts. *Kidney Int* 1987;32:395–398, with permission.)

cular access site. Studies comparing PTA with surgical revision have yielded conflicting results (123,124), and one approach cannot be recommended over the other.

PTA is effective for the treatment of vein-graft anastomotic lesions (Fig. 4.7), proximal vein lesions, central vein lesions (Fig. 4.8), and intragraft lesions. In addition, PTA may correct multiple venous stenoses, long (6- to 40-cm) venous stenoses, and complete venous occlusions (64). Initial technical success is achieved in 82% to 94% of cases. In a large and carefully studied series, a successful treatment was defined as one that maintained graft patency and that did not need to be repeated; success rates (unassisted patency rates) were 61% at 6 months and 38% at 1 year (64). Success rates for repeat treatments were no different than success rates for initial treatments. Other investigators have achieved similar results (60,63, 125–130).

Self-expandable endovascular stents, placed percutaneously, have been used in conjunction with PTA for the treatment of venous stenoses. A randomized trial comparing PTA with PTA plus endovascular stent placement for the treatment of vein-graft anastomotic lesions demonstrated that endovascular stent placement offered no advantage (131). The use of stents should be reserved for the treatment of elastic stenoses. A study performed at our institution examined the use of stents in the treatment of central venous stenoses (132). Endovascular stent placement was found to delay recurrences of elastic stenoses—lesions that readily compress on inflation of the balloon but readily

expand on its deflation. Elastic lesions account for roughly 20% of central lesions. Stents were not helpful in the treatment of nonelastic lesions. Endovascular stent placement should be reserved for the treatment of elastic lesions of the central veins and for the treatment of recurrent central vein stenoses. Self-eluting stents, such as those recently tested in coronary arteries, have not yet been tested in venous stenoses. In theory, they hold great promise because they may inhibit the hyperplasia that follows stent deployment.

Once thrombosis occurs, surgical thrombectomy, pharmacomechanical thrombolysis, or mechanical thrombolysis may be employed. No matter which technique is performed, correction of the venous stenosis should be performed to maintain access patency. Palder et al. (31) demonstrated that surgical thrombectomy combined with bypass of the venous stenosis (Fig. 4.9) produced significantly longer patency than did simple thrombectomy or patch angioplasty (31). It has recently been reported that surgical thrombectomy coupled with PTA is as effective as surgical thrombectomy coupled with surgical revision (133). Although surgical thrombectomy, pharmacomechanical thrombolysis, or mechanical thrombolysis are good options for thrombosed synthetic grafts, these approaches are not very good for the treatment of thrombosed primary fistulas (134). Nevertheless, they may be attempted.

In pharmacomechanical thrombolysis (pulse-spray thrombolysis) (121,135), angiography is performed to determine

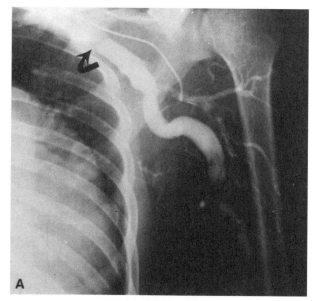

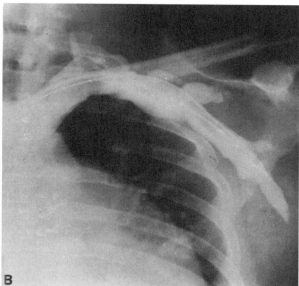

FIG. 4.8. Subclavian vein stenosis **(A)** before and **(B)** after percutaneous transluminal angioplasty. (From Schwab SJ, et al. Hemodialysis-associated subclavian vein stenosis. *Kidney Int* 1988;33:1156–1159, with permission.)

the extent of the clot and to visualize the graft and draining veins. Two catheters with closely spaced side holes are inserted into the midportion of the graft in a crossed manner (Fig. 4.10). A thrombolytic agent is "sprayed" into the clot under high pressure, and thrombolysis is achieved by both pharmacologic and mechanical means. An angioplasty balloon is then used to macerate residual clots and to dilate the venous stenosis.

The technique of mechanical thrombolysis (121) is similar to that of pharmacomechanical thrombolysis, but a thrombolytic

agent is not used. Saline is injected through a pulse-spray catheter to macerate the clot. An angioplasty balloon is used to further macerate the clot and dilate the venous stenosis. An embolectomy catheter is used to remove the arterial plug, and a saline flush is used to clear any residual clot.

These techniques may be performed in 1 to 2 hours, and the graft may be used immediately for dialysis. Comparative studies have demonstrated that these techniques are equally effective (136–138); both techniques yield excellent initial success rates and 90-day unassisted patency rates of roughly 30% to 48% (121,135–138). Surgical thrombectomy and revision may yield a similar patency rate (139,140), but surgical treatment generally entails delays, hospitalization, and extension of the access up the extremity.

One approach cannot be recommended over the others. Instead, the decision as to whether an individual patient should be treated by surgical thrombectomy or by a nonsurgical technique should be guided by the expertise of the treating institution's vascular surgeons and vascular radiologists.

Other Methods for the Prevention of Access Thrombosis

Two studies have reported that the antiplatelet agent ticlopidine reduces thrombosis rates of primary arteriovenous fistulas in the first postoperative month (141,142). A prospective, randomized trial suggested that dipyridamole decreases the thrombosis rate in patients with new PTFE grafts but that aspirin does not (143). Neither agent was found to be beneficial in patients with previously thrombosed grafts. Fish oil, by inhibiting cyclooxygenase or preventing intimal hyperplasia, may prove to be useful. In a small randomized study, fish oil at a dose of 4,000 mg daily was found to increase the patency rate for synthetic grafts (144). Angiotensin-converting enzyme (ACE) inhibitors may also hold promise. In animal models, angiotensin II induces smooth muscle proliferation, and ACE inhibitors prevent myointimal proliferation. In a retrospective analysis of synthetic graft survival, it was found that ACE inhibitor therapy was associated with a higher access survival rate (145). Large randomized controlled trials are being planned to assess the efficacy of clopidogrel in maintaining primary fistula patency and to assess the efficacy of dipyridamole/aspirin in maintaining graft patency.

SUMMARY

Double-lumen central venous catheters are the preferred form of vascular access for acute hemodialysis. Insertion complications become less likely as the operator gains experience. Several measures may be undertaken that will reduce the likelihood of catheter-related infection. Catheter thrombosis remains a major problem but may be managed by instillation of human tissue plasminogen activator into the catheter lumens or by replacement of the catheter over a guidewire. Because of the association of subclavian vein catheterization

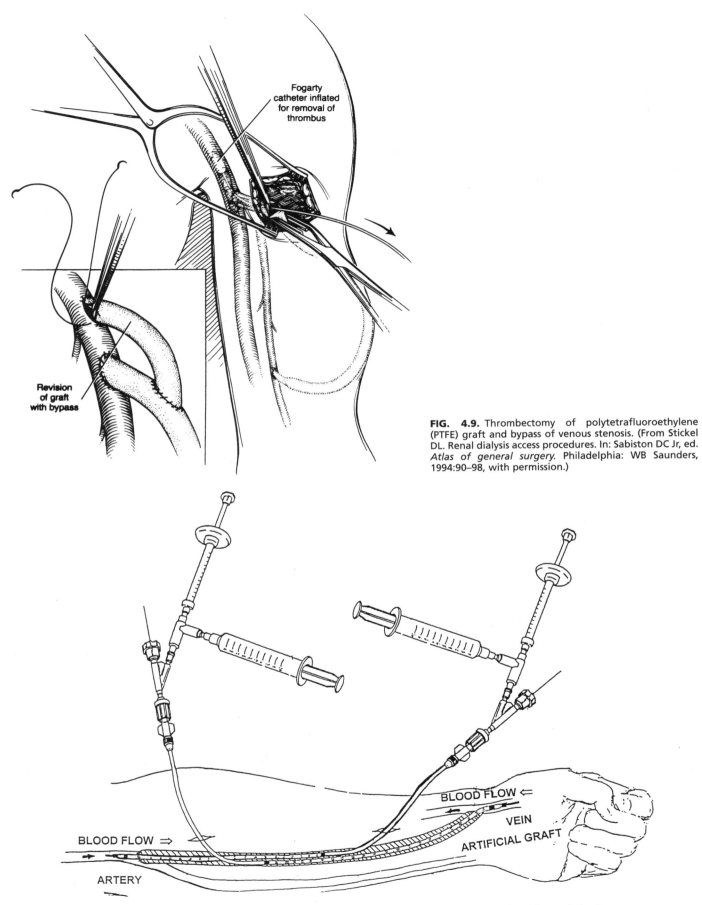

FIG. 4.9. Thrombectomy of polytetrafluoroethylene (PTFE) graft and bypass of venous stenosis. (From Stickel DL. Renal dialysis access procedures. In: Sabiston DC Jr, ed. *Atlas of general surgery.* Philadelphia: WB Saunders, 1994:90–98, with permission.)

FIG. 4.10. Pulse-spray thrombolysis. (From AngioDynamics Inc., Glens Falls, New York, with permission.)

with subsequent development of subclavian vein stenosis, subclavian vein catheters should be avoided in those patients in whom fistula placement is anticipated.

Because primary arteriovenous fistulas are most likely to provide long-term complication-free access, they remain the preferred form of chronic vascular access. Careful planning months before the anticipated need for hemodialysis will maximize the chance for successful primary arteriovenous fistula creation. If a native fistula cannot be created, a PTFE graft should be placed. The use of cuffed catheters as permanent vascular access is discouraged. Once permanent vascular access is established, maintenance of its patency presents a continual challenge to the nephrologist, dialysis staff, vascular surgeon, and vascular radiologist.

Thrombosis is the leading cause of vascular access loss, and venous stenoses are the leading cause of vascular access thrombosis. Prospective detection and correction of venous stenoses will prolong access patency. Several methods for the prospective detection of venous stenoses are employed today, but it is anticipated that serial, on-line measurement of access blood flow by hemodialysis machines will one day be the standard method.

REFERENCES

1. Quinton W, et al. Cannulation of blood vessels for prolonged hemodialysis. *ASAIO Trans* 1960;6:104.
2. Gravenstein N, et al. In vitro evaluation of relative perforating potential of central venous catheters. *J Clin Monit* 1991;7:1–6.
3. Cohen AM, et al. Simplified technique for placement of long-term central venous silicone catheters. *Surg Gynecol Obstet* 1982;154:721–724.
4. Kelber J, et al. Factors affecting the delivery of high-efficiency dialysis using temporary vascular access. *Am J Kidney Dis* 1993;22:24–29.
5. Sznajder JI, et al. Central vein catheterization: failure and complication rates by three percutaneous approaches. *Arch Intern Med* 1986;146:259–261.
6. Stuart RK, et al. Incidence of arrhythmia with central venous catheter insertion and exchange. *JPEN* 1990;14:152–155.
7. Brother TE, et al. Experience with subcutaneous infusion ports in three hundred patients. *Surg Gynecol Obstet* 1988;166:295–301.
8. Goldfarb G, et al. Percutaneous cannulation of the internal jugular vein in patients with coagulopathies: an experience based on 1,000 attempts. *Anesthesiology* 1982;56:321–323.
9. Vanholder R, et al. Morbidity and mortality of central venous catheter hemodialysis: a review of 10 years' experience. *Nephron* 1987;47:274–279.
10. Vanherweghem JL, et al. Complications related to subclavian catheters for hemodialysis. *Am J Nephrol* 1986;6:339–345.
11. Uldall PR. Temporary vascular access for hemodialysis. In: Nissenson AR, et al., eds. *Dialysis therapy*, 2nd ed. Philadelphia: Hanley and Belfus, 1993:5–10.
12. Briscoe CE, et al. Extensive neurological damage after cannulation of the internal jugular vein. *BMJ* 1984;288:1195–1196.
13. Blitt CD, et al. An unusual complication of percutaneous internal jugular vein cannulation: puncture of an endotracheal cuff. *Anesthesiology* 1974;40:306–307.
14. Butsch JL, et al. Bilateral vocal cord paralysis: a complication of percutaneous cannulation of the internal jugular vein. *Arch Surg* 1976;111:828–829.
15. Hartle E, et al. Ultrasound guided cannulation of the femoral vein for acute hemodialysis access. *J Am Soc Nephrol* 1993;4:352(abst).
16. Cheesbrough JS, et al. A prospective study of the mechanisms of infection associated with hemodialysis catheters. *J Infect Dis* 1986;154:579–589.
17. Maki DG, et al. A semiquantitative culture method for identifying intravenous-catheter–related infection. *N Engl J Med* 1977;296:1305–1309.
18. Oliver MJ, et al. Risk of bacteremia from temporary hemodialysis catheters by site of insertion and duration of use: a prospective study. *Kidney Int* 2000;58:2543–2545.
19. Maki DG, et al. Prospective randomised trial of povidone-iodine, alcohol, and chlorohexidine for prevention of infection associated with central venous and arterial catheters. *Lancet* 1991;338:339–343.
20. Levin A, et al. Prevention of hemodialysis subclavian vein catheter infection by topical povidone-iodine. *Kidney Int* 1991;40:934–938.
21. Conly JM, et al. A prospective, randomized study comparing transparent and dry gauze dressings for central venous catheters. *J Infect Dis* 1989;159:310–319.
22. Ponec D, et al. Recombinant tissue plasminogen activator (alteplase) for restoration of flow in occluded central venous access devices—a double-blind placebo-controlled trial: the cardiovascular thrombolytic to open occluded lines (COOL) efficacy trial. *J Vasc Interv Radiol* 2001;12:951–955.
23. Brismar B, et al. Diagnosis of thrombosis by catheter phlebography after prolonged central venous catheterization. *Ann Surg* 1981;194:779–783.
24. Davis D, et al. Subclavian venous stenosis: a complication of subclavian dialysis. *JAMA* 1984;252:3404–3406.
25. Fant GF, et al. Late vascular complications of the subclavian dialysis catheter. *Am J Kidney Dis* 1986;3:225–228.
26. Barrett N, et al. Subclavian stenosis: a major complication of subclavian dialysis catheters. *Nephrol Dial Transplant* 1988;3:423–425.
27. Cimochowski GE, et al. Superiority of the internal jugular over the subclavian access for temporary dialysis. *Nephron* 1990;54:154–161.
28. Schillinger F, et al. Post catheterisation vein stenosis in haemodialysis: comparative angiographic study of 50 subclavian and 50 internal jugular accesses. *Nephrol Dial Transplant* 1991;6:722–724.
29. Schwab SJ, et al. Hemodialysis associated subclavian vein stenosis. *Kidney Int* 1988;33:1156–1159.
30. Brescia MJ, et al. Chronic hemodialysis using venipuncture and a surgically created arteriovenous fistula. *N Engl J Med* 1966;275:1089–1092.
31. Palder SB, et al. Vascular access for hemodialysis: patency rates and results of revision. *Ann Surg* 1985;202:235–239.
32. Winsett OE, et al. Complications of vascular access for hemodialysis. *South Med J* 1985;78:513–517.
33. DeMeester J, et al. Factors affecting catheter and technique survival in permanent silicone single lumen dialysis catheters. *J Am Soc Nephrol* 1992;3:361(abst).
34. Moss AH, et al. Use of a silicone dual lumen catheter with a Dacron cuff as a long-term vascular access for hemodialysis patients. *Am J Kidney Dis* 1990;16:211–215.
35. Suhocki PV, et al. Silastic cuffed catheters for hemodialysis vascular access: thrombolytic and mechanical correction of malfunction. *Am J Kidney Dis* 1996;28:379–386.
36. Beathard GA, et al. Initial clinical results with the LifeSite hemodialysis access system. *Kidney Int* 2000;58:2221–2227.
37. Levin NW, et al. Initial results of a new access device for hemodialysis. *Kidney Int* 1998;54:1739–1745.
38. Schwab SJ, et al. Multicenter clinical trial results with the LifeSite hemodialysis access system. *Kidney Int* 2002;62:1026–1033.
39. Canaud B, et al. Dialock: a new vascular access device for extracorporeal renal replacement therapy—preliminary clinical results. *Nephrol Dial Transplant* 1999;14:692–698.
40. Stone WJ, et al. Therapeutic options in the management of end-stage renal disease. In: Jacobson HR, et al., eds. *The principles and practice of nephrology.* Philadelphia: BC Decker, 1991:736–739.
41. NKF-K/DOQI Clinical practice guidelines for vascular access. New York: National Kidney Foundation, 2001:24–27.
42. Oliver MJ, et al. Comparison of transposed brachiobasilic fistulas to upper arm grafts and brachiocephalic fistulas. *Kidney Int* 2001;60:1532–1539.
43. Anderson CB, et al. Blood flow measurements in arteriovenous dialysis fistulas. *Surgery* 1977;81:459–461.
44. Moran MR, et al. Flow of dialysis fistulas. *Nephron* 1985;40:63–66.

45. Burdick JF, et al. Experience with Dacron graft arteriovenous fistulas for dialysis access. *Ann Surg* 1978;187:262–266.
46. Rittgers SE, et al. Noninvasive blood flow measurement in expanded polytetrafluoroethylene grafts for hemodialysis access. *J Vasc Surg* 1986;3:635–642.
47. Shackleton CR, et al. Predicting failure in polytetrafluoroethylene vascular access grafts for hemodialysis: a pilot study. *Can J Surg* 1987; 30:442–444.
48. Strauch BS, et al. Forecasting thrombosis of vascular access with Doppler color flow imaging. *Am J Kidney Dis* 1992;19:554–557.
49. Depner TA, et al. Longevity of peripheral A-V grafts and fistulae for hemodialysis is related to access blood flow. *J Am Soc Nephrol* 1996;7: 1405(abst).
50. Kherlakian GM, et al. Comparison of autogenous fistula versus expanded polytetrafluoroethylene graft fistula for angioaccess in hemodialysis. *Am J Surg* 1986;152:238–243.
51. Munda R, et al. Polytetrafluoroethylene graft survival in hemodialysis. *JAMA* 1983;249:219–222.
52. Tordoir JHM, et al. Long-term follow-up of the polytetrafluoroethylene (PTFE) prosthesis as an arteriovenous fistula for haemodialysis. *Eur J Vasc Surg* 1987;2:3–7.
53. Raju S. PTFE grafts for hemodialysis access: techniques for insertion and management of complications. *Ann Surg* 1987;206:666–673.
54. Tellis VA, et al. Expanded polytetrafluoroethylene graft fistula for chronic hemodialysis. *Ann Surg* 1979;189:101–105.
55. Shusterman NH, et al. Successful use of double-lumen, silicone rubber catheters for permanent hemodialysis access. *Kidney Int* 1989;35: 837–890.
56. Gibson SP, et al. Five years experience with Quinton Permcath for vascular access. *Nephrol Dial Transplant* 1991;6:269–274.
57. Lund GB, et al. Outcome of tunneled hemodialysis catheters placed by radiologists. *Radiology* 1996;198:467–472.
58. Schwab SJ. Hemodialysis vascular access. In: Jacobson HR, et al., eds. *The principles and practice of nephrology.* Philadelphia: BC Decker, 1991:766–772.
59. Etheredge EE, et al. Salvage operations for malfunctioning polytetrafluoroethylene hemodialysis access grafts. *Surgery* 1983;94:464–470.
60. Beathard GA. Percutaneous angioplasty for the treatment of venous stenosis: a nephrologist's view. *Semin Dial* 1995;8:166–170.
61. Beathard GA. Percutaneous therapy of vascular access dysfunction: optimal management of access stenosis and thrombosis. *Semin Dial* 1994;7:165–167.
62. Bone GE, et al. Management of dialysis fistula thrombosis. *Am J Surg* 1979;138:901–906.
63. Schwab SJ, et al. Prevention of hemodialysis fistula thrombosis: early detection of venous stenoses. *Kidney Int* 1989;36:707–711.
64. Beathard GA. Percutaneous transvenous angioplasty in the treatment of vascular access stenosis. *Kidney Int* 1992;42:1390–1397.
65. Carty GA, et al. Mid-graft stenosis in expanded polytetrafluoroethylene hemodialysis conduits. *Dial Transplant* 1990;19:486–489.
66. NKF-K/DOQI clinical practice guidelines for vascular access. New York: National Kidney Foundation, 2001:70.
67. Bhat DJ, et al. Management of sepsis involving expanded polytetrafluoroethylene grafts for hemodialysis access. *Surgery* 1980;87: 445–450.
68. Keane WF, et al. Incidence and type of infections occurring in 445 chronic hemodialysis patients. *ASAIO Trans* 1977;23:41–46.
69. Dobkin JF, et al. Septicemia in patients on chronic hemodialysis. *Ann Intern Med* 1987;88:28–33.
70. Higgins RM. Infections in a renal unit. *QJM* 1989;70:41–51.
71. Kaplowitz LG, et al. A prospective study of infections in hemodialysis patients: patient hygiene and other risk factors for infection. *Infect Control Hosp Epidemiol* 1988;9:534–541.
72. O'Brien TF. Infection in dialysis and transplant patients. In: Tilney NL, et al., eds. *Surgical care of the patient with renal failure.* Philadelphia: WB Saunders, 1982:67–97.
73. Morgan AP, et al. Femoral triangle sepsis in dialysis patients. *Ann Surg* 1980;191:460–464.
74. NKF-K/DOQI clinical practice guidelines for vascular access. New York: National Kidney Foundation, 2001:69.
75. Marr KA, et al. Catheter-related bacteremia and outcome of attempted catheter salvage in patients undergoing hemodialysis. *Ann Intern Med* 1997;127:275–280.
76. Kovalik EC, et al. A clustering of epidural abscesses in chronic hemodialysis patients: risks of salvaging access catheters in cases of infection. *J Am Soc Nephrol* 1996;7:2264–2267.
77. Berkoben M, et al. A hemodialysis patient with excruciating back pain. *Semin Dial* 1996;9:286–288.
78. Robinson DL, et al. Bacterial endocarditis in hemodialysis patients. *Am J Kidney Dis* 1997;30:521–524.
79. Rosen AB, et al. Cost-effectiveness of transesophageal echocardiography to determine the duration of therapy for intravascular catheter-associated *Staphylococcus aureus* bacteremia. *Ann Intern Med* 1999; 130:810–820.
80. Shaffer D. Catheter-related sepsis complicating long-term, tunneled central venous dialysis catheters: management by guidewire exchange. *Am J Kidney Dis* 1995;25:593–596.
81. Beathard GA. Management of bacteremia associated with tunneled-cuffed hemodialysis catheters. *J Am Soc Nephrol* 1999;10:1045–1049.
82. NKF-K/DOQI clinical practice guidelines for vascular access. New York: National Kidney Foundation, 2001:71–72.
83. Krishnasami Z, et al. Management of hemodialysis catheter-related bacteremia with an adjunctive antibiotic lock solution. *Kidney Int* 2002;61:1136–1142.
84. Barth RH, et al. Use of vancomycin in high-flux hemodialysis: experience with 130 courses of therapy. *Kidney Int* 1996;50:929–936.
85. Marx MA, et al. Cefazolin as empiric therapy in hemodialysis-related infections: efficacy and blood concentrations. *Am J Kidney Dis* 1998; 32:410–414.
86. Smith TL, et al. Emergence of vancomycin resistance in *Staphylococcus aureus.* *N Engl J Med* 1999;340:493–501.
87. Sieradzki K, et al. The development of vancomycin resistance in a patient with methicillin-resistant *Staphylococcus aureus* infection. *N Engl J Med* 1999;340:517–523.
88. Anderson CB, et al. Cardiac failure and upper extremity arteriovenous dialysis fistulas. *Arch Intern Med* 1976;136:292–297.
89. West JC, et al. Arterial insufficiency in hemodialysis access procedures: correction by "banding" technique. *Trans Proc* 1991;23: 1838–1840.
90. Rivers SP, et al. Correction of steal syndrome secondary to hemodialysis access fistulas: a simplified quantitative technique. *Surgery* 1992; 112:593–597.
91. Kirkman RL. Technique for flow reduction in dialysis access fistulas. *Surg Gynecol Obstet* 1991;172:231–233.
92. Tawa NE, et al. Angioaccess in the renal failure patient. In: Maher JF, ed. *Replacement of renal function by dialysis,* 3rd ed. Boston: Kluwer Academic, 1989:218–228.
93. Bell PRF, et al. Vascular access for hemodialysis. In: Nissenson AR, et al., eds. *Clinical dialysis,* 2nd ed. Norwalk, CT: Appleton & Lange, 1990:26–44.
94. NKF-K/DOQI clinical practice guidelines for vascular access. New York: National Kidney Foundation, 2001:74.
95. NKF-K/DOQI clinical practice guidelines for vascular access. New York: National Kidney Foundation, 2001:36–45.
96. Besarab A, et al. Utility of intra-access pressure monitoring in detecting and correcting venous outlet stenoses prior to thrombosis. *Kidney Int* 1995;47:1364–1373.
97. Burger H, et al. Percutaneous transluminal angioplasty improves longevity in fistulae and shunts for hemodialysis. *Nephrol Dial Transplant* 1990;5:608–611.
98. Tordoir JHM, et al. The correlation between clinical and duplex ultrasound parameters and the development of complications in arterio venous fistulae for hemodialysis. *Eur J Vasc Surg* 1990;4:179–184.
99. Sands JJ, et al. Prolongation of hemodialysis access survival with elective revision. *Clin Nephrol* 1995;44:329–333.
100. Anderson CB, et al. Venous angiography and surgical management of subcutaneous hemodialysis fistulas. *Ann Surg* 1978;187:194–204.
101. Trerotola SO, et al. Screening for access graft malfunction: comparison of physical examination with US. *J Vasc Interv Radiol* 1996;7: 15–20.

102. NKF-K/DOQI clinical practice guidelines for vascular access. New York: National Kidney Foundation, 2001:41.

103. Safa AA, et al. Detection and treatment of dysfunctional hemodialysis access grafts: effects of a surveillance program on graft patency and the incidence of thrombosis. *Radiology* 1996;199:653–657.

104. NKF-K/DOQI clinical practice guidelines for vascular access. New York: National Kidney Foundation, 2001:39–40.

105. Sherman RA. The measurement of dialysis access recirculation. *Am J Kidney Dis* 1993;22:616–621.

106. Sherman RA. Recirculation revisited. *Semin Dial* 1991;4:221–223.

107. Depner TA, et al. High venous urea concentrations in the opposite arm: a consequence of hemodialysis-induced compartment disequilibrium. *ASAIO J* 1991;37:M141–M143.

108. Schneditz D, et al. Cardiopulmonary recirculation in dialysis—an under-recognized phenomenon. *ASAIO J* 1992;38:M194–M196.

109. Depner T, et al. Peripheral urea disequilibrium during hemodialysis is temperature-dependent. *J Am Soc Nephrol* 1991;2:321(abst).

110. NKF-K/DOQI clinical practice guidelines for vascular access. New York: National Kidney Foundation, 2001:48.

111. Besarab A, et al. The relationship of recirculation to access blood type. *Am J Kidney Dis* 1997;29:223–229.

112. Tattersall JE, et al. Haemodialysis recirculation detected by the three-sample method is an artefact. *Nephrol Dial Transplant* 1995;8:60–63.

113. Depner TA, et al. Hemodialysis access recirculation measured by ultra-sound dilution. *ASAIO J* 1995;41:M749–M753.

114. Windus DW, et al. Optimization of high-efficiency hemodialysis by detection and correction of fistula dysfunction. *Kidney Int* 1990;38:337–341.

115. Collins DM, et al. Fistula dysfunction: effect on rapid hemodialysis. *Kidney Int* 1992;41:1292–1296.

116. Oudenhoven LFIJ, et al. Magnetic resonance, a new method for measuring blood flow in hemodialysis fistulae. *Kidney Int* 1994;45:884–889.

117. Krivitsky NM. Theory and validation of access flow measurement by dilution technique during hemodialysis. *Kidney Int* 1995;48:244–250.

118. Depner TA, et al. Clinical measurement of blood flow in hemodialysis access fistulae and grafts by ultrasound dilution. *ASAIO J* 1995;41:M745–M749.

119. Schwab SJ, et al. Hemodialysis arteriovenous access: detection of stenosis and response to treatment by vascular access blood flow. *Kidney Int* 2001;59:358–362.

120. Katz SG, et al. The percutaneous treatment of angioaccess graft complications. *Am J Surg* 1995;170:238–242.

121. Beathard GA. The treatment of vascular access graft dysfunction: a nephrologist's view and experience. *Adv Ren Replace Ther* 1994;1:131–147.

122. Trerotola SO. Pulse-spray thrombolysis of hemodialysis grafts: not the final word. *AJR* 1995;164:1501–1503.

123. Brooks JL, et al. Transluminal angioplasty versus surgical repair for stenosis of hemodialysis grafts: a randomized study. *Am J Surg* 1987;153:530–531.

124. Dapunt O, et al. Transluminal angioplasty versus conventional operation in the treatment of hemodialysis fistula stenosis: results from a 5-year study. *Br J Surg* 1987;74:1004–1005.

125. Kanterman RY, et al. Dialysis access grafts: anatomic location of venous stenosis and results of angioplasty. *Radiology* 1995;195:135–139.

126. Glanz S, et al. The role of percutaneous angioplasty in the management of chronic hemodialysis fistulas. *Ann Surg* 1987;206:777–781.

127. Glanz S, et al. Dialysis access fistulas: treatment of stenoses by transluminal angioplasty. *Radiology* 1984;152:637–642.

128. Mori Y, et al. Stenotic lesions in vascular access: treatment with transluminal angioplasty using high-pressure balloons. *Intern Med* 1994;33:284–287.

129. Gmelin E, et al. Insufficient hemodialysis access fistulas: late results of treatment with percutaneous balloon angioplasty. *Radiology* 1989;171:657–660.

130. Turmel-Rodrigues L, et al. Insufficient dialysis shunts: improved long-term patency rates with close hemodynamic monitoring, repeated percutaneous balloon angioplasty, and stent placement. *Radiology* 1993;187:273–278.

131. Beathard GA. Gianturco self-expanding stent in the treatment of stenosis in dialysis access grafts. *Kidney Int* 1993;43:872–877.

132. Kovalik EC, et al. Correction of central venous stenoses: use of angioplasty and vascular Wallstents. *Kidney Int* 1994;45:1171–1181.

133. Schwartz CI, et al. Thrombosed dialysis grafts: comparison of treatment with transluminal angioplasty and surgical revision. *Radiology* 1995;194:337–341.

134. NKF-K/DOQI clinical practice guidelines for vascular access. New York: National Kidney Foundation, 2001:66.

135. Valji K, et al. Pharmacomechanical thrombolysis and angioplasty in the management of clotted hemodialysis grafts: early and late clinical results. *Radiology* 1991;178:243–247.

136. Beathard GA. Mechanical versus pharmacomechanical thrombolysis for the treatment of thrombosed dialysis access grafts. *Kidney Int* 1994;45:1401–1406.

137. Trerotola SO, et al. Thrombosed dialysis access grafts: percutaneous mechanical declotting without urokinase. *Radiology* 1995;191:721–726.

138. Middlebrook MR, et al. Thrombosed hemodialysis grafts: percutaneous mechanical balloon declotting versus thrombolysis. *Radiology* 1995;196:73–77.

139. Summers S, et al. Urokinase therapy for thrombosed hemodialysis access grafts. *Surg Gynecol Obstet* 1993;176:534–538.

140. Beathard GA. Thrombolysis versus surgery for the treatment of thrombosed dialysis access grafts. *J Am Soc Nephrol* 1995;6:1619–1624.

141. Grontoft K, et al. Thromboprophylactic effect of ticlopidine in arteriovenous fistulas for hemodialysis. *Scand J Urol Nephrol* 1985;19:55–57.

142. Fiskerstrand CE, et al. Double-blind randomized trial of the effect of ticlopidine in arteriovenous fistulas for hemodialysis. *Artif Organs* 1985;9:61–63.

143. Sreedhara R, et al. Antiplatelet therapy in graft thrombosis: results of a prospective randomized double blind study. *Kidney Int* 1994;45:1477–1483.

144. Schmitz PG, et al. Prophylaxis of hemodialysis graft thrombosis with fish oil: double-blind, randomized, prospective trial. *J Am Soc Nephrol* 2002;13:184–190.

145. Gradzki R, et al. Use of ACE inhibitors is associated with prolonged survival of arteriovenous grafts. *Am J Kidney Dis* 2001;38:1240–1244.

5

RECIRCULATION IN THE HEMODIALYSIS ACCESS

RICHARD A. SHERMAN AND TOROS KAPOIAN

For dialysis to be optimally efficient, blood entering the dialyzer should contain urea and other uremic solutes in concentrations similar to those of the body as a whole. However, solute concentrations in dialyzer inflow blood are commonly lower than those in systemic blood, a difference that has usually been attributed to dialyzed blood flowing retrograde from the "venous" needle to the "arterial" needle. When this blood is circulated again through the dialyzer *recirculation* is said to be present. Recirculation most often occurs when vascular access blood flow is less than dialyzer blood flow. However, differences in solute concentration between "systemic" and dialyzer inflow blood are not usually due to recirculation.

EFFECT OF RECIRCULATION ON DIALYSIS EFFICIENCY

Dialysis of recirculated blood will reduce the overall efficiency of the hemodialysis treatment. The extent of the reduction in dialytic efficiency depends on the fractional clearance by the dialyzer of the solute in question. For a poorly cleared, large-molecular-weight uremic toxin, the venous-line (postdialyzer) concentration of this solute differs little from the arterial-line (predialyzer) concentration. Recirculation will result in little loss of dialytic efficiency for such a solute because dialysis of recirculated venous-line blood is almost as efficient as dialysis of arterial-line blood. However, for a small-molecular-weight solute (e.g., urea) with a high dialytic fractional clearance (i.e., a high ratio of dialytic clearance to dialyzer blood flow), dialysis of recirculated blood is much less efficient and has a much greater impact on the solute's effective clearance.

The extent to which recirculation reduces effective dialytic clearance can be approximated by multiplying the percentage recirculation by the percentage extraction of the solute by the dialyzer. This method is reasonably accurate at other than very high levels of recirculation. The effect of recirculation on dialytic efficiency is illustrated in the following examples.

EXAMPLE 1

A recirculation of 25% is found in a patient treated using a dialyzer that clears urea at 210 mL/min and vitamin B_{12} at 42 mL/min with a blood flow of 300 mL/min. What is the approximate loss of dialytic efficiency for these solutes?

ANSWER

The percentage extractions of urea and vitamin B_{12} are 70% (210 mL/min divided by 300 mL/min) and 14% (42 mL/min divided by 300 mL/min), respectively. The approximate reduction in effective urea clearance is 25% × 70%, or 17.5%; effective vitamin B_{12} clearance is reduced by 25% × 14%, or 3.5%.

The reduction in effective solute clearance is actually greater than that indicated by this approximation. The simplified approach does not take into account the blood that is making multiple short circuits through the dialyzer, reducing solute concentrations in the arterial line to values below those calculated. For example, with a 25% recirculation, 6.25% of the recirculated blood (25% of 25%) is on its second circuit and 1.6% is on its third circuit through the dialyzer. The actual fractional reduction in clearance is

$$R/(R + ((1 - R)/Fe)$$

where R is the fraction of recirculated blood, and Fe is the fractional solute extraction (1).

EXAMPLE 2

What is the actual reduction in urea clearance for the patient described in Example 1?

ANSWER

$$R/(R + ((1 - R)/Fe) = 0.25$$

$$0.25/(0.25 + ((1 - 0.25)/0.7) = 0.19$$

Thus, the actual reduction in urea clearance with a 25% recirculation rate (and 70% extraction of urea by the dialyzer) is 19% (rather than 17.5%).

PATHOPHYSIOLOGY OF RECIRCULATION

Recirculation will occur when access blood flow is insufficient to meet the demands of the blood pump, resulting in retrograde flow from the venous to the arterial needle. Because blood flow in a well-functioning access typically exceeds 1,000 mL/min (2,3) and dialyzer blood flow typically ranges from 350 to 500 mL/min, the presence of recirculation usually indicates severe impairment of access blood flow. In some cases, recirculation results from the combination of closely placed needles and turbulent flow at the venous needle site facilitating uptake of venous blood flow at the arterial needle. However, this is only seen when access blood flow is marginal (i.e., exceeding dialyzer blood flow by <150 mL/min) (4). Recirculation may also occur as a result of unusual access anatomy (5) or, more commonly, misdirected or reversed needles, typically a result of insufficient information about access anatomy (Table 5.1).

Until recent years, recirculation was not measured accurately and was routinely overestimated. This problem obscured recognition of the fact that recirculation is rare (4,6–8) and has prevented clinicians from understanding its pathophysiology. Recirculation does not occur in a properly cannulated access unless the access blood-flow rate is less than the dialyzer blood-flow rate (9). The converse statement, recirculation must occur when dialyzer blood flow exceeds access blood flow, is usually but not always the case. An important exception is when a stenotic lesion between the needles limits access flow while also preventing recirculation (Table 5.2).

The relationship that has been noted between recirculation rates and dialyzer blood flow is largely an artifactual one (10–12) and exists only in patients whose access blood-flow rates are less than their dialyzer blood-flow rates (9,13). Most patients do not have such low blood-flow rates. The observed relationship between measured recirculation (by the peripheral-vein technique) and dialyzer blood flow (13) was based in part on the accentuation in arteriovenous (AV) urea disequilibrium accompanying the more efficient dialysis associated with the higher blood flow.

When recirculation is truly present, it is always of concern. Its presence indicates a problem with dialysis delivery as well as with access blood flow and/or needle placement.

TABLE 5.1. CAUSES OF AN ELEVATED ACCESS RECIRCULATION RATE

Arteriovenous Access
Access blood-flow rate less than dialyzer blood-flow rate
Reversed needle placement
Excessively close needle placement with marginal access blood flow
Central Venous Access
Low blood flow in accessed vein
Reversed blood lines
Single-needle access
Catheter dysfunction (because of fibrin sheath?)
Transient retrograde blood flow in SVC?

SVC, superior vena cava.

TABLE 5.2. RELATIONSHIP BETWEEN RECIRCULATION AND BLOOD-FLOW RATE

Recirculation Present
Implication: ABFR < DBFR
Exceptions:
1. Error in measurement of recirculation
2. Arterial and venous needles reversed
3. Arterial and venous needles positioned closely and ABFR marginally greater (<150 mL/min) than DBFR
4. Single-needle dialysis
Recirculation Absent
Implication: ABFR > DBFR
Exceptions:
1. Error in measurement of recirculation
2. Stenotic lesion between needles
3. Venous needle in minor branch of native-vein fistula

ABFR, access blood flow rate; DBFR, dialyzer blood flow rate.

MEASUREMENT OF RECIRCULATION

A number of tests and maneuvers can detect the presence of recirculation. Recirculation is diagnosed when venous-line blood is demonstrated to be present in the dialyzer inflow (arterial) line. Most commonly, the concentration of a dialyzable solute (usually urea) is examined in arterial-line blood and compared with that in systemic blood; when the systemic value exceeds the arterial-line value it is assumed that venous-line blood is recirculating and reducing arterial-line blood urea nitrogen (BUN). However, as will be discussed later, this assumption is often incorrect—dramatically so when a peripheral vein is the source for the systemic sample and to a lesser extent with most other urea-based tests. The accuracy of these tests largely depends on the degree to which the chosen systemic sample truly reflects recirculation-free, dialyzer inflow blood. The revised slow-stop flow urea method, discussed later, uses a systemic sample that meets this criterion.

The fractional recirculation is calculated as follows.

$$R = (C_s - C_a)/(C_s - C_v)$$

where C_s, C_a, C_v are the concentrations (C) of the measured solute (urea) in systemic (s), arterial-line (a), and venous-line (v) blood. An example of the application of this formula is listed in the following.

EXAMPLE 3

The BUN in arterial-line blood is 70 mg/dL, venous-line blood, 25 mg/dL, and systemic blood 90 mg/dL. What fraction of dialyzer blood flow is recirculated from the venous line?

ANSWER

$$R = (C_s - C_a)/(C_s - C_v)$$
$$C_s = 90 \text{ mg/dL}$$
$$C_a = 70 \text{ mg/dL}$$
$$C_v = 25 \text{ mg/dL}$$
$$R = (90 - 70)/(90 - 25) = 20/65 = 0.31 \text{ (or 31\%)}$$

More sophisticated techniques for measuring recirculation are coming into clinical use. Techniques that are being developed or have recently become available alter venous-line blood in some way and detect that alteration using a sensor in the arterial line. The techniques use one of the following approaches:

■ Venous blood is cooled, and recirculation is determined by measuring the temperature drop in arterial-line blood (14).
■ Saline is injected in the venous line, with recirculation determined by changes in light transmission (15) or ultrasound dilution (16) in the arterial line.
■ Hypertonic saline is injected into the venous line, and recirculation is detected by changes in electrical conductivity in the arterial line (6).

These methods of measuring recirculation are generally more accurate than urea-based methods. Recirculation may also be measured by using glucose- (17), hematocrit- (18), and potassium- (19) based techniques.

Another new approach to the recognition of recirculation is Doppler ultrasound detection of retrograde flow within the access during dialysis. Of particular interest is the observation that transient, cyclical retrograde flow will be seen without recirculation in patients with low (e.g., <650 mL/min) but not severely reduced (e.g., less than dialyzer blood-flow rate) access blood flows (20). This cyclical pattern reflects cardiac cycle related flow variations.

The increasing sophistication of tests for recirculation should not obscure the value of a bedside assessment for recirculation using the arterial and venous pressure monitors on the dialysis machine (21–23). When recirculation is present, all flow between the needles is retrograde (i.e., from the venous to the arterial needle). Interruption of this retrograde flow by temporary access occlusion (using finger pressure) between the needles will sharply increase either venous pressure (when a venous stenosis is present) or the negative prepump "arterial" pressure (when an arterial stenosis is present). When recirculation is occurring due to reversed needle placement, this occlusion maneuver will immediately interrupt dialysis, with both the venous and negative arterial pressure rising sharply. When recirculation is absent and interneedle flow is from the arterial to the venous end of the access, occlusion tends to lower venous pressure (depending on the amount of "excess" flow) with little effect on arterial pressure.

Problems with the Peripheral-Vein Recirculation Test

The peripheral-vein recirculation test is no longer considered an appropriate means of assessing recirculation (24). The reason is that peripheral venous blood is not appropriate as a "systemic" sample to be compared with the "predialyzer" sample (C_a), which has an arterial source (25). Arterial and venous BUN values differ negligibly under normal circumstances, but they differ significantly during hemodialysis (26–28).

The basis for this AV disequilibrium can be understood by considering the means by which urea in the interstitial and intracellular spaces is cleared from the body during dialysis. The blood leaving the dialyzer has a BUN that is about 60% to 70% less

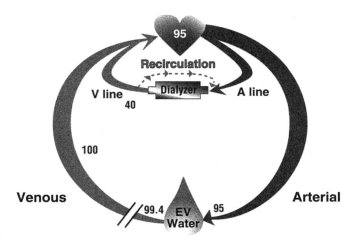

FIG. 5.1. A simplified sketch of the dialysis circuit with an arteriovenous (AV) access (inner loop) depicting local access recirculation and cardiopulmonary recirculation. (Blood flow through the AV access that does not go through the dialyzer is not shown.) To best follow the sequence, move clockwise from the breakpoint at the lower left. Dialyzed blood with a blood urea nitrogen (BUN) of 40 mg/dL is added to venous blood with a BUN of 100 mg/dL, resulting in a lower BUN in cardiac and arterial blood (95 mg/dL); thus, an AV urea difference is produced. The BUN rises from 95 mg/dL to almost 100 mg/dL after it passes through the capillaries where blood is "refilled" with urea. (From Sherman RA, et al. Recirculation, urea disequilibrium, and dialysis efficiency: peripheral arteriovenous versus central venovenous vascular access. *Am J Kidney Dis* 1997;29:479–489, with permission.)

than that of blood entering the dialyzer. This low urea blood enters the large veins and then the central veins where it reduces the urea concentration of blood returning to the heart from elsewhere in the body. The extent of the reduction in central vein (and, subsequently, arterial) urea depends on dialyzer extraction of urea and the dialyzer blood flow (urea clearance) as well as the cardiac output (29). The resultant differences in arterial and venous BUN—AV disequilibrium—can be viewed to be a result of dialyzed blood short-circuiting the systemic circulation (Fig. 5.1) in a manner analogous to recirculation in the access (30,31). Thus, it has also been termed cardiopulmonary recirculation (32,33). An example of this effect is provided in the following.

EXAMPLE 4

Early in dialysis the BUN in a peripheral vein is 100 mg/dL. What BUN might be expected in an artery of the same arm drawn simultaneously? Assume a cardiac output of 5 L/min, a dialyzer blood flow of 350 mL/min, and a postdialyzer venous-line BUN of 30 mg/dL. It should also be assumed that the BUN of 100 mg/dL in the peripheral vein is representative of venous blood in the patient's circulation (other than that of veins draining the vascular access).

ANSWER

Blood is leaving (and returning to) the heart at 5 L/min. Of this 5 L, 350 mL will be blood with a BUN of 30 mg/dL (3.5 dL ×

30 mg/dL = 105 mg) and 4.65 L will be blood with BUN of 100 mg/dL (46.5 dL × 100 mg/dL = 4,650 mg). As a result, arterial and mixed central-vein BUN will be about 5 mg/dL lower than that of the peripheral vein, or about 95 mg/dL.

$$(105 \text{ mg} + 4,650 \text{ mg})/50 \text{ dL} = 95.1 \text{ mg/dL}$$

The arterial blood with a reduced BUN now enters the arterioles and then the body's capillaries where a urea gradient will exist between cellular and interstitial water and blood. Urea will move down this gradient, perhaps to equilibrium, raising the concentration of urea in the venous effluent almost to its initial value. Only a minute or so is required for blood to complete its vein-artery-capillary-vein circuit. Fig. 5.1 illustrates the answer for Example 4 as well as the equilibration process in the capillaries.

Thus, a difference in BUN between arterial and venous blood is expected during dialysis. This AV disequilibrium will be increased by high-efficiency dialysis and by a low cardiac output, because the former adds more blood with a lower BUN to the circuit whereas the latter results in the dialyzed blood being a greater proportion of the blood returning to the heart. Example 5 illustrates the calculation of "recirculation" in a patient being dialyzed using both arms for access.

EXAMPLE 5

A patient with a cardiac output of 2.5 L/minute is receiving dialysis with arterial and venous lines in separate arms. The arterial- and venous-line BUN values are 90 mg/dL and 27 mg/dL, respectively. The BUN in the femoral vein is 100 mg/dL. What is the percentage recirculation?

ANSWER

Clearly, access recirculation must be 0%, given the arrangement of the dialysis circuit. However, a calculated recirculation of 14% is found as a consequence, most likely, of AV disequilibrium.

$$(100 - 90)/(100 - 27) = 0.14 \text{ (or 14\%)}$$

Another problem to be considered when blood from a peripheral vein is used for the systemic sample is that the BUN may not be the same in all venous compartments (27,29,34). Consider the distal portion of a nonfistula arm during dialysis under conditions of peripheral vasoconstriction. Even though the urea concentration in venous blood draining the arm may have achieved urea equilibration with the cells and interstitial fluid during its passage through the capillaries, the total amount of urea removed from the tissues may be minimal if blood flow through the arm is low. The urea concentration in the poorly perfused compartment (the arm) and its venous drainage will remain closer to the high value present at the start of dialysis than it will in a better perfused compartment in which the BUN rapidly falls as dialysis time passes. The BUN difference in the veins draining the well-perfused and poorly perfused compartments will tend to increase as dialysis progresses.

This venovenous disequilibrium may be significant clinically. In a 12-patient study, BUN concentrations in peripheral arm veins differed from arterial values by about 10% at 5 minutes into dialysis (consistent with the expected AV disequilibrium) but differed by a mean of 26% at 60 minutes and by 36% at 120 minutes of treatment (22). This disequilibrium could be eliminated (with the venous BUN in the nondialysis arm approaching arterial values) when perfusion of the extremity was increased by direct warming of the arm and an increase in dialysate temperature to 39°C (34). An increase in blood flow resulting in enhanced tissue urea removal probably accounted for the finding.

The peripheral-vein recirculation method will be most accurate when performed within the first 30 minutes of dialysis to minimize the error produced by venovenous disequilibrium (35). However, given its inherent inaccuracy and its requirement for a venipuncture, there appears to be little justification for its continued use. Use of a peripheral artery "systemic" specimen will yield a definitive recirculation measurement because it avoids the effect of both venovenous and AV disequilibrium (36). However, it entails significant risk to the patient and thus is also not recommended.

Two-Needle Methods for the Measurement of Recirculation

Even before the recognition of AV and venovenous disequilibrium, alternative methods were sought to avoid intradialytic venipuncture for sampling systemic blood. Such methods were desirable because accessible veins for such sampling in dialysis patients are often poor or nonexistent. Venipuncture in patients receiving heparin also increases the likelihood of hematoma formation. Site compression is, therefore, often prolonged and typically requires significant nursing time because the patient may not be able to perform this task while the opposite arm is being used for dialysis.

A number of methods for the measurement of recirculation have been reported that do not require venipuncture. In all of these two-needle methods, blood from a peripheral vein (for the systemic sample) is replaced by blood from the arterial line after dialytic conditions have been altered to minimize contamination of this line with recirculated blood. The standard arterial-line (C_a) and venous-line (C_v) samples are obtained in the usual fashion.

A major problem in evaluating two-needle methods is that reports of their accuracy have generally been made by comparing them to the "definitive" peripheral-vein method. The two-needle methods use an arterial-line specimen for the systemic sample (C_s), so they actually offer the advantage of eliminating venovenous and potentially eliminating AV disequilibrium. Thus, whether recirculation calculated using a two-needle method matches results obtained using the peripheral-vein method is not the appropriate standard to judge the accuracy of two-needle methods. A two-needle method that successfully avoids contamination of the systemic sample with venous-line blood will more accurately reflect true access recirculation than does the peripheral-vein method. It should be noted, however, that the clinical correlations of elevated recirculation levels have, until recent years, been made using results obtained with the peripheral-vein method.

Several approaches have been used to achieve the goal of briefly eliminating (or at least minimizing) recirculation so that blood from the arterial line will approximate systemic (C_s) values. Reports have been published in which this substitute arterial-line sample is obtained before (37) or after (37,38) dialysis, after slowing (39–43) or stopping (37,38) blood flow, after occluding the graft between the arterial and venous needles (23,44), or after stopping dialysate flow (45).

The stop-dialysate, the stop-blood-flow, and the low-(blood)-flow methods all incorporate a delay before obtaining the arterial-line systemic sample to eliminate the effect of recirculated blood already in the dialysis circuit. Any delay in obtaining the systemic sample after effective dialysis has been halted has a potential impact on the result of the study. AV disequilibrium, present while dialysis is underway, will rapidly dissipate once the addition of dialyzed blood to the central blood compartment ends. Thus, the BUN in an arterial-line systemic sample obtained within 30 to 50 seconds after the addition of dialyzed blood to the circuit has ceased will be significantly lower than the one obtained at 1 to 3 minutes (44–46), when arterial and venous blood are reaching equilibration. It is now recognized that arterial-line urea rebound begins within 15 seconds after dialysis is slowed or stopped (28). As a result, a higher calculated recirculation may be present when arterial-line systemic sampling is delayed than when it is prompt (46). Prompt sampling, however, risks a falsely low recirculation resulting from possible contamination of the arterial line with recirculated blood that remains in the circuit. To obtain an accurate determination of access recirculation, the substitute arterial-line sample must be obtained after a risk of contamination has passed but before the abrupt rise in arterial-line BUN (because of dissipation of AV disequilibrium) occurs. For the sake of completeness, it should be noted that after dialysis stops, a portion of the early rise (1 to 3 minutes) and most of the late rise (3 to 12 minutes) in BUN is due to dissipation of venovenous disequilibrium (i.e., urea washout from poorly perfused compartments).

Two-needle methods may or may not eliminate the effect of AV disequilibrium on the calculation of recirculation (depending on sample timing), but they do eliminate most of the problems from venovenous disequilibrium. As a result, these methods can be used at any time during treatment. Because access recirculation may increase as dialysis proceeds in patients with marginal access blood flow resulting from a fall in cardiac output, hypotension, and/or volume depletion resulting in diminished access flow (11,43), it may be desirable to increase the sensitivity of the recirculation test by using it later in dialysis. However, with any urea-based test, the low BUN values present late in dialysis will increase the frequency of false-positive results.

Recommended Technique for the Measurement of Recirculation

Our increased understanding of intradialytic urea kinetics and the pathophysiology of access recirculation has required modification of prior approaches to urea-based recirculation measurement. Recirculation is generally absent when access blood flow

TABLE 5.3. REVISED SLOW-STOP FLOW UREA RECIRCULATION METHOD

1. Set pump speed to desired rate for at least 3 minutes
2. Obtain venous and arterial-line samples
3. Reduce pump speed to 120–150 mL/min for exactly 10 seconds then stop pump
4. Clamp above arterial sampling port
5. Obtain systemic sample from arterial port
6. Calculate recirculation

exceeds dialyzer blood flow. As a result, recirculation is rare at very low dialyzer blood-flow rates because very low access blood-flow rates (i.e., <150 mL/min) are rare. Thus, contamination of the arterial-line systemic sample, previously avoided in two-needle low-flow recirculation techniques by use of a dialyzer blood-flow rate of 50 mL/min, is unlikely to be a problem even at significantly higher dialyzer blood-flow rates (e.g., 150 mL/min). This is fortunate, because the arterial-line systemic sample must be obtained earlier after dialysis is slowed than was previously believed to avoid urea rebound. However, the dead space between the needle and sampling port still must be cleared. Obtaining the "low-flow" systemic sample 10 seconds after reducing dialyzer blood flow to 120 to 150 mL/min will accomplish both objectives (41) (Table 5.3).

Using the method shown in Table 5.3 yields an average recirculation value very similar to that obtained with the highly accurate ultrasound dilution method. Mean values in 43 patients without recirculation (0%) by ultrasound dilution averaged 1.9% with the modified slow-stop flow method (41). However, significant variability exists in urea determination (47) such that recirculation could not be reliably recognized (i.e., present on ultrasound dilution) unless the slow-stop flow value exceeded 10%. (Duplicate abnormal values, each more than 5%, will probably be equally reliable.)

CLINICAL UTILITY OF RECIRCULATION MEASUREMENTS

Recirculation measurements provide useful information and are valuable in a number of clinical settings (Table 5.4).

TABLE 5.4. MEASUREMENT AND EVALUATION OF RECIRCULATION

Indications
  New vascular access
  Unexplained shortfalls in dialysis delivery
  Screening for vascular access stenosis
Method
  Revised slow-stop flow method
  Non-urea-based method
Interpretation
  Abnormal measurement that usually indicates ABFR < DBFR:
    Recirculation >10% by recommended urea-based method
    Recirculation >0–5% by non-urea-based method

Access Blood-Flow Rate

The level of access recirculation provides an indirect estimate of access blood-flow rate, although its accuracy is far less than that of more routine measurement techniques (48).

EXAMPLE 6

Patient A has 25% recirculation at a dialyzer blood flow of 400 mL/min. What is the approximate access blood-flow rate?

ANSWER

Of the 400 mL/min entering the dialyzer, 100 mL/min (25% of 400 mL/min) is recirculated blood. Recirculation is not usually present until access blood-flow rate falls below dialyzer blood-flow rate, implying that all the blood entering the access must be taken up by the arterial needle before any blood flowing retrograde from the venous needle (recirculation) is used. Therefore, access blood flow in this patient is approximately 300 mL/min. To generalize the point, access blood flow equals dialyzer blood flow X (1 − R), where R is the recirculation fraction. This relationship obviously applies only when significant levels of recirculation are present.

New Vascular Access

Measurement of recirculation in a newly placed vascular access provides some assurance that needle placement is correct. Reversal of arterial and venous needles may not be readily apparent clinically. Significant recirculation (usually greater than 25% to 30%) in a new, otherwise satisfactory appearing and functioning access should prompt consideration of needle reversal as the cause of the abnormal finding.

Knowledge of the level of recirculation can be incorporated into the dialysis prescription. The reduction in dialysis efficiency resulting from recirculation can be calculated and included in urea kinetic modeling. An example of this is provided in the following.

EXAMPLE 7

In Example 1, a dialyzer with a urea clearance of 210 mL/min (at a 300 mL/min blood flow) was used. A 25% recirculation rate resulted in a 19% decrease in dialysis efficiency in that case. Assuming a body weight of 69 kg, how does the calculated dialysis time required to deliver a *Kt/V* of 1.2 compare when recirculation is and is not included in the determination of the dialysis prescription?

ANSWER

$$\text{Dialyzer clearance (K)} = 210 \text{ mL/min}$$

$$\text{Urea distribution volume (V)} = 0.58 \times 69 \text{ kg} = 40 \text{ L}$$

$$Kt/V = 1.2$$

Thus

$$Kt = 1.2 \text{ V}$$

$$t = 1.2 \times \frac{40{,}000 \text{ mL}}{210 \text{ mL/min}}$$

$$t = 229 \text{ minutes}$$

If recirculation equals 25% and dialysis efficiency is reduced by 19% (as calculated earlier), then the expected reduction in dialytic urea clearance is 0.19 × 210 mL/min = 40 mL/min. Thus

$$t = \frac{1.2 \times 40{,}000 \text{ mL}}{(210 \text{ mL/min} - 40 \text{ mL/min})}$$

$$t = 282 \text{ minutes}$$

More simply, one can see that 229 minutes is 19% shorter than 282 minutes.

As can be seen in the example, recirculation can dramatically alter required dialysis time.

Unexplained Shortfalls in Dialysis Delivery

Dialysis delivery is now widely followed in chronic hemodialysis patients, either with urea kinetic modeling or by monitoring the urea reduction ratio (URR). Decreased dialysis delivery is often caused by relatively obvious problems involving dialysis time and dialyzer blood flows (49). An elevated recirculation is the most common cause of a reduction in dialysis delivery that does not have an obvious cause.

Recirculation should be measured when an unexplained reduction in *Kt/V* or URR occurs or when the prescribed *Kt/V* differs substantially and without explanation from the delivered *Kt/V*. When formal urea kinetic modeling is used, recirculation can be suspected when an inordinately high V or a low effective K is found.

Vascular Access Stenoses

Measurement of recirculation has been advocated as a screening test for vascular access stenosis. Gotch (25) found recirculation measured at a mean blood flow of 194 mL/min to average 4.2% in 24 patients but noted values of 65% and 75% in two patients with severe arterial and venous stenoses, respectively. Seidman et al. (50) screened 75 hemodialysis patients and found that 7% (five patients) had more than 20% recirculation. Two of these five patients were noted to have subsequent graft closure or to require access revision.

Nardi et al. (51) found recirculation (peripheral-vein technique) to be <10% in all 20 patients with well-functioning accesses. In contrast, two patients with suspected distal access stenoses had values of 17% and 46%, respectively. Levy et al. (52) found all 11 patients with recirculation over 15% (peripheral-vein technique) to have significant venous or arterial stenoses.

Windus et al. (53) measured recirculation (peripheral-vein technique) in 103 patients usually (i.e., in 75% of patients) because of unexplained shortfalls in dialysis delivery. Eighteen of 22 patients (82%) with recirculation rates of more than 15% who underwent fistulograms were found to have clinically significant abnormalities. In a study of 52 unselected patients, Collins et al. (12) found that 33 patients had recirculation values of more than 20% (peripheral-vein technique) and that 26 of them (79%) had significant venous stenoses.

The measurement of recirculation is largely an indirect measure of access blood flow—when recirculation is present, access blood flow is usually less than dialyzer blood flow and when recirculation is absent access blood flow usually exceeds dialyzer blood flow. Important exceptions to this generalization exist and are listed in Table 5.2.

With developing technology and the ability to monitor access blood flow regularly (e.g., by indicator velocity dilution methodology), the need for routine use of recirculation as a screening tool for vascular access stenosis will eventually be obviated. Until such time as this technology is widely used, however, recirculation measurements, along with access pressure measurements, have an important role in access monitoring.

Data suggest that the utility of recirculation measurements differs in native-vein and prosthetic AV accesses because of the differing relationship between access flow and thrombosis risk in these two forms of vascular access (6,54). The risk of thrombosis resulting from venous stenosis in a prosthetic access graft appears to increase sharply when access blood-flow rates decline below 600 to 800 mL/min (55–59). In contrast, native-vein fistulae tend to remain patent until blood flows decline to substantially lower levels. Therefore, the presence of recirculation in an AV graft is usually a relatively late marker for an access at risk of clotting because recirculation will not be noted until access blood-flow rate is less than the usual dialyzer blood-flow rate (i.e., 350 to 500 mL/min). In native-vein fistulae, however, recirculation is an earlier marker for an increased risk of thrombosis.

The measurement of access pressures (both venous pressures at 200 mL/min and intraaccess pressures) in native-vein fistulae is of limited value as a screening tool for venous stenosis. Although increasingly severe venous stenosis is associated with increasing access pressures in prosthetic grafts, pressures often do not rise substantially in native-vein fistulae (perhaps because of collateral drainage around a stenotic lesion). As a result, one must rely on recirculation measurements to a greater extent in native-vein fistulae.

RECOMMENDATIONS FOR THE CLINICAL USE OF RECIRCULATION MEASUREMENTS IN AV ACCESSES

The measurement of recirculation is useful in detecting reversed needle placement, a problem that occurs more frequently than is acknowledged, particularly in new AV accesses. Therefore, this measurement should be obtained as a routine test after initiation of dialysis using a new AV access.

The measurement of recirculation as a routine screening test for vascular access stenosis in patients with AV grafts is of little value, given the rarity of recirculation in this setting. However, it remains a valuable test in selected circumstances—confirming a suspicion of very low access flow (particularly with arterial disease in which venous pressures are often low) and with unexplained declines in dialysis delivery. When recirculation is present in an AV graft, the graft is at very high risk of thrombosis,

indicating the need for accelerated evaluation and intervention. This point suggests that measuring recirculation in some patients with other evidence of serious AV graft pathology (e.g., high and rising venous or intraaccess pressures) might alter clinical management of the patient.

Recirculation is more likely to occur with native-vein fistulae than with AV grafts. In addition, recirculation is much more likely to be the sole indicator of access stenosis with native-vein fistulae. However, in native-vein fistulae stenoses are much less common than in grafts, so screening for stenotic lesions has a much lower yield. The cost-risk-benefit issues have yet to be clarified. Until such time as they are, measuring recirculation in native-vein fistulae every 2 to 3 months should be considered. As previously noted, however, measurement of access blood flow makes recirculation measurements (for access screening) unnecessary.

RECIRCULATION DURING SINGLE-NEEDLE DIALYSIS

Recirculation during single-needle dialysis is substantial even at the low blood-flow rates characteristic of these systems. In the older, single-pump systems, recirculation ranged from 17% to 22%, whereas a somewhat lower level of recirculation was seen when double-pump systems were used (9% to 17%) (60). When single-needle central-vein catheters are used, even higher levels of recirculation will be seen because of the larger dead space of the system. Questions regarding the accuracy of the measurements exist because of the methodology employed to measure recirculation.

Double-lumen fistula needles in the well-functioning access have been reported to have low (less than 5%) recirculation rates at low blood flows (61). A mean recirculation of 3.8% at a 200 mL/min blood flow was found in 42 patients dialyzed with a coaxial needle (using a stop-blood-flow technique). Mean recirculation doubled when blood flow was increased to 300 mL/min. These needles are probably more susceptible to excessive recirculation in patients with poorly functioning accesses or when the higher blood flows characteristic of current dialysis practice are used.

RECIRCULATION WITH DOUBLE-LUMEN CENTRAL-VEIN CATHETERS

Double-lumen central-vein catheters are becoming more widely used, both for temporary and permanent vascular access. With the close proximity of the inflow and outflow ports on these catheters, concern about the extent of recirculation is appropriate. However, the basis for the recirculation commonly observed in these catheters may be related, at least in part, to the retrograde blood flow present in the central veins following atrial contraction (62).

Recirculation in these catheters should be measured by a two-needle technique. Neither AV nor venovenous disequilibrium is at issue, because central-vein blood is used for all sam-

TABLE 5.5. RECIRCULATION IN DOUBLE-LUMEN CENTRAL-VEIN HEMODIALYSIS CATHETERS

Source	Catheter (No.)	Recirculation	Method
Tapson et al., 1985 (69)	Shiley (18)	5.9%	Peripheral vein
	Quinton-Mahurkar (11)	7.6%	Peripheral vein
Bregman et al., 1986 (63)	VasCath (10)	1.7%	Peripheral vein
Canaud et al., 1986 (70)	Twin Cath (50)	7.7%	Peripheral vein
Schanzer et al., 1986 (68)	HemoCath (4)	8.6%	Peripheral vein
	Raaf (6)	7.1%	Peripheral vein
Schwab et al., 1988 (74)	Permcath (10)	all <5%	Not reported
Shusterman et al., 1989 (66)	Permcath (7)	5.5%	Not reported
Moss et al., 1990 (67)	Permcath (7)	7.5.%	Not reported
Blake et al., 1990 (72)	Permcath (11)	5.9%	Peripheral vein
Kelber et al., 1992 (64)	VasCath (8)	5.4%	30-sec slow flow
Twardowski et al., 1992 (73)	Permcath (13) VasCath (5)	>2%	1-min slow flow
Uldall et al., 1993 (71)	Cook (24)	11.9%	Peripheral vein
Leblanc et al., 1996 (65)	Quinton (24)		

ples. Inadvertent contamination of the systemic samples with dialyzed blood using a two-needle technique is also less likely than with peripheral accesses because of the typically high central-vein blood flows.

In a peripheral vascular access, an inability to achieve adequate blood flow is likely to be associated with an increased level of recirculation. In a central-vein double-lumen access, however, poor blood flows are not typically associated with increased recirculation. This difference reflects the typical underlying cause of the impaired blood flow—an anatomic problem in the former and an intraluminal catheter obstruction in the latter.

Recirculation rates in central-vein catheters are typically low, usually less than 10% (63–74) (Table 5.5). When such catheters are used in vessels with low intrinsic blood-flow rates such as the femoral vein, recirculation levels rise dramatically and become dependent on dialyzer blood flow. When blood flow was increased from 250 to 400 mL/min, recirculation rose from 18% to 38% in 15-cm femoral-vein double-lumen catheters (64). However, recirculation did not rise with the increase in blood-flow rate in 24-cm femoral catheters (64). Similarly, recirculation averaged 22.8% in nine 13.5-cm femoral catheters but only 12.6% in seventeen 19.5-cm catheters (64). A similar difference was noted in femoral catheters greater than 20 cm (8.3%) and less than 20 cm (26.3%) (75). The most likely explanation for this catheter-length-related recirculation is the blood-flow rate in the accessed vessel. The longer catheters probably reach the common iliac vein, where blood flows are sufficient to meet the demand of the blood pump with little recirculation.

When central-vein catheters malfunction, it is not unusual to reverse the inflow and outflow lines to achieve adequate blood-flow rates. In this setting, recirculation levels increase only modestly (5% to 12%) (60,66,76) compared with the consequences of reversing lines in a double-needle fistula setting. The much lower ratio of dialyzer flow to access flow in central veins versus peripheral veins very likely accounts for this difference. Rarely, markedly high levels of recirculation may occur when a communication develops between the two catheter lumens (77).

REFERENCES

1. Ilstrup K, et al. Examining the foundations of urea kinetics. *Trans Am Soc Artif Intern Organs* 1985;31:164–168.
2. Depner TA, et al. Clinical measurement of blood flow in hemodialysis access fistulae and grafts by ultrasound dilution. *ASAIO J* 1995;41: M745–M749.
3. Oudenhoven L, et al. Magnetic resonance, a new method for measuring blood flow in hemodialysis fistulae. *Kidney Int* 1994;45:884–889.
4. MacDonald JT, et al. Identifying a new reality: zero vascular access recirculation using ultrasound dilution. *ANNA J* 1996;23:603–608.
5. Krisper P, et al. Access recirculation in a native fistula in spite of a seemingly adequate access flow. *Am J Kidney Dis* 2000;35:529–532.
6. Lindsay RM, et al. A device and a method for rapid and accurate measurement of access recirculation during hemodialysis. *Kidney Int* 1996; 41:1152–1160.
7. George TO, et al. Access recirculation (AR) by ultrasound dilution compared to a 20 sec flow urea method. *J Am Soc Nephrol* 1996;6:489(abst).
8. Depner TA, et al. Hemodialysis access recirculation measured by ultrasound dilution. *ASAIO J* 1996;41:M749–M753.
9. Besarab A, et al. The relationship of recirculation to access blood flow. *Am J Kidney Dis* 1997;29:223–229.
10. Sherman R, et al. Rate-related recirculation: the effect of altering blood flow on dialyzer recirculation. *Am J Kidney Dis* 1991;17:170–173.
11. Ukponmwan O, et al. The effects of blood flow rate and dialysis time on recirculation. *J Am Soc Nephrol* 1991;2:352.
12. Collins DM, et al. Fistula dysfunction: effect on rapid hemodialysis. *Kidney Int* 1992;41:1292–1296.
13. Sherman RA, et al. Recirculation reassessed: the impact of blood flow rate and the low-flow method reevaluated. *Am J Kidney Dis* 1992;23: 846–848.
14. Kaufman AM, et al. Haemodialysis access recirculation measurement by blood temperature monitoring—a new technique. *J Am Soc Nephrol* 1991;2:332.
15. Hester RL, et al. Non-invasive determination of recirculation in the patient on dialysis. *ASAIO J* 1992;38:M190–M193.
16. Depner TA, et al. Hemodialysis access recirculation measured by ultrasound dilution. *ASAIO J* 1995;41:M749–M753.
17. Magnasco A, et al. Glucose infusion test: a new screening test for vascular access recirculation. *Kidney Int* 2000;57:2123–2128.
18. Lindsay RM, et al. A comparison of methods for the measurement of hemodialysis access recirculation: an update. *ASAIO J* 1998;44:191–193.
19. Brancaccio D, et al. Potassium-based dilutional method to measure hemodialysis access recirculation. *Int J Artif Organs* 2001;24:606–613.
20. Weitzel WF, et al. Retrograde hemodialysis access flow during dialysis as a predictor of access pathology. *Am J Kidney Dis* 2001;37:1241–1246.
21. Depner TA. Diagnostic value of vascular access compression. *Semin Dial* 1993;6:271–272.

22. Depner TA. Techniques for prospective detection of venous stenosis. *Adv Ren Replace Ther* 1994;1:119–130.
23. Besarab A, et al. Prospective evaluation of vascular access function: the nephrologist's perspective. *Semin Dial* 1996;9[Suppl 1]:S21–S29.
24. Sherman A. The measurement of dialysis access recirculation. *Am J Kidney Dis* 1993;22:616–621.
25. Gotch FA. Hemodialysis: technical and kinetic considerations. In: Brenner BM, et al., eds. *The kidney.* Philadelphia: WB Saunders, 1976: 1672–1704.
26. VanStone J, et al. Peripheral venous blood is not the appropriate specimen to determine recirculation rate. *J Am Soc Nephrol* 1991;2:354.
27. Depner TA, et al. High venous urea concentrations in the opposite arm. *ASAIO J* 1991;37: M141–M143.
28. Schneiditz D, et al. Systemic recirculation in dialysis: an under-recognized phenomenon. *ASAIO J* 1992;21:84.
29. Sherman RA. Recirculation revisited. *Semin Dial* 1991;4:221–223.
30. Sherman RA. The regional blood flow model: a revisitation. *Semin Dial* 1995;8:12–14.
31. Ginn HE. Removal of serum components by hemodialysis. *Proceedings of the 4th International Congress of Nephrology.* Basel/Munchen/New York: Karger, 1970;3:174–187.
32. Schneditz D, et al. Cardiopulmonary recirculation in dialysis—an under-recognized phenomenon. *ASAIO J* 1992;38:M194–M196.
33. Schneditz D, et al. Cardiopulmonary recirculation during hemodialysis. *Kidney Int* 1992;42:1450–1456.
34. Depner T, et al. Peripheral urea disequilibrium during hemodialysis is temperature-dependent. *J Am Soc Nephrol* 1991;2:321.
35. Sherman RA. Dialysis access recirculation. In: Nissenson AR, et al., eds. *Dialysis therapy,* 2nd ed. Philadelphia: Hanley & Belfus, 1992:19–21.
36. Burr T, et al. Haemodialysis recirculation measured using a femoral artery sample. *Nephrol Dial Transplant* 1994;9:395–398.
37. Kobrin SM, et al. Measurement of hemodialysis access recirculation: a two-needle method at the start of dialysis. *ASAIO J* 1989;35:508–510.
38. Pederson JA, et al. Two-needle calculations of recirculation compared with the standard three-needle method. *Clin Nephrol* 1990;33:203–206.
39. Gibson SM, et al. Reproducible measurement of recirculation without peripheral venipuncture. *Kidney Int* 1990;37:297.
40. Sherman RA, et al. Assessment of a two-needle technique for the measurement of recirculation during hemodialysis. *Am J Kidney Dis* 1991; 18:80–83.
41. Kapoian T, et al. Validation of a revised slow-stop flow recirculation method. *Kidney Int* 1977;52:839–842.
42. Sherman RA. The regional blood flow model: a revisitation. *Semin Dial* 1995;8:12–14.
43. Emovon O, et al. Urea recirculation: result variability with three different techniques. *J Am Soc Nephrol* 1992;3:363.
44. Schnediz D, et al. Impact of cardiopulmonary recirculation on measurement of access recirculation. *J Am Soc Nephrol* 1992;3:393.
45. Depner TA, et al. Effect of urea rebound on stop-flow measurements of hemodialysis access recirculation. *J Am Soc Nephrol* 1992;3:362.
46. Kirschbaum B. Recirculation measures with urea and mannitol during hemodialysis. *Artif Organs* 1994;18:547–551.
47. Hester RL, et al. The determination of hemodialysis blood recirculation using blood urea nitrogen measurements. *Am J Kidney Dis* 1992;20:598–602.
48. Lindsay RM, et al. Estimation of hemodialysis access blood flow rates by a urea method is a poor predictor of access outcome. *ASAIO J* 1998; 44:818–822.
49. Parker TF, et al. Delivering the prescribed dialysis. *Semin Dial* 1993; 6:13–15.
50. Seidman MS, et al. Extent of blood recirculation during two-needle hemodialysis. *ASAIO J* 1979;8:56.
51. Nardi L, et al. Recirculation: review, techniques for measurement and ability to predict hemoaccess stenosis before and after angioplasty. *Blood Purif* 1988;6:85–89.
52. Levy SS, et al. Value of clinical screening for detection of asymptomatic hemodialysis vascular access stenoses. *Angiology* 1992;43:421–424.
53. Windus DW, et al. Optimization of high-efficiency hemodialysis by detection and correction of fistula dysfunction. *Kidney Int* 1990;38: 337–341.
54. Besarab A, et al. Utility of intra-access pressure monitoring in detecting venous outlet stenoses prior to thrombosis. *Kidney Int* 1995;47: 1364–1373.
55. Sands Y, et al. The effect of Doppler flow screening studies and elective revisions in dialysis access failure. *ASAIO J* 1992;38:M524–M527.
56. Strauch BS, et al. Forecasting thromboses of vascular access with Doppler color flow imaging. *Am J Kidney Dis* 1992;19:554–557.
57. Besarab A, et al. The relation of intra-access pressure to intra-access flow. *J Am Soc Nephrol* 1995;6:483(abst).
58. Koksoy C, et al. Predictive value of colour Doppler ultrasonography in detecting failure of vascular access grafts. *Br J Surg* 1995;82:50–52.
59. Sands JJ, et al. Prolongation of hemodialysis access survival with elective revision. *Clin Nephrol* 1995;44:334–337.
60. VanHolder R, et al. Single needle hemodialysis. In: Maher JF, ed. *Replacement of renal function by dialysis,* 3rd ed. Dordrecht, the Netherlands: Kluwer, 1986:382–399.
61. Ogden DA, et al. Blood recirculation during hemodialysis with a coaxial counterflow single needle blood access catheter. *Trans Am Soc Artif Organs* 1979;25:325–327.
62. Sherman RA, et al. Recirculation, urea disequilibrium, and dialysis efficiency: peripheral arteriovenous versus central venovenous vascular access. *Am J Kidney Dis* 1997;29:479–489.
63. Bregman H, et al. Minimum performance standards for double-lumen subclavian cannulas for hemodialysis. *Trans Am Soc Artif Organs* 1986; 32:500–502.
64. Kelber J, et al. The effects of double lumen catheter placement site and blood flow rate on effective clearance in hemodialysis. *J Am Soc Nephrol* 1992;3:373.
65. Leblanc M, et al. Blood recirculation in temporary central catheters for acute hemodialysis. *Clin Nephrol* 1996;45:315–319.
66. Shusterman NH, et al. Successful use of double-lumen, silicone rubber catheters for permanent hemodialysis access. *Kidney Int* 1989;35: 887–890.
67. Moss AH, et al. Use of a silicone dual-lumen catheter with a Dacron cuff as a long-term vascular access for hemodialysis patients. *Am J Kidney Dis* 1990;16:211–215.
68. Schanzer H, et al. Double-lumen, silicone rubber, indwelling venous catheters. *Arch Surg* 1986;121:229–232.
69. Tapson JS, et al. Dual lumen subclavian catheters for haemodialysis. *Int J Artif Organs* 1985;8:195–200.
70. Canaud B, et al. Internal jugular vein cannulation with two silicone rubber catheters: a new and safe temporary vascular access for hemodialysis—thirty months' experience. *Artif Organs* 1986;10:397–403.
71. Uldall R, et al. A new vascular access catheter for hemodialysis. *Am J Kidney Dis* 1993;21:270–277.
72. Blake PG, et al. The use of dual lumen jugular venous catheters as definitive long-term access for haemodialysis. *Int J Artif Organs* 1990;13: 26–31.
73. Twardowski ZJ, et al. Blood recirculation in intravenous catheters for hemodialysis. *J Am Soc Nephrol* 1992;3:399.
74. Schwab SJ, et al. Prospective evaluation of a Dacron cuffed hemodialysis catheter for prolonged use. *Am J Kidney Dis* 1988;11:166–169.
75. Little MA, et al. Access recirculation in temporary hemodialysis catheters as measured by the saline dilution technique. *Am J Kidney Dis* 2000;36:1135–1139.
76. Crespo R, et al. Blood recirculation in malfunctioning catheters for haemodialysis. *EDTNA ERCA J* 1999;25:38–39.
77. Sarnak MJ, et al. Severe access recirculation secondary to free flow between the lumens of a dual-lumen dialysis catheters. *Am J Kidney Dis* 1999;33:1168–1170.

ANTICOAGULATION STRATEGIES DURING HEMODIALYSIS PROCEDURES

RICHARD A. WARD AND GEORGE R. ARONOFF

Unfractionated heparin is the most frequently used anticoagulant for preventing thrombosis of the extracorporeal circuit during hemodialysis. This mixture of glycosaminoglycans prevents clotting by increasing inhibition of serine proteases (1). The intent of anticoagulation with unfractionated heparin is to decrease thrombosis in the dialyzer and blood lines without inducing excessive bleeding. However, the therapeutic window for heparin is narrow.

Too much heparin results in excessive or prolonged bleeding. Inadequate heparin allows thrombosis of the extracorporeal circuit, leads to increased blood loss in the dialyzer, and reduces the amount of dialysis delivered to the patient. There remains neither an ideal strategy for preventing clotting of the extracorporeal circuit without anticoagulation nor a completely satisfactory dosing strategy for unfractionated heparin. This chapter describes approaches to anticoagulation during dialysis and discusses barriers to a satisfactory outcome despite the selection of an appropriate anticoagulant and dose. The emphasis is on use of unfractionated heparin (referred to as heparin throughout the chapter), although alternative anticoagulants are considered briefly.

COAGULATION IN DIALYSIS PATIENTS

Although dialysis requires anticoagulation to prevent thrombosis of the dialyzer, uremia paradoxically causes a bleeding diathesis. Although the exact pathogenesis remains unclear, this bleeding tendency may result from abnormal platelet adhesion to the subendothelium (2–4). Correction of anemia with erythropoietin improves bleeding times (5–7) and platelet adhesion and aggregation (8). Desmopressin (1-deamino-8-D-arginine vasopressin) also reverses the uremic bleeding diathesis by increasing von Willebrand factor (9). However, excessive anticoagulation during the dialysis procedure may exacerbate the bleeding tendency of dialysis patients, increasing the risk of bleeding after invasive procedures, gastrointestinal hemorrhage, and fatal subdural hematomas or intracerebral hemorrhages.

Dialysis patients are also susceptible to thrombotic events (4). Evidence of a hypercoagulable state in these patients includes increased plasma concentrations of fibrinogen (10–12), increased factor VII activity (11,13), and increased fibrinolytic activity (10,12,14). In addition, plasma levels of inhibitors of coagulation, such as antithrombin III (10–12) and free protein S (12), are reduced. Insufficient heparinization during dialysis allows activation of the intrinsic coagulation pathway, leading to production of thrombin and the formation of fibrin clots. Platelet adhesion and activation follow. On the background of a procoagulant state, this activation of the coagulation system may predispose to thrombosis of the vascular access. Access thrombosis is an important barrier to adequate dialysis, results in substantial morbidity, and increases cost.

MEASURING THE ANTICOAGULANT EFFECT OF HEPARIN

The heparin dose regimen is an important part of the dialysis prescription. An ability to measure the level of heparin in blood is necessary to determine the best heparin dose. Because heparin used for hemodialysis is a mixture of components, heparin formulations are standardized in terms of international units (IU), using a United States Pharmacopeia (USP) standard heparin as a reference. In clinical practice, it is not pragmatic to measure blood levels of heparin. Instead, the dose of heparin is managed by measuring its anticoagulant effect.

The anticoagulant effect of heparin is measured as the increased time taken for clot formation under controlled conditions. For hemodialysis, the clotting time assay must be convenient to use in the dialysis unit and give a result within a few minutes, allowing adjustment of the heparin dose during dialysis. These requirements limit the choice of an assay to one using whole blood and incorporating an activating agent to accelerate clotting. Examples include the activated clotting time (ACT), which uses contact activating agents such as kaolin, glass, or diatomaceous earth, and the whole blood partial thromboplastin time (WBPTT), which uses a phospholipid reagent to mimic platelet factor 3 activity. Traditional clinical laboratory assays are not suitable. For example, the partial thromboplastin time uses plasma, and the Lee-White clotting time has a response time of 20 to 30 minutes for the doses of heparin usually used during hemodialysis.

Following enactment of the Clinical Laboratory Improvement Amendments (CLIA) of 1988, automated clotting time measurement systems replaced the manually performed WBPTT

TABLE 6.1. SELECTION CRITERIA FOR AUTOMATED CLOTTING TIME SYSTEMS

Magnitude of clotting time at clinically relevant concentrations of heparin
Sensitivity of the assay to changes in heparin concentration
Ease of use
Availability of quality assurance and proficiency testing programs
Cost of consumables

From Ward RA. Heparinization for routine hemodialysis. *Adv Renal Replace Ther* 1995;2:362–370, with permission.

as the means of monitoring anticoagulation during hemodialysis in the United States. That law requires that any laboratory testing of human specimens be performed in a certified laboratory that incorporates quality control, proficiency testing, and calibration verification in its testing program. Such procedures are difficult to establish for a manual test in a hemodialysis unit.

Several automated clotting time systems that incorporate quality control and proficiency testing procedures are commercially available and suitable for use in hemodialysis units. Although the general operating principles of these systems are similar, including use of an activator and detection of clot formation, a number of factors must be considered in choosing between them (Table 6.1). The clotting time obtained for a given level of heparin depends on the test system used (15–17). Some of these differences are illustrated by the data in Fig. 6.1, which shows ACT measurements as a function of heparin concentration for three different automated systems (15). The HemoTec and TriMed systems exhibited similar increases in clotting time with increasing heparin dose. Lesser increases in clotting times were obtained with the Hemochron system. A heparin dose of 0.5 IU/mL increased clotting time 190 seconds above baseline as

measured with the HemoTec and TriMed systems but only 75 seconds with the Hemochron system. The latter system seems more useful, because a result is obtained more quickly than with the other two systems. However, systems that yield a greater increase in clotting time per unit of heparin provide better discrimination between heparin concentrations than do systems with a smaller increase in clotting time per unit of heparin.

In choosing a system, a balance must be struck between the magnitude of the clotting time and the sensitivity of the assay. The baseline clotting time and range of values expected for a therapeutic dose of heparin must be established for the particular test system used.

ESTABLISHING AN APPROPRIATE LEVEL OF ANTICOAGULATION

The purpose of anticoagulation during hemodialysis is to prevent clotting in the extracorporeal circuit without causing excessive bleeding. The target clotting time depends on the clotting time assay and the clinical situation. An increase in ACT to 140% to 180% of the baseline value provides adequate anticoagulation. Increases of this amount prevent visible clotting in the dialyzer and blood tubing and initiation of coagulation as measured by changes in the plasma levels of thrombin-antithrombin III complex and fibrinopeptide A (18–20). An increase in WBPTT to 200% to 250% of the baseline value results in equivalent anticoagulation. A smaller increase in clotting time, 125% to 150% of the baseline value for ACT assays, may be used in patients with increased risk of bleeding.

Fig. 6.2 shows the ideal anticoagulation profile for hemodialysis. Immediately before initiating blood flow in the extracorporeal circuit, the patient's clotting time is increased to the level

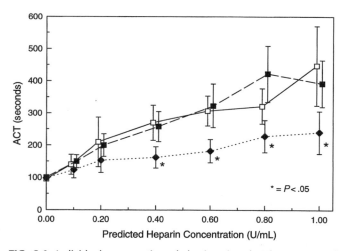

FIG. 6.1. Individual mean activated clotting time (ACT) responses of three different ACT test instruments at varying predicted heparin concentrations. Error bars represent standard deviation of plotted mean values. □ HemoTec Automated Coagulation Timer (HemoTec Inc., Englewood, Colorado); ◆ Hemochron 400 System with P214/P215 test tubes (International Technidyne, Edison, New Jersey); ■ TriMed ACTivator (Kendall McGaw, Santa Ana, California). (From Uden DL, et al. The effect of heparin on three whole blood activated clotting tests and thrombin time. *ASAIO Trans* 1991;37:88–91, with permission.)

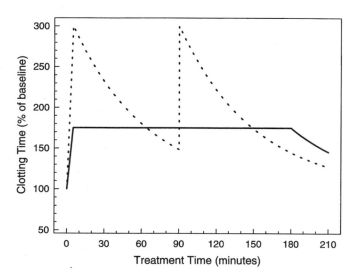

FIG. 6.2. Idealized anticoagulation profiles during hemodialysis. The solid line shows the clotting time profile obtained with a loading dose and constant infusion of heparin; the broken line shows the profile obtained with a loading dose and midtreatment bolus of heparin. (From Ward RA. Heparinization for routine hemodialysis. *Adv Ren Replace Ther* 1995;2:362–370, with permission.)

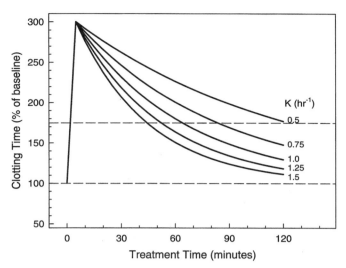

FIG. 6.3. Effect of increasing values of the elimination rate constant (K) on the level of anticoagulation following a single loading dose of heparin. The lower broken line represents the baseline clotting time; the upper broken line represents the desired level of anticoagulation during hemodialysis. (From Ward RA. Heparinization for routine hemodialysis. *Adv Ren Replace Ther* 1995;2:362–370, with permission.)

required to prevent clotting in the circuit. The clotting time is maintained at that level throughout dialysis, before being allowed to decrease toward the baseline value at the end of dialysis. Allowing the clotting time to decrease at the end of dialysis minimizes bleeding when the access needles are withdrawn. This clotting time profile can only be obtained using a loading dose and constant infusion of heparin.

An alternative anticoagulation strategy uses intermittent dosing. An initial loading dose of heparin is administered, followed by one or more additional bolus doses during dialysis. Intermittent dosing is simple and eliminates the need for an infusion pump and syringe. However, as Fig. 6.2 shows, this approach results in periods of over- and under-anticoagulation compared with the loading dose and constant infusion method. Furthermore, the use of intermittent dosing is time-consuming and requires the constant attention of dialysis personnel to ensure that timely heparin boluses are given.

Finally, the magnitude and frequency of the bolus doses depends on the patient's ability to eliminate heparin. Fig. 6.3 illustrates this dependency. As the patient's rate of heparin elimination increases, periods of under-heparinization will be more pronounced unless more frequent bolus doses of heparin are used. The narrow therapeutic window for heparin means that intermittent dosing increases the exposure of patients to the adverse consequences of inadequate heparinization, such as dialyzer clotting during periods of low clotting times, and hemorrhage when the clotting time is high. For these reasons, the loading dose and constant infusion method is preferred.

DETERMINING THE HEPARIN DOSE

Most dialysis units use an empirical approach to estimate the heparin dose for an individual patient. The dose of heparin is

chosen without regard to patient-to-patient differences or is adjusted on some semiquantitative assessment of blood loss in the dialyzer. However, pharmacokinetic studies of heparin dosing demonstrate that patients vary widely in their response to heparin (21,22), suggesting that empirical dosing of heparin is unsatisfactory.

Heparin Pharmacokinetics and Pharmacodynamics

Pharmacokinetic studies suggest that heparin is distributed in a volume approximating the whole blood volume. Elimination kinetics follows a combination of zero- and first-order processes (23). The half-life of heparin is prolonged in patients with end-stage renal disease (ESRD) (24) and the half-life, volume of distribution, and clearance of heparin vary considerably in hemodialysis patients (22).

Pharmacodynamic studies of the anticoagulant activity of heparin have produced conflicting results. Using clotting time assays to study the pharmacodynamic response, the volume of distribution has been shown to approximate the plasma volume, whereas elimination is reported to follow first-order kinetics (25) or a combination of zero- and first-order kinetics (26).

The different results obtained in pharmacokinetic and pharmacodynamic studies may reflect the heterogeneity of heparin preparations. Only a fraction of heparin preparations possess anticoagulant activity, and the anticoagulant effect depends on the availability of other endogenous proteins such as antithrombin III. In the relatively narrow therapeutic range used for hemodialysis, the zero-order component of heparin elimination is of little clinical significance (22). Therefore, heparin elimination during hemodialysis can be described as a first-order process.

A Pharmacodynamic Model for Heparin Dosing in Hemodialysis

A pharmacodynamic model for heparin offers the most utility in the clinical practice of hemodialysis. The anticoagulant properties of heparin are of primary interest and heparin is conveniently assayed by its anticoagulant activity. A simplified pharmacodynamic model has been developed to predict individual heparin dosing during hemodialysis (21). This model is based on the assumptions that heparin is distributed in a single pool corresponding to the plasma space and removed by first-order elimination. The anticoagulant effect of heparin is defined as the increase in clotting time above the baseline value, or response R (seconds).

$$R = \text{Clotting time} - \text{Baseline clotting time} \qquad [1]$$

The response, R, is described in terms of sensitivity (S, the response per unit dose of heparin in seconds per IU) and the elimination rate constant K (hour^{-1}) by the following equation.

$$R_t = R_0 e^{-Kt} + (I_R S/K)(1 - e^{-Kt}) \qquad [2]$$

where R_0 and R_t are the responses before and after an elapsed time, t (hour), and I_R is the infusion rate of heparin (IU/hour).

The parameters S and K can be determined by obtaining serial clotting times during three or four dialysis treatments and solving the model equations as described in the following. The loading dose and constant infusion of heparin needed to yield a desired increase in clotting time can then be calculated for a given patient using average values of S and K for that patient.

Determining the Model Parameters

A blood sample is drawn to measure the baseline clotting time following insertion of the first access needle. The loading dose of heparin is administered through the needle, followed by a saline rinse to ensure that all the heparin enters the circulation. Five minutes are allowed to elapse to ensure that the heparin loading dose is uniformly distributed in the plasma space. A sample for a second clotting time is then obtained, either through the other access needle or through the same needle after first withdrawing 5 to 10 mL to clear the needle of saline. Dialysis is initiated and the constant infusion of heparin started. Clotting time samples are obtained from the arterial blood line at hourly intervals throughout dialysis, and the volume of heparin infused between successive clotting times is noted from the volume remaining in the heparin infusion syringe. At the end of dialysis, a set of clotting times and heparin doses, similar to those shown in Table 6.2, will have been determined. These data are used to calculate the model parameters.

The sensitivity, S, is determined by dividing the increase in clotting time between the baseline and 5-minute samples by the loading dose of heparin. In the example given in Table 6.2

$$S = (175 \text{ seconds} - 113 \text{ seconds})/1,875 \text{ IU} = 0.033 \text{ seconds/IU}$$

Equation 2 cannot be solved directly for the elimination rate constant K, and an iterative procedure must be used. Equation 2 is rearranged as follows.

$$K' = (I_R S (1 - e^{-Kt}))/(R_t - R_0 e^{-Kt}) \quad [3]$$

An initial estimate of K of 1.0 hour^{-1} is entered into the right-hand side of Eq. 3 and a second estimate, K', is calculated. Using the period between the 60-minute and 120-minute clotting times in Table 6.2 as an example

$$I_R = 1,250 \text{ IU/hour}$$

$$S = 0.033 \text{ second/IU}$$

$$t = 1 \text{ hour}$$

$$R_t = 48 \text{ seconds}$$

$$R_0 = 42 \text{ seconds}$$

Substituting these values into Eq. 3 gives

$$K' = (1,250 \times 0.033 \times (1 - e^{-1.0 \times 1}))/ \\ (48 - 42e^{-1.0 \times 1}) = 0.80 \text{ hour}^{-1} \quad [4]$$

This process is repeated until consecutive estimates of K agree to within ±0.02 hour^{-1}. Convergence is usually obtained within two to four iterations. This process is easily accomplished using a personal computer. Alternatively, nomograms for estimating S and K are available (21). In this manner, a value of K is calculated for each interval during dialysis as shown in Table 6.2.

Calculating the Heparin Doses

The calculated value of S and the mean of the values of K are used to determine improved estimates of the loading dose and infusion rate from the following equations.

$$\text{Desired increase in clotting time}/S = \text{Loading dose} \quad [5]$$

$$\text{Desired increase in clotting time} \times K / S = \text{Infusion rate} \quad [6]$$

For the example in Table 6.2, S is 0.033 second/IU and the mean value of K is 0.92 hour^{-1}. For a desired increase in clotting time of 70 seconds, these values yield a loading dose of 70/0.033 = 2,121 IU and an infusion rate of 70 × 0.92/0.033 = 1,951 IU/hour.

Values of loading dose and infusion rate calculated from Eqs. 5 and 6 should be rounded off to practical levels. For example, some heparin infusion pumps allow the infusion rate to be changed in 250 IU/hour increments. Thus, the calculated infusion rate of 1,951 IU/hour should be rounded up to 2,000 IU/hour. To prevent inadvertent under-anticoagulation in the first few minutes of dialysis if there is a delay in starting the constant infusion of heparin, the loading dose should always be rounded up, in this case to 2,200 IU.

Using these improved estimates of loading dose and infusion rate, the modeling process is repeated during the next dialysis treatment. Experience has shown that average values of S and K obtained over three to four modeling sessions will provide satis-

TABLE 6.2. TYPICAL CLOTTING TIME AND HEPARIN ADMINISTRATION DATA AND CALCULATED VALUES OF THE MODEL PARAMETERS

Baseline RACT[a] = 113 Sec		Heparin Loading Dose = 1875 IU		Sensitivity = (175 – 113)/1875 = 0.033 Sec/IU	
Time (Minutes)	Infusion Syringe Volume (mL)	Heparin Infusion Rate (IU/hr)[b]	RACT[a] (Seconds)	Response (Seconds)	Elimination Rate Constant (Hr^{-1})
5	7.5	—	175	62	—
60	6.25	1250	155	42	1.23
120	5.0	1250	161	48	0.85
180	3.75	1250	165	52	0.74
240	2.5	1250	160	47	0.86

Data obtained during pharmacodynamic modeling of anticoagulation.
[a]Recalcified ACT, HemoTec Automated Coagulation Timer (HemoTec Inc., Englewood, CO).
[b]Calculated from the change in syringe volume, elapsed time, and heparin concentration (1,000 IU/mL).

factory estimates of heparin loading dose and infusion rates for most patients.

ESTIMATING HEPARIN DOSES IN THE ABSENCE OF FORMAL KINETIC MODELING

Pharmacodynamic modeling provides the best method for estimating heparin doses. However, implementation of traditional pharmacodynamic modeling is labor intensive and costly to implement. As such, it is poorly suited to busy dialysis units with limited resources. Recently, more sophisticated statistical and computer modeling approaches to individualizing anticoagulation during hemodialysis have been investigated (27,28). Using a nonlinear mixed effects population kinetic model, we developed the following expressions for dose prediction (28).

$$\text{Loading dose (IU)} = 1{,}600 + 10 \times (\text{Wgt} - 76) - 300 \times \text{Fd} - 100 \times \text{Fs} \qquad [7]$$

$$\text{Infusion rate (IU/hour)} = 1{,}750 \qquad [8]$$

where Wgt is the patient's weight (kg), Fd indicates the presence (Fd = 1) or absence (Fd = 0) of diabetes, and Fs indicates that the patient is (Fs = 1) or is not (Fs = 0) a smoker. Eqs. 7 and 8 were used to predict initial heparin doses in a controlled clinical study using dialyzer reuse rate and delivered dose of dialysis as outcome measures (29). The initial doses were adjusted over three to four treatments using clotting time measurements obtained before and after the administration of the loading dose

and at the midpoint of dialysis. A significant improvement in dialyzer reuse rates, with no decrease in the delivered dose of dialysis, was obtained for most but not all patients. Techniques, such as this, offer an approach intermediate between formal pharmacodynamic modeling, which is expensive and time-consuming, and completely empirical dosing, which does not account for the known variability between patients.

When it is necessary to estimate heparin doses in the absence of any modeling data, the experience gained in modeling large numbers of patients can provide some guidance in estimating doses. One such case may be estimating the initial dose and infusion rate for a new dialysis patient. Pharmacodynamic modeling of large numbers of patients has demonstrated that the values of model parameters and the doses of heparin required to achieve a given level of anticoagulation vary widely (21,22). Fig. 6.4 illustrates the variability of S and K, and the doses of heparin required to achieve a WBPTT during dialysis of 250% of baseline in 160 hemodialysis patients. The loading doses and infusion rates of heparin vary from 400 to 6,500 IU and 500 to 5,250 IU/hour.

The sensitivity to heparin, S, correlates with body weight (30). The correlation is weaker in dialysis patients than in normal subjects, possibly because of the wider range of hematocrits and differences in the state of hydration in the former group. These data, together with those of Low et al. (31), suggest that a dose of 25 to 30 IU/kg would be appropriate as an initial estimate of loading dose for routine hemodialysis. To date, no similar method of estimating the elimination rate constant, K, has been developed. In

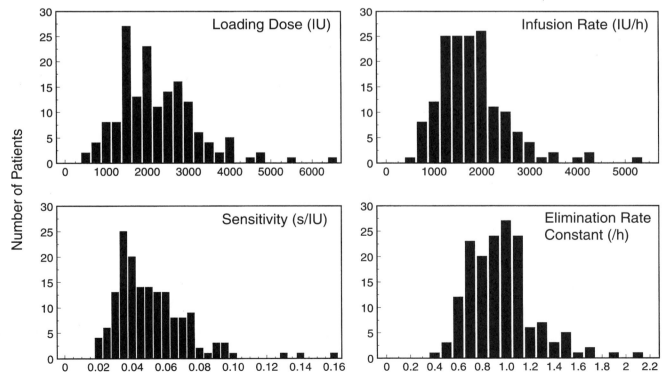

FIG. 6.4. Variability in sensitivity and elimination rate constant, and the doses of heparin required to produce an intradialytic whole blood partial thromboplastin time (WBPTT) of 250% of the baseline value in 160 hemodialysis patients. (From Ward RA. Heparinization for routine hemodialysis. *Adv Ren Replace Ther* 1995;2:362–370, with permission.)

particular, there is no correlation between K and body weight. In the absence of any predictor of K, it seems appropriate to use the average infusion rate for a large group of patients—that is, a dose in the range of 1,500 to 2,000 IU/hour—and to refine that value based on measured clotting times.

ALTERNATIVE ANTICOAGULATION STRATEGIES

Alternative strategies to the routine heparinization described in the previous sections are aimed largely at providing anticoagulation for patients who are at high risk of bleeding. These patients include those with acute illnesses or gastrointestinal bleeding or before and after surgery. Several methods have been demonstrated to be effective in preventing clotting in the extracorporeal circuit (Table 6.3). However, with the possible exception of low molecular weight heparins (LMWHs), none of these methods has proven superior to conventional heparinization for routine hemodialysis. Their application should be limited to situations of high bleeding risk or to those rare patients with heparin allergy.

Traditionally, patients at high risk of bleeding were anticoagulated using regional heparinization in which heparin was infused proximal to the dialyzer, followed by protamine distal to the dialyzer. This procedure, which is rarely used today, offers no advantage over dialysis with low doses of systemic heparin.

Anticoagulation with very low doses of heparin is an effective means of providing anticoagulation in high bleeding risk patients. Heparinization is effected by a small initial dose, 10 to 25 IU/kg, followed by either a low-dose continuous heparin infusion, 11 to 22 IU/kg/hour, or small intermittent doses (32–34). The dose of heparin administered may be adjusted based on clotting times (33,35). The success of low-dose heparin does not seem to be influenced by the choice of dialyzer membrane (36,37). However, with low doses of heparin increases in clotting time have been observed to vary by ±50% from day to day in individual patients given the same dose of heparin (38). Also, because target clotting times are low, errors in technique during heparin administration are more likely to result in complications than during standard heparinization. Thus, low-dose heparin should be reserved for patients at risk of bleeding and with the understanding that minimizing the bleeding risk may result in increased clotting of the extracorporeal circuit on some occasions.

LMWH consists of saccharide chains with a mean molecular size of about 5 kD that are derived from enzymatic or chemical depolymerization of unfractionated heparin. LMWH enhances the inhibition of factor Xa but does not inhibit thrombin activity. For this reason, traditional clotting time assays cannot be

used to measure the effect of LMWHs. Instead, their bioactivity is measured in terms of anti-factor Xa activity using a chromogenic substrate (39). LMWHs offer some advantages over unfractionated heparin. The longer half-life of LMWH allows these preparations to be given as a single predialysis dose, usually based on body weight (40–43). Visual assessment of dialyzer clotting (40,42,44) and measurement of biochemical markers of coagulation (45) suggest that LMWH should be dosed to give an anti-factor Xa activity of greater than 0.4 to 0.5 U/mL at the end of dialysis. Decreased bleeding and more favorable lipid profiles have been reported in chronic dialysis patients treated with LMWH (44,46,47), although the advantage with respect to lipid profiles remains controversial (48). Increased cost and the lack of regulatory approval remain barriers to the widespread use of LMWH in the United States.

Type II heparin-induced thrombocytopenia (HIT) is a serious complication of heparin therapy that necessitates discontinuing the use of unfractionated heparin. The antibody involved in HIT also reacts with LMWH in many cases (49–51). Danaparoid is an antithrombotic agent that consists of a mixture of heparan sulfate, dermatan sulfate, and chondroitin sulfate; it does not contain heparin or LMWH species and has a low cross-reactivity with heparin-associated antibodies (52). Danaparoid has been used successfully to anticoagulate patients with HIT for hemodialysis (50,53). Danaparoid is reported to allow successful dialysis without clotting or bleeding complications when administered as a single predialysis dose of 35 U/kg (54,55). However, the half-life of danaparoid is prolonged in patients with renal failure, and anti-factor Xa activities remain significantly increased 24 hours after administration of the drug for hemodialysis (53,55). For that reason, the dose should be adjusted progressively based on the predialysis anti-factor Xa activity in patients receiving danaparoid for routine hemodialysis (52). Even with dose adjustment, these patients must be considered at risk for bleeding complications.

Regional anticoagulation with citrate has been demonstrated to be an effective alternative to the use of heparin. Trisodium citrate infusion into the blood entering the dialyzer chelates calcium and prevents coagulation. Anticoagulation is reversed, and ionized calcium levels restored, through a combination of citrate loss into the dialysate and infusion of calcium into the venous blood line or calcium influx from the dialysate. Multiple protocols have been described for citrate anticoagulation (56–59). The simplest method involves infusion of concentrated trisodium citrate solution into the arterial blood line, coupled with the use of dialysate containing normal levels of calcium and magnesium (57,59). The citrate infusion rate is adjusted to provide a 25% to 75% increase in ACT at the entry to the dialyzer (57–59). Other methods use calcium- and magnesium-free dialysate and reinfuse calcium into the venous blood line (56,60). Citrate anticoagulation may be useful in patients with heparin allergy, but problems with hypocalcemia, hypernatremia, and metabolic alkalosis render this technique more cumbersome than routine heparin anticoagulation (61,62). The dialysate bicarbonate concentration should be reduced to 25 to 30 mM to guard against metabolic alkalosis, which may develop if the bicarbonate generated from citrate metabolism is added to the normal influx of bicarbonate from the dialysate (63). In extreme cases, failure to adequately

TABLE 6.3. ALTERNATIVES TO STANDARD ANTICOAGULATION WITH UNFRACTIONATED HEPARIN

Low-dose unfractionated heparin
Low molecular weight heparin
Regional anticoagulation with citrate
No anticoagulation

correct ionized calcium levels has been reported to result in electrolyte imbalance and cardiac arrest (64), and an ability to monitor ionized calcium concentrations during hemodialysis is considered essential for patient safety.

Hemodialysis can also be successfully performed without anticoagulants (65,66). Higher blood flow rates and flushing the dialyzer frequently with saline help prevent clotting.

FACTORS PREVENTING ADEQUATE ANTICOAGULATION

Even when pharmacodynamic modeling individualizes heparin dosing, the results may be unsatisfactory. Dialyzer clotting or bleeding from the needle puncture sites may be persistent or occur only on isolated occasions. Reasons for an unsatisfactory outcome relate to the patient or to technical problems in therapy delivery.

Patient-Related Issues

Heparin exerts its major influence through antithrombin III. Thus, the ability of heparin to inhibit coagulation will be impaired in patients deficient in antithrombin III. Antithrombin III concentrations may be slightly decreased in hemodialysis patients (10–12), but patients with a severe antithrombin III deficiency are rare and antithrombin III deficiency is an unlikely cause of dialyzer clotting.

Intercurrent illness may change a patient's coagulation status and affect the elimination of heparin (67,68). It is advisable to measure some random clotting times in patients with an intercurrent illness such as an infection and to be prepared to temporarily increase the heparin infusion rate if these clotting times are below the target range.

Heparin can physically interact with a number of drugs (69). However, with the possible exception of nitroglycerin (70,71), there is little evidence that drugs alter the anticoagulant effect of heparin. Smoking increases the elimination rate of heparin (72), and a history of smoking was found to be a significant covariate in population pharmacodynamic models of heparin dosing in hemodialysis patients (28).

Patients treated with erythropoietin require more heparin to prevent dialyzer clotting (73,74). Whether the increased heparin requirement reflects an ability of erythropoietin to improve the hemostatic disorders of uremia (6) or is a consequence of an increased hematocrit is unclear. Whatever the reason, it may be necessary to increase the level of anticoagulation following the initiation of erythropoietin therapy.

Technical Problems in Therapy Delivery

Dialyzers sometimes clot unexpectedly in apparently stable patients, giving rise to questions about the appropriateness of their anticoagulation regimen. Usually, these isolated events result from some technical problem in the delivery of therapy rather than an inadequate heparin prescription.

As shown in Table 6.4, errors in the administration of heparin are a common problem. After administration of the heparin load-

TABLE 6.4. PROBLEMS IN THERAPY DELIVERY THAT MAY RESULT IN INADEQUATE ANTICOAGULATION OR FAILURE TO PREVENT CLOTTING OR BLEEDING

Errors in administration of the heparin dose
  Heparin doses drawn up incorrectly
  Insufficient time allowed for loading dose to distribute
  Failure to deliver the prescribed constant infusion of heparin
Problems associated with the blood circuit
  Failure to adequately prime the dialyzer
  Excessive turbulence in the arterial drip chamber
  Excessive recirculation
  Failure to rotate needle sites

From Ward RA. Heparinization for routine hemodialysis. *Adv Renal Replace Ther* 1995;2:362–370, with permission.

ing dose into the access needle, sufficient saline must be used to ensure that the complete heparin dose enters the circulation. Three to 5 minutes are required for the heparin to distribute in the plasma before extracorporeal circulation is commenced. Failure to follow these steps results in clotting as unheparinized blood enters the dialyzer during the first minutes of dialysis. Once administered, the loading dose begins to be eliminated. If the constant infusion of heparin is not started immediately, this elimination will result in a steadily decreasing clotting time.

A number of factors may prevent the timely administration of the infused heparin. The line from the heparin syringe to the blood line must be primed with heparin during the setup for dialysis to avoid infusing either saline or air during the first 30 minutes of dialysis. In addition, clamps should not be left on the line. Some heparin pumps have a maximum operating pressure. Beyond this pressure, they will not infuse accurately. Post-blood-pump pressures greater than 400 mm Hg should be avoided, particularly when high blood-flow rates are used in conjunction with high hematocrits and small-bore access needles.

Care must be taken to eliminate all air bubbles from the dialyzer during the priming process and to avoid excessive turbulence in the drip chambers during dialysis. Blood-air interfaces predispose to clotting, particularly if they are associated with turbulence and foam formation (36,75–77).

Recirculation in the vascular access may cause clotted dialyzers in the presence of apparently adequate clotting times. As blood passes through the dialyzer, ultrafiltration causes hemoconcentration. Blood of increased hematocrit then returns to the access. Recirculation results in some of this blood being returned to the dialyzer where it is concentrated further. In this manner, the hematocrit of the blood in the dialyzer progressively increases above systemic levels. In extreme circumstances, such as when the arterial access needle is inadvertently placed downstream of the venous needle and ultrafiltration rates are high, the hematocrit in the dialyzer will reach very high levels (greater than 60%), and the dialyzer will clot.

Prolonged bleeding from the access needle sites after dialysis is often blamed on excessive anticoagulation. Although the level of anticoagulation may play a role in this bleeding, mechanical problems related to venipuncture are also frequently a factor. In particular, failure to rotate needle sites with a synthetic graft will lead to destruction of the graft material and make it very difficult to stop bleeding, regardless of the level of heparin.

SUMMARY

Because of wide patient-to-patient variability, individualization of heparin dosing is necessary to reach an appropriate balance between clotting in the extracorporeal circuit and bleeding complications during hemodialysis. This goal can be achieved best by a loading dose and constant infusion of heparin, in which the doses are determined using whole blood clotting times and a pharmacodynamic model. Because the magnitude of the whole blood clotting time depends on the method of measurement, care must be taken to establish the baseline clotting time and desired therapeutic range for the particular test to be used. Despite careful pharmacodynamic modeling, the results of anticoagulation may be unsatisfactory. When this situation occurs, other aspects of therapy delivery, such as errors in heparin delivery, inadequate preparation of the dialyzer, and access dysfunction, should be considered as possible contributory factors.

REFERENCES

1. Rosenberg RD, et al. The heparin-antithrombin system: a natural anticoagulant mechanism. In: Colman RW, et al., eds. *Hemostasis and thrombosis: basic principles and clinical practice,* 3rd ed. Philadelphia: JB Lippincott, 1994:837–860.
2. Jubelirer SJ. Hemostatic abnormalities in renal disease. *Am J Kidney Dis* 1985;5:219–225.
3. Carvalho AC. Acquired platelet dysfunction in patients with uremia. *Hematol Oncol Clin North Am* 1990;4:129–143.
4. Eberst ME, et al. Hemostasis in renal disease: pathophysiology and management. *Am J Med* 1994;96:168–179.
5. Vigano G, et al. Recombinant human erythropoietin to correct uremic bleeding. *Am J Kidney Dis* 1991;18:44–49.
6. Moia M, et al. Improvement in the haemostatic defect of uraemia after treatment with recombinant human erythropoietin. *Lancet* 1987;2:1227–1229.
7. Akizawa T, et al. Effects of recombinant human erythropoietin and correction of anemia on platelet function in hemodialysis patients. *Nephron* 1991;58:400–406.
8. Zwaginga JJ, et al. Treatment of uremic anemia with recombinant erythropoietin also reduces the defects in platelet adhesion and aggregation caused by uremic plasma. *Thromb Haemost* 1991;66:638–647.
9. Mannucci PM, et al. Deamino-8-D-arginine vasopressin shortens the bleeding time in uremia. *N Engl J Med* 1983;308:8–12.
10. Nakamura Y, et al. Enhanced coagulation-fibrinolysis in patients on regular hemodialysis treatment. *Nephron* 1991;58:201–204.
11. Gris J-C, et al. Increased cardiovascular risk factors and features of endothelial activation and dysfunction in dialyzed uremic patients. *Kidney Int* 1994;46:807–813.
12. Vaziri ND, et al. Blood coagulation, fibrinolytic, and inhibitory proteins in end-stage renal disease: effect of hemodialysis. *Am J Kidney Dis* 1994;23:828–835.
13. Kario K, et al. Factor VII hyperactivity in chronic dialysis patients. *Thromb Res* 1992;67:105–113.
14. Mezzano D, et al. Hemostatic disorder of uremia: the platelet defect, main determinant of the prolonged bleeding time, is correlated with indices of activation of coagulation and fibrinolysis. *Thromb Haemost* 1996;76:312–321.
15. Uden DL, et al. The effect of heparin on three whole blood activated clotting tests and thrombin time. *ASAIO Trans* 1991;37:88–91.
16. Ward RA. Precise anticoagulation for hemodialysis: importance of whole blood coagulation time test reagent. *Dial Transplant* 1979;8:606–607.
17. Brill-Edwards P, et al. Establishing a therapeutic range for heparin therapy. *Ann Intern Med* 1993;119:104–109.
18. Wilhelmsson S, et al. Whole-blood activated coagulation time for evaluation of heparin activity during hemodialysis: a comparison of administration by single-dose and by infusion. *Clin Nephrol* 1983;19:82–86.
19. Ireland H, et al. Heparin as an anticoagulant during extracorporeal circulation. In: Lane DA, et al., eds. *Heparin: chemical and biological properties, clinical applications.* London: Edward Arnold, 1989:549–574.
20. Ward RA, et al. Prevention of blood loss in dialysers with DEAE-cellulose membranes does not require increased doses of heparin. *Nephrol Dial Transplant* 1993;8:1140–1145.
21. Farrell PC, et al. Precise anticoagulation for routine hemodialysis. *J Lab Clin Med* 1978;92:164–176.
22. Kandrotas RJ, et al. Pharmacokinetics and pharmacodynamics of heparin during hemodialysis: interpatient and intrapatient variability. *Pharmacotherapy* 1990;10:349–356.
23. Kandrotas RJ. Heparin pharmacokinetics and pharmacodynamics. *Clin Pharmacokinet* 1992;22:359–374.
24. Teien AN, et al. Heparin elimination in uraemic patients on haemodialysis. *Scand J Haematol* 1976;17:29–35.
25. Estes JW, et al. Pharmacokinetics of heparin: distribution and elimination. *Thromb Diathes Haemorrh* 1974;33:26–37.
26. de Swart CAM, et al. Kinetics of intravenously administered heparin in normal humans. *Blood* 1982;60:1251–1258.
27. Jannett TC, et al. Adaptive control of anticoagulation during hemodialysis. *Kidney Int* 1994;45:912–915.
28. Smith BP, et al. Prediction of anticoagulation during hemodialysis by population kinetics and an artificial neural network. *Artif Organs* 1998;22:731–739.
29. Ouseph R, et al. Improved dialyzer reuse after use of a population pharmacodynamic model to determine heparin doses. *Am J Kidney Dis* 2000;35:89–94.
30. Ward RA, et al. Precise heparinization for hemodialysis of nonuremic subjects. *ASAIO J* 1980;3:147–152.
31. Low CL, et al. Effect of a sliding scale protocol for heparin on the ability to maintain whole blood activated partial thromboplastin times within a desired range in hemodialysis patients. *Clin Nephrol* 1996;45:120–124.
32. Swartz RD, et al. Preventing hemorrhage in high-risk hemodialysis: regional versus low-dose heparin. *Kidney Int* 1979;16:513–518.
33. Swartz RD. Hemorrhage during high-risk hemodialysis using controlled heparinization. *Nephron* 1981;28:65–69.
34. Ward DM. Extracorporeal management of acute renal failure patients at high-risk of bleeding. *Kidney Int* 1993;43[Suppl 41]:S237–S244.
35. Gotch FA, et al. Precise control of minimal heparinization for high bleeding risk hemodialysis. *ASAIO Trans* 1977;23:168–175.
36. Ward RA, et al. Low-dose heparinization can be used with DEAE-cellulose hemodialysis membranes. *ASAIO Trans* 1990;36:M321–M324.
37. Wright MJ, et al. Low thrombogenicity of polyethylene glycol-grafted cellulose membranes does not influence heparin requirements in hemodialysis. *Am J Kidney Dis* 1999; 34:36–42.
38. Ward RA. Effects of haemodialysis on coagulation and platelets: are we measuring membrane biocompatibility? *Nephrol Dial Transplant* 1995; 10[Suppl 10]:12–17.
39. Teien AN, et al. Assay of heparin in plasma using a chromogenic substrate for activated factor X. *Thromb Res* 1976;8:413–416.
40. Grau E, et al. Low molecular weight heparin (CY-216) versus unfractionated heparin in chronic hemodialysis. *Nephron* 1992;62:13–17.
41. Simpson HK, et al. Long-term use of the low molecular weight heparin tinzaparin in haemodialysis. *Haemostasis* 1996;26:90–97.
42. Sagedal S, et al. A single dose of dalteparin effectively prevents clotting during haemodialysis. *Nephrol Dial Transplant* 1999;14:1943–1947.
43. Saltissi D, et al. Comparison of low-molecular-weight heparin (enoxaparin sodium) and standard unfractionated heparin for haemodialysis anticoagulation. *Nephrol Dial Transplant* 1999;14:2698–2703.
44. Schrader J, et al. Comparison of low molecular weight heparin to standard heparin in hemodialysis/hemofiltration. *Kidney Int* 1988;33:890–896.
45. Hafner G, et al. Laboratory control of minimal heparinization during haemodialysis in patients with a risk of haemorrhage. *Blood Coagul Fibrinolysis* 1994;5:221–226.

46. Suzuki T, et al. Clinical application of Fragmin (FR-860) in hemodialysis: multicenter cooperative study in Japan. *Semin Thromb Hemost* 1990;16[Suppl]:46–54.
47. Deuber HJ, et al. Reduced lipid concentrations during four years of dialysis with low molecular weight heparin. *Kidney Int* 1991;40:496–500.
48. Kronenberg F, et al. Influence of various heparin preparations on lipoproteins in hemodialysis patients: a multicenter study. *Thromb Haemost* 1995;74:1025–1028.
49. Greinacher A, et al. Heparin-associated thrombocytopenia: the antibody is not heparin specific. *Thromb Haemost* 1992;67:545–549.
50. Magnani HN. Heparin-induced thrombocytopenia (HIT): an overview of 230 patients treated with Orgaran (ORG 10172). *Thromb Haemost* 1993;70:554–561.
51. Ramakrishna R, et al. Heparin-induced thrombocytopenia: cross-reactivity between standard heparin, low molecular weight heparin, dalteparin (Fragmin) and heparinoid, danaparoid (Organon). *Br J Haematol* 1995;91:736–738.
52. Wilde MI, et al. Danaparoid: a review of its pharmacology and its clinical use in the management of heparin-induced thrombocytopenia. *Drugs* 1997;54:903–924.
53. Rowlings PA, et al. The use of low molecular weight heparinoid (Org 10172) for extracorporeal procedures in patients with heparin dependent thrombocytopenia and thrombosis. *Aust N Z J Med* 1991;21:52–54.
54. Henny CP, et al. The effectiveness of a low molecular weight heparinoid in chronic intermittent hemodialysis. *Thromb Haemost* 1985;54:460–462.
55. Polkinghorne KR, et al. Pharmacokinetic studies of dalteparin (Fragmin), enoxaparin (Clexane), and danaparoid sodium (Orgaran) in stable chronic hemodialysis patients. *Am J Kidney Dis* 2002;40:990–995.
56. Pinnick RV, et al. Regional citrate anticoagulation for hemodialysis in the patient at high risk for bleeding. *N Engl J Med* 1983;308:258–261.
57. Von Brecht JH, et al. Regional anticoagulation: hemodialysis with hypertonic trisodium citrate. *Am J Kidney Dis* 1986;8:196–201.
58. Flanigan MJ, et al. Regional hemodialysis anticoagulation: hypertonic tri-sodium citrate or anticoagulant citrate dextrose-A. *Am J Kidney Dis* 1996;27:519–524.
59. Evenepoel P, et al. Regional citrate anticoagulation for hemodialysis using a conventional calcium-containing dialysate. *Am J Kidney Dis* 2002;39:315–323.
60. Apsner R, et al. Simplified citrate anticoagulation for high-flux hemodialysis. *Am J Kidney Dis* 2001;38:979–987.
61. Kelleher SP, et al. Severe metabolic alkalosis complicating regional citrate hemodialysis. *Am J Kidney Dis* 1987;9:235–236.
62. Silverstein FJ, et al. Metabolic alkalosis induced by regional citrate hemodialysis. *ASAIO Trans* 1989;35:22–25.
63. Van der Meulen J, et al. Citrate anticoagulation and dialysate with reduced buffer content in chronic hemodialysis. *Clin Nephrol* 1992;37:36–41.
64. Charney DI, et al. Cardiac arrest after hypertonic citrate anticoagulation for chronic hemodialysis. *ASAIO Trans* 1990;36:M217–M219.
65. Sanders PW, et al. Hemodialysis without anticoagulation. *Am J Kidney Dis* 1985;5:32–35.
66. Schwab SJ, et al. Hemodialysis without anticoagulation: one-year prospective trial in hospitalized patients at risk for bleeding. *Am J Med* 1987;83:405–410.
67. Farrell PC, et al. Precise anticoagulation during coronary care management. *ASAIO J* 1979;8:71(abst).
68. Hirsh J, et al. Heparin kinetics in venous thrombosis and pulmonary embolism. *Circulation* 1976;53:691–695.
69. Colburn WA. Pharmacologic implications of heparin interactions with other drugs. *Drug Metab Rev* 1976;5:281–293.
70. Pizzulli L, et al. Nitroglycerin inhibition of the heparin effect. *Dtsch med Wschr* 1988;113:1837–1840.
71. Bode V, et al. Absence of drug interaction between heparin and nitroglycerin: randomized placebo-controlled crossover study. *Arch Intern Med* 1990;150:2117–2119.
72. Cipolle RJ, et al. Heparin kinetics: variables related to disposition and dosage. *Clin Pharmacol Ther* 1981;29:387–393.
73. Spinowitz BS, et al. Impact of epoetin beta on dialyzer clearance and heparin requirements. *Am J Kidney Dis* 1991;18:668–673.
74. Veys N, et al. Influence of erythropoietin on dialyzer reuse, heparin need, and urea kinetics in maintenance hemodialysis patients. *Am J Kidney Dis* 1994;23:52–59.
75. Osada H, et al. Microbubble elimination during priming improves biocompatibility of membrane oxygenators. *Am J Physiol* 1978;234:H646–H652.
76. Keller F, et al. Risk factors of system clotting in heparin-free haemodialysis. *Nephrol Dial Transplant* 1990;5:802–807.
77. Sperschneider H, et al. Impact of membrane choice and blood flow pattern on coagulation and heparin requirement—potential consequences on lipid concentrations. *Nephrol Dial Transplant* 1997;12:2638–2646.

APPROACH TO HEMODIALYSIS KINETIC MODELING

VICTORIA A. KUMAR AND THOMAS A. DEPNER

HISTORICAL PERSPECTIVE

Hemodialysis was first used to sustain life in patients with acute renal failure during the 1940s. Despite many shortcomings and initial failures it was clear that life could be prolonged when previously death from uremia was certain. When it was first used to sustain life in patients with end-stage renal disease (ESRD) during the 1960s, the frequency and intensity of treatments were limited by availability and by adverse reactions. Early in the development, limited membrane permeability and patient intolerance of high blood flows necessitated prolonged treatments often of 8 or 10 hours.

In the late 1970s a National Cooperative Dialysis Study (NCDS) sponsored by the U.S. National Institutes of Health (NIH) showed that a minimum clearance per dialysis was required (1–3). This represented a change from the previous reliance on solute levels and shifted the focus from dialyzer surface area to solute clearance (4). Tolerance of dialysis improved as membranes were made more permeable, bicarbonate was substituted for acetate in the dialysate, and better control of fluid removal was achieved. Tolerance was also aided by the reversal of severe anemia afforded by recombinant erythropoietin and by improved biocompatibility of dialysis membranes permitting increased solute flux and shortening of the dialysis treatment—a goal sought by many, especially the patients (5,6).

Over the past 15 years concerns have been raised about unacceptably high mortality rates in patients maintained with hemodialysis in the United States compared with other countries, causing the focus to turn to prescribing practices and reimbursement (7–10). As a result, the practice of quantifying dialysis by estimating solute removal has moved from the realm of scientific curiosity to acceptance by the dialysis community and then to a mandated requirement by dialysis sponsors.

This chapter reviews what is known about urea modeling—how to implement it and how to interpret the patient-specific parameters that it provides. Definitions of the symbols used throughout this chapter and their common units of measurement are displayed in Table 7.1.

UREA, A MARKER FOR CLEARANCE AND PROTEIN CATABOLISM

Table 7.2 lists the properties that qualify urea as an indicator of dialysis efficiency and adequacy. Urea is the most abundant organic solute to accumulate in patients with renal failure, so its concentration is usually high and relatively easy to measure. Urea is easily dialyzed across synthetic extracorporeal membranes primarily because of its small molecular size; it moves easily across living membranes along preestablished pathways for facilitated transport (e.g., in red cells) (11–16). Because it diffuses easily, measurement of clearance across dialysis membranes is a sensitive index of solute removal, a fundamental goal of dialysis.

Measurement of urea generation is an index of protein catabolism which, in stable patients, reflects protein intake and can provide assistance with dietary management. A relatively precise relationship between urea generation and protein catabolism was found several years ago in two separate metabolic studies of a small number of dialyzed and nondialyzed patients (17,18). Both studies showed essentially the same result.

$$nPCR = 5,420 \times G/V + 0.17 \text{ (18)} \qquad [1]$$

where G is the urea nitrogen generation rate (mg/minute), nPCR is the normalized protein catabolic rate (g/kg/day), and V is the urea distribution volume (mL).

Protein catabolism is expressed per kilogram of ideal or normalized body weight. The latter is derived from V, assuming that V is 58% of body weight.

Paradoxically, patients with low urea generation rates have poorer outcomes. Reduced protein-derived urea generation results from poor nutritional intake. Suppression of the appetite can be caused either by inadequate dialysis or comorbid diseases such as infection or cardiovascular complications, the leading causes of death in ESRD (2,3,19,20). This means that urea levels in the patient are difficult to interpret. Decreases resulting from dialysis are beneficial, whereas decreases because of poor nutrition are harmful. Attempts to demonstrate a toxic effect of urea have led to the conclusion that urea is at best a mild toxin (21–23). Other easily dialyzed

TABLE 7.1. SYMBOLS USED IN THIS CHAPTER

Symbol	Units of Measure	Definition
B	mL/min	Fluid gain (loss) between (during) dialyses
BUN	mg/mL, mg/dL	Blood urea nitrogen concentration
BW	any units	Body weight
C	mg/mL	Concentration (e.g., of urea or urea N)
CAPD	NA	Continuous ambulatory peritoneal dialysis
C_{Av}	mg/mL	Average concentration
C_0	mg/mL	Initial (predialysis) concentration
C_1	mg/mL	Concentration in the proximal compartment
C_2	mg/mL	Concentration in the remote compartment
C_D	mg/mL	Concentration in the dialysate
C_E	mg/mL	Postdialysis concentration after equilibration
C_i	mg/mL	Concentration in blood entering the dialyzer
C_S	mg/mL	Concentration in systemic blood
C_T	mg/mL	Concentration at time T
e	none	Natural logarithm base (2.718)
eKt/V	fraction per dialysis	equilibrated Kt/V
F_{CPR}	fraction	Fractional cardiopulmonary recirculation
G	mg/min	Urea generation rate
K	mL/min	Total urea clearance
k	/min	Solute elimination (rate) constant
K_0A	mL/min	Mass transfer area coefficient
Kt/V	fraction per dialysis	Fractional clearance index for urea
K_C	mL/min	Intercompartment mass-transfer area coefficient
K_D	mL/min	Dialyzer urea clearance
K_R	mL/min	Residual (native kidney) urea clearance
1n	none	Natural logarithm
nPCR	g/kg/day	Protein catabolic rate normalized to V
Q_B	mL/min	Dialyzer blood flow
Q_D	mL/min	Dialysate flow
Q_F	mL/min	Ultrafiltration rate during dialysis
QS	mL/min	Systemic blood flow (CO minus access flow)
R	fraction per dialysis	Postdialysis BUN/predialysis BUN
RG	mg	Correction factor for K_R and urea generation
t	min	Time
TAC	mg/mL, mg/dL	Time-averaged BUN
t_i	min	Time interval between two dialyses
UF	liters/ dialysis	Ultrafiltrate volume
URR	fraction per dialysis	Urea reduction ratio $(C_1 - C_2)/C_1$
V_0	mL, liters	Predialysis volume of urea distribution
V, V_D, V_T	mL, liters	Postdialysis volume of urea distribution
ΔV	mL, liters	Change in V during dialysis
V_1	mL, liters	Volume of the proximal (dialyzed) compartment
V_2	mL, liters	Volume of the remote compartment
W	kg	Patient weight
ΔWt	fraction/ dialysis	Fractional weight loss during dialysis

CO, cardiac output; NA, not applicable.

TABLE 7.2. PROPERTIES OF UREA THAT AFFECT KINETIC MODELING

Most abundant of organic solutes that accumulate in renal failure
Distribution volume is total body water
Easily dialyzed
   Molecular weight = 60 daltons
   Polar, water soluble
   Uncharged
Source
   Produced by the liver
   End-product of protein nitrogen metabolism
Transport
   Passive diffusion in vitro and in vivo
   Facilitated diffusion in vivo
Relatively nontoxic

solutes must be responsible for the uremic syndrome, much more so than urea. Alternatively, an indirect effect of urea such as carbamylation of protein may mediate its toxicity (24–27).

An inescapable conclusion from these observations, and one that guides the clinical application of urea modeling today, is that urea is a poor marker of uremia but a good marker of dialysis. Frequent measurements of urea concentration before and following dialysis, when combined with an appropriate model of urea kinetics, provide vital clinical information about both the adequacy of dialysis and the nutritional status of the patient.

FACTORS THAT DETERMINE THE REQUIREMENT FOR DIALYSIS

Several patient-specific factors that determine how much dialysis is needed are listed in Table 7.3. These include the patient's size (body water volume), residual urea clearance, and fluid gain between dialyses. Another factor that may dictate the need for more dialysis is pregnancy (28,29).

TABLE 7.3. HEMODIALYSIS PRESCRIPTION COMPONENTS

Patient Variables
Urea distribution volume (total body water)
Urea generation rate from protein catabolism
Residual (native kidney) urea clearance
Fluid accumulation
Solute compartmentalization
Center-controlled variables
Dialysis Variables
Dialyzer clearance components
   Model of dialyzer (urea mass-transfer-area coefficient)
   Blood flow
   Dialysate flow
Duration of dialysis
Schedule or frequency of dialysis

Protein Catabolism

Adjusting the dose to the urea generation rate has been considered less important in recent years because of the emphasis on higher minimum doses of dialysis (30–32). The higher doses have caused mean urea concentrations to fall below the safe ceiling that was suggested by the NCDS; thus, the additional adjustment of the dose for urea generation is less critical and is usually unnecessary (3). In addition, there is increasing evidence that nutrition has a strong influence on patient outcome; thus, the emphasis has shifted from restricting protein to encouraging more protein and caloric intake (33–35). The United States Multicentered Modification of Diet in Renal Disease (MDRD) study also raised concerns about protein restriction adversely influencing survival of patients approaching end-stage (36,37).

Several investigators have reported a correlation between nPCR and the dose of dialysis expressed as Kt/V suggesting that increasing the dose of dialysis will improve the appetite (38–41). This conclusion is subject to error for several reasons. First, if the dose of dialysis is not strictly controlled by urea modeling, physicians may simply give more dialysis to patients with high protein intake, creating a correlation that reflects a physician response to appetite rather than vice versa. Second, both nPCR and Kt/V are determined from the same set of blood urea nitrogen (BUN) values (see later); thus, an artifactual mathematical correlation resulting from coupling is expected, the magnitude of which depends on the total error in the BUN measurements (42,43). Third, as pointed out by Nolph and others, the real correlation is probably curvilinear with a plateau effect above a certain dose breakpoint; thus, comparing two populations with different Kt/V doses may falsely exaggerate the effect of increasing Kt/V above the breakpoint (39,44).

Residual Native Kidney Clearance

Seemingly insignificant levels of residual urea clearance (e.g., 1 or 2 mL/min) can markedly decrease the need for dialysis, but most nephrologists do not compensate for residual function by decreasing the dialysis dose. Reasons for omitting this practice include the inconvenience and expense associated with collecting and measuring urine and calculating the residual clearance, and the common negative psychologic effect on the patient from subsequent increases in the dialysis dose (usually translated to prolonging time on dialysis) as native kidney function inevitably declines.

Body Size

Body size is an obvious modulator of dialysis need, but the precise denominator to use as an index of size is debated (45,46). The urea distribution volume, equated to total body water, is a mathematically convenient denominator but it may not be appropriate, especially when body surface area has been used for several decades to normalize the native creatinine or inulin clearance (47). The concentration of uremic toxins in body fluids is thought to modulate toxicity and, therefore, the need for dialysis, but for first-order processes the concentration is a function of generation and removal and does not depend on the space of

distribution. For a patient whose clearance (K) is constant, and whose toxin generation rate (G) is equal to the removal rate, changes in the volume of distribution (V) have no effect on concentration in the steady state (C = G/K). For example, an increase in V from edema formation or a decline in V from muscle loss would not affect toxin concentrations if all else is constant. Instead, the toxin generation rate is the factor that determines concentration and toxicity and is, therefore, the most logical variable to which the dose should be normalized in patients of differing size. It is unlikely that edema fluid is a source of uremic toxins and recent theory suggests that muscle is also an unlikely source (48,49). Unfortunately, because the critical toxic compounds have not been identified, the precise relationship between their generation rates and body size remains speculative.

Reanalysis of NCDS data in terms of Kt/V instead of urea concentration suggested that morbidity and mortality increased sharply as Kt/V fell below a threshold of 0.8 (3). As a result, dialysis therapy was deemed adequate when clearance × time per dialysis equaled total body water (TBW or V). Here V serves as a surrogate for body mass that correlates with toxin generation but there are concerns about this association as noted previously. Use of V as a normalizing denominator for dose was additionally confounded by the discovery that V independently predicts and correlates positively with survival (50–52). Patients with lower body mass have both a higher Kt/V and a higher mortality risk. African Americans with ESRD tend to have a higher body mass and both a lower Kt/V and a lower mortality risk (53,54). These paradoxical effects of V have led some to recommend using the product of clearance and treatment time (Kt) as the index of dose instead of Kt/V (50). However, to do so ignores the obvious requirement for lower clearances in smaller patients, especially pediatric patients or much smaller animals (elephant vs. mouse argument). The notion that all patients require the same dose of dialysis regardless of body mass is both counterintuitive and contradictory to the standards for prescription of most therapies. Larger patients have higher solute generation rates and require more clearance than smaller patients to achieve the same blood concentration. The higher risk of mortality in smaller dialysis patients may result from malnutrition instead of underdialysis. Although malnutrition alone portends a poor prognosis in the dialysis patient, it can also result from comorbid conditions including inflammatory states that may independently affect survival (55).

Table 7.3 also lists fluid accumulation between dialyses as a component of the dialysis prescription. Although it increases the requirement for fluid removal during each treatment, fluid accumulation actually decreases the need for dialysis both because of a dilution effect and because removing fluid during hemodialysis increases the efficiency of solute removal (56).

Prescribed Compared to Delivered Dose

The dialysis center controls the amount of dialysis provided by manipulating the center-controllable variables (listed in Table 7.3). Although it is helpful to be able to measure each of these parameters precisely, standard urea kinetic modeling gives a retrospective estimate of the amount of dialysis delivered to the patient without the need for measuring the prescribed dialyzer clearance, flow rates, or even treatment time. This closes the loop of quality control by allowing a comparison between the amount of dialysis prescribed and that actually delivered (57). How urea modeling accomplishes this is explained in more detail in the following.

TARGETING THE AMOUNT OF DIALYSIS

How to Measure Dialysis: How Much Is Enough?

The amount of dialysis required to keep patients healthy and relatively symptom-free is probably greater than the amount required to keep them alive for a year. The morbidity experienced by patients enrolled in the NCDS demonstrated the importance of controlling average urea concentrations and it also showed that measuring and controlling the urea concentration was not enough (2,58). A statistical analysis of the NCDS data showed that patient outcome correlated best with the time-averaged concentration (TAC) of BUN; it also correlated strongly with protein catabolism (nPCR) (2). Putting these two findings together in a later mechanistic analysis of the data the investigators showed that providing a minimum amount of dialysis—expressed as a clearance of urea per dialysis—factored for patient size (Kt/V) would ensure the best outcome (3).

The relationships among time-averaged BUN, Kt/V, and nPCR are shown in Fig. 7.1. The "safe zone" is shown in the heavy line representing the isopleth for a Kt/V of 1.2 per dialysis. The curvilinear surface represents the mathematical relationship among the three variables TAC, nPCR, and Kt/V, for patients dialyzed three times weekly. Note that only two of the three variables are required to find a point on the surface plot, which means that the three variables are mathematically interdependent and that arguments favoring one as more accurate

than another are trivial. Note also that Kt/V is specifically given for dialysis three times weekly. For twice weekly or another schedule, the Kt/V axis must be changed.

The NCDS showed that to achieve optimal patient outcome one must guarantee that the dose of dialysis delivered to each patient (Kt/V) is constant and relatively independent of BUN (2,3). These findings reflect the failure of the serum urea concentration as an indicator of both dialysis adequacy and uremia. This should not be surprising to nephrologists, who have long held a double-standard interpretation of the BUN in patients who do not yet require dialysis. The BUN has been considered important to measure, but when the patient is symptomatic and the BUN is low, it is ignored (58). Some patients have died a uremic death with a BUN as low as 50 mg/dL. Clearly, dialyzable toxins other than urea account for a major part if not all of the uremic syndrome; thus, control of urea concentration is not enough to guarantee adequate dialysis (21–23,59).

A safety net, expressed as Kt/V, guarantees that each patient will receive a minimum amount of dialysis, relatively independent of BUN levels and protein catabolism. If the patient is not improving or is failing for unknown reasons, it behooves the nephrologist to increase the dose of dialysis unless he or she is confident that the dose is already well above the level currently considered a safe minimum. This recommendation acknowledges our current inability to define the uremic state more precisely, our ignorance of factors that may mediate individual requirements for dialysis and our concerns, based on historical data, about the contribution of protein catabolism to uremia (60–64).

Interpreting Kt/V: Limitations

The term KtV describes the fractional clearance of urea during a single hemodialysis. The fraction can be greater than one because blood flow recirculates during hemodialysis, diluting the concentration gradient and allowing the body water compartment to be dialyzed more than once during a single treatment. Because the BUN falls during a single hemodialysis, removal of urea also falls and would eventually fall to zero, effectively extinguishing the dialysis even though clearance remains constant. This self-limiting or self-defeating aspect of intermittent hemodialysis is important to recognize when expressing the dose as Kt/V.

Modeled Kt/V is a measure of the amount or dose of dialysis received by the patient, and it correlates with outcome; however, the expected correlation is nonlinear, as demonstrated by the NCDS and other outcome studies (2,3,65,66). Part of the reason for this nonlinearity is the curvilinear relationship between solute removal and Kt/V as shown in Fig. 7.2. Once the dose reaches a minimum standard, increasing Kt/V further does not necessarily improve outcome. Kt/V is not a direct measure of outcome or the effectiveness of the dose but is simply a stopgap method of assuring dialysis adequacy in the absence of knowledge about the critical toxins removed. Because dialysis is a self-limiting process, the amount of solute removed diminishes exponentially as the amount of dialysis is increased. In other words, doubling Kt/V does not double the amount of solute removed and may accomplish very little if the critical solutes

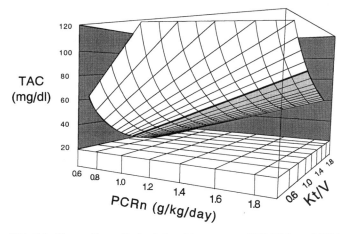

FIG. 7.1. The mathematical relationships among nPCR, TAC, and Kt/V form a curvilinear plane in three dimensions. Lines running diagonally across the plane are Kt/V isopleths; the line at $Kt/V = 1.2$ represents the currently accepted minimum standard, and the region of the plane below this is the "safe" domain. Data were derived from the single-compartment model; all scales are linear.

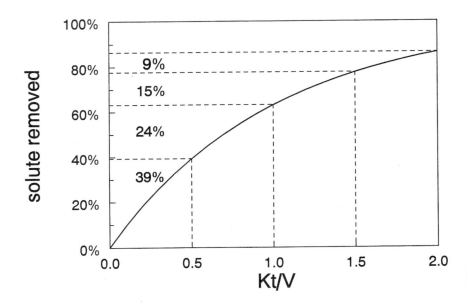

FIG. 7.2. For each increment in *Kt/V* the removal rate falls and will ultimately plateau. Further increases in *Kt/V* beyond the break in the plateau for this particular solute afford no benefit to the patient.

have already fallen to low levels or disequilibrium prevents further solute removal.

SINGLE-COMPARTMENT KINETIC MODELING

Clearance, a Better Measure of Dialysis

The clearance concept is intuitive but its precise definition, origin, and application often escape nephrologists and even physiologists. It is probably best understood as a measure of the elimination process unencumbered by other variables. The solute removal rate is itself a measure of elimination but for both filtration and dialysis the rate is a linear function of the concentration. Expressing the elimination process as a clearance takes the effect of concentration out of the rate term.

$$\text{Clearance} = (\text{removal rate})/\text{concentration}$$

Because the removal rate is directly proportional to the concentration, clearance is constant over a wide range of concentrations and removal rates, an effective measure of the elimination process unencumbered by these two variables.

When the removal rate is proportional to the concentration, the process is called "first order," meaning that the removal rate is proportional to the first power of the concentration. In comparison, for zero-order processes the removal rate is constant, independent of the concentration (e.g., urea generation by the liver). For both the native kidney and dialysis, a generalized equation for a first-order process is

$$dC/dt = -kC \qquad [2]$$

where C is the solute concentration at any time (t) and k is the elimination constant expressed as a fraction per unit of time.

Rearranging Eq. 2 and multiplying by the volume of solute distribution (V), clearance is defined as

$$dCV/dt/C = -kV \qquad [3]$$

where dCV/dt is the solute removal rate and kV is the clearance.

Because the removal rate divided by concentration is a flow, clearance is often described as the flow equivalent to complete removal of the solute. This definition is intuitive but it bypasses the previous steps in the derivation of the clearance concept. Clearance is a useful expression only for first-order processes. We do not calculate the clearance of sodium, for example, a non-first-order process.

Determinants of dialyzer clearance include the flow rates of blood and dialysate and properties of the membrane, primarily its size, permeability, and geometry. Similar to the clearance concept, these encumbering variables in the elimination expression can be removed mathematically by expressing elimination as a mass transfer coefficient (67).

$$K_0A = \frac{Q_B \cdot Q_D}{Q_B - Q_D} \ln\left(\frac{Q_B\,(Q_D - K_D)}{Q_B\,(Q_D - K_D)}\right) \qquad [4]$$

where K_0A is the mass transfer area coefficient, Q_B is the blood flow rate, Q_D is the dialysate flow rate, and K_D is the dialyzer clearance.

The mass transfer coefficient, sometimes called the dialyzer intrinsic clearance, is also expressed as a flow that can be considered the maximum clearance possible at infinite flow rates for the particular dialyzer model. A rearrangement of Eq. 4 has practical value for determining the prescribed dialyzer clearance from the machine settings of blood and dialysate flow and is a vital input parameter during the kinetic modeling process described later.

Three-BUN Method

Because removal of urea by the dialyzer is a first-order process, the rate of removal is expressed mathematically in Eq. 2. Integration of this simple equation gives a familiar expression that describes the removal of drugs by a single exponential process (68).

$$C = C_0 e^{-kt} \qquad [5]$$

where C_0 is the initial urea concentration and e is the base for natural logarithms (2.718).

The rate of elimination falls with time because the concentration falls with time; that is, the process eventually extinguishes itself. However, the fractional change in concentration, $(dC/C)/dt$, is constant ($-k$) and can be determined simply by measuring two timed concentrations, C_0 and C.

$$\ln (C_0/C) = kt \qquad [6]$$

where t is the time interval between measurements of C_0 and C. When the fractional removal rate (k) is multiplied by the urea volume of distribution (V), the result is a clearance (K).

$$K = kV \text{ or } k = K/V \qquad [7]$$

By substituting Eq. 7 into Eq. 6 and rearranging, another familiar expression appears.

$$Kt/V = \ln (C_0/C) \qquad [8]$$

This equation shows that the log ratio of the starting urea concentration (C_0) to the ending concentration (C) can be used as an index of the amount of dialysis delivered, circumventing the necessity for measuring each of the three components of the expression Kt/V. Fig. 7.3 shows the relationship between time and C expressed as BUN on a linear scale to the left and on a logarithmic scale to the right [69]. The slope of the logarithmic line is $-k$ or $-K/V$. Note that this simplified graphic analysis of urea kinetics gives the *ratio* of clearance to urea volume (K/V). To resolve K, V must be determined independently and vice versa. Note also that the absolute values for C_0 and C are not important; their relative values determine Kt/V. For example, if the BUN falls from 150 to 75 mg/dL or from 50 to 25 mg/dL

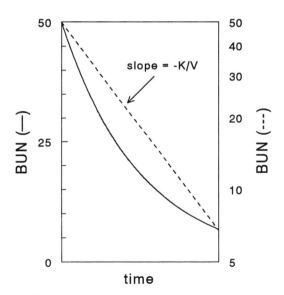

FIG. 7.3. Blood urea nitrogen (BUN) falls logarithmically during hemodialysis treatments. The slope of the log decline (right axis) is $-K/V$. K is total urea clearance, and V is the volume of urea distribution. (Adapted from Depner TA. Quantification of dialysis: urea modeling—the basics. *Semin Dial* 1991;4:179–184, with permission.)

during dialysis, Kt/V is the same. Because Kt/V is determined from BUN measurements in the patient, it is a patient-specific parameter, not a machine parameter; Kt/V is a measure of response to dialysis rather than a measure of the amount of dialysis prescribed [70].

Urea generation in milligrams is the product of the change in urea concentration between dialyses in milligrams per milliliter multiplied by the urea volume in milliliters. Because the nPCR is factored for patient volume (Eq. 1), net protein catabolism can be determined from changes in BUN between dialyses, provided there is no residual renal function or volume changes [70,71].

$$nPCR = 5,420 \,((C'_0 - C_T)/t_i) + 0.17 \qquad [9]$$

where nPCR is the normalized protein catabolic rate (g/kg body wt/day), C'_0 is the second predialysis BUN (mg/mL), C_T is the postdialysis BUN (mg/mL), and t_i is the time interval between dialyses (min).

It is important to note that the simplifications included in Eqs. 5 through 9 help illustrate fundamental relationships but preclude their use in the clinical setting. These equations should not be used to model urea kinetics in patients because they fail to include several important patient variables already mentioned, the most important of which are residual urea clearance and the change in body fluid content during and between dialyses. Both factors lower the predialysis BUN and reduce the required change in BUN during dialysis, complicating the computation of nPCR. A third parameter that has a slight but significant effect on Kt/V and V is the amount of urea generated during dialysis. A more precise mathematical expression of urea concentrations during dialysis includes these additional three parameters.

$$d(VC)/dt = G - (K_D + K_R)C \qquad [10]$$

where V is the volume of urea distribution, G is the urea generation rate (presumed constant), K_D is the dialyzer urea clearance, and K_R is the patient's residual urea clearance.

Integration of Eq. 10 gives a better, although more complex, expression of urea concentration during and between dialyses [56,72].

$$C = C_0 \left(\frac{V_0 + Bt}{V_0}\right)^{-\left(\frac{K+B}{B}\right)} + \left(\frac{G}{K+B}\right)\left(1 - \left(\frac{V_0 + Bt}{V_0}\right)^{-\left(\frac{K+B}{B}\right)}\right) \qquad [11]$$

where V_0 is the volume of urea distribution before dialysis, K during dialysis is the sum of $K_D + K_R$, K between dialyses is K_R, and B is the rate of fluid gain between or during dialyses (negative during).

Equation 11 describes single-compartment variable-volume urea kinetics and can generate a more accurate profile of BUN versus time, such as that shown in Fig. 7.4.

Kt/V is derived primarily from the fall in BUN during a single dialysis, and nPCR is determined primarily from the change in BUN between dialyses, as indicated in Fig. 7.4. To measure nPCR, the third BUN can be omitted; a technique for accomplishing this is described later.

Total protein catabolism exceeds nPCR, often by several fold [73]. Protein breakdown releases free amino acids that are mostly reincorporated into new protein. This anabolic resynthe-

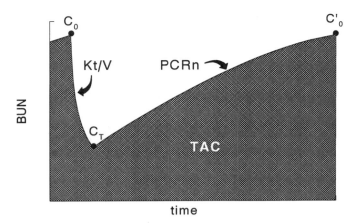

FIG. 7.4. Single-pool blood urea nitrogen (BUN) profile. *Kt/V* is derived from the fall in BUN during dialysis, nPCR from the rise between dialyses, and time-averaged concentration BUN from the shaded area under the curve. The rise from C_T to C'_0 is nonlinear when fluid is gained and/or when significant residual function exists. (Adapted from Hakim RM, et al. In depth review: adequacy of hemodialysis. *Am J Kidney Dis* 1992;20:107–123, with permission.)

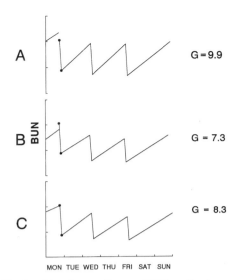

FIG. 7.5. The two-blood urea nitrogen (BUN) method approximates G using a trial-and-error approach. **A:** G is too high, predicting an inordinately high predialysis BUN 1 week later. **B:** G is too low. The computer reproduces the BUN/time profile using different values for G until the calculated predialysis BUN 1 week later matches the measured BUN (as in **C**). (From Depner TA, et al. Modeling urea kinetics with two vs. three BUN measurements: a critical comparison. *ASAOI Trans* 1989;35:499–502, with permission.)

sis of protein is a large fraction of the total catabolic rate, the difference representing a smaller net rate of irreversible nitrogen loss from breakdown of amino acids to urea (74). Thus, nPCR determined from urea modeling is a measure of *net protein catabolism*. Net protein catabolism is equal to protein intake in stable patients who are in nitrogen balance.

Two-BUN Method

As illustrated in Fig. 7.4, nPCR is derived mainly from the change in BUN between dialyses, implying that a third BUN is necessary to complete the modeling process. When nPCR is determined from a postdialysis BUN and a subsequent predialysis BUN, only the difference between these values enters into the calculation (Eq. 9); their absolute values are ignored (69). Similarly *Kt/V* is derived mainly from the ratio of predialysis to postdialysis BUN (Eq. 8). If the absolute values of the predialysis and postdialysis BUN are also included in the calculations, the third BUN measurement can be eliminated (56,58,75). This simplifies the urea modeling process without detracting from its accuracy.

The technique for resolving G from only two BUN measurements is shown in Fig. 7.5. The method requires a weekly steady state of nitrogen balance—that is, a constant dialysis prescription and a constant dietary nitrogen intake from day to day for at least a week (three dialyses). Naturally, protein intake varies widely from day to day in most people. Paradoxically, the two-BUN technique for measuring nPCR is less influenced by a dietary binge than is the three-BUN method, because the absolute value of the predialysis BUN (the major determinant of nPCR) is determined by more than a single interdialysis interval (75). The two-BUN method also offers the patient less opportunity to influence the result by altering his or her diet during the interval between the second and third blood samplings. However, even when nPCR is carefully measured, the variance is at least twice that of *Kt/V*.

How to Implement Single-Compartment Modeling with Two BUNs

The single-compartment, variable-volume model is the most commonly applied clinical tool for quantifying hemodialysis. Two of the modeling assumptions, single-pool distribution during dialysis and absence of rebound, cause errors that are offsetting (see section on comparison with the single-compartment model that follows); thus, the final calculations of V and *Kt/V* closely match those of more complex models (76).

The only two unknown variables in Eq. 11 are G and V; K is measurable and is required to start the modeling process. As shown later, the value chosen for K need not be precisely accurate to determine *Kt/V*. To start the modeling process, arbitrary values for G and V are chosen and the predialysis BUN is substituted for C_0 in Eq. 11. V is then adjusted until the calculated value for C matches the measured postdialysis BUN using a repetitive (iterative) approach. Then the postdialysis BUN is substituted for C_0 in Eq. 11, and G is adjusted until C matches the predialysis BUN, using the technique described in Fig. 7.5 for two-BUN modeling. The iterations are then repeated with the new values for G and V. The accuracy of V and G will depend on the accuracy of the chosen value for K, but K/V and G/V will be affected little by inaccuracies in K or V. nPCR can be calculated from G/V using Eq. 1, and *Kt/V* is the product of K and t divided by V. K between dialyses consists of K_R only. Care should be taken to adjust B for changing interdialysis intervals.

This entire mathematical process can be easily automated with a computer, the slowest of which usually requires less than 1 second to complete the calculations. The computer will quickly show that the values chosen for K and t have relatively little effect on the final calculated value of *Kt/V*.

MULTIPLE-COMPARTMENT KINETIC MODELING

As the intensity of hemodialysis is increased and time is shortened, the potential for development of solute concentration gradients, called *solute disequilibrium,* increases. Evidence that disequilibrium develops during hemodialysis derives mainly from the rebound in solute concentration following dialysis (76,77). Even urea, which is a highly diffusible solute, has an easily detected rebound, indicating that the simple, single-compartment model has shortcomings. Fig. 7.6 shows a series of BUN measurements in a patient undergoing high-flux hemodialysis. The dashed line, representing the best fit of a single-compartment model, misses the data points by a significant margin, especially early in the treatment and immediately following dialysis.

Two kinds of solute disequilibrium have been described: diffusion-dependent disequilibrium and flow-dependent disequilibrium; both reduce the effectiveness of hemodialysis.

Diffusion-Dependent Disequilibrium

Diffusion-dependent disequilibrium is the type of disequilibrium described by the classic two-compartment model and at one time was thought to be the only type of disequilibrium (78). The classic model, which is described in detail later, is patterned after the extracellular and intracellular separation of body water compartments where the primary resistance to diffusion is located at the cell membrane (Fig. 7.7). This type of disequilibrium is also called "membrane dependent" and is analogous to the membrane-dependent resistance to diffusion in the extracorporeal dialyzer.

The Classic Two-Compartment Diffusion Model of Urea Kinetics

To improve the agreement of modeled predictions with the actual data, an additional compartment can be added as shown

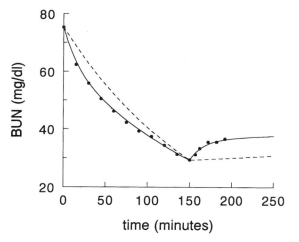

FIG. 7.6. A two-compartment model *(solid line)* predicts the blood urea nitrogen (BUN) values *(solid dots)* measured in a patient during and following high-flux hemodialysis. A single-compartment variable-volume model *(dashed line)* overestimates the BUN during dialysis and fails to predict the rebound postdialysis. (From Depner TA. Refining the model of urea kinetics: compartment effects. *Semin Dial* 1992;5:147–154, with permission.)

Two compartments, variable V$_1$

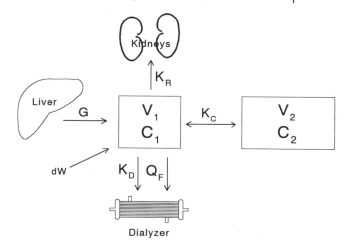

FIG. 7.7. Two-compartment variable-volume diffusion model. A mass-balance diagram of urea kinetics assuming two compartments, V$_1$ and V$_2$. The rate of intercompartment urea transfer is expressed as K$_C$, a mass transfer area coefficient. K$_R$ is residual native kidney clearance of urea, K$_D$ is dialyzer clearance, Q$_F$ is ultrafiltration during dialysis, and dW is fluid gain between dialyses. (Adapted from Depner TA. *Prescribing hemodialysis: a guide to urea modeling.* Boston: Kluwer Academic, 1991, with permission.)

in Fig. 7.7 (76,78). The two compartments, V$_1$ that equilibrates with the dialyzer and V$_2$, are separated by a resistance to diffusion that limits urea flux. The resistance is represented as K$_C$, the intercompartment mass transfer area coefficient, a permeability factor that correlates positively with the membrane surface area and inversely with resistance to diffusion between compartments. Addition of another compartment requires modification of Eq. 10.

$$d(V_1 C_1)/dt = G - C_1(K_D + K_R) - K_C(C_1 - C_2) \quad [12]$$

$$d(V_2 C_2)/dt = K_C(C_1 - C_2) \quad [13]$$

where V$_1$ is the proximal (dialyzed) compartment volume, V$_2$ is the remote compartment volume, C$_1$ is the urea nitrogen concentration in V$_1$, and C$_2$ is the urea nitrogen concentration in V$_2$.

Several assumptions are usually made to reduce the complexity of this model. Because urea is generated in the liver and then diffuses into the blood, G is considered to apply only to the proximal dialyzed compartment. Salt and water intake in the interval between treatments causes V$_1$ to expand and to shrink during dialysis, but, like the intracellular space, V$_2$ is considered constant. By ignoring changes in the volume of both compartments, early developers of this model were able to obtain explicit solutions (to Eq. 12 and Eq. 13) by simple iteration, like the formal single-compartment model.

In contrast to Eq. 10, Eqs. 12 and 13 are not easily solved when V is allowed to vary. Several techniques for solution have been reported, including numerical approximation methods that require a high-speed computer to resolve the four unknown variables, V$_1$, V$_2$, G, and K$_C$ (79–83). When this model is applied to clinical data, a better fit between measured and predicted values is observed, as shown in Fig. 7.6. The ratio $V_1:V_2$ is usually close to 1:2 when fitted by this two-compartment modeling technique, which adds support to the validity of the model.

Flow-Dependent Disequilibrium

In 1990 another type of disequilibrium was found within the blood compartment during high-flux treatments that could not be explained by the classic model (84). Urea concentration differences averaging 10 mg/dL and as high as 20 mg/dL were found in blood drawn simultaneously from both arms in a series of patients undergoing hemodialysis. The concentration gradient slowly dissipated over a 20- to 30-minute postdialysis period. Dependence on blood flow was suggested by a response to both central and superficial warming (84,85).

To explain the dialysis-induced intravascular concentration gradients, another model of hemodialysis urea kinetics was proposed, as shown in Fig. 7.8 (70). Later studies of the early response to dialysis and of exercise during dialysis, and documentation of cardiopulmonary recirculation using thermal and ultrasound dilution techniques confirmed the existence of

blood-flow-related solute disequilibrium during hemodialysis (86—89). This convective type of resistance to dialysis has been quantified and is much better understood today. Flow-dependent disequilibrium has the potential to accentuate diffusion-dependent disequilibrium, which is highly dependent on the nature of the solute as well as the membrane. In contrast, flow-related disequilibrium, as described by the model, should not be affected by the molecular weight or size of the solute. No studies to date have tested this theory.

Cardiopulmonary Recirculation

A specific subtype of flow-dependent disequilibrium, probably accounting quantitatively for more than half of hemodialysis-induced convective disequilibrium, has been called *cardiopulmonary recirculation* (86). Cardiopulmonary recirculation represents the fraction of blood returning from the dialyzer that is rapidly returned to the dialyzer through the heart and lungs. It is found only during dialysis conducted through peripheral arteriovenous (AV) shunts (Fig. 7.8) and, accordingly, is absent in patients dialyzed through central venous catheters lacking a peripheral AV access.

As discussed in more detail in Chapter 5, the recirculation fraction is simply the ratio of access flow to cardiac output.

$$F_{CPR} = \frac{Q_{Ac}}{Q_{Ac} + Q_S} \qquad [14]$$

where F_{CPR} is the recirculation fraction (fraction of blood entering the dialyzer that is recirculated blood), Q_{Ac} is access blood flow, and Q_S is systemic blood flow (cardiac output minus Q_{Ac}).

Part of the deviation from single-pool kinetics shown in Fig. 7.6 can be attributed to cardiopulmonary recirculation, which reduces urea concentration entering the dialyzer to levels below that returning from the systemic circuit (90).

$$C_i = Q_S \ominus_S K_D \qquad [15]$$

where C_i is the urea concentration in blood entering the dialyzer and C_S is the urea concentration in blood returning from the systemic circuit.

The reduced concentration C_i can be substituted for C_0 in Eq. 11 or for C_1 in Eq. 12. Because the magnitude of this effect is predictable, based on estimates of cardiac output and dialyzer clearance, even simpler single-compartment models can incorporate a correction for cardiopulmonary recirculation.

Solute disequilibrium may also be caused by differences in blood flow among capillary beds (84,91) as shown in Fig. 7.8. When the transit of blood through a particular circuit is delayed (e.g., the skin in a cold environment or during episodes of hypotension), urea removal from the organ served by the capillary system is delayed. This causes urea concentrations to fall more rapidly in the central well-perfused compartment (reducing dialyzer efficiency), while higher urea concentrations persist in more peripheral, less well-perfused compartments. Viewed from the most peripheral compartment, flow through the remainder of the body consists of several parallel circuits, each of which could be considered a path for recirculation of dialyzed blood. The distinction between recirculation and solute disequilibrium

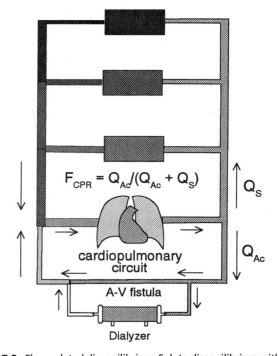

Flow-related Disequilibrium

$$F_{CPR} = Q_{Ac}/(Q_{Ac} + Q_S)$$

Q_S

Q_{Ac}

cardiopulmonary circuit

A-V fistula

Dialyzer

FIG. 7.8. Flow-related disequilibrium. Solute disequilibrium within the blood compartment is explained by this model of multiple parallel circuits, each with a different blood flow/tissue volume. Blood leaving the heart is distributed to all tissue compartments at the same solute concentration, whereas solute concentrations in the blood leaving each compartment are different. The fraction of dialyzer venous blood that reenters the dialyzer by passing through the heart and lungs (F_{CPR}) is called *cardiopulmonary recirculation*. Q_{Ac} is access blood flow and Q_S is systemic blood flow.

is lost in this case because, from the vantage point of the most peripheral compartment, blood that bypasses the compartment is recirculating. The recirculated blood is simply blood that has not equilibrated with the compartment in question before returning to the dialyzer. The cardiopulmonary circuit represents only one of these parallel circuits.

How to Implement Multiple-Compartment Modeling

More than two BUN measurements are required for formal two-compartment modeling. The best times for obtaining these are midway during dialysis and midway during and at the end of the rebound phase. Numerical solutions to Eqs. 12 and 13 are used in place of Eq. 11. Urea concentrations in each compartment are computed at small time intervals, then adjustments are made in V_1, V_2, G, and K_C, similar to the single-pool technique, until the computed profile fits the measured data points. C_1 in Eq. 12 can be adjusted for cardiopulmonary recirculation using Eq. 15 as shown previously. A high-speed computer is required for this type of modeling.

Schneditz et al. (92) has developed an analogous model (with an analytical solution) from flow considerations alone, a pure convectional model based on differences in regional organ perfusion during hemodialysis. Although the pattern of fall in BUN is slightly different, the rebound is indistinguishable from predictions of the classic model. The effect of flow disequilibrium on the concentration pattern and removal of other solutes has not been measured; thus, it is not yet possible to determine the relative roles of these two radically different models.

Comparison with the Single-Compartment Model

Although the single-compartment variable-volume model fails to estimate intradialysis and postdialysis urea concentrations (Fig. 7.6), it predicts V and, therefore, Kt/V with reasonable accuracy (76,81). The reason for this unexpected performance is the offsetting direction of errors in the numerator and the denominator of the equation for V. If G and ultrafiltration are ignored, V can be calculated during dialysis as the amount of urea removed divided by the change in urea concentration.

$$\frac{= K_D \int\limits_{t=0}^{t=T} Cdt}{C_0 - C_E} \qquad [16]$$

where C_0 is the predialysis BUN and C_E is the equilibrated postdialysis BUN.

The amount of urea removed during a single dialysis is the product of K_D and the area under the time versus BUN curve (numerator of Eq. 16). Fig. 7.9 shows the error in that calculation as the shaded area between the two-compartment prediction and the single-compartment prediction of urea nitrogen concentrations. The error in the denominator is the difference between the immediate postdialysis BUN (C_T) and the equilibrated BUN (C_E). For the usual 3- to 4-hour dialysis with a Kt/V of 1.2 to 1.3, the errors are of similar magnitude and off-

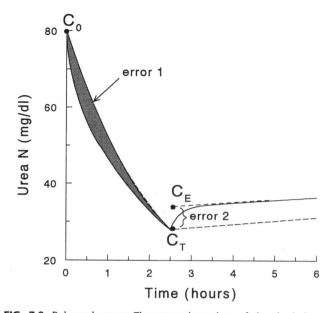

FIG. 7.9. Balanced errors. The upper boundary of the shaded area shows the single-compartment prediction of BUN during hemodialysis. The lower boundary is the two-compartment model line. C_T is the blood urea nitrogen (BUN) measured immediately after dialysis. C_E is the equilibrated BUN extrapolated to the postdialysis time. The single-compartment model overestimates the BUN during dialysis and consequently overestimates the amount of urea removed shown as the shaded area (error 1) and in the numerator of Eq. 14. It also underestimates the equilibrated BUN (C_T) causing a false overestimate of the change in concentration (error 2) in the denominator of Eq. 14.

set each other (81,93). The result is a fairly accurate prediction of V by the single-compartment model, depending to some extent on the rate of ultrafiltration during dialysis. Urea generation (G) and nPCR, however, are overestimated by the single-compartment model because there is no compensating error.

Because of its complexity, multicompartment modeling is not recommended for routine clinical application. This type of modeling should be used when an accurate profile of BUN during and immediately after dialysis is required or when an accurate measure of G is required and to model the kinetics of solutes other than urea.

Both single-compartment and multiple-compartment models overestimate the amount of dialysis *received* by the patient. The "K" in Kt/V by convention is effective *dialyzer* clearance of urea (Table 7.4). More important for the therapeutic effect is the *patient's* clearance, often termed the *whole body* clearance, defined in Table 7.4. For patients with significant urea disequilibrium, whole body clearance is significantly less than dialyzer clearance because some of the patient's urea is compartmentalized and only slowly released to the dialyzer. Whole body Kt/V, often called eKt/V, can be resolved by applying the single-compartment model to the *equilibrated* postdialysis BUN instead of the *immediate* postdialysis BUN (81). Two-compartment models are capable of determining both the effective dialyzer clearance and the patient's whole body clearance because these models either require measurement of the equilibrated postdialysis BUN or they estimate it. A more direct measurement of whole body clearance can be obtained using the dialysate method as explained later.

TABLE 7.4. UREA CLEARANCES DEFINED

Residual Clearance
Clearance by the patient's native kidneys, often negligible or absent
  Contributes little to total clearance during dialysis
  Major effect on urea kinetics occurs between dialyses
Dialyzer Clearance
Instantaneous: measured across the dialyzer from simultaneous inlet
  and outlet BUN
Integrated: modeled from predialysis and immediate postdialysis
    blood samples
  Average dialyzer clearance for an entire dialysis
  Not affected by urea disequilibrium
Patient Clearance
Also called *whole body clearance*
  Derived from the predialysis and equilibrated postdialysis BUN
  Always lower than dialyzer clearance: difference due to urea
    disequilibrium, recirculation
  Includes the small contribution from residual clearance
Continuous Equivalent of Intermittent Clearance (EKR)
Derived from G/TAC
  Always lower than *patient clearance*
  Allows comparison of different schedules including continuous
    treatment

G/TAC, urea generation rate/time-averaged BUN.

Urea modeling is primarily used to quantify dialysis and allow tailoring of the dose to the individual patient's needs. Concern has been raised about patients who may rebound more than others and may be underdialyzed because the single-compartment model fails to consider the rebound when calculating their delivered dose. Recent studies have found that rebound is highly predictable and that such outliers may not actually exist (94,95). Based on measurements of the postdialysis BUN up to 60 minutes, eKt/V was estimated best by a simple equation, called the *rate equation,* that predicts rebound from the intensity or rate of solute removal during dialysis (94,96):

$$eKt/V = spKt/V - 0.6\ K/V + 0.03 \qquad [17]$$

Although Eq. 17 was empirically derived, it is predictable from current knowledge of the genesis of rebound from solute gradients in the patient. These gradients are highly dependent on the fractional rate of solute removal, expressed in Eq. 17 as K/V.

DIALYSATE METHOD

The models of urea kinetics discussed previously compute the effective urea clearance indirectly by analyzing *blood* urea concentrations. Other parameters computed from blood-side modeling such as G and V depend on adjustments for ultrafiltration, assumed blood and plasma water content, estimation of urea removal, and corrections for disequilibrium. Urea clearance can be measured in a more direct way by measuring *dialysate* urea concentrations (97–101). Advantages of dialysate sampling are listed in Table 7.5. Dialysate pumps and flow are subject to less variation than blood flow and can be calibrated during a patient treatment using direct volumetric methods. Sampling and analysis are simpler and expose both dialysis and laboratory personnel to less risk from bloodborne infectious agents. Dialysate

TABLE 7.5. ADVANTAGES OF DIALYSATE SAMPLING AND ANALYSIS

Sampling
No need for sterile equipment, needles
Less risk to dialysis, lab personnel
Waste product, no limit to sample size
Flow is directly measurable using volumetric techniques
Analysis
Simpler, more economical
No cells or plasma to separate
No interference with assay technique from:
  Hemolysis
  Lipemia
  Clot formation
  Protein (e.g., electrode drift)
No correction for water content

methods give a more direct measure of whole-body clearance and of fractional urea removal from the whole patient unhampered by variances in blood flow, time, or dialyzer clearance resulting from clotting in the dialyzer or manufacturing defects and other factors. In addition, the problems with disequilibrium discussed previously are eliminated because routine measurement of the postdialysis BUN is not required. However, the precision of Kt/V determined by the dialysate method has recently been questioned; this is discussed further later.

Theoretical Basis of the Dialysate Method

A limited amount of data is required when the dialysate method is used to quantify hemodialysis as shown in Table 7.6. The postdialysis volume of urea distribution (V) need be measured only once or whenever the patient's dry weight changes significantly. It can be measured by sampling blood after equilibration is reestablished, usually 30 minutes to an hour after dialysis, and applying the following mass-balance equation, a variant of Eq. 16

$$V = \frac{Q_D C_D t - \Delta V C_0 - RG}{C_0 - C_E} \qquad [18]$$

where Q_D is total dialysate flow including Q_F, C_D is the dialysate urea nitrogen concentration, ΔV is the fluid lost during dialysis, C_0 is the predialysis BUN, RG is a correction for K_R and urea generation, and C_E is the equilibrated postdialysis BUN.

Both C_0 and C_E must be corrected for plasma water content. RG is the amount of urea generated during the dialysis minus the amount removed by the patient's native kidneys.

$$RG = t(G - K_R C_{Av}) \qquad [19]$$

TABLE 7.6. REQUIRED INPUT FOR THE DIALYSATE METHOD

Dialysate urea concentration (C_D)
Dialysate flow (Q_D)
Predialysis BUN (C_0)
Volume of urea distribution (V)

These terms usually contribute very little and in most patients can be ignored. If included, C_{Av} can be approximated as the log mean $C = (C_0 - C_E)/\ln(C_0/C_E)$. Total body urea content at the start of dialysis is $C_0(V + \Delta V)$. The amount of urea removed is $Q_D C_D t$.

When solute removal is measured directly, the total effect of a single dialysis can be expressed also directly as the solute removal index (SRI) (102,103). SRI is the fractional solute removal, the amount removed divided by the initial total body content.

$$SRI = \frac{Q_D C_D t}{C_0(V + \Delta V)} \qquad [20]$$

Although SRI is a fraction of the initial solute content, the fraction may be greater than one because of ongoing solute generation during dialysis. For urea, a direct mathematical relationship between Kt/V and SRI may be demonstrated from Eq. 8.

$$Kt/V = -\ln(1 - SRI) \qquad [21]$$

Equation 22 is a rearrangement of Eq. 21.

$$SRI = (1 - e^{-Kt/V}) \qquad [22]$$

Equation 8 can be used here instead of the more complex equations that include G, Q_F, and two compartment adjustments, because the amount of urea removed ($Q_D C_D t$) is measured directly; it includes the contribution of ultrafiltration and requires no correction for G or solute disequilibrium. SRI is easier to conceptualize and has been considered by some to be a better index of small solute removal and a better overall measure of dialysis than Kt/V. Unfortunately, there are no standards of adequacy for SRI. Until such standards are available, SRI can be converted to Kt/V using Eq. 21 with the understanding that K represents whole body clearance as discussed previously. Because whole body clearance is always lower than dialyzer clearance, Kt/V determined from Eq. 21 is lower than Kt/V estimated from one- or two-compartment modeling (104).

Limitations of the Dialysate Method

Despite the advantages listed in Table 7.5, dialysate methods that compare measurements of the quantity removed to estimates of the total urea present at the start of dialysis suffer from an inherently larger error when measuring the dose of dialysis compared with blood-side methods (105). Although the primary goal may be to calculate SRI rather than Kt/V, dialysate methods inject more error into either measurement because they rely on subtraction of two relatively large quantities to obtain the desired measurement. To determine eKt/V using the dialysate method, one must subtract the measured amount of urea removed during dialysis from $C_0 V$ and divide by V to calculate C_E. The resulting percentage error in C_E is considerably larger than usual measurement errors and is higher at higher doses of dialysis when C_E is low. The resulting relatively large error in eKt/V, as shown in Fig. 7.10, is avoided by blood-side methods that estimate eKt/V, for example, by using Eq. 17 from BUN levels measured during or shortly after dialysis. The magnified subtraction error inherent in the dialysate method can be minimized by measuring the dialysate concentrations multiple

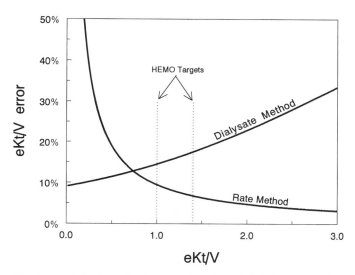

FIG. 7.10. Dialysate method error. As the dose of dialysis, measured as eKt/V, increases, the error in eKt/V determined using the dialysate method increases significantly, whereas the error from blood-side methods (rate equation) decreases slightly. HEMO Project target values are shown as vertical dotted lines.

times throughout the dialysis and fitting a curve to the resulting concentration profile. As current investigators of dialysate methods appear to be moving in that direction—that is, providing a profile of the dialysate urea concentration—this limitation of the method may not be a stumbling block (100,101,106,107).

How to Quantify Dialysis Using the Dialysate Method

Total dialysate collections have been used in research facilities to measure dialysate urea (97). This is a cumbersome procedure that cannot be easily adapted for routine clinical use. Dialysate can also be sampled using a partial dialysate collector. A small percentage of spent dialysate is continuously sampled and collected. The total quantity removed can then be easily calculated from the aggregate concentration, treatment time, and dialysate flow rate.

Methods that analyze BUN readings on multiple samples of dialysate throughout the dialysis treatment appear promising for clinical application (100,101). These techniques measure urea nitrogen concentrations in multiple timed dialysate samples throughout the dialysis session. If dialysate flow is constant, the total amount of urea removed can be determined by summing the flow × concentration products using a trapezoidal function or by fitting the data to an exponential elimination curve (100, 101,103,108).

Once the amount of urea removed is measured, Eq. 18 can be used to calculate V. If V is valid and confirmed, it need not be measured again unless the patient's postdialysis (dry) volume is suspected to have changed. Subsequent quantitation by the dialysate method can be accomplished with only a predialysis BUN and measurement of dialysate urea as described previously. Kt/V is obtained from Eq. 21. Urea clearance (K) is extracted from Kt/V from knowledge of time (t) and V. The term K, which for blood-side urea modeling is defined as effective dialyzer clearance, must be redefined for the dialysate method as patient clearance, as described in Table 7.4.

An attractive practical feature of the dialysate method is that no measurement of equilibrated postdialysis BUN (C_E) is required, except for the one-time calculation of V. However, C_E can be calculated at any time by rearranging Eq. 18.

$$C_E = \frac{C_0 (V + \Delta V) - Q_D C_D t + RG}{V} \qquad [23]$$

The dialysate method is critically dependent on accurate measurement of dialysate urea concentrations that are often low, especially toward the end of dialysis. Bacterial contamination of dialysate can also lead to urea degradation and erroneous dialysate urea concentration.

Bedside urea monitors using urea-sensitive electrodes can be used to model urea kinetics in real time instead of retrospectively (101,106,107,109). Real-time monitoring can ensure the adequacy of each treatment by targeting removal of a predetermined amount of urea, instead of targeting a predetermined time interval as is currently done.

Another inexpensive and noninvasive method for monitoring the delivered dialysis dose is on-line conductivity or ionic dialysance (110–112). Urea and sodium are both small molecules with roughly equivalent clearances across dialyzer membranes. Because sodium and its anions are quantitatively the only significant ionized solutes in dialysate, changes in dialysate electrical conductivity can be used to measure sodium diffusion across the membrane. These measurements can be made automatically with meters placed in the dialysate inflow and outflow lines. To create a significant sodium gradient between blood and dialysate, the sodium concentration in dialysate is abruptly increased for a few minutes by altering dialysate and water proportioning. The resulting change in conductivity from dialysate inlet to outlet reflects movement of sodium into the patient, a function of sodium dialysance (113).

$$D = [Q_d + Q_f]\left[1 - \frac{(Co_1 - Co_2)}{(Ci_1 - Ci_2)}\right] \qquad [24]$$

Co and Ci are dialysate outlet and inlet conductivities (mS/cm), D is dialysance (mL/min), Q_d is dialysate flow, Q_f is ultrafiltration flow, and subscripts 1 and 2 indicate measurements before and after the step-up in conductivity.

Several short measurements of conductivity or ionic dialysance can be measured and averaged over the course of a treatment to improve the measurement precision. If V is estimated and updated periodically, the actual delivered spKt/V can be calculated in real time for each treatment. Ionic dialysance closely correlates with standard blood and dialysate-side measurements of clearance but is approximately 5% lower than blood urea clearance (112). The conductivity method has several advantages including on-line and more frequent determinations of delivered dose, decreased cost, and elimination of invasive blood sampling. Although the influence of dialysis membranes on the clearance of charged electrolytes is still debated, the difference between ionic clearance and blood urea clearance actually appears less pronounced for charged membranes (112).

THE DIALYSIS SCHEDULE: LESS FREQUENT IS LESS EFFICIENT

The patient presents a barrier to intermittent dialysis that is greater than had been anticipated in the past. Even for urea, one of the most diffusible solutes, resistance to removal can be easily demonstrated as multiple concentration gradients develop within the patient during both standard and high efficiency dialysis. Increasing the frequency tends to diminish this effect and allows more efficient removal of solute despite no change in the weekly Kt/V as shown in Fig. 7.11. Increasing the frequency improves the efficiency of dialysis by reducing the amplitude of oscillations in solute concentration and by diminishing patient-dependent disequilibrium. Advances in dialysis technology have improved the dialyzer and dialyzer membranes but not the resistance to diffusion in patients. If the dose of dialysis is held constant and the frequency of treatments is decreased from the accepted standard of three treatments per week, morbidity is increased. As frequency increases to six to seven treatments per week, morbidity and mortality should improve based on the improvements in efficiency that lower the concentration of toxic solutes (114).

Recently, both ESRD patients and dialysis caregivers have expressed a growing interest in more frequent dialysis schedules, including short daily treatments using standard blood and dialysate flow rates and long nocturnal treatments using lower flow regimens. Both techniques are reported to improve extracellular volume control, blood pressure, anemia, and nutritional

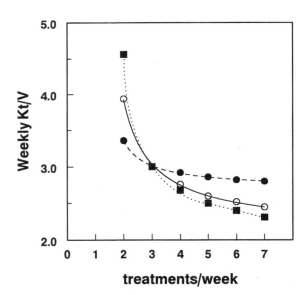

FIG. 7.11. *Kt/V* required to achieve the same time-averaged concentration (TAC). As the frequency of hemodialysis treatments increases, the efficiency of each treatment increases. The vertical axis shows the total weekly dose (*Kt/V*) required to maintain the average blood urea nitrogen (BUN) (TAC) constant. ¥, prediction of the single-compartment model; ○, two-compartment model predictions for urea (K_C = 500 mL/min); ■, a theoretical molecule with K_C = 200 mL/min. (Adapted from Depner TA. Quantifying hemodialysis and peritoneal dialysis: examination of the peak concentration hypothesis. *Semin Dial* 1994;7:315–317, with permission).

status. Nocturnal hemodialysis, when performed six to seven times per week, also has been reported to lower the concentrations of both small and larger molecular weight solutes, including phosphorus and β_2-microglobulin (115). Quantification of dose becomes problematic for daily dialysis because dialyzer Kt/V does not reflect patient clearance and summation of daily single pool Kt/V to give a weekly spKt/V does not account for the improved efficiency of more frequent treatments. Several methods that have been reported to better quantify the dose when dialysis is performed at different frequencies and intensities are discussed in the following.

Continuous Equivalent of Urea Clearance (EKR)

Because uremia is caused by toxic concentrations of solutes in the body and the major therapeutic goal is solute removal, some measure of the residual solute level in the patient is a logical yardstick of uremia and the adequacy of dialysis. If, in the absence of changes in generation rate, urea can be used as a surrogate toxin, then equivalent states of toxicity are theoretically reflected in the mean or time-averaged BUN. This is the premise of a method for assessing the equivalency of treatments in patients undergoing intermittent treatments according to different weekly schedules (56,116). This approach also acknowledges that the mean serum urea concentration (TAC) is a linear function of the urea generation rate when clearance is held constant as shown in Fig. 7.1.

The mathematical relationship among the three variables shown in Fig. 7.1 is fixed by a plane, so only two variables can vary randomly (within limits). The third variable is defined by the other two. Another way of formulating the recommendation that urea clearance (Kt/V) should be held constant according to accepted guidelines [e.g., Dialysis Outcomes Quality Initiative (DOQI)] is to recommend that the ratio of G/TAC should be held constant. If G is fixed, then the entire effort is reduced to maintaining TAC constant. This goal seems logical, as noted previously, and is perhaps a bit more intuitive and clinically satisfying, because G and TAC are patient parameters in contrast to the machine parameter, K. Instead of holding Kt/V constant, if the real goal of dialysis is to maintain G/TAC constant, then dialysis at different frequencies and continuous dialysis can be compared with intermittent dialysis by comparing G/TAC.

A method for calculating both the target and the delivered dose of dialysis from the constant relationship between TAC and nPCR, independent of the dialysis schedule and day of the week, was advocated several years ago (56). Note that this approach is different from the previous antiquated practice of using the BUN in a cross section of patients to determine dialysis adequacy. Instead, the patient is compared with himself or herself in a theoretical identical state of protein nutrition and nitrogen balance—only the dialysis is changed. Note also that if the urea removal rate is substituted for G in the expression G/TAC, the result is the conventional expression of continuous urea clearance used for continuous replacement therapies and for native kidney function.

Clearance can be expressed as a removal rate divided by solute concentration. In a steady state of nitrogen balance, the rate of urea removal is equal to the urea generation rate (G), so the clearance for a continuously dialyzed patient can be approximated as G/C, where C is the serum urea concentration. For intermittently hemodialyzed patients, because G and TAC can be calculated using formal kinetic modeling, an equivalent clearance (EKR) can be calculated as (116)

$$EKR = G/TAC \qquad [25]$$

If EKR is normalized to a typical V of 40 L, the result can be expressed in terms of nPCR and TAC using the equation of Borah et al. (Eq. 1) for nPCR (18,117)

$$nEKR = \frac{40(nPCR - 0.17)}{5.42\,TAC} \qquad [26]$$

where EKR is the continuous equivalent of the patient's intermittent urea clearance. Calculated in this manner, EKR is a total clearance that includes the effect of residual native function, but the dialyzer component can be extracted from it simply by subtracting K_R.

For intermittently dialyzed patients, the dialyzer component of EKR is always lower than the measured dialyzer clearance and lower than the modeled patient clearance. The difference reflects the inefficiency of intermittent compared with continuous dialysis (117,118). Intermittent clearance requires a higher weekly clearance to achieve the same TAC, as shown in Fig. 7.11. EKR in a hemodialyzed patient is the continuous clearance necessary to maintain the equivalent TAC at the patient's protein catabolic rate (nPCR).

Note that EKR is expressed in the usual units of clearance (mL/min) and, like dialyzer clearance, it can be normalized to V or, like native kidney clearance, it may be normalized to surface area. When normalized to a 40-L patient, the consensus-derived minimum Kt/V of 1.2 per dialysis for thrice weekly dialysis translates to an EKR of approximately 12 mL/min when corrected for serum water content. This could be any combination of residual and dialyzer clearances. For example, if residual clearance is 3.0 mL/min, then the dialyzer clearance need only be 10 mL/min to meet the minimum standard.

Standards for EKR do not change with dialysis frequency, so the EKR of intermittent hemodialysis can be directly compared with standardized clearances obtained with continuous replacement therapy like continuous ambulatory peritoneal dialysis (CAPD), with the EKR of patients dialyzed daily or with the clearance of continuously functioning native kidneys. This universal applicability to patients before starting dialysis and after starting any mode of dialysis or transplantation is an attractive feature. It also allows the familiar expression of clearance, commonly used to quantify native kidney function, to describe the function of the artificial kidney.

In continuously dialyzed patients Kt/V, SRI, and normalized EKR are all equivalent (the same number). As the minimum dose of dialysis considered necessary to maintain health in hemodialyzed patients has increased, the practice of delaying the initiation of maintenance dialysis in patients with progressive renal failure is less rational (119). Data from the MDRD study suggested that it may be necessary to begin dialysis treatments sooner to avoid a deterioration in health that in some patients is irreversible (36,37).

Limitations of EKR

Although substitution of EKR for *Kt/V* as a measure of dialysis is appealing from several points of view, implementation is problematic. EKR is a simple concept but is not simple to calculate; it requires a measure of TAC and either G or nPCR, three variables that are not easily obtained without modeling urea kinetics. In addition, the single-compartment model overestimates G and underestimates TAC, causing a significant overestimation of EKR.

At the current time there are no standards for EKR, and regulatory agencies in the United States currently demand either *Kt/V* or URR to document dialysis adequacy.

Although G has a larger variance than V or *Kt/V* there are no data on the variance in EKR, which may be more stable than G but less stable than *Kt/V*.

When the minimum standard dose of dialysis is not achieved, EKR does not offer a method to correct the problem. For hemodialyzed patients, *Kt/V* must be calculated to predict the necessary adjustment in K or t.

When compared with the currently accepted minimum standard dose of hemodialysis, the accepted minimum standard for peritoneal dialysis, expressed as EKR, is closer than comparable values expressed as *Kt/V*, but EKR remains significantly lower for peritoneal dialysis. It is possible that the requirement for peritoneal dialysis should be raised further, or that peritoneal dialysis patients enjoy some additional unidentified benefit from dialysis that reduces their risk of death independent of EKR (120). Another likely possibility is that urea clearance and TAC are not the appropriate parameters for comparing the two modalities and that another solute with a lower K_C (higher resistance to diffusion in the patient) would demonstrate equivalent EKR values. This is the basis for another method for quantifying dialysis, described later, that is independent of the daily treatment schedule.

Normalized *Kt/V*

Calculation of normalized *Kt/V* is based on the observation that disequilibrium for many small dialyzable solutes is greater than urea. The concept is similar to that of the continuous equivalent clearance described previously and Eq. 25 is used to calculate normalized clearance except that TAC is determined from two pool formal urea modeling. The solute behaves in every way like urea except with regard to disequilibrium as reflected in lower values for KC—the intercompartment diffusion constant. The bottom tracing of Fig. 7.11 shows that solutes with low KC (Eq. 12) have a steeper decline in the clearance required to maintain a constant TAC when dialysis frequency varies over a range from one to seven per week (118). Solutes exhibiting greater disequilibrium among body compartments are affected more by changes in frequency than urea. When a lower KC value is entered into the two compartment model, greater benefit is seen when frequency increases from three per week to six per week (121). The concentrations of solutes with low KC fall more than urea as frequency increases. This approach requires a formal two compartment, variable volume mathematical model that is not practical for current use in the dialysis clinic, but it demonstrates a fundamental principle that may be useful if the technique can be simplified.

This technique and the standard *Kt/V* method described later give similar results that have been used to explain the difference in the minimum weekly *Kt/V* currently recommended for hemodialysis compared with peritoneal dialysis (122). Although there are no data to validate either, the models are supported clinically by experience with CAPD. Based on a consensus on outcomes, the minimum *Kt/V* recommended by the DOQI committee for patients treated with CAPD is 2.0 per week, much lower than the minimum sp*Kt/V* of 3.6 per week recommended for patients treated with hemodialysis thrice weekly (123). For both normalized and standard methods but not for EKR, the minimum *Kt/V* is 2.0 per week when weekly sp*Kt/V* is 3.6, thus removing the discrepancy in dose recommendations among modalities of treatment.

Standard *Kt/V*

Another recently developed method to measure and compare dialysis dose regardless of schedule uses the predialysis BUN (124). This method also requires calculation of G and uses the mean predialysis BUN, as opposed to the peak BUN or TAC, as the denominator in the expression of steady state clearance (Eq. 25). Like EKR and normalized *Kt/V*, expressing the dose as an equivalent continuous clearance permits simple addition of native kidney function to both measures of intermittent and continuous renal replacement therapy. Because the mean predialysis BUN is used to define the standard *Kt/V*, the resulting value is always lower than sp*Kt/V*, e*Kt/V*, or EKR.

Limitations of Blood-Side Modeling as Frequency Increases

It is important to consider that blood-based methods of dose quantification lose some of their power when applied to more frequent prolonged treatments because the difference between the predialysis and postdialysis urea concentration is reduced leading to greater errors in the calculation of their ratio. As the frequency increases approaching continuous dialysis, blood-side modeling is no longer possible. Measuring the dose of more frequent hemodialysis may require measurement of cross-dialyzer clearances or dialysate methods, similar to measurements of continuous peritoneal dialysis.

SIMPLIFIED APPROACHES TO QUANTIFYING DIALYSIS

Because the relationships among time, solute removal, and clearance are logarithmic and influenced by multiple variables, the mathematical expressions of urea kinetics are often complex. Inclusion of all the pertinent variables using formal modeling requires a programmable calculator or a computer. To circumvent the need for complex mathematical programs and equipment and to provide tools for quick bedside estimates, simplified approaches to urea modeling have been proposed (63,96,125,126). Two approaches are used: algebraic formulas that provide explicit solutions and nomograms.

Simplified Mathematical Formulas

Simplified mathematical formulas eliminate the stepwise or iterative solutions for *Kt/V* and nPCR by ignoring the lesser variables. Eq. 8 is a simplified formula that ignores ultrafiltration, urea generation, and disequilibrium during dialysis. A more accurate formula, derived empirically by Daugirdas (127), is shown here.

$$Kt/V = -\ln(R - 0.03) + (4 - 3.5R)UF/W \qquad [27]$$

where R is the ratio of postdialysis/predialysis BUN, UF is the total ultrafiltrate volume in liters/dialysis, and W is the patient's weight in kilograms.

Equation 27 approximates the contributions of urea generation and ultrafiltration during dialysis in the first and second terms, respectively. It requires use of a scientific calculator or log table, but no iterative programming is required.

A similar equation has been developed from a mathematical analysis of urea kinetics by Garred et al. (128), who used an approximation of G to eliminate the requirement for iteration.

$$Kt/V = \ln(R)\left[1 + \frac{1}{1-R}\frac{\left(\frac{\Delta V}{V}\right)}{1-0.01786t}\right] \qquad [28]$$

where t is dialysis time in hours. A simpler, although slightly less accurate, version of Eq. 28 requires only body weight measurements (BW) instead of V (128).

$$Kt/V = \frac{\left[3\left(\frac{\Delta BW}{BW}\right) - \ln(R)\right]}{1-0.01786t} \qquad [29]$$

The protein catabolic rate is more difficult to approximate with simple formulas because the dialysis schedule, residual clearance, and fluid gain play significant roles (129,130). Equation 9 is an example of a simplified formula that ignores fluid gain and residual clearance and also requires a third BUN measurement. To include the latter variables, and reduce the requirement to two BUN measurements, equations have been derived for hemodialysis given three times and two times weekly, with and without residual clearance (131):

For dialysis 3 times a week
start of week

$$nPCR = C_0/(36.3 + 5.48 \times Kt/V + (53.5/Kt/V)) + 0.168$$

midweek

$$nPCR = C_0/(25.8 + 1.15 \times Kt/V + (56.4/Kt/V)) + 0.168$$

end of week

$$nPCR = C_0/(16.3 + 4.3 \times Kt/V + (56.6/Kt/V)) + 0.168$$

For dialysis 2 times a week
start of week

$$nPCR = C_0/(48.0 + 5.14 \times Kt/V + (79.0/Kt/V)) + 0.168$$

end of week

$$nPCR = C_0/(33.0 + 3.60 \times Kt/V + (83.2/Kt/V)) + 0.168$$

C_0 is the predialysis BUN. If the patient has significant residual native kidney function (K_R >1.0 mL/min), the following formulas should be used to adjust C_0 upward before calculating nPCR from the previous formulas.

For dialysis 3 times a week

$$C_0 = C_0[1 + (((0.70 + 3.08)/Kt/V)K_R/V)]$$

For dialysis 2 times a week

$$C_0 = C_0[1 + (((1.15 + 4.56)/Kt/V)K_R/V)]$$

Urea Reduction Ratio (URR)

Another parameter mathematically related to *Kt/V* is the URR, which is the fractional fall in BUN during a single dialysis (63,125,132). The denominator is the predialysis BUN and the numerator is the difference between predialysis and postdialysis BUN. If urea volume remains constant during dialysis and no disequilibrium occurs, URR approximates SRI, a parameter that can be directly measured using the dialysate method (see previous). Unfortunately, URR does not include the effects of ultrafiltration, a process that removes (clears) urea without affecting urea concentrations, and can be a significant part of the total removed (Fig. 7.12). In addition, URR is zero for native kidney

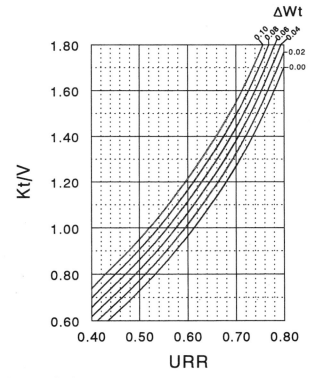

FIG. 7.12. The logarithmic relationship between the urea reduction ratio and *Kt/V* derived from formal urea modeling. This relationship is significantly affected by fluid removal during dialysis. ΔWt is the change in weight during dialysis expressed as a fraction of the postdialysis weight. (From Depner TA. Estimation of *Kt/V* from URR for varying levels of weight loss: a bedside graphic aid. *Semin Dial* 1993; 6:242, with permission.)

function and in continuously dialyzed patients; in hemodialyzed patients URR does not correlate linearly with clearance or Kt/V, as shown in Fig. 7.12. Because it is simple to calculate, URR is widely used to quantify hemodialysis and assess its adequacy. If the standards are set conservatively in centers where URR is the only measure of dialysis, patients should be protected from underdialysis and are far better off than patients who have no yardstick of dialysis regularly applied. However, the majority of the time and effort required for formal modeling is also required for measurement of URR (see the section on a comparison of simplified methods of formal modeling later in the chapter).

Nomograms

To avoid complex mathematics that deal with nonlinear relationships, graphical representation of the data can be used to measure the amount of dialysis delivered and its adequacy. Nomograms are more satisfying to some because they give visual relationships among the important variables and are more adaptable to teaching (133). Nomograms are limited because a maximum of three variables can be represented on one three-dimensional graph. Usually the three most important variables are graphed and the others are held constant or ignored.

A Comparison of Simplified Methods to Formal Modeling

The previous simplified formulas and graphics are helpful instructional tools and allow quick estimates when a computer is not immediately available. For routine application in a clinic, however, little is gained by short-cutting formal urea modeling. The most time-consuming and expensive aspects of urea modeling are collecting the blood samples, serum analysis, and entry of data into the computer. Once the data is entered, it can be stored and evaluated by computer programs that require a fraction of a second to complete each analysis. The data can be compared with previous analyses, and permanent hard copies can be generated for chart storage and communication. The terms "quick" and "bedside" sometimes, applied to simplified formulas, are misleading because the time lag between sampling the blood and return of data from the laboratory is ignored. A major goal of urea modeling is to individualize therapy; ignoring critical variables such as a volume change during dialysis, or assuming a mean value for all patients, defeats this purpose.

PRACTICE GUIDELINES AND STANDARDS

Until recently, the guidelines for dosing hemodialysis were derived almost entirely from data accumulated by the NCDS (134). A consensus conference sponsored by the NIH in 1994 concluded that the minimum Kt/V should be raised to 1.2 per dialysis, three treatments per week (31). Subsequent efforts sponsored by industry and government, including the Renal Physicians Association and the National Kidney Foundation, echoed and supported this goal (30–32,135). Although the NCDS supported a lower minimum, the practice of dialysis has changed significantly, including the patient population.

Hemodialysis is also better tolerated so more dialysis can be given with fewer adverse effects of the treatment itself. However, because contemporary data were lacking, another national cooperative study (the HEMO study) was instituted to evaluate potential benefits from further increases in the dialysis dose and flux (136). The method chosen to quantify and control the dose of hemodialysis in this study was formal urea modeling. The equilibrated Kt/V (eKt/V) that accounts for urea disequilibrium and is considered a more accurate reflection of patient urea clearance was used to quantify the dialysis dose. Use of the simple rate equation to measure eKt/V as mentioned previously eliminated the need for a postdialysis blood sample. The equation was validated before the HEMO study and correlated well with standard blood side methods for determining eKt/V in the HEMO study (95).

In the HEMO study, randomized patients received either the "standard" dose of dialysis (target eKt/V of 1.05 per treatment) or a "high" dose (target eKt/V of 1.45 per treatment). The two randomized prescriptions were tightly controlled by study investigators so that midway through the study, less than 4% of patients who received the standard dose of dialysis fell below the current minimum recommended $spKt/V$ of 1.20.

No significant difference in mortality between treatment groups was found at the conclusion of the study, although women who received the higher dialysis dose had a slightly lower risk of death and hospitalization compared with men. The HEMO study provides strong evidence that the minimum thrice weekly hemodialysis dose recommended by DOQI is adequate. The study results are not inconsistent with an expectation of improved outcomes with increases in dialysis frequency. Although the high Kt/V averaged 36% higher than the standard dose in this study, the separation, when expressed as standard or normalized Kt/V, was about 17%. On the practical side, it appears that we have reached a limit to delivering dialysis thrice weekly. Large increases in the weekly effective Kt/V can only be accomplished by increasing the frequency to a daily regimen or by continuous dialysis. Prolongations of treatment time and increases in dialyzer clearance have less impact when the treatment is given infrequently.

PITFALLS OF UREA MODELING

When urea modeling produces unexpected results, a troubleshooting routine should be initiated. The most common sources of error are listed in Table 7.7. A frequent source of error and probably the greatest source of scatter in the data generated by single-compartment modeling is the postdialysis BUN. Current consensus favors drawing the blood specimen at the immediate end of dialysis (see the section on comparison with the single-compartment model and Fig. 7.9) while taking precautions against dilution of the blood urea because of access recirculation (32,137,138). To prevent an error from access recirculation, the specimen should be drawn 10 seconds after slowing the blood pump to approximately 100 mL/min. If the delay is longer than 15 seconds, substantial rebound will occur because of cardiopulmonary recirculation. (More detailed discussions of the pitfalls of urea modeling can be found in references 32 and 139.)

TABLE 7.7. PITFALLS OF UREA MODELING

Errors that Affect the Delivery or Adequacy of Dialysis
Predialysis BUN: most reliable of the two measurements
  Avoid any delay (even 30 seconds) after starting the blood pump
  Avoid dilution from saline or heparin
Postdialysis BUN: most subject to error
  Avoid local recirculation (see Chapter 5)
  Consider urea rebound from cardiopulmonary recirculation and
    other sources of disequilibrium
Errors that Affect the Assessment of Equipment Function
Clearance errors: clearance is almost always overestimated
  Blood flow errors
    Low prepump pressure (140)
    Poor flow calibration
    Poor pump segment occlusion
  Failure to correct for serum and whole blood water content
  Loss of surface area from reuse or clotting
  Inflated manufacturer's in vitro clearances
  Recirculation (refer to above)
Timing errors: wall clock syndrome (141)
Volume errors: patients may not conform to the anthropometric
  formulas
Errors that Affect the Measurement of nPCR
Predialysis and postdialysis BUN errors (see above)
Residual clearance errors

nPCR, protein catabolic rate normalized to volume.

Despite the mathematical complexities outlined previously, the implementation of urea modeling is relatively simple. For instance, the most popular methods for assessing dialysis adequacy require only two BUN measurements. As a consequence, potential errors that might result from measuring more complex functions, such as dialyzer clearance or urea distribution volume, are minimized. Efforts to maintain or improve the reliability of the tests of dialysis adequacy should, therefore, focus on sampling techniques and accuracy of laboratory measurements. On the other hand, when urea modeling is used to evaluate equipment function, to determine, for example, why the prescribed amount of dialysis does not match that delivered, accurate estimates of dialyzer clearance, urea volume, and dialysis duration are required. Table 7.7 separates the pitfalls of urea modeling into these two major categories, those impacting on adequacy assessment caused by errors in BUN measurement and those affecting assessment of equipment function caused by errors in the prescription or in V.

SUMMARY

It is fortunate and gratifying that an empirically derived treatment such as hemodialysis is so successful in reversing the life-threatening effects of uremia, but because the cause of uremia is inadequate native kidney function, the amount of dialysis delivered should be quantified to ensure adequate replacement function. Because the major effect of dialysis is solute removal, it seems reasonable to use solute removal as a yardstick, and the best measure of solute removal by dialysis is clearance.

Carefully controlled studies have shown that the clearance obtained from urea kinetic modeling predicts outcome and, therefore, can be used to judge the adequacy of each treatment.

Urea kinetic modeling is a mathematical simulation of urea flux that helps to predict urea removal and urea levels both during and between hemodialyses. Established and proven clinical techniques for quantifying dialysis allow tailoring of prescriptions to each patient's need. The goals of urea modeling are first to maintain a uniform quantity of treatment in all patients and second to identify potential problems that impair dialysis efficiency in each patient. The parameters *Kt/V*, nPCR, and EKR, obtained from single- or multiple-compartment modeling help dialysis caregivers focus on patients whose prescriptions (including their dialysis schedule, time on dialysis, dialyzer clearance, and dietary protein) need adjustment.

Nephrologists today have accepted the need for measuring dialysis, and a tentative consensus has been reached about minimum doses expressed as a normalized clearance. Controversy continues to exist about the measuring techniques, and new insights and methods continue to appear in the dialysis forums and literature. Fortunately, the amount of dialysis a patient receives can be accurately determined from a limited number of simple measurements of BUN and other parameters. Without applying some form of mathematical modeling, however, focus on the BUN alone can be misleading. Use of simplified formulas and nomograms is far better than relying on the BUN alone, but formal urea modeling using a programmable calculator or computer provides the most precise analysis with which to individualize therapy. Recent considerations of the effects of solute disequilibrium and recirculation have helped to sharpen the accuracy and usefulness of urea kinetic modeling, which is now accepted and expected as part of dialysis care.

REFERENCES

1. Lowrie EG, et al. Clinical example of pharmacokinetic and metabolic modeling: quantitative and individualized prescription of dialysis therapy. *Kidney Int* 1980;18[Suppl 10]:S11–S16.
2. Laird NM, et al. Modeling success or failure of dialysis therapy: the National Cooperative Dialysis Study. *Kidney Int* 1983;23[Suppl 13]:101–106.
3. Gotch FA, et al. A mechanistic analysis of the National Cooperative Dialysis Study (NCDS). *Kidney Int* 1985;28:526–534.
4. Lowrie EG, et al. Effect of the hemodialysis prescription on patient morbidity: report from the National Cooperative Dialysis Study. *N Engl J Med* 1981;305:1176–1181.
5. Hakim RM, et al. Effects of acetate and bicarbonate dialysate in stable chronic dialysis patients. *Kidney Int* 1985;28:535–540.
6. Keshaviah P, et al. Rapid high-efficiency bicarbonate hemodialysis. *Trans Am Soc Artif Intern Organs* 1986;32:17.
7. Hull AR, et al. Proceedings from the morbidity, mortality and prescription of dialysis symposium: introduction and summary. *Am J Kidney Dis* 1990;15:375–383.
8. Held PJ, et al. Mortality and duration of hemodialysis treatment. *JAMA* 1991;265:871–875.
9. Hakim RM, et al. Report of a workshop on technique and technology. *Am J Kidney Dis* 1993;21:109–110.
10. Kopple JD, et al. Recommendations for reducing the high morbidity and mortality of United States maintenance dialysis patients. The National Kidney Foundation. *Am J Kidney Dis* 1994;24:968–973.
11. Macey RI, et al. Inhibition of water and solute permeability in human red cells. *Biochim Biophys Acta* 1970;211:104–106.
12. Hunter FL. Facilitated diffusion in human erythrocytes. *Biochim Biophys Acta* 1970;211:216–221.
13. Mayrand RR, et al. Urea and ethylene glycol facilitated transport system in the human red cell membrane. *J Gen Physiol* 1983;81:221–237.

14. Brahm J. Urea permeability of human red cells. *J Gen Physiol* 1983; 82:1–23.
15. Yousef LW, et al. A method to distinguish between pore and carrier kinetics applied to urea transport across the erythrocyte membrane. *Biochem Biophys Acta* 1989;984:281–288.
16. Sands JM, et al. Urea transporters in kidney and erythrocytes. *Am J Physiol* 1997;273(3 Pt 2):F321–F339.
17. Cottini EP, et al. Urea excretion in adult humans with varying degrees of kidney malfunction fed milk, egg, or an amino acid mixture: assessment of nitrogen balance. *J Nutr* 1973;103:11–21.
18. Borah MF, et al. Nitrogen balance during intermittent dialysis therapy of uremia. *Kidney Int* 1978;14:491–500.
19. Anderstam B, et al. Middle-sized molecule fractions isolated from uremic ultrafiltrate and normal urine inhibit ingestive behavior in the rat. *J Am Soc Nephrol* 1996;7:2453–2460.
20. Foley RN, et al. Clinical epidemiology of cardiovascular disease in chronic renal disease. *Am J Kidney Dis* 1998;32[5 Suppl 3]:S112–S119.
21. Merrill JP, et al. Observations on the role of urea in uremia. *Am J Med* 1953;14:519–520.
22. Johnson WJ, et al. Effects of urea loading in patients with far-advanced renal failure. *Mayo Clin Proc* 1972;47:21–29.
23. Bergstrom J, et al. Uraemic toxins. In: Drukker W, et al., eds. *Replacement of renal function by dialysis,* 2nd ed. Boston: Martinus Nijhoff, 1983:354–390.
24. Fluckiger R, et al. Hemoglobin carbamylation in uremia. *N Engl J Med* 1981;304:823–827.
25. Smith WGJ, et al. Carbamylated haemoglobin in chronic renal failure. *Clin Chim Acta* 1988;178:297–304.
26. Kwan JT, et al. Carbamylated haemoglobin, urea kinetic modelling and adequacy of dialysis in haemodialysis patients. *Nephrol Dial Transpl* 1991;6:38–43.
27. Davenport A, et al. Carbamylated hemoglobin: a potential marker for the adequacy of hemodialysis therapy in end-stage renal failure. *Kidney Int* 1996;50:1344–1351.
28. Hou S. Pregnancy in women requiring dialysis for renal failure. *Am J Kidney Dis* 1987;9:368–373.
29. Gipson D, et al. Principles of dialysis: special issues in women. *Semin Nephrol* 1999;19:140–147.
30. Renal Physicians Association. *Clinical practice guideline on adequacy of hemodialysis.* Washington, DC: Renal Physicians Association, 1993.
31. Consensus development conference panel. Morbidity and mortality of renal dialysis: an NIH consensus conference statement. *Ann Intern Med* 1994;121:62–70.
32. DOQI. National Kidney Foundation—Dialysis Outcomes Quality Initiative: clinical practice guidelines for hemodialysis adequacy. *Am J Kidney Dis* 1997;30:S22–S63.
33. Hakim RM, et al. Malnutrition in hemodialysis patients. *Am J Kidney Dis* 1993;21:125–137.
34. Ikizler TA, et al. Spontaneous dietary protein intake during progression of chronic renal failure. *J Am Soc Nephrol* 1995;6:1386–1391.
35. Bergstrom J. Why are dialysis patients malnourished? *Am J Kidney Dis* 1995;26:229–241.
36. Walser M. Does prolonged protein restriction preceding dialysis lead to protein malnutrition at the onset of dialysis? *Kidney Int* 1993;44: 1139–1144.
37. Effects of dietary protein restriction on the progression of moderate renal disease in the Modification of Diet in Renal Disease Study. *J Am Soc Nephrol* 1996;7:2616–2626.
38. Lindsay RM, et al. Which comes first, Kt/V or PCR—chicken or egg? *Kidney Int* 1992;38[Suppl]:S32–S36.
39. Nolph KD. Small solute clearances and clinical outcomes in CAPD [editorial; comment]. *Perit Dial Int* 1992;12:343–345.
40. Ronco C, et al. Adequacy of continuous ambulatory peritoneal dialysis: comparison with other dialysis techniques. *Kidney Int* 1994;46 [Suppl]:18–24.
41. Hakim RM, et al. Effects of dose of dialysis on morbidity and mortality. *Am J Kidney Dis* 1994;23:661–669.
42. Uehlinger DE. Another look at the relationship between protein intake and dialysis dose. *J Am Soc Nephrol* 1996;7:166–168.
43. Greene T, et al. Mathematical coupling and the association between Kt/V and PCRn. *Semin Dial* 1999;12[Suppl 1]:S20–S28.
44. Gotch FA, et al. Clinical outcome relative to the dose of dialysis is not what you think: the fallacy of the mean. *Am J Kidney Dis* 1997; 30:1–15.
45. Sherman RA. Quantitating peritoneal dialysis: the problem with V. *Semin Dial* 1996;9:381–383.
46. Chertow GM, et al. Exploring the reverse J-shaped curve between urea reduction ratio and mortality. *Kidney Int* 1999;56:1872–1878.
47. Levey AS. Measurement of renal function in chronic renal disease [clinical conference]. *Kidney Int* 1990;38:167–184.
48. Depner TA. Uremic toxicity: urea and beyond. *Semin Dial* 2001;14: 246–251.
49. Levin N, et al. A hypothesis to account for the inverse relationship of relative risk of mortality to urea distribution volume in dialysis patients. *J Am Soc Nephrol* 2002;13:12:452.
50. Lowrie EG, et al. The urea [clearance × dialysis time] product (Kt) as an outcome-based measure of hemodialysis dose. *Kidney Int* 1999; 56:729–737.
51. Kopple JD, et al. Body weight-for-height relationships predict mortality in maintenance hemodialysis patients. *Kidney Int* 1999;56: 1136–1148.
52. Port FK, et al. Dialysis dose and body mass index are strongly associated with survival in hemodialysis patients. *J Am Soc Nephrol* 2002; 13:1061–1066.
53. Owen WF Jr, et al. Dose of hemodialysis and survival: differences by race and sex. *JAMA* 1998;280:1764–1768.
54. U.S. Renal Data System. *USRDS 2001 annual report.* Bethesda, MD: National Institutes of Health, National Institute of Diabetes and Digestive and Kidney Diseases, 2002.
55. Kaysen GA, et al. Determinants of albumin concentration in hemodialysis patients. *Am J Kidney Dis* 1997;29:658–668.
56. Depner TA. *Prescribing hemodialysis: a guide to urea modeling.* Boston: Kluwer Academic, 1991.
57. Delmez JA, et al. Hemodialysis prescription and delivery in a metropolitan community. *Kidney Int* 1992;41:1023–1028.
58. Gotch FA. Kinetic modeling in hemodialysis. In: Nissenson AR, et al., eds. *Clinical dialysis,* 3rd ed. Norwalk, CT: Appleton & Lange, 1995:156–188.
59. Vanholder R, et al. Hippuric acid as a marker. In: Ringoir S, et al., eds. *Uremic toxins.* New York: Plenum, 1987:59–67.
60. Schreiner GE, et al. *Uremia: biochemistry, pathogenesis, and treatment.* Springfield, IL: Charles C Thomas, 1961.
61. Giovannetti S, et al. A low nitrogen diet with proteins of high biological value for severe chronic uraemia. *Lancet* 1964;1:1000–1001.
62. Giordano C, et al. Loss of large amounts of amino acids in hemodialysis. *Biochemic Applicata* 1968;15:373.
63. Lowrie EG, et al. Principles of prescribing dialysis therapy: implementing recommendations from the National Cooperative Dialysis Study. *Kidney Int* 1983;23[Suppl 13]:S113–S122.
64. Richet G. Early history of uremia. *Kidney Int* 1988;33:1013–1015.
65. Owen WF Jr, et al. The urea reduction ratio and serum albumin concentration as predictors of mortality in patients undergoing hemodialysis. *N Engl J Med* 1993;329:1001–1006.
66. Teraoka S, et al. Current status of renal replacement therapy in Japan. *Am J Kidney Dis* 1995;25:151–164.
67. Michaels AS. Operating parameters and performance criteria for hemodialyzers and other membrane-separation devices. *Trans Am Soc Artif Intern Organs* 1966;12:387–392.
68. Gibaldi M, et al. *Pharmacokinetics.* New York: Marcel Dekker, 1982.
69. Depner TA. Hemodialysis urea modeling: the basics. *Semin Dial* 1991;4:179–184.
70. Depner TA. Standards for dialysis adequacy. *Semin Dial* 1991;4: 245–252.
71. Hakim RM, et al. In depth review: adequacy of hemodialysis [see comments]. *Am J Kidney Dis* 1992;20:107–123.
72. Sargent JA, et al. Which mathematical model to study uremic toxicity—National Cooperative Dialysis Study. *Clin Nephrol* 1982;17: 303–314.
73. Mitch WE. Nutritional therapy and the progression of renal insuffi-

ciency. In: Mitch WE, et al., eds. *Nutrition and the kidney.* Boston: Little, Brown, 1988:154–179.

74. Lim VS, et al. The effect of hemodialysis on protein metabolism: a leucine kinetic study. *J Clin Invest* 1993;91:2429–2436.

75. Depner TA, et al. Modeling urea kinetics with two vs. three BUN measurements: a critical comparison. *ASAIO Trans* 1989;35:499–502.

76. Depner TA. *Multicompartment models: prescribing hemodialysis—a guide to urea modeling.* Boston: Kluwer Academic, 1991:91–126.

77. Pedrini LA, et al. Causes, kinetics, and clinical implications of post-hemodialysis urea rebound. *Kidney Int* 1988;34:817–824.

78. Sargent JA, et al. Principles and biophysics of dialysis. In: Maher JF, ed. *Replacement of renal function by dialysis,* 3rd ed. Dordrecht, the Netherlands: Kluwer Academic, 1989:87–143.

79. Heineken FG, et al. Intercompartmental fluid shifts in hemodialysis patients. *Biotechnol Progr* 1987;3:69–73.

80. Evans JH, et al. Mathematical modelling of haemodialysis in children. *Pediatr Nephrol* 1992;6:349–353.

81. Depner TA. Refining the model of urea kinetics: compartment effects. *Semin Dial* 1992;5:147–154.

82. Grandi F, et al. Analytic solution of the variable-volume double-pool urea kinetics model applied to parameter estimation in hemodialysis. *Comput Biol Med* 1995;25:505–518.

83. Burgelman M, et al. Estimation of parameters in a two-pool urea kinetic model for hemodialysis. *Med Engl Phys* 1997;19:69–76.

84. Depner TA, et al. High venous urea concentrations in the opposite arm: a consequence of hemodialysis-induced compartment disequilibrium. *ASAIO J* 1991;37:M141–M143.

85. Depner T, et al. Peripheral urea disequilibrium during hemodialysis is temperature-dependent. *J Am Soc Nephrol* 1991;2:321.

86. Schneditz D, et al. Cardiopulmonary recirculation during hemodialysis. *Kidney Int* 1992;42:1450–1456.

87. Kong CH, et al. The effect of exercise during haemodialysis on solute removal. *Nephrol Dial Transpl* 1999;14:2927–2931.

88. Depner TA, et al. Hemodialysis access recirculation measured by ultrasound dilution. *ASAIO J* 1995;41:M749–M753.

89. Sombolos K, et al. Urea concentration gradients during conventional hemodialysis. *Am J Kidney Dis* 1996;27:673–679.

90. Schneditz D, et al. Impact of cardiopulmonary recirculation on measurement of access recirculation. *J Am Soc Nephrol* 1992;3:393.

91. Sherman RA. Recirculation revisited. *Semin Dial* 1991;4:221–223.

92. Schneditz D, et al. Formal analytical solution to a regional blood flow and diffusion based urea kinetic model. *ASAIO J* 1994;40:M667–M673.

93. Daugirdas JT, et al. Effect of a two-compartment distribution on apparent urea distribution volume. *Kidney Int* 1997;51:1270–1273.

94. Daugirdas JT, et al. Overestimation of hemodialysis dose depends on dialysis efficiency by regional blood flow but not by conventional two pool urea kinetic analysis. *ASAIO J* 1995;41:M719–M724.

95. Daugirdas JT, et al. Comparison of methods to predict equilibrated Kt/V in the HEMO Pilot Study. *Kidney Int* 1997;52:1395–1405.

96. Daugirdas JT. Simplified equations for monitoring Kt/V, PCRn, eKt/V, and ePCRn. *Adv Ren Replace Ther* 1995;2:295–304.

97. Malchesky PS, et al. Direct quantification of dialysis. *Dial Transpl* 1982;11:42–44.

98. Ellis P, et al. Comparison of two methods of kinetic modeling. *Trans Am Soc Artif Intern Organs* 1984;30:60–64.

99. Garred LJ. Urea kinetic modeling by partial dialysate collection. *Int J Artif Organs* 1989;12:96–102.

100. Garred LJ. Dialysate-based kinetic modeling. *Adv Ren Replace Ther* 1995;2:305–318.

101. Depner TA, et al. Multicenter clinical validation of an on-line monitor of dialysis adequacy. *J Am Soc Nephrol* 1996;7:464–471.

102. Keshaviah P, et al. A new approach to dialysis quantification: an adequacy index based on solute removal. *Semin Dial* 1994;7:85–90.

103. Keshaviah P. The solute removal index—a unified basis for comparing disparate therapies [editorial]. *Perit Dial Int* 1995;15:101–104.

104. Flanigan MJ, et al. Quantitating hemodialysis: a comparison of three kinetic models [see comments]. *Am J Kidney Dis* 1991;17:295–302.

105. Depner TA, et al. Imprecision of the hemodialysis dose when measured directly from urea removal. Hemodialysis Study Group. *Kidney Int* 1999;55:635–647.

106. Alloatti S, et al. On-line dialysate urea monitor: comparison with urea kinetics. *Int J Artif Organs* 1995;18:548–552.

107. Chauveau P, et al. Adequacy of haemodialysis and nutrition in maintenance haemodialysis patients: clinical evaluation of a new on-line urea monitor. *Nephrol Dial Transpl* 1996;11:1568–1573.

108. Sternby J. Whole body Kt/V from dialysate urea measurements during hemodialysis. *J Am Soc Nephrol* 1998;9:2118–2123.

109. Keshaviah PR, et al. On-line monitoring of the delivery of the hemodialysis prescription. *Pediatr Nephrol* 1995;9:S2–S8.

110. Petitclerc T, et al. A model for non-invasive estimation of in vivo dialyzer performances and patient's conductivity during hemodialysis. *Int J Artif Organs* 1993;16:585–591.

111. Polaschegg HD. On-line dialyser clearance using conductivity. *Pediatr Nephrol* 1995;9[Suppl]:S9–S11.

112. Mercadal L, et al. Is ionic dialysance a valid parameter for quantification of dialysis efficiency? *Artif Organs* 1998;22:1005–1009.

113. Petitclerc T, et al. Non-invasive monitoring of effective dialysis dose delivered to the haemodialysis patient. *Nephrol Dial Transpl* 1995;10: 212–216.

114. Clark WR, et al. Quantifying the effect of changes in the hemodialysis prescription on effective solute removal with a mathematical model. *J Am Soc Nephrol* 1999;10:601–609.

115. Mucsi I, et al. Control of serum phosphate without any phosphate binders in patients treated with nocturnal hemodialysis. *Kidney Int* 1998;53:1399–1404.

116. Casino FG, et al. The equivalent renal urea clearance: a new parameter to assess dialysis dose. *Nephrol Dial Transpl* 1996;11:1574–581.

117. Depner TA. Benefits of more frequent dialysis: lower TAC at the same Kt/V. *Nephrol Dial Transpl* 1998;13:20–24.

118. Depner TA. Quantifying hemodialysis and peritoneal dialysis: examination of the peak concentration hypothesis. *Semin Dial* 1994;7: 315–317.

119. Hakim RM, et al. Initiation of dialysis [editorial]. *J Am Soc Nephrol* 1995;6:1319–1328.

120. Paniagua R, et al. Effects of increased peritoneal clearances on mortality rates in peritoneal dialysis: ADEMEX, a prospective, randomized, controlled trial. *J Am Soc Nephrol* 2002;13:1307–1320.

121. Depner T, et al. Solute seclusion: an alternative to the peak concentration hypothesis. *J Am Soc Nephrol* 2001;12:447A.

122. Depner TA. Why daily hemodialysis is better: solute kinetics. *Semin Dial* 1999;12:462–471.

123. DOQI. I. NKF-K/DOQI Clinical practice guidelines for hemodialysis adequacy: update 2000. *Am J Kidney Dis* 2001;37[Suppl 1]:S7–S64.

124. Gotch FA. The current place of urea kinetic modelling with respect to different dialysis modalities. *Nephrol Dial Transpl* 1998;13[Suppl 6]: 10–14.

125. Jindal KK, et al. Percent reduction in blood urea concentration during hemodialysis (PRU): a simple and accurate method to estimate Kt/V urea. *Trans Am Soc Artif Intern Organs* 1987;33:286–288.

126. Daugirdas JT. The post: pre dialysis plasma urea nitrogen ratio to estimate Kt/V and NPCR: validation [see comments]. *Int J Artif Organs* 1989;12:420–427.

127. Daugirdas JT. Second generation logarithmic estimates of single-pool variable volume Kt/V: an analysis of error. *J Am Soc Nephrol* 1993;4: 1205–1213.

128. Garred LJ, et al. Simple Kt/V formulas based on urea mass balance theory. *ASAIO J* 1994;40:997–1004.

129. Depner TA, et al. Equations for normalized protein catabolic rate based on two-point modeling of hemodialysis urea kinetics. *J Am Soc Nephrol* 1996;7:780–785.

130. Garred LJ, et al. Simple equations for protein catabolic rate determination from predialysis and postdialysis BUN. *ASAIO J* 1995;41: 889–895.

131. Depner TA. Quantifying hemodialysis. *Am J Nephrol* 1996;16:17–28.

132. Lowrie EG, et al. The urea reduction ratio (URR): a simple method for evaluating hemodialysis treatment. *Contemp Dial Nephrol* 1991; 12:11–20.

133. Daugirdas JT. Chronic hemodialysis prescription: a urea kinetic approach. In: Daugirdas JT, et al., eds. *Handbook of dialysis,* 2nd ed. Boston: Little, Brown, 1994:92–120.

134. Keen M, et al. Current standards for dialysis adequacy. *Adv Ren Replace Ther* 1995;2:287–294.

135. Blake P, et al. Recommended clinical practices for maximizing peritoneal dialysis clearances [see comments]. *Perit Dial Int* 1996;16:448–456.

136. Eknoyan G, et al. The hemodialysis (HEMO) study: rationale for selection of interventions. *Semin Dial* 1996;9:24–33.

137. Depner TA. Assessing adequacy of hemodialysis: urea modeling. *Kidney Int* 1994;45:1522–1535.

138. Sherman RA, et al. Recirculation reassessed: the impact of blood flow rate and the low-flow method reevaluated. *Am J Kidney Dis* 1994;23:846–888.

139. Depner TA. Pitfalls in quantitating hemodialysis. *Semin Dial* 1993;6:127–133.

140. Depner TA, et al. Pressure effects on coller pump blood flow during hemodialysis. *ASAIO J* 1990;36:456–459.

141. Gotch FA, et al. Care of the patient on hemodialysis. In: Cogan MG, et al., eds. *Introduction to dialysis*. New York: Churchill Livingstone, 1985:73–143.

CHOOSING THE BEST DIALYSIS OPTIONS IN THE PATIENT WITH CHRONIC RENAL FAILURE

ROCHELLE CUNNINGHAM

OVERVIEW OF TREATMENT OPTIONS

There are three treatment modalities available for patients with chronic renal failure. Although these treatment modalities have proven to be life sustaining, patients with end-stage renal disease (ESRD) still have significant morbidity and mortality. Ideally, the dialysis modality of choice would be cost effective, associated with the lowest morbidity and mortality, and result in the highest quality of life.

In terms of overall efficacy, renal transplantation is the modality of choice for patients with ESRD. After the first year, it is the most cost-efficient modality and long term provides the highest quality of life with the longest life expectancy (1). Living donor kidney transplantation by far offers the best form of renal replacement therapy with a half-life greater than 25 years depending on the haplotype match (2). Recently, there has been a 7% increase in the number of organ donors (3). This increase has been attributed mainly to an increase in the number of living donations. Despite the increase, there are still many more patients awaiting kidney transplants than available cadaveric donors. In 2001, over 12,000 kidney transplants were performed in the United States, but more than 52,000 patients remain on the wait list (3). During this same period, there were 70,000 new patients with advanced renal failure identified and there are now more than 300,000 patients with ESRD (3). Although experience in renal transplantation has grown with the newer agents and more palatable immunosuppressive regimens, it is still not appropriate or available to all patients with chronic renal failure. As a result, most patients with chronic renal failure will require dialysis therapy, and dialysis therapy per se will remain the most commonly used method of renal replacement therapy. Chapter 42 provides a discussion of the preparation of dialysis patients who are thought to be candidates for renal transplants.

Although most ESRD patients are suitable for either hemodialysis (HD) or peritoneal dialysis (PD), certain considerations must be taken into account in choosing a replacement modality. This chapter gives a brief overview of the various treatment modalities and the factors involved in choosing the best dialysis therapy for the patient with chronic renal failure.

DIALYSIS MODALITY DISTRIBUTION

Although HD remains the most common form of renal replacement therapy worldwide, in certain areas such as, Mexico, Hong Kong, and New Zealand, PD is the modality of choice (4). Recently, there has been a disconcerting trend toward decreasing use of PD in the United States and abroad (5). In the United States, PD use has continued to decline over the last 8 years from its peak of 14.7% in 1993 to approximately 9.4% in 1999 (4). Although PD use is much higher in Canada (approximately 23.6% of prevalent patients), it has also seen a decline over the last 7 years (4,6). There appears to be general agreement among nephrologists as to preferences of ESRD treatment modalities, yet disparities persist between preferences and practices even among and between different geographic regions (7). The reason for the difference between preference and practice remains unclear, especially in light of the potential cost savings of PD.

MODALITY SELECTION

In choosing a dialysis therapy for a particular patient several variables factor into the decision-making process. These factors include the type of treatment modality, financial and reimbursement constraints, and patient variables such as motivation and physical limitations. Physician factors, such as experience and preferences of the nephrologist, also influence modality selection. Table 8.1 details several of the critical considerations in selecting a modality. Fig. 8.1 provides an algorithm to aid in the selection of particular type of renal replacement therapy. Although there are few absolute medical contraindications to either PD or HD, modality selection is, to a large extent, determined by nonmedical factors, and it is likely these factors that explain the marked variability in dialysis modality distribution (5,8).

Physician opinion was once thought to be the major determinant of modality selection (9). In the United States and Canada, nephrologists were surveyed and found to be in agreement as to the mix of patients on HD versus PD, 69% and 63% versus 31% and 37%, respectively (10). This differed greatly

TABLE 8.1. FACTORS THAT INFLUENCE MODALITY CHOICE

Physician factors
   Physician bias and experience
   Physician reimbursement
   Resource availability
Financial and reimbursement factors
   Fee for service
   Public vs. private ownership
   Resource availability/existing infrastructure
Patient factors
   Physical limitations
   Patient social or living conditions
   Geographic location
   Predialysis education
   Social or cultural influences

from the actual mix, at least in the United States, of 9.4%; Canada, however had a closer approximation with 23% of prevalent patients on PD (4,6). Financial and reimbursement factors may also be important considerations. For example, countries in which remuneration for PD is low relative to HD tend to have lower rates of PD use (11). On the other hand, in the United States, physician fees for PD and HD are identical, but HD use is five times as common as that of PD (9). Clearly, other influences exist.

An immediate issue for many physicians is the availability of an existing infrastructure to support a specific modality. There is greater ease in initiating a particular patient with a preexisting infrastructure. Along with having the available support system is the issue of cost versus profitability. The marginal cost of an additional HD patient is less than the cost associated with the addition of a PD patient, especially if there is a limited PD infrastructure or a relatively small PD program. In this regard, it may be more cost effective to choose HD for a particular patient than to have a patient start PD.

It is unclear to what extent patient factors influence modality selection; however, a very important patient factor is the ability of the patient to perform PD safely. Patients with certain physical limitations will have difficulties performing PD at home. In addition, with the increase in the average age and comorbidity of patients initiating renal replacement therapy in the United States, it may seem simpler in such instances to direct the patient to HD, in which the procedure is performed by dialysis personnel. Therefore, many of the older and sicker patients may not be considered candidates for PD. This may have also contributed to the recently observed decline in PD use in the United States (12). In addition, other considerations, such as occupation, race, family support, the importance of autonomy, and other social or cultural factors also exert some influence on a patient's preference for a particular dialysis modality.

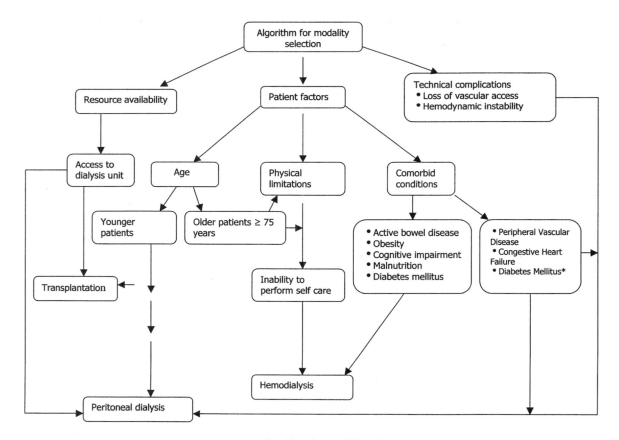

FIG. 8.1. Algorithm for modality selection.

Geography is another factor that may influence dialysis modality selection. The use of PD is higher in areas where population density is low and where there is a relatively long distance between HD units. This observation may explain the variation of PD even within a particular country. For example, PD use in the United States had been as high as 18% to 20% in the rural Midwest but significantly lower in the more densely populated Northeast (13). This gap, although still evident, is now much smaller (3).

Recently, there has been an increase in the number of proprietary dialysis centers and, thus, the number of HD facilities in both the United States and Canada. This increase may explain why there is less incentive to choose PD as a form of renal replacement therapy. In reference to cost, ESRD is the only disease-based entitlement program for Medicare. As a result of the federal government's involvement, several attempts have been made to control health care costs in this population, most notably the establishment of a capitated fee for outpatient dialysis (the composite rate) and fixed fees for the nephrologists supervising the dialysis. Because Medicare reimburses facilities and nephrologists through partially capitated payments, it has imposed on the provider some of the same financial incentives as health maintenance organizations (HMOs) and, as with other health care providers, has led to industry consolidation of outpatient dialysis services. Multicenter dialysis companies operating on a for-profit basis are now replacing not-for-profit and sole proprietorship facilities. Currently, approximately 75% of all for-profit facilities are affiliated with a chain (3).

The concern for this growth is not only for its effect on PD use but also for its effect on the quality of care of ESRD patients. It has been suggested that in an attempt to contain cost, the quality of care may be adversely affected. A recent study by Garg et al. (14) reported a 20% higher mortality among patients treated at for-profit facilities than not-for-profit facilities. In addition, there was also a 26% lower likelihood of being placed on the kidney transplant waiting list (14). Although these findings remain controversial, they highlight the practical importance of the effect of cost containment on quality of care. For PD patients, there is cost savings in performing the dialysis, because PD patients perform the procedure at home reducing the labor costs in providing therapy. Several studies have suggested that PD when efficiently managed may represent a highly cost-effective modality of ESRD care (15,16).

Predialysis education and early referral also affect modality selection. Although currently an underused tool, the use of predialysis education is likely to improve as a result of the recent development of K/DOQI guidelines for chronic kidney disease (CKD). A recent study found that given free choice and predialysis education, 50% of patients would select PD (17). Predialysis education may not always be an option for some patients, especially those who are late referrals or noncompliant, however, when available may improve PD use (18–20).

HEMODIALYSIS VERSUS PERITONEAL DIALYSIS: WHICH IS BETTER?

After the introduction of PD, there was speculation as to whether it would prove to be an effective and viable long-term alternative to HD, particularly in terms of patient and technique survival. It has passed the test of time and is considered an effective form of renal replacement therapy. The debate now is which dialytic modality provides the best patient outcome. To answer this question a prospective, randomized clinical trial would need to be performed, a study difficult to construct mainly because of the process of modality selection and the tremendous heterogeneity within the HD and PD populations, which may in many instances preclude the use of a specific modality. Therefore, any attempt to perform a comparative study will remain difficult and inherently flawed to some extent. Most comparative studies are either small and lack the statistical strength to detect a difference or involve registry data, which usually lack important patient information. This may explain the conflicting results of many studies performed since the introduction of PD.

As to which modality is superior, it has been suggested that HD is superior to PD. Bloembergen et al. (21) in a large epidemiologic comparative study of prevalent HD and PD dialysis found a 19% higher adjusted mortality risk (all-cause mortality) for peritoneal patients with the greatest risk in women and older patients (older than 55 years). Another study by Held et al. (22), which made adjustments for patient characteristics including the presence of comorbid conditions at the onset of ESRD, also found a higher adjusted mortality risk for PD patients with diabetes compared with HD patients with diabetes.

In contrast, a study by Nelson et al. (15) using the Michigan Kidney Registry found no significant difference in mortality risk of nondiabetic hypertensive ESRD patients, and a lower mortality among PD patients with ESRD secondary to glomerulonephritis or diabetes. Furthermore, young diabetic PD patients 20 to 52 years old had the lowest mortality rates, and mortality increased significantly with age in all groups (15). Fenton et al. (23), analyzing Canadian incident patients, found a 27% lower risk an effect concentrated in the first 2 years postinitiation.

In an attempt to reconcile these differences, a recent analysis by Collins et al. (16) evaluated incident Medicare patients from 1994 through 1996. In this study, PD was associated with a significantly lower risk of death in all patients except diabetics 55 years of age or older in whom there was a 21% greater mortality risk for women, particularly death resulting from infection (16). It appears that there may be a survival advantage for PD over the first 2 years of dialysis, a finding also recently confirmed by a Danish study (24) that showed a substantial advantage of PD over HD during the first 1 to 2 years of dialysis. However, after the first 2 years, there was no difference except for in diabetic patients in whom the survival advantage subsequently disappeared (24).

The more recent results of a survival advantage with PD may be explained by the presence of potential confounders such as the selection bias of younger, more healthy patients for PD, the presence of a greater dialysis dose resulting from residual renal function in PD patients, or the recent technologic advances that have resulted in better catheters and safer transfer delivery systems and thus lower infectious complication rates. In any case, the more recent results have not reconciled the issue of which modality is best but rather highlight the need for future studies. Further studies with longer follow-up periods may help to clarify these conflicting results.

PERITONEAL DIALYSIS

Description and Rationale

PD involves using the peritoneum as a dialysis and ultrafiltration membrane (see Chapters 14 and 15). Dialysate is instilled into the peritoneal space and removed at various intervals taking with it nitrogenous wastes, fluid, and electrolytes. The concentration gradient between the plasma and dialysate drives solute removal. In comparison to conventional dialysis membranes, PD is generally more effective at removal of larger molecular weight molecules, such as β_2-microglobulin than smaller molecular weight molecules, such as urea (25). Ultrafiltration is accomplished by establishing a hydroosmotic gradient with glucose from relatively high glucose concentrations in the dialysate.

There are various forms of PD. Continuous ambulatory peritoneal dialysis (CAPD) involves exchange of peritoneal fluid every 4 to 6 hours during the day. Continuous cycling peritoneal dialysis (CCPD) is an automated form of PD that involves using a cycler, usually at night to perform exchanges while the patient sleeps. There are advantages and disadvantages to each form of PD therapy. CAPD is more efficacious for patients with slow lymphatic reabsorption and solute clearance rates. CCPD is a preferred modality for those patients with higher lymphatic reabsorption and solute clearance rates. Some patients will need to combine both modalities to achieve adequate clearances (26).

Access

Chronic PD catheters are cuffed catheters inserted into the peritoneal space, and unlike the uncuffed acute catheters used for HD, the PD catheters can function successfully for 2 years or more. It is recommended that catheter use after placement be delayed for 2 to 3 weeks to allow for proper healing, although under certain conditions earlier use may be allowed. If earlier use is indicated, low volume exchanges are encouraged for the first 2 to 3 weeks.

Dialysis Prescription

PD generally produces lower clearance rates for low molecular weight solutes compared with HD using cuprophane or cellulose acetate membranes and higher clearance rates for larger molecular weight solutes. Generally, creatinine clearance rates obtained when combining PD and residual renal function greater than 60 L/week are felt to represent an adequate dialysis prescription. A *Kt/V* exceeding 2.0, using urea as a marker, also represents adequate delivery of PD. Although dialysis dose has been shown to affect mortality in PD patients, it is likely that dialysis dose along with nutritional status combined are better predictors of patient survival (27,28).

The kinetics of solute and fluid removal are unique to each individual dialysis patient and are subject to change over time. The rate at which fluid is removed depends on the dialysate glucose concentration, the rapidity with which glucose is dialyzed across the peritoneal membrane, and the rate of lymphatic reabsorption. Because the transport properties of the peritoneal membrane and the rate of lymphatic reabsorption cannot be modified, the use of either higher tonicity dwells, i.e., higher glucose concentrations, shorter dialysate dwell times, or higher dwell volumes, will enhance fluid removal.

Solute flux, on the other hand, is less consistent with PD. PD, in general, provides a low level of clearance delivered continuously as compared with HD that provides a high level of clearance delivered intermittently. The removal of solute is influenced by the same factors that influence fluid removal. Therefore, peritoneal solute clearance can be increased by either increasing the time on PD, the frequency of exchanges, or by using larger dwell volumes. The peritoneal equilibration test (PET) allows clinicians to measure and follow the peritoneal membrane solute transport characteristics in their patients and determine if a patient has rapid, average, or slow solute flux. Once the transport characteristics are determined for a particular patient, a more effective dialysis regimen can be prescribed. For a detailed discussion on PD adequacy see Chapter 14.

Complications

The complications associated with PD include those associated with the placement of access as well as those associated with the actual procedure. Unusual complications, such as the perforation of a major blood vessel or bowel after placement of a catheter, can lead to hemorrhage, sepsis, and, on rare occasions, death. More commonly, PD complications include infections, such as peritonitis, exit-site infections, protein malnutrition secondary to protein losses within the peritoneal fluid, and lipid derangements. Inadequate dialysis, although not necessarily a complication, is often the reason for technique failure and occurs as a result of changes in the characteristics of the peritoneal membrane.

Infections

The frequency of peritonitis has decreased dramatically over the past decade secondary to improved catheter and tubing connectors. Gram-positive organisms especially, *Staphylococcus* sp., still remain the most commonly isolated organisms. Infections with gram-negative organisms and fungal infections also occur. Although rare these infections can be life threatening and usually require removal of the peritoneal catheter for adequate treatment (29). Exit-site and tunnel infections are not uncommon and can be treated effectively with local or with systemic antibiotic therapy and only rarely requiring catheter removal (30). See Chapter 41 for a more detailed discussion of infections in dialysis patients.

Protein Malnutrition

Protein loss with PD can be significant, ranging from 4 to 20 g/day through the dialysate and may be exacerbated during an episode of peritonitis (30,31). An additional factor to be considered is the amount of calories administered using glucose dialysate. This can often lead to protein malnutrition. The alternatives to the glucose-containing dialysate are the amino-acid-based solutions that have been offered as a method for the treatment of protein malnutrition. Unfortunately, the amino-acid-based solutions have been shown to be only modestly effective in nutritionally compromised patients (see Chapter 30) (32).

Lipid Derangements

Lipid abnormalities are another complication of using dextrose-containing dialysate and result from the high glucose absorption. The exact mechanism of uremic dyslipidemia remains unclear but has been associated with decreased catabolism of apoprotein-B-containing lipoproteins (apo B) as a result of the decreased activity of lipolytic enzymes and altered lipoprotein composition (33). The most common lipid abnormalities are a high total and low-density lipoprotein (LDL) cholesterol, low high-density lipoprotein (HDL) cholesterol, high apo B, low apo A-I, high triglycerides, and high lipoprotein (a) Lp(a) levels. In comparison to HD patients, PD patients have higher apo B protein and LDL cholesterol levels that are markedly atherogenic (34). The hypertriglyceridemia often observed in PD patients results from the overproduction of the very low density lipoproteins and a deficiency of lipoprotein lipase as well as a partial deficiency of hepatic lipase (34). Polyglucose preparations, such as icodextrin, have been associated with a reduction in glucose-induced lipid abnormalities and may be an acceptable alternative in certain patients (35).

Hyperinsulinemia and Hyperglycemia

The use of glucose dialysate can result in hyperinsulinemia and hyperglycemia. Hyperinsulinemia occurs as a result of increased insulin secretion and results in plasma insulin levels that are persistently high. This has been found to be an independent risk factor for the development of atherosclerosis (34). In addition, the use of glucose dialysate can lead to the de novo development of hyperglycemia in some patients and the loss of glycemic control in those patients previously well controlled. As a result, oral hypoglycemics as well as insulin may often be required.

Hernia Formation

Hernia formation is a mechanical complication of PD that occurs as a result of the increased intraabdominal pressure from instillation of dialysis fluid into the peritoneal cavity. Approximately 10% to 20% of patients develop hernias at some time on PD with the risk factors for development being large dialysate volumes and activities that involve isometric straining or the Valsalva maneuver (36). Inguinal (direct and indirect), pericatheter, ventral, umbilical, and femoral are common hernias that occur and can be further delineated with ultrasonography or computed tomography (CT) scanning. Surgical intervention is required to repair the defect.

Inadequate Dialysis

An inability to achieve adequate dialysis usually becomes apparent with progressive loss of residual renal function. Failure to achieve dialysis adequacy can also occur as a result of the impaired transport characteristics of the peritoneal membrane from recurrent episodes of peritonitis (see Chapter 15). Excluding other complications, these are the major reasons for failure of this form of renal replacement therapy.

Advantages and Disadvantages of Peritoneal Dialysis Therapy

PD's greatest advantages are its portability and low cost. Although easy to learn, it requires several weeks of training before initiating. In addition, PD allows for greater hemodynamic stability and proves useful in patients with severe cardiomyopathy (37). The major disadvantages are those related to the complications listed previously and the burden of increased patient participation with this form of renal replacement therapy. For some patients, the increased patient participation may be unappealing.

HEMODIALYSIS

Description and Rationale

HD involves removal of toxins and waste product with dialysis. Solutes are removed largely by diffusion down a chemical gradient and ultrafiltration results from the hydrostatic pressure gradient. HD was first used in the 1940s for the treatment of acute renal failure. It is now the most common form of renal replacement for patients with ESRD in the United States. There are currently more than 300,000 patients receiving some form of dialytic therapy (3).

Access

The advent of the Scribner shunt facilitated the development of HD as a form of renal replacement therapy (38). Vascular access can be obtained by either placement of a central venous catheter or by the surgical creation of an arteriovenous (AV) shunt. The most common complications associated with access placement are infections and clotting (see Table 8.2 for comparisons of the

TABLE 8.2. ADVANTAGES AND DISADVANTAGES OF HEMODIALYSIS ACCESS

	Advantages	Disadvantages
Venous catheters	Quick and easy to insert and use	Complications associated with central line placement
		Central venous system stenosis
AVF	Best long-term function	Complications associated with central line placement
	Lower risk of infection and thrombosis	Central venous system stenosis
		Infection
		Thrombosis
AVG	Good long-term function	Surgery required
	Lower risk of infection and thrombosis	Not ready for immediate use

AVF, arteriovenous fistula.

advantages and disadvantages of different forms of HD access and Chapter 4 for a more detailed discussion).

Venous Catheters

Venous catheters are placed transcutaneously with or without a subcutaneous tunnel. Subcutaneous catheters have a reportedly greater longevity. Clotting and infections are also frequent complications associated with this form of access. Internal jugular catheter placement is now the preferred site as a result of the increasing frequency of central venous stenosis associated with subclavian vein catheters. The occurrence of subclavian vein stenosis may have long-lasting consequences since the placement of an AV shunt or longevity of an existing AV shunt may be affected.

Arteriovenous Shunts

AV shunts can be classified as fistulas (entirely autologous anastomoses between the patient's own artery and vein) or grafts (which involve an interposition of synthetic material, usually Gore-Tex) between an artery and vein. They are usually placed in the upper extremity, but an AV shunt may also be placed in the thigh. In general, arteriovenous fistulas (AVFs) have greater durability and have a lower rate of infection and thrombotic complications compared with grafts (39). The placement of an AVF requires veins of sufficient caliber. It is recommended that in preparation for access placement, a general rule is to prohibit blood draws from the nondominant arm. Patients with diabetes mellitus or peripheral vascular disease may have difficulty obtaining adequate access in light of the degree of atherosclerotic involvement. As a result, more synthetic grafts are placed. In general, less than 20% of all surgical shunts are AVFs (40).

Access Complications

The major complications with all forms of dialysis access are infection and thrombosis. Although adherence to strict sterile technique can greatly reduce the incidence of access infections, when systemic infections occur removal of the venous catheter or Gore-Tex is often required for successful treatment.

Dialysis Prescription

The prescription for HD has evolved over the past two decades and now is based on urea kinetics and generally shorter treatments (see Chapters 7 and 11 for discussion). This has to some extent also led to underdialysis for many patients. To ensure adequate dialysis most facilities use a "minimum time" and Kt/V (41). The optimal dialysis prescription is still unclear, although recent evidence has suggested better clinical outcomes with higher frequency and longer duration of HD (42,43). The main considerations in optimizing HD prescription are economic considerations; cost associated with longer dialysis; and patient preferences, such as willingness to increase dialysis time. Current K/DOQI recommendations are a minimum of 3 to 4 hours and a minimum delivered Kt/V greater than 1.2 per treatment.

Complications

Equipment-related Complications

Acute HD-associated complications include those related to machine malfunction such as overheating of dialysate producing delayed hemolysis, misproportioning of dialysate concentrate causing acute hyperosmolarity or hypoosmolarity, bubble detector failure allowing for air embolus, and excessive or inadequate ultrafiltration, now less of a problem since the development of volumetric HD machines.

Operator error and water treatment failure are other HD-associated complications. Water treatment failure that leads to bacterial contamination can result in the release of endotoxins (44–47). Copper or chloramine intoxication leading to hemolysis is a rare but important cause of hemolysis and results from improper water treatment. In addition, hemolysis can also result from excessive amounts of formaldehyde entering the circulation after dialyzer reprocessing. Although a large dose of formaldehyde will acutely lead to symptoms, smaller doses produce a form of delayed hemolysis.

Aluminum intoxication is another example of water treatment failure. Aluminum intoxication from contaminated water results in a chronic syndrome of dialysis encephalopathy, aluminum osteodystrophy, and microcytic anemia (48,49). Although a significant problem in the past, aluminum intoxication is now less of a problem secondary to adequate procedures for water treatment and the replacement of aluminum-containing phosphate binders with calcium phosphate binders.

Acute HD reactions can occur and are membrane-related complications such as the first-use syndrome, bradykinin-related hypotension, bronchospasm in patients receiving angiotensin-converting enzyme (ACE) inhibitors, and dialysis hypoxia associated with pulmonary leukostasis (50).

Dialysis Hypotension (see Chapter 19)

Dialysis hypotension is the most common acute complication associated with chronic HD. The cause is likely multifactorial and includes either excessive or rapid ultrafiltration; lack of vasoconstriction; or cardiac factors, such as failure to increase cardiac output from underlying cardiac disease (30). Treatment involves monitoring the rate of ultrafiltration as well as other therapeutic measures, such as the use of bicarbonate solutions and higher dialysate sodium concentrations (51).

Advantages and Disadvantages of Hemodialysis

In-center dialysis has the advantage of being relatively straightforward and simple to initiate. It can adequately substitute normal renal function for extended periods of time although it has the disadvantage of being associated with a certain amount of expense and complexity. In addition, HD requires adequate staffing and supervision; this has been a tremendous hurdle for many centers given the shortage of qualified personnel. Perhaps the greatest disadvantage is the underemployment and unemployment rate of HD patients. Few patients remain actively employed once HD is initiated. Although this trend has improved over recent years, the rate

TABLE 8.3. COMPARISON OF DIFFERENT TREATMENT MODALITIES

	Cost	Quality of Life	Availability	Complications
Living related transplant	++	++++	+	++[a]
Cadaveric renal transplant	++	+++	++	+
Peritoneal dialysis	+	+++	+++	+++
Hemodialysis	+++	++	++++	+++
Home hemodialysis	+++	+++	+	++

[a]Risk to donor.

of employment still remains dismally low. Recent reports indicate the percentage of employed chronic dialysis patients of working age varies between 11% and 31% (52). A recent international study coordinated by the Dialysis Outcomes and Practice Patterns Study Group (53) of 4,123 prevalent HD patients of working age found 21%, 30%, and 55% of patients in the United States, Europe, and Japan, respectively, currently employed. Perhaps more interesting is the relatively small proportion of ESRD patients employed at the start of dialysis, approximately 20% to 35% (54,55). Therefore, it is apparent that many patients become unemployed before starting dialysis and efforts to improve employment should focus on pre-ESRD education and rehabilitation.

Home Hemodialysis

PD and home HD fall into this category. The advantages and disadvantages of PD have been discussed previously. Home nocturnal hemodialysis (HND) as a form of renal replacement therapy developed as a result of evidence that suggested greater frequency and longer duration of HD provided better clinical outcomes (42,43). HND is performed six to seven nights per week for 8 to 10 hours at night while the patient sleeps, and venous catheters are required for vascular access. Certain precautions are taken to prevent accidental disconnection and air embolization, and dialysis functions are monitored constantly via modem.

Home HD has been found to be associated with improved clinical parameters, such as improved hemodynamic stability and β_2-microglobulin clearance and markedly improved blood pressure control (13). Protein intake was improved and patients were able to reduce their requirement for phosphate binders (13). Patients also report an enhanced quality of life (13).

Although annually HND is associated with higher costs, cost per treatment is less than in-center HD treatment. The disadvantage of home HD is that it does require training before initiating and longer treatment schedules; therefore, patient motivation may be a factor. In addition, catheter-related complications and difficulty with sleep are still notable disadvantages.

RECOMMENDATIONS

There is no one dialysis modality clearly superior (56). Although it has been suggested that patient outcomes are better with HD, there are no randomized controlled trials that definitively answer this question and each modality has its associated advantages and disadvantages (Table 8.3) (57). Many factors influence modality selection. Issues that affect modality selection such as

whether a dialysis facility is publicly or privately owned, the availability of an existing infrastructure, and the profitability or remuneration for a particular dialysis modality are likely to remain. These important considerations should not replace the need for adequate patient education about renal replacement therapy. It is important to note that the aging of the dialysis population may have also exerted some influence on the current trends of modality selection and along with other factors may help to explain the decrease in PD use. Although dialysis modality selection should continue to be individualized, clearly most nephrologists elect HD for most patients. Ultimately, predialysis education and timing of referral will be the best determinants of dialysis modality selection.

REFERENCES

1. Becker BN, et al. Using renal transplantation to evaluate a simple approach for predicting the impact of end-stage renal disease therapies on patient survival: observed/expected life span. *Am J Kidney Dis* 2000; 35:653–659.
2. Washburn WK, et al. A single-center experience with six-antigen-matched kidney transplants. *Arch Surg* 1995;130:277–282.
3. U.S. Renal Data System. USRDS 2001 Annual Data Report. The National Institutes of Health, National Institutes of Diabetes and Digestive and Kidney Diseases. Bethesda, MD: 2001.
4. Mendelssohn DC. Reflections on the optimal dialysis modality distribution: a North American perspective. *NNI* 2002;16(4):26–30.
5. Mendelssohn DC, et al. Dialysis modality distribution in the United States. *Am J Kidney Dis* 2001;37:1330–1331.
6. Canadian Organ Replacement Registry (CORR). 1997 annual report. Don Mills, Ontario: Canadian Institute for Health Information.
7. Mattern WD, et al. Selection of ESRD treatment: an international study. *Am J Kidney Dis* 1989;13:457–464.
8. Nissenson AR, et al. ESRD modality selection into the 21st century: the importance of non-medical factors. *ASAIO J* 1997;43:143–150.
9. Blake PG. Factors affecting international utilization of peritoneal dialysis: implications for increasing utilization in the United States. *Semin Dial* 1999;12:365–369.
10. Mendelssohn DC, et al. What do American nephrologists think about dialysis modality selection? *Am J Kidney Dis* 2001;37:22–29.
11. Nissenson AR, et al. Non-medical factors that impact on ESRD modality selection. *Kidney Int* 1993;43[Suppl 40]:S120–S127.
12. Blake PG, et al. Changes in the demographics and prescription of peritoneal dialysis during the last decade. *Am J Kidney Dis* 1998;32[Suppl 4]:S44–S51.
13. Pierratos A, et al. Nocturnal hemodialysis: three-year experience. *J Am Soc Nephrol* 1998;9:859–868.
14. Garg PP, et al. Effect of the ownership of dialysis facilities on the patient's survival and referral for transplantation. *N Engl J Med* 1999; 341:1653–1660.
15. Nelson CB, et al. Comparison of continuous ambulatory peritoneal dialysis and hemodialysis: patient survival with evaluation of trends during the 1980s. *J Am Soc Nephrol* 1992;3:1147–1155.

16. Collins AJ, et al. Mortality risks of peritoneal dialysis and hemodialysis. *Am J Kidney Dis* 1999;34:1065–1074.
17. Prichard SS. Treatment modality selection in 150 consecutive patients starting ESRD therapy. *Perit Dial Int* 1996;16:69–72.
18. Obrador GT, et al. Early referral to the nephrologist and timely initiation of renal replacement therapy: a paradigm shift in the management of patients with chronic renal failure. *Am J Kidney Dis* 1998;31:398–417.
19. Lameire N, et al. The referral of patients with ESRD is a determinant in the choice of dialysis modality. *Perit Dial Int* 1997;17[Suppl 12]: S161–S166.
20. Schmidt RJ, et al. Early referral and its impact on emergent first dialyses, health care costs, and outcome. *Am J Kidney Dis* 1998;32:278–283.
21. Bloembergen WE, et al. Comparison of mortality between patients treated with hemodialysis and peritoneal dialysis. *J Am Soc Nephrol* 1995;6:177–183.
22. Held PJ, et al. Continuous ambulatory peritoneal dialysis and hemodialysis: comparison of patients with adjustment for comorbid conditions. *Kidney Int* 1994;45:1163–1169.
23. Fenton SS, et al. Hemodialysis vs. peritoneal dialysis: a comparison of adjusted mortality rates. *Am J Kidney Dis* 1997;30:334–342.
24. Hiat JG, et al. Initial survival advantage of peritoneal dialysis relative to hemodialysis. *Nephrol Dial Transpl* 2002;17:112–117.
25. Kreidiet RT. The rise and fall of the Kt/V concept in CAPD. *Dial Transplant* 2002;17:970–972.
26. Diaz-Buxo JA. Enhancement of peritoneal dialysis: the PD Plus concept. *Am J Kidney Dis* 1996;27:92–98.
27. Churchill DN, et al. Adequacy of dialysis and nutrition in continuous peritoneal dialysis: association with clinical outcomes. *J Am Soc Nephrol* 1996;7:198–207.
28. Fung L, et al. Dialysis adequacy and nutrition determine prognosis in continuous ambulatory peritoneal dialysis patients. *J Am Soc Nephrol* 1996;7:737–744.
29. Tzamaloukas AH. Peritonitis in peritoneal dialysis patients: an overview. *Adv Ren Replace Ther* 1996;3:232–236.
30. Leehey DJ, et al. Peritonitis and exit site infection. In: Daugirdas JT, et al., eds. *Handbook of dialysis.* Philadelphia: Lippincott Williams & Wilkins, 2001:373–398.
31. Malhotra D, et al. Serum albumin in continuous peritoneal dialysis: its predictors and relationship to urea clearance. *Kidney Int* 1996;50: 243–249.
32. Sorkin MI, et al. Apparatus for peritoneal dialysis. In: Daugirdas JT, et al., eds. *Handbook of dialysis.* Philadelphia: Lippincott Williams & Wilkins, 2001:297–332.
33. Attman PO, et al. Lipoprotein metabolism and renal failure. *Am J Kidney Dis* 1993;21:573–592.
34. Prichard SS. Metabolic complications of peritoneal dialysis. In: Daugirdas JT, et al., eds. *Handbook of dialysis.* Philadelphia: Lippincott Williams & Wilkins, 2001:405–410.
35. Bredie SJ, et al. Effects of peritoneal dialysis with an overnight icodextrin dwell on parameters of glucose and lipid metabolism. *Perit Dial Int* 2001;21:275–281.
36. Baugman JM. Mechanical complications of peritoneal dialysis. In: Daugirdas JT, et al., eds. *Handbook of dialysis.* Philadelphia: Lippincott Williams & Wilkins, 2001:399–401.
37. Kawaguchi Y, et al. Current issues of continuous ambulatory peritoneal dialysis. *Artif Organs* 1995;19:1204–1209.
38. Boger MP. A brief historical development of vascular access for hemodialysis. *J Vasc Nurs* 1990;8:13–16.
39. Palder SB, et al. Vascular access for hemodialysis: patency rates and results of revision. *Ann Surg* 1985;202:235–239.
40. Venkatesan J, et al. Dialysis considerations in the patient with chronic renal failure. In: Henrich WL, ed. *Principles and practices of dialysis.* Baltimore: Williams & Wilkins, 1994:549–555.
41. Hornegerger JC. The hemodialysis prescription and cost effectiveness. Renal Physicians Association Working Committee on Clinical Guidelines. *J Am Soc Nephrol* 1993;4:1021–1027.
42. Charra B, et al. Importance of treatment time and blood pressure control in achieving long-term survival on dialysis. *Am J Nephrol* 1996;16: 35–44.
43. Held PJ, et al. Mortality and duration of hemodialysis treatment. *JAMA* 1991;265:871–875.
44. Klein E. Effects of disinfectants in renal dialysis patients. *Environ Health Perspect* 1986;69:45–47.
45. Neilan BA, et al. Prevention of chloramines-induced hemolysis in dialyzed patients. *Clin Nephrol* 1978;10:105–108.
46. Said R, et al. Acute hemodialysis due to profound hypo-osmolality: a complication of hemodialysis. *J Dial* 1977;1:447–452.
47. Orringer EP, et al. Formaldehyde-induced hemolysis during chronic hemodialysis. *N Engl J Med* 1976;294:1416–1420.
48. Hodsman AB, et al. Bone aluminum and histomorphometric features of renal osteodystrophy. *J Clin Endocrinol Metab* 1982;54:539–546.
49. Alfrey AC. Dialysis encephalopathy syndrome. *Ann Rev Med* 1978;29: 93–98.
50. Schaefer RM, et al. Role of bradykinin in anaphylactoid reactions during hemodialysis with AN69 dialyzers. *Am J Nephrol* 1993;13:473–477.
51. Henrich WL. Hemodynamic instability during hemodialysis. *Kidney Int* 1986;30:605–612.
52. Theorell T, et al. The role of paid work in Swedish chronic dialysis patients—a nationwide survey: paid work and dialysis. *J Intern Med* 1991;230:501–509.
53. Dickinson DM, et al. International variation in the employment status of hemodialysis patients: results from the DOPPS. *J Am Soc Nephrol* 2000;11:229A(abst).
54. Holley JL, et al. An analysis of factors affecting employment of chronic dialysis patients. *Am J Kidney Dis* 1994;23:681–685.
55. Patient characteristics at the start of ESRD: data from the HCFA medical evidence form. *Am J Kidney Dis* 1999;34[Suppl 2]:S63–S73.
56. Blake PG. Do mortality rates differ between hemodialysis and CAPD? A look at the Canadian vs. U.S. data. *Neph Dial Transpl* 1996;25:75–100.
57. Bloembergen WE, et al. A comparison of mortality between patients treated with hemodialysis and peritoneal dialysis. *J Am Soc Nephrol* 1995;6:177–183.

9

HEMODIALYSIS ADEQUACY AND THE TIMING OF DIALYSIS INITIATION

ANDREW S. O'CONNOR AND JAY BARRY WISH

Since the advent of chronic renal replacement therapy in the 1960s, nephrologists have investigated various means of determining the appropriate delivery of dialysis. A review of the relevant literature reveals a considerable evolution during this period and a discernible trend toward a consensus on what parameters determine adequacy. The concept of adequate dialysis has shifted from the minimum amount of dialysis needed to sustain life into a more complete expression of the amount of dialysis that will be beneficial for optimal patient survival while balancing available resources for maximal efficiency. Hence adequate dialysis is now closer to "optimal dialysis."

The issue of what parameters constitute appropriate treatment of end-stage renal disease (ESRD) with dialysis therapy has assumed an increasingly important role, as more than 259,000 patients in the United States were being treated with chronic hemodialysis at the end of 2001, according to data from the Centers for Medicare and Medicaid Services (CMS) (1). While the death rate for ESRD patients remains quite high (approximately 67,000 hemodialysis patients alone died in 1999), the continued aging of the U.S. population, the increase in the incidence of diseases such as diabetes and hypertension, and numerous other factors have led to the development of ESRD in more than 88,000 patients in this same time period. At the current rate of growth, it is estimated that the hemodialysis population will increase to more than 500,000 by the year 2010, with Medicare expenditures expected to increase to more than $28 billion (2).

Despite this increase in the overall size of the ESRD population, there has been a markedly slower increase in the number of nephrologists (3). For instance, the ratio of dialysis patients to nephrologists in 1995 was approximately 50:1; in 1999 this ratio increased to 54.7:1. Based on the current growth of physicians and the projections of numbers of patients, it is expected that this ratio will further increase to 80:1 by the year 2010 (4). With this imbalance in the number of patients to physicians, as well as the financial constraints related to the provision of dialysis therapy, it is necessary to define just what constitutes "adequate" dialysis therapy in order to streamline therapies and establish appropriate clinical guidelines for practice.

Payers, including CMS (formerly known as the Health Care Financing Administration, or HCFA) and private insurers, are increasingly demanding the demonstration of cost-effective care as a primary criterion in contracting with health care providers such as dialysis facilities. As more than $12.7 billion was spent in 1999 by Medicare alone for the treatment of patients with ESRD (2), it is not surprising that the quality of care provided to this vulnerable population has come under increased scrutiny and economic strain. Obviously, a pivotal aspect of the quality of this care is the "adequacy" of dialysis provided.

Beginning in the early 1970s, with the implementation of "Medicare entitlement" relating to payment for dialysis services, CMS/HCFA has systematically collected facility-specific data regarding the provision of dialysis care. To assist in the collection and monitoring of this patient-specific information, 18 ESRD networks were established. One goal of these networks is to establish an oversight system for the provision of dialysis care. Since 1991, the ESRD networks have also been involved in continuous quality improvement (CQI) projects. Such activities allow individual providers within each network to examine their own practices, define areas for improvement, and develop plans to meet these areas of improvement. One such CQI initiative has been the monitoring and improvement in the adequacy of hemodialysis treatment.

This chapter reviews the key literature in an attempt to define adequate dialysis: how to prescribe it, how to deliver it, how to monitor it, and how to incorporate it into a cycle of CQI to achieve better patient outcomes. This discussion may touch on many aspects of hemodialysis that impact on adequacy, including membrane characteristics, dialysis modality selection, dialysate composition, intradialytic events, vascular assess function, and other important topics that are discussed in better detail elsewhere in this book.

Our understanding of hemodialysis adequacy is still evolving. Nephrology journals and national meetings continue to devote significant attention to the subject, and a National Institutes of Health (NIH)–sponsored multicenter prospective randomized study, the HEMO study, addressing the issue has recently been completed. The results of the HEMO study and existing studies provide a framework for further refinement of the two practice guidelines that have already been written on the subject of hemodialysis adequacy (5,6).

HISTORICAL PERSPECTIVE

Until 1974, nephrologists frequently prescribed hemodialysis regimens based on clinical judgment, often paying more attention to fluid balance than to the need to remove metabolic waste products. Amelioration of uremic signs and symptoms was the goal of the latter, but this was invariably subjective. The pathogenesis of the uremic syndrome was not clearly understood, although the paradigm that dialysis clears the blood of a responsible metabolic waste product(s) provided the framework of therapy (7). Multiple toxins have been proposed (Table 9.1) (8), some being linked to specific manifestations of the uremic syndrome; yet the correlation of uremic symptoms to blood levels of these substances has not been clearly demonstrated. Even today the true nature of the uremic syndrome remains incompletely understood.

Although it is inherently not a very toxic molecule (9), urea, a 60-dalton solute widely distributed in total body water, has been used as the surrogate for other uremic toxins because of its size, abundance, and dialyzability. This has often led to confusion by nephrologists and nonnephrologists alike, believing that the blood urea nitrogen (BUN) level causes uremic signs and symptoms and that dialysis is essential for BUN levels above 100 mg/dL. Historically, the clearance of urea has formed the cornerstone of measuring the efficacy and, by inference, the adequacy of dialysis therapy.

Poor outcomes, despite intensive dialysis treatments and "adequate" urea removal, led researchers familiar with solute kinetics to theorize that larger molecules with molecular weights of 500 to 2,000 daltons, "middle molecules," may be responsible for the uremic syndrome (10). The smaller pores of standard cellulosic membranes of the 1960s and 1970s were able to clear urea, but urea clearance did not invariably predict actual outcomes. Despite the removal of urea by these membranes, many patients continued to experience symptoms attributable to the lack of removal of some undefined toxic metabolite (11,12). Furthermore, peritoneal dialysis patients seemed to fare better than hemodialysis patients despite increased levels of BUN and, by inference, less dialysis. This was ascribed to the larger pore size of the peritoneal membrane as compared with cellulosic hemodialysis membranes and the removal of some larger, ill-defined, middle molecule. These observations evolved into what is now known as the "middle molecule hypothesis" (10).

In 1974, under the guidance of the National Institutes of Health, a consensus conference was held in Monterey, California, to discuss the nature of the uremic syndrome, as well as the development of a clinically useful and meaningful marker of dialysis therapy. During this conference, various aspects of dialysis care were examined, including the nature and pathogenesis of the uremic syndrome, quantification of dialysis therapy, nutritional status, renal osteodystrophy, and several other abnormalities commonly observed in hemodialysis patients.

The stage was set to test whether the clearance of urea or the as yet unidentified middle molecule correlated better with outcomes in hemodialysis patients. With the sponsorship of the National Institutes of Health (NIH), a multicenter prospective randomized study was designed and implemented to target BUN levels by varying dialysate and blood flows while affecting the clearance of hypothetical middle molecules by varying the dialysis duration. This landmark study is known as the National Cooperative Dialysis Study (NCDS) (12).

National Cooperative Dialysis Study

A total of 160 patients were randomized into four groups, with each group targeting either a low or high BUN level (50 mg/dL versus 100 mg/dL average) measured over a time averaged period ("TAC-urea") and a short or long dialysis time (3 ± 0.5 hours versus 4.5 to 5.0 hours). After a follow-up of 6 months, medical dropouts and hospitalization rates were measured. Subsequently, 12-month mortality rates were measured in follow-up studies (13). The results demonstrated that patients dialyzed with high BUNs and short times clearly had poor outcomes, with up to a 70% hospitalization rate (Fig. 9.1) (14). Overall, this initial analysis of the data suggested that BUN was the major factor leading to morbidity. As a result of the findings of this study, for several years after the publication of this study, many nephrologists focused on control of BUN and did not

TABLE 9.1. UREMIC SOLUTES WITH POTENTIAL TOXICITY

Urea	Middle molecules
Guanidines	Ammonia
Methylguanidine	Alkaloids
Guanidine	Trace metals
β-Guanidinopropionic acid	Uric acid
Guanidinosuccinic acid	Cyclic AMP
γ-Guanidinobutyric acid	Amino acids
Taurocyamine	Myoinositol
Creatinine	Mannitol
Creatine	Oxalate
Arginic acid	Glucuronate
Homoarginine	Glycols
N-α-acetylarginine	Lysozyme
Phenols	Hormones
O-cresol	Parathormone
P-cresol	Natriuretic factor
Benzylalcohol	Glucagon
Phenol	Growth hormone
Tyrosine	Gastrin
Phenolic acids	Xanthine
P-hydroxyphenylacetic acid	Hypoxanthine
β-(m-hydroxyphenyl)-hydracrilic acid	Furanpropionic acid
Hippurates	Amines
P-(OH)hippuric acid	Putrescine
O-(OH)hippuric acid	Spermine
Hippuric acid	Spermidine
Benzoates	Dimethylamine
Polypeptides	Polyamines
β₂-microglobulin	Endorphins
Indoles	Pseudouridine
Indol-3-acetic acid	Potassium
Indoxy sulfate	Phosphorus
5-Hydroxyindol acetic acid	Calcium
Indol-3-acrylic acid	Sodium
5-Hydroxytryptophol	Water
N-acetyltryptophan	Cyanides
Tryptophan	

Adapted from Vanholder RC, et al. Adequacy of dialysis: a critical analysis. *Kidney Int* 1992;42:540–558.

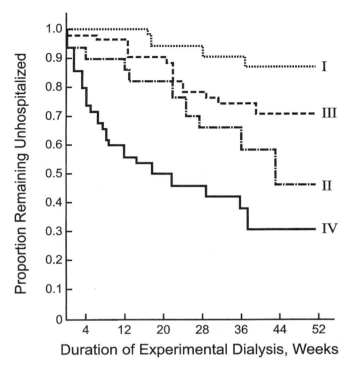

FIG. 9.1. Proportion of patients in the NCDS remaining unhospitalized, shown as a function of time in the four study groups. The proportion was lower in the high-BUN groups (II and IV) than in the low-BUN groups (I and III). (Reprinted with permission from Lowrie EG, et al. Effect of hemodialysis prescription on patient morbidity: report from the National Cooperative Dialysis Study. *N Engl J Med* 1981;305: 1176–1181.)

consider the dose of dialysis when prescribing and delivering dialysis therapy (15).

Despite a number of aspects of the NCDS that persist as controversial, it was the largest multicenter trial for determining dialysis adequacy before the HEMO study. Its enduring lesson, which was not learned until subsequent analyses of the NCDS data were published over several years following the study, is that quantifying and providing an adequate delivered dose of dialysis is of utmost importance if we are to make a positive impact on outcome. The NCDS also validated the importance of small molecule clearance, which forms the basis of current standards of adequacy (5).

The enormous contribution of the NCDS and its subsequent reanalysis to the current thinking regarding hemodialysis therapy cannot be overstated. Several weaknesses of the NCDS, however, preclude our applying the results universally into clinical practice. These issues point out the need for caution in the interpretation of the NCDS results, and a review of these should help place the study in proper perspective.

Age of the NCDS Cohort

The NCDS study population had an average age range of 18 to 70, with a mean age of 51 ± 12.9 years (13). The dialysis population has since grown older, with approximately 50% of incident patients more than 65 years old in 1999 (2). The elderly

population has different causes of ESRD (16), have varied and more comorbid conditions (17), and have been shown to die sooner regardless of dialysis prescription (18). In fact, after a mean age of 59 years, each year of advancing age has been associated with an approximately 3% increase in the odds ratio for death (18). Elderly patients generally have poorer nutrition, less opportunity for social rehabilitation, and less physical activity. They also have a greater chance of being demented and unable to influence their own treatment, let alone follow prescribed therapy (19,20). All these factors highlight the changing demographics of the "typical" American dialysis patient and limit the application of the NCDS in determining how to dialyze an aging population.

Comorbid Conditions

Patients who had advanced atherosclerotic cardiovascular disease, pulmonary disease, recurrent infections, cancer, or other significant comorbid conditions were excluded from the NCDS to achieve the expected follow-up period of 1 to 3 years (13). However, comorbidity with multiple conditions has increased among ESRD patients from 1976 to the present. Figure 9.2 is a graphical demonstration of the overall increasing illness of the hemodialysis population from 1996 to 2001. The first graph in this figure demonstrates that overall the number of comorbidities in the incident dialysis population is increasing. The second demonstrates that the actual comorbid illnesses within these groups are growing increasingly severe (2). For instance, the majority of incident hemodialysis patients starting therapy in 1999 had two or more comorbid illnesses, the most common being congestive heart failure and ischemic heart disease (2). Interestingly, a survey of the primary causes of death of dialysis patients highlights cardiovascular disease as the leading cause of death among dialysis patients (21). Internationally, this pattern of acceptance of older patients with increasing numbers and severity of comorbid illness also holds true (22). Thus the application of the NCDS data to patients with multiple comorbidities is questionable.

Diabetes Mellitus

Patients with diabetes were excluded from the NCDS. Today diabetic nephropathy is the single most common cause of ESRD in the United States, accounting for 43% of incident patients (2,23). The effect of diabetes on survival has been suggested in a report by Collins et al. (17), where higher doses of dialysis may be beneficial in diabetic patients. The application of the NCDS data to a diabetic population is limited, as these patients may require a dose of dialysis that approaches that provided for pregnant patients with ESRD (15).

Duration of Dialysis

The patients entering the NCDS had a mean duration of dialysis of 4.3 hours; the range studied was 2.5 to 5.5 hours (13). There are no data points below 2.5 hours and few data points below 3 hours. As a result of the NCDS findings, duration of dialysis was not considered as important as the BUN. In

Percent of Incident Dialysis Patients by Comorbid Illness 1996-2001

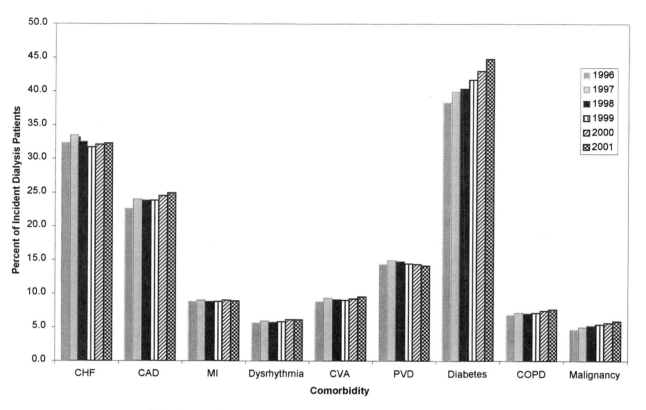

Number of Comorbidities at the Initiation of Dialysis 1996-2001

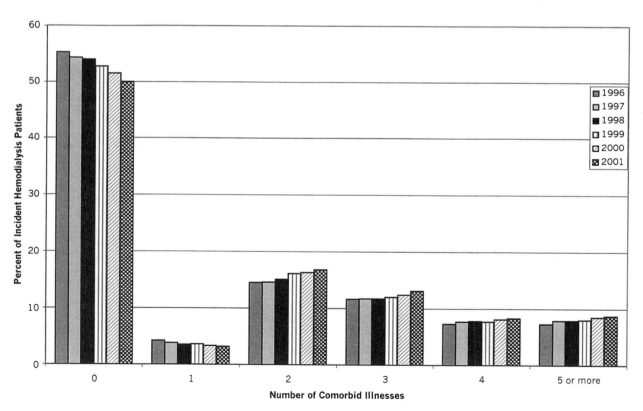

FIG. 9.2. Distribution and number of comorbidities in incident hemodialysis patients from 1996 to 2001. Top figure relates the total number of comorbid illnesses in hemodialysis patients by year. Bottom figure relates the growth of specific comorbid illnesses in all hemodialysis patients. (Data compiled from USRDS annual data report 2001.)

response to this, manufacturers of dialysis membranes began developing ways to achieve better urea clearance with shorter dialysis duration, as the dialysis facilities preferred to treat more patients for shorter time periods to maximize the efficiency of the facility and personnel (23,24).

It is predictable that as time for diffusion (i.e., dialysis) is shortened, there will be a point at which highly diffusible substances such as urea cease to predict adequate removal of other uremic waste products and an increase in morbidity, if not mortality, may result. Consequently, the role of duration of dialysis as an independent determinant of adequacy is being revisited. Studies have demonstrated a decreased survival in patients with dialysis time shorter than 3.5 hours (23,25). The NCDS data also revealed a trend toward increased morbidity with shorter dialysis times, although the correlation was not as strong as with high BUN levels (14). The NCDS data do not address how to weigh the independent effect of dialysis duration in a setting of current high-efficiency and high-flux dialysis membrane technology.

On the other extreme of duration of dialysis treatment, the Centre de Rein Artificiel in Tassin, France, has reported excellent 10-year survival rates, as well as unparalleled anemia and hypertension control in their patient population. The directors of this unit attribute their success primarily to the technique of prolonged daily dialysis treatments (26,27). This form of dialysis therapy, so-called prolonged hemodialysis (PHD), does offer several documented advantages to the prevalent form of in-center, three-times-per-week therapy practiced in the United States. However, the findings of the recently completed HEMO study (discussed in further detail later) point out that simply increasing the delivered dose of dialysis may not lead to improved outcomes among hemodialysis patients (28). Instead, to achieve patient outcomes similar to those in Tassin, what may be required is a fundamental rethinking of how to deliver dialysis therapy on a more consistent basis than three times per week.

Dialyzer Membrane

The NCDS was performed using purely cellulosic membranes (13), which have been replaced in up to 80% of facilities with newer, large-pore, high-flux, more biocompatible membranes. Applicability of dialysis prescription in the NCDS to current synthetic membranes such as polysulfone, polyacrilonitrite, or polymethylmethacrylite may be limited. This has been discussed elsewhere in the book (see Chapter 1).

Quantity of Dialysis

The retrospectively computed dialysis dose (Kt/V, to be discussed later in this chapter) for the NCDS cohort in groups I and III, with target BUN levels of 50 mg/dL on average, was between 0.9 and 1.3. Given that no groups in the NCDS received a greater dialysis dose, it is difficult to determine from the NCDS alone whether this dose is adequate, and impossible to determine whether this dose is optimal.

In a more recent study using the urea reduction ratio (URR) to quantify dialysis dose, it was demonstrated that patients receiving a URR of 60% or more had a lower mortality than patients receiving the NCDS URR of 50% or more (18). How-

ever, another study failed to demonstrate an improvement in mortality with higher dialysis doses among diabetic patients (29). Likewise, the HEMO study confirmed that doses of dialysis significantly greater (a single pool Kt/V of 1.71) than those currently recommended by the National Kidney Foundation–Kidney Disease Outcome Quality Initiative (NKF–K/DOQI) guideline (i.e., a spKt/V of 1.2) failed to provide additional survival benefit in a representative group of hemodialysis patients on a three-times-per-week treatment regimen. Specifically, what was shown was that with a "standard dose" of dialysis (achieved spKt/V of 1.32) the overall mortality was 17.1%. In the "high-dose" group (achieved spKt/V of 1.71) the mortality was 16.2%, a nonsignificant change. Reviewing these findings, it is notable that these excellent clearance rates were achieved with mean dialysis times of 190 ± 23 min (standard dose) and 219 ± min (high dose) (30). This finding speaks to the ability of modern dialysis technology to deliver adequate clearance of small molecules with only a modest increase in dialysis time.

Duration of the Study

The patients in the NCDS were studied for approximately 48 weeks, and most of the data were analyzed at 26 weeks (13). This may not have been enough longitudinal follow-up (17), especially as mortality actually increased approximately 1 year after the study was terminated (25,31). Again, the report by Eknoyan et al. from the HEMO study suggests that in a subgroup of female patients, a higher dose of dialysis may lead to a decrease in the risk of death and hospitalization, but this benefit of increased dose of dialysis did not appear for almost 3 years. Also in a separate subgroup of patients who had been on dialysis for more than 3.5 years at the start of the trial, the use of a high-flux dialysis filter appeared to reduce the risk of death. Further analyses of these groups will need to be completed before definitive conclusions can be drawn, however (28,30).

The influence of vintage (i.e., number of years on dialysis therapy) in the HEMO study, as well as duration of follow-up in analyses of the United States Renal Data System (USRDS) Case Mix Adequacy Study and Waves 1, 3, and 4 of the Dialysis Morbidity and Mortality Study (32), suggest that survival benefits from increased doses of dialysis may not be realized for a significant period of time, often greater than 3 or more years.

Other Issues

The hemodialysis techniques employed today—including ultrafiltration control, variable dialysate sodium programming, and bicarbonate dialysate—were not in widespread use during the NCDS era. The NCDS outcome measured was morbidity, not mortality (14), as is more commonly used in recent studies.

NUTRITION AND THE TIMING OF DIALYSIS INITIATION

Notwithstanding the previously held misconception that a low BUN is always good, it was elegantly shown in the NCDS that the protein catabolic rate (PCR), which is computed to represent dietary protein intake, is a strong and independent predictor of poor outcome (13). This became evident despite the NCDS protocol, which was designed to provide patients with a constant protein intake of 1.1. ± 0.3 g/day/kg body weight. In the final analysis the actual PCR range was more in the range of 0.6 to 1.5 g/day/kg body weight. Within this range a strong negative correlation between the PCR and probability of failure (*p*-failure—i.e., morbidity such as hospitalization) became evident, as demonstrated graphically in Fig. 9.3. This relationship of increasing *p*-failure with declines in PCR, held true irrespective of randomization to the low-BUN (50 mg/dL) or long-duration (4.5 hours) dialysis groups. Figure 9.3 shows how patients with very low PCR (0.6 g/day/kg body weight) will have at least a 35% probability of failure despite 4.5-hour dialysis treatment and a low (40 mg/dL) time-averaged concentration of urea (TAC urea). Conversely, a patient with a high PCR (1.2 g/day/kg body weight) will have less than a 15% probability of failure, even with a higher TAC urea of 60 mg/dL and the same duration of dialysis.

Subsequent studies have demonstrated how nutrition affects survival in dialysis patients when serum albumin is used as a marker for prognosis. Lowrie reported this with his National Medical Care (now FMC) database in 1990 (33) and again in 1994 (34) (Fig. 9.4), which demonstrated a marked increase in mortality as the serum albumin falls. This albumin/mortality relationship was also noted by Owen and colleagues in 1993 (18), as well as by several other authors. More recently, several authors and investigators have given increasing attention to the role that malnutrition plays in the survival of dialysis patients, as well as the link between the adequacy of dialysis therapy and overall nutritional fitness.

One such aspect of this nutrition/mortality relationship that has been explored by Chertow et al. (35) is the complexity of the relationship between dialysis dose, as measured by urea removal, and mortality. As is discussed later in this chapter, one of the

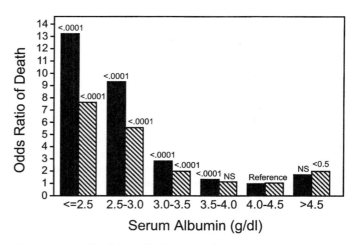

FIG. 9.4. Mortality risk profile for serum albumin concentration. *Solid bars* represent case mix adjustment; *cross-hatched bars* represent case mix plus laboratory adjustments. (Reprinted with permission from Lowrie EG. Chronic dialysis treatment: clinical outcome and related process of care. *Am J Kidney Dis* 1994;24:255–266.)

most important aspects of the NCDS study came not from the study itself, but from a reanalysis of the data several years later by Drs. Gotch and Sargent (36). In this mechanistic analysis of the data, a method of quantifying dialysis treatment by means of a dynamic measure, rather than the static measure of urea removal, was developed and verified as a valid measure of dialysis dose. However, even with the use of this dynamic measure, a complex relationship between dialysis dose and mortality is evident. Specifically, several authors have independently noted a "reverse J"–shaped relationship between the dose of hemodialysis, as measured by either URR or *Kt/V* (both terms are defined below). "Reverse J" means that with both extreme low and high values of urea removal, as measured by URR or *Kt/V,* there is an unexpected increase in the relative mortality of patients (37–39). This complexity of the dose/mortality relationship has led some authors to propose that urea distribution volume, *V,* is a surrogate marker for nutritional fitness. As such, urea distribution volume may possess survival characteristics of its own (35,40,41).

The fine line between trying to delay progression of renal disease versus inducing malnutrition and the consequent adverse effects on mortality has created substantial confusion and variation in clinical practice, especially with regard to the appropriate timing of initiation of chronic dialysis therapy. Although the Modification of Diet in Renal Disease (MDRD) study (42) provided some support for the hypothesis that dietary protein restriction slowed the progression of renal disease, the preceding studies have raised concern regarding the effects of pre-ESRD dietary protein restriction on patient mortality after ESRD supervenes. Kopple et al. (43) have concluded that 0.8 g/day/kg body weight of protein is safe for at least 2 to 3 years but recommend that additional indices of nutritional status such as serum transferrin, body weight, urine creatinine, and caloric intake be monitored regularly. The NIH Consensus in 1994 (44) recommended an initial diet of 0.7–0.8 g/day/kg body weight in pre-ESRD patients but cautioned to regularly assess for signs of malnutrition. Should such signs become evident, an

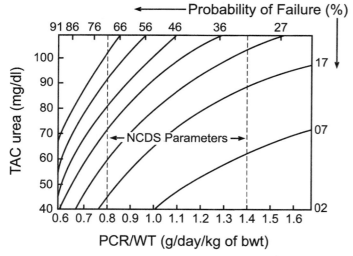

FIG. 9.3. A comparison of TAC urea, PCR, and probability of mortality for 4.5-hour dialysis in the NCDS. [Reprinted with permission from Lowrie EG, et al., ed. The National Dialysis Cooperative Study. *Kidney Int* 1983;23(Suppl 13):S1–S122.]

increase of protein intake to 1 to 1.2 g/day/kg body weight as well as increased caloric intake is recommended. The confusion is compounded by the multitude of factors affecting nutrition in the dialysis patient, such as anorexia due to uremia or under-dialysis, comorbid conditions such as diabetic gastroparesis, hormonal factors, and frequent hospitalizations (45). Because the adverse effects of protein malnutrition may last for months to years even after target protein intake has been restored, our institution favors a dietary protein intake of 1.0 to 1.2 g/day/kg body weight in our ESRD patients as well as patients who are thought to be within 1 to 2 years of developing ESRD. DeOreo (46), from our institution, has suggested that when the dose of dialysis is sufficient, nutrition becomes the major factor affecting mortality. Lowrie (33) has demonstrated a strong correlation between higher serum creatinine levels and improved survival in hemodialysis patients, reflecting better muscle mass, which is likely a marker for nutritional status and may be independent of dialysis dose. All these studies complement the NCDS and are reflections of the changing emphasis on nutrition in dialysis patients (47–51).

The appropriate timing of initiation of chronic dialysis therapy is closely tied to nutritional markers in dialysis patients. This relationship has been demonstrated in a number of observational studies in which spontaneous dietary protein restriction was observed with declining glomerular filtration rates (52–54). Concern regarding the long-term consequences of such dietary restriction, as well as the long-term effects of long-standing uremic toxicity has prompted several groups to investigate the appropriate timing of initiation of dialysis therapy. Initially, multiple investigators showed that earlier initiation of dialysis therapy led to prolonged duration of life, increased potential for rehabilitation, and decreases in hospitalization (55–57). The Canada–USA (CANUSA) study likewise showed that for patients with weekly creatinine clearances less than 38 L/week 12- and 24-month survival was 82% and 74%, respectively. However, in a group of patients with creatinine clearance greater than 38 L/week, 94.7% of patients survived 12 months and 90.8% of patients survived 24 months (58). Prompted by these studies, as well as expert opinion, the National Kidney Foundation's K/DOQI guidelines advise the initiation of dialysis therapy of some type when the weekly renal (residual) *Kt/V* falls below a level of 2.0 (an approximate creatinine clearance of 9 to 14 mL/min/1.73 m²). Clinical considerations that dialysis may not need to be imminently initiated are (a) stable or increasing edema-free body weight or (b) complete absence of clinical signs or symptoms attributable to uremia (5). Despite these convincing arguments that earlier initiation of dialysis leads to improvements in patient outcomes, three recent pieces of evidence have called this early initiation of dialysis therapy into question. The Dialysis Outcomes and Practice Patterns (DOPPS) study, which compares a large cohort of American dialysis patients to groups of patients from Europe (France, Germany, United Kingdom, Italy, Spain) and Japan, has shown that despite earlier initiation of dialysis among the American cohort of patients, the survival of this group of patients was actually worse than that of the groups from Europe and Japan. Even after consideration of potential confounding factors such as coexistent comorbidities and nutritional status as measured by albumin level, this

increase in mortality persisted (59). The NECOSAD-2 is a large, multicenter study in the Netherlands. In this prospective analysis, patient's health-related quality of life was measured by means of the Kidney Disease Quality of Life (KDQOL) Short Form repeatedly over the first year of dialysis therapy. Of 237 patients who had measurements of residual renal function measured between 0 and 4 weeks before the initiation of dialysis therapy, 38% were classified as late starters based on the K/DOQI guidelines. At baseline the Health Related Quality of Life (HRQOL) for this group of patients was statistically lower in the realms of physical role functioning, bodily pain, and vitality than that for patients who initiated timely dialysis per the K/DOQI guidelines. However, after a follow-up of 12 months, the differences among groups disappeared (60). A third study examined the effects of lead time bias in perceived increased longevity with an earlier start of dialysis (i.e., a perceived prolongation of survival due to longer monitoring of those patients who initiated dialysis at an earlier time in their disease process). To overcome the potential effects of lead time bias these authors assembled their cohort of patients on the basis of a residual creatinine clearance of 20 mL/min. Early and late start of hemodialysis was defined by a creatinine clearance cutoff of 8.0 mL/min. This analysis clearly showed that lead time bias is a real phenomenon in dialysis patients and that by monitoring patients from a defined starting point that predates the initiation of dialysis there was no difference in 10-year survival among the two groups of patients (61).

Although these studies do bring up interesting points, it should be kept in mind that approximately 60% of patients who initiate dialysis therapy suffer from some symptoms of uremia that are very often subtle. Keeping this in mind as well as the documented improvement in survival and decrease in health expenditures among patients who are referred for early nephrologic care, the initiation of dialysis therapy should be such that patients suffer no untoward effects due to depletion of bodily nutritional stores and maintain a reasonable quality of life. The previously cited NECOSAD study clearly shows that HRQOL at the time of initiation of dialysis is significantly lower in those patients who are maintained off of dialysis therapy. Given this and the often subtle symptoms of uremic toxicity, patients with impending dialysis needs should be monitored closely to avoid untoward effects of uremia and to make the transition to dialysis therapy as smooth as possible.

DIALYSIS QUANTIFICATION

The most important contribution of the NCDS is the concept that the delivered dose of dialysis can and should be quantified. With urea as the marker for most uremic toxins, the NCDS targeted the dose of dialysis by maintaining a certain TAC urea or midweek predialysis BUN, with the caveat that protein nutrition must be maintained. The duration of dialysis was found to be of marginal significance during the 6-month study but may have been more of a factor had the follow-up been extended for 12 to 24 months (23,45,62).

The lasting impact of the NCDS came from the analysis of Gotch and Sargent (36), which made the conceptual shift from viewing urea not from a static model (single midweek or averaged blood levels) but from a kinetic model (the change in urea during the course of a hemodialysis procedure). The most familiar kinetic urea model today is Kt/V, but it should be remembered that the NCDS did not use the Kt/V as its guide in dialysis prescription. The Kt/V paradigm evolved from a retrospective analysis of the data consisting of the actual delivered dose of dialysis from the patients in the NCDS (36).

K is the dialyzer urea clearance in milliliters per minute
t is the time (i.e., duration) of the dialysis therapy in minutes
V is representative of the volume of distribution of urea (approximately equal to total body water)

This expression attempts to express the dose of dialysis as fractional urea clearance and is analogous to the effects of normal body clearance mechanisms on the blood level of an administered drug.

Measuring the Dose of Hemodialysis

Many methods have been proposed to measure the dose of dialysis a patient receives. The square meter hour hypothesis and dialysis index was intended to address this issue (63) but did not take into consideration the volume of distribution of solute (e.g., urea). In the 1970s Teschan proposed a target dialytic clearance of 3,000 mL/week/L of body water (64). This took into consideration urea distribution volume and, at a regime of three dialyses per week, a target of 1,000 mL/dialysis/L body water translating to the dialysis index of 1, which was used as the reference point. Certainly, other terms have been devised such as probability of failure (13) in the NCDS, URR (65), and, as discussed earlier, the Kt/V (36). The latter two are currently the methods of choice for most institutions. As mentioned previously, however, the relationship between both Kt/V and URR and hemodialysis patient mortality is complex. Several recent studies have identified this complexity and have proposed other measures of dialysis dose, such as urea product (Kt) (39) and the hemodialysis product (HDP), which is defined as the hours of dialysis/session × (number of sessions/week)^2 (62). Whether these measures of dialysis dose are "better" in terms of being more valid predictors of patient outcomes remains to be proven. For instance, we have recently shown, in a large cohort of incident dialysis patients representative of the United States hemodialysis population, that the overall predictive ability of URR, spKt/V, double pool Kt/V, and Kt are all essentially the same (66).

Urea Reduction Ratio

The URR is an approximation of the fraction of BUN removed in a single dialysis session. The numerator is the difference between the pre- and postdialysis BUN, and the denominator is the predialysis BUN:

$$URR = (\text{Predialysis BUN} - \text{Postdialysis BUN}) \div \text{Predialysis BUN}$$

The URR has the advantage of simplicity, and has been used extensively to measure hemodialysis adequacy in large patient populations, including the FMC data set reported by Lowrie (33,34,65) and Owen (18) and the ESRD Core Indicator Project reported by CMS (67–69).

However, the URR has several very important shortcomings. Most important, like the static time-averaged urea concentration (TAC urea) used in the NCDS, the URR cannot be used to assess the patient's nutritional status, which is an independent predictor of outcome perhaps more powerful than the dose of dialysis (18,29,45). Furthermore, the URR does not account for urea removal that occurs with ultrafiltration.

Because of the URR's shortcomings, the Renal Physicians Association (6) and the NKF–K/DOQI (5) have both recommended against the use of URR to measure dialysis adequacy, favoring instead the Kt/V methods. Both FMC and the ESRD Core Indicator Project (now the ESRD Clinical Performance Measures Project) have recently changed to measuring and reporting the dose of dialysis to Kt/V.

Kt/V

Kt/V has become the preferred method for measuring delivered dialysis dose because it more accurately reflects urea removal than does URR, it can be used to assess the patient's nutritional status by permitting calculation of the normalized protein catabolic rate (nPCR), and it can be used to modify the dialysis prescription for a patient who has residual renal function. (See Chapter 7 for another discussion of this topic.)

Formal Urea Kinetic Modeling

Formal urea kinetic modeling (UKM) is the most accurate method for determining Kt/V and is preferred by both the Renal Physicians Association (RPA) (6) and NKF–K/DOQI (5) clinical practice guidelines on hemodialysis adequacy. However, formal UKM requires the use of a computer capable of solving differential equations to compute the following variables:

V, the volume of distribution of urea, which is approximately equivalent to total body water
K, by extrapolating a KoA (urea mass transfer area coefficient) value for the dialyzer that can be applied within a range of blood and dialysate flows
G, the urea generation rate, from which the nPCR can be computed

Once K and V are determined, one can arithmetically compute the time (t) required to deliver a target Kt/V. For example, if the target Kt/V is 1.4 and formal UKM has determined that K is 250 mL/min and V is 40 L, then the time required to deliver the target Kt/V of 1.4 would be $(40 \div 0.25) \times 1.4 = 224$ minutes.

The use of the formal iterative UKM model of determining V has been shown to be more accurate than anthropomorphic formulas proposed by Hume (70) and Watson (71) because these formulas were derived from analysis of healthy individuals and are probably not applicable to ESRD patients. More recently, Chertow et al. (72,73) has developed an ESRD-population-specific equation for calculating total body water based on bioelectrical impedance (BEI) monitoring. While determination of V by this method, which utilizes several readily available patient-specific anthropometric parameters, is fairly simple, whether it leads to significant differences in the ability to predict patient outcomes is subject to speculation.

Daugirdas II

Although formal UKM is preferred by the RPA and NKF-K/DOQI clinical practice guidelines for the reasons outlined earlier, its computational complexity has been a barrier to its widespread adoption. Many facilities have chosen instead to employ the more user-friendly second-generation natural logarithm formula for *Kt/V* proposed by Daugirdas (74), commonly known as Daugirdas II, which takes into account urea removed via ultrafiltration as well as urea generation during the dialysis treatment:

$$Kt/V = -\ln(R - 0.008 \times t) + (4 - 3.5 \times R) \times UF/W$$

where

ln is the natural logarithm
R is the postdialysis BUN/predialysis BUN
t is the duration of the dialysis session in hours
UF is the ultrafiltration volume in liters
W is the patient's postdialysis weight in kg

The Daugirdas II formula has been shown to approximate the formal UKM-derived result over the full range of single-pool, variable-volume *Kt/V* values (74–76) and has been endorsed by the NKF–K/DOQI clinical practice guidelines as the dialysis adequacy measurement of choice for providers unable or unwilling to perform formal UKM.

Postdialysis BUN Sampling

A number of technical issues involved in measuring dialysis adequacy have raised a great deal of controversy. The foremost is the timing and methodology for drawing the postdialysis BUN sample. This procedure is particularly important because inconsistency tends to overestimate the dose of dialysis delivered. In a review of national ESRD Clinical Performance Measures (CPM) Project data from 2000, Rocco et al. showed that such overestimation of the delivered dose of dialysis occurs in up to 31% of dialysis treatments. This extremely high rate of potential blood sampling error points out the need for continued quality improvement education efforts at the network and, even more important, facility/provider, level (77).

Following the conclusion of a hemodialysis treatment, the BUN precipitously rises due to three factors: vascular access recirculation, cardiopulmonary recirculation, and compartmental disequilibrium (Fig. 9.5) (78) (see Chapter 5).

Vascular Access Recirculation

The first BUN rise after a hemodialysis treatment, which occurs within 10 to 20 seconds, is due to vascular access recirculation, if present. Vascular access recirculation occurs when the blood flow rate through the extracorporeal circuit exceeds the arterial blood flow into the access, making the retrograde flow of blood back through the arterial circuit inevitable. Access recirculation is often the result of downstream venous stenoses at the prosthetic graft venous anastomosis, or the subclavian vein (see Chapter 5).

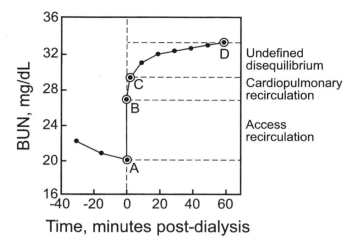

FIG. 9.5. A typical example of urea rebound, with more than half secondary to access recirculation (**A,B**), 15% from cardiopulmonary recirculation (**B,C**), and the remainder due to the resolution of perfusion and/or compartmental disequilibrium. (Reprinted with permission from Depner T. Assessing the adequacy of hemodialysis: urea modeling. *Kidney Int* 1994;45:1522–1535.)

The effects of access recirculation on the postdialysis BUN disappear within 10 to 20 seconds of the conclusion of the hemodialysis treatment. If the blood pump is turned down to 50 to 100 mL/min, it is extremely unlikely that access recirculation will occur, as arterial inflow into the graft or fistula invariably exceeds this level. Therefore the NKF–K/DOQI clinical practice guideline for hemodialysis adequacy recommends that the blood pump be slowed to 50 to 100 mL/min for at least 15 seconds before drawing the postdialysis BUN sample from the arterial port closest to the patient (5).

Cardiopulmonary Recirculation

The second component of the rise in BUN immediately after the conclusion of the hemodialysis treatment is cardiopulmonary recirculation, which is completed in 2 to 3 minutes. Cardiopulmonary recirculation refers to that small portion of blood that returns to the patient through the venous limb of the extracorporeal circuit, then circulates through the heart, lungs, and back to the arterial limb of the extracorporeal circuit without passing through any urea-rich tissues.

Cardiopulmonary recirculation typically accounts for only 15% of urea rebound following the conclusion of the hemodialysis treatment and does not occur when venous catheters are used for angioaccess.

Compartmental Disequilibrium

The third component of urea rebound, due to compartment disequilibrium, is not complete until at least 30 minutes after the conclusion of the hemodialysis treatment.

Originally, this phase was thought to represent the resolution of a disequilibrium between intra- and extracellular urea: extracellular urea is removed effectively during the hemodialysis treatment; then urea is released from the intracellular to the extracellular compartment at the conclusion of the treatment due to the gradient between the two pools.

More recently, it has been suggested that the compartment disequilibrium that occurs during a hemodialysis treatment is not between intracellular and extracellular fluid, but between high-blood-flow vascular beds (such as the kidney, lungs, brain, and other viscera), where relatively little urea is generated, and lower-blood-flow vascular beds (such as muscle, skin, and bone), where most urea is generated and which are more subject to vasoconstriction during hemodialysis (79). Once the hemodialysis treatment has concluded and blood flow increases to these organs, sequestered urea is "washed out" and the BUN concentration rebounds.

Equilibrated Kt/V

The magnitude of disequilibrium and urea rebound is proportional to the efficiency of the hemodialysis treatment, which can be described as K/V. In other words, the more efficient (shorter t for a given Kt/V) the hemodialysis treatment, the lower the BUN measured immediately after the hemodialysis treatment, and the more the Kt/V based on this BUN will overestimate the equilibrated Kt/V (eKt/V).

Daugirdas and Schneditz (80) have developed a relatively simple formula to estimate the eKt/V, based on the "single-pool" postdialysis BUN sample (drawn as described earlier at the conclusion of the hemodialysis treatment) and the treatment time:

$$eKt/V = spKt/V - 0.6 \times spKt/V / \text{hours} + 0.03$$

where $spKt/V$ is the single-pool Kt/V calculated from the Daugirdas II formula.

This formula, which obviates the need to draw a 30-minute postdialysis BUN to calculate eKt/V, was able to predict the eKt/V (based on actual 30-minute postdialysis BUN) better than models that use on-line dialysate urea monitoring (81,82) or intradialysis BUN measurement according to the Smye technique (83). The Smye technique is based on the fact that urea rebound disequilibrium (the degree to which the equilibrated postdialysis BUN exceeds the single-pool postdialysis BUN) will equal urea inbound disequilibrium (the degree to which measured BUN during the hemodialysis treatment is less than that predicted by its pharmacokinetics, based on dialyzer clearance and volume of distribution).

Adherence to the NKF–K/DOQI practice guidelines for postdialysis blood draw and the use of formal UKM or the Daugirdas II formula will yield a single-pool Kt/V that eliminates the effects of access recirculation but not of cardiopulmonary recirculation or of urea disequilibrium. The NKF–K/DOQI hemodialysis workgroup made this recommendation based on the small contribution of cardiopulmonary recirculation to urea rebound and the impracticality of detaining patients for 30 minutes after the conclusion of the hemodialysis treatment to draw the postdialysis BUN.

Furthermore, the $spKt/V$ was favored over a calculated eKt/V by the NKF–K/DOQI work group because the former is more familiar to most practitioners, because it was the model for the previous RPA clinical practice guidelines on adequacy of hemodialysis (6), and because most of the literature that correlates hemodialysis dose with patients' outcomes uses $spKt/V$.

HEMODIALYSIS DOSE AND OUTCOME

Given the more than 250,000 patients undergoing chronic hemodialysis and the total spending in 1999 for ESRD treatment in the United States of $12.7 billion (2), the outcome of this therapy is of significant concern. The survival of patients on hemodialysis tends to be better than that of lung cancer patients but is worse than that for both colon and prostate cancer patients (34). It is significant that the mortality rate of American ESRD patients is greater than that of their counterparts in other countries, notably those in Europe and Japan (84). Analysts have tried to explain these data in terms of patient differences, especially with regard to age and comorbidity (17), nutritional status (18,33), dialyzer reuse policy (85,86), incomplete data in the registry (87), and less than adequate dialysis dose delivery (17,88). However, even with adjustment of some of the preceding factors, a comparable hemodialysis population from Lombardy, Italy, had a better relative risk of survival than patients in the database of the United States Renal Data System (USRDS) (89). The authors could only postulate that this may be related to a difference in the quality of hemodialysis therapy.

Numerous publications have demonstrated that the delivered dose of hemodialysis is a significant predictor of patient outcome (14,16–18,90). Furthermore, many authors have concluded that the dialysis dose provided to American patients can and should be increased (18,25,88). The adjusted death rate among dialysis patients in the United States has fallen slightly during the past decade but remains greater than 20% (20.4% in 1998) (2). Data from the USRDS have demonstrated that for each increase in Kt/V of 0.1 up to around 1.2, mortality decreases by 7%; for each increase in URR of 0.05 up to around 0.65, mortality decreases by 11% (91). Likewise, the FMC database demonstrates a decrease in mortality with higher URRs, but a flattening of the curve with URRs above 0.65 (18). Even when the USRDS and the FMC data are converted to eKt/V by the appropriate equations, there appears to be a flattening of the mortality curve above an eKt/V of 1.05 (92). Likewise, the recently completed HEMO trial demonstrated that above a $spKt/V$ of 1.4, there did not appear to be a continuous decline in mortality (30).

HCFA/CMS's ESRD Core Indicators/Clinical Performance Measures Projects were developed to assess several key markers of quality of care in the hemodialysis population of the United States, including hemodialysis adequacy (measured by URR), anemia management, and nutritional status (1). Each year since 1994, a random sample of around 400 hemodialysis patients has been drawn from each of the 18 regional ESRD networks, and information regarding four key care indicators (adequacy of dialysis, hematocrit, nutritional status, and blood pressure control) has been reported. In 1999, the Core Indicators Project was merged with the ESRD Clinical Performance Measures (CPM) Project. The current CPMs reported for hemodialysis patients include hemodialysis adequacy, vascular access, anemia management, and serum albumin (Fig. 9.6). For the 2002 report on adequacy of hemodialysis, it was found that during the last quarter of 2001, of adult in-center hemodialysis patients who had been on dialysis for 6 months or longer, 91% had a mean delivered hemodialysis dose of 1.2 or more. For all patients, regard-

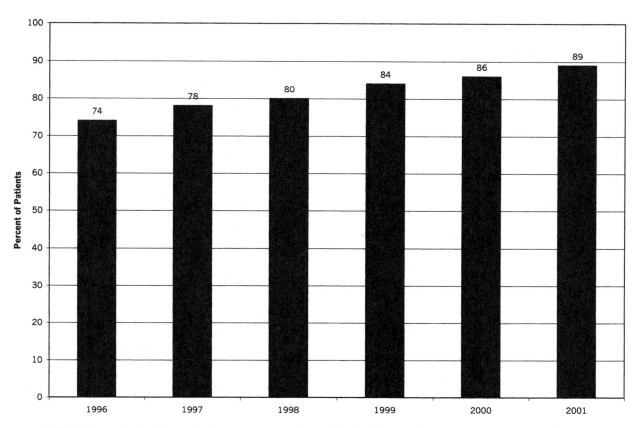

FIG. 9.6. Percent of adult (aged ≥18 years) in-center hemodialysis patients with mean *Kt/V* in October to December 2001 compared with previous study years. (Data from 2002 Annual Report. ESRD Core Indicators Project. Department of Health and Human Services, Centers for Medicare and Medicaid Services Office of Clinical Standards and Quality, December, 2002.)

less of length of time since starting dialysis, this figure was 89%, an increase of 3% from the same period in 2000 and an increase of approximately 15% since 1996 (1).

RPA Clinical Practice Guideline

The high prevalence of low hemodialysis dose as well as the relatively high mortality among hemodialysis patients in the United States prompted the 1993 publication of the Renal Physicians Association's Clinical Practice Guideline on Adequacy of Hemodialysis (6). The RPA guideline was the first clinical practice guideline that addressed the care of the patient with ESRD, and its dissemination likely contributed to the decline in patients with URRs of less than 0.65 between 1993 and 1996.

The RPA guideline recommended a minimum *Kt/V* of 1.2, based on a probabilistic model to assess how variation in the hemodialysis prescription affected quality-adjusted life expectancy (QALE). The RPA guideline noted that, though QALE increased with raising *Kt/V* above 1.2, the significant increase in costs required to achieve this higher dose of dialysis must be considered. The RPA guideline's final recommendation reflected a balance of concerns regarding decreasing incremental QALE and marginal cost-effectiveness. For facili-

ties using URR rather than *Kt/V,* a minimum value of 0.65 was recommended.

NKF–K/DOQI Clinical Practice Guideline

The NKF–K/DOQI clinical practice guideline on hemodialysis adequacy (K/DOQI guideline) (5) was published in 1997 and revised in 2001. The revised guideline includes recommendations for the treatment of pre-ESRD patients with chronic kidney disease as a reflection of the knowledge that appropriate referral and planning for dialysis therapy translate into improved patient outcomes (93,94). The authors of the K/DOQI guideline reviewed the RPA guideline as well as additional studies (16–18,38,95–97) that suggested that patients might benefit from hemodialysis doses greater than those recommended by the RPA guideline. However, those additional studies had many limitations, including comparison with historical standards (16,95), lack of patient randomization (17,38,96), lack of a standard collection of BUN samples (17,96), use of a broad range of categories of *Kt/V* or URR when grouping for analysis (17,38), or major differences in clinical practice or patient behavior compared with the American population (16). Furthermore, a retrospective analysis of a study from the USRDS database found no improvement in survival for a sp*Kt/V* of 1.2

to 1.4 or an e*Kt/V* of 1.0 to 1.2 (98). As a result, the authors of the K/DOQI guideline could not advise that the minimum hemodialysis dose recommended by the RPA guideline (sp*Kt/V* of 1.2 or URR of 0.65) be changed for adult patients with ESRD. However, the K/DOQI guideline did not discourage dialysis care teams from establishing greater minimum levels of hemodialysis dose for their patients.

NIH HEMO Study

The lower mortality rates reported for hemodialysis patients outside the United States and the extremely low mortality rates reported from Tassin, France, where patients undergo 24 m² hours of dialysis weekly (16,26), raise several nagging questions:

1. Is dialysis duration an independent factor in dialysis adequacy (a return to the middle-molecule hypothesis)?
2. Are shorter dialysis treatments to achieve a comparable (i.e., more efficient) *Kt/V* associated with adverse outcomes because they increase urea disequilibrium and therefore underestimate the equilibrated dose of dialysis delivered (which can be corrected for by using a double-pool e*Kt/V* target)? Or is the adverse outcome due to other factors, such as cardiovascular instability or rapid transcellular molecule fluxes?
3. Is there any cost-effective benefit to increasing the dose of dialysis above that recommended by the RPA and K/DOQI guideline?

In an attempt to answer these types of questions, the NIH sponsored and recently completed the HEMO study, a multi-center, prospective, randomized trial designed to assess the effects of hemodialysis dose (i.e., small-molecule clearance) and flux (i.e., middle-molecule clearance) (99) on morbidity and mortality.

The sweep of this study was comparable to that of the NCDS, but with turn-of-the-millennium technology. Like the NCDS, the HEMO study had four arms in a 2 × 2 matrix:

1. Arm 1: Standard urea clearance (URR about 0.67, sp*Kt/V* about 1.25, e*Kt/V* about 1.05) and a "high-efficiency" poly-sulfone dialysis membranes
2. Arm 2: Higher urea clearance (URR about 0.75, sp*Kt/V* about 1.65, e*Kt/V* about 1.45) and a high-efficiency membrane
3. Arm 3: Standard urea clearance and a "high-flux" polysul-fone dialysis membrane
4. Arm 4: Higher urea clearance and a high-flux membrane (100)

The main outcome measure of the HEMO trial was mortality, but with several important secondary outcomes also being monitored, specifically cardiac hospitalizations or deaths, infection-related hospitalizations or deaths, declines in albumin, and all-cause hospitalizations. These main and secondary outcomes indicate the principal causes of morbidity and mortality within the U.S. hemodialysis population.

The results of the HEMO trial confirm that the minimum dose of hemodialysis recommended by the previously mentioned guidelines is safe. Higher doses of dialysis and the use of "high-flux" membranes offer no specific morbidity or mortality advantage to the groups receiving these treatments. However, the preliminary reports of the trial do suggest that higher dialysis dose among women and high-flux membrane use in a group of patients who had been on dialysis for more than 3.5 years on entry to the trial may decrease morbidity, hospitalizations, and mortality in those subgroups (28,30). The benefit of higher dialysis dose in women but not men was also reported in an observational study from the Medicare database (101). At the time of this writing the full analyses of the HEMO trial, as well as those of selected subgroups, are still pending. Examples of further data that will be of interest will be the effects of high-dose and high-flux dialysis on (a) parameters of nutrition; (b) costs of dialysis-related medications such as erythropoietin and vitamin D analogs; (c) dialysis access–related procedures; and (d) health-related quality-of-life (HRQOL) measures. The apparent inconsistency between the results of the HEMO study, a prospective intervention trial, and other reports demonstrating improved outcomes with higher hemodialysis dose may be due to the fact that observational or cross-sectional analysis may be unable to adjust completely for confounding factors that may affect dialysis dose (e.g., sicker patients have more intradialytic hypotensive episodes or poorer blood flow) and its variability. In other words, above a minimum dialysis dose (such as sp*Kt/V* 1.20), the factor that is more predictive of outcome is not the average *Kt/V* but the percentage of treatments that fall below the minimum value (102).

BARRIERS TO ADEQUATE HEMODIALYSIS

The discussion of hemodialysis adequacy must not obscure the fact that other parameters, such as nutrition (18,29,33,45,46) and patient-assessed functional health status (103–106), have been shown to have an even stronger correlation with patient outcomes. Accordingly, appropriate care of the hemodialysis patient should not be focused on any single indicator such as dialysis dose. However, the clinician has more direct control over dialysis dose than over some of the other factors affecting outcomes, so it may constitute the greatest opportunity for physician behavior to influence patient survival.

Underprescription

Since the 1993 publication of the RPA guideline recommending a minimum URR of 0.65 or *Kt/V* of 1.2, a discernible trend toward improvements in the delivery of adequate dialysis to all ESRD patients can be seen (1). However, despite these marked improvements, 11% of patients did not meet minimum adequacy standards for the 3 months of study. Likewise, the use of central venous catheters remains unacceptably high, with up to 19% of patients in the ESRD CPM sample being dialyzed with a chronic venous catheter for 90 days or more (107). Among these patients who required the use of central venous catheters, the overall mean dialysis session length was actually shorter than among patients with native vein arteriovenous (AV) fistulas (219 versus 214 minutes), potentially leading to underprescription of dialysis. Underprescription remains a significant problem, accounting for 55% of underdialyzed patients reported by Delmez et al. (108) and 14% of all patients reported by Sehgal et al. (105).

As might be expected, underprescription of dialysis *(Kt/V)* is most likely to occur in a patient with a large urea volume of distribution *(V)*, in whom the dialysis variables *(Kt)* have not been increased in proportion to patient size (109). This is most apparent in patients with the heaviest quartile of body weight (>81 kg) who, despite longer treatment times, have an odds ratio of being underdialyzed (URR <65) of 3.2 [95% confidence interval (CI), 2.8 to 3.7] compared with the three lower quartiles (110).

The relationship between patient size and the likelihood of underprescription of dialysis therapy was also recently explored by Leon et al. in a group of dialysis patients drawn randomly from 22 chronic dialysis units in northeast Ohio. Using a *Kt/V* criterion of 1.3 as "adequate" dialysis, they found that 15% of patients were underdialyzed. Prescribed *Kt* (that portion of dialysis therapy that is modifiable by the prescribing physician) was strongly associated with patient volume, *V*. However, for every 10-L increment of *V*, *Kt* was only increased by a factor of 8.3, rather than 13 L, which would be required to maintain a *Kt/V* of 1.3. Because of this reduction in prescription, as patient size increased, the proportion of patients with a low prescription also increased, from 2% of patients with *V* <35 L to 42% of patients with *V* > 50 L (111).

To address the issue of adequate time of therapy, DeOreo performed a regression analysis of dry weight versus sp*Kt/V* among over 600 patients dialyzed in our affiliate facilities, and found a strong negative correlation, also suggesting a tendency for underprescription to heavier patients. Reworking the regression, DeOreo calculated that to achieve a sp*Kt/V* of 1.2 to 1.3 on a Fresenius polysulfone F8 or F80 dialysis membrane at a blood flow rate of 400 mL/min, the average patient would require 2.7 minutes of dialysis per kilogram of dry weight. A 100-kg individual would therefore require 270 minutes, or 4.5 hours, of dialysis with this regimen. Even if the physician extends the treatment prescription time accordingly, there may be facility or patient barriers to its fulfillment. Returning to the data from the HEMO study, this estimate of 2.7 minutes of dialysis/kg of body weight is exactly what was required to achieve the sp*Kt/V* demonstrated in the "standard dose" arm of the study (100). In other words, dialysis providers should use this estimate as a baseline dose when establishing the dialysis needs of new hemodialysis patients.

Other demographic factors likely to be associated with a higher *V*, and therefore a significant odds ratio for underdialysis, include:

Male gender (odds ratio 2.7, 95% CI 2.4 to 3.1) (112,113)
Young age, 18 to 44 (odds ratio 1.5, 95% CI 1.3 to 1.8) (112)
Black race (odds ratio 1.5, 95% CI 1.3 to 1.8) (112)

Whether the underdialysis of black patients is due exclusively to a larger urea volume of distribution is controversial. All the ESRD Core Indicator Projects as well as CPM annual reports have demonstrated a lower URR for blacks (63% ≥0.65 in 1996) (114) than for whites (70% ≥0.65 in 1996) despite longer treatment times for the former group. This was confirmed with data from the USRDS (115), which, however, failed to demonstrate a difference in volume for race and attributed the lower

hemodialysis dose in black patients to lower blood flow rates and smaller dialyzers. Pei et al. (116), however, attributed the racial differences to body size. This relationship between patient size, race, dose of dialysis, and dialysis-related mortality has also been explored by Owen et al., using the FMC database. In this retrospective analysis, the relative survival advantage that African American patients enjoy despite lower doses of hemodialysis, as measured by URR, was attributed to confounding of this measure by differences in patient size. Specifically, despite similar URRs, patients who are larger, in terms of urea distribution volume, would require a greater overall dose of dialysis (i.e., *Kt*) in order to achieve a similar URR (117). This analysis again points out that hemodialysis dose, whether measured by URR, *Kt/V*, or *Kt*, is only one of the factors that contributes to patient survival.

Inadequate Vascular Access

The second most important barrier to achieving the target-delivered hemodialysis dose is inadequate vascular access, which decreases the efficiency of dialysis due to both inadequate blood flow and access recirculation (see Chapters 4 and 5). Coyne et al. (118) found among 146 patients with a decline in *Kt/V* over a 3-month period. Twenty-four percent were due to decreased blood flow rates and 25% were due to recirculation. Sehgal et al. (105) found that 11% of their prevalent sample of 722 patients used catheters and that catheter use decreases the delivered *Kt/V* by 0.2. Erbeck et al. (119) similarly found that temporary catheter use decreases the delivered dose of dialysis by 8%, compared with patients with arteriovenous access or permanent catheters, and that treatment time should be increased by 30 minutes for patients with temporary catheters to achieve the same dose of dialysis as patients with other types of vascular access. Athirakul et al. (120) recommend that large patients (>85 kg) using cuffed dialysis catheters be prescribed extended treatment times. As mentioned previously, though, the use of catheters has not uniformly been associated with increases in treatment time, as demonstrated by the most recent ESRD CPM reports (107).

Shortened Treatment Time

Patient noncompliance with treatment time was observed in 3% of the treatments reported by Sehgal et al. (105) in which adequacy was measured, and accounted for 18% of the declines in *Kt/V* reported by Coyne et al. (118). Patient noncompliance reduced *Kt/V* by a factor of 0.1 in the Sehgal study, which is less significant than underprescription (0.5) or catheter use (0.2). In wave 2 of their Dialysis Morbidity and Mortality Study (DMMS), the USRDS reported that approximately 15% of hemodialysis patients shortened at least one session per month, 6% shortened two to three sessions, 1.5% shortened four to six sessions, and 0.9% shortened seven to 13 sessions (2). Skipped hemodialysis treatments are obviously an issue in total dialysis dose but would not be reflected by a decreased *Kt/V* or URR because no blood would be drawn from an absent patient. In a survival analysis of skipped treatments and dialysis prescription noncompliance, Leggat et al. demonstrated an approximate

10% increase in the risk of death for each hemodialysis session that is missed. In this analysis the authors also found that approximately 8.5% of patients skipped HD treatments at least once per month and that 20% shortened treatment times (121).

In an attempt to improve patient awareness of the issues related to hemodialysis adequacy, and thereby increase patient buy-in to the process, in 1995 the Health Care Financing Administration published and distributed a patient-oriented brochure entitled "Know Your Number." The "number" referred to the URR or *Kt/V*, encouraging patients to understand what the number means, to track it from month to month, and to become a partner in achieving adequacy targets of 0.65 or 1.2, respectively. In 1997, the Office of the Inspector General of the Department of Health and Human Services published two reports regarding the effectiveness of the "Know Your Number" initiative (122,123). Despite the HCFA's intention to achieve universal hemodialysis patient distribution of the brochure, two-thirds of patients surveyed did not receive it, and most of those who did were not familiar with their facility's use of URR or *Kt/V* tests and had no idea of what the appropriate target number for either of these tests should be. Interestingly, 60% of patients thought potassium was the index of adequacy. Nonetheless, 84% of the patients who received the brochure reported it to be easy to understand, and more than two-thirds reported it to be helpful. Facilities noted that 50% of their patients expressed an interest in the adequacy of their dialysis, and 29% were willing to track their numbers from month to month.

A survey administered to patients in two urban freestanding hemodialysis facilities in northeast Ohio, reported by Sehgal et al. (124), demonstrated that only 5% of subjects thought they were getting less dialysis than they needed, despite the fact that 41% had a *Kt/V* of less than 1.2. The authors concluded that these patient assessments were based on subjective factors and that targeted educational efforts to familiarize patients with the objective issues related to hemodialysis adequacy and outcomes have a long way to go.

As observed by Sehgal et al. in a separate study (19), patient education efforts were confounded in 22% of patients due to mild mental impairments, as measured by scores of 18 to 23 on the Mini-Mental State Examination (MMSE, perfect score = 30). An additional 8% of the sample had results indicating severe mental impairment, with MMSE scores of 0 to 17. This underscores the importance of involving patients' families and significant others in dialysis treatment, forming partnerships to maximize compliance and improve outcomes.

Clotting

Clotting during hemodialysis occurred in 1% of the treatments reported by Sehgal et al. (105) in a study that measured adequacy, resulting in a decrease in *Kt/V* of 0.3. As a general rule, the treatment duration was not extended to compensate for the "down" time of changing the extracorporeal circuit. Also notable is that the overall efficiency of the dialysis procedure decreased due to loss of dialyzer surface area to clotting. Adequate anticoagulation is obviously the most effective method to overcome this barrier to adequacy, but clearly there are patients whose bleeding risk precludes this approach. Further investigation is needed to determine the best course of action for this small subset of patients.

Reuse

The role of dialyzer reuse (see Chapter 2) as a barrier to hemodialysis adequacy is not clear-cut. Sehgal et al. (105) examined reuse in their model and did not find it to be an independent barrier. However, because the removal of urea is a function of the surface area of the membrane across which it diffuses and the surface area declines with the decrease in total cell volume (TCV) that occurs with reuse, it seems inevitable that a detectable decrease in dialysis adequacy will occur as the TCV decrease approaches the maximum of 20% that is allowed by the Association for the Advancement of Medical Instrumentation (AAMI) in their guidelines for reuse of hemodialysis membranes.

Fontoura et al. (125) found a highly significant linear regression between TCV and *Kt/V* ($p < 0.0003$), yet there was satisfactory preservation of *Kt/V* with up to 70 reuses. David-Neto et al. (126) found that the decrease in *Kt/V* correlated better with the number of reuses than the TCV, a finding also suggested by the data from Sehgal et al. Because the number of reuses at the time that adequacy of dialysis is measured is random, and additional reuses of that dialyzer may lead to a small reduction in the delivered dialysis dose from the measured value, it seems prudent to target the measured sp*Kt/V* or URR at a level slightly higher than the values recommended by the RPA and K/DOQI guideline so that every hemodialysis treatment, including the last reuse, will exceed the minimum target values.

Other Variables

Tables 9.2 and 9.3, adapted from Parker (127), illustrate the plethora of variables that may confound the provision of an ade-

TABLE 9.2. REASONS FOR COMPROMISED UREA CLEARANCE

I. Patient-related reasons
A. Decreased effective time on dialysis (breakdown on Table 9.3)
B. Decreased blood-flow rates (BFR)
  1. Access clotting
  2. Use of catheters
  3. Inadequate flow through vascular access
C. Recirculation
  1. Use of catheters
  2. Inadequate access for prescribed BFR
  3. Stenosis/clotting of access
II. Staff-related reasons
A. Decreased effective time (Table 9.3)
B. Decreased blood-flow rate
  1. Less than prescribed
  2. Difficult cannulation
C. Decreased dialysate flow rate
  1. Less than prescribed
  2. Inappropriately set
D. Dialyzer
  1. Inadequate quality of control of "reuse"
III. Mechanical problems
A. Dialyzer clotting during reuse
B. Blood pump calibration error
C. Dialysate pump calibration error
D. Inaccurate estimation of dialyzer performance by the manufacturer
E. Variability in blood tubing

Modified and adapted from Parker TF. Trends and concepts in the prescription and delivery of dialysis in the United States. *Semin Nephrol* 1992;12:271.

TABLE 9.3. REASONS FOR DECREASED EFFECTIVE TIME ON DIALYSIS

I. Patient-related reasons
A. Late start (patient tardy)
B. Early sign-off
  1. With consent (i.e., symptoms)
  2. Against advice (i.e., social)
C. Medical complications (e.g., hypotension)
D. "No show"
II. Staff-related reasons
A. Late start (staff tardy)
B. Wrong patient taken off
C. Time calculated incorrectly
D. Time on/off read incorrectly
E. Clinical deficiencies (e.g., no time registered)
F. Premature discontinuation for unit convenience
  1. Scheduling conflicts
  2. Emergencies
G. Incorrect assumptions of continuous treatment time (e.g., failure to account for interruptions of treatment like repositioning needles or accidental removal)
H. Inaccurate assessment of effective time by using variable time pieces
III. Mechanical reasons
A. Clotting of dialyzer
B. Dialyzer leaks
C. Machine malfunction

Modified and adapted from Parker TF. Trends and concepts in the prescription and delivery of dialysis in the United States. *Semin Nephrol* 1992;12:271.

quate dialysis dose. It is clearly not an exact science, and a normal distribution of delivered dialysis from a given prescribed dialysis dose will lead to a significant fraction of patients receiving less than the prescribed dose (92). Therefore for 90% of patients to receive a delivered Kt/V of 1.2 or greater, the K/DOQI guideline recommends a prescribed Kt/V of ≥ 1.3 (URR ≥ 0.70) (5).

CONCLUSION

Looking forward, it seems that we should, first and foremost, evaluate the patient while evaluating the adequacy of dialysis. Understanding the interaction of the multiple factors that affect overall survival and quality of life will heighten our awareness of specific issues that need to be addressed. We must evaluate nutritional status, physical activity, comorbid conditions, fluid and electrolyte balance, social and home conditions, and specific barriers to adequate hemodialysis. We must aim for Kt/V of ≥ 1.3 (URR $\geq 70\%$) with a delivered Kt/V of 1.2 or greater measured monthly, along with other laboratory values within target ranges. Although a third of the declines in Kt/V reported by Coyne et al. (118) could not be explained and returned spontaneously to adequate levels, the majority were real and therefore should be investigated and corrected.

Increasing recognition of the underprescription of hemodialysis for heavier patients has necessitated treatment duration exceeding 5 hours and caused facilities to reshuffle station allocation and turnover. Increased patient education to improve buy-in of longer treatment times when appropriate needs to occur at the facility level, but physicians can and should use the

materials and media that have been developed regionally and nationally for this purpose. Peer education by other patients through local, regional, or national patients' advocacy groups can also prove to be highly effective in increasing patients' participation in their care. An exploration of the patient's home, family, and socioeconomic situation can provide valuable insights that help to break down barriers to patient partnership.

It is still surprising that in the last 30 years we have not gone beyond urea in identifying specific toxins responsible for the uremic syndrome. Although urea is a good surrogate marker, identifying the responsible toxins and then removing them more efficiently remains a formidable challenge. The continued disparity in mortality rates between the United States and Europe points out the need for continued investigation regarding the most appropriate methods of delivering renal replacement therapy.

Further analysis of the NIH's HEMO study may help to clarify some of these issues and provide guidance in applying hemodialysis technology to achieve the best patient outcomes. We must deal with the fact that 11% of patients in the 2002 ESRD CPM Project (1) random sample did not have today's target Kt/V of 1.2 or greater. We have the quality improvement tools to identify the barriers to adequate hemodialysis in each of our facilities and the human capital to overcome them.

REFERENCES

1. Centers for Medicare and Medicaid Services. 2002 Annual Report, ESRD Clinical Performance Measures Project. Department of Health and Human Services, Centers for Medicare and Medicaid Services, Center for Beneficiary Choices, Baltimore, 2002.
2. U.S. Renal Data System. Excerpts from the USRDS 2001 annual data report: atlas of end-stage renal disease in the united states. *Am J Kidney Dis* 2001;38(Suppl 3):S1–S248.
3. Kletke PR, et al. The supply of renal physicians: an analysis of data from the American Medical Association Physician Masterfile. *Am J Kidney Dis* 1991;18:384–391.
4. Xue JL, et al. Forecast of the number of patients with end-stage renal disease in the United States to the year 2010. *J Am Soc Nephrol* 2001; 12:2753–2758.
5. National Kidney Foundation. K/DOQI clinical practice guidelines for hemodialysis adequacy, 2000. *Am J Kidney Dis* 2001;37:S7–S64.
6. Renal Physicians Association. Clinical practice guideline on adequacy of hemodialysis: clinical practice guideline 1. Dubuque, IA: Kendal/ Hunt, 1996.
7. Wolf AV, et al. Artificial kidney function: kinetics of hemodialysis. *J Clin Invest* 1951;30:1062–1070.
8. Vanholder RC, et al. Adequacy of dialysis: a critical analysis. *Kidney Int* 1992;42:540–558.
9. Luke RG. Uremia and the BUN. *N Engl J Med* 1981;305:1213–1215.
10. Scribner BH, et al. Evolution of the middle molecule hypothesis. In: Villareal H, ed. *Proceeding of the Fifth International Congress of Nephrology*. Basel: Karger, 1974:190–199.
11. Ginn HE. Neurobehavioral dysfunction in uremia. *Kidney Int* 1975; 8:S217–S221.
12. Ginn HE, et al. Neurotoxicity of uremia. *Kidney Int* 1975;8: S357–S360.
13. Lowrie EG, et al., ed. The National Dialysis Cooperative Study. *Kidney Int* 1983;23(Suppl 13):S1–S122.
14. Lowrie EG, et al. Effect of hemodialysis prescription on patient morbidity: report from the National Cooperative Dialysis Study. *N Engl J Med* 1981;305:1176–1181.
15. Depner TA. Optimizing the treatment of the dialysis patient: a painful lesson. *Semin Nephrol* 1997;17:285–297.
16. Charra B, et al. Survival as an index of adequacy of dialysis. *Kidney Int* 1991;41:1286–1291.

17. Collins AJ, et al. Urea index and other predictors of hemodialysis patient survival. *Am J Kidney Dis* 1994;23:272–282.
18. Owen WF, et al. The urea reduction ratio and serum albumin concentration as predictors of mortality in patients undergoing hemodialysis. *N Engl J Med* 1993;329:1001–1006.
19. Sehgal AR, et al. The prevalence, recognition and implication of mental impairment among hemodialysis patients. *Am J Kidney Dis* 1997; 30:41–49.
20. Muto Y, et al. Metabolic encephalopathy in the aged. *Nippon Naika Gakkai Zasshi* 1990;74:468–474.
21. Keane WF, et al. Influence of co-morbidity on mortality and morbidity in patients treated with hemodialysis. *Am J Kidney Dis* 1994;24: 1010–1018.
22. Krishnan M, et al. Epidemiology and demographic aspects of treated end-stage renal disease in the elderly. *Semin Dial* 2002;15:79–83.
23. Berger EE, et al. Mortality and length of dialysis. *JAMA* 1991;265: 909–910.
24. Levine DZ. Divided loyalties: relationships between nephrologists and industry. *Am J Kidney Dis* 2001;37:210–221.
25. Held PJ, et al. Mortality and duration of hemodialysis treatment. *JAMA* 1991;265:871–875.
26. Charra B, et al. Importance of treatment time and blood pressure control in achieving long-term survival on dialysis. *Am J Nephrol* 1996;16:35–44.
27. Raj DSC, et al. In search of ideal hemodialysis: is prolonged frequent dialysis the answer? *Am J Kidney Dis* 1999;34:597–610.
28. Mitka M. How to reduce mortality in hemodialysis patients still a puzzle. *JAMA* 2002;287:2643–2644.
29. Ward RA, et al. Predictors of short-term mortality in diabetic hemodialysis patients. *J Am Soc Nephrol* 1995;6:567(abst).
30. Eknoyan G, et al. Effect of dialysis dose and membrane flux in maintenance hemodialysis. *N Engl J Med* 2002;347:2010–2019.
31. Hakim RM. Assessing the adequacy of dialysis. *Kidney Int* 1990;37: 822–832.
32. Okechukwu CN, et al. Impact of years of dialysis therapy on mortality risk and the characteristics of longer term dialysis survivors. *Am J Kidney Dis* 2002;39:533–538.
33. Lowrie EG, et al. Death risk in hemodialysis patients: the predictive value of commonly measured variables and an evaluation of death rate differences between facilities. *Am J Kidney Dis* 1990;15:458–482.
34. Lowrie EG. Chronic dialysis treatment: clinical outcome and related process of care. *Am J Kidney Dis* 1994;24:255–266.
35. Chertow GM, et al. Exploring the reverse J-shaped curve between urea reduction ratio and mortality. *Kidney Int* 1999;56:1872–1878.
36. Gotch FA, et al. A mechanistic analysis of the National Cooperative Dialysis Study (NCDS). *Kidney Int* 1985;28:526–534.
37. Owen WF, et al. Dose of dialysis and survival: differences by race and sex. *JAMA* 1998;280:1764–1768.
38. Held PJ, et al. The dose of hemodialysis and patient mortality. *Kidney Int* 1996;50:550–556.
39. Lowrie EG, et al. The urea (clearance × dialysis time) product (Kt) as an outcome-based measure of hemodialysis dose. *Kidney Int* 1999;56: 729–737.
40. Sternby J. Significance of distribution volume in dialysis quantification. *Semin Dial* 2001;14:278–283.
41. Owen WF, et al. Explaining counter-intuitive clinical outcomes predicted by *Kt/V*. *Semin Dial* 2001;14:268–270.
42. Klahr S, et al. The effects of dietary protein restriction and blood pressure control on the progression of chronic renal disease: the Modification of Diet in Renal Disease Study. *N Engl J Med* 1994;330:877–884.
43. Kopple JD, et al. Effect of dietary protein restriction on nutritional status in the Modification of Diet in Renal Disease Study. *Kidney Int* 1997;52:778–791.
44. Consensus Development Conference Panel. Morbidity and mortality of renal dialysis: an NIH consensus conference statement. *Ann Intern Med* 1994;121:62–70.
45. Hakim RM, et al. Malnutrition in hemodialysis patients. *Am J Kidney Dis* 1993;21:125–137.
46. DeOreo PB. Analysis of time, nutrition and *Kt/V* as risk factors for mortality in dialysis patients. *J Am Soc Nephrol* 1991;2:231(abst).
47. Port FK, et al. Dialysis dose and body mass index are strongly associated with survival in hemodialysis patients. *J Am Soc Nephrol* 2002; 13:1061–1066.
48. Bergstrom J. Nutrition and mortality in hemodialysis. *J Am Soc Nephrol* 1995;6:1329–1341.
49. Leavey SF, et al. Simple nutritional indicators as independent predictors of mortality in hemodialysis patients. *Am J Kidney Dis* 1998;31: 997–1006.
50. Wolfe RA, et al. Body size, dose of hemodialysis, and mortality. *Am J Kidney Dis* 2000;35:80–88.
51. Mitch WE. Malnutrition: a frequent misdiagnosis for hemodialysis patients. *J Clin Invest* 2002;110:437–439.
52. Kopple JD, et al. Relationship between GFR and nutritional status: results from the MDRD study. *J Am Soc Nephrol* 1994;5:335a(abst).
53. Pollock CA. Protein intake in renal disease. *J Am Soc Nephrol* 1997;8:777–783.
54. Ikizler TA, et al. Spontaneous dietary protein intake during progression of chronic renal failure. *J Am Soc Nephrol* 1995;6:1386–1391.
55. Bonomini V, et al. Residual renal function and effective rehabilitation in chronic dialysis. *Nephron* 1976;16:89–102.
56. Bonomini V, et al. Benefits of early initiation of dialysis. *Kidney Int* 1985(Suppl 2);17:S57–S59.
57. Tattersall J, et al. Urea kinetics and when to commence dialysis. *Am J Nephrol* 1995;15:283–289.
58. Churchill DN, et al. Lower probability of patient survival with continuous peritoneal dialysis in the United States compared with Canada. Canada–USA (CANUSA) Peritoneal Dialysis Study Group. *J Am Soc Nephrol* 1997;8:965–971.
59. Goodkin DA, et al. The dialysis outcomes and practice patterns study (DOPPS): how can we improve the care of hemodialysis patients? *Semin Dial* 2001;14:157–159.
60. Korevaar JC, et al. Evaluation of DOQI guidelines: early start of dialysis treatment is not associated with better health-related quality of life. *Am J Kidney Dis* 2002;39:108–115.
61. Traynor JP, et al. Early initiation of dialysis fails to prolong survival in patients with end-stage renal disease. *J Am Soc Nephrol* 2002;13: 2125–2132.
62. Scribner BH, et al. The hemodialysis product (HDP): a better index of dialysis adequacy than *Kt/V*. *Dial Transplant* 2002;31:13–15.
63. Babb AL, et al. The genesis of the square meter hour hypothesis. *ASAIO Trans* 1971;17:80–91.
64. Teschan PE, et al. Quantitative indices of clinical uremia. *Kidney Int* 1979;15:676–697.
65. Lowrie EG, et al. The urea reduction ratio (URR): a simple method for evaluating hemodialysis treatments. *Contemp Dial Nephrol* 1991; 12:11–20.
66. O'Connor AS, et al. The relative predictive ability of four different measures of hemodialysis dose. *Am J Kidney Dis* 2002;40:1289–1294.
67. McClellan WM, et al. Data driven approach to improving care of incenter hemodialysis patients. *Health Care Finance Rev* 1995;16: 15–23.
68. Helgerson SD, et al. Improvement in the adequacy of delivered dialysis for adult in-center hemodialysis patients in the United States, 1993–1995. *Am J Kidney Dis* 1995;6:851–861.
69. McClellan WM, et al. Can dialysis therapy be improved? A report from the ESRD core indicators project. *Am J Kidney Dis* 1999;34: 1075–1082.
70. Hume R, et al. Relationship between total body water and surface area in normal and obese subjects. *J Clin Pathol* 1971;24:234–238.
71. Watson PE, et al. Total body water volumes for adult males and females estimated from simple anthropometric measurements. *Am J Clin Nutr* 1980;33:27–39.
72. Chertow GM, et al. Bioimpedance norms for the hemodialysis population. *Kidney Int* 1997;52:1617–1621.
73. Chertow GM, et al. Development of a population specific equation to estimate total body water in hemodialysis patients. *Kidney Int* 1996;51:1578–1582.
74. Daugirdas JT. Second generation logarithmic estimates of single pool variable volume *Kt/V*: an analysis of error. *J Am Soc Nephrol* 1993;4: 1205–1213.

75. Flanigan MJ, et al. Quantitating hemodialysis: a comparison of three kinetic models. *Am J Kidney Dis* 1993;17:295–302.

76. Bankhead MM, et al. Accuracy of urea removal estimated by kinetic models. *Kidney Int* 1995;48:785–793.

77. Rocco MV, et al. Comparison of predicted and calculated Kt/v values: results from the HCFA ESRD hemodialysis clinical performance measures project. *J Am Soc Nephrol* 2001;12:455A–456A (abst).

78. Depner T. Assessing the adequacy of hemodialysis: urea modeling. *Kidney Int* 1994;45:1522–1535.

79. Alquist M, et al. Development of a urea concentration gradient between muscle interstitium and plasma during hemodialysis. *Int J Artif Organs* 1999;22:811–815.

80. Daugirdas JT, et al. Overestimation of hemodialysis dose (delta *Kt/V*) depends upon dialysis efficiency *(K/V)* by regional blood flow and conventional 2 pool urea kinetic analyses. *ASAIO J* 1995;41:M719–M724.

81. HEMO Study Group. Comparison of methods to predict equilibrated *Kt/V* in the HEMO pilot study. *Kidney Int* 1997;52:1395–1405.

82. Depner TA, et al. Multicenter clinical validation of an on-line monitor of dialysis efficiency. *J Am Soc Nephrol* 1996;7:464–471.

83. Smye SW, et al. Estimation of treatment dose in high-efficiency dialysis. *Nephron* 1994;67:24–29.

84. Held PJ, et al. Five-year survival for end-stage renal patients in the United States, Europe and Japan, 1982–1987. *Am J Kidney Dis* 1990; 15:451–457.

85. Feldman HI, et al. Association of dialyzer reuse and hospitalization rates among hemodialysis patients in the U.S. *Am J Nephrol* 1999;19: 641–648.

86. Hull AR. Predictors of the excessive mortality rates of dialysis patients in the United States. *Curr Opin Nephrol Hypertens* 1994;3:286–291.

87. Wolfe RA, et al. Patient mix and mortality in chronic hemodialysis. *J Am Soc Nephrol* 1995;6:568(abst).

88. Parker TF, et al. Delivering the prescribed dialysis. *Semin Dial* 1993; 6:13–15.

89. Marcelli D, et al. ESRD patient mortality with adjustment of comorbid conditions in Lombardy (Italy) versus the United States. *Kidney Int* 1996;50:1013–1018.

90. Sehgal AR, et al. Improving the quality of hemodialysis treatment: a community-based randomized controlled trial to overcome patient-specific barriers. *JAMA* 2002;287:1961–1967.

91. U.S. Renal Data System. USRDS 1996 Annual Data Report. Bethesda, MD: National Institutes of Health, National Institute of Diabetes and Digestive and Kidney Diseases, 1996.

92. Gotch FA, et al. Clinical outcome relative to the dose of dialysis is not what you think: the fallacy of the mean. *Am J Kidney Dis* 1997;30:1–5.

93. Roderick P, et al. Late referral for dialysis: improving the management of chronic renal disease. *QJM* 2002;95(6):363–370.

94. Jungers P, et al. Longer duration of predialysis nephrological care is associated with improved long-term survival of dialysis patients. *Nephrol Dial Transplant* 2001;16:2357–2364.

95. Parker T, et al. Survival of hemodialysis patients in the United States is improved with a greater quantity of dialysis. *Am J Kidney Dis* 1994;23:670–680.

96. Hakim RM, et al. Effects of dose of dialysis on morbidity and mortality. *Am J Kidney Dis* 1994;23:661–669.

97. Hakim RM, et al. Adequacy of hemodialysis. *Am J Kidney Dis* 1992; 20:107–123.

98. Levin NW, et al. Comparison of mortality risk by *Kt/V* single pool versus double pool analysis in diabetic and non-diabetic hemodialysis patients. *J Am Soc Nephrol* 1995;6:606(abst).

99. Leypoldt JK, et al. Removal of middle molecules enhances survival in hemodialysis patients. *J Am Soc Nephrol* 1995;6:606(abst).

100. Eknoyan G, et al. The hemodialysis (HEMO) study: rationale for selection of interventions. *Semin Dial* 1996;9:24–33.

101. Wolfe RA, et al. URR >75% is associated with lower mortality among females but not among males. *J Am Soc Nephrol* 2002;13:20a(abst).

102. Port FK, et al. Dialysis dose and body mass index are strongly associ-

ated with survival in hemodialysis patients. *J Am Soc Nephrol* 2002; 13:1061–1066.

103. Kimmel PL, et al. Compliance with dialysis prescription, social support, quality of life and decreased depression level are associated with enhanced survival in inner city hemodialysis patients. *J Am Soc Nephrol* 1996;7:1451(abst).

104. Golper T. Patient education: can it maximize the success of therapy? *Nephrol Dial Transplant* 2001;16:S20–S24.

105. Sehgal AR, et al. Barriers to adequate delivery of hemodialysis. *Am J Kidney Dis* 1998;31:593–601.

106. Sherman RA, et al. Deficiencies in delivered hemodialysis therapy due to missed and shortened treatments. *Am J Kidney Dis* 1994;24:921–923.

107. Centers for Medicare and Medicaid Services. 2001 Annual Report, End-Stage Renal Diseases Clinical Performance Measures Project. Department of Health and Human Services, Centers for Medicare and Medicaid Services, Center for Beneficiary Choices, Baltimore, December 2001.

108. Delmez JA, et al. Hemodialysis prescription and delivery in a metropolitan community. *Kidney Int* 1992;41:1023–1028.

109. Port FK, et al. Optimizing the dialysis dose with consideration of patient size. *Blood Purif* 2000;18:295–297.

110. 1995 Core Indicators Project. Association of body weight with adequacy of dialysis (Suppl 1). Baltimore: Department of Health and Human Services, Health Care Financing Administration, Health Standards and Quality Bureau, August 1996.

111. Leon JB, et al. Identifying patients at risk for hemodialysis underprescription. *Am J Nephrol* 2001;21:200–207.

112. 1996 Core Indicators Project. Association of body weight with adequacy of dialysis (Suppl 1). Department of Health and Human Services, Health Care Financing Administration, Health Standards and Quality Bureau, March 1997.

113. Kuhlman M. Inadequacy of dialysis is more frequent in male vs. female patients. *J Am Soc Nephrol* 1996;7:1517(abst).

114. Department of Health and Human Services. ESRD Core Indicators Project, 1996 Annual Report. Baltimore: Health Care Financing Administration and the Health Standards and Quality Bureau, 1997.

115. Carroll CE, et al. Patient factors associated with delivered *Kt/V* in the U.S. *J Am Soc Nephrol* 1995;6:594(abst).

116. Pei Y, et al. Racial differences in dialysis adequacy related to body size. *J Am Soc Nephrol* 1997;8:208(abst).

117. Owen WF, et al. Dose of hemodialysis and survival, differences by race and sex. *JAMA* 1998;280:1764–1768.

118. Coyne DW, et al. Impaired delivery of hemodialysis prescriptions: an analysis of causes and an approach to evaluation. *J Am Soc Nephrol* 1997;8:1315–1318.

119. Erbeck KM, et al. Effect of hemodialysis access on delivered dose of dialysis *(Kt/V)*. *J Am Soc Nephrol* 1995;6:487(abst).

120. Athirakul K, et al. Cuffed central venous hemodialysis catheters and adequacy of dialysis. *J Am Soc Nephrol* 1996;7:1402–1403(abst).

121. Leggat JE, et al. Noncompliance in hemodialysis: predictors and survival analysis. *Am J Kidney Dis* 1998;32:139–145.

122. Adams M, et al. Experience of dialysis facilities (know your number brochure). Report of the Office of the Inspector General, January 1997:1–21.

123. Adams M, et al. Perspectives of dialysis patients (know your number brochure). Report of the Office of the Inspector General, January 1997:1–24.

124. Sehgal AR, et al. Patient assessments of adequacy of dialysis and protein nutrition. *Am J Kidney Dis* 1997;30:514–520.

125. Fontoura GR, et al. Multireprocessed dialyzers: correlations between *Kt/V* and fiber bundle volume. *J Am Soc Nephrol* 1997;8: 280A–281a(abst).

126. David-Neto E, et al. The impact of biocompatible dialyser reuse on *KtV*. *J Am Soc Nephrol* 1997;8:280A–281a (abst).

127. Parker TF. Trends and concepts in the prescription and delivery of dialysis in the United States. *Semin Nephrol* 1992;12:271.

10

HIGH-FLUX, HIGH-EFFICIENCY PROCEDURES

EDITH M. SIMMONS, B. BLAKE WEATHERSBY, THOMAS A. GOLPER, AND ALLAN J. COLLINS

The vast majority of hemodialysis procedures now performed in the United States can be considered both high-efficiency (HE) and high-flux (HF). Since their introduction in the 1980s they have become increasingly accepted as the standard of care in this country, and technological advances have made their application safer and more cost-effective. At the same time that HE–HF dialysis has become increasingly common, overall survival rates have improved among dialysis patients in spite of an aging population with increasing comorbidities. HE–HF dialysis membranes have made shorter dialysis times feasible in selected patients while maintaining adequate small solute clearance. In addition, HF membranes may proffer advantages to patients due to their superior removal of middle-molecular-weight substances.

This chapter will address the technical requirements, possible complications, and current clinical application of HE–HF treatments. In addition, we will discuss recent data on adequacy of dialysis and dialysis outcomes as they relate to HE–HF treatments.

DEFINITION OF HIGH-EFFICIENCY AND HIGH-FLUX DIALYSIS

The definitions of HE and HF procedures were formed primarily from the historical development of dialysis and the technical needs of each treatment. Currently, more than 70% of dialysis treatments in the United States can be classified as both HE and HF; however, it is important to define them separately to better understand their uses (1). Table 10.1 provides a comparison of the various characteristics of conventional, HE, and HF membranes.

Efficiency of dialysis refers to the rate of small solute transfer across the membrane. This is expressed as the urea mass transfer coefficient (KoA urea). KoA urea is the theoretical maximum urea clearance at infinite blood and dialysate flow rates. Once the KoA for a given dialyzer is known, the urea clearance under any given blood and dialysate flows can be calculated or located on a nomogram (2). HE dialysis is achieved primarily by increasing the surface area of the dialysis membrane. By most conventions, HE dialyzers have a KoA urea of greater than 450 mL/min, which translates to in vivo urea clearance rates of greater than 200 mL/min. This value is not entirely arbitrary. In the 1980s, when acetate was used as the buffering system, the use of more efficient dialyzers with KoA urea of more than 450 mL/min was associated with an increased incidence of intradialytic symptoms and complications. Because of their more rapid diffusion of small solutes, HE dialyzers allowed acetate from the dialysate to accumulate in the patient faster than it could be metabolized (3). High levels of acetate contributed to hypoxemia, decreased cardiac output, and hypotension (4). These complications while using the new HE membranes helped to usher in bicarbonate as the dialysate buffer of choice.

Figure 10.1 shows a key characteristic of HE membranes. In low-efficiency dialyzers, urea clearance plateaus at relatively low blood-flow rates. By contrast, urea clearance in HE dialyzers continues to rise with higher blood flows and does not plateau until blood flow exceeds 400 mL/min. Therefore a functioning access is important to take full advantage of HE membranes.

HF membranes are all HE as defined by KoA urea. In addition, their larger pore size and water permeability lead to a high ultrafiltration (UF) coefficient, which is defined as the volume removed (in milliliters) per hour per mm Hg of applied trans-

TABLE 10.1. COMPARISON OF CONVENTIONAL, HIGH-EFFICIENCY, AND HIGH-FLUX MEMBRANES

Characteristic	Conventional	High-Efficiency	High-Flux
KoA urea	<450 mL/min	>450 mL/min	>450 mL/min
Urea clearance	<200 mL/min	>200 mL/min	>200 mL/min
KUF	<15 mL/mm Hg/h	Variable	>15 mL/mm Hg/h
β_2-microglobulin clearance	<10 mL/min	Variable	>20 mL/min

KoA urea, mass transfer coefficient × area; KUF, ultrafiltration coefficient.

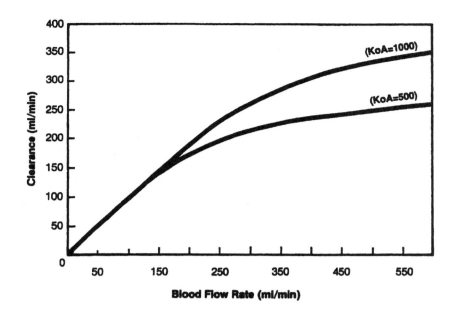

FIG. 10.1. Dialyzer urea clearance as a function of dialyzer mass transfer coefficient (KoA) and blood-flow rate (Q_b). (Reprinted with permission from Nissenson AR, et al. *Clinical dialysis,* 3rd ed. New York: McGraw-Hill, 1995:851.)

membrane pressure (TMP). HF membranes are usually defined as those having UF coefficients of greater than 15 mL/h/mm Hg TMP. Again, this value is of historical significance, as precise UF systems were required to prevent UF errors when using dialyzers with UF coefficients greater than 15. Precise UF control is a standard feature in most currently available dialysis machines. An additional way to characterize flux in dialysis membranes is by their β_2-microglobulin clearance. β_2-microglobulin is an 11.8-kD molecule implicated in the development of dialysis-related amyloidosis (DRA) (see Chapter 23).

Table 10.2 lists technical specifications of selected hemodialysis membranes (5).

TECHNICAL REQUIREMENTS FOR HIGH-EFFICIENCY AND HIGH-FLUX TREATMENTS

The discussion that follows outlines the technical requirements for HE–HF dialysis. As HE–HF treatments have become increasingly common in the United States, these requirements

have become standard features in the machines and systems of dialysis facilities. However, there are different systems of UF control and water treatment as well as controversy regarding water quality. This section is intended to help clinicians ask specific questions of manufacturers and dialysis providers to investigate which systems are best for a particular facility.

Ultrafiltration Control Systems

Many of the features of currently available dialysis machines have been created in large part to meet the needs of HE–HF treatments. It can be immediately appreciated, for example, that in HF dialyzers, with UF coefficients as high as 60 mL/h/mm Hg, considerable UF will occur, causing subsequent hypotension if the TMP is not carefully controlled.

The most extreme example of HF treatments reflects back on the clinical application of intermittent hemofiltration between 1975 and 1984 (6). During this interval, polyamide membranes of large surface area were used during hemofiltration with UF coefficients between 100 and 200 mL/h/mm Hg. To control the

TABLE 10.2. SELECTED HEMODIALYSIS MEMBRANES

Manufacturer	Model	Membrane	KoA Urea	KUF	Surface Area
Baxter	Tricea 210G	Cellulose acetate	1713	39	2.0
Baxter	PSN-210	Polysynthane	1044	10	2.0
Fresenius	F80A	Polysulfone	945	65	1.8
Fresenius	F8	Polysulfone	716	7	1.0
Fresenius	Optiflux F160	Polysulfone	1063	45	1.0
Gambro	Lundia Pro 800	Polycarbonate copolymer	583	11	1.0
Gambro	Polyflux 21S	Polyamide	1238	83	2.0
Toray	BK 2.1 U	Polymethylacrylate	903	40	2.0
Toray	B3 1.6 A	Polymethylacrylate	718	8	1.0

Modified from Ronco C, et al. *Membranes and filters for hemodialysis 2001.* Basel, Switzerland: S. Karger Publishers, 2001.
Units: KoA urea, mL/min; KUF, mL/h/mm Hg; surface area, m².

fluid balance, many investigators used sophisticated computerized UF control equipment to match UF and reinfusion of fluid, thereby maintaining patient stability. This historical perspective is important, since the outgrowth of HE and HF treatments came from the clinical comparison of HE hemodialysis and hemofiltration in a short treatment time (6). The technological advances required to use hemofilters were subsequently applied to HE dialyzers and ultimately to the HF dialyzers that evolved in the mid-1980s, necessitating more careful fluid balance. In this context it is important to discuss the types of UF control systems utilized to maintain fluid balance, since it is clear that an error of 10 mm Hg, using a HF dialyzer, can yield a net fluid volume loss of as much as 600 mL/h or 1.8 L in a 3-hour treatment.

The initial UF control systems applied during the era of hemofiltration were the forerunners of the systems applied in clinical practice today. The original microprocessor-based hemofiltration equipment, produced by Gambro Healthcare (Lakewood, Colorado), utilized a sophisticated strain gauge attached to a load cell that measured the rate of weight change from the 35-L containers used to collect ultrafiltrate and provide reinfusion fluid. This was, in fact, the first true volumetric UF control system. This type of system was not directly applicable to an on-line, single-pass dialysis system in which approximately 100 to 120 L of fluid were utilized during a dialysis treatment.

Microprocessor-based Electronic Systems

Further improvements in the UF control systems for hemofiltration led to a continuous on-line system that used electromagnetic flow sensors to measure dialysate inflow and outflow. This system was microprocessor controlled and had no mechanical flow components. This is classified as the first microprocessor-based electronic UF control system and is still used in hemodialysis machines manufactured by Gambro.

Electronic Flow Sensor Systems

A secondary application of these microprocessor-based electronic UF control systems centered on the development of a bearingless rotor placed in a centrifugal flow path, which spun a ring where the optical characteristics were sensed through a fiber-optic network that then determined flow rates. Instead of being electromagnetically based, they are a combination of mechanical and electronic sensing. Typical examples of this type of equipment are produced by Baxter Healthcare Corporation (Deerfield, Illinois) in their 1550 dialysis machines.

Volumetric Control Systems

The third major type of UF control system, developed in the early 1980s, utilizes a mechanical-based system to control the very high KUF of hemofilters (100 to 200 mL/h/mm Hg) and hemodiafilters. These so-called volumetric control systems are based on the creation of a closed inflow and outflow loop by multiple-valve isolation systems, with a secondary UF pump that removes fluid from the relatively closed circuit at a fixed rate. The closed-circuit system matches dialysis inflow and outflow by bellows displacement pumps as the UF control pump generates the appropriate TMP needed to limit UF during the dialysis treatment. Examples of this type of equipment are the Cobe Century III (Cobe Renal Intensive Care Division of Gambro Healthcare, Lakewood, Colorado), the Fresenius series of hemodialysis machines (Fresenius Medical Care, Lexington, Massachusetts), the System 1000 by Althin Medical, Inc. (Miami Lakes, Florida), the Toray UF control system (Houston, Texas), and the Italian Bellco machine (Bellco S.P.A., Saluggia, Vercelli, Italy). The UF control achieved by these mechanical bellows systems is compatible with both HE and HF dialyzers.

Proper System Maintenance

In the sensor-based systems, multiple sensor arrays provide monitoring systems to allow for adequate control of flow variance between the dialysate sensors picked up by the microprocessors. The bellows balancing systems have parallel, closed-loop circuits that are tested before dialysis for pressure leaks to determine whether there is appropriate seating of valves. When properly maintained, these systems, as indicated earlier, provide excellent UF control across all dialyzer KUF ranges. The critically important issue, however, is the maintenance needed to achieve optimal functioning of each of these dialysis delivery systems, for it is clear that without adequate maintenance each system can fail to provide adequate fluid balance control.

Microbiologic Contamination

Both electromagnetic and bearingless rotor systems can develop microbiological contaminants and film that can disrupt the flow sensor paths. This biofilm is secreted by the bacteria growing in the bicarbonate dialysate and is a glycopolysaccharide that helps the bacteria stick to the surface of the dialysate flow path (7,8). At times it sheds small white particulate matter that, when traveling through the bearingless rotor systems, can give false signals to the optical sensing system. In the electromagnetic system, the biofilm coating of the flow path can disrupt the magnetic field so that actual flow can be miscalculated.

Routine sterilization procedures with either formaldehyde, peracetic acid, or heat sterilization do not strip biofilm from dialysis machines, since the biochemical structure of biofilm makes it highly resistant to all neutral and acidic solutions. Biofilm is, however, exceedingly sensitive to alkaline solutions, best exemplified by sodium hypochlorite (bleach), sodium hydroxide, or Formula 409-type alkaline detergents. The most practical solution applied in the field, therefore, has been a 1:10 dilution of 5.25% bleach, typically through both dialysate inflow and outflow sensors and through the flow path. This is particularly important in the outflow sensors, since additional nutrients that diffuse across the membrane from the patient during the dialysis procedure encourage bacterial growth in the outflow path.

In the mechanical-based, so-called volumetric control systems, the multiplicity of valves requires ongoing maintenance to ensure the integrity of the closed-loop circuit. Proper seating of these valves is required to maintain the pressure gradient within the dialysate circuit, thus providing adequate positive pressure and TMP for the UF control. These valves can be sensitive to biofilm but, in fact, are more sensitive to crystal deposition of calcium carbonate within the dialysis circuit with the use of bicarbonate dialysate. In this context, the crystalline deposition interferes with the valve closures, causing loss of the pressures in the circuit. The deposits can be avoided by the careful application of pH sensors, which monitor the dialysate proportioning of sodium bicarbonate and calcium chloride. The ratios of acid and bicarbonate concentrates must be maintained within close limits to prevent precipitation if the pH of the dialysate exceeds 7.4. Additionally, to reduce precipitation, the dialysis-proportioning system can be initiated with acid concentrate to allow an acidic dialysate solution to bathe the flow path, thereby assisting the dissolution of crystalline precipitates before adding the bicarbonate concentrate.

The bellows valve UF control systems also require the same type of bleaching procedures as the sensor-based systems to strip the biofilm, the presence of which can cause valve failure. An alternative precipitate procedure uses acetic acid/vinegar solutions to dissolve calcium carbonate precipitates in the dialysis machines, thus appropriately cleaning the valves.

Bicarbonate Dialysate

Bicarbonate dialysate has become the predominant buffer in the era of HE–HF dialysis. In the mid-1980s as HE–HF dialyzers were introduced, reports of hemodynamic instability during HE–HF dialysis using acetate dialysate surfaced. It is believed that HE–HF membranes allow acetate to diffuse from dialysate to blood at a rate faster than the body can metabolize (9,10). At high levels, acetate has been shown to be a negative inotrope and peripheral vasodilator, contributing to hypotension (11,12). In addition, acetate dialysate has a low partial pressure of carbon dioxide, which leads to net carbon dioxide removal. By removing the respiratory drive of carbon dioxide, patients were found to hypoventilate, and hypoxemia was a common problem that may have contributed to acetate intolerance (13). However, the pathophysiology of "acetate intolerance" is not fully understood and likely multifactorial (see Chapter 3). Nevertheless, hemodynamic instability was not seen as frequently in HE–HF treatments that used bicarbonate dialysate, and it is now used in the vast majority of dialysis facilities in the United States.

Bicarbonate dialysis is not without its own complications and technical difficulties. In contrast to acetate dialysate, which is prepared from a single concentrate that inhibits bacterial growth, bicarbonate dialysate must be prepared from two concentrates to prevent precipitation of cations such as calcium and magnesium. One of these concentrates is pH neutral and supports bacterial growth, which can lead to contaminated dialysate.

Contaminated dialysate can lead to both short- and long-term complications. Acute pyrogenic reactions (PR) from bacterial contamination or endotoxin exposure may occur in one of 10,000 dialysis sessions, and approximately 20% of all dialysis centers report more than one PR per year (14). Less obvious reactions to contaminated dialysate include cytokine release that can contribute to hypotension, sedation, and anorexia (15). Chronic complications are less well understood or documented. Chronic inflammation due to contaminated dialysate may contribute to the pathogenesis of β-2 microglobulin amyloidosis,

catabolic loss of muscle proteins, erythropoietin-resistant anemia, and atherosclerotic cardiovascular disease (16–18).

Controversy exists regarding whether HE—and more so, HF—dialyzers are more permeable to endotoxin fragments and therefore lead to more PR. Many investigators have demonstrated that bacterial products can diffuse across dialysis membranes (19,20). It follows that the larger surface areas, pore size, and dialysate flow rates used in HE–HF dialysis would lead to greater potential diffusion of bacterial products across the membrane. However, in vitro studies have demonstrated that cellulosic low-flux membranes are actually more permeable to endotoxin fragments than synthetic HF membranes, which have high pyrogen-adsorbing capacity (21). This perceived benefit may be countered in vivo by endotoxin transfer across HF membranes due to back-filtration. There are conflicting data on the risk of PR with HE–HF membranes. Bicarbonate dialysate and HF membranes have been associated with a higher risk of PR (22). Some studies have shown that the practice of reuse, in which water comes into direct contact with the blood compartment, may be of more importance than membrane type (19). Gordon et al. showed no statistical difference in PR rates by treatment modality (conventional, HE, and HF) (23). Despite this controversy, it is accepted that dialysis membranes are permeable to bacterial products, though not uniformly, and important short-term and long-term effects of contaminated dialysate are likely.

Water Treatment

Each dialysis facility has its own strategy for water treatment. Any water treatment strategy must begin with guidelines for acceptable levels of bacteria and endotoxin. The Association for the Advancement of Medical Instrumentation (AAMI) allows bacterial growth of no more than 200 colony-forming units (CFU)/mL in water and 2,000 CFU/mL in dialysate; the AAMI standards also limit water and dialysate endotoxin units (EU) to 5/mL (14). However, some have advocated the use of "ultrapure" dialysate (24). For example, the European Pharmacopoeia sets the upper level of bacteria and endotoxin in dialysate at 100 CFU/mL and 0.250 EU/mL (25). Studies have shown that many dialysis units do not even achieve the less stringent AAMI guidelines. A study of water quality in hemodialysis units in 1994 revealed compliance with AAMI requirements for water on monthly surveys of only 70% for bacteria and 56% for pyrogens (26). A survey of water quality in 1992 showed compliance with AAMI standards for water; however, the average dialysate bacterial concentration was 19,000 CFU/mL, far exceeding AAMI criteria (22). Acceptable levels of bacteria and endotoxin are beyond the scope of this chapter and require further investigation.

A typical water treatment system is shown in Fig. 10.2. The first step involves pumping the source water through softeners to remove most of the calcium and magnesium. The water then travels through a carbon filter for removal of chlorine. Sediments are extracted in a series of filters before entering the reverse osmosis (RO) systems, which remove most of the remaining impurities by pumping the water through a small-pore semipermeable membrane. Ultraviolet lights help control microbiologic contamination. Mixed-bed deionization systems are often used to complete the removal of aluminum and other

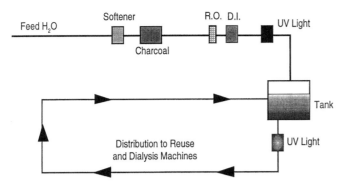

FIG. 10.2. Schematic of the typical water treatment and distribution systems in the RKDP metropolitan dialysis units. (DI, deionization tanks; RO, reverse osmosis; UV, ultraviolet lights.)

metals. The water is then deposited into a holding tank, where it is repressurized and distributed to each dialysis station and to the reuse area if applicable.

Special note must be made of the distribution system in which treated water is transferred from the storage tank to the individual dialysis machines. It is important in the design of the distribution system that stagnant areas are kept to a minimum to prevent bacterial adhesion to the piping. This can be achieved by shortening the connection distance from distribution loop to dialysis machine, minimizing pipe diameter to keep flow rates high, continuously circulating water through the distribution loop, and avoiding dead space and lateral arms (27).

Periodic disinfection of the water treatment and distribution system is important to maintain water quality and system efficiency. The water softeners, sediment filters, and carbon filters are particularly prone to microbiologic growth and biofilm and require periodic bleach disinfection. RO and deionization systems also require periodic chemical disinfection in accordance with manufacturer recommendations. To prevent biofilm deposition in the distribution system, a preparation of bleach, sodium hydroxide, and peroxyacetic acid is periodically flushed through the system (27).

Finally, systems of quality control must be in place to ensure that guidelines for water quality are met and exceeded (28). Samples of dialysis water should be obtained at least weekly and tested for bacteria and endotoxin. Water samples should be taken from critical areas in the water treatment and distribution system where contamination is more likely.

CLINICAL APPLICATIONS OF HIGH-EFFICIENCY, HIGH-FLUX THERAPIES

High-efficiency and high-flux therapies offer many advantages over conventional hemodialysis techniques, several of which have been associated with improved patient outcomes. Because of their large membrane surface areas that lead to high KoAs for low-molecular-weight solutes exceeding that of conventional dialyzers, both HE and HF dialyzers are capable of delivering adequate dialysis to large patients with high volumes of distribution for urea. High-flux dialyzers may confer additional bene-

fits due to their porosity for middle- and large-molecular-weight toxins, such as β_2-microglobulin, which has been implicated in the development of dialysis-related amyloidosis in long-term dialysis patients (see Chapter 23). Several studies have revealed significantly decreased plasma β_2-microglobulin levels in patients undergoing HF therapies (29–32). In a prospective, multicenter study of 380 patients randomized to four different dialysis techniques for 24 months, Locatelli et al. demonstrated substantial reductions in pretreatment β_2-microglobulin levels in patients receiving hemodialysis (23% reduction) or hemodiafiltration (16% reduction) using HF polysulfone membranes. In contrast, there were no changes in β_2-microglobulin levels in the patients assigned to cuprophane and low-flux polysulfone hemodialysis (29). These results support the hypothesis that removal, as a consequence of membrane flux, may have a greater impact on β_2-microglobulin levels than a lower rate of generation due to biocompatibility. Though a direct relationship between predialysis β_2-microglobulin levels and DRA has not been established, Kuchle et al. noted a significantly lower incidence of carpal tunnel syndrome and/or osteoarticular lesions among 20 long-term dialysis patients randomized to HF polysulfone membranes versus low-flux cuprophane membranes after an 8-year follow-up (30,31). These findings could have important clinical implications, given the significant morbidity related to DRA in long-term dialysis patients.

In addition to convective clearance, the enhanced removal of β_2-microglobulin and other large molecules can be related to the hydrophobic nature of the HF membrane surface, resulting in adsorption of certain circulating putative uremia-associated toxins (33). This mechanism may contribute to the removal of activated complement and cytokines, thus abating inflammation. Furthermore, most HF dialysis membranes are composed of synthetic material, though there are examples of modified cellulose-based HF membranes such as cellulose triacetate. These dialyzers tend to be more biocompatible than pure cellulose membranes in that they provoke less of an inflammatory reaction upon contact of blood with the membrane surface (see Chapter 1). The net effect is less activation of complement and cytokines, less granulocytopenia and thrombocytopenia, and less generation of free oxygen radicals (34). Outcomes attributed to improved membrane biocompatibility that have been supported by retrospective studies include reduced overall mortality as well as reduced mortality due to coronary artery disease and infection, decreased protein catabolic rate, improved nutrition, and fewer dialysis-related symptoms such as hypotension (35–39). However, because most of the biocompatible membranes employed in these studies were also HE and HF, it is difficult to determine the relative contributions of each of these factors to the specified outcomes.

Other potential benefits of high-flux membranes include a reduction in erythropoietin resistance, improved lipid profiles, specifically increased HDL cholesterol and lowered triglyceride levels, as well as removal of advanced glycosylation end-products, which have been implicated in the pathogenesis of atherosclerosis and DRA (40–45). The use of HF polysulfone dialyzers may even delay loss of residual renal function compared with conventional dialyzers, particularly when the underlying etiology of renal failure is nondiabetic parenchymal renal disease

(46,47). Furthermore, HE and HF therapies may allow for shorter dialysis times, and this has been a key motivating force behind their use.

SHORT HEMODIALYSIS

Over the past 30 years, the United States has experienced an overall tendency toward shorter dialysis treatments, with individual sessions reduced from 7 to 10 hours in the 1960s to as low as 2 to 3 hours in the 1980s and 1990s (48). Many factors have contributed to this drive for short hemodialysis, including patient preference for less time on dialysis, economic incentives, availability of HE therapies, and results of the National Cooperative Dialysis Study (NCDS), which suggested that treatment time had no significant effect on patient outcome (49).

Before the introduction of HE therapies in the mid-1980s, early attempts at short dialysis using standard modalities resulted in Kt/Ws urea of ≤ 3 mL/min/kg, which translated into Kt/Vs below 1, values considered insufficient by current National Kidney Foundation–Kidney Disease Outcomes Quality Initiative (NKF–K/DOQI) standards (50,51). The NCDS in 1983 was the first quantitative study to correlate dose of hemodialysis with patient outcomes. In a mechanistic reanalysis of the NCDS data in 1985, Gotch and Sargent noted a reduction in the probability of hospitalization and death from 57% when Kt/V was less than 0.8, to 13% when Kt/V was greater than 1.0. (52). Since then, several studies have demonstrated survival benefits with delivered single-pool (sp) Kt/Vs of at least 1.2, and this remains the minimum dose recommended by 2000 NKF–DOQI guidelines (51,53–56).

Requirements for Short Hemodialysis

With the advent of more efficient dialysis membranes with higher KoAs for urea, it has become feasible to provide adequate small solute removal using thrice-weekly dialysis sessions under 3 to 4 hours in carefully selected patients. Since treatment dose can no longer be defined by the amount of time an individual spends on dialysis in HE therapies, strict adherence to the recommended guidelines for urea clearance is essential for short hemodialysis to be safe and effective. Specifically, any reduction in treatment time must be counterbalanced by a proportionate increase in the dialyzer clearance of low-molecular-weight substances to maintain Kt constant and prevent underdelivery of dialysis. To achieve this, blood flow rates should be maintained at 350 to 450 mL/min to optimize dialyzer performance. Hence a properly functioning access with minimal recirculation is a prerequisite for HE therapies. In addition, up to 10% more clearance can be obtained by increasing dialysate flow from 500 mL/min to 800 mL/min (50).

Another requirement for successful short hemodialysis is sufficient removal of interdialytic weight gain (IDWG) without causing cardiovascular instability or patient discomfort. Rapid ultrafiltration rates (UFR) can be associated with hypotension and hemodynamic instability, especially if the UFR exceeds the rate of vascular refilling from the extracellular space. Patients at particular risk for hemodynamic complications include those

with underlying cardiac disease—namely, cardiac ischemia, arrhythmias, systolic or diastolic dysfunction—as well as those with autonomic dysfunction and persistent excessive IDWG (see Chapter 19). In a stable dialysis patient without other risk factors, an UFR of less than 20 mL/kg/h is generally well tolerated (57). Thus educating patients about weight gain is essential when utilizing short hemodialysis.

Concerns with Short Hemodialysis

Despite innovations in dialysis membrane technology and systems capable of delivering short dialysis, duration of treatment remains controversial. A fundamental concern surrounds the ability of short dialysis to provide consistently effective urea clearance. Because delivered dialysis dose appears to be a critical determinant of patient survival, it is imperative to consider any conditions that may interfere with the provision of prescribed therapy. This becomes particularly important as session length is shortened, since there is less margin for error. A number of studies of chronic outpatient dialysis patients in the last decade have uncovered substantial differences between the dialysis prescription and the measured Kt/V when session lengths averaged less than 3.5 hours (58–60).

Factors accounting for underdelivery of dialysis in the setting of shortened treatments are frequently patient related, such as tardiness or early sign-offs. Common staff-related issues include using less than the prescribed blood flow and overestimation of treatment time as a result of failure to account for interruptions in blood flow. Other causes for suboptimal delivery of therapy may be linked to technical difficulties or inadequacy of the dialysis prescription itself. Technical complications may include access recirculation, clotting within the dialyzer, and postdialysis urea rebound that occurs as urea equilibrates from peripheral compartments to the central circulation after dialysis is completed. The amount of urea rebound depends on the intensity of dialysis and can be more pronounced in patients with low urea volumes undergoing highly efficient short therapies, resulting in a measured spKt/V that may significantly overestimate the true urea clearance (61) (see Chapter 7). Thus, although providing an adequate initial prescription is important, the actual in vivo therapy may be considerably less than what has been prescribed. Careful monitoring and the education of staff and patients on the necessity of adhering to the prescribed treatment time are extremely important factors in adequate dialysis delivery. Whenever possible, treatment times should be increased to compensate for interruptions in therapy, and consideration should be given to targeting higher Kt/V and/or utilizing equilibrated Kt/V measurements in patients at risk for substantial urea rebound. Furthermore, urea kinetic modeling should be measured at least once a month to ensure that adequate delivery of therapy is maintained (51).

The rate-limiting factor for short hemodialysis is generally related to patient tolerance of ultrafiltration, specifically, the ability to correct IDWG while maintaining cardiovascular stability. There is concern that suboptimal volume removal with short therapies due to intradialytic symptoms may contribute to the high incidence or persistence of hypertension and ultimately to cardiovascular mortality, which underlies approximately 50% of the deaths in the dialysis population (48). The prevalence of hypertension has been reported in at least 50% to 80% of chronic hemodialysis patients in the United States, and there have been reports of increased antihypertensive medication requirements and a higher prevalence of left ventricular hypertrophy in patients dialyzed for shorter times (62–65). Thus caution must be exercised when selecting patients for short therapies. A number of investigators describe favorable experiences with short dialysis in patients without excessive IDWG (66,67). For instance, a prospective study by Dumler et al. found no changes in pre- or postdialysis blood pressures in a group of patients dialyzed less than 3 hours compared with conventional times of between 3 and 4 hours when interdialytic weight gains were kept below 4 kg (66). Likewise, shorter treatment times were not associated with an increase in intradialytic complications, and the frequency of nausea, vomiting, headaches, and back pain was decreased. However, there are recent reports of centers incorporating unconventionally long dialysis times in which most patients were able to discontinue antihypertensive medications (68,69). Extended hemodialysis was also associated with near normalization of left ventricular mass and improvement in left ventricular systolic function (70,71) (see Chapter 11).

It is uncertain whether, for a given value of *Kt/V*, short, high-efficiency, high-flux hemodialysis provides the same therapy as standard or longer treatment times. The removal of middle- and large-molecular-weight substances is predominantly time-dependent, and even with the currently available HF dialyzers, clearance of these substances will be greater with longer therapies. There are also reports of improved phosphorus control without the use of binders as well as better control of anemia with concomitant decreases in erythropoietin requirements when very long treatment times are employed (68,69,72).

Studies addressing outcomes with short therapies have also reported conflicting results. In a retrospective analysis of more than 12,000 U.S. hemodialysis patients, Lowrie and Lew noted a progressive increase in the risk of death when treatment times were 3 hours or less as compared with those lasting longer than 4 hours (73). Similarly, Held et al. observed 3-year relative mortality risks of 1.17 versus 2.18 in patients dialyzed under 3.5 hours per session compared with those treated more than 3.5 hours in a national random sample of 600 chronic hemodialysis patients (74). However, neither of these studies exclusively incorporated HE therapies or controlled for the dose of dialysis. On the other hand, a number of investigators have reported favorable short-term experiences with short dialysis when HE methods were employed to maintain adequate urea clearance. For example, Keshaviah and Collins were able to successfully shorten treatment times to less than 3 hours in most of their chronic hemodialysis population without any increase in morbidity at close to 1 year of follow-up (75). Nevertheless, given the limitations of the current studies, it remains difficult to discriminate between the effects of dose versus time on morbidity and mortality, as large-scale trials addressing these specific issues are lacking.

Short hemodialysis is attractive because it offers the potential for reduced labor costs as well as patient and staff conve-

nience. However, the same requirements for adequacy must apply to these shortened treatments as with conventional hemodialysis: to ensure effective solute removal and volume control without compromising patient well-being. At present, most studies evaluating the adverse effects of shortened dialysis time on morbidity and mortality are limited by confounding issues, such as delivery of inadequate dialysis; inconsistencies among membrane characteristics with regard to efficiency, flux, and biocompatibility, as well as lack of long-term follow-up. Furthermore, data in support of extended dialysis sessions are accumulating and suggest that these modalities may offer significant advantages over conventional therapies. Nevertheless, using an individualized approach to dialysis prescription, short HE, HF dialysis is generally well tolerated in the short term when individual patient characteristics regarding cardiovascular stability, blood pressure, and IDWG are considered. Additional studies addressing length of therapy and long-term outcomes are needed to better define not only adequate dialysis, but also optimal dialysis.

LONG-TERM SURVIVAL OF PATIENTS ON HIGH-EFFICIENCY AND HIGH-FLUX DIALYSIS

The true test of high-efficiency and high-flux dialysis therapy is the comparison of the long-term survival of these patients to that of patients on standard therapies. A number of studies have suggested a mortality benefit for patients undergoing HE–HF hemodialysis, though the exact mechanisms accounting for this improved survival remain controversial (32,35,36,76,77). In a retrospective cross-over study of 253 chronic dialysis patients, Hornberger et al. showed that the annual mortality rate was substantially lower in 107 patients switched to HF polysulfone biocompatible membranes (7% versus 20%) as compared with 146 patients who remained on conventional cellulosic membranes. Additionally, infection-related hospital admissions were twice as high in the patients treated with cellulosic membranes (35). Results from the United States Renal Data System (USRDS) Dialysis Morbidity and Mortality Study also support the beneficial effects of HF membranes on mortality. This study evaluated a random sample of 12,791 patients treated in 1,391 dialysis facilities across the United States. Among all membranes, mortality was lowest for patients treated with HF synthetic membranes. Furthermore, among the synthetic membranes, death rates were 25% greater for low-flux than for HF membranes when adjusted for *Kt/V*, suggesting that clearance of middle molecules may be a key factor in the improved outcomes seen with HF membranes (76).

The recently completed HEMO study, a National Institutes of Health–National Institute of Diabetes and Digestive Kidney Diseases (NIH–NIDDK)-sponsored prospective, randomized, multicenter trial of more than 1,800 U.S. chronic hemodialysis patients, was designed to specifically address the influences of a higher-dialysis dose and membrane flux on morbidity and mortality. Flux assignment was based on quarterly assessments of the clearance of β_2-microglobulin and controlled for dialyzer reuse. Low-flux dialyzers were defined as those with β_2-microglobulin clearance of less than 10 mL/min (mean, 3.4 mL/min), whereas

HF dialyzers had β_2-microglobulin clearances in excess of 20 mL/min (mean, 33.6 mL/min). Though the study failed to show a statistical difference in all-cause mortality with regard to either membrane flux or dose of dialysis during a mean follow-up of approximately 3 years, patients treated with HF membranes had a significantly lower rate of cardiovascular mortality as compared with those treated with low-flux membranes. Additionally, subgroup analysis revealed that patients who had been on hemodialysis for greater than the median of 3.7 years at study entry had a significantly lower relative risk of death if they were treated with HF rather than low-flux membranes (78). These findings suggest that HF membranes may offer advantages due to their improved clearance of middle-molecular-weight toxins, particularly those contributing to cardiovascular disease in end-stage renal failure (ESRD) patients.

In the USRDS 2002 Annual Data Report using CDC national surveillance data, Figure 11.32 illustrates that the number of dialysis facilities reporting conventional dialysis has markedly decreased whereas those reporting use of HE–HF therapies has increased (79). Indeed, when entire units utilize a therapy, the center effect has to be considered and major adjustments factored into the examination of outcomes. The problems that arise from such an analysis are further compounded by the impression of practicing nephrologists in favor of HE–HF dialysis. In the Dialysis Outcome and Practice Patterns Study (DOPPS), international comparisons are potentially insightful in examining survival by different dialysis techniques, but such studies are confounded by other differences in the populations when related to U.S. dialysis patients. Thus a contemporary study designed to compare outcomes between conventional versus HE–HF therapies will be difficult to perform.

CONCLUSION

HE–HF dialysis has become the predominant mode of dialysis in the United States. The technical needs of HE–HF dialysis have driven many of the advances in UF control and water treatment systems. While the earlier attempts at drastically reducing dialysis times have largely been abandoned, HE dialysis has allowed for shorter dialysis times in selected patients while maintaining adequate small solute clearance. Early evidence exists that HF dialyzers improve survival, perhaps by superior middle-molecule clearance or improved biocompatibility.

Continued technologic advances will likely require that current definitions and terms be modified, as HE–HF dialysis can now accurately be considered "conventional" hemodialysis.

REFERENCES

1. U.S. Renal Data System. *USRDS 2001 annual data report: atlas of end-stage renal disease in the United States.* Bethesda, MD: National Institutes of Health, National Institute of Diabetes and Digestive and Kidney Diseases, 2001.
2. Daugirdas JT, et al. *Handbook of dialysis,* 3rd ed. Philadelphia: Lippincott Williams & Wilkins, 2001:670–676.
3. Gonzalez FM, et al. On the effects of acetate during hemodialysis. *Trans Am Soc Artif Intern Organs* 1974;20A:169–174.
4. Novello AC, et al. Is bicarbonate dialysis better than acetate dialysis? *ASAIO J* 1983;6:103–107.
5. Ronco C, et al. *Membranes and filters for hemodialysis 2001.* Basel: Karger, 2001.
6. Keshaviah P, et al. Reduced treatment time: hemodialysis versus hemofiltration. *Trans Am Soc Artif Inter Organs* 1985;31:176–182.
7. Bland LA, et al. Potential bacteriologic and endotoxin hazards associated with liquid bicarbonate concentrate. *Trans Am Soc Artif Intern Organs* 1987;33:542–545.
8. Ebben JP, et al. Microbiologic contamination of liquid bicarbonate concentrate for hemodialysis. *Trans Am Soc Artif Intern Organs* 1987;33: 269–273.
9. Viljoen M, et al. Danger of hemodialysis using acetate dialysate in combination with a large surface area dialyser. *S Afr Med J* 1979;56:170–172.
10. Kaiser BA, et al. Acid-base changes and acetate metabolism during routine and high-efficiency hemodialysis in children. *Kidney Int* 1981;19: 70–79.
11. Ruder MA, et al. Comparative effects of acetate and bicarbonate hemodialysis on left ventricular function. *Kidney Int* 1985;27:768–773.
12. Vincent JL, et al. Acetate-induced myocardial depression during hemodialysis for acute renal failure. *Kidney Int* 1982;22:653–657.
13. Henrich WL, et al. High sodium bicarbonate and acetate hemodialysis: double-blind crossover comparison of hemodynamic and ventilatory effects. *Kidney Int* 1983;24:240–245.
14. Ismail N, et al. Water treatment for hemodialysis. *Am J Nephrol* 1996; 16:60–72.
15. Brunet P, et al. Water quality and complications of haemodialysis. *Nephrol Dial Transplant* 2000;15:578–580.
16. Baz M, et al. Using ultrapure water in hemodialysis delays carpal tunnel syndrome. *Int J Artif Organs* 1991;14:681–685.
17. Bistrian BR, et al. Protein-energy malnutrition in dialysis patients. *Am J Kidney Dis* 1999;33:172–175.
18. Mattila KJ, et al. Role of infection as a risk factor for atherosclerosis, myocardial infarction, and stroke. *Clin Infect Dis* 1998;26:719–734.
19. Pereira BJ, et al. Diffusive and convective transfer of cytokine-inducing bacterial products across hemodialysis membranes. *Kidney Int* 1995; 47:603–610.
20. Bommer J, et al. Potential transfer of endotoxin across high-flux polysulfone membranes. *J Am Soc Nephrol* 1996;7:883–888.
21. Lonnemann G, et al. Permeability of dialyzer membranes to TNF alpha-inducing substances derived from water bacteria. *Kidney Int* 1992;42:61–68.
22. Alter MJ, et al. National surveillance of dialysis-associated diseases in the United States, 1989. *ASAIO Transplant* 1991;37:97–109.
23. Gordon SM, et al. Pyrogenic reactions in patients receiving conventional, high-efficiency, or high-flux hemodialysis treatments with bicarbonate dialysate containing high concentrations of bacteria and endotoxin. *J Am Soc Nephrol* 1992;2:1436–1444.
24. Lonnemann G. Should ultra-pure dialysate be mandatory? *Nephrol Dial Transplant* 2000;15(Suppl 1):55–59.
25. Anonymous. Water for dilution of haemodialysis solutions, 3rd ed. *Eur Pharmacopoeia* 1997;1545–1546.
26. Laurence RA, et al. Quality of hemodialysis water: a 7-year multicenter study. *Am J Kidney Dis* 1995;25:738–750.
27. Canaud BJ, et al. Water treatment for contemporary hemodialysis. In: Jacobs C, et al., eds. *Replacement of renal function by dialysis,* 4th ed. Dordrecht, The Netherlands: Kluwer Academic, 1996:231–255.
28. Lonnemann G. The quality of dialysate: an integrated approach. *Kidney Int* 2000;76:S112–S119.
29. Locatelli F, et al. Effects of different membranes and dialysis technologies on patient treatment tolerance and nutritional parameters. The Italian Cooperative Dialysis Study Group. *Kidney Int* 1996;50: 1293–1302.
30. Kuchle C, et al. High-flux hemodialysis postpones clinical manifestation of dialysis-related amyloidosis. *Am J Nephrol* 1996;16:484–488.
31. Kuchle C, et al. Biocompatibility, β_2-microglobulin, and dialysis-associated amyloidosis. *Nephrology* 1997;3(Suppl 1):S404(abst).
32. Koda Y, et al. Switch from conventional to high-flux membrane reduces the risk of carpal tunnel syndrome and mortality of hemodialysis patients. *Kidney Int* 1997;52:1096–1101.

33. Birk HW, et al. Protein adsorption by artificial membrane materials under filtration conditions. *Artif Organs* 1995;19:411–415.

34. Hakim RM. Clinical implications of hemodialysis biocompatibility. *Kidney Int* 1993;44:484–494.

35. Hornberger JC, et al. A multivariate analysis of mortality and hospital admissions with high-flux dialysis. *J Am Soc Nephrol* 1992;3:1227–1237.

36. Hakim RM, et al. Effect of dialysis membrane on mortality of chronic hemodialysis patients. *Kidney Int* 1996;50:566–570.

37. Bloembergen WE, et al. Relationship of dialysis membrane and cause-specific mortality. *Am J Kidney Dis* 1999;33:1–10.

38. Gutierrez A, et al. Effect of in vivo contact between blood and dialysis membranes on protein catabolism in humans. *Kidney Int* 1990;38:487–494.

39. Parker TF III, et al. Effect of membrane biocompatibility on nutritional parameters in chronic hemodialysis patients. *Kidney Int* 1996;49:551–556.

40. Kobayashi H, et al. Removal of high molecular substances with large pore size membrane (BK-F). *Kidney Dial* 1993;34(Suppl):154–157.

41. Kawano Y, et al. Effect on alleviation of renal anemia by hemodialysis using high-flux dialyzer (BK-F). *Kidney Dial* 1994;200–203.

42. Seres DS, et al. Improvement of plasma lipoprotein profiles during high-flux dialysis. *J Am Soc Nephrol* 1993;3:1409–1415.

43. Blankestijn PJ, et al. High-flux dialysis membranes improve lipid profile in chronic hemodialysis patients. *J Am Soc Nephrol* 1995;5:1703–1708.

44. Josephson MA, et al. Improved lipid profiles in patients undergoing high-flux hemodialysis. *Am J Kidney Dis* 1992;20:361–366.

45. Makita Z, et al. Efficiency of removal of circulating advanced glycosylation end-products and mode of treatment in patients with ESRD. *Am Soc Nephrol* 1992;3:335(abst).

46. McCarthy JT, et al. Improved preservation of residual renal function in chronic hemodialysis patients using polysulfone dialyzers. *Am J Kidney Dis* 1997;29:576–583.

47. Hartmann J, et al. Biocompatible membranes preserve residual renal function in patients undergoing regular hemodialysis. *Am J Kidney Dis* 1997;30:366–373.

48. United States Renal Data System. *USRDS 1998 annual data report.* Bethesda, MD: U.S. Department of Health and Human Services. The National Institutes of Health, National Institute of Diabetes and Digestive and Kidney Diseases, 1998.

49. Lowrie EG. Effect of the hemodialysis prescription on patient morbidity. Report from the National Cooperative Dialysis Study. *N Engl J Med* 1981;305:1176–1181.

50. Collins A, et al. High-efficiency, high-flux therapies in clinical dialysis. In: Nissenson A, et al., eds. *Clinical dialysis,* 3rd ed. Norwalk, CT: Appleton & Lange, 1995:848–863.

51. *NKF-KDOQI clinical practice guidelines for hemodialysis adequacy.* New York: National Kidney Foundation, 2001:45–54.

52. Gotch FA, et al. A mechanistic analysis of the National Cooperative Dialysis Study (NCDS). *Kidney Int* 1985;28:526–534.

53. Hakim RM, et al. Effects of dose of dialysis on morbidity and mortality. *Am J Kidney Dis* 1994;23:661–669.

54. Collins AJ, et al. Urea index and other predictors of hemodialysis patient survival. *Am J Kidney Dis* 1994;23:272–282.

55. Parker TF, et al. Survival of hemodialysis patients in the United States is improved with a greater quantity of dialysis. *Am J Kidney Dis* 1994;23:670–680.

56. Held PJ, et al. The dose of hemodialysis and patient mortality. *Kidney Int* 1996;50:550–556.

57. Ahmad S. Complications of hemodialysis. *Manual of clinical dialysis.* London: Science Press, 1999:31–43.

58. Delmez JA, et al. Hemodialysis prescription and delivery in a metropolitan community. *Kidney Int* 1992;41:1023–1028.

59. Held PJ, et al. USRDS: hemodialysis prescription and delivery in the U.S.—results from USRDS case mix study. *J Am Soc Nephrol* 1991;2:328(abst).

60. Coyne DW, et al. Impaired delivery of hemodialysis prescriptions: an analysis of causes and an approach to evaluation. *J Am Soc Nephrol* 1997;8:1315–1318.

61. Daugirdas JT, et al. Overestimation of hemodialysis dose depends on dialysis efficiency by regional blood flow but not by conventional two-pool urea kinetic analysis. *ASAIO J* 1995;41:M719–M724.

62. Salem MM. Hypertension in the hemodialysis population: a survey of 649 patients. *Am J Kidney Dis* 1995;26:461–468.

63. Mailloux LU, et al. Hypertension in the ESRD patient: pathophysiology, therapy, outcomes and future directions. *Am J Kidney Dis* 1998;32:705–719.

64. Mittal SK, et al. Prevalence of hypertension in a hemodialysis population. *Clin Nephrol* 1999;51:77–82.

65. Wizemann V, et al. Short-term dialysis—long-term complications: ten years' experience with short-duration renal replacement therapy. *Blood Purif* 1987;5:193–201.

66. Dumler F, et al. Clinical experience with short-time hemodialysis. *Am J Kidney Dis* 1992;19:49–56.

67. Velasquez MT, et al. Equal levels of blood pressure control in ESRD patients receiving high-efficiency hemodialysis and conventional hemodialysis. *Am J Kidney Dis* 1998;31:618–623.

68. Charra B, et al. Importance of treatment time and blood pressure control in achieving long-term survival on dialysis. *Am J Nephrol* 1996;16:35–44.

69. Pierratos A. Nocturnal home hemodialysis: an update on a 5-year experience. *Nephrol Dial Transplant* 1999;14:2835–2840.

70. Chan CT, et al. Regression of left ventricular hypertrophy after conversion to nocturnal hemodialysis. *Kidney Int* 2002;61:2235–2239.

71. Chan C, et al. Improvement in ejection fraction by nocturnal hemodialysis in end-stage renal failure patients with coexisting heart failure. *Nephrol Dial Transplant* 2002;17:1518–1521.

72. Vos PF, et al. Clinical outcome of daily dialysis. *Am J Kidney Dis* 2001;37(Suppl 2):S99–S102.

73. Lowrie EG, et al. Death risk in hemodialysis patients: the predictive value of commonly measured variables and an evaluation of death rate between facilities. *Am J Kidney Dis* 1990;15:458–482.

74. Held PJ, et al. Mortality and duration of hemodialysis treatment. *JAMA* 1991;265:871–875.

75. Keshaviah P, et al. Rapid high-efficiency bicarbonate hemodialysis. *ASAIO Transplant* 1986;32:17–23.

76. Port FK, et al. Mortality risk by hemodialyzer reuse practice and dialyzer membrane characteristics: results from the USRDS dialysis morbidity and mortality study. *Am J Kidney Dis* 2001;37:276–286.

77. Woods HF, et al. Improved outcomes for hemodialysis patients treated with high-flux membranes. *Nephrol Dial Transplant* 2000;15(Suppl 1):36–42.

78. Eknoyan G, et al. Effect of dialysis dose and membrane flux in maintenance hemodialysis. *N Engl J Med* 2002;347:2010–2019.

79. U.S. Renal Data System. *USRDS 2002 annual data report: atlas of end-stage renal disease in the united states.* Bethesda, MD: National Institutes of Health, National Institute of Diabetes and Digestive and Kidney Diseases, 2002.

LONGER TIME DIALYSIS–NOCTURNAL DIALYSIS

ANDREAS PIERRATOS

DAILY HOME NOCTURNAL HEMODIALYSIS

Daily nocturnal hemodialysis began approximately 9 years ago in an effort to provide a well-tolerated high-dose dialysis modality, performed at home. It combines the benefits of long intermittent hemodialysis and short daily hemodialysis.

BACKGROUND INFORMATION

History

Daily home nocturnal hemodialysis was started in Toronto by the late Dr. Robert Uldall in 1994 with the assistance of a grant from the Ministry of Health of the province of Ontario, Canada (1,2). His source of inspiration was the smoothness and effectiveness of the continuous venovenous hemodialysis in the intensive care unit.

Long Intermittent Hemodialysis

By necessity, in the early years of dialysis, when using the inefficient dialyzers, hemodialysis had to be long to achieve adequate results. At that time the usual dialysis regimen was 8 hours, three times a week (3), often at night at home. This regimen changed with the development of higher-efficacy dialyzers. However, several dialysis centers have persevered with long intermittent 8-hour dialysis until now. The best-known center is the Hemodialysis Unit at Tassin, France (4), although other centers used the same regimen (5). During most of this 30-year period, cuprophane dialyzers and acetate-containing dialysate were used in the Tassin unit. Long intermittent dialysis has been performed both in center and at home, either during the day or at night. Usual blood flow was 250 mL/min and dialysate flow 500 mL/min. Average Kt/V was 1.85 and PCR was 1.4 g/kg (6). Several publications have described the benefits of this approach (4,6–9). The two main characteristics of long intermittent hemodialysis are

- Excellent blood pressure control
- Improved patient survival

Blood Pressure Control

Antihypertensives were withheld as soon as the patients were started on long intermittent hemodialysis even if this resulted in high blood pressure. Blood pressure (BP) was then controlled by decreasing the "dry weight" of the patient. This was well tolerated due to the increased length of dialysis. Low salt intake complemented this approach and was necessary for blood pressure control (10). More than 90% of the patients were off antihypertensives. Blood pressure control was not achieved in a few of the patients until several weeks later. This delay in BP control was described as the "lag" phenomenon (11).

Survival

Patient survival as described by the Tassin group has been higher than the survival of patients on hemodialysis in the large databases (United States Renal Data System [USRDS], European Dialysis and Transplantation Association [EDTA]). The reported 10-year survival was 75% (6). Similarly high survival rates were reported on long intermittent hemodialysis by the group in the U.K (5). The parameters correlating to survival were examined by the Tassin group (6). Dialysis dose in the form of Kt/V did not correlate with patient survival. On the other hand, the blood pressure control as well as Babb's Dialysis Index (12) and serum albumin did correlate with patient survival. The high survival of the patients on long intermittent hemodialysis was attributed by some to the patient selection bias reflecting the patient recruitment more than 20 years ago. Most of the selected patients were younger and relatively healthy. Indeed, the Tassin group reported higher mortality in the cohorts of patients who were admitted to the program at a later stage. The 5-year patient survival decreased from 89% to 54% when the pre-1979 patient cohort was compared with the one after 1990. The patients were older and had a larger number of comorbidities, including diabetes mellitus (6). Despite these poorer outcomes of the later cohorts, their survival rate was higher than the survival reported by the USRDS (6).

In earlier studies a high prevalence of left ventricular hypertrophy (LVH) at 76% has been reported on long intermittent hemodialysis (13,14) despite the good control of BP. It should be noted that there was a good correlation between the presence of anemia and LVH. Erythropoietin (EPO) was not available during most of the study observation period, and this may be relevant to the lack of regression of cardiac hypertrophy. No recent information has been published on the status of cardiac hypertrophy. There has been a beneficial effect of long intermittent hemodialysis on erythropoiesis since these patients were not transfusion-dependent despite the lack of availability of EPO (6).

Although long intermittent hemodialysis is characterized by increased removal of middle molecules (15,16), the Tassin patients were not spared from dialysis-related amyloidosis (17). This cannot be ascribed to the use of cuprophane membranes or to acetate-containing dialysate used in Tassin, since a similar incidence of amyloidosis was also seen among patients on long intermittent hemodialysis who were dialyzed using bicarbonate-containing dialysate and noncuprophane membranes (18). Although phosphate control is better on long intermittent hemodialysis than on conventional hemodialysis, phosphate binders are still needed.

Long intermittent hemodialysis in center at night is becoming more popular, as is the use at home, often in the form of every-other-day dialysis (19). A significant advantage of this approach is the decreased cost associated with the intermittent form of hemodialysis with the added benefit from the extended length of the treatment.

Daily Hemodialysis

Short daily hemodialysis was reported for the first time by DePalma in 1969 (20) [reprinted in 1999 (21)]. Sporadic use of short daily hemodialysis was practiced by several centers (22–24). The results of all published studies were very positive, including improved symptoms, better control in the blood pressure, and increase in hemoglobin. Despite these positive results, most of the initial efforts were abandoned for financial reasons. Most of the data on short daily hemodialysis during the last 20 years were generated in Italy, led by Buoncristiani's group (25–28). There has been a resurgence of the clinical interest as well as research activity over the last few years (29–33). Several dialysis units in Europe and North America and elsewhere are utilizing this method (30,34). It includes high efficacy hemodialysis for 2 to 2.5 hours 6 or 7 days per week. It is utilized in in-center facilities or at home. In view of the financial constraints due to the daily schedule, the in-center use of short daily hospital hemodialysis is at this time usually reserved as a "rescue" treatment (35).

By increasing the frequency of dialysis while maintaining the same weekly time, solute removal is enhanced. Both small and larger molecule removal are affected. Standard Kt/V (stdKt/V), a new yardstick of urea kinetic modeling was proposed by Gotch (36) to help compare the dose offered by the different dialysis regimens. StdKt/V is the same for all methods characterized by the same midweek predialysis BUN. This value, following the DOQI guidelines, is equal to 2.0 for all dialysis modalities. The stdKt/V on short daily hemodialysis is much higher than the equivalent value offered by conventional hemodialysis of the same weekly duration (37). For example, stdKt/V was calculated by Galland et al. (38) at 3.4 ± 0.1 per week on short daily hemodialysis, higher than on conventional hemodialysis at 2.1 ± 0.05. Urea kinetic modeling on frequent dialysis is discussed elsewhere in this book (Chapter 7). Larger molecule removal is also enhanced by daily hemodialysis even if the total weekly dial-

ysis time remains stable (16,39–41). The high frequency dialysis allows for the rebound of the serum levels of toxins that diffuse slowly across intercompartmental barriers and their more effective removal.

The benefits of short daily hemodialysis include improvement in the quality of life (27,30,42,43) with better tolerance of the dialysis procedure. The improvement is quite striking, especially in patients with significant comorbidities. Blood pressure control improves on short daily hemodialysis leading to regression of cardiac hypertrophy (28,44). There is evidence of improved nutrition characterized by increased appetite, weight gain and improvement in other nutritional parameters (45). Anemia control leads to a decrease in the dose of EPO (28,46). Although there is some improvement in phosphate control, the need for phosphate binders decreases only slightly, probably due to increased phosphate intake with improving appetite (47,48).

DAILY HOME NOCTURNAL HEMODIALYSIS

Daily home nocturnal hemodialysis combines the benefits of long intermittent hemodialysis and short daily hemodialysis.

Technique Description

Daily nocturnal hemodialysis involves long hemodialysis for the duration of sleep, six or seven nights a week. The option of dialysis seven nights per week is encouraged in patients with severe cardiomyopathy. The length of dialysis was adjusted according to the patient's sleep pattern. It varied between 6 and 10 hours, usually 8 hours. Any hemodialysis machine can be used for daily nocturnal hemodialysis. Blood flow varied from 200 to more than 400 mL/min (usually 250 mL/min) and dialysate flow from 100 to more than 500 mL/min (usually 300 mL/min). The blood flow provided by a single-needle system was adequate. Although any dialyzer can be used, most of the experience to date includes the use of high-flux dialyzers. Low-surface-area dialyzers were adequate (0.7 m², Fresenius F40) but large-surface-area dialyzers have not been harmful (1.7 m² Fresenius F80). In view of the hemodynamic stability of the patients, no partners were required. This is particularly important, since patients without partners have previously been denied the opportunity to perform home hemodialysis. Safety features include two inexpensive moisture sensors placed strategically on the floor to detect possible blood or dialysate leaks. No patient death related to the dialysis procedure has taken place since the inception of the program. Usual dialysate composition includes Na, 140 mEq/L; K, 2 mEq/L; bicarbonate, 28 to 35 mEq/L; and calcium, 3 to 3.5 mEq/L. Most of the patients add sodium phosphate in the form of Fleet enema into the acid (or bicarbonate) concentrate to prevent hypophosphatemia. The role of "ultrapure" dialysate has not been established, and most of the clinical experience has been derived by using conventional dialysate. In view of the long and frequent dialysis regimen, the use of "ultrapure" dialysate is encouraged. This is currently feasible through the inclusion of an "ultrafilter" as part of the hemodialysis machine setting.

Dialyzer Reuse

Delayed dialyzer reprocessing has been utilized for daily nocturnal hemodialysis (49). Using this technique, dialyzers were rinsed with heparinized saline after the end of dialysis, and subsequently were stored in a small refrigerator at home. Once a week, these membranes were transported to the center and exchanged with a set of the patients' own reprocessed dialyzers. When the patient residence was a long distance from the center, an existing laboratory specimen transportation network was used for the transportation of the dialyzers. Dialyzer reuse is not currently practiced at the Humber River Regional Hospital because of improved financial arrangements.

Remote Monitoring

The patients at Humber River Regional Hospital have been monitored "live" remotely using the DAX software developed by Cybernius Medical (Edmonton, Alberta) (50). Similar software has also been produced by some dialysis machine manufacturers. An observer at the dialysis center awakens the patients who do not attend to their machine alarms, by calling them through a separate telephone line. All the dialysis parameters available to the patient at home such as alarms, flow rates, and ultrafiltration rates are also available to the observer. Remote monitoring is useful to monitor the compliance to the treatment and lastly has been utilized to warn patients about incorrect machine settings. The connection to the dialysis machines is achieved via telephone or Internet (51,52). The use of the Internet for dialysis monitoring allows for the utilization of regional monitoring centers capable of servicing wider areas (state, province, country). The need for live remote monitoring is still debated, and at this point most consider it optional.

Access

Although initially only central venous catheters were used for daily nocturnal hemodialysis, AV fistulas and grafts are now used routinely. Safety is of paramount importance. The Inter-Link system and a "locking box" provides a safe catheter connection and prevents disconnection or air embolism at night (Fig. 11.1). Steel needles (15 to 17 gauge, 1 to 1.25 inch) or plastic cannulas are used for cannulation following the "buttonhole technique" (53). The buttonhole technique includes the insertion of the dialysis needle into the same puncture hole in every dialysis. Usually one or two pairs of buttonholes are utilized. Extra care should be taken to prepare the "buttonhole" site before the insertion of the needle. This should be done after removing the "scab" using a sterile needle or sterile tweezers before the needle insertion using an antiseptic technique. "Blunt" needles have recently been introduced providing the additional advantage of minimizing the risk of blood leak around the needle. An inexpensive enuresis alarm sensor is taped on each of the dialysis needles to awaken the patient in case of blood leak (Fig. 11.2). Using a single-needle configuration and the buttonhole technique in an AV fistula is the preferable approach for daily home nocturnal hemodialysis. Daily home nocturnal hemodialysis is the only modality for which a single-needle configuration provides adequate blood flow (average about 200 mL/min). The advantages of this technique are that the number of cannulations per week is similar to that of conventional hemodialysis and that it offers additional safety. This safety is related to the fact that dislodgement of the needle will lead to dialysis machine alarm when the air entering the needle and the blood tubing is sensed by the machine.

Anticoagulation

Anticoagulation during dialysis is similar to the method used in conventional hemodialysis. Most patients utilizing central venous catheters were maintained on oral warfarin. Catheter malfunction is addressed with instillation of TPA (2 mg/port) into the catheter. The dose of warfarin is adjusted to prevent recurrence with the target INR set higher with each subsequent clotting. If two doses of TPA are ineffective in the presence of INR above 2.5, the catheter is replaced over a guidewire. This has been a rare occurrence. Use of citrate-containing locking solutions (ACD-A, Neutrolin) eliminates the problem of the falsely elevated INR values often caused by the sample contamination with heparin. Most patients are on a subtherapeutic dose of coumadin with an average INR of 1.3.

Infection

Access-related infections are encountered when either CVC or fistulas/grafts are utilized. All patients are provided with blood culture media at home as well as antibiotics in the form of vancomycin, tobramycin, or ceftazidime, with ceftazidime used in patients with residual kidney function. The expiration dates of the supplies are monitored at each clinic visit.

Catheters

The incidence of catheter-induced bacteremias with nocturnal hemodialysis is in our experience relatively low (approximately 1.5/1,000 days). In the presence of infections the usual symptoms included fever and chills, frequently presenting at the time of preparation for dialysis in the evening. Unless patients are very symptomatic and require a hospital visit, they obtained blood cultures at home and begin empiric treatment with intravenous antibiotics (usually a dose of vancomycin and tobramycin if they have previously tolerated such agents). Usually, they do not dialyze during that night. They bring the blood culture bottles and receive more antibiotic supplies at the hospital the following morning. The treatment is subsequently modified based upon the blood culture results and is continued for 2 weeks. Vancomycin dose is usually 1 g every second dialysis session. Tobramycin dose includes a loading dose of 1.7 to 2.0 mg/kg followed by 1.2 mg/kg post each session, usually 80 mg. Vancomycin is usually replaced by cephalothin 1 to 2 g/d in the case of susceptible Gram-positive organisms. If the infection relapses, the catheter is replaced over a guidewire after restarting or continuing the antibiotic coverage. Exit site infections are distinctly unusual and require replacement of the catheter if a prolonged 3- to 4-week antibiotic treatment fails.

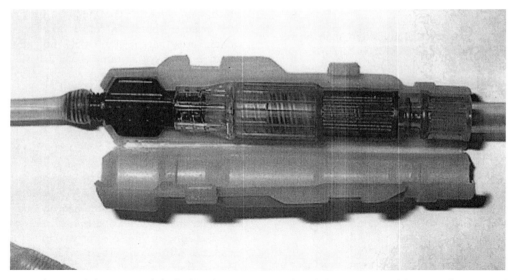

FIG. 11.1. The InterLink system and the locking box prevent accidental disconnection of the central venous catheter from the dialysis tubing.

Rare complications of catheter infections included catheter tunnel infections, septic pulmonary emboli, endocarditis, mycotic brain aneurysms leading to cerebral bleed and septic arthritis.

Fistulas/Grafts

Fistula infections are infrequent. They are associated with local redness, difficulty of cannulation, and signs of blood overcoagulability. They should be recognized readily and treated aggressively, since they may lead to rapid access loss, bacteremia, and septic emboli. If there is a suspicion of such complication, blood cultures are obtained and treatment with antibiotics as well as low-molecular-weight heparin subcutaneously are initiated. In selected cases, urgent fistulograms and angioplasty have salvaged the access. It is conceivable that the use of the buttonhole technique has led to fistula infections in cases where the proper antiseptic technique with antisepsis was not followed adequately.

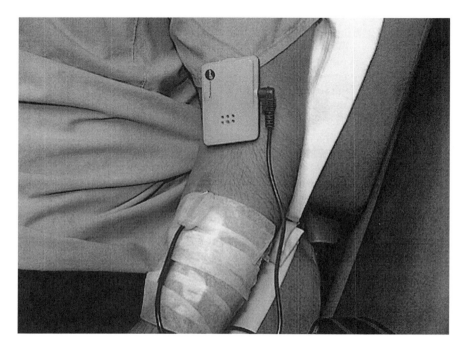

FIG. 11.2. The Enuresis alarm placed on the dialysis needle insertion site gives warning when there is a blood leak.

Central Vein Stenosis/Thrombosis

Central vein stenosis is a common complication of the use of central venous catheters. It is usually asymptomatic or presents with jugular vein distention, facial edema, mild headache, decreased hearing, or symptoms reminiscent of upper respiratory tract infections (stuffed nose, watery eyes, etc.). Superior vena cava venogram confirms the diagnosis. It is done either through the femoral route or by simultaneous bilateral rapid dye infusion into the antecubital veins of both arms. Balloon dilatation of the stenosis with or without stenting has been successful. In the case of acute thrombosis, continuous infusion of thrombolytics (TPA) usually in the intensive care unit overnight followed by balloon angioplasty restores the patency.

Patient Selection Criteria/Training

The patient selection criteria are liberal. Any patient who can be trained on home hemodialysis, has no contraindication to systemic heparinization, and has adequate space at home is eligible for daily home nocturnal hemodialysis. Presence of comorbidities is not a contraindication, nor is the remote residence of the patient from the center. Patients with terminal heart failure, coronary artery disease, ascites, and hemodynamic instability are particularly suited for daily nocturnal hemodialysis. Incident end-stage renal disease (ESRD) patients followed in the chronic kidney disease (CKD) clinic are likely to be the main source of patients in the future. Patients with comorbidities or who failed CAPD represent good candidates for recruitment. The patient training (54) is usually done while on conventional hemodialysis three times a week. Other training regimens, including short daily hemodialysis, have been explored. The length of training depends on the previous experience of the patient, with a typical length of 5 weeks for previously untrained patients followed by three overnight treatments in the training center. A nurse-to-patient ratio of 1:1 during training is usual, although a ratio of one nurse to two patients for at least part of the training is possible.

At the Humber River Regional Hospital in Toronto, 84 patients started and 75 completed training over an 8.5-year period. Nine patients failed training. The patients who completed training included 52 males and 23 females aged 19 to 65 years with an average of 48 ± 11 years. Out of the 75 patients 12 were transplanted; six left the program, usually for medical reasons; seven died; and 50 continue on daily home nocturnal hemodialysis. The total experience has been 180 patient years and the average time on daily home nocturnal hemodialysis was 29 months. The number of patients on daily home nocturnal hemodialysis in Ontario is about 90 to 100, with about 200 patients in North America.

Results

Table 11.1 outlines the benefits of daily nocturnal hemodialysis when compared with conventional hemodialysis.

Quality of Life

All patients reported significant improvement in well-being and level of energy. The changes were apparent sometimes within days in significantly symptomatic patients. Within a month, at the first clinic appointment, the patients reported softer skin, disappearance of pruritus, disappearance of nausea, and improved appetite. Moreover, many patients showed a noticeable and at times impressive change in complexion, with disappearance of the sallow complexion of uremia. Another impressive change was the hemodynamic stability with disappearance of hypotensive episodes, cramping, and shortness of breath as well as unsolicited reports of improved libido. A small number of patients complained of headaches during or after the dialysis procedure that improved and disappeared over a few weeks. Quality-of-life questionnaires in the form of MOS SF-36, sickness impact profile (SIP), and Beck Depression Index showed significant improvement of quality of life in several of the measured parameters (43,55). Even patients with frequent alarms declined offers to return to conventional hemodialysis. Five out of six patients who were temporarily switched to short daily dialysis were anxious to convert back to daily nocturnal hemodialysis. Seven out of 75 patients elected to dialyze seven nights a week either because they felt better or wished to maintain their liberal fluid intake. Vocational rehabilitation improved on daily home nocturnal hemodialysis. Of the current 50 patients below the age of 65, 27 had some type of employment before the conversion to daily home nocturnal hemodialysis. Thirty-two patients were employed after the conversion. Furthermore, in this group of patients the number of patients who had full employment increased from 13 to 22.

Dialysis Dose (Urea /Phosphate/β_2-Microglobulin)

Using dialysate collection, the measured urea Kt/V was 0.99 ± 0.3 per session when using dialysate flow of 100 mL/min (50). By increasing blood and dialysate flow, Kt/V can exceed 2.0 per session (56). The best approach to dialysis quantitation on daily hemodialysis is still under debate (57). Daily nocturnal hemodialysis offers a standard Kt/V of about 5 (58). Therefore the ability of daily nocturnal hemodialysis to provide small-mol-

TABLE 11.1. BENEFITS OF DAILY NOCTURNAL HEMODIALYSIS AS COMPARED WITH CONVENTIONAL HEMODIALYSIS

Improves quality of life and aids vocational rehabilitation
Provides high small-molecule clearance
Provides high phosphate clearance leading to normal serum phosphate without binders
Increases middle-molecule clearance, including β_2-microglobulin
Improves blood pressure control, usually without the need for antihypertensives
Decreases left ventricular hypertrophy
Improves ventricular function in patients with cardiac dysfunction
Is associated with lower homocysteine levels
Improves sleep apnea
Improves cognitive function
Improves anemia control and decreases erythropoietin utilization
Decreases parathyroid hormone and dissolves extraosseous tumoral calcifications
Offers unrestricted diet
Improves nutrition
Is associated with lower hospitalization rate

ecule clearance is unparalleled, and therefore best suited for the treatment of large patients.

Phosphate control has been uniformly excellent (59). The weekly phosphate removal in the dialysate was twice as high as that with conventional hemodialysis (4.8 ± 1.7 g versus 2.2 ± 0.6 g). Serum predialysis phosphate levels were significantly lower with nocturnal hemodialysis (4.0 versus 6.5 mg/dL) than with conventional hemodialysis ($p < 0.001$). The serum phosphate normalized within 1 to 2 weeks after the initiation of the treatment, and phosphate binders were discontinued in all patients. Despite the high-phosphate diet, about 75% of the patients required the addition of sodium phosphate into the acid or bicarbonate dialysate concentrates to avoid hypophosphatemia. The amount varied, depending on the dialysis intensity, diet, and need for phosphate during the repair phase of renal osteodystrophy or anabolic phase (e.g., pregnancy). We have utilized Fleet enema added to the "acid" concentrate at doses between 30 and 120 mL/4 L dialysate jug. The addition of phosphate to the bicarbonate solution has also been used, as has the oral Fleet preparation. Serum phosphate levels with the aid of the phosphate dialysate additive were as follows: predialysis, 3.6 ± 0.6 mg/dL; postdialysis, 2.6 ± 0.3 mg/dL.

β_2-microglobulin (β_2-m) removal is four times as high as on conventional hemodialysis, and long-term serum β_2-m levels are lower than during conventional hemodialysis (60). The mass of β_2-m removed was significantly higher with daily home nocturnal hemodialysis (127 ± 48 versus 585 ± 309 mg, $p < 0.001$), with a percentage reduction in serum level of 20.5 ± 5.8 versus $38.8 \pm 7.1\%$ ($p < 0.0001$) and a $Kt/V \beta_2$-m of 0.21 ± 0.09 versus 0.56 ± 0.17 ($p < 0.0006$). The increased β_2-m removal corresponds to the fourfold increase in the weekly duration of hemodialysis. At this point it is unclear if this improved efficacy will affect the prevalence or the course of dialysis-related amyloidosis (see Chapter 23).

Cardiovascular Effects

Blood Pressure Control

In a controlled study, after conversion from conventional hemodialysis to daily nocturnal hemodialysis there was a decline of systolic, diastolic, and pulse pressure (from 145 ± 20 to 122 ± 13 mm Hg, $p < 0.001$; from 84 ± 15 to 74 ± 12 mm Hg, $p < 0.02$; from 61 ± 12 to 49 ± 12 mm Hg, $p \leq 0.002$, respectively) (61). The need for antihypertensive medications decreased from 1.8 to 0.3 medications ($p < 0.001$). This effect is only partially related to decrease in the extracellular fluid volume (ECFV). ECFV as measured by bioelectrical impedance (BIA) following dialysis remained unchanged after the conversion of the patients from conventional to daily home nocturnal hemodialysis. The patients predictably came off all antihypertensives with the exception of a small dose of a beta blocker (usually atenolol 25 mg every other day) which was necessary for about 30% of the patients. If the blood pressure was not well controlled the patients are requested to lower their "dry weight." Conversely, if they were hypotensive, they decreased or discontinued the antihypertensives or they increased their dry weight. We have also observed the "lag phenomenon" described by the Tassin group

(11) in a few patients who were able to stop their last antihypertensive medication only several months later. Blood pressure control worsened transiently in several patients during periods when they developed other complications or they were under emotional stress.

Left Ventricular Hypertrophy

In the same study (61) the left ventricular mass index decreased on daily nocturnal hemodialysis from 147 ± 42 to 114 ± 40 g/m^2 ($p < 0.004$), whereas it did not change in the control group. Preliminary data suggest that daily nocturnal hemodialysis is associated with decrease in systemic peripheral resistance as well as improved endothelial function (62). In this study, the posthypoxemia or postnitroglycerin administration brachial artery vasodilatation improved after the conversion to daily home nocturnal hemodialysis.

Cardiac Function

Daily home nocturnal hemodialysis improved the cardiac function in patients with ventricular dysfunction. Indeed, the ejection fraction of the six patients with impaired cardiac function increased significantly from 28% $\pm$ 12% to 41% $\pm$ 18% as measured by radionucleotide angiography (63). Two of these patients were accepted for kidney transplantation whereas they were not eligible for the procedure before their conversion to daily home nocturnal hemodialysis.

Homocysteine

Increased plasma homocysteine is a risk factor for atherosclerosis. It is seen in 85% of hemodialysis patients. Predialysis plasma total homocysteine levels in 23 patients on daily nocturnal hemodialysis were compared with those in 31 patients undergoing conventional hemodialysis. Geometric mean total homocysteine levels for the daily nocturnal hemodialysis patients were significantly lower [12.7 versus 20.0 μmol/L, ($p < 0.0001$)], as was the prevalence of mild-to-moderate hyperhomocysteinemia of more than 12 μmol/L [DHNHD, 57%; CHD, 94% ($p < 0.002$)]. The mechanism leading to the decrease in serum homocysteine levels is unclear.

Sleep

Tolerance of dialysis during the night has been better than expected. Sleep studies were done before as well as several weeks or months after the conversion of the first 14 patients to daily home nocturnal hemodialysis (64). Out of the 14 patients seven were found to have sleep apnea. The conversion was associated with a reduction in the frequency of apnea and hypopnea from 25 ± 25 to 8 ± 8 episodes per hour of sleep ($p = 0.03$). This reduction occurred predominantly in seven patients with sleep apnea, in whom the frequency of episodes fell from 46 ± 19 to 9 ± 9 per hour ($p = 0.006$), accompanied by increases in the minimal oxygen saturation [from 89.2% $\pm$ 1.8% to 94.1% $\pm$ 1.6%, ($p = 0.005$)], transcutaneous partial pressure of carbon dioxide [from 38.5 ± 4.3 to 48.3 ± 4.9 mm Hg ($p = 0.006$)], and serum bicarbonate concentration [from 23.2 ± 1.8 to 27.8 ± 0.8 mmol/L ($p < 0.001$)]. There was no improvement in the frequency of involuntary leg movements.

Cognitive Function

Psychological studies were done prior and after conversion to daily home nocturnal hemodialysis. There was a significant improvement upon conversion to daily home nocturnal hemodialysis by an average of 16%. The tests included the "choice reaction" (p <0.01), logical reasoning (p <0.02), serial addition/subtraction (p <0.05) and the Stroop test (p <0.01) (65).

Anemia Control

Conversion to daily home nocturnal hemodialysis is associated with an increase in hemoglobin (Hb) leading to a decrease in the dose of erythropoietin. In a cohort of 23 patients followed for at least 2 years Hb increased from 10.7 ± 1.3 to 11.8 ± 1.6 g/dL (61). EPO dose decreased from 10,372 to 8,090 units per week. It is conceivable that the meticulous attention to the iron replenishment via the intravenous route has contributed to this improvement. The patients self-administered intravenous iron preparations or in some centers they visited the hospital for the intravenous iron administration. In a group of 50 patients currently on daily home nocturnal hemodialysis at the Humber River Regional Hospital, 34% are not on EPO.

Calcium Metabolism/Bone Disease

The calcium phosphate product normalized in all patients. This led to the dissolution of tumoral extraosseous calcifications in one patient (66).

Serial bone density measurements every 6 to 12 months in all patients were used to determine the ideal dialysate calcium. They showed progressive decrease in bone density during the early phase of the study (67). This led to the use of increased dialysate calcium, which prevented further bone loss and restored bone density. Dialysate calcium, currently used, is 3.26 ± 0.20 mEq/L. Fixed dialysate concentrations of 3 or 3.5 mEq/L were used or the patients were asked to add the extra prescribed amount of calcium chloride in a powder form into the acid concentrate. The average serum calcium levels were as follows: before dialysis, 9.85 ± 0.28 mg/dL; after dialysis, 10.7 ± 0.25 mg/dL. Parathyroid hormone (PTH) was easily suppressed by increasing dialysate calcium. PTH levels decreased from 610 ± 620 to 240 ± 310 pg/mL (p = 0.007) within 6 months.

Bone density studies performed monthly for 6 months followed by yearly studies are very useful in adjusting dialysate calcium concentrations and ensuring that negative calcium balance is avoided. They should be considered an important parameter for the management of these patients. The role of calcitriol is currently unknown. Suppression of very high levels of PTH has been achieved by increasing the dialysate calcium rather than using vitamin D analogs intravenously.

Preliminary results from bone biopsies on 17 patients on daily nocturnal hemodialysis revealed a high prevalence of low bone turnover (67). This may be partially due to the high dialysate calcium aiming to maintain calcium balance. Obvi-

ously, further research is needed to establish the ideal dialysate calcium concentration on daily home nocturnal hemodialysis.

Nutrition

Diet is unrestricted on daily home nocturnal hemodialysis. No restriction in dietetic sodium, potassium, phosphate, or water has been imposed. High phosphate and protein intake has been encouraged. Amino acid losses were substantial on daily nocturnal hemodialysis in the range of 10 to 15 g/d (68). Both serum essential and nonessential serum amino acids increased on daily home nocturnal hemodialysis, but the ratio remained abnormal (69). Twenty-four patients were followed with total body nitrogen and potassium measurements using in vivo neutron activation analysis. There was a nonsignificant increase in total body nitrogen (70). Serum albumin did not change significantly (3.95 ± 0.42 g/dL to 3.87 ± 0.37 g/dL) over an average of 28 months. Over a similar length of time body weight increased by 1.86 ± 5.35 kg (p = 0.026).

Survival and Hospitalization Rates

The relatively small number of patients currently on daily home nocturnal hemodialysis does not allow for final conclusions in these areas. The 5-year survival rate of the patient population of 75 patients was 80%.

In a prospective controlled study, 56 patients were enrolled, 33 on daily home nocturnal hemodialysis and a control group of 23 on conventional hemodialysis. The hospitalization rate of the patients on daily nocturnal hemodialysis was lower at 1.8 days versus 6.8 days per year in the control group, although the difference was not significant (71).

Cost

The cost of daily hemodialysis was examined in a retrospective as well as a prospective study. Mohr et al. (43) compared the cost of conventional hemodialysis three times a week to the cost of short daily hemodialysis in center or at home and daily nocturnal hemodialysis at home. The cost included expense of hospitalizations as well as medications including EPO. Despite the higher cost of the dialysis procedure on the daily therapies, the overall cost of daily hemodialysis was lower, mainly due to the decreased hospitalization rates and decreased dose of medications including EPO. In comparison with conventional hemodialysis, the savings were $6,400 (USD) per patient per year for in-center short daily hemodialysis, $9,800 for home short daily hemodialysis, and $9,500 for daily home nocturnal hemodialysis. The savings were lower if "live" remote patient monitoring and single use of dialyzers were included in the cost for daily home nocturnal hemodialysis (72).

In a prospective controlled study, McFarlane et al. (71) compared the cost of total care of 23 patients on conventional hemodialysis to the cost of the care of 33 patients on daily home nocturnal hemodialysis. The control group was selected to include patients that, given the opportunity, were willing and capable of being trained on daily home nocturnal hemodialysis. The two patient groups were followed prospectively for 1 year.

The costing analysis determined a mean annual cost of health care of $35,084 for daily home nocturnal hemodialysis, and $42,930 for conventional hemodialysis ($p = 0.003$). The main reason for the financial benefit of the daily home nocturnal hemodialysis group was the decreased labor cost, the lower hospitalization rate, and the lower medication use.

A cost utility study was also performed using the same costing values (73). Utility scores were generated using the standard gamble (SG) technique and a willingness-to-pay (WTP) technique (74). The SG technique tries to establish the risk of death that the patient would accept in order to return to excellent health. Obviously, a patient with good quality of life would not accept such a high risk. Mean SG scores were 0.70 ± 0.26 for daily home nocturnal hemodialysis and 0.51 ± 0.36 for conventional hemodialysis ($p = 0.046$) favoring daily nocturnal hemodialysis. The WTP technique tries to establish the percentage of a defined annual income that a patient would sacrifice to return to excellent health. Patients enjoying a good quality of life would sacrifice a lower percentage of their income. Mean WTP scores were 0.42 ± 0.23 for conventional hemodialysis and 0.73 ± 0.19 for conventional hemodialysis ($p <0.001$), both favoring daily home nocturnal hemodialysis. The cost utility by SG was $50,041/QALY (quality-adjusted life years) for daily home nocturnal hemodialysis, and $83,556/QALY for conventional hemodialysis. This study demonstrated that daily home nocturnal hemodialysis offers improved quality at lower cost.

Although the total cost of patients on daily home nocturnal hemodialysis is lower than that of conventional hemodialysis, the direct cost to the hemodialysis units is usually higher, because of the increased frequency of dialysis. Depending on the method and the amount of reimbursement paid to the dialysis providers, there can be financial incentives or disincentives for the provision of such therapies.

Obstacles

Despite the significant evidence that daily hemodialysis offers significant advantages, its utilization remains limited. The main obstacles are lack of hard outcome data, financial aspects of the daily treatments, lack of infrastructure for home hemodialysis, and lack of user-friendly hemodialysis machines.

Lack of Hard Outcome Data

Obviously, data showing better survival rates derived from controlled studies are important and are not available. In view of the difficulties and the cost involved in such studies it is unlikely they will be forthcoming.

Financial Aspects of the Daily Treatments

Disincentives

Since the direct cost of daily hemodialysis seems to be higher than conventional hemodialysis, the payers are reluctant to fund such methods. The dialysis providers have difficulty absorbing the cost of dialysis if the reimbursement rates stay at the current levels. Another financial disincentive is the decreased need for EPO and intravenous vitamin D analog use. Depending on the reimbursement method for the provision of dialysis, the use of these medications can be profitable to the provider, thereby providing a disincentive to pursue the therapy.

Incentives

With capitated care there may be financial incentives for the organization providing the dialysis treatment to adopt the daily hemodialysis regimens. The benefits from the lower hospitalization rate and decreased dose of medications including EPO can be higher than the increased direct costs of providing dialysis (75).

Lack of Infrastructure for Home Hemodialysis

The decline of utilization of home hemodialysis has led to a decrease in the familiarity of the nurses and physicians with these methods. This has created a significant inertia in exploring these new avenues. There is a need for the university centers as well as industry to help with the training of the dialysis providers so that they can establish the proper patient training facilities (76).

Lack of User-friendly Hemodialysis Machines

There is renewed activity in this area with several manufacturers offering machines adapted for home use or new machines specifically being designed for home daily treatments (77).

The Future

The need for improvement of outcomes will encourage the use of these alternative dialysis modalities. In the presence of the current dialysis reimbursement difficulties one would expect increased utilization of long intermittent hemodialysis. Also, one would expect a slow growth of in-center short daily hemodialysis for patients with significant comorbidities. Increased reimbursement would lead to an accelerated growth of both short daily home hemodialysis as well as daily home nocturnal hemodialysis. It is expected that about 20% of the patients would select these home modalities. The introduction of simpler hemodialysis machines will increase their utilization further. The growth of daily therapies at home will be important in the face of significant nursing shortages. The shortage of nurses as well as nephrologists will also provide an impetus for the creation of the appropriate financial environment for the growth of home daily therapies.

ACKNOWLEDGMENTS

The development of daily home nocturnal hemodialysis was supported by grants from the Ministry of Health of Ontario, Canada.

REFERENCES

1. Uldall PR, et al. Simplified nocturnal home hemodialysis (SNHHD): a new approach to renal replacement therapy. *J Am Soc Nephrol* 1994;5: 428.

2. Uldall R, et al. Slow nocturnal home hemodialysis at the Wellesley Hospital. *Adv Ren Replace Ther* 1996;3:133–136.

3. Barber S, et al. Adequate dialysis. *Nephron* 1975;14:209–227.

4. Charra B, et al. Survival as an index of adequacy of dialysis. *Kidney Int* 1992;41:1286–1291.

5. Covic A, et al. Long-hours home haemodialysis—the best renal replacement therapy method? *QJM* 1999;92:251–260.

6. Laurent G, et al. The results of an 8 h thrice weekly haemodialysis schedule. *Nephrol Dial Transplant* 1998;13(Suppl 6):125–131.

7. Charra B, et al. Control of hypertension and prolonged survival on maintenance hemodialysis. *Nephron* 1983;33:96–99.

8. Charra B, et al. Importance of treatment time and blood pressure control in achieving long-term survival on dialysis. *Am J Nephrol* 1996;16:35–44.

9. Charra B, et al. Long, slow dialysis. *Miner Electrolyte Metab* 1999;25:391–396.

10. Charra B, et al. Survival in dialysis and blood pressure control. *Contrib Nephrol* 1994;106:179–185.

11. Charra B, et al. Blood pressure control in dialysis patients: importance of the lag phenomenon. *Am J Kidney Dis* 1998;32:720–724.

12. Babb AL, et al. Quantitative description of dialysis treatment: a dialysis index. *Kidney Int Suppl* 1975;Jan(2):23–29.

13. Covic A, et al. Echocardiographic findings in long-term, long-hour hemodialysis patients. *Clin Nephrol* 1996;45:104–110.

14. Huting J, et al. Asymmetric septal hypertrophy and left atrial dilatation in patients with end-stage renal disease on long-term hemodialysis. *Clin Nephrol* 1989;32:276–283.

15. Chapman GV, et al. Uremic middle molecules: separation and quantitation. *Artif Organs* 1981;4(Suppl):160–165.

16. Clark WR, et al. Quantifying the effect of changes in the hemodialysis prescription on effective solute removal with a mathematical model. *J Am Soc Nephrol* 1999;10:601–609.

17. Laurent G, et al. Dialysis related amyloidosis. *Kidney Int* 1988;24 (Suppl):S32–S34.

18. Goldsmith DJ, et al. Prolonged slow dialysis and better survival. *Am J Kidney Dis* 2000;35:361–362.

19. Kurella M, et al. Intermittent nocturnal in-center hemodialysis: UCSF–Mt. Zion experience. *J Am Soc Nephrol* 2002;13:410A.

20. DePalma JR, et al. A new automatic coil dialyser system for "daily" dialysis. *Proc EDTA* 1969;6:26–34.

21. DePalma JR, et al. A new automatic coil dialyser system for "daily" dialysis. *Semin Dial* 1999;12:410–418.

22. Snyder D, et al. Clinical experience with long-term brief, "daily" haemodialysis. *Proc EDTA* 1975;11:128–135.

23. Bonomini V, et al. Daily-dialysis programme: indications and results. *Nephrol Dial Transplant* 1998;13:2774–2777.

24. Louis BM, et al. Clinical experience with long-term 5-days-a-week hemodialysis. *Proc Clin Dial Transplant Forum* 1975;5:58–60.

25. Buoncristiani U. Fifteen years of clinical experience with daily haemodialysis. *Nephrol Dial Transplant* 1998;13(Suppl 6):148–151.

26. Buoncristiani U, et al. Daily dialysis: long-term clinical metabolic results. *Kidney Int* 1988;24:S137–S140.

27. Buoncristiani U, et al. Dramatic improvement of clinical-metabolic parameters and quality of life with daily dialysis. *Int J Artif Organs* 1989;12:133–136.

28. Woods JD, et al. Clinical and biochemical correlates of starting "daily" hemodialysis. *Kidney Int* 1999;55:2467–2476.

29. Pierratos A. Daily hemodialysis: why the renewed interest? [see comments]. *Am J Kidney Dis* 1998;32(Suppl 4):S76–S82.

30. Kooistra MP, et al. Daily home haemodialysis in The Netherlands: effects on metabolic control, haemodynamics, and quality of life. *Nephrol Dial Transplant* 1998;13:2853–2860.

31. Ting G. Future role of short daily hemodialysis: an opinion based on a California study. *Semin Dial* 1999;12:448–450.

32. Ting G. The strategic role of daily hemodialysis in managed care in the United States. *Semin Dial* 2000;13:385–388.

33. Kjellstrand C, et al. Daily hemodialysis: dialysis for the next century. *Adv Ren Replace Ther* 1998;5:267–274.

34. Traeger J, et al. Daily versus standard hemodialysis: one year experience. *Artif Organs* 1998;22:558–563.

35. Ting GO. The case for short daily hemodialysis, why sDHD will be the predominant modality for frequent dialysis. *ASAIO J* 2001;47:443–445.

36. Gotch FA. The current place of urea kinetic modelling with respect to different dialysis modalities. *Nephrol Dial Transplant* 1998;13(Suppl 6):10–14.

37. Galland R, et al. Daily hemodialysis versus standard hemodialysis: urea TAC, TAD, weekly e*Kt/V*, Std(*Kt/V*) and nPCR. *Home Hemodial Int* 1999;3:33–36.

38. Galland R, et al. Chronic renal replacement therapy by short daily hemofiltration. *J Am Soc Nephrol* 2001;12:266A.

39. Pierratos A. Effect of therapy time and frequency on effective solute removal. *Semin Dial* 2001;14:284–288.

40. Fagugli RM, et al. Behavior of non-protein-bound and protein-bound uremic solutes during daily hemodialysis. *Am J Kidney Dis* 2002;40:339–347.

41. Floridi A, et al. Daily haemodialysis improves indices of protein glycation. *Nephrol Dial Transplant* 2002;17:871–878.

42. Mohr PE, et al. *The quality of life and economic implications of daily dialysis*. Bethesda, MD: The Project HOPE Center for Health Affairs, 1999:8.

43. Mohr PE, et al. The case for daily dialysis: its impact on costs and quality of life. *Am J Kidney Dis* 2001;37:777–789.

44. Fagugli RM, et al. Short daily hemodialysis: blood pressure control and left ventricular mass reduction in hypertensive hemodialysis patients. *Am J Kidney Dis* 2001;38:371–376.

45. Galland R, et al. Short daily hemodialysis rapidly improves nutritional status in hemodialysis patients. *Kidney Int* 2001;60:1555–1560.

46. Fagugli RM, et al. Anemia and blood pressure correction obtained by daily hemodialysis induce a reduction of left ventricular hypertrophy in dialysed patients. *Int J Artif Organs* 1998;21:429–431.

47. Lugon JR, et al. Effects of in-center daily hemodialysis upon mineral metabolism and bone disease in end-stage renal disease patients. *Sao Paulo Med J* 2001;119:105–109.

48. Chan CT, et al. Improvement in phosphate control with short daily in-center hemodialysis (SDHD). *J Am Soc Nephrol* 2001;12:262A.

49. Pierratos A, et al. Delayed dialyzer reprocessing for home hemodialysis. *Home Hemodial Int* 2000;4:51–54.

50. Pierratos A, et al. Nocturnal hemodialysis: three-year experience [see comments]. *J Am Soc Nephrol* 1998;9:859–868.

51. Pierratos A. Nocturnal home haemodialysis: an update on a 5-year experience. *Nephrol Dial Transplant* 1999;14:2835–2840.

52. Hoy CD. Remote monitoring of daily nocturnal hemodialysis. *Hemodialysis Int* 2001;5:8–12.

53. Twardowski Z, et al. Different sites versus constant sites of needle insertion into arteriovenous fistulas for treatment by repeated dialysis. *Dial Transplant* 1979;8:978–980.

54. Ouwendyk M, et al. Daily hemodialysis: a nursing perspective. *Adv Ren Replace Ther* 2001;8:257–267.

55. Brissenden JE, et al. Improvements in quality of life with nocturnal hemodialysis. *J Am Soc Nephrol* 1998;9:168A.

56. O'Sullivan DA, et al. Improved biochemical variables, nutrient intake, and hormonal factors in slow nocturnal hemodialysis: a pilot study [see comments]. *Mayo Clin Proc* 1998;73:1035–1045.

57. Depner TA. Daily hemodialysis efficiency: an analysis of solute kinetics. *Adv Ren Replace Ther* 2001;8:227–235.

58. Gotch FA. Is *Kt/V* urea a satisfactory measure for dosing the newer dialysis regimens? *Semin Dial* 2001;14:15–17.

59. Mucsi I, et al. Control of serum phosphate without any phosphate binders in patients treated with nocturnal hemodialysis. *Kidney Int* 1998;53:1399–1404.

60. Raj DS, et al. beta-microglobulin kinetics in nocturnal haemodialysis. *Nephrol Dial Transplant* 2000;15:58–64.

61. Chan CT, et al. Regression of left ventricular hypertrophy after conversion to nocturnal hemodialysis. *Kidney Int* 2002;61:2235–2239.

62. Chan CT, et al. Impact of nocturnal hemodialysis on blood pressure and endothelially mediated vasodilation. *J Am Soc Nephrol* 2002;13:60A.

63. Chan CT, et al. Improvement in left ventricular systolic function with long-term nocturnal hemodialysis. *J Am Soc Nephrol* 2001;12:262A.

64. Hanly PJ, et al. Improvement of sleep apnea in patients with chronic

renal failure who undergo nocturnal hemodialysis. *N Engl J Med* 2001; 344:102–107.

65. Pierratos A, et al. Nocturnal hemodialysis (NHD) improves daytime cognitive function. *J Am Soc Nephrol* 1998;9:180A.
66. Kim SJ, et al. Resolution of massive uremic tumoral calcinosis with daily nocturnal home hemodialysis. *Am J Kidney Dis* 2003;41:E12.
67. Pierratos A, et al. Calcium, phosphorus metabolism and bone pathology on long term nocturnal hemodialysis. *J Am Soc Nephrol* 2001;12:274A.
68. Ikizler TA, et al. Amino acid and albumin losses during hemodialysis. *Kidney Int* 1994;46:830–837.
69. Raj DS, et al. Plasma amino acid profile on nocturnal hemodialysis. *Blood Purif* 2000;18:97–102.
70. Pierratos A, et al. Total body nitrogen increases on nocturnal hemodialysis. *J Am Soc Nephrol* 1999;10:299A.
71. McFarlane PA, et al. The cost savings of home nocturnal versus conventional in-centre hemodialysis. *Kidney Int* 2002;62:2216–2222.
72. Mohr PE. The economics of daily dialysis. *Adv Ren Replace Ther* 2001; 8:273–279.
73. McFarlane PA, et al. Cost-utility of home nocturnal hemodialysis and conventional in-centre hemodialysis. *J Am Soc Nephrol* 2001;12: 339A.
74. Morimoto T, et al. Utilities measured by rating scale, time trade-off, and standard gamble: review and reference for health care professionals. *J Epidemiol* 2002;12:160–178.
75. Hannah RG. The role of managed care in daily dialysis. *ASAIO J* 2001; 47:462–463.
76. Nissenson AR. Daily hemodialysis: challenges and opportunities in the delivery and financing of end-stage renal disease patient care. *Adv Ren Replace Ther* 2001;8:286–292.
77. Kenley RS. Tearing down the barriers to daily home hemodialysis and achieving the highest value renal therapy through holistic product design. *Adv Ren Replace Ther* 1996;3:137–146.

12

PRESCRIBING DRUGS FOR DIALYSIS PATIENTS

GEORGE R. ARONOFF AND MICHAEL E. BRIER

Uremia affects every organ system in the body. Changes in the absorption, distribution, metabolism, and excretion of drugs and their active or toxic metabolites must be taken into account when dosing patients on hemodialysis or peritoneal dialysis. The problems of end-stage renal disease (ESRD) are often superimposed on underlying hypertension, diabetes, and heart disease, compounding the complexity of management.

The kidney is the major regulator of the internal fluid environment. Therefore the physiologic changes associated with severe renal disease have pronounced effects on the pharmacology of many drugs. Improvements in the management of patients with renal failure have created a large patient population for which special understanding of drug disposition is important. The development of new dialysis membranes, the wide acceptance of chronic peritoneal dialysis, and the popularity of continuous renal replacement therapies add to the need for detailed understanding of drug transport across biological and synthetic membranes. Physicians caring for these patients must possess a basic understanding of the biochemical and physiologic effects of uremia on drug disposition, and the effects of dialysis on drug and metabolite removal. This chapter deals with these problems and offers suggestions on how to deal effectively with pharmacotherapy in the dialysis patient.

INITIAL PATIENT ASSESSMENT

Clinical evaluation always begins with a careful history and physical examination. Knowledge of previous medication history, drug-related allergy or toxicity, and concurrent medicines is important in the initial evaluation of patients on dialysis. Reviewing the possibility of drug interactions before choosing a drug regimen reduces potentially adverse drug effects. On average, dialysis patients routinely receive 11 different medications and have three times the incidence of adverse drug events as patients with normal renal function (1–3). Focusing therapy on specific diagnoses allows the clinician to limit the number of drugs the patient is taking and lessens the chances of untoward drug interactions. When possible, drug therapy should be individualized to take advantage of the fact that one drug can be used to treat several conditions. For example, a calcium channel antagonist can be used to treat hypertension and angina.

Estimating extracellular fluid volume is necessary to determine the distribution volume of drugs. Edema or ascites increases the distribution volume of many drugs, whereas volume depletion shrinks this space.

Individualization of the drug regimen requires measurements of body height and weight. For obese patients, ideal body weight (IBW) should be calculated. For men, IBW is 50 kg plus 2.3 kg for each inch more than 5 feet. For women, IBW is 45.5 kg plus 2.3 kg for each inch more than 5 feet. Many clinicians use the average of the measured body weight and the ideal body weight as the value on which to base drug doses (4).

Evaluating functional impairment of other excretory organs is also important. The failure of other organs limits the possibilities for alternate pathways of drug and metabolite elimination. For instance, the stigmata of liver disease suggest the potential need to alter drug dosages further in patients with renal failure.

MEASURING RESIDUAL RENAL FUNCTION

The rate of drug and metabolite elimination by the kidneys is proportional to the glomerular filtration rate. Some dialysis patients have residual renal function that substantially contributes to the elimination of drugs and their metabolites. Estimating residual renal function in dialysis patients still making urine is difficult because the serum creatinine reflects the adequacy of dialysis and muscle mass as well as residual glomerular filtration rate. Creatinine clearance measurements less accurately reflect the glomerular filtration rate in patients with renal failure severe enough to require dialysis. Changing serum creatinine over the duration of the clearance measurement, the contribution of tubular creatinine secretion, and the accumulation of chromagens contribute to the difficulty in measuring residual renal function. Serum creatinine measurements alone should not be used to estimate intrinsic renal function in dialysis patients. The plasma clearance rate of certain radioisotopes more accurately estimates residual renal function in these patients; however, the use of radioisotopes is complicated by the need to dispose of radioactive materials.

Conventional quantification of residual renal function in hemodialysis patients is measured by urea clearance, creatinine clearance, or the combination of both. This approach requires a

24-hour urine collection, which is often difficult to perform and inaccurate. It requires that serum measurements of urea and creatinine be measured before and after the urine collection to estimate the average values during the collection. Measuring the elimination of iohexol after an intravenous dose with a single blood measurement of iohexol has been reported to be an accurate and safe measure of residual renal function in dialysis patients and can simplify drug dosing (5). However, at present, iohexol clearances are not routinely performed to measure residual renal function. Residual renal function decreases over time and is usually less than 5 mL/min after 1 year on hemodialysis (6).

EFFECTS OF UREMIA ON DRUG DISPOSITION

Bioavailability

The bioavailability of a drug is the amount that enters the central circulation and the rate at which it appears. Drugs given intravenously enter the venous circulation directly and generally demonstrate rapid onset of action. Drugs given by other routes must first traverse a series of membranes and need to pass through important organs of elimination before entering the systemic circulation. Only a fraction of the administered dose reaches the site of drug action. Even drugs given intravenously and by inhalation must pass though the lungs before reaching arterial blood flow. Like other organs, the lungs remove substantial amounts of the agents.

For drugs given orally, the rate and extent of gastrointestinal absorption are important considerations. Once an orally administered drug is absorbed into the portal circulation, it must pass through the liver. Therefore the bioavailability of an orally administered drug is also dependent on the extent of its metabolism during its first pass through the liver.

Generally, uremia decreases gastrointestinal absorption of drugs. Gastrointestinal symptoms are common in uremia, but little specific information about bowel function is available in patients with renal failure. When urea accumulates in the plasma, the salivary concentration of urea increases as well. Ammonia forms in the presence of gastric urease and buffers gastric acid, increasing gastric pH. The ammonia is absorbed and converted to urea again by the liver. The gastric alkalinizing effect of this internal urea–ammonia cycle decreases the absorption of drugs that are best absorbed in an acidic environment. For example, iron salts must be hydrolyzed by gastric acid for absorption. Dialysis patients malabsorb these compounds if acid hydrolysis in the stomach is impaired. In addition, the dissolution of many tablet dosage forms requires the acid environment normally found in the stomach. Absorption of these products is incomplete and occurs more slowly in an alkaline environment (7).

The ingestion of multivalent cations frequently used in antacids also diminishes drug absorption (8,9). Patients with renal impairment often ingest large quantities of antacids to bind dietary phosphate. Chelation and the formation of nonabsorbable complexes reduce bioavailability of some drugs. This effect is particularly important on the absorption of some antibiotics and digoxin.

Craig and colleagues have demonstrated impaired gastrointestinal absorptive function by showing that the absorption of the simple sugar D-xylose is reduced by nearly 30% in patients with renal failure requiring dialysis (10). However, the processes of gastrointestinal drug absorption are complex, may be saturable and dose dependent, and are more variable in patients with renal failure than in those with normal renal function (11). Gastroparesis, commonly observed in diabetic patients with renal failure, prolongs gastric emptying and delays drug absorption. Similarly, diarrhea decreases gut transit time and diminishes drug absorption by the small bowel.

Uremia alters first-pass hepatic metabolism. Decreased biotransformation leads to the appearance of increased amounts of active drug in the systemic circulation and enhanced bioavailability of some drugs. Conversely, impaired protein binding allows more free drug to be available at the site of hepatic metabolism, thereby increasing the amount of drug removed during the hepatic first pass. With the complex interaction of absorption and first-pass hepatic metabolism, it is not surprising that drug bioavailability is more variable in patients with renal impairment than in patients with normal renal function.

Distribution

After a drug is administered, it is dispersed throughout the body at a given rate. At equilibrium, the apparent volume of distribution is calculated by dividing the amount of the drug in the body by its plasma concentration. This apparent volume of distribution does not correspond to a specific anatomic space. Rather, the volume of distribution is a mathematical construct used to estimate the dose of a drug required to achieve a therapeutic plasma concentration. Agents that are highly protein bound, or those that are water-soluble, tend to be restricted to the extracellular fluid space and have small volumes of distribution. On the other hand, highly lipid-soluble drugs penetrate body tissues and exhibit large volumes of distribution.

Renal insufficiency frequently alters drug distribution volume. Edema and ascites increase the apparent volume of distribution of highly water-soluble or protein-bound drugs. Usual doses of such drugs given to edematous patients will result in inadequate, low plasma levels. Conversely, dehydration or muscle wasting tends to decrease the volume of distribution. In these cases, usual doses result in unexpectedly high plasma concentrations.

The alteration of plasma protein binding in patients with renal insufficiency is an important factor affecting eventual drug action. The volume of distribution of a drug, the quantity of free drug available for action, and the degree to which the agent can be eliminated by hepatic or renal excretion are all influenced by protein binding. Drugs that are protein-bound attach reversibly either to albumin or glycoprotein in plasma. Organic acids are thought to bind to a single binding site, whereas organic bases probably have multiple sites of attachment (12).

Protein-bound organic acids such as hippuric acid, indoxyl sulfate, and 3-carboxy-4-methyl-5-propyl-2-furanpropionic acid (CMPF) accumulate in renal failure and decrease protein binding of many acidic drugs (13–15). Altered protein binding affects organic bases less than organic acids. A combination of decreased serum albumin concentration and a reduction in albumin affinity for the drug reduces protein binding in uremia. Even when the plasma albumin concentration is normal, the

Protein Binding Defect in Uremia

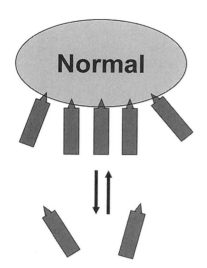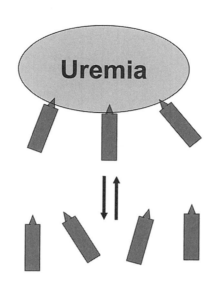

FIG. 12.1. Protein-binding defect in uremia. Displacement of drug from its binding site by the accumulation of undefined uremic toxin or a uremia-induced conformational change in the binding site geometry results in more free drug in plasma.

protein binding defect of some drugs correlates with the level of azotemia and may be corrected with dialysis (16–19). As illustrated in Fig. 12.1, affinity is influenced by uremia-induced changes in the structural orientation of the albumin molecule or by the accumulation of endogenous inhibitors of protein binding that competes with drugs for their binding sites.

The consequences of impaired plasma protein binding in uremia are important since the unbound fraction of several acidic drugs is substantially increased. Serious toxicity can occur if the total plasma concentration of these drugs is pushed into the therapeutic range by increasing the dose. For such drugs, total and unbound plasma concentrations should be measured.

Predicting the clinical consequences of altered protein binding in uremia is difficult. Although decreased binding results in more free drug being available at the site of drug action or toxicity, the distribution volume is increased, resulting in lower plasma concentrations after a given dose. In addition, more unbound drug is available for metabolism and excretion and decreases the half-life of the drug in the body. Table 12.1 lists drugs with decreased protein binding in dialysis patients.

Metabolism

Renal failure substantially affects drug biotransformation. Uremia slows the rate of reduction and hydrolysis reactions. Glucuronidation, sulfate conjugation, and microsomal oxidation usually occur at normal rates in patients with uremia (20,21). Peptide and ester hydrolysis are substantially reduced.

Uremia may also alter the disposition of drugs metabolized by the liver through changes in plasma protein binding. The systemic clearance of a highly protein-bound drug with a low hepatic extraction ratio depends on the simultaneous effects of renal disease on protein binding and intrinsic metabolic drug clearance. Protein binding of such a drug is related to creatinine clearance in an inverse hyperbolic relationship, whereas the

unbound intrinsic metabolic clearance declines linearly with creatinine clearance. Because the effects of renal failure on these two factors offset each other in terms of total systemic clearance, the lowest total systemic clearance will be seen in patients with more moderate renal impairment, not in dialysis patients. The systemic clearance of drugs with a high hepatic extraction ratio is not as susceptible to the effect of renal disease as that of low-extraction-ratio drugs (22).

The production of active or toxic metabolites is an important aspect of drug metabolism in patients with renal failure. Many of these metabolites depend on the kidneys for their removal from the body. The accumulation of active metabolites can explain, in part, the high incidence of adverse drug reactions seen in renal failure. Table 12.2 lists some drugs that form active or toxic metabolites in dialysis patients.

TABLE 12.1. DRUGS WITH DECREASED PROTEIN BINDING IN DIALYSIS PATIENTS

Barbiturates
Cardiac glycosides
Dicloxacillin
Cephalosporins
Clofibrate
Doxepin
Loop diuretics
Oxazepam
Penicillins
Pentobarbital
Phenobarbital
Phenytoin
Sulfonamides
Salicylate
Temazepam
Theophyline
Valproic acid
Warfarin

TABLE 12.2. DRUGS THAT HAVE ACTIVE OR TOXIC METABOLITES IN DIALYSIS PATIENTS

Acetaminophen	Isosorbide
ACE inhibitors	Levodopa
Angiotensin	Lorcainide
Receptors	Meperidine
Blockers	Metronidazole
Adriamycin	Methyldopa
Allopurinol	Miglitol
Amiodarone	Minoxidil
Amoxapine	Morphine
Azathioprine	Nitrofurantoin
Benzodiazepines	Nitroprusside
β-blockers	Procainamide
Bupropion	Primidone
Buspirone	Propoxyphene
Cardiac glycosides	Pyrimethamine
Cephalosporines	Quinidine
Chloral hydrate	Serotonin reuptake inhibitors
Chlorazepate	Spironolactone
Clofibrate	Sulfanylureas
Desipramine	Sulindac
Diltiazem	Thiazolidinediones
Encainide	Triamterene
Esmolol	Trimethadione
H₂ blockers	Verapamil
Hydroxyzine	Vidarabine
Imipramine	

Drug dosing guidelines for dialysis patients are usually derived from studies in patients with stable, chronic renal failure. However, these recommendations are often extrapolated to seriously ill patients with acutely decreased renal function. The preservation of nonrenal metabolic clearance has been demonstrated in patients with acute renal failure (21). The preservation of metabolic clearance observed early in the course of acute renal failure suggests that drug dosing schemes extrapolated from individuals with stable chronic renal failure could result in ineffectively low drug concentrations in patients with acute renal dysfunction.

Calculating Drug Doses

The goal of the initial drug dose is to achieve therapeutic drug concentrations rapidly. A loading dose equivalent to the dose given to a patient with normal renal function should be given to patients with renal impairment, if the physical examination suggests normal extracellular fluid volume. If the loading dose of a drug is not known, it can be calculated from the following expression:

$$\text{Loading Dose} = V_d \times \text{IBW} \times C_p$$

where V_d is the drug's volume of distribution in liter per kilogram, IBW is the patient's ideal body weight in kilograms, and C_p is the desired steady-state plasma drug concentration.

Several methods can be used to determine subsequent drug doses. The fraction of the normal dose recommended for a patient with renal failure can be calculated as follows:

$$D_f = t_{1/2} \text{ normal} / t_{1/2} \text{ renal failure}$$

where D_f is the fraction of the normal dose to be given; $t_{1/2}$ normal is the elimination half-life of the drug in a patient with normal renal function; and $t_{1/2}$ renal failure is the elimination half-life of the drug in a patient with renal failure. To maintain the normal dose interval in patients with renal impairment, the amount of each dose, following the loading dose, can be determined from the following relationship:

$$\text{Dose in Renal Impairment} = \text{Normal Dose} \times D_f$$

The resulting dose is usually given at the same dose interval as that for patients with normal renal function. This method is effective for drugs with a narrow therapeutic range and short plasma half-life. Figure 12.2 illustrates plasma concentrations following an initial loading dose and reduction of the individual doses.

Prolonging the dose interval in dialysis patients is frequently a convenient method to reduce drug dosage. This method is particularly useful for drugs with a broad therapeu-

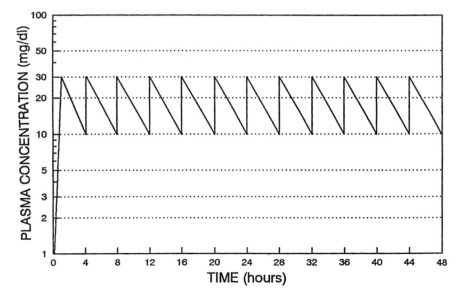

FIG. 12.2. Plasma concentrations following a normal loading dose and reduced maintenance doses. This approach avoids high peak and low trough concentrations and is best for drugs with a narrow range between the therapeutic and toxic concentrations.

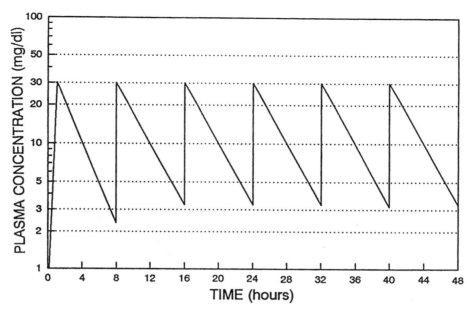

FIG. 12.3. Plasma concentrations following a normal loading dose and repeated normal doses at a prolonged dose interval. Higher peak and lower trough concentrations result.

tic range and long plasma half-life. If prolonging the dose interval, rather than decreasing the individual doses, is desirable, the dose interval in renal impairment can be estimated from the following expression:

Dose Interval in Renal Impairment = Normal Dose Interval/D_f

If the range between therapeutic and toxic levels is too narrow, either potentially toxic or subtherapeutic plasma concentrations result. Figure 12.3 shows the resulting plasma concentrations from prolonging the dose interval in an individual with impaired renal function.

A combined approach using both the dose reduction and interval prolongation methods is often practical. The dosage is modified by multiplying the usual daily maintenance dose by the dose fraction. Once the average daily dose is calculated, it can be divided into convenient dosing intervals. The decision to extend the dosing interval beyond a 24-hour period should be based on the need to maintain therapeutic peak or trough levels. The dosing interval may be prolonged if the peak level is most important. When the minimum trough level must be maintained, it is preferable to modify the individual dose or use a combination of dose and interval methods to determine the correct dosing strategy. Drugs removed by dialysis given once daily should be given after the dialysis treatment.

DRUG REMOVAL BY DIALYSIS

Drug removal by conventional hemodialysis occurs primarily by the process of drug diffusion across the dialysis membrane. Diffusion proceeds down a concentration gradient from the plasma to the dialysate. Drug removal by conventional hemodialysis is most effective for drugs that are less than 500 daltons and are less than 90% protein bound. Drugs that have small volumes of

distribution are more effectively removed by dialysis than those compounds that are distributed in adipose tissue or that have extensive tissue binding. Removal of small-molecular-weight drugs is enhanced by increasing the blood and dialysate flow rates and by using large surface area dialyzers. Larger molecules require more porous membranes for increased removal. The hemodialysis clearance of a drug can be estimated from the following relationship:

$$Cl_{HD} = Cl_{urea} \times (60/MW_{drug})$$

where Cl_{HD} is the drug's clearance by hemodialysis, Cl_{urea} is the clearance of urea by the dialyzer, and MW_{drug} is the molecular weight of the drug (23). The urea clearance for most standard dialyzers varies between 150 and 200 mL/min (24).

The use of porous dialysis membranes to perform high-flux dialysis decreases the importance of drug molecular mass in determining drug removal during extracorporeal circulation. During high-flux dialysis, the volume of distribution and percent protein binding of the drug are more important determinants of dialysis drug clearance. Recent studies suggest that for drugs that are not highly protein bound and have relatively small volumes of distribution, drug removal occurs by diffusion and parallels urea clearance, despite a very large molecular mass (25,26). The removal of drugs during high-flux dialysis will depend more on treatment time, blood and dialysate flow rates, and distribution volume and binding of the drug to serum proteins. The consequence of these observations is that much more drug will be removed during high-flux dialysis than previously estimated for conventional hemodialysis. Furthermore, substantial amounts of drug may be removed if the agent is given during high-flux dialysis treatments (27).

Peritoneal dialysis is much less efficient at removing drugs than is hemodialysis (28). As with conventional hemodialysis, drug removal by peritoneal dialysis is most effective for smaller-molecular-weight drugs that are not extensively bound to serum proteins. Larger-molecular-weight drugs may be somewhat more removed by peritoneal dialysis because of secretion into peritoneal lymphatic fluid. Similarly, drugs that have small volumes of distribution are more effectively removed than those that are distributed in adipose tissue or have extensive tissue binding. Removal of small-molecular-weight drugs depends on the number of peritoneal dialysis exchanges done daily. Peritoneal drug clearance can be estimated from the relationship:

$$Cl_{PD} = Cl_{urea} \times \frac{\sqrt{60}}{\sqrt{MW_{drug}}}$$

where Cl_{PD} is the peritoneal drug clearance, Cl_{urea} is the peritoneal urea clearance, and MW_{drug} is the molecular weight of the drug. Peritoneal urea clearance is approximately 20 mL/min. In general, if a drug is not removed by hemodialysis, it will not be removed by peritoneal dialysis.

Table 12.3 lists drugs frequently used in dialysis patients and the appropriate dosage adjustments. Suggestions for reduction of the individual doses, prolonging of the dose interval, or a combination of the methods are included. Recommendations for supplemental doses following hemodialysis and during CAPD are listed.

Drug transport by the peritoneal membrane is unidirectional (29). Although peritoneal dialysis does not rapidly remove drugs, many are well absorbed when placed in peritoneal dialysate. Table 12.4 includes some commonly used antibiotics for patients performing CAPD with suggestions for dosages used to treat ambulatory peritonitis and systemic infections.

Molecular weight, membrane characteristics, blood-flow rate, and the addition of dialysate determine the rate and extent of drug removal during continuous renal replacement therapies (CRRT). Molecular weight affects drug removal by diffusion

TABLE 12.3. DOSE ADJUSTMENT FOR DRUGS FREQUENTLY USED IN DIALYSIS PATIENTS

Drug	Half-life (Hours)	Protein Binding (%)	Volume of Distribution (L/kg)	Method	Renal Failure Dose	Dose After Hemodialysis	Dose During CAPD	Dose During CRRT
	Normal/Renal Failure							
Acarbose	3–9/Prolonged	15	0.32	D	Avoid	Unknown	Unknown	Avoid
Acebutolol	7–9/7	20	1.2	D	30% to 50%	None	None	50%
Acetazolamide	1.7–5.8/Unknown	70–90	0.2	I	Avoid	Unknown	Unknown	Avoid
Acetohexamide	1–1.3/Unchanged	65–90	0.21	I	Avoid	Unknown	None	Avoid
Acetohydroxamic acid	3.5–5/15–23	Unknown	Unknown	D	Avoid	Unknown	Unknown	Unknown
Acetaminophen	2/2	20–30	1–2	I	q8h	None	None	q6h
Acetylsalicylic acid (Aspirin)	2–3/Unchanged	80–90	0.1–0.2	I	Avoid	Dose after dialysis	None	q4–6h
Acrivastine	1.4–2.1/Unknown	50	0.6–0.7	D	Unknown	Unknown	Unknown	Unknown
Acyclovir	2.1–3.8/20	15–30	0.7	D,I	2.5 mg/kg q24h	Dose after dialysis	Dose for renal failure	3.5 mg/kg/d
Adenosine	<10 sec/Unchanged	0	?	D	100%	None	None	100%
Albuterol	2–4/4	7	2–2.5	D	50%	Unknown	Unknown	75%
Alcuronium	3–3.5/16	40	0.28–0.36	D	Avoid	Unknown	Unknown	Avoid
Alfentanil	1–3/Unchanged	88–95	0.3–1	D	100%	NA	NA	NA
Allopurinol	2–8/Unchanged	<5	0.5	D	25%	1/2 dose	Unknown	50%
Alprazolam	9.5–19/Unchanged	70–80	0.9–1.3	D	100%	None	Unknown	NA
Alteplase (tPA)	0.5	Unknown	0.1	D	100%	Unknown	Unknown	100%
Altretamine	7/Unknown	Unknown	Unknown	D	Unknown	Unknown	Unknown	Unknown
Amantadine	12/500	60	4–5	I	q7d	None	None	q48–72h
Amikacin	1.4–2.3/17–150	<5	0.22–0.29	D,I	20% to 30% q24–48h	2/3 normal dose after dialysis	15–20 mg/l/d	30% to 70% q12–18h
Amiloride	6–8/10–144	30–40	5–5.2	D	Avoid	NA	NA	NA
Amiodarone	14–120 d/Unchanged	96	70–140	D	100%	None	None	100%
Amitriptyline	24–40/Unchanged	96	6–36	D	100%	None	Unknown	NA
Amlodipine	35–50/50	>95	21	D	100%	None	None	100%
Amoxapine	8–30/Unknown	90	Unknown	D	100%	Unknown	Unknown	NA
Amoxicillin	0.9–2.3/5–20	15–25	0.26	I	q24h	Dose after dialysis	250 mg q12h	NA
Amphotericin	24/Unchanged	90	4.0	I	q24–36h	None	Dose for renal failure	q24h
Amphotericin B colloidal dispersion	24–30/? Unchanged	90	4.0	I	q24–36h	None failure	Dose for renal	q24h
Amphotericin B lipid complex	19–45/? Unchanged	90	1.7–3.9	I	q24–36h	None failure	Dose for renal	q24h
Ampicillin	0.8–1.5/7–20	20	0.17–0.31	I	q12–24h	Dose after dialysis	250 mg q12h	q6–12h
Amrinone	2.6–8.3/Unknown	20–40	1.3–1.6	D	50% to 75%	Unknown	Unknown	100%
Anistreplase	1.2	Unknown	0.08	D	100%	Unknown	Unknown	100%
Astemizole	20 d/Unchanged	97	Unknown	D	100%	Unknown	Unknown	NA
Atenolol	6.7/15–35	3	1.1	D,I	30% to 50% q96h	25–50 mg	None	50% q48h
Atovaquone	55–77/Unknown	99	Unknown		Unknown: 100%	Unknown: None	Unknown	Unknown
Atracurium	0.3–0.4/Unchanged	82	0.15–0.18	D	100%	Unknown	Unknown	100%

(continued)

TABLE 12.3. *(continued)*

Drug	Half-life (Hours) Normal/Renal Failure	Protein Binding (%)	Volume of Distribution (L/kg)	Method	Renal Failure Dose	Dose After Hemodialysis	Dose During CAPD	Dose During CRRT
Auranofin	70–80 d/Unknown	60	Unknown	D	Avoid	None	None	None
Azathioprine	0.16–1/Increased	20	0.55–0.8	D	50%	Yes	None	None
Azithromycin	10–60/?	8–50	18	D	100%	None	Unknown	75%
Azlocillin	0.8–1.5/5–6	30	0.18–0.27	I	q8h	Dose after dialysis	Dose for renal failure	q6–8h
Aztreonam	1.7–2.9/6–8	45–60	0.5–1.0	D	25%	0.5 g after dialysis	Dose for renal failure	50% to 75%
Benazepril	22/30	95	0.15	D	25% to 50%	None	None	50% to 75%
Bepridil	24–48/24–48	Unknown	Unknown		Unknown	None	None	Unknown
Betamethasone	5.5/Unknown	65	1.4	D	100%	Unknown	Unknown	100%
Betaxolol	15–20/30–35	45–60	5–10	D	50%	None	None	100%
Bezafibrate	2.1/7.8	95	0.24–0.35	D	25%	Unknown	Unknown	50%
Bisoprolol	9–13/18–24	30–35	3	D	50%	Unknown	Unknown	75%
Bleomycin	9/20	Unknown	0.3	D	50%	None	Unknown	75%
Bopindolol	4–10/Unchanged	Unknown	2–3	D	100%	None	None	100%
Bretylium	6–13.6/16–32	6	8.2	D	25%	None	None	25% to 50%
Bromocriptine	3/Unknown	90–96	Unknown	D	100%	Unknown	Unknown	Unknown
Brompheniramine	6/Unknown	Unknown	12	D	100%	Unknown	Unknown	NA
Budesonide	2–2.7/Unknown	88	4.3	D	100%	Unknown	Unknown	100%
Bumetanide	1.2–1.5/1.5	96	0.2–0.5	D	100%	None	None	NA
Bupropion	10–21/Unknown	82–88	27–36	D	100%	Unknown	Unknown	NA
Buspirone	2–3/5.8	95	5.0	D	100%	None	Unknown	NA
Busulfan	2.5–3.4/Unknown	3–15	1.0	D	100%	Unknown	Unknown	100%
Butorphanol	2–4/Unknown	80	9–11	D	50%	Unknown	Unknown	NA
Capreomycin	2	Unknown	Unknown	I	q48h	Give dose after HD only	None	q24h
Captopril	2–3/21–32	25–30	0.7–3	D,I	50% q24h	25% to 30%	None	75% q12–18h
Carbamazepine	24 single; 4–6 chronic dosing	75	0.8–1.6	D	100%	None	None	None
Carbidopa	2/Unknown	Unknown	Unknown	D	100%	Unknown	Unknown	Unknown
Carboplatin	6/Increased	15–24	0.23–0.28	D	25%	1/2 dose	Unknown	50%
Carmustine	1.5/Unknown	Unknown	3.3	D	Unknown	Unknown	Unknown	Unknown
Carteolol	7/33	20–30	4.0	D	25%	Unknown	None	50%
Carvedilol	5–8/5–8	95	1–2	D	100%	None	None	100%
Cefaclor	1/3	25	0.24–0.35	D	50%	250 mg after dialysis	250 mg q8–12h	NA
Cefadroxil	1.4/22	20	0.31	I	q24–48h	0.5–1.0 g after dialysis	0.5 g/d	NA
Cefamandole	1/6–11	75	0.16–0.25	I	q12h	0.5–1.0 g after dialysis	0.5–1.0 g q12h	q6–8h
Cefazolin	2/40–70	80	0.13–0.22	I	q24–48h	0.5–1.0 g after dialysis	0.5 g q12h	q12h
Cefepime	2.2/18	16	0.3	I	q24–48h	1.0 g after dialysis	Dose for renal failure	Not recommended
Cefixime	3.1/12	50	0.6–0.11	D	50%	300 mg after dialysis	200 mg/d	Not recommended
Cefmenoxime	0.8–1.3/6–12	43–75	0.27–0.37	D,I	0.75 g q12h	0.75 g after dialysis	0.75 g q12h	0.75 g q8h
Cefmetazole	1.2/21	75	0.18	I	q48h	Dose after dialysis	Dose for renal failure	q24h
Cefonicid	4/17–59	96	0.09–0.18	D,I	0.1 g/d	None	None	None
Cefoperazone	1.6–2.5/2.9	90	0.14–0.20	D	100%	1 g after dialysis	None	None
Ceforanide	3/25	80	0.17	I	q24–48h	0.5–1.0 g after dialysis	None	1.0 g/d
Cefotaxime	1/15	37	0.15–0.55	I	q24h	1 g after dialysis	1 g/d	1 g q12h
Cefotetan	3.5/13–25	85	0.15	D	25%	1 g after dialysis	1 g/d	750 mg q12h
Cefoxitin	1/13–23	41–75	0.2	I	q24–48h	1 g after dialysis	1 g/d	q8–12h
Cefpodoxime	2.5/26	26	0.6–1.2	I	q24–48h	200 mg after dialysis only	Dose for renal failure	NA
Cefprozil	1.7/6	40	0.65	D,I	250 mg q24h	250 mg after dialysis	Dose for renal failure	Dose for renal failure
Ceftazidime	1.2/13–25	17	0.28–0.4	I	q48h	1 g after dialysis	0.5 g/d	q24–48h
Ceftibutin	1.5–2.7/22	70	0.2	D	25%	300 mg after dialysis only	Dose for renal failure	50%
Ceftizoxime	1.4/35	28–50	0.26–0.42	I	q24h	1 g after dialysis	0.5–1.0 g/d	q12–24h
Ceftriaxone	7–9/12–24	90	0.12–0.18	D	100%	Dose after dialysis	750 mg q12h	100%
Cefuroxime axetil	1.2/17	35–50	0.13–1.8	D	100%	Dose after dialysis	Dose for renal failure	NA
Cefuroxime sodium	1.2/17	33	0.13–1.8	I	q12h	Dose after dialysis	Dose for renal failure	1 g q12h

(continued)

TABLE 12.3. *(continued)*

Drug	Half-life (Hours)	Protein Binding (%)	Volume of Distribution (L/kg)	Method	Renal Failure Dose	Dose After Hemodialysis	Dose During CAPD	Dose During CRRT
	Normal/Renal Failure							
Celiprolol	4–5/5	Unknown	Unknown	D	75%	Unknown	None	100%
Cephalexin	0.7/16	20	0.35	I	q12h	Dose after dialysis	Dose for renal failure	NA
Cephalothin	0.5–1/3–18	65	0.26	I	q12h	Dose after dialysis	1 g q12h	1 g q8h
Cephapirin	0.4/2.5	45–60	0.22	I	q12h	Dose after dialysis	1 g q12h	1 g q8h
Cephradine	0.7–1.3/6–15	10	0.25–0.46	D	25%	Dose after dialysis	Dose for renal failure	NA
Cetirizine	7–10/20	93	0.4–0.6	D	30%	None	Unknown	NA
Chloral hydrate	7–14/Unknown	70–80	0.6	D	Avoid	None	Unknown	NA
Chlorambucil	1/Unknown	Unknown	0.86	D	Unknown	Unknown	Unknown	Unknown
Chloramphenicol	1.6–3.3/3–7	45–60	0.5–1.0	D	100%	None	None	None
Chlorazepate	39–85/36	Unknown	1.3	D	100%	Unknown	Unknown	NA
Chlordiazepoxide	5–30/Unchanged	94–97	0.3–0.5	D	50%	None	Unknown	100%
Chloroquine	2–4/5–50 d	50–65	Large	D	50%	None	None	None
Chlorpheniramine	14–24/Unknown	72	6–12	D	100%	None	Unknown	NA
Chlorpromazine	11–42/Unchanged	91–99	8–160	D	100%	None	None	100%
Chlorpropamide	24–48/50–200	88–96	0.09–0.27	D	Avoid	Unknown	None	Avoid
Chlorthalidone	44–80/Unknown	76–90	3.9	I	Avoid	NA	NA	NA
Cholestyramine	Not absorbed	None	None	D	100%	None	None	100%
Cibenzoline	7/22	50	4–5	D,I	66% q24h	None	None	100% q12h
Cidofovir	2.5/Unknown	<6%	0.3–0.8	D	Unknown: Avoid	Unknown	Unknown	Unknown, avoid
Cilastin	1/12	44	0.22	D	Avoid	Avoid	Avoid	Avoid
Cilazapril	40–50/>60	Unknown	0.5–0.8	D,I	10% to 25% q72h	None	None	50% q24–48h
Cimetidine	1.5–2/5	20	0.8–1.3	D	25%	None	Avoid	50%
Cinoxacin	1.2/12	63	0.25	D	Avoid	Avoid	Avoid	Avoid
Ciprofloxacin	3–6/6–9	20–40	2.5	D	50%	250 mg q12h (200 mg if iv)	250 mg q8h (200 mg if iv)	200 mg iv q12h
Cisapride	7–10/Unchanged	98	2.4	D	50%	Unknown	Unknown	50% to 100%
Cisplatin	0.3–0.5/Unknown	90	0.5	D	50%	Yes	Unknown	75%
Cladribine	7–14/Unknown	Unknown	50–80	D	Unknown	Unknown	Unknown	Unknown
Clarithromycin	2.3–6/?	70	2–4	D	50% to 75%	Dose after dialysis	None	None
Clavulanic acid	1/3–4	30	0.3	D	50% to 75%	Dose after dialysis	Dose for renal failure	100%
Clindamycin	2–4/3–5	60–95	0.6–1.2	D	100%	None	None	None
Clodronate	13/Increased	36	0.25	D	Avoid	Unknown	Unknown	Unknown
Clofazamine	10–70 days (?)/ Unknown	Unknown	Unknown		Unknown: 100%	Unknown: None	Unknown: None	Unknown
Clofibrate	15–17.5/30–110	92–97	0.14	I	Avoid	None	Unknown	q12–18h
Clomipramine	19–37/Unknown	97	Unknown	D	Unknown	Unknown	Unknown	NA
Clonazepam	18–50/Unknown	47	1.5–4.5	D	100%	None	Unknown	NA
Clonidine	6–23/39–42	20–40	3–6	D	100%	None	None	100%
Codeine	2.5–3.5/Unknown	7	3–4	D	50%	Unknown	Unknown	75%
Colchicine	19/40	31	2.2	D	50%	None	Unknown	100%
Colestipol	Not absorbed	None	None	D	100%	None	None	100%
Cortisone	0.5–2/3.5	90	Unknown	D	100%	None	Unknown	100%
Cyclophosphamide	4–7.5/10	14–20	0.5–1	D	75%	1/2 dose	Unknown	100%
Cycloserine	0.5	Unknown	0.11–0.26	I	q24h	None	None	q12–24h
Cyclosporine	3–16/Unchanged	96–99	3.5–7.4	D	100%	None	None	100%
Cytarabine	0.5–3/Unchanged	13	2.6	D	100%	Unknown	Unknown	100%
Dapsone	20–30/Unknown	70–90	1–1.5		Unknown	Unknown: None	Dose for renal failure	Unknown
Daunorubicin	18–27/Unknown	Unknown	Unknown	D	100%	Unknown	Unknown	Unknown
Delavirdine	5.8 h	98	0.5		Unknown: 100%	Unknown: None	Unknown	Unknown
Desferoxamine	6/Unknown	Unknown	2–2.5	D	100%	Unknown	Unknown	100%
Desipramine	18–26/Unknown	92	10–50	D	100%	None	None	NA
Dexamethasone	3–4/Unknown	70	0.8–1	D	100%	Unknown	Unknown	100%
Diazepam	20–90/Unchanged	94–98	0.7–3.4	D	100%	None	Unknown	100%
Diazoxide	17–31/30–60	>90	0.2–0.3	D	100%	None	None	100%
Diclofenac	1–2/Unchanged	>99	0.12–0.17	D	100%	None	None	100%
Dicloxacillin	0.7/1–2	95	0.16	D	100%	None	None	NA
Didanosine	0.6–1.6/4.5	<5%	1.0	I	q24–48h	Dose after dialysis	Dose for renal failure	Dose for renal failure
Diflunisal	5–20/62	>99	0.1–0.13	D	50%	None	None	50%
Digitoxin	144–200/210	94	0.6	D	50% to 75%	None	None	100%
Digoxin	36–44/80–120	20–30	5–8	D,I	10% to 25% q48h	None	None	25% to 75% q36h
Dilevalol	8–12/19–30	75	25	D	100%	None	None	Unknown
Diltiazem	2–8/3.5	98	9–10	D	100%	None	None	100%
Diphenhydramine	3.4–9.3/Unknown	80	3.3–6.8	D	100%	None	None	None

(continued)

TABLE 12.3. *(continued)*

Drug	Half-life (Hours) Normal/Renal Failure	Protein Binding (%)	Volume of Distribution (L/kg)	Method	Renal Failure Dose	Dose After Hemodialysis	Dose During CAPD	Dose During CRRT
Dipyridamole	12/Unknown	99	2.4	D	100%	Unknown	Unknown	NA
Dirithromycin	30–44/Unknown	15–30	>10	D	100%	None	Unknown	100%
Disopyramide	5–8/10–18	54–81	0.8–2.6	I	q24–40h	None	None	q12–24h
Dobutamine	2 min/Unknown	Unknown	0.25	D	100%	Unknown	Unknown	100%
Doxacurium	1.2–1.6/3.7	28–34	0.12–0.22	D	50%	Unknown	Unknown	50%
Doxazosin	16–22/16–22	98	1–1.7	D	100%	None	None	100%
Doxepin	8–25/10–30	95	9–33	D	100%	None	None	100%
Doxorubicin	35/Unchanged	80–85	2–5	D	100%	None	Unknown	100%
Doxycycline	15–24/18–25	80–90	0.75	D	100%	None	None	100%
Dyphylline	1.8–2.3/12	<3	0.8	D	25%	1/3 dose	Unknown	50%
Enalapril	11–24/34–60	50–60	Unknown	D	50%	20% to 25%	None	75% to 100%
Epirubicin	35/35	80–85	10–40	D	100%	None	Unknown	100%
Erbastine	13–16/23–26	98	1–2	D	50%	Unknown	Unknown	50%
Erythromycin	1.4/5–6	60–95	0.6–1.2	D	50% to 75%	None	None	None
Esmolol	7–15 min/Unchanged					None	None	Unknown
Estazolam	8–24/Unknown	93	Unknown	D	100%	Unknown	Unknown	NA
Ethacrynic acid	2–4/Unknown	90	0.1	I	Avoid	None	None	NA
Ethambutol	4/7–15	10–30	1.6–3.2	I	q48h	Dose after dialysis	Dose for renal failure	q24–36h
Ethchlorvynol	10–20	35–50	3–4	D	Avoid	None	None	NA
Ethionamide	2.1	30	Unknown	D	50%	None	None	None
Ethosuximide	35–55/Unchanged	10	0.6–0.9	D	100%	None	Unknown	Unknown
Etodolac	5–7/Unchanged	>99	0.4	D	100%	None	None	100%
Etomidate	4–5/Unchanged	75	2–4.5	D	100%	Unknown	Unknown	100%
Etoposide	4–8/19	74–94	0.17–0.5	D	50%	None	Unknown	75%
Famciclovir	1.6–2.9/10–22	<25%	1.5	I	50% q48h	Dose after dialysis	Unknown	Unknown
Famotidine	2.5–4/12–19	15–22	0.8–1.4	D	10%	None	None	25%
Fazadinium	1/Unchanged	17	0.18–0.23	D	100%	Unknown	Unknown	100%
Felodipine	10–14/21–24	99	9–10	D	100%	None	None	100%
Fenoprofen	2–3/Unchanged	>99	0.1	D	100%	None	None	100%
Fentanyl	2.5–3.5/Unchanged	79–87	2–5	D	100%	Unknown	Unknown	100%
Fexofenadine	14/19–25	70	Unknown	I	q24h	Unknown	Unknown	q12–24h
Flecainide	12–19.5/19–26	52	8.4–9.5	D	50% to 75%	None	None	100%
Fleroxacin	13/21–28	20	1.1–2.4	D	50%	400 mg after dialysis	400 mg/d	NA
Fluconazole	22/Unknown	12	0.7	D	100%	200 mg after dialysis	Dose for renal failure	100%
Flucytosine	3–6/75–200	<10	0.6	I	q24h	Dose after dialysis	0.5–1.0 g/d	q16h
Fludarabine	7–12/24	Unknown	5–40	D	50%	Unknown	Unknown	75%
Flumazenil	0.7–1.3/Unknown	40–50	0.6–1.1	D	100%	None	Unknown	NA
Flunarizine	17–18 d/Unknown	99	43–78	D	100%	None	None	None
Fluorouracil	0.1/Unchanged	10	0.25–0.5	D	100%	Yes	Unknown	100%
Fluoxetine	24–72/Unchanged	94.5	12–42	D	100%	Unknown	Unknown	NA
Flurazepam	47–100/Unchanged	Unknown	3.4	D	100%	None	Unknown	NA
Flurbiprofen	3–5/Unchanged	99	0.1	D	100%	None	None	100%
Flutamide	4–6/Unknown	Unknown	Unknown	D	100%	Unknown	Unknown	Unknown
Fluvastatin	0.5–1/Unknown	Unknown	0.42	D	100%	Unknown	Unknown	100%
Fluvoxamine	12–15/Unchanged	77	25	D	100%	None	Unknown	NA
Foscarnet	3/Prolonged (up to 100 h)	17	0.3–0.6	D	6 mg/kg	Dose after dialysis	Dose for renal failure	15 mg/kg
Fosinopril	12/14–32	95	0.15	D	75% to 100%	None	None	100%
Furosemide	0.5–1.1/2–4	95	0.07–0.2	D	100%	None	None	NA
Gabapentin	5–7/132	Unbound	0.7	D,I	300 mg qd	300 mg load, then 200–300		300 q12–24h
Gallamine	2.3–2.7/6–20	30–70	0.21–0.24	D	Avoid	NA	NA	Avoid
Ganciclovir	3.6/30	Unknown	0.47	I	q48–96h	Dose after dialysis	Dose for renal failure	2.5 mg/kg/d
Gancicloviroral				D,I	Unknown: 500 mg q48–96h	Unknown: Dose after dialysis	Dose for renal failure	NA
Gemfibrozil	7.6/Unchanged	97–99	Unknown	D	100%	None	Unknown	100%
Gentamicin	1.8/20–60	<5	0.23–0.26	D,I	20% to 30% q24–48h	2/3 normal dose after dialysis	3–4 mg/L/d	30% to 70% q12h
Glibornuride	5–12/Unknown	95	0.25	D	Unknown	Unknown	Unknown	Avoid
Gliclazide	8–11/Unknown	85–95	0.24	D	Unknown	Unknown	Unknown	Avoid
Glipizide	3–7/Unknown	97	0.13–0.16	D	100%	Unknown	Unknown	Avoid
Glyburide	1.4–2.9/Unknown	99	0.16–0.3	D	Avoid	None	None	Avoid
Gold sodium thiomalate	250 d/Unknown	95	5–9	D	Avoid	None	None	Avoid
Griseofulvin	14/20	Unknown	1.6	D	100%	None	None	None

(continued)

TABLE 12.3. *(continued)*

Drug	Half-life (Hours)	Protein Binding (%)	Volume of Distribution (L/kg)	Method	Renal Failure Dose	Dose After Hemodialysis	Dose During CAPD	Dose During CRRT
	Normal/Renal Failure							
Guanabenz	12–14/Unknown	90	10–12	D	100%	Unknown	Unknown	100%
Guanadrel	4–10/19	20	11.5	I	q24–48h	Unknown	Unknown	q12–24h
Guanethidine	120–140/Unknown	<5	Unknown	I	q24–36h	Unknown	Unknown	Avoid
Guanfacine	12–23/15–25	65	4–6.5	D	100%	None	None	100%
Haloperidol	10–19/Unknown	90–92	14–21	D	100%	None	None	100%
Heparin	0.3–2/Unchanged	>90	0.06–0.1	D	100%	None	None	100%
Hexobarbital	3.5–4/Unknown	65	1.1	D	100%	None	Unknown	NA
Hydralazine	2–4.5/7–16	87	0.5–0.9	I	q8–16h	None	None	q8h
Hydrocortisone	1.5–2/Unknown	Unknown	Unknown	D	100%	Unknown	Unknown	100%
Hydroxyurea	Unknown	Unknown	0.5	D	20%	Unknown	Unknown	Unknown
Hydroxyzine	14–20/Unknown	Unknown	19.5	D	Unknown	100%	100%	100%
Ibuprofen	2–3.2/Unchanged	99	0.15–0.17	D	100%	None	None	100%
Idarubicin	36–70/Unknown	Unknown	Unknown		Unknown	Unknown	Unknown	Unknown
Ifosfamide	4–10/Unknown	Unknown	0.4–0.64	D	75%	Unknown	Unknown	100%
Iloprost	0.3–0.5	Unknown	0.7	D	50%	Unknown	Unknown	100%
Imipenem	1/4	13–21	0.17–0.3	D	25%	Dose after dialysis	Dose for renal failure	50%
Imipramine	12–24/Unknown	96	10–20	D	100%	None	None	NA
Indapamide	14–18/Unchanged	76–79	0.3–1.3	D	Avoid	None	None	NA
Indinavir	1.8 hr/Unknown	60	Unknown		Unknown: 100%	Unknown: None	Dose for renal failure	Unknown
Indobufen	6–7/27–33	>99	0.18–0.21	D	25%	Unknown	Unknown	NA
Indomethacin	4–12/Unchanged	99	0.12	D	100%	None	None	100%
Insulin	2–4/Increased	5	0.15	D	50%	None	None	75%
Ipratropium	1.6/Unknown	Unknown	4.6	D	100%	None	None	100%
Isoniazid	0.7–4/8–17	4–30	0.75	D	50%	Dose after dialysis	Dose for renal failure	Dose for renal failure
Isosorbide	0.15–0.5/4	72	1.5–4	D	100%	10–20 mg	None	100%
Isradipine	1.9–4.8/10–11	97	3–4	D	100%	None	None	100%
Itraconazole	21/25	99	10	D	50%	100 mg q12–24h	100 mg q12–24h	100 mg q12–24h
Kanamycin	1.8–5/40–96	<5	0.19–0.23	D,I	20% to 30% q24–48h	2/3 normal dose after dialysis	15–20 mg/L/d	30% to 70% q12h
Ketamine	2–3.5/Unchanged	Unknown	1.8–3.1	D	100%	Unknown	Unknown	100%
Ketanserin	14–19/25–35	95	3–6	D	100%	None	None	100%
Ketoconazole	1.5–3.3/3.3	99	1.9–3.6	D	100%	None	None	None
Ketoprofen	1.5–4/Unchanged	99	0.11	D	100%	None	None	100%
Ketorolac	4–6/10	>99	0.13–0.25	D	50%	None	None	50%
Labetolol	3–9/Unchanged	50	5.6	D	100%	None	None	100%
Lamivudine	5–11/20	36	0.83	D,I	25 mg qd (50 mg first dose)	Dose after dialysis	Dose for renal failure	50–150 mg qd (full first dose)
Lamotrigine	25–30/Unchanged	40–60	0.9–1.3	D	100%	Unknown	Unknown	100%
Lansoprazole	1.3–2.9/Unchanged	>98	Unknown	D	100%	Unknown	Unknown	Unknown
Levodopa	0.8–1.6/Unknown	5–8	0.9–1.6	D	100%	Unknown	Unknown	100%
Levofloxacin	4–8/76	24–38	1.1–1.5	D	25% to 50%	Dose for renal failure	Dose for renal failure	50%
Lidocaine	2–2.2/1.3–3	60–66	1.3–2.2	D	100%	None	None	100%
Lincomycin	4–5/10–20	70–80	0.31–0.6	I	q12–24h	None	None	NA
Lisinopril	30/40–50	0–10	0.13–0.15	D	25% to 50%	20%	None	50% to 75%
Lispro insulin	1/Prolonged	Unknown	0.26–0.36	D	50%	None	None	None
Lithium carbonate	14–28/40	None	0.5–0.9	D	25% to 50%	Dose after dialysis	None	50% to 75%
Lomefloxacin	8/44	15	1.8–3.1	D	50%	Dose for renal failure	Dose for renal failure	NA
Loracarbef	0.8–1.3/32	25	0.3–0.4	I	q3–5d	Dose after dialysis	Dose for renal failure	q24h
Lorazepam	5–10/32–70	87	0.9–1.3	D	100%	None	Unknown	100%
Losartan	3/4–6	30	0.4	D	100%	Unknown	Unknown	100%
Lovastatin	1.1–1.7/Unchanged	>95	Unknown	D	100%	Unknown	Unknown	100%
Low-molecular-weight heparin	2.2–6/3.6–5	Unknown	0.06–0.13	D	50%	Unknown	Unknown	100%
Maprotiline	48/Unknown	Unknown	Unknown	D	100%	Unknown	Unknown	NA
Meclofenamic acid	3/Unchanged	>99	Unknown	D	100%	None	None	100%
Mefenamic acid	3–4/Unchanged	Unknown	Unknown	D	100%	None	None	100%
Mefloquine	15–33 d/Unknown	98	20		Unknown: 100%	Unknown: None	Unknown: None	Unknown
Melphalan	1.1–1.4/4–6	90	0.6–0.75	D	50%	Unknown	Unknown	75%
Meperidine	2–7/7–32	70	4–5	D	50%	Avoid	None	Avoid
Meprobamate	9–11/Unchanged	0–30	0.5–0.8	I	q12–18h	None	Unknown	NA
Meropenem	1.1/6–8	Low	0.35	D,I	250–500 mg q24h	Dose after dialysis	Dose for renal failure	250–500 mg q12h
Metaproterenol	2–6/Unknown	10	7.6	D	100%	Unknown	Unknown	100%
Metformin	1–5/Prolonged	Negligible	1–4	D	Avoid	Unknown	Unknown	Avoid

(continued)

TABLE 12.3. *(continued)*

Drug	Half-life (Hours) Normal/Renal Failure	Protein Binding (%)	Volume of Distribution (L/kg)	Method	Renal Failure Dose	Dose After Hemodialysis	Dose During CAPD	Dose During CRRT
Methadone	13–58/Unknown	60–90	3–6	D	50% to 75%	None	None	NA
Methenamine mandelate	4/Unknown	Unknown	Unknown	D	Avoid	NA	NA	NA
Methicillin	0.5–1/4	35–60	0.31	I	q8–12h	None	None	q6–8h
Methimazole	3–6/Unchanged	None	0.6	D	Unknown	Unknown	100%	
Methotrexate	8–12/Increased	45–50	0.76	D	Avoid	Yes	None	50%
Methyldopa	1.5–6/6–16	<15	0.5	I	q12–24h	250 mg	None	q8–12h
Methylprednisolone	1.9–6/Unchanged	40–60	1.2–1.5	D	100%	Yes	Unknown	100%
Metoclopramide	2.5–4/14–15	40	2–3.4	D	50%	None	Unknown	50% to 75%
Metocurine	3.5–5.8/11.3	70	0.42–0.57	D	50%	Unknown	Unknown	50%
Metolazone	4–20/Unknown	95	1.6	D	100%	None	None	NA
Metoprolol	3.5/2.5–4.5	8	5.5	D	100%	50 mg	None	100%
Metronidazole	6–14/7–21	20	0.25–0.85	D	50%	Dose after dialysis	Dose for renal failure	100%
Mexiletine	8–13/16	70–75	5.5–6.6	D	50% to 75%	None	None	None
Mezlocillin	0.6–1.2/2.6–5.4	20–46	0.18	I	q8h	None	None	q6–8h
Miconazole	20–24/Unchanged	90	Large	D	100%	None	None	None
Midazolam	1.2–12.3/Unchanged	93–96	1.0–6.6	D	50%	NA	NA	NA
Midodrine	0.5/Unknown	Unknown	Unknown		Unknown	5 mg q8h	Unknown	5–10 mg q8h
Miglitol	3–5/Prolonged	Unknown	Unknown	D	Avoid	Unknown	Unknown	Avoid
Milrinone	1/1.5–3	Unknown	0.25–0.35	D	50% to 75%	Unknown	Unknown	100%
Minocycline	12–16/12–18	70	1.0–1.5	D	100%	None	None	100%
Minoxidil	2.8–4.2/Unchanged	0	2–3	D	100%	None	None	100%
Mitomycin C	0.5–1/Unknown	Unknown	0.5	D	75%	Unknown	Unknown	Unknown
Mitoxantrone	23–40/Unknown	75	200–300	D	100%	Unknown	Unknown	100%
Mivacurium	1.5–3	Unknown	0.1	D	50%	Unknown	Unknown	Unknown
Moricizine	2/3	95	>5.0	D	100%	None	None	100%
Morphine	1–4/Unchanged	20–30	3.5	D	50%	None	Unknown	75%
Moxalactam	2.3/18–23	35–59	0.18–0.4	I	q24–48h	Dose after dialysis	Dose for renal failure	q12–24h
Nabumetone	24/Unchanged	>99	0.11	D	100%	None	None	100%
N-Acetylcysteine	2.3–6/Unknown	50	0.33–0.47	D	75%	Unknown	Unknown	100%
N-Acetylprocainamide	6–8/42–70	10–20	1.5–1.7	D,I	25% q12–18h	None	None	50% q8–12h
Nadolol	19/45	28	1.9	D	25%	40 mg	None	50%
Nafcillin	0.5/1.2	85	0.35	D	100%	None	None	100%
Nalidixic acid	6/21	90	0.25–0.35	D	Avoid	Avoid	Avoid	NA
Naloxone	1–1.5/Unknown	54	3	D	100%	NA	NA	100%
Naproxen	12–15/Unchanged	99	0.1	D	100%	None	None	100%
Nefazodone	2–4/Unchanged	99	0.22–0.87	D	100%	Unknown	Unknown	NA
Nelfinavir	1.8–3.4/Unknown	Unknown	Unknown		Unknown	Unknown	Unknown	Unknown
Neostigmine	1.3/3.0	None	0.5–1.0	D	25%	Unknown	Unknown	50%
Netlimicin	1–3/35–72	<5	0.16–0.30	D,I	10% to 20% q24–48h	2/3 normal dose after dialysis	3–4 mg/L/d	20% to 60% q12h
Nevirapine	40/?	60%	1.2–1.4	D	Unknown: 100%	Unknown: None	Dose for renal failure	Unknown
Nicardipine	5/5–7	98–99	0.8	D	100%	None	None	100%
Nicotinic acid	0.5–1/Unknown	Unknown	Unknown	D	25%	Unknown	Unknown	50%
Nifedipine	4–5.5/5–7	97	1.4	D	100%	None	None	100%
Nimodipine	1–2.8/22	98	0.9–2.3	D	100%	None	None	100%
Nisoldipine	6.6–7.9/6.8–9.7	99	2.3–7.1	D	100%	None	None	100%
Nitrazepam	18–36/Unknown	Unknown	Unknown	D	100%	Unknown	Unknown	NA
Nitrofurantoin	0.5/1	20–60	0.3–0.7	D	Avoid	NA	NA	NA
Nitroglycerine	2–4 min/Unchanged	Unknown	2–3	D	100%	Unknown	Unknown	100%
Nitroprusside	<10 min/<10 min	0	0.2	D	100%	None	None	100%
Nitrosoureas	Short/Unknown	Unknown	Unknown	D	25% to 50%	None	Unknown	Unknown
Nizatidine	1.3–1.6/5.3–8.5	28–35	0.8–1.3	D	25%	Unknown	Unknown	50%
Norfloxacin	3.5–6.5/8	14	<0.5	I	Avoid	NA	NA	NA
Nortriptyline	25–38/15–66	95	15–23	D	100%	None	None	NA
Ofloxacin	5–8/28–37	25	1.5–2.5	D	25% to 50%	100 mg bid	Dose for renal failure	300 mg/d
Omeprazole	0.5–1/Unchanged	95	Unknown	D	100%	Unknown	Unknown	Unknown
Ondansetron	2.5–5.5/Unchanged	75	2	D	100%	Unknown	Unknown	Unknown
Orphenadrine	16/Unknown	Unknown	Unknown	D	100%	Unknown	Unknown	NA
Ouabain	21/60–70	40	Unknown	I	q36–48h	None	None	q24–36h
Oxaproxin	50–60/Unchanged	>99	0.2	D	100%	None	None	100%
Oxatomide	20/Unknown	91	Unknown	D	100%	None	None	NA
Oxazepam	5–10/25–90	97	0.6–1.6	D	100%	None	Unknown	100%
Oxcarbazepine	8–9/Unknown	40	0.7–0.8	D	100%	Unknown	Unknown	Unknown
Paclitaxel	9–30/Unknown	Unknown	30–60	D	100%	Unknown	Unknown	100%

(continued)

TABLE 12.3. *(continued)*

Drug	Half-life (Hours) Normal/Renal Failure	Protein Binding (%)	Volume of Distribution (L/kg)	Method	Renal Failure Dose	Dose After Hemodialysis	Dose During CAPD	Dose During CRRT
Pancuronium	1.7–2.2/4.3–8.2	70–85	0.15–0.38	D	Avoid	Unknown	Unknown	50%
Paroxetine	10–16/30	95	13	D	50%	Unknown	Unknown	NA
PAS	1.0	15–50	0.11–24	D	50%	Dose after dialysis	Dose for renal failure	Dose for renal failure
Penbutolol	22/24	>95	Unknown	D	100%	None	None	100%
Penicillamine	1.5–3/Increased	80	Unknown	D	Avoid	1/3 dose	Unknown	Avoid
Penicillin G	0.5/6–20	50	0.3–0.42	D	20% to 50%	Dose after dialysis	Dose for renal failure	75%
Penicillin VK	0.6/4.1	50–80	0.5	D	100%	Dose after dialysis	Dose for renal failure	NA
Pentamidine	29/118	69	55–462	I	q48h	None	None	None
Pentazocine	2–5/Unknown	50–75	5	D	50%	None	Unknown	75%
Pentobarbital	18–48/Unchanged	60–70	1.0	D	100%	None	Unknown	100%
Pentopril	2–3/10–14	60	0.8	D	50%	Unknown	Unknown	50% to 75%
Pentoxifylline	0.8/Unchanged	None	2.4–4.2	D	100%	Unknown	Unknown	100%
Perfloxacin	10/15	25–43	2.0	D	100%	None	None	100%
Perindopril	5/27	20	0.6–0.8	D	50%	25% to 50%	Unknown	75%
Phenelzine	1.5–4/Unknown	Unknown	Unknown	D	100%	Unknown	Unknown	NA
Phenobarbital	60–150/117–160	40–60	0.7–1	I	q12–16h	Dose after dialysis	1/2 normal dose	q8–12h
Phenylbutazone	50–100/Unchanged	99	0.09–0.17	D	100%	None	None	100%
Phenytoin	24/Unchanged	90	1.0	D	100%	None	None	None
Pindolol	2.5–4/3–4	50	1.2	D	100%	None	None	100%
Pipecuronium	2.3/4.4	Unknown	0.31	D	25%	Unknown	Unknown	50%
Piperacillin	0.8–1.5/3.3–5.1	30	0.18–0.30	I	q8h	Dose after dialysis	Dose for renal failure	q6–8h
Piretanide	1.4/1.6–3.4	94	0.3	D	100%	None	None	NA
Piroxicam	45–55/Unchanged	>99	0.12–0.15	D	100%	None	None	100%
Plicamycin	2/Unknown	Low	Unknown	D	50%	Unknown	Unknown	Unknown
Pravastatin	0.8–3.2/Unchanged	Unknown	Unknown	D	100%	Unknown	Unknown	100%
Prazepam	36–200/36	Unknown	Unknown	D	100%	Unknown	Unknown	NA
Prazosin	2–3/2–3	97	1.2–1.5	D	100%	None	None	100%
Prednisolone	2.5–3.5/Unchanged	Saturable	2.2	D	100%	Yes	Unknown	100%
Prednisone	2.5–3.5/Unchanged	Saturable	2.2	D	100%	None	Unknown	100%
Primaquine	4–7/Unknown	Unknown	3–4		Unknown: 100%	Unknown	Unknown	Unknown
Primidone	5–15/Unchanged	20–30	0.4–1	I	q12–24h	1/3 dose	Unknown	Unknown
Probenecid	5–8/Unchanged	85–95	0.15	D	Avoid	Avoid	Unknown	Avoid
Probucol	23–47 d/Unknown	Unknown	Unknown	D	100%	Unknown	Unknown	100%
Procainamide	2.5–4.9/5.3–5.9	15	2.2	I	q8–24h	200 mg	None	q6–12h
Promethazine	12/Unknown	93	13.5	D	100%	None	None	100%
Propafenone	5/Unknown	>95	3.0	D	100%	None	None	100%
Propofol	3–4.5/Unchanged	Unknown	3.0–14.4	D	100%	Unknown	Unknown	100%
Propoxyphene	9–15/12–20	78	16	D	Avoid	None	None	NA
Propranolol	2–6/1–6	93	2.8	D	100%	None	None	100%
Propylthiouracil	1–2/Unchanged	80	0.3–0.4	D	100%	Unknown	Unknown	100%
Protryptyline	54–98/Unknown	92	15–31	D	100%	None	None	NA
Pyrazinimide	9/26	5	0.75–1.3	D	Avoid	Avoid	Avoid	Avoid
Pyridostigmine	1.5–2/6	Unknown	0.8–1.4	D	20%	Unknown	Unknown	35%
Pyrimethamine	80/Unchanged	27	2.9	D	100%	None	None	None
Quazepam	20–40/Unknown	95	Unknown	D	Unknown	Unknown	Unknown	NA
Quinapril	1–2/6–15	97	1.5	D	75%	25%	None	75% to 100%
Quinidine	6/4–14	70–95	2–3.5	D	75%	100–200 mg	None	100%
Quinine	5–16/Unchanged	70	0.7–3.7	I	q24h	Dose after dialysis	Dose for renal failure	q8–12h
Ramipril	5–8/15	55–70	1.2	D	25% to 50%	20%	None	50% to 75%
Ranitidine	1.5–3/6–9	15	1.2–1.8	D	25%	1/2 dose	None	50%
Reserpine	46–168/87–323	96	Unknown	D	Avoid	None	None	100%
Ribavirin	30–60/Unknown	0	9–15	D	50%	Dose after dialysis	Dose for renal failure	Dose for renal failure
Rifabutin	16–69/Unchanged	71–89	8.2–9.3		100%	None	None	Unknown
Rifampin	1.5–5/1.8–11	60–90	0.9	D	50% to 100%	None	Dose for renal failure	Dose for renal failure
Ritonavir	3/Unknown	98–99	0.4		Unknown: 100%	Unknown: None	Dose for renal failure	Unknown
Saquinavir	12/?	98%	10		Unknown: 100%	Unknown: None	Dose for renal failure	Unknown
Secobarbital	20–35/Unknown	44	1.5–2.5	D	100%	None	None	NA
Sertraline	24/Unchanged	97	25	D	100%	Unknown	Unknown	NA
Simvastatin	Unknown	>95	Unknown	D	100%	Unknown	Unknown	100%
Sodium valproate	6–15/Unchanged	90	0.19–0.23	D	100%	None	None	None
Sotalol	7.5–15/56	<1	1.3	D	15% to 30%	80 mg	None	30%

(continued)

TABLE 12.3. *(continued)*

Drug	Half-life (Hours) Normal/Renal Failure	Protein Binding (%)	Volume of Distribution (L/kg)	Method	Renal Failure Dose	Dose After Hemodialysis	Dose During CAPD	Dose During CRRT
Sparfloxacin	15–20/38.5	35–55	4.5	D,I	50% q48h	Unknown: Dose for GFR <10	Unknown	50% to 75%
Spectinomycin	1.6/16–29	5–20	0.25	D	100%	None	None	None
Spironolactone	10–35/Unchanged	98	Unknown	I	Avoid	NA	NA	Avoid
Stavudine	1.0–1.4/5.5–8	<1%	0.5	D,I	50% q24h	Dose after dialysis	Unknown	Unknown
Streptokinase	0.6–1.5/Unknown	Unknown	0.02–0.08	D	100%	NA	NA	100%
Streptomycin	2.5/100	35	0.26	I	q72–96h	1/2 normal dose after dialysis	20–40 mg/L/d	q24–72h
Streptozotocin	0.25/Unknown	Unknown	0.5	D	50%	Unknown	Unknown	Unknown
Succinylcholine	3/Unknown	Unknown	Unknown	D	100%	Unknown	Unknown	100%
Sufentanil	1–2/Unchanged	92	1.7–5.2	D	100%	Unknown	Unknown	100%
Sulbactam	1/10–21	30	0.25–0.5	I	q24–48h	Dose after dialysis	0.75–1.5 g/d	750 mg q12h
Sulfamethoxazole	10/20–50	50	0.28–0.38	I	q24h	1 g after dialysis	1 g/d	q18h
Sulfinpyrazone	2.2–5/Unchanged	>95	0.06	D	Avoid	None	None	100%
Sulfisoxazole	3–7/6–12	85	0.14–0.28	I	q12–24h	2 g after dialysis	3 g/d	NA
Sulindac	8–16/Unchanged	95	Unknown	D	100%	None	None	100%
Sulotroban	0.7–3/9–39	Unknown	Unknown	D	10%	Unknown	Unknown	Unknown
Tamoxifen	18/Unknown	>98	20	D	100%	Unknown	Unknown	100%
Tazobactam	1/7	22	0.21	D	50%	1/3 dose after dialysis	Dose for renal failure	75%
Teicoplanin	33–190/62–230	60–90	0.5–1.2	I	q72h	Dose for renal failure	Dose for renal failure	q48h
Temazepam	4–10/Unknown	96	1.3–1.5	D	100%	None	None	NA
Teniposide	6–10/Unknown	99	0.2–0.7	D	100%	None	None	100%
Terazosin	9–12/8–12	90–94	0.5–0.9	D	100%	Unknown	Unknown	100%
Terbutaline	3/Unknown	15–25	0.9–1.5	D	Avoid	Unknown	Unknown	50%
Terfenadine	16–23/Unknown	97	Unknown	D	100%	None	None	NA
Tetracycline	6–10/57–108	55–90	>0.7	I	q24h	None	None	q12–24h
Theophylline	4–12/Unchanged	55	0.4–0.7	D	100%	1/2 dose	Unknown	100%
Thiazides	6–8/12–20	40	3.0	D	Avoid	NA	NA	NA
Thiopental	3.8/6–18	72–86	1–1.5	D	75%	NA	NA	NA
Ticarcillin	1.2/11–16	45–60	0.14–0.21	D,I	1–2 g q12h	3 g after dialysis	Dose for renal failure	1–2 g q8h
Ticlopidine	24–33/Unknown	98	Unknown	D	100%	Unknown	Unknown	100%
Timolol	2.7/4	60	1.7	D	100%	None	None	100%
Tobramycin	2.5/27–60	<5	0.22–0.33	D,I	20% to 30% q24–48h	2/3 normal dose after dialysis	3–4 mg/L/d	30% to 70% q12h
Tocainide	14/22–27	10–20	3.2	D	50%	200 mg	None	100%
Tolazamide	4–7/Unknown	94	Unknown	D	100%	Unknown	Unknown	Avoid
Tolbutamide	4–6/Unchanged	95–97	0.1–0.15	D	100%	None	None	Avoid
Tolmetin	1–1.5/Unchanged	>99	0.1–0.14	D	100%	None	None	100%
Topiramate	19–23/48–60	9–17	0.6–0.8	D	25%	Unknown	Unknown	50%
Topotecan	4–6/Prolonged	Unknown	40	D	25%	Unknown	Unknown	50%
Torsemide	2–4/4–5	97–99	0.14–0.19	D	100%	None	None	NA
Tranexamic acid	1.5/Unknown	3	Unknown	D	10%	Unknown	Unknown	Unknown
Tranylcypromine	1.9–3.5/Unknown	Unknown	Unknown	D	Unknown	Unknown	Unknown	NA
Trazodone	6–11/Unknown	89–95	1–2	D	Unknown	Unknown	Unknown	NA
Triamcinolone	1.9–6/Unchanged	Unknown	1.4–2.1	D	100%	Unknown	Unknown	100%
Triamterene	2–12/10	40–70	2.2–3.7	I	Avoid	NA	NA	Avoid
Triazolam	2–4/Unchanged	85–95	Unknown	D	100%	None	None	NA
Trihexyphenidyl	10/Unknown	Unknown	Unknown	D	Unknown	Unknown	Unknown	Unknown
Trimethadione	12–24/Unknown	None	Unknown	I	q12–24h	Unknown	Unknown	q8–12h
Trimethoprim	9–13/20–49	30–70	1–2.2	I	q24h	Dose after dialysis	q24h	q18h
Trimetrexate	4–22/Unknown	95	0.6 (10–31 L/m²)	D	Unknown: Avoid?	Unknown	Unknown	Unknown
Trimipramine	24/Unknown	90–96	31	D	100%	None	None	NA
Tripelennamine	3–4.5/Unknown	Unknown	10	D	Unknown	Unknown	Unknown	NA
Triprolidine	5/Unknown	Unknown	Unknown	D	Unknown	Unknown	Unknown	NA
Tubocurarine	0.5–4/5.5	30–50	0.22–0.39	D	Avoid	Unknown	Unknown	50%
Urokinase	Unknown	Unknown	Unknown	D	Unknown	Unknown	Unknown	Unknown
Valacyclovir				D,I	0.5 g q24h	Dose after dialysis	Dose for renal failure	Unknown
Vancomycin	6–8/200–250	10–50	0.47–1.1	D,I	500 mg q48–96h	Dose for renal failure	Dose for renal failure	500 mg q24–48h
Vecuronium	0.5–1.3/Unchanged	30	0.18–0.27	D	100%	Unknown	Unknown	100%
Venlafaxine	4/6–8	27	6–7	D	50%	None	Unknown	NA
Verapamil	3–7/2.4–4	83–93	3–6	D	100%	None	None	100%
Vidarabine	1.5/Unknown	25	0.7	D	75%	Infuse after dialysis	Dose for renal failure	100%
Vigabatrin	5–7/13–15	None	0.8	D	25%	Unknown	Unknown	50%

(continued)

TABLE 12.3. *(continued)*

Drug	Half-life (Hours) Normal/Renal Failure	Protein Binding (%)	Volume of Distribution (L/kg)	Method	Renal Failure Dose	Dose After Hemodialysis	Dose During CAPD	Dose During CRRT
Vinblastine	1–1.5/Unknown	75	13–40	D	100%	Unknown	Unknown	100%
Vincristine	1–2.5/Unknown	75	5–11	D	100%	Unknown	Unknown	100%
Vinorelbine	20–40/Unknown	15	75	D	100%	Unknown	Unknown	100%
Warfarin	34–45/Unchanged	99	0.15	D	100%	None	None	None
Zafirlukast	10/Unchanged	99	Unknown	D	100%	Unknown	Unknown	100%
Zalcitabine	1–2/>8 h	<4%	0.54	I	q24h	Unknown	Unknown	Unknown
Zidovudine	1.1–1.4/1.4–3	10–30	1.4–3	D,I	100 mg q8h	Dose for renal failure	Dose for renal failure	100 mg q8h
Zileuton	2.3/Unchanged	>90	2.3		100%	None	Unknown	100%

Note: Method refers to changing the dose (D) or the dose interval (I). Percentages are the percent of the dose for normal renal function. NA is listed for drugs where dosing is not applicable during renal replacement therapy.

during dialysis more than during convection during CRRT because of the large pore size of membranes used for CRRT. Since most drugs are less than 1,500 daltons, drug removal by CRRT does not depend greatly on molecular weight.

The volume of distribution of a drug is the most important factor determining removal by CRRT. Drugs with a large volume of distribution are highly tissue bound and not accessible to extracorporeal circuit in quantities sufficient to result in substantial removal by CRRT. Even if the extraction across the artificial membrane is 100%, only a small amount of a drug with a large volume of distribution is removed. A volume of distribution greater than 0.7 L/kg substantially decreases CRRT drug removal.

Drug protein binding also determines how much is removed during CRRT. Only unbound drug is available for elimination by CRRT. Protein binding of more than 80% provides a substantial barrier to drug removal by convection or diffusion.

During continuous hemofiltration, an ultrafiltration rate of 10 to 30 mL/min is achieved. The addition of diffusion by continuous dialysis increases drug clearance, depending on blood and dialysate flow rates. As during high-flux dialysis, drug removal parallels the removal of urea and creatinine. The simplest method for estimating drug removal during CRRT is to estimate urea or creatinine clearance during the procedure (30).

DRUG LEVEL MONITORING

Measurement of plasma drug concentrations is helpful in assessing a particular dosage regimen when the relationship between drug levels and efficacy or toxicity has been established. These measurements are clearly most important for drugs with a narrow therapeutic range or difficult to measure pharmacological effects.

Serum levels are determined after an appropriate loading dose has been given. In the absence of a loading dose, three or four doses of the drug should be administered before serum lev-

TABLE 12.4. ANTIBIOTIC DOSAGES FOR PATIENTS ON CAPD

Drug	Loading Dose	Maintenance Dose
Amikacin	7.5 mg/kg	25 mg/L
Ampicillin	1 g	60 mg/L
Aztreonam	15 mg/kg	250 mg/L
Carbenicillin	5 g	250 mg/L
Cefazolin	1 g	125 mg/L
Cefoperazone	—	2 g every other bag
Ceftazidime	1 g	125 mg/L
Ceftriaxone	—	1 g in one bag/d
Clindamycin	—	150 mg/L
Gentamicin	2 mg/kg	4 mg/L
Imipenem/cilastatin	500 mg	250 mg every other bag
Moxalactam	1 g	125 mg/L
Penicillin	500,000 U	100,000 U/L
Piperacillin	—	4 g every other bag
Ticarcillin/clavulante	1.2 g	120 mg/L
Tobramycin	2 mg/kg	4 mg/L
Vancomycin	30 mg/kg	20 mg/L

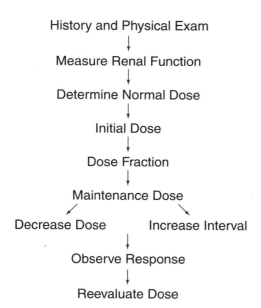

History and Physical Exam

↓

Measure Renal Function

↓

Determine Normal Dose

↓

Initial Dose

↓

Dose Fraction

↓

Maintenance Dose

↙   ↘

Decrease Dose   Increase Interval

↓

Observe Response

↓

Reevaluate Dose

FIG. 12.4 A practical schema for drug dosing in dialysis patients.

els are measured. This ensures that a steady-state serum concentration has been established. For some drugs, both maximum and minimum concentrations are relevant. Peak levels are most meaningful when measured after rapid drug distribution has occurred. Conversely, minimum concentrations are usually measured just before giving the next scheduled dose. Figure 12.4 shows a practical schema for drug prescribing in patients with renal impairment.

The heterogeneity of renal disease makes responses to drug therapy quite variable. Dosage nomograms, drug tables, and computer-assisted dosing recommendations provide guidelines for deriving an initial approach to drug administration in patients with decreased renal function. Continuing evaluation of the therapeutic response and modification of the regimen individualized for each patient and each clinical situation ensure effective clinical management of dialysis patients.

REFERENCES

1. Manley HJ, et al. Comparing medication use in two hemodialysis units against national dialysis databases. *Am J Health Syst Pharm* 2000;57: 902–906.
2. Jick H. Adverse drug effects in relation to renal function. *Am J Med* 1977;62:514–517.
3. Pearson TF, et al. Factors associated with preventable adverse drug reactions. *Am J Hosp Pharm* 1994;51:2268–2272.
4. Aronoff GR, et al. Principles of administering drugs to patients with renal failure. In: Bennett WM, et al., eds. *Contemporary issues in nephrology: pharmacotherapy of renal diseases and hypertension.* New York: Churchill-Livingstone, 1987:1.
5. Swan SK, et al. Determination of residual renal function with iohexal clearance in hemodialysis patients. *Kidney Int* 1996;49:232–235.
6. Lang SM, et al. Preservation of residual renal function in dialysis patients: effects of dialysis-technique-related factors. *Perit Dial Int* 2001;21:52–57.
7. Anderson RJ, et al. *Clinical use of drugs in renal failure.* Springfield, IL: Charles C Thomas, 1976.
8. Hurwitz A. Antacid therapy and drug kinetics. *Clin Pharmacokin* 1977;2:269–280.
9. Maton PN, et al. Antacids revisited: a review of their clinical pharmacology and recommended therapeutic use. *Drugs* 1999;57:855–870.
10. Craig RM, et al. Kinetic analysis of D-xylose absorption in normal subjects and in patients with chronic renal failure. *J Lab Clin Med* 1983; 101:496–506.
11. Craig RM, et al. D-xylose kinetics and hydrogen breath tests in functionally anephric patients using 15-gram dose. *J Clin Gastroenterol* 2000;31:55–59.
12. Reidenberg MN. The binding of drugs to plasma proteins and the interpretation of measurements of plasma concentration of drugs in patients with poor renal function. *Am J Med* 1977;62:482–485.
13. Dromgoole SH. The binding capacity of albumin and renal disease. *J Pharmacol Exp Ther* 1974;191:318–323.
14. Niwa T. Organic acids and the uremic syndrome: protein metabolite hypothesis in the progression of chronic renal failure. *Semin Nephrol* 1996;16:167–182.
15. McNamara PJ, et al. Endogenous accumulation products and serum protein binding in uremia. *J Lab Clin Med* 1981;98:730–740.
16. Boobis SW. Alteration of plasma albumin in relation to decreased drug binding in uremia. *Clin Pharmacol Ther* 1977;22:147–153.
17. Reidenberg MM, et al. Influence of disease on binding of drugs to plasma proteins. *Ann NY Acad Sci* 1973;226:115–126.
18. Reidenberg MM, et al. Protein binding of diphenylhydantoin and desmethylimipramine in plasma from patients with poor renal function. *N Engl J Med* 1971;285:264–267.
19. Kovacs SJ, et al. Pharmacokinetics and protein binding of eprosartan in hemodialysis-dependent patients with end-stage renal disease. *Pharmacotherapy* 1999;19:612–619.
20. Reidenberg MN. The biotransformation of drugs in renal failure. *Am J Med* 1977;62:482–485.
21. Macias WL, et al. Vancomycin pharmacokinetics in acute renal failure; preservation of nonrenal clearance. *Clin Pharmacol Ther* 1991;50: 688–694.
22. Yuan R, et al. Effect of chronic renal failure on the disposition of highly hepatically metabolized drugs. *Int J Clin Pharmacol Ther* 2000;38: 245–253.
23. Maher JF. Pharmacokinetics in patients with renal failure. *Clin Nephrol* 1984;21:39–46.
24. Oosterhuis WP, et al. In vivo evaluation of four hemodialysis membranes: biocompatibility and clearances. *Dial Transplant* 1995;24:450–454.
25. Scott MK, et al. Vancomycin mass transfer characteristics of high-flux cellulosic dialysers. *Nephrol Dial Transplant* 1997;12:2647–2653.
26. Schaedeli F, et al. Urea kinetics and dialysis treatment time predict vancomycin elimination during high-flux hemodialysis. *Clin Pharmacol Ther* 1998;63:26–38.
27. Scott MK, et al. Effects of dialysis membrane on intradialytic vancomycin administration. *Pharmacotherapy* 1997;17:256–262.
28. Paton TW, et al. Drug therapy in patients undergoing peritoneal dialysis: clinical pharmacokinetic considerations. *Clin Pharmacokin* 1985;10:404–426.
29. Bunke CM, et al. Cefazolin and cephalexin kinetics in continuous ambulatory peritoneal dialysis. *Clin Pharm Ther* 1983;33:66–72.
30. Keller F, et al. Individualized drug dosage in patients treated with continuous hemofiltration. *Kidney Int* 1999;72(Suppl):S29–S31.

13

CONTINUOUS DIALYSIS THERAPEUTIC TECHNIQUES

THAWEE CHANCHAIRUJIRA AND RAVINDRA L. MEHTA

Over the last decade significant advances have been made in the availability of different dialysis methods for replacement of renal function. Although most of these have been developed for patients with end-stage renal disease (ESRD), they are being applied increasingly to the treatment of acute renal failure (ARF). The availability of highly permeable membranes has allowed development of continuous renal replacement techniques (CRRT), which remove fluids and solutes gradually, resulting in better hemodynamic stability and better fluid and solute control (1). These techniques are rapidly gaining acceptance worldwide as the treatment of choice for ARF in critically ill, hemodynamically unstable patients (2–7). This chapter serves as a framework for future reference, providing a description of the basic techniques, an outline of the key areas of application, and a summary of the results with these therapies.

TERMINOLOGY

Continuous therapies encompass a variety of modalities that vary in terminology. Recently, an international group of experts has developed the Acute Dialysis Quality Initiative (8) and has proposed adopting previously developed standardized terms for these therapies. The basic goal was to link the nomenclature to the operational characteristics of the different techniques (9). Each letter in the acronym represents a specific characteristic related to the duration, driving force, and operational features. The letter *C* is used in all the terms to describe the continuous nature. The letters *AV* or *VV* in the terminology identify the technique's driving force—that is, the mean arterial pressure for arteriovenous (AV) circuits, and external pumps for venovenous (VV) circuits. Solute removal in these techniques is achieved by convection, diffusion, or a combination of these methods. Thus the letters *UF, H, HD,* and *HDF* identify the technique's operational characteristics:

Convective techniques, including ultrafiltration (UF) and hemofiltration (H), depend on solute removal by solvent drag (10).

Diffusion-based techniques, similar to intermittent hemodialysis (HD), are based on the principle of a solute gradient between the blood and the dialysate (11).

Hemodiafiltration (HDF) processes use both diffusion and convection in the same technique. In this instance, both dialysate and a replacement solution are used, and both small and middle molecules can be removed easily (12).

The only exception to this nomenclature system is the acronym SCUF (slow continuous UF), which remains as a reminder of these therapies' origins as simple techniques to har-

TABLE 13.1. CONTINUOUS RENAL REPLACEMENT THERAPY: COMPARISON OF TECHNIQUES

Access	SCUF AV	CAVH AV	CVVH VV	CAVHD AV	CAVHDF AV	CVVHD VV	CVVHDF VV	PD Peritoneal Catheter
Pump	No	No	Yes	No	No	Yes	Yes	No[b]
Filtrate (mL/h)	100	600	1,000	300	600	300	800	100
Filtrate (L/d)	2.4	14.4	24	7.2	14.4	7.2	19.2	2.4
Dialysate flow (L/h)	0	0	0	1.0	1.0	1.0	1.0	0.4
Replacement fluid (L/d)	0	12	21.6	4.8	12	4.8	16.8	0
Urea clearance (mL/min)	1.7	10	16.7	21.7	26.7	21.7	30	8.5
Simplicity[a]	1	2	3	2	2	3	3	2
Cost[a]	1	2	4	3	3	4	4	3

Modified from Mehta RL. Renal replacement therapy for acute renal failure: matching the method to the patient. *Semin Dial* 1993;6:253–259.
[a]1 = most simple and least expensive; 4 = most difficult and expensive.
[b]Cycler can be used to automate exchanges but adds to the cost and complexity.
Abbreviations: CAVH, continuous arteriovenous hemofiltration; CAVHD, continuous arteriovenous hemodialysis; CAVHDF, continuous arteriovenous hemodiafiltration; CVVH, continuous venovenous hemofiltration; CVVHD, continuous venovenous hemodialysis; CVVHDF, continuous venovenous hemodiafiltration; PD, peritoneal dialysis; SCUF, slow continuous ultrafiltration.

ness the power of AV circuits (13). Table 13.1 illustrates the terminology applied to CRRT therapies.

COMPONENTS

The key components of any CRRT method include the access and circuit, the membrane, an anticoagulant, solutions for replacement fluid and dialysate, and the pumps. Each of these elements can be manipulated to achieve a particular therapeutic goal.

Access and Circuit

The circuit, the characteristics of each CRRT component, and the operation influence the success of any CRRT procedure. Among these factors, the access and circuit that are used are key (14–16); this is especially true with AV circuits, where the driving force is the patient's mean arterial pressure. Because blood flow rates vary, there is a higher risk for periods of extremely low flow, which predispose the patient to thrombosis. For AV procedures (CAVH, CAVHD, CAVHDF), large-bore, small-length catheters generally are preferred to permit a high blood flow rate. Arterial access has been associated with a significantly high complication rate (17), and AV procedures are uncommonly used now. With the recent development of the double-lumen venous catheter, a new generation of blood pump modules and circuit designs with sensors interfaced to more intelligent software in the CRRT machine, application of CRRT in the intensive care unit is now safer and easier (18). There is now a clear preference for pump-driven CRRT. This is largely based on the fact that it is considered to be a more user-friendly technique with less vascular access-related morbidity compared with the spontaneous arteriovenous technique.

In pumped systems (CVVH, CVVHD, CVVHDF), double-lumen catheters are commonly used, the size of which should be selected based on the site of insertion (femoral, subclavian, jugular) to optimize flow. If femoral catheters are used, the tip should optimally be in the inferior vena cava. Since CRRT is likely to be continued for several days at a time, some centers recommend changing the access site on a periodic basis. However, a recent clinical trial did not find any evidence to support this practice (19). CRRT is often required for patients who already have an AV fistula or graft for vascular access. In these circumstances the fistula or graft can be used for access; however, this requires the use of plastic needles that must be taped securely to prevent inadvertent tears in the access site. In pumped systems, the circuit characteristics are determined by the manufacturer's specifications and machine parameters. Two issues are particularly relevant in monitoring the delivered blood flow rate: (a) pump speed setting does not necessarily equate with a delivered blood flow, and (b) most instances of filter clotting are accompanied by access clotting. Newer-generation pumps (Gambro/Hospal Prisma, Braun Diapact, and Baxter Accura) have built-in pressure sensors for access and filter pressures that can inform about reductions in blood flow. However, such reductions may not always be predictive (20).

Pumps

All CRRT circuits use pumps to regulate the flow of replacement fluid, dialysate, and anticoagulant. Pumped CRRT methods also use pumps to regulate the blood flow and control the ultrafiltrate, replacement fluid, and dialysate flow rates. Standard intravenous pumps are often used to deliver the replacement fluid, dialysate, and anticoagulant and to control UF (21–26). Although such standard systems work very well, they are not linked to each other. Thus an alarm condition in one pump does not influence the operation of the other pumps—a particular disadvantage in pumped CRRT. For example, when an infusion pump is used to control the ultrafiltrate, the ultrafiltrate pump will continue to run even after an alarm stops the blood flow pump; the result is a marked increase in the viscosity of blood emerging from the filter. Additionally, the inaccuracy of the infusion pumps, which may range from 5% to 15%, results in significant errors in fluid balance when the infusion pumps are used for controlling fluid (25,27).

Newer systems (Gambro/Hospal Prisma; Braun Diapact, Baxter Accura) have integrated pumps to control blood flow and infusion of replacement fluid, dialysate, and ultrafiltrate. Because the pumps are linked, an alarm condition in one of the pumps results in all the pumps stopping simultaneously, thus reducing the potential for circuit problems.

Several centers have used standard dialysis machines for CRRT (28). The key difference between existing dialysis machines used for intermittent dialysis and these newer CRRT systems is the speed at which dialysate flow is regulated. Traditional dialysis machines have dialysate flow rates set at 500 to 800 mL/min, whereas CRRT systems control dialysate flow rates at 1 to 2 L/h (17 to 34 mL/min). The Fresenius dialysis machines have now been modified to allow a dialysate flow rate of 100 mL/min, thereby permitting a lower diffusive clearance than standard intermittent hemodialysis (IHD). These systems have been used for continuous therapies or extended daily dialysis (EDD) or slow, low-efficiency dialysis procedures (29). No comparisons of dedicated CRRT machines to standard dialysis machines have been made; however, it is clear that several configurations of pumped CRRT exist. In general, pumped CRRT systems offer regulation of blood flow and standardized monitoring of factors such as venous pressures, which are not available in nonpumped systems. Given the superiority of dedicated CRRT machines for CRRT treatment, substituting a standard dialysis machine is difficult; however, this may be necessary in some centers where CRRT machines are unavailable.

Membrane

A variety of membranes are currently available in different configurations for CRRT (30,31). The choice of a membrane for CRRT depends upon the desired operational parameters. In most settings small solute removal is dependent upon the membrane pore size, surface area, and flow characteristics. Middle and large molecules are additionally influenced by adsorptive characteristics of the membrane and flow rates (12,31–33). A key feature of nonpumped CRRT systems is a highly permeable membrane that permits adequate UF with a low mean arterial pressure. This type of membrane is particularly important in AV circuits, where the filtration pressure, which drops across the length of the filter, is opposed by the rising oncotic pressure from the removal of ultrafiltrate. Synthetic membranes—such as polysulfone, polyamide, and polyacrylonitrile (PAN) membranes—maximize the efficiency of nonpumped CRRT. However, these membranes differ in their permeability characteristics. Ultrafiltration rates tend to decrease with time, even when other factors are constant (11). The decline in filter permeability may be related to protein coating the membrane, a phenomenon termed *concentration repolarization* (34); however, it may also be influenced by membrane characteristics (14,35,36).

A large exponential decay in permeability within the first 6 hours is followed by a more gradual decay. Polysulfone membrane permeability appears to decrease most markedly, both initially and in later periods, whereas PAN and polyamide membranes have minimal decays after the initial decline. Other investigators (14) also demonstrated that hydraulic membrane permeability (Lp) significantly affects UF rates; polyamide membranes had a higher UF rate (QF) than polysulfone membranes. More recently, the same group has shown stable hemofilter performance over 72 hours (36). Thus if the primary indication is fluid removal, a polyamide or polysulfone membrane would suffice; however, if solute control is desired, a membrane with better diffusive characteristics (such as the AN-69 PAN) is preferable. Membrane characteristics also determine removal of solutes (e.g., cytokines) by adsorption rather than by mass transfer across the membrane. In critically ill patients with sepsis or multiorgan failure, a state of enhanced complement activation with high levels of circulating cytokines, platelet-activating factor, kinins, and other inflammatory mediators is likely to be present, even before the start of the dialysis procedure. In recent years, several studies have emphasized that dialysis membrane adsorption may also participate significantly in the removal of inflammatory mediators such as cytokines (37,38). The PAN/AN69 membrane has been shown to efficiently adsorb anaphylatoxins (C3a, C5a), bradykinin, endotoxins, and cytokines (IL-1, TNF), the factors that play a role in pathophysiology of sepsis (38–40). For mediators such as TNF, adsorption may be the main clearance mechanism. Increasing the permeability of the membrane is another option for removal of mediators in sepsis and has been tried with some success in these therapies (41). Although membrane biocompatibility is a characteristic that is thought to influence outcomes from ARF (42), it has not been evaluated for CRRT, as most centers use synthetic membranes.

In pumped CRRT the choice of membrane depends less on the need to achieve an adequate UF. Cellulose acetate and cuprophane membranes could be used, but synthetic membranes generally are preferable, as clearances can be enhanced easily. An important consideration is matching the surface area of the membrane to the patient size, particularly for pediatric patients. Membranes specifically designed for pediatric and neonatal application are limited in their availability, but in most instances standard adult membranes can be adapted for pediatric application (43–47).

Anticoagulant

As in other extracorporeal circuits, anticoagulation is essential to prevent the activation of clotting mechanisms within the circuit (48,49). Adequate anticoagulation ensures efficacy of the filter in fluid and solute removal, overall filter longevity, and optimum patient management. When the anticoagulation is insufficient, filtration performance deteriorates and the filter may eventually clot (50), contributing to blood loss. Excessive anticoagulation, on the other hand, may result in bleeding complications, which have been reported to occur in 5% to 26% of treatments (51).

Several methods of anticoagulation are now available. Table 13.2 summarizes the key features of the most common methods. Heparin continues to be the most commonly used anticoagulant, although its use is associated with a high incidence of bleeding and in some instances heparin-induced thrombocytopenia (52,53). Regional citrate anticoagulation eliminates the bleeding risk but requires the use of a specialized dialysis solution and monitoring of ionized calcium (51,54–58). It provides effective regional anticoagulation by chelating calcium in the extracorporeal circuit. The anticoagulation is reversed by systemic infusion of calcium. The metabolism of citrate by the liver, kidney, and skeletal muscles generates bicarbonate. The principal metabolic side effect is hypocalcemia and metabolic alkalosis. Several protocols using trisodium citrate have been described (Table 13.3) (55–61). At present, there has been limited experience with low-molecular-weight heparin (62–65), prostacyclin analogs (65–71), and other anticoagulants such as orgaran (72) and high-molecular-weight dextran (73). Recombinant hirudin has also been utilized for CRRT with variable results; however, its major drawback is the lack of reversibility (53,74–76). Some patients may not require any anticoagulation, but filter patency is limited to 24 to 36 hours in most instances. Filter efficacy usually declines before the filters clot, and thus should be monitored routinely. Filter longevity in excess of 96 hours is fairly common with citrate anticoagulation, whereas 36 to 48 hours' patency is usually the norm with heparin or no anticoagulation (77–79).

In practice, most critically ill patients with renal failure have intrinsic clotting system activation, a reduction in the natural anticoagulants, and evidence of intravascular coagulation as assessed by prothrombin fragments and thrombin–antithrombin III complexes. Platelet activation can occur either because of interaction with the activated clotting cascade or from contact with the CRRT circuit. Circuit design can reduce the risk of clotting by careful thought to the vascular access, length and resistance of the lines, use of predilutional fluid, and geometry and fiber material used in the hemofilter membrane (77–79). The efficacy of the available anticoagulant techniques and their relative advantages and disadvantages are reviewed in detail elsewhere (49,62). At the current time, none of these methods is considered ideal, and selection is usually influenced by several factors (Table 13.4). Most important, technical factors and experience with anticoagulants are important determinants of the success of any anticoagulant regimen.

Solutions

All CRRT other than SCUF and hemodialysis requires replacement fluids to compensate for the ultrafiltrate removed. Hemodialysis and HDF techniques in addition use a dialysate. The composition of these solutions can be varied extensively to achieve specific metabolic goals (80). For example, bicarbonate-

TABLE 13.2. ANTICOAGULATION MODALITIES FOR CONTINUOUS RENAL REPLACEMENT

Method	Filter Prime	Initial Dose	Maintenance Dose	Monitoring	Advantages	Disadvantages
Saline solution	2 L saline	150–250 mL prefilter	100–250 mL/h prefilter	Visual check	No anticoagulant used	Poor filter patency
Heparin	2 L saline 2,500–10,000 U	5–10 U/kg	3–12/kg/h	ACT 200–250; PTT 1.5–2.0 times normal	Standard method; easy to use; inexpensive	Bleeding risk; thrombocytopenia
LMW heparin	2 L saline	40 mg	10–40 mg/6 h	Factor Xa levels maintained between 0.1 and 0.41 U/mL	Decreased risk of bleeding	Special monitoring; not available everywhere; expensive
Regional heparin	2,500 U/2 L saline	5–10 U/kg	3–12 U/kg/h; + protamine postfilter	PTT: postfilter ACT 200–250	Reduced bleeding risk	Complex; risk of thrombocytopenia; protamine effects; hypotension
Regional citrate	2 L saline	4% trisodium citrate 150–180 mL/h	100–180 mL/h 3% to 7% of BFR, Ca replaced by central line	ACT: 200–250 maintain ionized calcium 0.96–1.2 efficacy, mmo l/L	No bleeding; no thrombocytopenia; improved filter longevity	Complex; needs Ca monitoring; alkalosis
Prostacyclin	2 L saline + heparin	Heparin 2–4 U/kg 4–8 ng/kg/min	4–8 ng/kg/min	ACT, PTT, platelet aggregation	Reduced heparinization	Needs heparin addition; hypotension
Nafomostat mesilate	2 L saline	—	0.1 mg/kg/h	ACT	No heparin	New procedure (?), filter efficacy

Reprinted with permission from Mehta RL. New developments in continuous arteriovenous hemofiltration/dialysis. In: Andreucci VE, et al., eds. *International Yearbook of Nephrology*, 1992.
ACT, activated clotting time; BFR, blood-flow rate; LMW, heparin, low molecular weight heparin; PTT, partial thromboplastin time.

based solutions can be used to correct acidemia, and the electrolyte content can be altered to correct electrolyte imbalance (81–83). Table 13.5 shows the composition of the most commonly used solutions for replacement and dialysate.

In the absence of commercially available solutions most centers in the United States have used standard peritoneal dialysis solutions (Baxter Dianeal, 1.5%) as dialysate. Commercial H solutions available in Europe (Hospal Hemosol) and in the

United States (Baxter Hemofiltration solution) have largely been lactate based and have raised concerns that the capacity to convert these buffers to bicarbonate may be reduced in multiple organ failure (84–87). More recently, the use of bicarbonate-based solutions has been found to be beneficial, and bulk production using standard dialysis machines has been described (88). These solutions are likely to be nonsterile and thus there is a risk of transferring infectious particles across the highly per-

TABLE 13.3. COMPARISON OF CITRATE PROTOCOLS

	Modality	Blood-Flow Rate	Citrate Delivery	Dialysate	Replacement Fluid	Patency at 48 h
Mehta et al.	CAVHD	52–125 mL/min	23.8 mmol/hr[a]	Na$^+$ 117 mEq/L Cl$^-$ 122.5 mEq/L K$^+$ 4 mEq/L Mg^{2+} 1.5 mEq/L Dextrose 2.5%	0.9% saline	~50%
Palsson et al.	CVVH	180 mL/min	18.6 mmol/hr[b]	N/A	Na$^+$ 117 mEq/L Cl$^-$ 122.5 mEq/L Mg^{2+} 1.5 mEq/L Citrate 40 mEq/L Dextrose 0.2%	
Kutsogiannis et al.	CVVHDF	125 mL/min	25 mmol/hr	Na$^+$ 110 mEq/L Cl$^-$ 110 mEq/L Mg^{2+} 1.5 mEq/L	Na$^+$ 110 mEq/L Cl$^-$ 110 mEq/L Mg^{2+} 1.5 mEq/L Varied NaHCO$_3^-$	~70%
Tolwani et al.	CVVHD	125–150 mL/min	17.5 mmol/hr	0.9% saline	N/A K$^+$ 3 mEq/L Mg^{2+} 2 mEq/L	61%

[a]Initial citrate infusion rate.
[b]Average citrate infusion rate.

TABLE 13.4. FACTORS AFFECTING ANTICOAGULANT REQUIREMENT IN CRRT

Variable	Parameters	Comments
Technical	Access and circuit	Most important factor. Catheter internal diameter and length influence blood flow. Kinks in catheter promote clotting. Air–blood interface in bubble trap is common site for clotting to start.
	Membrane	No significant differences in membrane type and frequency of clotting. Membrane geometry may be a factor in nonpumped systems.
	Operating characteristics	Site of delivery of anticoagulant at vascular access exit prolongs circuit life. Filtration fraction less than 20% is an important determinant of filter life as higher values increase viscosity of blood. Pumped UF without linkage to blood pump may increase tendency for filter clotting. Predilution with replacement fluid and use of dilute anticoagulant solution allow proper mixing of anticoagulant.
Patient	Coagulopathies	Thrombocytopenia and liver dysfunction reduce need for anticoagulant.
	Antithrombin III	Acquired deficiency of AT III is common in multiorgan failure and increases filter clotting.
	Underlying disease	Sepsis and multiorgan failure associated with DIC influence choice of anticoagulant and efficacy of anticoagulant.
Logistics	Experience	Experience with different anticoagulant regimens for chronic dialysis is often main factor for determining use. Heparin is commonest anticoagulant.
	Availability of anticoagulants	An important barrier to use of newer anticoagulant regimens is the ease with which components are available (e.g., orgaran and prostacyclin not commonly used in U.S.).
	Monitoring	**ACT, PTT commonly used for heparin effect. May be subject to regulations from CLIA in the U.S. Specific measures for other methods (e.g., factor Xa levels for low-molecular-weight heparin).**

CLIA, Clinical Laboratory Information Act; DIC, disseminated intravascular coagulation.

TABLE 13.5. COMPOSITION OF REPLACEMENT FLUID AND DIALYSATE FOR CRRT

Replacement Fluid

	Golper	Kierdorf	Lauer	Paganini	Mehta (Heparin)	Mehta (Citrate)
Na+	147	140	140	140	140.5	154
Cl	115	110	—	120	115.5	154
HCO^3	36	34	—	6	25	—
K+	0	0	2	2	0	—
Ca^{2+}	1.2	1.75	3.5	4	4	—
Mg^{2+}	0.7	0.5	1.5	2	—	—
Glucose	6.7	5.6	—	10	—	—
Acetate	—	41	40	—	—	—

Dialysate

	1.5% Dianeal	Hemosol AG 4D	Hemosol LG 4D	Baxter	UCSD Citrate	PrismaSate BK0/3.5	PrismaSate BK2/0
Na (mEq/L)	132	140	140	140	117	140	140
K (mEq/L)	—	4	4	2	4	0	2
Cl (mEq/L)	96	119	109.5	117	121	109.5	108
Lactate (mEq/L)	35	—	40	30	—	3	3
Acetate (mEq/L)	—	30	—	—	—	—	—
Bicarb (mEq/L)	—	—	—	—	Variable	32	32
Ca (mEq/L)	3.5	3.5	4	3.5	—	3.5	0
Mg (mEq/L)	1.5	1.5	1.5	1.5	1.5	1	1
Dextrose (G/dL)	1.5	0.8	0.11	0.1	0.1–0.5	0	0.11

meable filters. Newer solutions (DSI Normocarb, Gambro Prismasate) being introduced worldwide are bicarbonate based; however, experience with these solutions is limited (61,88–91).

The volume of replacement solutions used largely depends on the goals for fluid management and can be tailored for each individual patient as described in the following discussion of fluid management. In general, H techniques (CAVH/CVVH) require a significant amount of replacement fluid. Hemodialysis techniques (CAVHD/CVVHD) have no need for replacement solutions, and HDF methods (CAVHDF/CVVHDF) use moderate amounts of replacement fluid. The volume of dialysate solutions ranges from 1 to 2 L/h.

OPERATIONAL CHARACTERISTICS

The success of any CRRT procedure depends on an understanding of the operational characteristics unique to these techniques and appropriate use of specific components to deliver the therapy. Solute removal and fluid management, the major requirements of any CRRT procedure, are achieved by alterations in the key components.

Solute Removal

Solute removal in CRRT is achieved either by convection, diffusion, or a combination of both these methods.

Convective Techniques

Convective techniques include UF and H, and they depend on solute removal by solvent drag. As solute removal depends solely on convective clearance, it can only be enhanced by increasing the volume of ultrafiltrate produced. Ultrafiltration requires fluid removal only. Hemofiltration necessitates partial or complete replacement of the fluid removed to prevent significant volume loss and resulting hemodynamic compromise. Larger molecules are more efficiently removed by this process; hence middle molecular clearances are superior. In most situations, UF rates of 1 to 3 L/h are used. Recently, however, high-volume H with 6 L of ultrafiltrate produced every hour has been used to remove middle- and large-molecular-weight cytokines in sepsis (92,93). Fluid balance is achieved by replacing the ultrafiltrate removed by a replacement solution. The composition of the replacement fluid can be varied, and the solution can be infused before or after the filter.

Diffusion Techniques

Diffusion-based techniques are similar to intermittent hemodialysis in that both are based on the principle of a solute gradient between the blood and the dialysate. However, unlike in intermittent hemodialysis, diffusion-based CRRT methods have dialysate flow rates that are significantly lower than the blood flow rates, resulting in complete saturation of the dialysate. (Typically, the blood flow rates are 100 to 200 mL/min, and the dialysate flow rates are 1 to 2 L/h, or 17 to 34

mL/min.) As a consequence, dialysate flow rates become the limiting factor for solute removal and provide an opportunity for clearance enhancement. Small molecules are preferentially removed by these methods.

Combination Techniques

If both diffusion and convection are used in the same technique, as in HDF, both dialysate and a replacement solution are used and small and middle molecules can both be removed easily.

Process of Solute Removal

Sigler et al. (11,12) significantly enhanced our current understanding of the processes involved in solute removal in CRRT systems. In CAVH and CVVH, solutes are removed purely by convective transport. CAVHDF and CVVHDF use additional diffusive transfer. In CAVHD and CVVHD diffusive transfer is the main force for solute removal. The total solute clearance in CAVHDF and CVVHDF is the sum of the convective and diffusive clearances. As the molecular weight cutoff for the membranes is greater than 20,000 daltons, most low- and middle-molecular-weight substances have sieving coefficients (SC) of 1. Clearance is equal to Q_{eff} (the effluent flow rate) $\times$ SC for most middle molecules and is directly proportional to the amount of filtrate produced. Small molecules are less dependent on convective clearance and are more effectively transferred by diffusion.

CAVHD and CAVHDF (CVVHD/CVVHDF) dialysate flow rates are between 16.7 and 33.2 mL/min (1 to 2 L/h), which is much lower than the blood flow rate (50 to 120 mL/min). This allows for complete saturation of the dialysate fluid with solutes. Thus the limiting factor for solute removal by diffusion is the dialysate flow rate, not the blood flow rate, as it is with conventional hemodialysis. Blood-flow rates are not limiting until they are below 50 mL/min (94). Dialysate flow rates of up to 3 L/h do not appear to affect the UF rate, in spite of higher pressure within the dialysate compartment. Such low dialysate flow rates usually prevent backfiltration of fluid to the blood compartment (95).

Enhancing Solute Clearance

Several methods can be used to enhance solute clearance. In CAVH, Kaplan (72,96) demonstrated that suction applied to the ultrafiltrate port enhanced filtrate volumes, increased effective filter life, and was even more efficacious in conjunction with predilution. When replacement fluid is infused, postfilter solute clearance is equal to SC $\times$ Q_{eff}, where Q_{eff} is the effluent flow rate out of the device (equal to the UF flow rate across the filter membrane and dialysate flow rate). When replacement fluid is administered on the inlet side of the filter (predilution), this will result in a reduced solute concentration in the blood entering the filter. The effective small solute clearance for predilutional H is equal to Q_{eff} $\times$ (Q_b/[Q_b + Q_r]), where Q_b and Q_r represent blood and replacement fluid rates. Clearance in predilution H is less than that in postdilutional H for the same Q_{eff}. However, because of the dilution of blood entering the filter, much higher filtration fractions (larger Q_{eff} and Q_r) are feasible in predilutional H. Thus higher effective clearances are achievable in predilutional H, but at the expense of increased replacement fluid requirements (97). This reduces the viscosity of blood within the filter, promotes superior filtration rates, and increases urea clearances by facilitating transfer of BUN from the intraerythrocytic compartment.

If an external pump is applied to the circuit (as in CVVH), the limitation of low UF rates is overcome, as 20 to 40 L of filtrate can be easily produced in 24 hours (98,99). Dialysate used across the membrane markedly improves clearances and retains the simplicity of the procedure. Solute clearances can be further enhanced in CAVHDF and CVVHDF by increasing the dialysate flow rate to 2 L/h (11).

Combining convection and diffusion allows flexibility in enhancing clearances by increasing the volume of ultrafiltrate or the dialysate flow rates. Using this method, we have had mean BUN clearances in the range of 23 to 30 mL/min even in hypotensive patients (100). The advantage of this approach over diffusive techniques alone is that convective transfer contributes to middle-molecule clearance, an important factor in removing the mediators seen in ARF, such as tumor necrosis factor (TNF) and interleukin 1 (IL-1) (38,101,102).

An additional consideration is that, unlike intermittent techniques, the dose of dialysis delivered in CRRT is not time dependent. In intermittent techniques, hemodynamic instability, shortened dialysis times, and logistic factors often impact adversely on the dose delivered. In patients with ARF, Paganini et al. (103) found that 65.4% of all intermittent hemodialysis treatments resulted in lower Kt/V than prescribed. In a subsequent study the same group reported that nonsurvivors had a significantly lower dose of dialysis delivered than survivors (104). In practice, this shortcoming largely goes unrecognized, and probably contributes to decreased solute clearance.

Drug Removal

Because convective transfer is the main mechanism of solute removal in CAVH and CVVH, the disposition of patients on drugs largely depends on the sieving coefficient of the drug, the degree of protein binding, and the UF rate. Several investigators have described the pharmacokinetics of different drugs in CRRT and developed guidelines for dosing (105–108). The effect of these therapies on newer antibiotics, cardiac drugs, and other agents has also been studied (89-91,109–121). Table 13.6 lists current recommendations on drug dosing in CRRT (108).

Fluid Management

Continuous renal replacement techniques have two inherent characteristics that allow them to be used as highly effective methods for fluid control: (a) the use of highly permeable membranes and (b) the continuous nature of the techniques. Both of these factors permit fluid removal that is limited only by the primary driving force (mean arterial pressure for nonpumped systems, pump speed for pumped systems) and the efficacy of the filter over time.

TABLE 13.6. DRUG DOSING IN CRRT

Drug	Normal Dosage (mg/day)	Dose in CRRT (mg)
Amikacin	1,050	250 QD to BID
Netilmycin	420	100–150 QD
Tobramycin	350	100 QD
Vancomycin	2,000	500 QD to BID
Ceftazidime	6,000	1,000 BID
Cefotaxime	12,000	2,000 BID
Ceftriaxone	4,000	2,000 QD
Ciprofloxacin	400	200 QD
Imipenem	4,000	500 TID to QID
Metronidazole	2,100	500 TID to QID
Piperacillin	24,000	4,000 TID
Digoxin	0.29	0.10 QD
Phenobarbital	233	100 BID to QID
Phenytoin	524	250 QD to BID
Theophylline	720	600–900 QD

Modified from Kroh UF, et al. Management of drug dosing in continuous renal replacement therapy. *Semin Dial* 1996;9:161–165.
Note: Reflects doses for CVVH with UFR 20–30 mL/min.

Fluid Balance

The ability to remove large volumes of fluid can be manipulated in several different ways for fluid balance (122). There are three levels of intervention, each with its advantages and disadvantages (Table 13.7). In level 1 the ultrafiltrate volume obtained is limited to match the anticipated needs for fluid balance. This calls for an estimate of the amount of fluid to be removed over 8 to 24 hours and subsequent calculation of the UF rate. This strategy is similar to that commonly used for intermittent hemodialysis and differs only in that the time to remove fluid is 24 hours instead of 3 to 4 hours. For example, if it is estimated that 4 L of fluid need to be removed over a 24-hour period, the UF rate is set at approximately 170 mL/h. With this method the CRRT technique is used essentially as a means of achieving a fixed output per hour but no attempt is made to manipulate the UF rate or accommodate changes in fluid intake. As a consequence, replacement fluid may not be used and net fluid balance achieved may vary significantly from desired balance at the end of the time period. In some instances no attempt is made to set a particular ultrafiltrate rate, and fluid removed at the end of each time period (8 to 24 hours) is simply tabulated and listed as an output. Thus there is minimal control for fluid management.

In level 2 the ultrafiltrate volume every hour is deliberately set to be greater than the hourly intake and net fluid balance is achieved by hourly replacement fluid administration. In this method a greater degree of control is possible and fluid balance can be set to achieve any desired outcome. The success of this method depends on the ability to achieve UF rates, which always exceed the anticipated intake. This allows flexibility in manipulation of the fluid balance so that for any given hour the fluid status could be net negative, positive, or even. A key advantage of this technique is that the net fluid balance achieved at the end of every hour is truly a reflection of the desired outcome. For instance, as described in the example previously, if 4 L of fluid are to be removed over 24 hours, the desired outcome

TABLE 13.7. APPROACHES FOR FLUID MANAGEMENT IN CRRT

	Level 1	Level 2	Level 3
UF volume	Limited	>intake	>intake
Replacement	Minimal	Adjusted to achieve fluid balance	Adjusted to achieve fluid balance
Fluid balance	8 hour	Hourly	Hourly targeted
UF pump	Yes	Yes/No	Yes/No
Examples	SCUF, CAVHD, CVVHD	CAVH, CVVH, CAV/VVHDF	CAVHDF, CVVHDF, CVVH
Advantages			
Simplicity	+++	++	+
Achieve fluid balance	+	+++	+++
Regulate volume changes	+	++	+++
CRRT as support	+	++	+++
Disadvantages			
Nursing effort	+	++	+++
Errors in fluid balance	+++	++	+
Hemodynamic instability	++	++	+

+, least; ++, intermediate; +++, greatest.

every hour is 170 mL/h. This implies that the UF rate should be ≥ 170 mL/h + intake every hour. The net fluid balance desired may or may not be achievable; however, this method permits control of overall fluid management using the CRRT technique. The amount of replacement fluid needed to achieve fluid balance is easily calculated using a flow sheet.

Level 3 extends the concept of the level 2 intervention to target the desired net balance every hour to achieve a specific hemodynamic parameter (e.g., central venous pressure [CVP], pulmonary artery wedge pressure [PAWP], or mean arterial pressure). Once a desired value for the hemodynamic parameter is determined, fluid balance can be linked to that value. For example, if it is desirable to keep a patient's PAWP between 14 and 16, a sliding scale for hourly fluid management can be formulated so that for PAWP values of 12 to 14, net fluid balance is maintained at zero; for values greater than 14, fluid is removed; and for values less than 12, fluid is replaced. In essence, this method maximally utilizes the capacity of CRRT techniques to control fluids. A key issue to recognize here is that by incorporating this level, CRRT techniques have tremendous flexibility and are not simply devices for fluid removal but allow overall control of fluid management as fluid regulatory devices. This external control is a key advantage over intermittent hemodialysis. Additionally, it can be viewed as an advantage over the normal kidney wherein limited control is possible. In general, greater control calls for more effort, however, and may result in improved outcomes.

We have used this method successfully in several cases to target intervention and fine-tune fluid removal without compromising cardiac output. By incorporating level 3 intervention, CRRT becomes tremendously flexible—not simply a device for fluid removal but a means of overall control of fluid management. Not only is this external control a key advantage over intermittent hemodialysis, but it approaches the filtration capacity of the normal kidney (with which only limited external control is possible).

CRRT versus Intermittent Techniques

Although CRRT uses the same forces for solute and fluid removal as intermittent techniques, operationally it is quite different. As shown in Table 13.8 the major difference is that time is no longer a limiting factor for blood purification. As a consequence, it is possible to use slower blood and dialysate flow rates to achieve weekly clearances that are equivalent, and often superior, to intermittent techniques. Recently, several investigators have used longer-duration intermittent hemodialysis with lower dialysate flow rates. The procedures are termed *extended daily dialysis* (EDD) (28) or *slow, low-efficiency dialysis* (SLED) (29). Both techniques rely on diffusive clearance and can easily achieve metabolic control; however, the intermittent nature of the procedure may not allow as efficient a fluid balance as with CRRT. No direct comparisons have been done of EDD and SLED and CRRT.

TABLE 13.8. FLUID MANAGEMENT IN CRRT: FLOWSHEET COMPUTATIONS

	06	07	08	09	10	11	12	13	14	8 Hour Total
1A. UF output	2,000	1,900	1,700	1,400						
1B. Dialysate infused	1,000	1,000	1,000	1,000						
1C. Actual UF out	1,000	900	700	400						
2. Additional out	400	200	200	200						
3. Total out	1,400	1,100	900	600						
4. All intake except replacement	200	400	400	600						
5. Hourly fluid balance	−1,200	−700	−500	0						
6. Desired outcome	−100	+200	0	−100						
7. Calculated replacement	1,100	900	500	0						
8. Actual net balance	**−100**	**+200**	**0**	**0**						

A major difference between these methods lies in their ability to dissociate solute removal (e.g., sodium) from fluid balance. As an example, with CRRT, varying the composition of the replacement fluid or dialysate can alter the solute balance, whereas the fluid balance can be kept net even, negative, or positive. This latter feature, the capacity to fine-tune fluid balance on an ongoing basis, makes CRRT far more versatile than intermittent techniques (122,123).

In contrast to intermittent techniques, in which, by necessity, the fluid balance depends on the time available to remove fluid, CRRT makes targeted intervention for fluid balance possible, to achieve any particular hemodynamic parameter. We have found that the flexibility provided by this method allows appropriate management of complex patients who could not be treated effectively by intermittent techniques.

APPLICATIONS

Continuous therapies provide all the common features of intermittent hemodialysis, but they are best used in the setting of an intensive care unit (ICU). Because fluid and solute removal is continuous and can be controlled easily, these methods have a significant advantage in the hemodynamically unstable patient. In addition to providing renal replacement, these techniques permit unlimited fluid administration, thereby allowing nutritional repletion in critically ill patients.

Patients with ARF in the presence of multiple organ failure, sepsis, burns, or cardiogenic shock are all likely to be better managed with these methods. With ARF, an important management consideration is defining the goals of therapy. Several issues must be considered, including the timing of the intervention, the amount and frequency of dialysis, and the duration of therapy. In practice, no set criteria are followed, and these decisions are based on individual preferences and experience

(124–126). Dialytic intervention in ARF is usually considered when there is clinical evidence of uremic symptoms or biochemical evidence of solute and fluid imbalance. Most nephrologists will intervene with dialysis if patients have BUN values greater than 100 mg/dL, hyperkalemia or marked acidosis, evidence of fluid overload unresponsive to diuretics, central nervous system manifestations, a pericardial rub, or gastrointestinal hemorrhage attributed to uremia (127). Unfortunately, there is no consensus on the timing of intervention for ARF.

In ESRD, dialysis is usually not initiated until creatinine clearances are less than 5 mL/min (range, 5 to 10 mL/min) or the patient is symptomatic. Although these criteria are often extrapolated to ARF, they are problematic; in treating ESRD the aim is to keep the patient off dialysis as long as possible, but in ARF the strategy is to minimize and avoid uremic complications. With ARF, therefore, it is not necessary to wait for progressive uremia before initiating dialytic support. Clearly, our current practices in this area need reappraisal.

Treatment must recognize that the patient with ARF is somewhat different than the one with ESRD. The rapid decline of renal function associated with multiple-organ failure does not permit the adaptive response that characterizes the course of the patient with ESRD. In consequence, the traditional indications for renal replacement may need to be redefined. For instance, excessive volume resuscitation, a common strategy used for multiple-organ failure, may be an indication for dialysis even in the absence of significant elevations in BUN.

It may be more appropriate to consider dialytic intervention in the ICU patient as a form of renal support rather than as renal replacement. This term distinguishes ICU intervention as providing support for all the organs, rather than replacing one organ's function. Table 13.9 lists some of the revised indications for dialytic intervention using this approach.

CRRT is particularly well suited to provide renal support in the ICU patient. The freedom to provide continuous fluid man-

TABLE 13.9. COMPARISON OF DIALYSIS PRESCRIPTION AND DOSE DELIVERED IN CRRT AND IHD

	IHD	CRRT
Dialysis Prescription		
Membrane characteristics	Variable permeability	High permeability
Anticoagulation	Short duration	Prolonged
Blood flow rate	≥200 mL/min	<200 mL/min
Dialysate flow	≥500 mL/min	17–34 mL/min
Duration	3–4 hours	Days
Clearance	High	Low
Dialysis Dose Delivered		
Patient factors		
Hemodynamic instability	+++	+
Recirculation	+++	+
Infusions	++	+
Technique factors		
Blood flow	+++	++
Concentration repolarization	+	+++
Membrane clotting	+	+++
Duration	+++	+
Other Factors		
Nursing errors	+	+++
Interference	+	+++

agement permits the application of unlimited nutrition, the adjustment of hemodynamic parameters, and the achievement of steady-state solute control, which are difficult with intermittent therapies. It is thus possible to widen the indications for renal intervention and provide a customized approach for the management of each patient.

Patient selection for CRRT should ideally be based on a careful consideration of multiple factors (124,128,129). The general principle is to provide adequate renal support without adversely affecting the patient. Some of the factors that should influence the selection of CRRT for any given patient are discussed in the next section.

Indications for Renal Replacement

The primary indication for dialytic intervention can be a major determinant of the therapy chosen, because different therapies vary in their efficacy for solute and fluid removal. In the ICU, indications for renal replacement are more diverse and more amenable to modification based on the clinical situation. For instance, if the indication for dialysis is to facilitate the removal of a drug such as theophylline in a patient with a drug overdose, intermittent hemodialysis is a logical choice, given its efficacy and rapidity of response. If the indication is fluid removal in a hemodynamically unstable postsurgical cardiac patient, CRRT is preferable.

In most patients, however, the indication for dialysis may not be as clear-cut, and both solute and fluid removal are desired. In such situations, the course of the desired response must also influence the decision. For example, life-threatening hyperkalemia in an otherwise stable patient is probably better treated with intermittent hemodialysis, whereas in a catabolic patient with ARF who is hemodynamically stable the selection would need to be based on other criteria.

Presence of Other Organ Failure

When ARF complicates the course of a critically ill patient in the ICU, it worsens the prognosis and increases mortality (45,130–135). In this setting, ARF is usually associated with multiple-organ failure, which can influence the choice of renal replacement therapy in two ways. First, multiple-organ failure may limit the choice of therapies. For example, patients with abdominal surgery may not be suitable for peritoneal dialysis because it increases the risk of wound dehiscence and infection (136–138). Patients who are hemodynamically unstable may not tolerate intermittent hemodialysis (4,139–141). Second, the requirement for anticoagulation depends on the presence of coagulation abnormalities. Peritoneal dialysis avoids anticoagulation, and intermittent hemodialysis can be performed with saline flushes. In contrast, CRRT is difficult without anticoagulation.

Additionally, the impact of the chosen therapy on compromised organ systems is an important consideration. In the patient with acute brain injury requiring renal replacement therapy, the conventional intermittent hemodialysis may exacerbate the injury by compromising cerebral perfusion pressure, either by a reduction in cerebral perfusion or because of increased cerebral edema (142). Rapid removal of solutes and fluid, as occurs with intermittent hemodialysis, can result in a disequilibrium

syndrome and worsen neurologic status. In acute peritoneal dialysis, the instillation of large volumes into the peritoneal cavity can have an adverse effect on pulmonary function, resulting in an increased alveolar–arterial oxygen gradient and basal atelectasis with a net reduction in PaO_2 (143). In addition, sudden changes in intraperitoneal volume, such as draining out, may result in cardiovascular instability because of changes in cardiac filling pressures and systemic vascular resistance (144). Peritoneal dialysis may be attractive in ARF that is a complication of acute pancreatitis, but it would contribute to additional protein losses in the hypoalbuminemia patient with liver failure (144). Continuous therapies provide better hemodynamic stability, but if they are not monitored carefully they can lead to significant volume depletion. As discussed earlier, providing overall support for the patient with multiple-organ failure should be the primary goal.

Access

Lack of appropriate vascular access limits the use of continuous therapies. If arterial access cannot be obtained, CAVH and CAVHD cannot be performed and CVVH or CVVHDF must be considered. Similarly, the availability of appropriate venous access is crucial for intermittent hemodialysis. The variety of vascular catheters now available obviates the need for surgical access. If vascular access cannot be obtained, peritoneal dialysis may be the only alternative, particularly in the pediatric patient (145). Using the appropriate type of catheter and insertion technique is important to minimize complications (146).

Patient Mobility

A major consideration in the choice of therapy is the patient's mobility requirements. If the patient must be moved on or from the bed for tests, procedures, or trips to the operating room, continuous therapies become more difficult. The use of arterial access for CAVH and CAVHD restricts patient ambulation. In pumped CRRT, the pumps currently available are not equipped with battery packs, thereby making patient transportation difficult.

Anticipated Duration of Treatment

Renal replacement for ARF is based on the premise that kidney function will return and that dialysis can be discontinued. However, this desired outcome does not always occur. This is particularly true for the patient with ARF and multiple-organ failure, in whom the ultimate prognosis depends on the recovery of other organ systems. In these patients, dialytic support may only prolong the time to death, so it must be instituted only when the goals and end point of therapy have been defined (45,131,147–149).

A "trial" of dialysis therapy should be negotiated with the patient's family and other critical care personnel. A trial period will facilitate the withdrawal of dialysis should there be no likelihood of recovery. For instance, an elderly patient with respiratory, cardiac, and liver failure secondary to sepsis who requires dialytic support for ARF should have a finite period of dialysis (1 to 2 weeks) and should be reassessed for evidence of improvement in all organ systems. If there is no likelihood of recovery,

TABLE 13.10. POTENTIAL APPLICATIONS FOR CONTINUOUS RENAL REPLACEMENT THERAPY

Renal Replacement	Renal Support	Nonrenal Applications
Acute renal failure	Fluid management	Cytokine removal, ? sepsis
Chronic renal failure	Solute control	Heart failure
	Acid–base adjustments	Cancer chemotherapy
	Nutrition	Liver support

withdrawal of dialysis must be considered. The location of the patient (ICU or non-ICU) is an additional determinant of therapy, because CRRT should only be performed where constant monitoring and one-to-one nursing is available.

Nonrenal Applications of CRRT

As shown in Table 13.10, there is increasing interest in using CRRT for indications other than renal failure (3,38,150). For example, CRRT may provide an important benefit to septic patients with multiple-organ failure as a method of renal support, but it remains to be seen if additional applications as a specific therapy for sepsis can be supported.

Using CRRT as a therapeutic technique for modulating the inflammatory response to sepsis has been the primary focus of research into additional applications (38,101,151–154). Although a fair amount of experimental evidence supports the potential role of hemofiltration in sepsis, the results with clinical trials exploring the use of CRRT and other combination methods for treating sepsis have largely been unsuccessful (92,155–159). At the current time use of these methods to treat sepsis in the absence of acute renal failure cannot be recommended. Other investigators have used CRRT for regional chemotherapy, harnessing the adsorptive capacity of the membrane to remove chemotherapeutic agents (160–164). This appears to be an emerging application of CRRT. Similar CRRT applications using antibody-coated microspheres or polymyxin-impregnated membranes to remove endotoxin are currently under development (165,166).

Another group of patients ideally suited to CRRT consists of those with significant cardiac disease and diuretic-resistant congestive heart failure. The fluid removal capacity of CRRT has been shown to restore dry weight, improve urinary output, decrease neurohumoral activation, and prolong symptom- and edema-free time. The possible mechanisms of action of such beneficial effects include decreased myocardial edema, a decrease in left ventricular end diastolic pressure with optimization of the Starling relationship and increased myocardial performance, and the removal of circulating myocardial depressant factors (167–172).

Another important area for application is the therapy of inborn errors of metabolism in infants (173,174). CRRT can be used more efficiently than intermittent hemodialysis to support metabolic function, allowing an opportunity for more definitive treatments.

RESULTS WITH CONTINUOUS TECHNIQUES

Currently, there is only limited information comparing CRRT with intermittent hemodialysis. Therefore the choice of inter-

mittent or continuous therapy is largely based on the availability of CRRT and the familiarity of the nephrologist and other personnel, particularly ICU staff, with the procedure. In centers where CRRT is routinely done, this choice is usually based on the nephrologist's experience. In general, the results obtainable by CRRT must be compared to those obtainable by intermittent hemodialysis, the gold standard.

Efficacy

Solute Control

Most patients with ARF in the ICU are hypercatabolic, with protein catabolic rates (PCR) greater than 2 g/kg; thus these patients have an extremely high urea generation rate. In such cases, standard alternate-day intermittent hemodialysis is usually insufficient to maintain BUN levels below 80 mg/dL (130,175,176). Because continuous therapies provide renal replacement 24 hours a day, BUN levels are significantly lower than with intermittent therapies (176). Clark et al. (177) reported steady-state BUN levels of 79 mg/dL on CVVH, in comparison to peak BUN levels of 101 mg/dL on intermittent hemodialysis.

Among the continuous therapies, CAVH alone is inadequate for small-solute removal (178–180), and it may not be able to maintain BUN concentrations below 120 to 150 mg/dL in severely catabolic patients. In our experience, continuous HDF techniques (CAVHDF, CVVHDF) provide better fluid and solute control than CAVHD or CVVHD. We have routinely achieved solute control with urea clearances ranging from 23 to 30 mL/min in hypercatabolic patients (181). Similar results have been obtained by other investigators using CVVH. Macias et al. (182) used CVVH in 25 patients and achieved solute control in all but one hypercatabolic patient. In a recent series of 250 CVVH patients treated over 10 years, no patient required additional hemodialysis for solute control (128). Van Bommel et al. similarly found lower steady-state solute levels in CVVHDF in contrast to intermittent hemodialysis.

Although it is clear that lower solute concentrations can be achieved with CRRT, whether this is an important criterion impacting on various outcomes from ARF still needs to be determined. In a recent retrospective analysis, van Bommel (183) found no difference in BUN levels among survivors and nonsurvivors with ARF. As discussed earlier, the findings of a lower Kt/V for BUN in nonsurvivors is intriguing; however, these findings should be considered preliminary, as the assumptions for computing Kt/V equivalents in ARF may not be valid (31). Ronco et al. (148) recently demonstrated an improved survival in critically ill patients with ARF treated with CVVH with UF rates of 35 mL/kg/h compared with 20 mL/kg/h. Their results are promising; however, they need to be confirmed at other centers.

Fluid Management

Fluid removal is a desirable component of any renal replacement therapy and is a major goal of renal replacement for ARF (184). There is some evidence that volume overload may be an independent contributor to mortality in ICU patients, thus making it an important factor even in the absence of uremia (185). Fluid removal in intermittent hemodialysis is easily achieved in most cases; however, the rate of fluid removal has to be high and the process must be completed in 3 to 4 hours every day. As a consequence, large shifts in fluid balance generally result, contributing to hemodynamic instability (122,141,186,187).

Additionally, fluid removal, and hence fluid balance, is limited to the period of dialysis. If the patient is hemodynamically unstable during this period, it may be difficult to remove any fluid. By contrast, CRRT has the advantage of providing renal replacement continuously, so fluid removal or replacement can be precisely adjusted for each patient (122,188). A mean UF rate of 3 to 4 mL/min will permit fluid losses of 4.3 to 5.7 L in 24 hours, which is usually sufficient to maintain fluid balance in most patients. We usually aim for UF rates of 17 to 20 mL/min to improve convective clearance and to replace part or all of this volume every hour to achieve a net fluid balance (123,124). Because the process is gradual, hemodynamic stability is easily maintained.

These therapies allow ongoing modulation of fluid balance and targeted fluid management. The high efficacy of these therapies in continuous fluid removal recommends them for use in other situations besides renal failure (38,150,189,190).

Hemodynamic Stability

Intermittent hemodialysis relies on diffusion to transport solutes and fluid across a semipermeable membrane. This type of transport usually results in large, rapid alterations in fluid and solutes over a short period, so hemodynamic instability, reflected by hypotension and cardiac arrhythmias, is encountered in approximately 25% to 50% of dialysis patients (191–193).

A major area of concern is that episodes of hypotension during dialysis can impact negatively on renal and patient outcome (194). This concern has largely arisen from observations that ARF patients who underwent intensive dialysis and were subsequently biopsied showed fresh lesions of tubular necrosis that were likely to have resulted during dialysis (195,196). With the availability of volumetric-controlled, precise UF, control is possible; however, dialysis-induced hypotension can still occur (see Chapter 19). Most patients treated with CRRT are more hemodynamically stable and tolerate the procedure well (197). Manns et al. (194) have shown that the incidence of hypotensive episodes during CRRT is significantly lower than comparable periods of intermittent hemodialysis. Additionally, these decreases in blood pressure appear to be associated with a decrease in renal function as measured by creatinine clearances.

In continuous therapies using arteriovenous circuits there will be an automatic decrease in UF if the patient becomes hypotensive because the driving force is the mean arterial pres-

sure. This decrease in UF tends to limit volume losses and improve hemodynamic stability. Pumped continuous therapy has a greater potential for hypotension, but most patients remain stable (95). Macias et al. (182) found four episodes of volume-responsive hypotension during 193.5 treatment days of CVVH. Similarly, Bellomo et al. (176) found no periods of hemodynamic instability in more than 9,000 hours of continuous hemodiafiltration. Although CRRT appears to have lower complication rates, these may be underestimated, since it is often difficult to ascertain if the complication was due to the therapy or to the patient's underlying hemodynamic state (123).

Effect on Nutrition

Continuous therapies have a major advantage over intermittent hemodialysis in permitting unlimited nutrition because fluid removal is not a limiting factor. Bartlett et al. (198) found that nutritional status was better in patients on CAVH. Similarly, Chima et al. (199) found that nutritional status improved in all 16 patients on CAVH, although 14 were in negative nitrogen. In our experience, CRRT allows better nutritional support—we were able to match or exceed the nutritional goals for patients treated with this modality—whereas this was not possible in patients on intermittent hemodialysis (100). Other investigators have had similar results (200,201). Urea kinetics in eight patients on CVVH revealed that the normalized protein catabolic rate (nPCR) was 1.46 ± 0.54 g/kg/d (mean ± SD) and that the nitrogen deficit was large (more than 8 g/d), reflecting deficiencies in nonprotein energy administration (202).

Recent studies have further explored the benefit of aggressive nutrition support using these techniques. Bellomo et al. (203) found that although it was possible to deliver protein in excess of 2.5 g/kg, there was no additional benefit on outcome, and steady-state BUN levels were higher.

In the overall nutritional balance of the patient, two other factors need to be recognized. The dialysate fluid used in CAVHD is 0.5% to 2.5% glucose, which can be absorbed during the procedure (154 to 270 g/d) and contributes to the caloric load (12,204,205). This glucose content is also associated with an increase in endogenous insulin secretion in most patients, and some patients may require exogenous insulin (204). We routinely modify the nutritional prescription to take into account the caloric contribution of CRRT (206).

A second nutritional factor is the loss of amino acids across the filter that range from 2.7 to 8.9 g at low flow rates (less than 102 g/d) to 30 g at higher flow rates (206,207). Losses appear to depend more on the serum levels than on the underlying clinical status of the patient. Other investigators have found that patients with ARF have low concentrations of several amino acids; further, losses that occur across the filter are predictably dependent on the dialysate flow rate. It is thus important to modify the nutritional prescription to provide enough amino acids to compensate for this loss (usually 14 to 16 g of nitrogen in total parenteral nutrition [TPN]) (207–209). Other investigators have reviewed this area and suggested guidelines for the nutritional support of the patient with ARF (210–212).

The composition of the dialysate and replacement fluid is an important factor to be considered. Lactate-based dialysis and hemofiltration solutions may result in hyperlactatemia and worsening of acid–base status. Additionally, the lactate-buffered substitution fluids used in CAVH tend to have higher urea generation rates than bicarbonate solutions (80,213,214).

Outcome

Despite significant advances in the management of ARF over the last four decades, the perception is that the associated mortality has not changed significantly (215–218). Recent publications suggest that there may have been some improvement during the last decade (219–221). Intermittent hemodialysis and peritoneal dialysis were the main therapies until a decade ago, and they improved the outcome from the 100% mortality of ARF to its current level.

The effect of continuous renal replacement therapy on overall patient outcome is still unclear. Table 13.11 summarizes the results from the major studies using CRRT and the actual mortality figures. Some investigators record hospital discharge as an outcome, whereas others have used a definition of ICU survival, resulting in differences in mortality statistics. The absence of an effect on mortality may represent an initial bias in patient selection because, in general, continuous therapies have until recently been given only to patients who were hemodynamically unstable and "too sick" to receive intermittent hemodialysis (1,124,222). In this situation CRRT is likely to be used infrequently at best and would result in an increased likelihood of failure purely from lack of expertise with the procedure.

A recent study of 250 patients treated with CAVH/CVVH from 1981 to 1991 found a significant relationship between outcome and the accession number marking entrance into the study. The authors used a logistic regression model with an odds ratio of mortality of 1.00 for the first 50 patients and found that the ratio dropped to 0.195 for the last 50 (95% confidence interval 0.06 to 0.61), suggesting that improvements in technique and its continued use may be responsible (128).

Critical evaluation of CRRT in comparison with intermittent hemodialysis is scanty (223). Sieberth (224) found that continuous therapies reduced mortality in high-risk patients but were not superior to intermittent therapy. However, there is little information regarding the impact of these therapies in a controlled trial. Kierdorf (225) retrospectively compared 73 patients

treated by continuous hemofiltration over 2 years with 73 patients treated with intermittent hemodialysis, and found a significantly lower mortality in the CVVH group (57 deaths) versus the intermittent hemodialysis group (68 deaths). Jakob et al. (226) have recently reviewed 15 studies comparing intermittent hemodialysis (522 patients) to CRRT (651 patients) and did not find any evidence for an improved outcome from CRRT. However, the same authors found that a review of 67 published studies using CRRT revealed a trend to decreasing mortality despite no change in the mean Apache II scores. Another retrospective study (227) from a single center also demonstrated a higher mortality with CVVH that was related to the choice of therapy in more severely ill patients.

We conducted a multicenter randomized controlled trial comparing intermittent hemodialysis to CRRT for the treatment of ARF in 166 patients (IHD = 82, CRRT = 84) (100). We found that intermittent hemodialysis resulted in a lower mortality (41.5%) than occurred with CRRT (59.5%). However, despite the randomization process, patients allocated to CRRT had a higher severity of illness scores at baseline. Adjusting for the differences in baseline characteristics resulted in both groups having similar mortality. Renal functional recovery overall was similar in both groups; however, complete renal recovery in survivors was significantly better in the CRRT group. Although we and others have been unable to demonstrate an advantage of these therapies in influencing mortality, we believe this may represent the difficulty in changing a global outcome that is impacted by several other factors (228). It is probably more relevant to focus on other outcomes, such as renal functional recovery, rather than mortality (229).

We believe that continued research is required in this area, but there appears to be enough evidence to support the use of CRRT as an alternative therapy, potentially preferable to intermittent hemodialysis, in treating ARF in the ICU. Recent meta-analysis of studies comparing CRRT to IHD support this concept (230).

Procedure-Related Complications

Complications associated with continuous therapies are mostly the result of the potential for volume depletion, particularly if monitoring is inadequate and calculations are inac-

TABLE 13.11. MORTALITY IN ARF: COMPARISON OF CRRT VERSUS IHD

Authors	Type of Study	IHD (N)	% Mortality	CRRT (N)	% Mortality	Change (%)	P Value
Mauritz 1986	Retrospective	31	90	27	70	−20	ns
Alarabi 1989	Retrospective	40	55	40	45	−10	ns
Mehta 1991	Retrospective	24	85	18	72	−13	ns
Kierdorf 1991	Retrospective	73	93	73	77	−16	<.05
Bellomo 1992	Retrospective	167	70	84	59	−11	ns
Bellomo 1993	Retrospective	84	70	76	45	−25	<.01
Kruczynski 1993	Retrospective	23	82	12	33	−49	<.01
Simpson 1993	Prospective	58	82	65	70	−12	ns
Kierdorf 1994	Prospective	47	65	48	60	−4.5	ns
Mehta 1996	Prospective	82	41.5	84	59.5	+18	ns

Modified from Kierdorf M, et al. Continuous treatment modalities in acute renal failure. *Nephrol Dial Transplant* 1995;10:2001–2008.

curate (6,123). Because large volumes of fluid can be removed quickly, meticulous monitoring is essential and requires a nurse-to-patient ratio of at least 1:1, if not more (122). Access-related problems with arterial catheters include peripheral embolism and dissection, resulting in limb ischemia. Fortunately, embolism and dissection are rare, but we emphasize that arterial catheters should be of appropriate size and should be placed by experienced personnel (17,19,190). Connections should be taped to prevent accidental disconnection. Because CRRT requires anticoagulation for longer periods, the risk for complications related to anticoagulation is higher, although this has not been the case in our experience (49,56,77,191).

Hypothermia is a common feature of CRRT, as the replacement fluids and dialysate are usually not warmed enough and lead to core temperature cooling (150,192,231–233). Cooler temperature fluids can be beneficial in some patients as a means of reducing body temperature (150,193). A major concern is that the continuous nature of these therapies provides a greater opportunity for manipulation by inexperienced personnel. In our experience, standardizing the protocols for use of these therapies and restricting their use to trained personnel can limit undesirable incidents of this nature.

Cost

Information on the costs of the two techniques is scanty. Most investigators have found that CRRT costs are somewhat greater than those for intermittent hemodialysis (149,183,234). Our experience suggests that the major difference is the cost of supplies for CRRT. For intermittent hemodialysis, the costs for supplies such as hemofilters, tubing, and dialysate are significantly discounted in most centers for bulk buying, because the same membranes are used for ESRD patients (100). In contrast, hemofilters for CRRT are usually priced three to four times higher than comparable intermittent hemodialysis filters. Recent randomized prospective studies give evidence of the true cost differences between CRRT and IHD. When comparing direct costs for randomized patients in the San Diego study, IHD led to an aggregate cost of $3,077, and CRRT had a cost of $3,946 for 8.4 treatments and 7.9 treatments, respectively. The cost analysis for labor and materials per treatment showed that the labor costs were comparable between these two therapies. There was a significant difference in material costs, with IHD costing $66 per treatment and CRRT costing $338. This study would suggest that cost differences are real and are approximately $250 to $300 per treatment. This disparity may be greatly reduced if continuous therapy is used more frequently, allowing for further reduction in filter prices. The advantages of better nutrition, better fluid balance, and easier management of hemodynamics should outweigh the additional cost (1,235–237). It has also been our experience that physician time is greater for CRRT, but this represents a learning curve in using these techniques. In our institution, we have standardized protocols and have found that as physicians become experienced with CRRT the time required is reduced. Whether these techniques are cost-effective still requires further research.

THE FUTURE

As experience with CRRT grows, innovations in technology will likely keep pace. Over the last decade, most of the major manufacturers of dialysis equipment have developed new pumps dedicated for these techniques. Most of these devices (Gambro/ Hospal Prisma; Baxter Accura) offer automated fluid balancing and sophisticated controls that are similar to those in standard dialysis machines (238). Membrane technology is also evolving, and antithrombogenic membranes are on the horizon. Recent work in the area of blood flow monitoring suggests that future CRRT machines may include ultrasound blood flow measurement. Such flow measurements can be computer-linked to the blood pump to ensure correct blood flow, and a screen display could represent this flow pictorially (239). Furthermore, on-line monitoring of filtrate may be used to indicate urea clearance as a continuous display to clinicians during therapy (240).

Finally, the application of these therapies is likely to expand to other areas, including the treatment of sepsis (7,241–244), congestive heart failure (190,245), and multiple-organ failure (150,246); a form of liver support (247,248); and cardiopulmonary bypass for cytokine manipulation (168,249–252). It remains to be seen how these therapies will change our current management of these patient groups.

SUMMARY

CRRT is rapidly emerging as a viable alternative to intermittent hemodialysis for the management of the critically ill patient with acute renal failure. Several different methods are now available and can be adapted to fit any given situation. We believe that these methods should be considered as part of the nephrologist's therapeutic tools in the management of ARF. Further research is required to identify the patient populations most likely to benefit, and to define criteria for appropriate timing of intervention with these therapies. It is apparent that the next few years will be an exciting time in the development of these therapies and will undoubtedly provide opportunities for exploring uncharted areas.

REFERENCES

1. Ronco C, et al. Continuous renal replacement techniques. *Contrib Nephrol* 2001;132:236–251.
2. Oda S, et al. Continuous hemofiltration/hemodiafiltration in critical care. *Ther Apher* 2002;6:193–198.
3. Kornecki A, et al. Continuous renal replacement therapy for non-renal indications: experience in children. *Isr Med Assoc J* 2002;4:345–348.
4. Flynn JT. Choice of dialysis modality for management of pediatric acute renal failure. *Pediatr Nephrol* 2002;17:61–69.
5. Weksler N, et al. Continuous venovenous hemofiltration improves intensive care unit, but not hospital survival rate, in nonoliguric septic patients. *J Crit Care* 2001;16:69–73.
6. Ronco C, et al. Continuous renal replacement therapy in critically ill patients. *Nephrol Dial Transpl* 2001;16(Suppl 5):67–72.
7. Bellomo R, et al. Blood purification in the intensive care unit: evolving concepts. *World J Surg* 2001;25:677–683.
8. Ronco C, et al. Acute dialysis quality initiative. *Blood Purif* 2001;19: 222–226.

9. Bellomo R, et al. Nomenclature for continuous renal replacement therapies. *Am J Kidney Dis* 1996;28:S32–S37.

10. Henderson L. Hemofiltration: from the origin to the new wave. *Am J Kidney Dis* 1996;28:S100–S104.

11. Sigler MH. Transport characteristics of the slow therapies: implications for achieving adequacy of dialysis in acute renal failure. *Adv Ren Replace Ther* 1997;4:68–80.

12. Sigler MH, et al. Solute transport in continuous hemodialysis: a new treatment for acute renal failure. *Kidney Int* 1987;32:562–571.

13. Kramer P. Continuous arteriovenous hemofiltration: a physiologic and effective kidney replacement therapy. *Contrib Nephrol* 1985;44: 236–247.

14. Olbricht CJ, et al. Continuous arteriovenous hemofiltration: in vivo functional characteristics and its dependence on vascular access and filter design. *Nephron* 1990;55:49–57.

15. Jenkins R, et al. Effects of access catheter dimensions on blood flow in continuous arteriovenous hemofiltration. *Contrib Nephrol* 1991; 93:171–174.

16. Ahmed Z. Introduction of percutaneous arteriovenous femoral shunt: a new access for continuous arteriovenous hemofiltration. *Am J Kidney Dis* 1990;16:115–117.

17. Tominaga GT, et al. Vascular complications of continuous arteriovenous hemofiltration in trauma patients. *J Trauma* 1993;35:285–288; discussion, 288–289.

18. Ronco C, et al. New CRRT systems: impact on dose delivery. *Am J Kidney Dis* 1997;30:S15–S19.

19. Wester JP, et al. Catheter replacement in continuous arteriovenous hemodiafiltration: the balance between infectious and mechanical complications. *Crit Care Med* 2002;30:1261–1266.

20. Ronco C, et al. Continuous renal replacement therapy: evolution in technology and current nomenclature. *Kidney Int* 1998;66(Suppl): S160–S164.

21. Sanchez C, et al. Continuous venovenous renal replacement therapy using a conventional infusion pump. *ASAIO J* 2001;47:321–324.

22. Moller Jensen D, et al. Continuous venovenous haemodialysis: a three-pump system. *Nephron* 1996;72:159–162.

23. Peachey TD, et al. Pump control of continuous arteriovenous haemodialysis. *Lancet* 1988;2:878.

24. Kitaevich Y, et al. Development of a high-precision continuous extracorporeal hemodiafiltration system. *Biomed Instrum Technol* 1993;27: 150–156.

25. Jenkins R, et al. Accuracy of intravenous infusion pumps in continuous renal replacement therapies. *ASAIO J* 1992;38:808–810.

26. Salifu MO, et al. A new method to control ultrafiltration in conventional continuous renal replacement therapy. *ASAIO J* 2001;47:389–391.

27. Baldwin IC, et al. Continuous hemofiltration: nursing perspectives in critical care. *New Horiz* 1995;3:738–747.

28. Kumar VA, et al. Extended daily dialysis: a new approach to renal replacement for acute renal failure in the intensive care unit. *Am J Kidney Dis* 2000;36:294–300.

29. Marshall MR, et al. Urea kinetics during sustained low-efficiency dialysis in critically ill patients requiring renal replacement therapy. *Am J Kidney Dis* 2002;39:556–570.

30. Sigler MH, et al. Membranes and devices used in continuous renal replacement therapy. *Semin Dial* 1996;9:98–106.

31. Clark WR, et al. CRRT efficiency and efficacy in relation to solute size. *Kidney Int* 1999;72(Suppl):S3–S7.

32. Brunet S, et al. Diffusive and convective solute clearances during continuous renal replacement therapy at various dialysate and ultrafiltration flow rates. *Am J Kidney Dis* 1999;34:486–492.

33. Relton S, et al. Dialysate and blood flow dependence of diffusive solute clearance during CVVHD. *ASAIO J* 1992;38:M691–M696.

34. Leypoldt J. Fouling of ultrafiltration and hemodialysis membranes by plasma proteins. *Blood Purif* 1994;12:285–291.

35. Jenkins RD, et al. Permeability decay in CAVH hemofilters. *ASAIO Trans* 1988;34:590–593.

36. Schaeffer J, et al. Long-term performance of hemofilters in continuous hemofiltration. *Nephron* 1996;72:155–158.

37. Journoris DSW. Continuous hemofiltration in patients with sepsis or multiorgan failure. *Semin Dial* 1996;9:173–178.

38. Sieberth HG, et al. Is cytokine removal by continuous hemofiltration feasible? *Kidney Int* 1999;72(Suppl):S79–S83.

39. Brophy PD, et al. AN-69 membrane reactions are pH-dependent and preventable. *Am J Kidney Dis* 2001;38:173–178.

40. Swinford RD, et al. Dialysis membrane adsorption during CRRT. *Am J Kidney Dis* 1997;30:S32–S37.

41. Barzilay E, et al. Use of extracorporeal supportive techniques as additional treatment for septic-induced multiple organ failure patients. *Crit Care Med* 1989;17:634–637.

42. Jaber BL, et al. Extracorporeal adsorbent-based strategies in sepsis. *Am J Kidney Dis* 1997;30:S44–S56.

43. Bunchman TE, et al. Continuous venovenous hemodiafiltration in infants and children. *Am J Kidney Dis* 1995;25:17–21.

44. Bishof NA, et al. Continuous hemodiafiltration in children. *Pediatrics* 1990;85:819–823.

45. Goldstein SL, et al. Outcome in children receiving continuous venovenous hemofiltration. *Pediatrics* 2001;107:1309–1312.

46. Headrick CL. Applications in continuous venous to venous hemofiltration: interactive pediatric case study. *Crit Care Nurs Clin North Am* 1998;10:215–217.

47. Zobel G, et al. Five years' experience with continuous extracorporeal renal support in paediatric intensive care. *Intensive Care Med* 1991; 17:315–319.

48. Webb AR, et al. Maintaining blood flow in the extracorporeal circuit. *Intensive Care Med* 1995;21:84–93.

49. Mehta RL. Anticoagulation during continuous renal replacement therapy. *ASAIO J* 1994;40:931–935.

50. Martin PY, et al. Anticoagulation in patients treated by continuous venovenous hemofiltration: a retrospective study. *Am J Kidney Dis* 1994;24:806–812.

51. Ward DM, et al. Extracorporeal management of acute renal failure patients at high risk of bleeding. *Kidney Int* 1993;41(Suppl): S237–S244.

52. Van de Wetering J, et al. Heparin use in continuous renal replacement procedures: the struggle between filter coagulation and patient hemorrhage. *J Am Soc Nephrol* 1996;7:145–150.

53. Schneider T, et al. Continuous haemofiltration with r-hirudin (lepirudin) as anticoagulant in a patient with heparin induced thrombocytopenia (HIT II). *Wien Klin Wochenschr* 2000;112:552–555.

54. Mehta RL, et al. Regional citrate anticoagulation for continuous arteriovenous hemodialysis: an update after 12 months. *Contrib Nephrol* 1991;93:210–214.

55. Palsson R, et al. Regional citrate anticoagulation in continuous venovenous hemofiltration in critically ill patients with a high risk of bleeding. *Kidney Int* 1999;55:1991–1997.

56. Thoenen M, et al. Regional citrate anticoagulation using a citrate-based substitution solution for continuous venovenous hemofiltration in cardiac surgery patients. *Wien Klin Wochenschr* 2002;114:108–114.

57. Hofmann RM, et al. A novel method for regional citrate anticoagulation in continuous venovenous hemofiltration (CVVHF). *Ren Fail* 2002;24:325–335.

58. Kutsogiannis DJ, et al. Regional citrate anticoagulation in continuous venovenous hemodiafiltration. *Am J Kidney Dis* 2000;35:802–811.

59. Tolwani AJ, et al. Simplified citrate anticoagulation for continuous renal replacement therapy. *Kidney Int* 2001;60:370–374.

60. Dworschak M, et al. Lifesaving citrate anticoagulation to bridge to danaparoid treatment. *Ann Thorac Surg* 2002;73:1626–1627.

61. Bunchman TE, et al. Pediatric hemofiltration: normocarb dialysate solution with citrate anticoagulation. *Pediatr Nephrol* 2002;17: 150–154.

62. Abramson S, et al. Anticoagulation in continuous renal replacement therapy. *Curr Opin Nephrol Hypertens* 1999;8:701–707.

63. Lorenzini JL, et al. Continuous hemofiltration with a low molecular weight heparin, enoxaparine: report on two cases. *Int J Clin Pharmacol Ther Toxicol* 1991;29:89–91.

64. Singer M, et al. Heparin clearance during continuous veno-venous haemofiltration. *Intensive Care Med* 1994;20:212–215.

65. Camici M, et al. Safety and efficacy anticoagulation in extracorporeal hemodialysis by simultaneous administration of low-dose prostacyclin and low molecular weight heparin. *Minerva Med* 1998;89:405–409.

66. Klotz KF, et al. Use of prostacyclin in patients with continuous hemofiltration after open heart surgery. *Contrib Nephrol* 1995;116: 136–139.

67. Zobel G, et al. Continuous arteriovenous hemofiltration in premature infants. *Crit Care Med* 1989;17:534–536.

68. Ponikvar R, et al. Use of prostacyclin as the only anticoagulant during continuous venovenous hemofiltration. *Contrib Nephrol* 1991;93: 218–220.

69. Langenecker SA, et al. Anticoagulation with prostacyclin and heparin during continuous venovenous hemofiltration. *Crit Care Med* 1994; 22:1774–1781.

70. Journois D, et al. Assessment of standardized ultrafiltrate production rate using prostacyclin in continuous venovenous hemofiltration. *Contrib Nephrol* 1991;93:202–204.

71. Davenport A, et al. Comparison of the use of standard heparin and prostacyclin anticoagulation in spontaneous and pump-driven extracorporeal circuits in patients with combined acute renal and hepatic failure. *Nephron* 1994;66:431–437.

72. Chong BH, et al. Orgaran in heparin-induced thrombocytopenia. *Haemostasis* 1992;22:85–91.

73. Palevsky PM, et al. Failure of low molecular weight dextran to prevent clotting during continuous renal replacement therapy. *ASAIO J* 1995; 41:847–849.

74. Kern H, et al. Bleeding after intermittent or continuous r-hirudin during CVVH. *Intensive Care Med* 1999;25:1311–1314.

75. Saner F, et al. Anticoagulation with hirudin for continuous venovenous hemodialysis in liver transplantation. *Acta Anaesthesiol Scand* 2001;45:914–918.

76. Frank RD, et al. Hirudin elimination by hemofiltration: a comparative in vitro study of different membranes. *Kidney Int* 1999;72 (Suppl):S41–S45.

77. Tan HK, et al. Continuous veno-venous hemofiltration without anticoagulation in high-risk patients. *Intensive Care Med* 2000;26: 1652–1657.

78. Stefanidis I, et al. Hemostatic alterations during continuous venovenous hemofiltration in acute renal failure. *Clin Nephrol* 1996;46: 199–205.

79. Davenport A. The coagulation system in the critically ill patient with acute renal failure and the effect of an extracorporeal circuit. *Am J Kidney Dis* 1997;30:S20–S27.

80. Davenport A. Dialysate and substitution fluids for patients treated by continuous forms of renal replacement therapy. *Contrib Nephrol* 2001;132:313–322.

81. Macias WA, et al. Acid base balance in continuous renal replacement therapy. *Semin Dial* 1996;9:145–151.

82. Palevsky P. Continuous renal replacement therapy component selection: replacement fluid and dialysate. *Semin Dial* 1996;9:107–111.

83. Zimmerman D, et al. Continuous veno-venous haemodialysis with a novel bicarbonate dialysis solution: prospective cross-over comparison with a lactate buffered solution. *Nephrol Dial Transpl* 1999;14: 2387–2391.

84. Thomas AN, et al. Comparison of lactate and bicarbonate buffered haemofiltration fluids: use in critically ill patients. *Nephrol Dial Transpl* 1997;12:1212–1217.

85. Wright DA, et al. Use of continuous haemofiltration to assess the rate of lactate metabolism in acute renal failure. *Clin Sci (Lond)* 1996;90: 507–510.

86. Morgera S, et al. Comparison of a lactate-versus acetate-based hemofiltration replacement fluid in patients with acute renal failure. *Ren Fail* 1997;19:155–164.

87. Levraut J, et al. Effect of continuous venovenous hemofiltration with dialysis on lactate clearance in critically ill patients. *Crit Care Med* 1997;25:58–62.

88. Leblanc M, et al. Bicarbonate dialysate for continuous renal replacement therapy in intensive care unit patients with acute renal failure. *Am J Kidney Dis* 1995;26:910–917.

89. Hilton PJ, et al. Bicarbonate-based haemofiltration in the management of acute renal failure with lactic acidosis. *QJM* 1998;91: 279–283.

90. Heering P, et al. The use of different buffers during continuous

91. hemofiltration in critically ill patients with acute renal failure. *Intensive Care Med* 1999;25:1244–1251.

91. Forni LG, et al. Continuous hemofiltration in the treatment of acute renal failure. *N Engl J Med* 1997;336:1303–1309.

92. Hoffmann JN, et al. Effect of hemofiltration on hemodynamics and systemic concentrations of anaphylatoxins and cytokines in human sepsis. *Intensive Care Med* 1996;22:1360–1367.

93. Grootendorst AF, et al. High volume hemofiltration improves right ventricular function in endotoxin-induced shock in the pig. *Intensive Care Med* 1992;18:235–240.

94. Siegler MH, et al. Continuous arteriovenous hemodialysis: an improved technique for treating acute renal failure in critically ill patients. In: Nissenson A, et al., eds. *Clinical dialysis.* Norwalk, CT: Appleton & Lange, 1989:720–734.

95. Golper TA, et al. Continuous venovenous hemofiltration for acute renal failure in the intensive care setting: technical considerations. *ASAIO J* 1994;40:936–939.

96. Kaplan AA. Predilution versus postdilution for continuous arteriovenous hemofiltration. *Trans Am Soc Artif Intern Organs* 1985;31: 28–32.

97. Garred LLP, et al. Urea kinetic modeling for CRRT. *Am J Kidney Dis* 1997;30:S2–S9.

98. Brocklehurst IC, et al. Creatinine and urea clearance during continuous veno-venous haemofiltration in critically ill patients. *Anaesthesia* 1996;51:551–553.

99. Bellomo R, et al. Adequacy of dialysis in the acute renal failure of the critically ill: the case for continuous therapies. *Int J Artif Organs* 1996;19:129–142.

100. Mehta RL, et al. A randomized clinical trial of continuous versus intermittent dialysis for acute renal failure. *Kidney Int* 2001;60: 1154–1163.

101. Van Bommel EF, et al. Impact of continuous hemofiltration on cytokines and cytokine inhibitors in oliguric patients suffering from systemic inflammatory response syndrome. *Ren Fail* 1997;19: 443–454.

102. Hoffmann JN, et al. Hemofiltration in human sepsis: evidence for elimination of immunomodulatory substances. *Kidney Int* 1995;48: 1563–1570.

103. Paganini EP, et al. Dialysis delivery in the ICU: are patients receiving the prescribed dialysis dose? *J Am Soc Nephrol* 1992;3:384.

104. Paganini EP, et al. Establishing a dialysis therapy/patient outcome link in intensive care unit acute dialysis for patients with acute renal failure. *Am J Kidney Dis* 1996;28:81–90.

105. Keller F, et al. Individualized drug dosage in patients treated with continuous hemofiltration. *Kidney Int* 1999;72(Suppl):S29–S31.

106. Bohler J, et al. Pharmacokinetic principles during continuous renal replacement therapy: drugs and dosage. *Kidney Int* 1999;72 (Suppl):S24–S28.

107. Kroh UF. Drug administration in critically ill patients with acute renal failure. *New Horiz* 1995;3:748–759.

108. Golper TA. Update on drug sieving coefficients and dosing adjustments during continuous renal replacement therapies. *Contrib Nephrol* 2001;132:349–353.

109. Traunmuller F, et al. Clearance of ceftazidime during continuous venovenous haemofiltration in critically ill patients. *J Antimicrob Chemother* 2002;49:129–134.

110. Thomson AH, et al. Flucytosine dose requirements in a patient receiving continuous veno-venous haemofiltration. *Intensive Care Med* 2002;28:999.

111. Robatel C, et al. Determination of meropenem in plasma and filtrate-dialysate from patients under continuous veno-venous haemodiafiltration by SPE-LC. *J Pharm Biomed Anal* 2002;29:17–33.

112. Kim MK, et al. Clearance of quinupristin-dalfopristin (Synercid) and their main metabolites during continuous veno-venous hemofiltration (CVVH) with or without dialysis. *Int J Artif Organs* 2002;25: 33–39.

113. Barrueto F, et al. Clearance of metformin by hemofiltration in overdose. *J Toxicol Clin Toxicol* 2002;40:177–180.

114. Valtonen M, et al. Elimination of the piperacillin/tazobactam combination during continuous venovenous haemofiltration and haemodi-

afiltration in patients with acute renal failure. *J Antimicrob Chemother* 2001;48:881–885.

115. Wallis SC, et al. Pharmacokinetics of ciprofloxacin in ICU patients on continuous veno-venous haemodiafiltration. *Intensive Care Med* 2001;27:665–672.

116. Kishino S, et al. Effective fluconazole therapy for liver transplant recipients during continuous hemodiafiltration. *Ther Drug Monit* 2001;23:4–8.

117. Hansen E, et al. Pharmacokinetics of levofloxacin during continuous veno-venous hemofiltration. *Intensive Care Med* 2001;27:371–375.

118. Bugge JF. Pharmacokinetics and drug dosing adjustments during continuous venovenous hemofiltration or hemodiafiltration in critically ill patients. *Acta Anaesthesiol Scand* 2001;45:929–934.

119. Van der Werf TS, et al. Cefpirome and continuous venovenous hemofiltration. *Intensive Care Med* 2000;26:831.

120. Taniguchi T, et al. Pharmacokinetics of milrinone in patients with congestive heart failure during continuous venovenous hemofiltration. *Intensive Care Med* 2000;26:1089–1093.

121. Shah M, et al. Rapid removal of vancomycin by continuous venovenous hemofiltration. *Pediatr Nephrol* 2000;14:912–915.

122. Mehta RL. Fluid management in CRRT. *Contrib Nephrol* 2001;132:335–348.

123. Mehta RL. Acid-base and electrolyte management in continuous renal replacement therapy. *Blood Purif* 2002;20:262–268.

124. Mehta RL. Indications for dialysis in the ICU: renal replacement vs. renal support. *Blood Purif* 2001;19:227–232.

125. Mehta RL. Continuous renal replacement therapies in the acute renal failure setting: current concepts. *Adv Ren Replace Ther* 1997;4:81–92.

126. Schrier RW, et al. Strategies in management of acute renal failure in the intensive therapy unit. In: Bihari D, et al., eds. *Current concepts in critical care: acute renal failure in the intensive therapy unit.* Berlin: Springer-Verlag, 1990:193–214.

127. Mehta R. Renal replacement therapy for acute renal failure: matching the method to the patient. *Semin Dial* 1993;6:253–259.

128. Barton IK, et al. Acute renal failure treated by haemofiltration: factors affecting outcome. *Q J Med* 1993;86:81–90.

129. Jorres A. Extracorporeal treatment strategy in acute renal failure. *Int J Artif Organs* 2002;25:391–396.

130. Bellomo R, et al. Changing acute renal failure treatment from intermittent hemodialysis to continuous hemofiltration: impact on azotemic control. *Int J Artif Organs* 1999;22:145–150.

131. Gopal I, et al. Out of hospital outcome and quality of life in survivors of combined acute multiple organ and renal failure treated with continuous venovenous hemofiltration/hemodiafiltration. *Intensive Care Med* 1997;23:766–772.

132. Holm C, et al. Acute renal failure in severely burned patients. *Burns* 1999;25:171–178.

133. Karlowicz MG, et al. Acute renal failure in the neonate. *Clin Perinatol* 1992;19:139–158.

134. Mehta RL, et al. Refining predictive models in critically ill patients with acute renal failure. *J Am Soc Nephrol* 2002;13:1350–1357.

135. Ronco C, et al. Acute renal failure in patients with kidney transplant: continuous versus intermittent renal replacement therapy. *Ren Fail* 1996;18:461–470.

136. Phu NH, et al. Hemofiltration and peritoneal dialysis in infection-associated acute renal failure in Vietnam. *N Engl J Med* 2002;347:895–902.

137. Daugirdas J. Peritoneal dialysis in acute renal failure—why the bad outcome? *N Engl J Med* 2002;347:933–935.

138. Steiner R. Continuous equilibration peritoneal dialysis in acute renal failure. *Perit Dial Int* 1989;9:5–7.

139. Geronemus RP. Slow continuous hemodialysis. *ASAIO Trans* 1988;34:59–60.

140. Hombrouckx R, et al. Go-slow dialysis instead of continuous arteriovenous hemofiltration. *Contrib Nephrol* 1991;93:149–151.

141. Manns M, et al. Continuous renal replacement therapies: an update. *Am J Kidney Dis* 1998;32:185–207.

142. Davenport A. Renal replacement therapy in the patient with acute brain injury. *Am J Kidney Dis* 2001;37:457–466.

143. DeBroe M, et al. Pulmonary aspects of dialysis patients. In: Jacobs C,

et al., eds. *Replacement of renal function by dialysis,* 4th ed. Boston: Kluwer Academic, 1996:1034–1048.

144. Davenport A. Is there a role for continuous renal replacement therapies in patients with liver and renal failure? *Kidney Int* 1999;72 (Suppl):S62–S66.

145. Golej J, et al. Low-volume peritoneal dialysis in 116 neonatal and paediatric critical care patients. *Eur J Pediatr* 2002;161:385–389.

146. Lewis MA, et al. Practical peritoneal dialysis: the Tenckhoff catheter in acute renal failure. *Pediatr Nephrol* 1992;6:470–475.

147. Than N, et al. Continuous haemofiltration in acute renal failure. *Lancet* 2000;356:1441; discussion, 1442.

148. Ronco C, et al. Effects of different doses in continuous veno-venous haemofiltration on outcomes of acute renal failure: a prospective randomised trial. *Lancet* 2000;356:26–30.

149. Gilman CM, et al. Continuous venovenous hemofiltration: a cost-effective therapy for the pediatric patient. *ANNA J* 1997;24:337–341.

150. Schetz M. Non-renal indications for continuous renal replacement therapy. *Kidney Int* 1999;72(Suppl):S88–S94.

151. Bellomo R, et al. Coupled plasma filtration adsorption. *Blood Purif* 2002;20:289–292.

152. Silvester W. Mediator removal with CRRT: complement and cytokines. *Am J Kidney Dis* 1997;30:S38–S43.

153. Wakabayashi Y, et al. Removal of circulating cytokines by continuous haemofiltration in patients with systemic inflammatory response syndrome or multiple organ dysfunction syndrome. *Br J Surg* 1996;83:393–394.

154. Hoffmann JN, et al. Removal of mediators by continuous hemofiltration in septic patients. *World J Surg* 2001;25:651–659.

155. Hanasawa K. Extracorporeal treatment for septic patients: new adsorption technologies and their clinical application. *Ther Apher* 2002;6:290–295.

156. Gomez A, et al. hemofiltration reverses left ventricular dysfunction during sepsis in dogs. *Anesthesiology* 1990;73:671–685.

157. Reeves JH, et al. Continuous plasma-filtration in sepsis syndrome. Plasma-filtration in Sepsis Study Group. *Crit Care Med* 1999;27:2096–2104.

158. Tetta C, et al. Endotoxin and cytokine removal in sepsis. *Ther Apher* 2002;6:109–115.

159. Toft P, et al. Effect of hemodiafiltration and sepsis on chemotaxis of granulocytes and the release of IL-8 and IL-10. *Acta Anaesthesiol Scand* 2002;46:138–144.

160. Curley SA, et al. Hepatic arterial infusion chemotherapy with complete hepatic venous isolation and extracorporeal chemofiltration: a feasibility study of a novel system. *Anticancer Drugs* 1991;2:175–183.

161. Saccente SL, et al. Prevention of tumor lysis syndrome using continuous veno-venous hemofiltration. *Pediatr Nephrol* 1995;9:569–573.

162. Muchmore JH, et al. Regional chemotherapy with hemofiltration: a rationale for a different treatment approach to advanced pancreatic cancer. *Hepatogastroenterology* 1996;43:346–355.

163. Muchmore J. Regional chemotherapy plus hemofiltration for the treatment of regionally advanced malignancy (editorial). *Cancer* 1996;78:941–943.

164. Gutman M, et al. Regional perfusion with hemofiltration (chemofiltration) for the treatment of patients with regionally advanced cancer. *Cancer* 1996;78:1125–1130.

165. Boldt J, et al. The effects of pentoxifylline on circulating adhesion molecules in critically ill patients with acute renal failure treated by continuous veno-venous hemofiltration. *Intensive Care Med* 1996;22:305–311.

166. Hirasawa H, et al. Blood purification for prevention and treatment of multiple organ failure. *World J Surg* 1996;20:482–486.

167. Iorio L, et al. Daily hemofiltration in severe heart failure. *Kidney Int* 1997;59:S62–S65.

168. Coraim FI, et al. Continuous hemofiltration for the failing heart. *New Horiz* 1995;3:725–731.

169. Dormans TP, et al. Chronic intermittent haemofiltration and haemodialysis in end-stage chronic heart failure with oedema refractory to high dose frusemide. *Heart* 1996;75:349–351.

170. Blake P, et al. Isolation of "myocardial depressant factor(s)" from the

ultrafiltrate of heart failure patients with acute renal failure. *ASAIO J* 1996;42:M710–M713.

171. Ramos R, et al. Outcome predictors of ultrafiltration in patients with refractory congestive heart failure and renal failure. *Angiology* 1996; 47:447–454.

172. Tsang GM, et al. Hemofiltration in a cardiac intensive care unit: time for a rational approach. *ASAIO J* 1996;42:M710–M713.

173. Summar M, et al. Effective hemodialysis and hemofiltration driven by an extracorporeal membrane oxygenation pump in infants with hyperammonemia. *J Pediatr* 1996;128:379–382.

174. Jouvet P, et al. Continuous venovenous haemodiafiltration in the acute phase of neonatal maple syrup urine disease. *J Inherit Metab Dis* 1997;20:463–472.

175. Bellomo R, et al. A comparison of conventional dialytic therapy and acute continuous hemodiafiltration in the management of acute renal failure in the critically ill. *Ren Fail* 1993;15:595–602.

176. Bellomo R, et al. Use of continuous haemodiafiltration: an approach to the management of acute renal failure in the critically ill. *Am J Nephrol* 1992;12:240–245.

177. Clark WR, et al. Urea kinetics during continuous hemofiltration. *ASAIO J* 1992;38:M664–M667.

178. Bartlett RH, et al. Continuous arteriovenous hemofiltration for acute renal failure. *ASAIO Trans* 1988;34:67–77.

179. Golper TA. Continuous arteriovenous hemofiltration in acute renal failure. *Am J Kidney Dis* 1985;6:373–386.

180. Maher ER, et al. Prognosis of critically ill patients with acute renal failure: APACHE II score and other predictive factors. *Q J Med* 1989;72:857–866.

181. Mehta RL, et al. Regional citrate anticoagulation for continuous arteriovenous hemodialysis in critically ill patients. *Kidney Int* 1990;38: 976–981.

182. Macias WL, et al. Continuous venovenous hemofiltration: an alternative to continuous arteriovenous hemofiltration and hemodiafiltration in acute renal failure. *Am J Kidney Dis* 1991;18:451–458.

183. Van Bommel E, et al. Acute dialytic support for the critically ill: intermittent hemodialysis versus continuous arteriovenous hemodiafiltration. *Am J Nephrol* 1995;15:192–200.

184. Mukau L, et al. Acute hemodialysis in the surgical intensive care unit. *Am Surg* 1988;54:548–552.

185. Lowell JA, et al. Postoperative fluid overload: not a benign problem. *Crit Care Med* 1990;18:728–733.

186. Zobel G, et al. Continuous extracorporeal fluid removal in children with low cardiac output after cardiac operations. *J Thorac Cardiovasc Surg* 1991;101:593–597.

187. Sodemann K, et al. Automated fluid balance in continuous hemodialysis with blood safety module BSM 22/VPM. *Contrib Nephrol* 1991;93:184–192.

188. Barton IK, et al. Haemofiltration: how to do it. *Br J Hosp Med* 1997;57:188–193.

189. Schelling JR, et al. Management of tumor lysis syndrome with standard continuous arteriovenous hemodialysis: case report and a review of the literature. *Ren Fail* 1998;20:635–644.

190. Sharma A, et al. Clinical benefit and approach of ultrafiltration in acute heart failure. *Cardiology* 2001;96:144–154.

191. Bellomo R, et al. The effect of intensive plasma water exchange by hemofiltration on hemodynamics and soluble mediators in canine endotoxemia. *Am J Respir Crit Care Med* 2000;161:1429–1436.

192. Cavalcanti S, et al. Numerical simulation of the hemodynamic response to hemodialysis-induced hypovolemia. *Artif Organs* 1999; 23:1063–1073.

193. Santoro A, et al. Blood volume regulation during hemodialysis. *Am J Kidney Dis* 1998;32:739–748.

194. Manns M, et al. Intradialytic renal haemodynamics: potential consequences for the management of the patient with acute renal failure. *Nephrol Dial Transpl* 1997;12:870–872.

195. Solez L, et al. The morphology of acute tubular necrosis in man: analysis of 57 renal biopsies and comparison with the glycerol model. *Medicine* 1979;58:362–367.

196. Conger J. Does hemodialysis delay recovery from acute renal failure. *Semin Dial* 1990;3:146–150.

197. Bellomo R, et al. Continuous versus intermittent renal replacement therapy in the intensive care unit. *Kidney Int* 1998;66(Suppl): S125–S128.

198. Bartlett RH, et al. Continuous arteriovenous hemofiltration: improved survival in surgical acute renal failure? *Surgery* 1986;100: 400–408.

199. Chima CS, et al. Nitrogen balance in postsurgical patients with acute renal failure on continuous arteriovenous hemofiltration and total parenteral nutrition. *Contrib Nephrol* 1991;93:39–41.

200. DiCarlo JV, et al. Continuous arteriovenous hemofiltration/dialysis improves pulmonary gas exchange in children with multiple organ system failure. *Crit Care Med* 1990;18:822–826.

201. Kuttnig M, et al. Parenteral nutrition during continuous arteriovenous hemofiltration in critically ill anuric children. *Contrib Nephrol* 1991;93:250–253.

202. Clark WR, et al. Quantification of creatinine kinetic parameters in patients with acute renal failure. *Kidney Int* 1998;54:554–560.

203. Bellomo R, et al. A prospective comparative study of moderate versus high protein intake for critically ill patients with acute renal failure. *Ren Fail* 1997;19:111–120.

204. Bellomo R, et al. Acute continuous hemofiltration with dialysis: effect on insulin concentrations and glycemic control in critically ill patients. *Crit Care Med* 1992;20:1672–1676.

205. Frankenfield DC, et al. Glucose dynamics during continuous hemodiafiltration and total parenteral nutrition. *Intensive Care Med* 1995;21:1016–1022.

206. Monson PT, et al. Nutrition in acute renal failure: a reappraisal for the 1990s. *J Ren Nutr* 1994;4:58–77.

207. Davenport A, et al. Amino acid losses during continuous high-flux hemofiltration in the critically ill patient. *Crit Care Med* 1989;17: 1010–1014.

208. Davies SP, et al. Amino acid clearances and daily losses in patients with acute renal failure treated by continuous arteriovenous hemodialysis. *Crit Care Med* 1991;19:1510–1515.

209. Kuttnig M, et al. Nitrogen and amino acid balance during total parenteral nutrition and continuous arteriovenous hemofiltration in critically ill anuric children. *Child Nephrol Urol* 1991;11:74–78.

210. Kopple JD. The nutrition management of the patient with acute renal failure. *J Parenter Enteral Nutr* 1996;20:3–12.

211. Macias WL, et al. Impact of the nutritional regimen on protein catabolism and nitrogen balance in patients with acute renal failure. *J Parenter Enteral Nutr* 1996;20:56–62.

212. Marin A, et al. Practical implications of nutritional support during continuous renal replacement therapy. *Curr Opin Clin Nutr Metab Care* 2001;4:219–225.

213. Marangoni R, et al. Lactate versus bicarbonate on-line hemofiltration: a comparative study. *Artif Organs* 1995;19:490–495.

214. Bellomo R. Bench-to-bedside review: lactate and the kidney. *Crit Care* 2002;6:322–326.

215. Koreny M, et al. Prognosis of patients who develop acute renal failure during the first 24 hours of cardiogenic shock after myocardial infarction. *Am J Med* 2002;112:115–119.

216. Andreoli SP. Acute renal failure. *Curr Opin Pediatr* 2002;14:183–188.

217. Abernethy VE, et al. Acute renal failure in the critically ill patient. *Crit Care Clin* 2002;18:203–222.

218. Silvester W, et al. Epidemiology, management, and outcome of severe acute renal failure of critical illness in Australia. *Crit Care Med* 2001;29:1910–1915.

219. Anderson RJ. Renal replacement therapy in intensive care: one size does not fit all. *Crit Care Med* 2001;29:2028–2029.

220. Guerin C, et al. Initial versus delayed acute renal failure in the intensive care unit: a Multicenter Prospective Epidemiological Study. *Am J Respir Crit Care Med* 2000;161:872–879.

221. Liano F, et al. Outcomes in acute renal failure. *Semin Nephrol* 1998;18:541–550.

222. Mendelssohn DC, et al. What do American nephrologists think about dialysis modality selection? *Am J Kidney Dis* 2001;37:22–29.

223. Kierdorf H, et al. Continuous treatment modalities in acute renal failure. *Nephrol Dial Transpl* 1995;10:2001–2008.

224. Sieberth HG, et al. Is continuous haemofiltration superior to inter-

mittent dialysis and haemofiltration treatment? *Adv Exp Med Biol* 1989;260:181–192.

225. Kierdorf H, et al. Continuous venovenous hemofiltration in acute renal failure: is a bicarbonate- or lactate-buffered substitution better? *Contrib Nephrol* 1995;116:38–47.

226. Jakob SM, et al. Does continuous renal replacement therapy favorably influence the outcome of patients? *Nephrol Dial Transpl* 1996;11:1235–1250.

227. Swartz RD, et al. Comparing continuous hemofiltration with hemodialysis in patients with severe acute renal failure. *Am J Kidney Dis* 1999;34:424–432.

228. DuBose TD Jr, et al. Acute renal failure in the 21st century: recommendations for management and outcomes assessment. *Am J Kidney Dis* 1997;29:793–799.

229. Mehta R. Acute renal failure in the intensive care unit: which outcomes should we measure? *Am J Kidney Dis* 1996;28:74–79.

230. Kellum JA, et al. Continuous versus intermittent renal replacement therapy: a metaanalysis. *Intensive Care Med* 2002;28:29–37.

231. Manns M, et al. Thermal energy balance during in vitro continuous veno-venous hemofiltration. *ASAIO J* 1998;44:M601–M605.

232. Seigler RS, et al. Continuous venovenous rewarming: results from a juvenile animal model. *Crit Care Med* 1998;26:2016–2020.

233. Ruzicka J, et al. Effects of ultrafiltration, dialysis, and temperature on gas exchange during hemodiafiltration: a laboratory experiment. *Artif Organs* 2001;25:961–966.

234. Moreno L, et al. Continuous renal replacement therapy: cost considerations and reimbursement. *Semin Dial* 1996;9:209–214.

235. Hoyt D. CRRT in the area of cost containment: is it justified? *Am J Kidney Dis* 1997;30(Suppl 4):S102–S104.

236. Bellomo R, et al. Continuous haemofiltration in the intensive care unit. *Crit Care* 2000;4:339–345.

237. Bent P, et al. Early and intensive continuous hemofiltration for severe renal failure after cardiac surgery. *Ann Thorac Surg* 2001;71:832–837.

238. Ronco C, et al. Machines for continuous renal replacement therapy. *Contrib Nephrol* 2001;132:323–334.

239. Baldwin I. Keeping pace with changes in technology and technique. *Blood Purif* 2002;20:269–274.

240. Ronco C, et al. Online monitoring in continuous renal replacement therapies. *Kidney Int* 1999;72:S8–S14.

241. Bellomo R, et al. Treatment of sepsis-associated severe acute renal failure with continuous hemodiafiltration: clinical experience and comparison with conventional dialysis. *Blood Purif* 1995;13:246–254.

242. Bellomo R. Continuous hemofiltration as blood purification in sepsis. *New Horiz* 1995;3:732–737.

243. Grootendorst AF, et al. The role of hemofiltration in the critically ill intensive care unit patient: present and future. *Blood Purif* 1993;11:209–223.

244. Schetz M. Removal of cytokines in septic patients using continuous veno-venous hemodiafiltration. *Crit Care Med* 1994;22:715–716; discussion, 719–721.

245. Canaud B, et al. Slow continuous ultrafiltration: a means of unmasking myocardial functional reserve in end-stage cardiac disease. *Contrib Nephrol* 1991;93:79–85.

246. Druml W. Nonrenal indications for continuous hemofiltration therapy in patients with normal renal function? *Contrib Nephrol* 1995;116:121–129.

247. Argibay PF, et al. Polyacrylonitrile membrane interposition between a xenograft and an animal in fulminant liver failure: the concept of xenohemodiafiltration. *ASAIO J* 1996;42:M411–M416.

248. Hammer GB, et al. Continuous venovenous hemofiltration with dialysis in combination with total hepatectomy and portocaval shunting: bridge to liver transplantation. *Transplantation* 1996;62:130–132.

249. Despotis GJ, et al. Hemofiltration during cardiopulmonary bypass: the effect on anti-Xa and anti-IIa heparin activity. *Anesth Analg* 1997;84:479–483.

250. Journois D, et al. High-volume, zero-balanced hemofiltration to reduce delayed inflammatory response to cardiopulmonary bypass in children. *Anesthesiology* 1996;85:965–976.

251. Kubota T, et al. Continuous haemodiafiltration during and after cardiopulmonary bypass in renal failure patients. *Can J Anaesth* 1997;44:1182–1186.

252. Paret G, et al. Continuous arteriovenous hemofiltration after cardiac operations in infants and children. *J Thorac Cardiovasc Surg* 1992;104:1225–1230.

ADEQUACY OF PERITONEAL DIALYSIS

JOHN M. BURKART

Chronic dialysis is certainly a remarkable medical success story, extending the lives of some patients with kidney failure for more than 20 years (1). This success routinely occurs despite the finding that typical urea clearances for patients on continuous ambulatory peritoneal dialysis (CAPD) are only approximately one-tenth that of the normal kidney (70 L urea clearance/week on CAPD versus 750 L/week for normal renal function) (Table 14.1) and the fact that dialysis itself replaces only some of the typical functions of the normal human kidney, typically not correcting anemia and renal osteodystrophy without additional medications.

Despite the success of our current renal replacement therapies, there is room for improvement. Mortality rates in the United States have historically been in the range of 10% to 25% per annum (2), on average, ten times higher than those of age- and sex-matched controls in the healthy population (3). Some have suggested that this increased rate of mortality in dialysis patients is due to inadequacies in the prescribed dose of dialysis (4,5). In an attempt to improve patient outcomes, nephrologists have focused on attempts to increase dialysis dose using small solute clearance as the yardstick for determining adequacy (6,7). Studies that have examined the relationship between relative risk of death and small solute clearance suggested that more (solute clearance) was better. This has led to the development of guidelines for adequacy of peritoneal dialysis (PD) (8), which were subsequently revised (9).

This chapter discusses adequacy for peritoneal dialysis in terms of total solute clearance, volume control, and other issues related to the peritoneal dialysis prescription. Although this chapter focuses on small solute clearance issues, the optimal treatment of a patient with end-stage renal disease (ESRD) must also address blood pressure control, treatment of acidosis, anemia, prevention of metabolic bone disease, and perhaps treatment/prevention of a chronic inflammatory state. Most of these issues are beyond the scope of this chapter.

WHAT YARDSTICK FOR ADEQUACY OF DIALYSIS SHOULD WE USE?

Some of the clinical manifestations of uremia are readily apparent to the clinician or patient (10). These include decreased appetite, metallic taste, nausea, vomiting, pericarditis, pleuritis, and encephalopathy. Unfortunately, uremia or "underdialysis" may also be associated with hypertension (11), lipid abnormalities (12), cardiovascular disease, and neuropathy (13). These and other signs and symptoms of uremia are not always readily apparent and at times may be very insidious in onset and potentially fatal or irreversible. Therefore nephrologists need a measurable laboratory parameter that can be obtained during the course of chronic kidney disease and when a patient is on dialysis that predicts the presence of uremic complications and patient outcome. There is no documented single substance that has been shown to be the "uremic toxin." Undoubtedly, the clinical manifestations of the uremic syndrome are the result of the synergistic effect of multiple retained solutes across a broad spectrum of molecular weights. The uremic syndrome results from the serum levels (body burden) of these solutes. These levels are the result of generation and removal of the individual solute. However, as mentioned, it is not known which ones to measure. Of the known retained solutes, urea reaches the highest concentrations, yet it is known that infusing urea into healthy volunteers results in little or no symptomatology. Consequently, any laboratory marker(s) for "adequacy of dialysis" will have to rely on a surrogate marker for efficacy of the treatment of uremia. Currently these tend to be clearances of urea nitrogen, creatinine, phosphorus, or β_2 microglobulin.

Historical data suggest that the outcome for patients on both hemodialysis (HD) (14) and PD (15) is related to total small solute clearance and to surrogates of nutritional status such as dietary protein intake, body mass, and serum albumin levels. The relationships between protein intake, solute clearance, and the manifestations of uremia or nutritional status are likely to be different in each patient, but in the absence of significant

TABLE 14.1. SOLUTE REMOVAL BY DIALYSIS AND THE NATURAL KIDNEY

	Natural Solute Kidney	HD— Standard Flux	HD— High Flux	CAPD
Urea (L/week)	750	130	130	70
Vitamin B$_{12}$ (L/week)	1,200	30	60	40
Insulin (L/week)	1,200	10	40	20
β_2-microglobulin	1,000	0	300	250

From Keshaviah P. Adequacy of CAPD: a quantitative approach. *Kidney Int* 1992;42(Suppl 28):S160–S164.
CAPD, continuous ambulatory peritoneal dialysis; HD, hemodialysis.

comorbid disease they tend to correlate positively with solute clearance (16).

Currently, recommended standard "yardsticks" for adequacy of peritoneal dialysis include urea clearance normalized to its volume of distribution (Kt/V_{urea}) and creatinine clearance (CCr) normalized to 1.73 m^2. However, as will be discussed later, contemporary data may suggest that one may also need to refocus on other known "yardsticks" of renal replacement therapy, such as sodium removal, volume control, and β_2-microglobulin clearance.

Measurement of Solute Clearance

Current guidelines recommend obtaining a 24-hour collection of both urine and peritoneal effluent for analysis of total solute clearance ($K_{renal} + K_{peritoneal} = K_{rp \ or \ total}$). Urea and creatinine clearances are obtained to calculate weekly Kt/V_{urea} and weekly CCr/1.73 m^2. It is recommended that residual renal and peritoneal clearances be added 1:1, assuming that the potential beneficial effects on patient outcome from 1 unit of residual renal and 1 unit of peritoneal clearances are equal. At the time these recommendations were made, there were no data to prove this.

Why Small Solute Clearance?

Multiple studies, all differing in methodology and the number of patients enrolled, have examined the relationship between patient outcomes in terms of relative risk of death or morbidity and the relationship to total small solute clearance, the significance of which has been reviewed elsewhere (17,18). All tend to conclude that outcomes such as relative risk of death and hospitalizations are in some way related to total small solute clearance. Minimal total solute clearance goals supported by data from each study are slightly different and briefly reviewed later. Data published before 1996 are the basis of the original National Kidney Foundation–Dialysis Outcomes Quality Initiative (NKF–DOQI) guidelines. Contemporary data and their potential implications for revisions of the guidelines will also be reviewed.

K/tV Data

Historical Publications

The original theoretical constructs for CAPD predicted that an anephric 70-kg patient (total body water or V = 42 L) would remain in positive nitrogen balance when prescribed five 2-L exchanges each day (19). Studies using *univariate* analysis of data correlating outcomes with small solute clearance suggested the following: in patients with residual renal function, maintain a total weekly Kt/V_{urea} target of more than 1.5 in one (20) and >2.0 in another (21). While a study in anuric patients suggested that patients with a Kt/V of more than 1.89 did best (22).

Studies using the statistically more correct *multivariate* analysis of data to determine the predictive value of Kt/V_{urea} on survival found the following: a survival advantage in patients with a weekly Kt/V_{urea} of more than 1.89 in one study (23); and, in another study of *prevalent* PD patients (mean baseline GFR 1.73 mL/min) followed for up to 3 years, the best survival was noted in patients with a total Kt/V_{urea} of at least 1.96 with no

incremental improvement in survival with higher small solute clearances in a group (24). Finally, the Canada–USA (CANUSA) study (15), a prospective, multicenter, observational cohort study of *incident* patients in North America and Canada (mean baseline GFR 3.8 mL/min), predicted that over the range of solute clearance studied, every 0.1-unit increase in Kt/V would be associated with a 6% decrease in the relative risk of death. The same effect was predicted for creatinine clearance and there was no evidence of a plateau effect.

Although performed in 1995, the CANUSA study provided the best historical evidence that survival on PD is related to total solute clearance. It is important to note that the results were based on theoretical constructs and two very important assumptions: (a) total solute clearance remained stable over time, and (b) 1 unit or mL/min of clearance due to residual renal function is equal to 1 unit or mL/min of clearance due to peritoneal dialysis. In fact, total solute clearance decreased over time as residual renal function decreased, with no corresponding increase in the peritoneal component. Therefore because the peritoneal component of total solute clearance tended not to change over the course of the study, one interpretation of CANUSA would be to say that the more residual renal function the patient has, the better the predicted outcome (25). Similar outcome data correlating patient outcome with small solute clearance in terms of creatinine clearance are available. In some publications, total weekly CCr/1.73 m^2 was more predictive of all cause outcomes than total weekly Kt/V_{urea}.

Based on historical studies published before 1996 and the possible association between solute clearance and dietary protein intake (reviewed later), the original NKF–DOQI working group on adequacy of peritoneal dialysis recommended the following total solute clearance goals for CAPD: a total weekly Kt/V_{urea} of more than 2.0/week and a total weekly CCr of more than 60 L/1.73 m^2 week. For continuous cyclic peritoneal dialysis (CCPD) and for nightly intermittent peritoneal dialysis (NIPD), slightly higher total weekly Kt/V_{urea} total weekly CCr/1.73 m^2 were recommended. It was acknowledged that the CAPD targets were only marginally evidence based and that there were no prospective randomized studies to support those recommendations. It was also acknowledged that targets for CCPD and NIPD were opinion based with little to no outcome data for the recommendations. Subsequently, other medical societies recommended targeting a total weekly Kt/V_{urea} of 2.0 (Canada guidelines) (26) and 1.7 (UK guidelines) (27) for all PD therapies.

Contemporary Studies

Contemporary studies have further examined the effect of increasing peritoneal clearance on survival. There are three studies from a group in China. Szeto et al. (28) retrospectively reviewed their experience in 168 prevalent CAPD patients followed for 1 year. Outcomes for patients with a total Kt/V_{urea} of more than 1.7/week (baseline mean total Kt/V_{urea} 2.03 ± 0.25 for patients with RRF (residual renal function) and baseline mean total Kt/V_{urea} was 1.93 ± 0.18 for patients without RRF) were compared with those for patients with a total Kt/V_{urea} of < 1.7/week (mean total Kt/V_{urea} was 1.38 ± 0.22). Overall mortality at 1 year was 8.3%; however, although there was no statistically significant difference between the groups, 9/14 deaths occurred in the anuric patients with a weekly Kt/V_{urea} <1.7/week. Based on this, one might infer that a weekly peritoneal Kt/V_{urea} of <1.7 in an anuric patient may be associated with an increased relative risk of death in the long term if these trends continued. In another study these authors showed an association between outcome and total solute clearance, mainly due to the residual renal component (29). In contrast, in an evaluation of 140 prevalent anuric patients, followed a mean of 22.0 + 11.9 months, they found a positive correlation between peritoneal clearance and survival (30). In these patients, the mean baseline peritoneal Kt/V_{urea} was 1.72 ± 0.31/week and 42% were prescribed three 2-L exchanges each day (patients whose prescription was modified if there were ultrafiltration [UF] problems). Each 0.1 unit decrease in Kt/V was associated with a 6% increase in mortality, similar to that predicted by CANUSA.

These data in Asian patients suggest that once a certain minimal peritoneal small solute clearance is achieved (perhaps a peritoneal Kt/V_{urea} >1.8/week) and the patient is on 24 h/d of peritoneal clearance, further incremental increases in small solute clearance result in little increase in short-term outcome.

Davies et al. (31,32) found an association between total solute clearance and survival, and as in other studies, this was all due to variations in residual renal clearance, not peritoneal. In a study of 122 anuric Canadian patients, Bhaskaran et al. (33) reported that the best survival, representing a 58% reduction in mortality, was found in the group of patients with a Kt/V_{urea} >1.8/week (creatinine clearance >50 L/1.73 m²/week.) There was no demonstrable incremental improvement for higher weekly clearances. However, the 95% CI of the study was 0.26 to 1.13, reflecting the low statistical power achieved in this study in a relatively small number of patients. Similarly, in a group of 205 incident patients new to PD since 1996, whose mean total Kt/V was always well above DOQI targets by replacing lost residual renal clearance with peritoneal clearance, there was no effect of small solute clearance (total, residual renal alone, peritoneal alone) with outcome (34).

There are two prospective, randomized trials that evaluated the effect of an increase in peritoneal clearance on survival. In the smaller of the two studies, Mak et al. (35) prospectively evaluated the effect of an increase in dialysis dose in a controlled trial in 82 CAPD patients. Baseline, all patients were prescribed three 2-L exchanges per day. They were then randomized to continue this regimen mean Kt/V_{urea} of 1.67 per week or increase their PD prescription to four 2-L exchanges per day (mean, Kt/V_{urea} 2.02 per week), and all were followed for 1 year. Over short-term follow-up (1 year) there was a difference in hospitalization rates. However, hospitalization rates increased in the control group and decreased in the intervention group, so this may be misleading.

A provocative prospective, randomized, interventional study evaluating the effect of an increase in peritoneal solute clearance in 965 CAPD patients in Mexico, the "ADEMEX" study, found no beneficial effect on outcome for patients who had a statistically significant increase in their peritoneal solute clearance (36). All patients had 24 hours per day of peritoneal dwell, and at baseline, all were on four 2-L exchanges per day; RRF was similar in the two groups. Averaged total solute clearances over the

course of that study were as follows: total Kt/V_{urea}, 1.80 ± 0.02 in controls versus 2.27 ± 0.02 in the interventional group, whereas peritoneal only Kt/V_{urea} was 1.62 ± 0.01 in controls versus 2.13 ± 0.01 in the intervention group. Corresponding CCr values in L/week/1.73 m² were 54.1 ± 1.0 versus 62.9 ± 0.7 and 46.1 ± 0.45 versus 56.9 ± 0.48, respectively. The distribution of prescriptions in the interventional group was 10 L/d in 37% of patients, 11 L/d in 20%, 12 L/d in 21%, 12.5 L/d in 8%, and 15 L/d in 14%. These data suggest that for the average patient on standard CAPD (24 h/d of peritoneal dwell time), once small solute clearance is above a certain minimal amount, further increases in small solute clearance result in no demonstrable incremental increase in patient outcome. As noted in the observational studies cited earlier, RRF was the main predictor of mortality, with an 11% increase in mortality for each 10 L/week/1.73 m² decrease in weekly renal creatinine clearance and a 6% increase in mortality for each 0.1 unit decrease in weekly renal Kt/V urea clearance. In this study, although there was a statistically significant increase in peritoneal UF volume in the intervention group (0.97 ± 0.05 L/d versus 0.84 ± 0.03 L/d, *p* <0.05) there was no demonstrable improvement in outcome with increasing peritoneal UF.

In summary, contemporary data would suggest that the original minimal weekly small solute clearance goals for urea in patients treated with continuous therapies such as CAPD *may need* to be revised. The data *do not* say that the recommended minimal total weekly small solute clearance goals should be lowered for all patients. They *do suggest* that nephrologists should be more comfortable with individualizing their prescriptions and, if a patient is not at goal but is eating well and feeling well, there is no reason to transfer the patient to HD due to inadequate dialysis. The data suggest that we need to consider focusing on additional "yardsticks" of adequacy of dialysis.

The European committee for adequacy of PD is expected to amend its guidelines and recommend a weekly peritoneal Kt/V_{urea} of more than 1.7/week with a UF volume of at least 1 L/d (verbal communication, Dr Ray Krediet). The NKF–DOQI guidelines for the United States are currently evaluating these contemporary data to determine if those guidelines need to be revised in response to these data. It is important to keep in mind that the influence of solute clearance on outcome may vary in different ethnic populations. In the United States Renal Data System (USRDS) experience African-Americans on HD tend to have a lower relative risk of death than whites, presumably with the same solute clearance. Similarly, in data reviewed earlier, Asians appeared to have better survival than North American patients despite lower relative total solute clearances. Why? Were there better normalized middle molecule clearances? Was there better blood pressure and volume control? Are the recommended minimal solute clearances dependent on metabolic rate, amount of dietary calories consumed as protein, or other unrecognized factors or differences in comorbid diseases? (37). More data are needed.

Creatinine Clearance Data

Most of the studies reviewed earlier that examined the predictive value of total Kt/V_{urea} on outcome also evaluated the effect of total CCr/1.73 m². In the CANUSA study total CCr predicted not only death, but also technique survival and hospitalization (15). Analysis of those data suggested that a total weekly CCr of more than 70 L/1.73 m² would predict a 78% 2-year patient survival. Other studies suggested that the minimal total weekly target should be >58 L/1.73 m² (24); or >50 L/1.73 m² (38), whereas anuric patients did best if clearance was >50 L/1.73 m² (33). In the ADEMEX study, there was no difference in outcome between the control group (mean total CCr of 54 L/1.73 m²/week) versus the intervention group (mean total CCr of 62.9 L/1.73 m²/week) (36).

These data suggest that as with Kt/V_{urea}, with lower values of total CCr/1.73 m², increases in CCr were associated with an improvement in symptoms and a decrease in the relative risk of death. However, at higher levels of total CCr, the predictive value of improving outcome with an incremental increase in clearance was minimal.

Some (39–41) but not all (36,42,43) studies have suggested that after controlling for urea clearance, outcomes in patients with slower rates of solute clearance by peritoneal diffusion ("low" transporters see the following section on Peritoneal Membrane Transport) do better than those with rapid rates of peritoneal solute clearance by diffusion ("high" transporters). Although with the same prescription (instilled volumes and dwell times) rapid and low transporters have similar urea clearances, they tend to have markedly different creatinine clearances. These differences are predicted by kinetic modeling. In fact, one could predict that once anuric, the average patient with a Kt/V_{urea} of 2.0 is unlikely to have a CCr/1.73 m² of more than 60 L/week (44), the targets recommended for minimal total solute clearances while on CAPD for urea and creatinine, respectively. It is because of these outcomes and physiologic differences between clearances of various solutes that the newer guidelines for continuous therapies such as CAPD have revised total creatinine clearance goals for low and low-average transporters.

How might one explain the observation that with similar urea clearances, low transporters (with lower delivered creatinine clearances) have a lower relative risk of death than rapid transporters? Perhaps this is because adequacy of dialysis and patient outcomes are related to more than small solute clearances. It is more difficult to maintain euvolemia through peritoneal UF in rapid transporters for reasons discussed later. Perhaps the increased risk is due to slight volume overload and an increase in the risk for cardiovascular mortality. Preliminary data suggest that patients who have a chronic inflammatory state are more likely to be rapid transporters. Rapid transporter status may be a marker for some other comorbid disease state such as chronic inflammation that is associated with an increase in the relative risk of death.

Importance of Residual Renal Clearance

In contrast to the conflicting data about the benefit of increasing peritoneal clearance on survival, studies have consistently shown that residual renal clearance is associated with a decrease in the relative risk of death both for patients on PD and for patients on hemodialysis (45).

Reanalysis of the CANUSA data (46) suggested that for each 5 L/week/1.73 m² increase in glomerular filtration rate (GFR),

there was a 12% decrease in the relative risk of death. There was no demonstrable benefit from peritoneal clearance. Estimates of net fluid removal suggested that a 250-mL/d increment in urine volume was associated with a 36% decrease in the relative risk of death, whereas net peritoneal UF and total fluid removed were not predictive of outcome. An evaluation of 673 patients followed for one year reported that decreasing renal clearance, not peritoneal clearance, was statistically associated with an increased mortality rate (47). Similar findings were reported in a review of 873 patients selected for evaluation in the 2000 Health Care Financing Administration Clinical Practice Management project database (48). Other smaller observational studies have also replicated these findings (49,50).

In the ADEMEX study reviewed earlier, residual renal function, not peritoneal, was a predictor of mortality, with an 11% increase in mortality for each 10 L/week/1.73 m² decrease in weekly renal creatinine clearance and a 6% increase in mortality for each 0.1-unit decrease in weekly renal Kt/V urea clearance. These data are consistent with the magnitude of the effects of residual renal function on mortality cited in other studies.

Reasons for these observations are unclear. In PD one reason may be that although 1 unit of residual renal clearance may be the same as 1 unit of peritoneal clearance when measured in terms of Kt/V_{urea}, this may not be true for other solutes. For instance, as will be discussed later, if a patient has a residual renal Kt/V_{urea} of 2.0, his or her residual renal CCr is likely to be about 120 L/week. In contrast, an anuric patient with a peritoneal Kt/V_{urea} of 2.0/week will likely have a CCr of about 55 L/week. This difference may be even more pronounced for middle-molecular-weight solutes such as β_2-microglobulin. A second reason may be that as one increases peritoneal Kt/V_{urea}, there may not be a corresponding increase in clearance of larger solutes such as β_2-microglobulin, whereas with residual renal clearance, as Kt/V_{urea} increases, the clearance of other solutes may increase to the same degree. Furthermore, residual renal clearance may allow better control of blood pressure and volume than what is typically achieved in anuric PD patients. Finally, it is important to remember that the effect of our dialysis is always a constant balance between benefit and toxicity. Is it possible that when increasing instilled volume or when attempting to increase UF with current therapies we increase the toxicity of the therapy? When using 2.5-L exchanges versus 2.0-L exchanges, there is increased glucose absorption from the peritoneal cavity. Is it possible that any possible benefit from the increased clearance is mitigated by the increased glucose absorption and its associated toxicity?

The implications of these observations on "adequacy" of PD are the following: These data suggest that small solute clearance is predictive of outcome. However, it may be most predictive of short-term outcome. It has been shown that increasing instilled volume is likely to relieve clinical signs and symptoms of uremia (51) even though the major effect is to increase small solute, not middle-molecular-weight solute clearances. With standard therapies available today, once on 24 h/d of peritoneal dwell and with a certain minimal small solute clearance, there is little incremental improvement in outcome as small solute clearance (Kt/V_{urea}) is further increased. Above these minimal small solute targets, if on standard PD therapies, once on 24 h/d of peri-

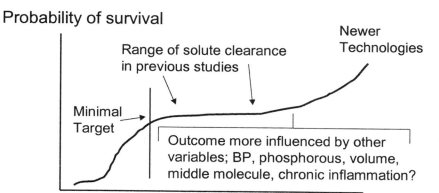

Probability of survival

Newer Technologies

Range of solute clearance in previous studies

Minimal Target

Outcome more influenced by other variables; BP, phosphorous, volume, middle molecule, chronic inflammation?

Total *Small* Solute Clearance?

FIG. 14.1. Possible relationship between total small solute clearance and patient survival for standard therapies.

toneal dwell time, maneuvers that result in a further increase in small solute clearance tend to have little influence on the clearance of other solutes (52,53) or improvement in the control of other parameters (middle-molecule clearance, volume, phosphate clearance, etc.) that may have an influential effect on long-term outcome (Fig. 14.1). It has been shown that as you increase the peritoneal component of the prescription, going from two 6-hour dwells per day (total dwell time, 12 hours) to two 12-hour dwells per day (total dwell time − 24 h) β_2-microglobulin clearance doubles. However, with further increases in the prescription such as to do four, 6-hour dwells per day (24 h/d of total dwell) there was no further increase in β_2-microglobulin clearances (52).

Perhaps alternative PD therapies such as those associated with continuous flow technologies, which appear to offer an increase in β_2-microglobulin clearance over standard technologies, will be beneficial (54).

RECOMMENDED ACCEPTABLE TOTAL SOLUTE CLEARANCE TARGETS FOR PERITONEAL DIALYSIS

The original 1996 NKF–DOQI working group on adequacy of peritoneal dialysis recommended the following total solute clearance goals: For CAPD, a total weekly Kt/V_{urea} of more than 2.0/week and a total weekly CCr of more than 60 L/1.73 m^2 week (Table 14.2). For continuous cyclic peritoneal dialysis (CCPD) a total weekly Kt/V_{urea} of more than 2.1/week and a

TABLE 14.2. MINIMAL RECOMMENDATIONS FOR DIALYSIS DOSE

Modality	Kt/V_{urea}	Creatinine Clearance
CAPD	>2.0 per week	>60 L/week/1.73 m^2
CCPD	>2.1 per week	>63 L/week/1.73 m^2
NIPD, DAPD	>2.2 per week	>66 L/week/1.73 m^2

CAPD, continuous ambulatory peritoneal dialysis; CCPD, continuous cyclic peritoneal dialysis; DAPD, daily intermittent peritoneal dialysis; NIPD, nightly intermittent peritoneal dialysis.

total weekly CCr of more than 63 L/1.73 m^2 week; and for nightly intermittent peritoneal dialysis (NIPD), a total weekly Kt/V_{urea} of more than 2.2/week and a total weekly CCr of more than 66 L/1.73 m^2 week. It was acknowledged that the CAPD targets were evidence based but that the evidence before 1996 did not include any prospective randomized studies to support the recommendation. It was also acknowledged that targets for CCPD and NIPD were opinion based with little or no outcome data for the recommendations.

Reasons for the higher recommended total small solute clearances for intermittent therapies are based on the following theoretical arguments: (a) the possibility that the peak concentration of retained solutes (55), not the time-averaged concentration of retained solutes, relates to uremic symptoms and perhaps inhibits appetite (Fig. 14.2); and (b) data that suggest that when one adjusts for differences in comorbid diseases and scales for differences in the dose of dialysis for peritoneal dialysis and hemodialysis, expected 2-year survival is the same (56,57).

As mentioned, for classic continuous cycling peritoneal dialysis (CCPD), the recommended targets were a weekly Kt/V_{urea} of more than 2.1 and a weekly creatinine clearance of more than 63 L/1.73 m^2. This slight increase in weekly total solute clearance goals for CCPD when compared with CAPD is based on the fact that the daytime dwell for CCPD (14 to 15 hours) tends to be longer than the nighttime dwell (9 to 10 hours) for CAPD. During the long daytime dwell for CCPD, diffusive transport tends to stop because equilibrium between dialysis and plasma has been reached in most patients and hence the therapy is less "continuous" than for CAPD. For more obvious "intermittent" therapies such as nightly intermittent peritoneal dialysis (NIPD) or daily intermittent peritoneal dialysis (DAPD), the recommended weekly Kt/V_{urea} is incrementally higher (58).

These initial minimal total solute clearance targets were met with skepticism (59,60). Furthermore, because of lack of data, these guidelines omitted targets for other solutes and for BP and volume control. As a result, nephrologists may have also focused only on small solute clearances, neglecting middle molecules and UF volume as important components of "adequacy of dialysis."

Subsequent outcome data and clinical experience reviewed above have resulted in a modification of the guidelines. In a group of anuric Canadian patients, only 57% of CAPD and

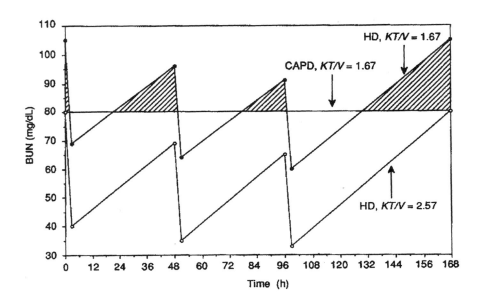

FIG. 14.2. Theoretical weekly BUN profiles for hemodialysis patients with a weekly Kt/V of 1.67 and 2.57 compared with the steady state BUN of CAPD with a weekly Kt/V of 1.67. (Keshaviah PR, et al. The peak concentration hypothesis: a urea kinetic approach to comparing the adequacy of continuous ambulatory peritoneal dialysis [CAPD] and hemodialysis. *Perit Dial Int* 1989;9:257–260.)

81% of APD patients had a weekly Kt/V_{urea} of more than 2.0 and 2.2, respectively, yet there was excellent survival even in anuric patients with a total Kt/V_{urea} of 1.8 (33). Additionally, only 35% of CAPD and 35% of APD patients reached the creatinine clearance of 60 and 66 L/1.73 m²/week, respectively. Others have found that in a group of PD patients thought to be doing well, only 38% of patients met both targets, whereas another 38% met neither target (61). As mentioned earlier, contemporary data are influencing a reevaluation of these targets, but at the time of this publication official revisions have not been published. What is clear, however, is that CCPD with a last bag fill and a mid-day exchange actually may represent a more "continuous" therapy than CAPD.

It appears that in new guidelines there will also be an increased emphasis on BP control and volume control by adjusting daily peritoneal UF. Medical societies are now reviewing these data and deciding if they justify modification of existing guidelines. The European committee for adequacy of PD is likely to not only lower their recommended small solute clearance target (PD alone Kt/V_{urea} of more than 1.7/week) but also add a guideline suggesting that one also have 1 L of peritoneal UF per day (Table 14.3) (personal communication).

IMPACT OF NUTRITIONAL STATUS ON PATIENT OUTCOME

It is well known that nausea, vomiting, and appetite suppression are symptoms of uremia and that uremic patients tend to have decreased dietary protein intake (DPI) (62). Furthermore, spontaneous DPI decreases as residual renal GFR decreases to less than 50 to 25 mL/min (63). These tendencies may be exacerbated during the period before the initiation of dialysis when many patients are not only anorexic but are also acidotic and are often treated with low-protein "renal protective" diets. As a result, patients may exhibit signs of protein malnutrition when they present for dialysis. A more "timely" start of dialysis (see

later) may prevent this. Studies in both ESRD (64–68) and non-ESRD (69) patients have shown that one of the most important predictors of outcome is the patient's underlying nutritional status. In hemodialysis patients, as the serum albumin decreases from the reference value of 4.5 to 4.0 g/dL to an albumin of less than 2.5 g/dL, the risk of death increased to 18 times that of the reference group (65). These data suggest that outcome is related to nutritional status, a parameter that may be influenced by total small solute clearance. However, it is important to remember that nutritional status is dependent not only on the prevention of or treatment of uremia, but also on many non-ESRD-related factors (comorbid diseases, depression, gastroparesis, etc.).

TABLE 14.3. RECOMMENDED TOTAL SMALL SOLUTE CLEARANCE GOALS FROM VARIOUS NATIONAL SOCIETIES

Society	Year	Kt/V_{urea} Goal	Creatinine Clearance Goal	UF Volume
NKF-DOQI, National Kidney Foundation–Dialysis Outcomes Quality Initiative	2000			
CAPD (Low and LA)		2.0	60 L/1.73 m²	NA
CAPD (High and HA)		2.0	50 L/1.73 m²	NA
CCPD		2.1	63 L/1.73 m²	NA
NIPD		2.0	66 L/1.73 m²	NA
Canadian	1998			
Low and LA		2.0	60 L/1.73 m²	NA
High and HA		2.0	50 L/1.73 m²	NA
United Kingdom	1997	1.7	NA	NA
European	2002[a]	1.7 (PD only)	NA	1 L

Raymond Krediet, personal communicaton. CAPD, continuous ambulatory peritoneal dialysis; CCPD, continuous cyclic peritoneal dialysis; HA, high average; LA, low average; NA, not available; NIPD, nightly intermittent peritoneal dialysis; PD, peritoneal dialysis; UF, ultrafiltration.

Dialysis itself is associated with unique metabolic and nutritional problems. Peritoneal dialysis patients are known to have a decreased appetite and early satiety (70,71). They typically lose 5 to 15 g of protein and 2 to 4 g of amino acids per day in their dialysate (72). These losses amount to a net loss equivalent to 0.2 g protein/kg/d and tend to be higher in rapid transporters than in low transporters. These losses are increased during episodes of peritonitis (73), at times doubling even after a mild episode. Although peritoneal losses of protein may correlate with serum albumin levels, they do not seem to correlate with the actual nutritional status of chronic peritoneal dialysis patients (74).

It is well known from clinical and experimental observations that overtly uremic patients are anorectic and tend to have decreased protein intake. Patients with chronic renal insufficiency tend to decrease their protein intake spontaneously. As a result of these observations, the working hypothesis has been that underdialysis or uremia leads to a decreased appetite, malnutrition, and decreased albumin synthesis. However, cross-sectional studies have provided contradictory results regarding the potential association between nutrition and dialysis dose (75–79). Some investigators believe that this relationship is simply mathematical coupling of data (80). Prospective studies, however, have demonstrated that increasing the dose of dialysis up to levels felt to be adequate resulted in an increase in nPNA values (77), in energy intake (81), and in percent lean body mass. These findings are in accord with the observation that the relationship between dose of dialysis and protein intake becomes flat at a Kt/V level greater than about 1.9 (82,83) and are the reason for the clinical recommendation that suggests that a malnourished dialysis patient may be malnourished because of "underdialysis."

It is now noted that malnutrition can be reflective of poor nutritional intake, inflammation (84–87), or both (88,89). Serum albumin levels are known to be an acute phase reactant, decreasing in the face of inflammation. C-reactive protein levels are abnormally high in most peritoneal dialysis patients, and there is a direct association between elevated CRP levels and increased rates of mortality (90,91) and cardiovascular disease (92–94).

Malnutrition is a significant risk factor for mortality and hospitalizations in chronic peritoneal dialysis patients (15,95,96). Estimates of malnutrition in chronic peritoneal dialysis patients range from 40% to 76%, with the variability in prevalence due to differing definitions of malnutrition as well as differences in the patient population studied (97–99). Few studies provide data on longitudinal changes in nutritional parameters. A prospective study performed in 118 patients who were started on peritoneal dialysis found that mean serum albumin levels increased by approximately 0.2 g/dL over 24 months, nPNA declined by approximately 0.1 g/kg/d, whereas BMI and body fat were essentially unchanged (100).

The link between malnutrition and poor clinical outcome was not established using serum albumin alone as a marker for nutritional status. Other surrogates for nutritional status such as loss of muscle mass, as indicated by lower serum creatinine levels, lower creatinine generation rates, or total body nitrogen levels as well as low serum albumin levels, low prealbumin levels,

and subjective global assessment score are all good predictors of morbidity and mortality. Hence for optimal PD therapy, the effect of total solute clearance on nutrition must be known and optimized.

MEASUREMENTS OF NUTRITIONAL STATUS

Of the readily available measures of nutritional status, serum albumin levels, protein equivalent of nitrogen balance (PNA) and subjective global assessment scores (SGA), have traditionally been used (see Chapter 30).

Serum Albumin Levels

Serum albumin levels, in part a reflection of visceral protein storage, predict patient outcome in ESRD populations, no matter if obtained at the initiation of therapy (15,101) over the duration of dialysis (102) or measured at a stable period while on dialysis (103,104). Different assays for serum albumin give markedly different results (105). The Bromocresol green assay is preferred. Using this, the mean serum albumin level in 1,202 PD patients in late 1994 and early 1995 was 3.5 g/dL (106). In an individual PD patient, the significance of an isolated serum albumin level must be viewed with caution. An isolated level does not necessarily predict nutritional status. Levels must be followed over time and interpreted in context of other patient related issues such as trends in the level, transport type, solute clearance, comorbid diseases, and so on.

We now have a better understanding of the causes of hypoalbuminemia. They are multifactorial (Table 14.4). When evaluating an individual patient, all causes must be considered, including the possibility that a chronic inflammatory state exists. Evolving data suggest that ESRD or perhaps the treatment of ESRD represents a chronic inflammatory state. During peritoneal dialysis, the peritoneal cavity is repeatedly exposed to unphysiologic fluids (107,108), which may (109) or may not (110) induce a chronic inflammatory state. Morphologic studies reveal that the morphology of the peritoneum changes over time on PD (111). The precipitating event leading to these changes is unknown but may be related to cytotoxicity, the hyperosmolality, low-pH byproducts of sterilization, or the plastic tubing or the lactate buffers of PD solutions, and is associated with glycosylation of protein, which may lead to changes at times altering peritoneal transport and resulting in the development of a sclerosing syndrome of the peritoneal cavity (112,113). Our current "standard" solutions may need to be modified to better maintain long-term viability of the peritoneal membrane in terms of clearance capacity and membrane durability. Once more is known, future discussions of adequacy may also

TABLE 14.4. CAUSES OF HYPOALBUMINEMIA

Dilutional (volume overload)
Decreased synthesis
Increased body losses
    Urine
    Dialysate
Chronic inflammatory states

involve discussions about controlling or modifying the chronic inflammatory state and its relationship to membrane viability and nutritional status.

Dietary Protein Intake

Most (95%) nitrogen intake in humans is in the form of protein. Therefore when the patient is in a steady state (not catabolic or anabolic), total nitrogen excretion multiplied by 6.25 (there are about 6.25 g of protein per gram of nitrogen) is thought to be an estimation of a person's dietary protein intake (DPI) (114). Estimated DPI is calculated from urea nitrogen appearance (UNA) in dialysate and urine. Multiple equations have been derived, some of which have been validated in CAPD (not NIPD) patients (PNA = PCR + protein losses) (Table 14.5). These estimations were initially called the protein catabolic rate (PCR). However, PCR actually represents the amount of protein catabolism exceeding synthesis required to generate an amount of nitrogen that is excreted. PCR is actually a net catabolic equivalent. Thus because these calculations are based on nitrogen appearance, the term is more appropriately called the protein equivalent of nitrogen appearance, or PNA.

Keshaviah and Nolph (115) have compared these formulas and recommended the Randerson equation (116), where PNA = 10.76 (UNA + 1.46), and UNA is in milligrams per minute, or PNA = 10.76 (UNA/1.44 + 1.46), and UNA is in grams per day. These equations assume that the patient is in a steady state where UNA = urea nitrogen output, which equals urea generation. The Randerson equation also assumes that the average daily protein loss in the dialysate is 7.3 g/d. In dialysis patients with substantial urinary or dialysate protein losses, these direct protein losses must be added to the equation to yield a true PNA. Most societies have recommended monitoring a patient's estimated DPI over time to assure adequate nutritional status. A baseline PNA should be obtained during training. These should then be recalculated every 4 to 6 months using the same 24-hour dialysate and urine collections used to monitor solute clearances. Decreasing values would then suggest a decreasing protein intake. One cause for this may be a suboptimal total solute clearance.

For comparison purposes, it is recommended that PNA be normalized for patient size (nPNA). What weight to use for that normalization is contested. Depending on what weight is used in calculating nPNA, there may or may not be a statistical relationship between clinical evidence of malnutrition and nPNA values below target. The PNA normalized by actual weight tends to be high or may appear to be increasing over time in malnourished individuals if normalized (divided) by a smaller malnourished weight when compared with the patient's baseline weight (117). This fact is important not only for evaluating patient-to-patient comparisons, but more important, when comparing serial measurements in an individual patient. The DOQI working group and others have recommended using standard weight or V/0.58 for normalization (118). In this case, the weight used for normalization does not change over time, so that nPNA is more likely to reflect actual changes in DPI. Although most guidelines recommend monitoring estimated nPNA over time, looking for changes, it has been suggested that in cross-sectional analysis the absolute amount of protein intake, not nPNA, correlated best with outcome and signs of malnutrition.

Data from the CMS-CPM project for the year 2000 found that in chronic peritoneal dialysis patients the mean protein equivalent of nitrogen appearance (nPNA) was 0.95 ± 0.31 g/kg/d, their normalized creatinine appearance rate was 17 ± 6.5 mg/kg/d, and the mean percent lean body mass (% LBM) was 64% ± 17% of actual body weight (119).

There is some controversy as to what amount of dietary protein intake (DPI), in terms of grams of protein per kilogram of body weight, is needed to maintain positive nitrogen balance in peritoneal dialysis patients. Early studies suggested that a dietary protein intake of at least 1.2 g/kg/d was needed to maintain nitrogen balance (120,121), a value considerably higher than that recommended for normal individuals. The National Kidney Foundation Clinical Practice Dialysis Outcomes Quality Initiative (DOQI) guidelines recently recommended a dietary protein intake for chronic peritoneal dialysis patients of: 1.2 to 1.3 g/kg/d (122). Cross-sectional studies by Bergstrom et al. (78) and Nolph (123) suggest that their patients who show no signs of malnutrition seem to eat less (0.99, 0.88 g protein/kg/d, respectively). The results are likely due to variations in the patient populations studied, historical dietary patterns, and amounts of residual renal function present. Therefore several investigators have proposed that the daily protein intake in these patients should be in the range of 0.9 to 1.1 g/kg/d (124,125).

Patients undergoing chronic peritoneal dialysis should have a total daily energy intake of 35 kcal/kg/d for patients who are less than 60 years of age and 30 kcal/kg for patients 60 years of age or more (122,126). This includes both dietary intake and the energy intake derived from glucose absorbed from the peritoneal dialysate. Many patients typically eat less (127,128). Food supplements, enteral tube feedings, and both intradialytic and total parenteral nutrition have been used to treat malnutrition (129). Percutaneous endoscopic gastrostomy tubes should be used cautiously, however, as their use has been associated with a high rate of peritonitis. In addition, bicarbonate supplementation can result in improvements in weight and body mass index (130).

Subjective Global Assessment Score

The subjective global assessment (SGA) score (131) modified for PD is a valid estimate of nutritional status in PD patients

TABLE 14.5. COMMONLY USED FORMULAS FOR CALCULATING PNA

Randerson I	PNA = 10.76 (UNA/1.44 + 1.46), where UNA is in g/day
Randerson II	PNA = 10.76 (UNA + 1.46), where UNA is in mg/min
Modified Borah	PNA = 9.35 G_{un} + .294 V + protein losses
Teehan	PNA = 6.25 (UN_{loss} + 1.81 + .031 B. Wt.)
Kjelldahl	PNA = 6.25 × N. loss
Bergstrom	PNA = 19 + 7.62 × UNA

Modified from Kopple JD, et al. A proposed glossary for dialysis kinetics. *Am J Kidney Dis* 1995;26:963–981 and Keshaviah P, et al. Protein catabolic rate calculations in CAPD patients. *ASAIO Trans* 1991;37:M400–M402. PNA, protein equivalent of nitrogen balance; UNA, urea nitrogen appearance.

(132). In the CANUSA study, a modified SGA using a seven-point scale addressing four items (weight change, anorexia, subcutaneous tissue, and muscle mass) predicted outcome (15). On multivariate analysis, poorer SGA scores were associated with a higher relative risk of death. It is recommended that this simple test be obtained sequentially (twice a year) in PD patients to evaluate nutritional status. If a decline is noted, evaluate for comorbid diseases and consider a suboptimal total solute clearance as the cause.

MAJOR DETERMINANTS OF TOTAL SOLUTE CLEARANCE

Small solute clearance is typically measured in terms of urea kinetics (Kt/V_{urea}) and creatinine clearance (CCr)/1.73 m². Guidelines recommend attaining certain target "total" (peritoneal and residual renal) clearances/week.

Residual Renal Function

Each 1 mL/min of corrected residual renal creatinine clearance adds approximately 10 L/week/1.73 m² of CCr for the average patient with a body surface area (BSA) of 1.73 m². Similarly, each 1 mL/min of residual renal urea clearance adds approximately 0.25 Kt/V_{urea} units to the total weekly Kt/V_{urea} urea for a 70-kg male. Creatinine and urea are used as surrogate markers for small-molecular-weight clearance. When calculating the CCr due to residual renal function, it is important to remember that at very low glomerular filtration rates (GFR) or creatinine clearances, much of the creatinine in the urine is due to proximal tubular secretion rather than to actual glomerular filtration. As a result, traditional measurements of creatinine clearance (24-hour collection) can significantly overestimate the true GFR. If using creatinine kinetics as the surrogate, it is recommended that the sum of the measured urea clearance and creatinine clearance divided by 2 be used to approximate underlying residual renal GFR. This amount in liters per day is then added to the daily peritoneal creatinine clearance to determine total daily CCr. The clearance of most other small-molecular-weight substances such as urea by the kidney only involves glomerular filtration and little to no tubular secretion. Therefore if one is measuring dialysis dose using urea kinetics, no adjustment for tubular secretion is needed.

At the initiation of dialysis, this often represents a significant amount of the recommended target solute clearances. In one report the residual renal component represented 39% of total clearance (133), while representing 25% of the total in another review (134). For instance, if a patient starts PD with a residual renal creatinine clearance of 5 mL/min (not an unusual scenario), the corrected renal creatinine clearance (GFR) would be about 4 mL/min, adding approximately 40 L/week of creatinine clearance to overall solute clearance, whereas the residual renal urea clearance might be about 3 mL/minute.

Some have suggested that residual renal function is better preserved with peritoneal dialysis than with hemodialysis (135–138). It is acknowledged that residual renal clearance is an important supplement to that provided by dialysis and is an important predictor of outcome. As residual renal function decreases, total clearance expressed as Kt/V_{urea} or CCr will decrease unless replaced by an increase in the peritoneal component. Tattersall et al. (139) and others (140) have shown that it was possible to compensate for declining residual renal function by increasing dialysis dose.

Peritoneal Membrane Transport Characteristics

The first step in tailoring an individual patient's peritoneal dialysis prescription is to know that patient's peritoneal membrane transport characteristics. Unlike hemodialysis, where the physician has a wide menu of dialyzers to choose from for each individual patient, peritoneal dialysis patients are "born" with their membrane. At present, there is no clinically proven way to favorably change membrane transport or predict transport type before beginning PD.

The peritoneal equilibration test (PET) (141) is the standard way to characterize peritoneal membrane transport properties of an individual patient. It is a standardized test in which, after an overnight dwell, 2 L of 2.5% dextrose dialysate is instilled (time 0) and allowed to dwell for 4 hours. Dialysate urea, glucose, sodium, and creatinine are measured at time 0, and after 2 and 4 hours of dwell time. Serum values are drawn after 2 hours. Dialysate is drained after 4 hours of dwell, and drain volume is measured. Dialysate to plasma ratios (D/P) of creatinine and urea are determined after 2 and 4 hours of dwell, as is the ratio of dialysate glucose at those drain times to the initial dialysate glucose concentration (D/Do) (Fig. 14.3). Based on published data, the patient's peritoneal membrane type is then characterized as high, high-average, low-average, and low. In a review of 806 patients, 10.4% were found to be high transporters; 53.1%, high average; 30.9%, low average; and 5.6%, low transporters (142). Once characterized, the peritoneal dialysis prescription that would best match the patient's transport characteristics can then be chosen.

These D/P ratios can be calculated for any solute. By doing so, one can appreciate the difference in expected clearances for various-sized solutes. For instance, as noted in Fig. 14.4, urea (mol wt 60 daltons) is transported faster than creatinine (mol wt 112 daltons). Most patients are greater than 90% equilibrated for urea after a 4-hour dwell, whereas for creatinine, the average patient is only 65% equilibrated at 4 hours. As noted in the figure, these differences are even more marked for low transporters and are clinically most noted when using a therapy that utilizes multiple short dwells (CCPD, NIPD).

Solute removal by PD is related to the D/P ratio of that solute times the dialysate *drain volume* (DV). Patients with small drain volumes tend to have lower clearances. UF during a dwell is related to osmotic forces induced by crystalloid (glucose, amino acid) or colloid (icodextrin) substances. It is important to point out that rapid transporters of creatinine/urea also tend to be rapid absorbers of dialysate glucose. Once the osmotic glucose gradient is mitigated by absorption, UF ceases and lymphatic absorption of fluid predominates (Fig. 14.5). Therefore, in rapid transporters, although the D/P ratios of urea and creatinine at 4-hour or longer dwells tend to be close to unity, their

PERITONEAL EQUILIBRATION TEST

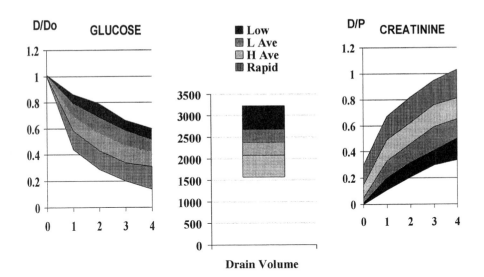

FIG. 14.3. Dialysate-to-plasma (D/P) ratio urea and ratios of dialysate glucose at time of sampling to dialysate glucose at time 0 during typical 4-hour dwell with 2.5% dextrose. (Modified from Twardowski ZJ, et al. Peritoneal equilibration test. *Perit Dial Bull* 1987;7: 138–147, and Twardowski ZJ, et al. Peritoneal dialysis modifications to avoid CAPD dropouts. In: Khanna R, et al., eds. *Advances in continuous ambulatory peritoneal dialysis.* Proceedings of the Seventh Annual CAPD Conference, Kansas City, Missouri, February 1987. Toronto: Peritoneal Dialysis Bulletin, 1987:171–178.)

drain volumes tend to be small and hence their solute removal is less than optimal due to the small drain volumes (143). In fact, during the long overnight dwell of CAPD (9 hours) or during the long daytime dwell of classic CCPD (15 hours), rapid transporters may have *drain* volumes that are actually less than the *instilled* volume. For these patients, short dwell times are needed to reduce or minimize fluid reabsorption and optimize clearances. In patients who are low transporters, intraperitoneal glucose is slowly absorbed, hence peak UF occurs later during the dwell and net UF can be obtained even after prolonged dwells. In these patients, the D/P ratio increases almost linearly during the dwell. It is not until 8 to 10 hours that the D/P ratio reaches unity.

To put these differences in perspective one can appreciate that after only a 2-hour dwell time, a rapid transporter likely will have achieved 2 L of creatinine clearance, whereas the creatinine clearance in a low-transport individual may be only 1 L or less,

despite a larger drain volume (Fig. 14.6). It may take the low transporter up to 7 or 8 hours of dwell time to achieve the same clearance that a rapid transporter achieves after only a 2-hour dwell. These differences must be taken into account when attempting to tailor an individual patient's peritoneal dialysis prescription.

The PET is the most practical and widely used method to classify peritoneal transport; however, other ways also exist. In these other tests, instead of using D/P ratios, these tests use mass transfer area coefficients (MTAC) (144,145), which are more precise and more succinctly define transport. The MTACs define transport independent of UF (convection-related solute removal), and hence in theory are not influenced by dwell volume or glucose concentration. The practical use of MTAC for modeling a peritoneal dialysis prescription requires additional laboratory measurements and computer models, but once obtained, MTAC can be easily used in the clinical setting (146).

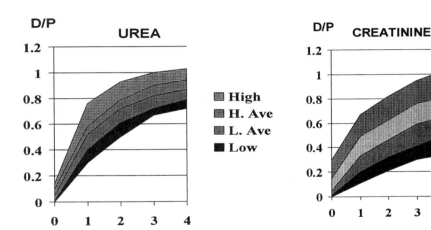

FIG. 14.4. Dialysate-to-plasma (D/P) ratios for urea and creatinine during the standard peritoneal equilibration test (PET). Exact values at 2 and 4 h are shown. (Modified from Twardowski ZJ, et al. Peritoneal equilibration test. *Perit Dial Bull* 1987;7:138–147, and Twardowski ZJ, et al. Peritoneal dialysis modifications to avoid CAPD dropouts. In: Khanna R, et al., eds. *Advances in continuous ambulatory peritoneal dialysis.* Proceedings of the Seventh Annual CAPD Conference, Kansas City, Missouri, February 1987. Toronto: Peritoneal Dialysis Bulletin, 1987:171–178.)

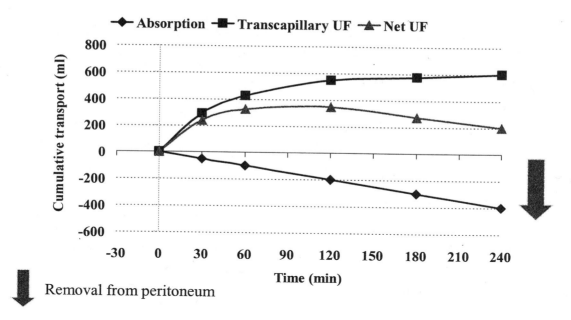

FIG. 14.5. Time profiles of opposing forces governing ultrafiltration (transcapillary ultrafiltration and lymphatic absorption. Lymphatic absorption, ◆; transcapillary ultrafiltration, ■; net ultrafiltration, ▲. (Modified from Mactier RA, et al. Contribution of lymphatic absorption to loss of ultrafiltration and solute clearances on continuous ambulatory peritoneal dialysis. *J Clin Invest* 1987;80:1311–1316.)

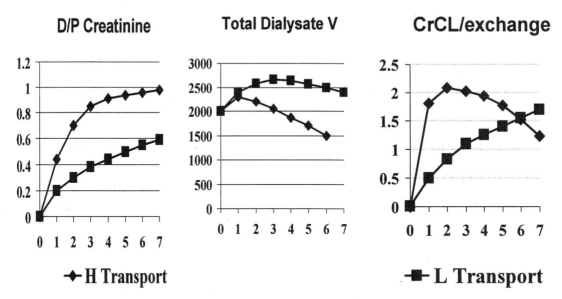

FIG. 14.6. Idealized curves of creatinine and water transport during an exchange with 2 L of 2.5% glucose dialysis solutions in patients with extremely low and high transport characteristics. (Twardowski ZJ. Nightly peritoneal dialysis [why? who? how? and when?]. *ASAIO Trans* 1990;36:8–16.)

The standard peritoneal permeability analysis is another, less often used test to follow transport and UF characteristics (147). The test not only determines transport characteristics, but also better evaluates lymphatic reabsorption. If one does a PET using 4.25% dextrose to maximize UF, one is better able to determine the amount of sodium sieving and can better differentiate the causes of UF failure (148,149).

Peritoneal membrane transport tends to remain stable over time. Rippe and Krediet reviewed nine cross-sectional and 16 longitudinal studies of peritoneal transport (150). In 14 of 25 studies, there tended to be no change in peritoneal transport over time on PD; in the other 11 studies, there was a slight increase in low- and medium-molecular-weight solute transport over time. Others found no change in peritoneal transport in 23 patients followed for at least 7 years (151), especially in patients with low peritonitis rates (152). In contrast, there was a tendency to increase in small solute transport and loss of UF, especially in patients with frequent peritonitis (153,154). Others have noted that up to 30.9% of patients developed UF failure (change in transport) after 6 years on PD (155). These data emphasize the importance of monitoring membrane transport (usually with PET testing) over time to optimize solute clearance, drain volumes, BP, and UF while minimizing hypertonic glucose use. If transport type changes, the prescription may need to be altered.

Normalization and Influence of Body Size on Solute Clearance

Removal of the same absolute amount of solute from a 55-kg elderly female as from an 80-kg muscular male may not result in the same control of uremia. These patients likely have different metabolic rates and protein intakes. Therefore the absolute amount of daily solute removed or cleared must be normalized for differences in body size [normalized by volume *(V)* of distribution for Kt/V_{urea} and by body surface area [BSA] for CCr/1.73 m^2).

Kt/V_{urea} is normalized by *V*, whereas CCr imL/week/1.73 m^2, by BSA. See Table 14.6 for recommended formulas. Total body water *(V)* can be estimated as a fixed percentage of body weight, or more accurately, by using anthropometric formulas based on sex, age, height, and weight such as the Watson (156) or Hume (157) formulas in adults. These equations provide unrealistic estimates for *V* in patients whose weights are markedly different from normal body weight (NBW). BSA is usually calculated using the formula by Dubois and Dubois (158).

In a review of 806 PD patients, the median BSA was 1.85 m^2 (not 1.73 m^2), whereas the 25th percentile was 1.71 m^2 and the 75th percentile was 2.0 m^2 (142), whereas data from the CMS–CPM project for the year 2000 found that chronic peritoneal dialysis patients had a mean body weight of 76 ± 19 kg and body mass index (BMI) of 27.5 ± 6.4 kg/ m^2 (119). Despite the finding that most PD patients are larger than the "standard" BSA of 1.73 m^2, a review of the predicted clearances for Kt/V_{urea} for an average transporter over a broad range of BSA, suggests that if you were able to individualize therapy (increased instilled volumes, daytime exchange for CCPD, nightly exchange device), one should be able to achieve the recommended acceptable target total Kt/V_{urea} clearances for most patients on peritoneal dialysis (159). Based on the

TABLE 14.6. EQUATIONS FOR NORMALIZATION: CALCULATING *V* FOR *Kt/V* OR BODY SURFACE AREA (BSA) FOR CREATININE CLEARANCE

Formula for Estimating BSA

For all formulas, Wt is in kg and Ht is in cm:
DuBois and Dubois method: BSA (m^2) = 0.007184 × Wt$^{0.425}$ × Ht$^{0.725}$
Gehan and George method: BSA (m^2) = 0.235 × Wt$^{0.51456}$ × Ht$^{0.42246}$
Haycock method: BSA (m^2) = 0.024265 × Wt$^{0.5378}$ × Ht$^{0.3964}$

Formulas for Estimating V

Watson Method
For men: *V* (liters) = 2.447 + 0.3362 × Wt (kg) + 0.1074 × Ht (cm) − 0.09516 × Age (years)
For women: *V* = 2.097 + 0.2466 × Wt + 0.1069 × Ht

Hume Method

For men: *V* (liters) = −14.012934 + 0.296785 × Wt + 0.194786 × Ht
For women: *V* = −35.270121 + 0.183809 × Wt + 0.344547 × Ht

Mellitis-Cheek Method for Children

For boys: *V* (liters) = −1.927 + 0.465 × Wt (kg) + 0.045 × Ht (cm), when Ht ≤ 132.7 cm
V = −31.993 + 0.406 × Wt + 0.209 × Ht, when height is ≥ 132.7 cm
For girls: *V* = 0.076 + 0.507 × Wt + 0.013 × Ht, when height is < 110.8 cm
V = −10.313 + 0.252 × Wt 0.154 × Ht, when height is ≥ 110.8 cm

From Dubois D, et al. A formula to estimate the approximate surface area if height and weight be known. *Arch Intern Med* 1916;17:863–871. Gehan E, et al. Estimation of human body surface area from height and weight. *Cancer Chemother Rep* 1970;54 (part 1):225–235. Haycock GB, et al. Geometric method for measuring body surface area: a height-weight formula validated in infants, children and adults. *J Pediatr* 1978;93:62–66. Watson PE, et al. Total body water volumes for adult males and females estimated from simple anthropometric measurements. *Am J Clin Nutr* 1980;33:27–39. Hume R, et al. Relationship between total body water and surface area in normal and obese subjects. *J Clin Pathol* 1971;24:234–238. Mellitis ED, et al. The assessment of body water and fatness from infancy to adulthood. *Monogr Soc Res Child Dev,* Serial 140 1970;35:12–26.

patient's body size, one can predict whether an individual patient who is an average transporter would meet NKF–DOQI targets for small solute clearance using four 2.0-L exchanges per day once they were anuric (160–162), and what instilled volume/prescription would be needed to achieve the small solute clearance targets. Only anuric patients who are low transporters and who have large body surface areas (>1.8 m^2) would be unlikely to achieve these targets.

For malnourished patients whose weight is more than 10% less than their ideal weight, the NKF–DOQI guidelines recommend adjusting total solute clearance targets by the ratio of ideal to actual weight. In this case you target a relatively higher target solute removal to promote anabolism and an increased protein intake. Jones (163) noted that when ABW was used for normalization, there was no difference in total solute clearance (*Kt/V* or CCr) between patients who were well nourished and those who were malnourished. However, when calculated *V* and BSA were determined using desired body weight (DBW), there was a statistically significant difference between the groups for both weekly Kt/V_{urea} (1.68 ± 0.46 versus 1.40 ± 0.41, *p* <0.05) and for CCr in L/1.73 m^2/wk (52.5 ± 10.3 versus 41.6 ± 19.0, *p* <0.01).

It is uncertain what to do in the case of an obese individual. Large patients (BMI >27.5) on PD tend to do as well as or better than patients who are within 10% of their ideal weight

TABLE 14.7. ADEQUACY CALCULATIONS: WHAT WEIGHT SHOULD YOU USE?

BW Ratio	<0.9	0.9–1.1	>1.1
%	*19%*	*33%*	*48%*
BWa/BWd	0.82	1.01	1.37
Kt/Va	1.95	2.08	1.94
Kt/Vd	1.74	2.08	2.25
CCra (L/week)	68.1	71.5	64.1
CCrd (L/week)	62.6	71.7	72.4

a, actual body weight; d, desired body weight; BW, body weight; V, volume of distribution; cc, creatinine clearance. From Satko SG, et al. Frequency and causes of discrepancy between *Kt*/V and creatinine. *Perit Dial Int* 1997;17:S23.

(164). If one uses actual weight there is a marked difference in adequacy calculations (Table 14.7). Others have managed their patients, adjusting the PD prescription based on *Kt*/V urea and CCr/1.73 m² where the normalization calculations were done using ideal weight when calculating *V* or BSA found no difference in survival for patients whose actual weights were more than 10% above their ideal weight when compared with those whose weights were within 10% of ideal weight (34). For now it is still unclear what weight to use when calculating *Kt*/V or CCr in obese individuals. National committees have not amended their guidelines. However, it is clear that many obese patients do very well on PD, and if you individualize clearances, most are able to achieve target. As the NKF–DOQI guidelines suggested, attempt to reach recommended targets. If you cannot, look at the individual and decide how they are doing clinically before you automatically transfer the patient to HD.

SPECIAL CONSIDERATIONS

Rapid Transporters

Rapid transporters tend to optimize both solute clearance and UF after a short dwell time (approximately 2 hours) and therefore are likely to do well on short dwell therapies such as NIPD, with or without one or two 2- to 4-hour daytime dwells. One would predict that they would easily reach total solute clearance goals for *Kt*/V and creatinine clearance. Despite this relative ease in the ability to achieve recommended total solute clearance goals, these patients have recently been shown to have an increased relative risk of death and a decreased technique survival (39,40). In the CANUSA study, patients with a 4-hour D/P creatinine of more than 0.65 (high) were compared with those with a 4-hour D/P creatinine of less than 0.65 (low). The 2-year probability for technique survival was 79% among low transporters compared with 71% for high transporters. The probability of 2-year patient survival was 82% among low transporters versus 72% for high transporters, with a relative risk of death of 2.18 for high versus low transporters. Heaf (41) noted increased morbidity in rapid transporters. The reason(s) for this increased relative risk while on CAPD are unclear.

Nolph et al. (165) noted that high transporters (D/P >0.81) had increased incidence of malnutrition and low serum albumin levels. One possible explanation is the following: Many have shown that as the D/P ratio at 4 hours increases, there tends to

be increased protein loss. As dialysate protein losses increase, serum albumin levels decrease, and serum albumin correlates inversely with peritoneal membrane transport (166–168); another possible explanation may be overt or subtle volume overload. The typical dwells associated with CAPD tend to be associated with problems with UF in these patients. This volume overload may lead to increased blood pressure and/or increased LVH with its associated increased risks of death. Furthermore, to optimize UF, these patients will likely increase their percent glucose in their fluids, leading to better UF but increased glucose absorption. This increased glucose absorption may (127,169–171) or may not (172) inhibit appetite. The most recent finding is that serum albumin levels may be a marker for chronic inflammation and the finding that rapid transporters tend to have evidence of chronic inflammation.

It has been recommended that these patients change to NIPD with or without a short daytime dwell. This change maintains total solute clearance while decreasing the need for hypertonic glucose exchanges and therefore decreasing the relative amount of glucose absorption (173). If one does change to NIPD, it is important to remember that it is recommended that one now increase total solute clearance goals to *Kt*/V >2.2. There may be a small but insignificant decrease in protein losses when changing from CAPD to NIPD (166).

Acid–Base Metabolism

An essential component of providing "optimal" dialysis is correction of acidosis. Chronic acidosis has a detrimental effect on protein, carbohydrate, and bone metabolism. In CAPD patients, body base balance is self-regulated by feedback between plasma bicarbonate levels and bicarbonate gain/loss (174). Dialysis must provide sufficient replenishment of buffers to compensate for the daily acid load. Lactate (concentration 35 to 40 mmol/L) is the standard buffer utilized in currently available PD solutions, although newer bicarbonate-based solutions are in use in some countries (141). Lactate is converted to pyruvate and oxygenated or used in gluconeogenesis with the consumption of H+ and the generation of bicarbonate (175). Some CAPD patients remain acidemic. With lactate-containing buffer solutions, buffer balance is governed by the relative amounts of H+ generation, bicarbonate loss, lactate absorption, and lactate metabolism (176–178).

Most CAPD patients have stable mean plasma bicarbonate levels of about 25.6 mmol/L using a dialysate lactate of 35 mmol/L. Increasing dialysate lactate results in a higher serum bicarbonate level (179). Control of acidosis is traditionally thought important to prevent protein catabolism (180,181); however, two studies have found no correlation between serum albumin levels and bicarbonate concentration (182,183). More data are needed to evaluate the effect of PD fluid lactate levels on outcome.

The Preferred Target: *Kt*/V or Creatinine Clearance?

Currently, both total *Kt*/V$_{urea}$ and total CCr/1.73 m² can be used to monitor solute clearance. There are no data to suggest that one index is better than the other. Although these two yardsticks do not fall on the same linear scale, the two values usually correlate (184). However, in up to 20% of patients there is a significant discrepancy between the two (61,185,186). In these situations, one is often presented with a clinical dilemma. For instance, one may find a *Kt/V* that appears adequate when CCr is not, yet the patient may seem to be doing well. Similarly, one may have seen a patient who is gaining weight and eating well, yet the parameters are below target. How can one explain these findings? What does one do?

The reasons for these discrepancies are multifactorial and include the amount of residual renal function present and its relative contribution to total *Kt/V* or CCr, the difference in peritoneal transport of urea and creatinine, and the influence of patient size on normalization. Residual renal clearance is the result of glomerular filtration and tubular manipulation of that filtrate. Creatinine clearance by the kidneys is due to glomerular filtration and proximal tubular secretion, especially in advanced stages of renal insufficiency where the absolute amount of tubular creatinine secretion can increase by as much as 30%, accounting for up to 35% of total urinary creatinine (187). In contrast, with urea, there is glomerular filtration but also tubular reabsorption. Therefore in advanced stages of renal disease residual renal clearance of creatinine will be relatively greater than that for urea. Peritoneal clearance is predominantly diffusion driven. (There is also a component of convective clearance due to UF, but this contribution is relatively smaller than that due to diffusion.) Therefore because urea is a smaller-molecular-weight solute than creatinine, the numerical value for peritoneal clearance of urea tends to be relatively greater than that for creatinine clearance. This difference is most pronounced in patients who are low transporters. In summary, the ratio of CCr/*Kt/V* (arbitrary reference 60/2.0 = 30) tends to be higher at the initiation of dialysis when patients tend to have a significant amount of residual renal function. However, once anuric, the ratio of CCr/*Kt/V* tends to be lower (Fig. 14.7).

Peritoneal membrane transport characteristics may also explain this discrepancy. The diffusive clearance for urea is relatively greater than that for creatinine. During the typical dwells associated with CAPD, the dialysate-to-plasma ratio (D/P) for urea tends to reach unity (equilibration between blood and dialysate) in all patients, whereas the D/P ratio for creatinine tends to reach unity only in high transporters. Therefore the urea clearance/dwell tends to be greater than that for creatinine. This is most pronounced in low transporters where the ratio of CCr to *Kt/V* tends to be lower than in high transporters. The NKF–DOQI guidelines for adequacy of peritoneal dialysis made the assumption that the ratio of dialysis creatinine clearance to dialysis urea clearance in CAPD was 0.8 when formulating solute clearance targets. This was likely for an average transporter on CAPD; however, the basis for this assumption is not noted in the document.

The guidelines do not differentiate between genders. As can be seen in Table 14.6, the patient's weight has a different effect on normalization (*V* or BSA) for male or female and for CCr versus *Kt/V*. In patients with similar BSAs, instilled volume, transport type, and gender all have a significant effect on *Kt/V* calculations but not on CCr calculations. The mathematical relationship between BSA and *V* is not fixed. It is disturbed by both gender and obesity. Furthermore, the actual *V* is different if "obesity" is due to a change in body fat versus a change in body water (overhydration) (188) and if the patient has had an amputation (189). Therefore in the average anuric patient on five 2-L exchanges per day with average peritoneal transport characteristics, peritoneal creatinine clearance will be 73% of urea clearance (190). Thus in an anuric average transporter with a weekly peritoneal *Kt/V* of 2.0, the expected creatinine clearance is about 55 L/1.73 m^2/week in males and 47 L/1.73 m^2/week in females. Similarly, for NIPD patients with average transport, the peritoneal creatinine clearance will be 64% of urea. Thus for an anuric average transporter on NIPD, with a weekly *Kt/V* of 2.2, the expected weekly creatinine clearance will be 53 L/1.73 m^2 in males and 45 L/1.73 m^2 in females. As one can see from Table 14.8, in anuric patients at *Kt/V* target, creatinine clearance is more often than not going to be below NKF–DOQI recommendations. The problems with current "normalization" prac-

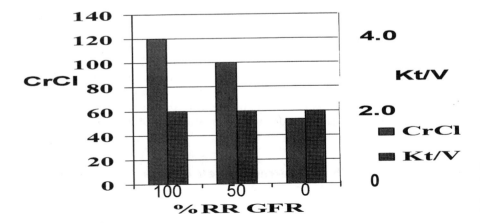

FIG. 14.7. Representative total weekly *Kt/V*$_{urea}$ and CCR/1.73 m^2 for an average 70-kg male, who is an average transporter with various amounts of RRF contributing to total solute clearance (100%, 50%, 0).

TABLE 14.8. CREATININE CLEARANCE (L) AT *Kt/V* OF 2.2 IN NIPD AND 2.0 IN CAPD

Transport Category	NIPD		CAPD	
	Females	Males	Females	Males
Minimal value	32.90	38.80	30.70	36.30
Low transporters	33.70	39.80	35.70	41.60
Mean (+ or –) SD	34.30	40.50	39.40	46.50
Low-average transporters	40.00	47.20	43.20	51.00
Mean	44.70	52.70	46.70	55.10
High-average transporters	48.00	56.60	50.10	59.10
Mean + SD	50.80	59.90	53.20	62.80[a]
High transporters	55.60	65.60	58.10	68.50[a]
Maximal value	59.40	70.00[a]	62.70[a]	73.90[a]

From Twardowski ZJ. Relationships between creatinine clearances and *Kt/V* in peritoneal dialysis patients: a critique of the DOQI document. *Perit Dial Int* 1998;18:252–255.
Assumptions: total body water in males = 41.7 L; total body water in females = 32.1 L; body surface area in males = 1.92 m^2; body surface area in females = 1.74 m^2.
CAPD, continuous ambulatory peritoneal dialysis (five 2-L exchanges.); NIPD, nocturnal intermittent peritoneal dialysis (hourly 2-L exchanges).
[a]Values are above the DOQI guidelines for creatinine clearance at recommended *Kt/V*.

tices were reviewed by Tzamaloukas et al. (191). These authors propose using *V* for normalization of both *Kt/V* and CCr despite the preceding descriptions, a practice not adapted by national guideline committees as of today.

There are no clinical outcome data to support the use of one solute clearance yardstick (CCr or *Kt/V*) over the other. Most of the published outcome data are related to *Kt/V*. These solute clearance goals are based on reported outcomes predicted by certain amounts of solute clearance. Based on this discussion, it is apparent that in most cases the two values correlate and that either could be used as an index of adequacy. As outlined earlier, at times it is not practical to achieve both targets. NKF–DOQI Guidelines and others (192) suggest that one should always strive to at least have *Kt/V* above target.

VOLUME AND BP CONTROL ISSUES

Cardiovascular disease continues to be the leading cause of death in ESRD patients. There is a high prevalence of left ventricular hypertrophy (LVH) and congestive heart failure (CHF) in patients initiating dialysis. The prevalence of LVH is higher in the elderly population and is increasing yearly (193). It is well known that predisposing factors for the development of LVH include volume overload and hypertension. In the reevaluation of the CANUSA study, it was shown that residual renal volume, not peritoneal UF, was predictive of outcome (35). In another study, both fluid and sodium removal were independent predictors of death (194). The survival rate increased linearly with both fluid and sodium removal. Elevated systolic blood pressure correlated positively with risk of death and negatively with salt and water removal. In a cohort of anuric APD patients all obtaining a certain minimal small solute clearance, peritoneal UF, not small solute clearance, was predictive of outcome (195). Some have shown that aggressive interventions directed at controlling blood volume using salt

restriction and if needed alterations of the peritoneal dialysis prescription to improve UF can result in control of blood pressure in most patients without the need to use antihypertensive medications (196). More data relating the effect of fluid removal on outcome are needed; however, these preliminary data do underscore the clinical significance of including blood pressure and volume control as part of adequacy of any dialysis therapy. As with small solute clearance issues, what is not as clear is whether the same volume removed by PD alone is as predictive as that removed by the native kidney. In 1995, when the initial NKF–DOQI guidelines were formulated, there were few data correlating outcome with UF. Hence the original publication had no guidelines that addressed UF other than to state that there were other components to adequacy of dialysis than small solute clearance.

New guidelines on adequacy are likely to include recommendations for salt and water removal. To optimize these parameters, one must attempt to preserve residual renal volume, initiate oral salt restriction, and individualize the PD prescription to optimize salt and water removal. When individualizing the prescription, most attention is directed toward the long dwell. A rational approach to fluid management in peritoneal dialysis has been reviewed elsewhere (197,198).

Classic peritoneal dialysis solutions contain glucose as the osmotic agent. Glucose is readily absorbed from the peritoneal cavity and as it is, the osmotic concentration of the intraperitoneal dialysate approaches that of blood. When there no longer is an osmotic gradient for crystalloid-induced UF, lymphatic reabsorption of fluid predominates and the intraperitoneal and eventual drain volume decreases. As a result, during the long dwell (overnight) in CAPD or during the long daytime dwell of APD, this phenomenon is likely to occur. Up to 30% of CAPD patients actually absorb fluid during their overnight dwell if using 1.5% dextrose PD solutions. Increasing the percent of dextrose to 2.5% or 4.25% decreases the percent of patients with negative net UF to

TABLE 14.9. LIKELY PATHWAYS FOR PERITONEAL FLUID AND SOLUTE REMOVAL

Glucose-Based Solutions Crystalloid-Induced Osmosis	Icodextrin-Based Solutions Colloid-Induced Osmosis
Water transport via Small and ultrasmall pores	Water transport via Small pores
Small solute movement By diffusion via small pores And by convection through small pores	Small solute transport By diffusion via small pores By convection via small pores
Macromolecule movement Across large pores and into lymphatics	Macromolecule movement Across large pores and into lymphatics
Osmotic agent (glucose) Rapidly absorbed by diffusion Across small and large pores	Osmotic agent (icodextrin) Slowly absorbed into peritoneal lymphatics

about 20% and 5%, respectively, whereas if on automated PD therapies, 80% of patients may have fluid adsorption during the overnight dwell if using 2.5% dextrose, versus 20% of patients using 4.25% dextrose (197). This means that in an anuric patient, the remaining dwells must first remove this "absorbed" fluid before removing any fluids taken by mouth during the day to maintain fluid balance. Because of the known effect of hypertension and volume overload on left ventricular function and risk of death, it is important to focus on maintaining positive UF during the long dwell. This can be done by increasing the tonicity of the dialysate; by modifying the dwell time, at times by breaking up the dwell; and by doing two dwells during that same time period or by just doing one short dwell with some dry time. Having dry time may solve the UF problem and maintain small solute clearance but will likely compromise peritoneal middle-molecular-weight clearance. If available, an alternative would be to use other osmotic agents that result in more sustained UF during the long dwell.

Polyglucose is an alternative osmotic agent available for use in Europe and Canada. Its pharmacokinetics have been reviewed elsewhere (199). Suffice it to say that polyglucose is a mixture of high-molecular-weight, water-soluble, glucose polymers isolated by fractionation of hydrolyzed starch ranging in molecular weight from 13,000 to 19,000 daltons. It is very slowly absorbed from the peritoneal cavity by direct absorption into the peritoneal lymphatics, not by diffusion, because it is too large to move across small pores. Because of the slow absorption there is sustained UF, even during long dwells of up to 15 hours. The differences between expected UF with the different solutions are especially apparent in patients who are high and high average transporters. This UF is achieved while using isotonic solutions (200). The reason one can obtain sustained UF with polyglucose solutions is because the force driving the UF is due to colloid osmotic differences between the peritoneal cavity and blood. These colloid osmotic forces are due to the difference between the number of large-molecular-weight solutes between the two compartments (polyglucose versus albumin). The clinical differences in UF profiles between dextrose solutions and polyglucose in CAPD and APD have been reviewed elsewhere (201–204). Table 14.9 outlines the reason for these differences and Fig. 14.8 illustrates the UF profiles of typically available dialysis fluids.

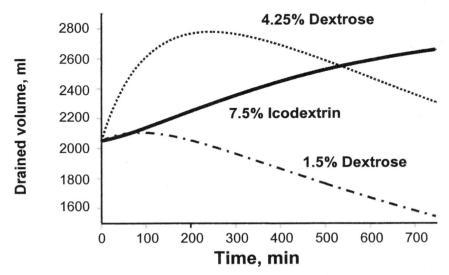

Rippe and Levin. Kidney Int 2000: 57(6): 2546-56

FIG. 14.8. Temporal profile of net ultrafiltration in high average transport patients with use of 1.5% dextrose (–·–·–), 4.25% dextrose (···), or 7.5% icodextrin (—) solutions. (From Mujias S, et al. Profiling of peritoneal UF. *Kidney Int* 2002;62[Suppl 81]:S17–S22.)

HOW TO MONITOR DIALYSIS DOSE

The most accurate way to measure dialysis dose is to measure the total amount of the solute in question cleared from the body during a specific time interval. In practice, for patients on PD, this means that 24-hour collections of dialysate and urine should be obtained. Total solute clearance is then calculated. An alternative would be to estimate the daily clearance either mathematically or with the use of computer-assisted kinetic modeling programs. However, although the estimations do tend to correlate with the actual clearance measured from 24-hour collections, there is a high degree of discordance (205,206). Therefore the gold standard for measurement of dialysis dose is to obtain 24-hour collections of both urine and dialysate to document the actual amount of solute removed. These studies should be obtained quarterly and within 1 month of any prescription change. Despite these recommendations, data from the United States suggest that adequacy studies are not done in many PD patients (207).

It is acknowledged from the review of outcome studies that total small solute clearance may not be the best yardstick for adequacy of dialysis. Uremic symptoms are related to serum concentrations. The measured clearance is the same if the BUN decreases from 150 to 75 mg/dL in one person as it is if it decreases from 50 to 25 mg/dL in another over the same amount of time. Does this represent the same amount of dialysis?

PET data are obtained to characterize the patient's peritoneal membrane transport characteristics (see earlier section on membrane transport), not to determine clearance. The two tests are complimentary to each other and are routinely used together for developing a patient's dialysis prescription and for problem solving. Several studies have documented that an individual patient's peritoneal membrane tends to be stable over time (208). However, in some patients it may change. Therefore peritoneal transport should be monitored to optimize clearance and UF. The PET is the most practical way to do this, and it is recommended that it be obtained twice a year. It has been shown that over time if there tends to be any change in transport characteristics, the D/P ratios were likely to increase slightly, associated with a small decrease in UF. Alternatively, one can estimate D/P values for PET from D/P values on 24-hour dialysate collections (*Dialysis Adequacy and Transport Test*, or DATT) when followed sequentially in an individual patient (209). Twenty-four-hour collections can also be used to calculate lean body mass (LBM), creatinine generation rates, and estimated protein intake (Table 14.10).

NONCOMPLIANCE

Noncompliance with a medical regimen is not uncommon. Because PD is a home therapy, it is not easy to document the degree of noncompliance with a patient's prescription. In contrast, the degree of noncompliance with the dialysis prescription itself is easily documented in in-center hemodialysis populations (5,210). Recent publications have suggested that a value above unity for the ratio of measured to predicted creatinine production may be an indication of recent periods of noncompliance (211–213). These authors speculated that, if the patient had been noncompliant before obtaining the 24-hour dialysate and urine collection but was compliant on the day of collection, then a "washout" effect would occur. In such a case, the creatinine production would be higher than would be predicted from standard equations, resulting in an elevated ratio of measured-to-predicted creatinine production. From these studies it has been estimated that only 78% of the prescribed therapy is actually delivered. Others have shown that the index is *not* a good indicator of compliance (214,215). More data are needed. Perhaps sequential rather than individual ratios will be helpful. Nevertheless, noncompliance with the prescription is a real issue as documented by patient questionnaires (216) and by looking at patient home inventories (217). Interestingly, noncompliance may be more of an issue in the United States than in other countries such as Canada.

At present, there is no definitive test short of asking patients and looking at home inventories to determine patient compliance. More important, one should discuss compliance with the patient and have a heightened awareness of the problem. Be sure to design PD prescriptions with the patients' lifestyle needs and abilities in mind. Five manual exchanges per day are not realistic for most patients. Automated therapies may help, and some of the newer devices may be able to track and document the number of exchanges actually carried out. Education and importance of compliance with prescription should be emphasized.

PRESCRIPTION DIALYSIS

Timing of Initiation

The NKF–DOQI guidelines (8,9) and others (218,219) have highlighted the need to treat patients throughout all the stages of chronic kidney disease (CKD) as a continuum. The tradi-

TABLE 14.10. USEFULNESS OF 24-HOUR COLLECTIONS OF DIALYSIS AND URINE

Creatinine Kinetics	Urea Kinetics
Creatinine clearance[D]	Urea clearance[D]
Creatinine clearance[U]	Urea clearance[U]
Total creatinine clearance[D+U]	Total urea clearance[D+U]
Creatinine production[D+U]	PNA[D+U]
Lean body mass[D+U]	Urea generation[D+U]
D/P creatinine[D]	
Ratio of measured to predicted creatinine generation	
Creatinine and Urea Kinetics	**24° Urine**
Estimated GFR (modified creat cl)	Drain volume—UF rates

Burkart JM, et al. Solute clearance approach to adequacy of peritoneal dialysis. *Perit Dial Int* 1996;16:457–470.
[D], dialysis only; [U], urine only; D/P, dialysis to plasma ratio; PNA, protein equivalent of nitrogen appearance.

tional indications for initiation of dialysis such as pericarditis, encephalopathy, refractory hyperkalemia, nausea, vomiting, and volume overload raise little controversy. Weight loss and signs of malnutrition are other, more subtle, "relative" indications for initiation. Interestingly, as opposed to ESRD when minimal target values for weekly total solute clearance have been established (i.e., Kt/V_{urea} >2.0, CCr >60 L/1.73 m², for CAPD), minimal values for solute clearance by residual renal function alone have not been established. This seems paradoxical. In fact, in the CANUSA study, the mean RR GFR at initiation was approximately 3.38 mL/min, an estimated RR CCr of 38 L/1.73 m²/week (15). A recent evaluation suggested that the median creatinine clearance level in 90,987 new dialysis patients in the United States was 8.9 mL/min, while the proportion of patients with a GFR >10, 5 to 10, and <5 mL/min was 14%, 63%, and 23%, respectively (220). There are indirect data to suggest that in general, patients who start dialysis with relatively more residual renal function have better outcomes and tend to be less malnourished.

The DOQI working group for PD adequacy has developed the following guideline: "Unless certain conditions are met, patients should be advised to initiate some form of renal replacement therapy when residual renal Kt/V_{urea} falls below 2.0/week." The conditions that indicate dialysis may not yet be needed are (a) stable to increasing edema-free body weight and (b) a nPNA of more than 0.8 g/kg/d and (c) complete absence of clinical signs and symptoms attributable to uremia (9).

This guideline does not preclude the importance of quality-of-life issues, blood pressure control, treatment of anemia and consideration of protein restriction and use of ACE inhibitors to prevent progression of disease. It still suggests individualization of therapy initiation. The recommendations are based on the following indirect evidence.

Baseline Nutritional Status Predicts Survival

Data suggest that baseline nutritional parameters such as serum albumin, lean body mass, nPNA, or subjective global assessment score are strong predictors of outcome. For instance, the predicted 2-year survivals for patients in the CANUSA study with baseline serum albumins of more than 35, 30 to 35, and less than 30 g/L were 85%, 75%, and 64%, respectively (15). Although these parameters increased over the first 6 months on dialysis, the baseline values, not those at 6 months, were what predicted outcomes.

As Residual Renal GFR Declines, So Does Spontaneous DPI

As GFR decreases (to below 25 to 50 mL/min), so does spontaneous dietary protein intake (221). In that report, patients with a CCr of more than 50 mL/min had a mean DPI of 1.01 g/kg/d, versus a DPI of 0.54 g/kg/d (less than currently recommended minimal requirements) in patients with a CCr of less than 10 mL/min. A similar statistically significant trend was also observed in the Modification of Diet in Renal Disease study (MDRD) (both the pilot and full-scale study) (222) and others (223).

Relationship Between Kt/V and DPI May Be the Same for CRI and for Continuous P

It has been demonstrated that the relationship between DPI and small solute clearance measured in terms of Kt/V is similar for CRI and CAPD patients (224).

Outcome Data

Some databases suggest that outcomes are better for patients who start dialysis early (in terms of GFR) than in those who start late (225–227). Others have reported that survival and hospitalization during the first 6 months after initiation of HD was related to baseline residual renal Kt/V (228,229). Data from the Danish ESRD registry on 4,291 patients who started dialysis between 1990 and 1999 were analyzed to determine the relative risk of death for patients on HD versus PD. They found that the relative risk of death changed over time, but favored PD over the first 2 years, with the survival advantage for PD decreasing with time on dialysis. After more than 1.5 years on dialysis, there was no longer a survival advantage to PD, but over the first 1.5 years there was (230).

Taken in aggregate, these studies suggest, at least in part, that outcome on dialysis is related to the level of residual renal function at the initiation of dialysis. One explanation for these observations may be the influence of residual renal solute clearance on the patient's nutritional status. The data suggest that the overall goal would be to keep total weekly Kt/V_{urea} >2.0 at all times. This can be achieved by the incremental use of either PD or HD with consideration of patient quality-of-life issues and minimal interruption of lifestyle or by initiating a full dose of dialysis once the RR Kt/V_{urea} is less than 2.0/week. More outcome data are needed and one needs to prove that any observed advantage is not just a result of lead time bias.

INITIAL PRESCRIPTION

When a patient presents with near ESRD or ESRD and peritoneal dialysis is elected, two alternatives for writing the initial prescription exist. For those patients with minimal residual renal function, the initial prescription should consist of a "full dose" of PD dialysis to meet minimal total solute clearance goals. If the patient has a significant amount of residual renal function (but residual renal Kt/V of less than 2.0), an "incremental" dosage of peritoneal dialysis can be used (231).

In both instances, the initial prescription is based on the patient's body size (BSA, and need for normalization) and amount of residual renal function (both potentially known variables at initiation of dialysis). At initiation, peritoneal transport is not known. Initial prescriptions are based on the assumption that the patient's peritoneal transport is average. Once stable on PD, a PET can be obtained, determining an individual patient's transport type, so that his/her prescription can be more appropriately tailored. During training, transport type can be predicted from drain volume during a timed (4-hour) dwell with 2.5% glucose and compared with those predicted by PET (107).

TABLE 14.11. EMPIRIC FULL-DOSE PD PRESCRIPTIONS

BSA	Residual Renal GFR	
	<2 mL/min	>2 mL/min
BSA > 1.71 m²	4 × 2.5 L CAPD	4 × 2.0 L CAPD
	5 × 2.0 L QUANTUM PD[a]	4 × 2.0 L + 2.0 L APD
	4 × 2.5 L + 2.5 L APD	
	3 × 2.5 L + 2.0 L + 2.0 L APD	
BSA 1.71 m²–2.0 m²	4 × 2.5 L CAPD	4 × 2.0 L CAPD
	3 × 2.5 L + 3.0 L CAPD	4 × 2.5 L + 2.0 L APD
	3 × 2.0 L + 2 × 2.5 L QUANTUM PD[a]	
	4 × 3.0 L + 2.5 L APD	
	3 × 2.5 L + 2.5 L + 2.5 L APD	
BSA > 2.0 m²	4 × 3.0 L CAPD	4 × 2.5 L CAPD
	5 × 2.5 L QUANTUM PD[a]	4 × 2.5 L + 2.5 L APD
	3 × 2.5 L + 2 × 3.0 L QUANTUM PD[a]	
	3 × 3.0 L + 3.0 L + 3.0 L APD	

Blake PG, et al. Peritoneal dialysis prescription management decision tree: a need for change. McGaw, IL: Baxter Healthcare Corporation, 1997.
[a]QUANTUM PD uses nightly exchange device to do a midnight exchange. APD, automated peritoneal dialysis; BSA, body surface area; GFR, glomerular filtration rate; PD, peritoneal dialysis.

Implementation

Examples of an empiric initial peritoneal dialysis prescription based on BSA and residual renal clearance for patients with minimal residual renal clearance are found in (Table 14.11) (232). These prescriptions are based on kinetic modeling and require 24-hour collections of dialysate and urine to confirm that targets are met.

Similarly, in patients with a significant amount of RRF, one can use empirical prescriptions based on kinetic modeling for implementing peritoneal dialysis using an incremental approach. These are also based on BSA and residual renal clearance (Table 14.12). Incremental dialysis requires close monitoring and proactive adjustment of dialysis prescriptions, twenty-four-hour collection of dialysate and urine to document clearances. Residual renal clearance should be obtained every 1 to 2 months so that the peritoneal component can be modified if indicated to make sure total weekly *Kt/V* is 2.0 or higher. The argument for incremental dialysis and the suggestions that this approach could be better or more practical for PD are reviewed elsewhere (225).

TABLE 14.12. EMPIRIC–INCREMENTAL–PD PRESCRIPTION

BSA	1.71 m²	1.86 m²	2.0 m²
Fill volume of bags	2.0	2.5	3.0
At indicated GFR, mL/min			
Start with one exchange	10	11	12
Switch to two	7	8	9
Full therapy	5	6	7

PITFALLS IN PRESCRIBING PERITONEAL DIALYSIS

There are some common pitfalls in prescribing the peritoneal component of total solute clearance. The following is a brief summary of some of these and should be considered whenever a patient appears underdialyzed. Because peritoneal dialysis is a home therapy, noncompliance with the prescription must always be considered as a reason for underdialysis. Certainly, patients may be compliant with their prescription when bringing in their 24-hour collections, but if the patient is noncompliant at home, he/she may be underdialyzed on a daily basis. Home visits to monitor the amount of supplies on hand and keep track of monthly orders may help sort this out.

Some issues to consider in patients on standard CAPD are (a) inappropriate dwell times (a rapid transporter would do better with short dwells), (b) failure to increase dialysis dose to compensate for loss of residual renal function, (c) inappropriate instilled volume (patient may only infuse 2 L of a 2.5-L bag) (233), (d) multiple rapid exchanges and one very long dwell (patient may do three exchanges between 9 a.m. and 5 p.m., and a long dwell from 5 p.m. to 9 a.m. (234); and (e) inappropriate selection of dialysate osmotic agent for long dwells that may not maximize UF and consequently clearance.

In general, when the goal is to increase total solute clearance, it is best to increase dwell volume, not number of exchanges. Increasing the number of exchanges decreases dwell time/exchange, making the therapy less effective for the average patient.

Other problems are specific for those patients on cycler therapy. The drain time may be inappropriately long (>20 min), thus increasing the time the patient must be connected to the cycler, perhaps limiting the number of exchanges a patient would tolerate. Inappropriately short dwell times may also be prescribed, making the therapy less effective for the average patient where length of dwell is crucial. Failure to augment total dialysis dose with a daytime dwell ("wet" day versus "dry" day) could also result in underdialysis. Cycler patients are typically on the cycler for 9 to 10 hours per night. Therefore the daytime dwell is long (14 to 15 hours). During this long dwell (longer than the long nighttime dwell for typical CAPD patients), diffusion stops and reabsorption often begins, minimizing clearance. Use of a midday exchange is an effective way to optimize both clearance and UF in these patients. Also, use of alternative osmotic agents such as icodextrin, which maintains UF during long dwells, will be helpful (235). These optimize both clearance and UF without hypertonic glucose. Finally, poor selection of dialysate glucose may not allow maximization of UF, resulting in less total clearance.

When changing from standard CAPD (long dwells) to cycler therapy (short dwells), it is important to remember the difference in transport rates of urea and creatinine and the effect that this change will have on the patient's overall clearance. These differences and their relevances for CAPD, CCPD, NIPD, and other modifications are reviewed by Twardowski (236). Transport of urea into the dialysate tends to occur faster than that for creatinine. Therefore if total solute clearance targets are measured using urea kinetics, keeping *Kt/V* constant going from long to short dwells may decrease creatinine clearance. In contrast, if creatinine clearance is the total solute clearance target, keeping creatinine clearance constant when changing from long to short dwells will keep Kt/V constant or even increase it. This concept has been termed *horizontal modeling* (237). Knowledge of the individual patient's peritoneal transport characteristics and familiarity with the differences in dialysis needs for rapid versus slow transporters is imperative to avoid problems or confusion.

ADJUSTING DIALYSIS DOSE

When determining an individual patient's prescription, one should aim for a total solute clearance that is above target but also allow for other indexes of adequate dialysis such as quality-of-life issues, blood pressure control, and dietary protein intake. If during routine monitoring or clinical evaluation of the patient the delivered dose of dialysis needs to be altered, this can easily be done in a scientific manner if you know the patient's present transport characteristics (PET), the present total clearance of urea or creatinine, and the relationship between dialysis clearance, drain volume, and dwell time based on the measured D/P ratios. It is important that these relationships be understood because increasing the instilled volume does not always result in an increase in clearance. For instance, in a patient who is a low transporter and in whom clearance is critically dependent on dwell time, changing from standard CAPD (infused volume—8 L) to a form of cycler therapy using 2-hour dwells, where the infused volume may be as high as 10 to 14 L may not always result in an overall increase in that patient's clearance.

Once familiar with these relationships, to adjust the dialysate prescription, you would need to know the D/P ratios at the anticipated dwell time and the patient's drain volume for that dwell time. By altering dwell time, you change the D/P ratio and the drain volume. By altering instilled volume, you also affect total drain volume and therefore clearance. In general, increasing the instilled volume without changing dwell time results in an increase in solute clearance.

Another means to tailor a dialysis prescription would be with the use of computer-assisted kinetic modeling programs (238,239), which allows for ease in adjusting a patient's dialysis prescription. Baseline PET data, drain volumes, and patient weights are needed for input data. Use of these programs usually allows one to set targets for solute clearance, glucose absorption, and anticipated dietary protein intake. These computer simulations then give one a menu of prescriptions that should achieve these targets, and one can choose the one that would best suit the patient's lifestyle.

Tidal peritoneal dialysis is a form of automated dialysis in which, after an initial dialysate fill, only a portion of the dialysate is drained from the peritoneum and is replaced with fresh dialysate after each cycle. This leaves the majority of the dialysate in constant contact with the peritoneal membrane. A typical tidal dialysis prescription usually requires 23 to 28 L of instilled volume, but preliminary studies suggest that tidal dialysis may be approximately 20% more efficient than nightly peritoneal dialysis at dialysate flow rates of about 3.5 L/h (240).

RISK OF COMPLICATIONS FROM INCREASED INTRAABDOMINAL PRESSURE

Intraperitoneal pressure increases almost linearly with increases in installed volumes (241). For any instilled volume, pressure is greatest sitting with the lowest pressures observed when supine. This increased pressure leads to increased tension of the abdominal wall and the potential for hernia formation in areas of weakness. Studies in individual units have reported an incidence of hernia formation of between 10% and 20% (242,243). Patients should be instructed to avoid activities that lead to increases in intraabdominal pressure, such as lifting. Theoretically, as one increases instilled volume to compensate for loss of RRF, the incidence of hernias should increase. At this time there are no definitive studies that state that as dialysis dose is increased by increasing instilled volume, the risk of hernias increases.

CLINICAL ASSESSMENT OF ADEQUACY

As mentioned in the beginning of this chapter, the clinical assessment of adequate dialysis does not just consist of any single laboratory measurement. It includes lack of signs or symptoms of uremia as well as a patient's feeling of well-being, control of blood pressure, anemia, and other biochemical parameters (244). The minimal target dialysis dose should be delivered and an adequate PNA should be achieved. If the clinical judgment is that the patient is manifesting signs of uremia despite what appears to be adequate laboratory measurements of "dialysis dose," it would be prudent to increase the patient's dialysis dose if no other cause for this symptomatology is found. Certainly, a patient could be very compliant with the prescription during the period of dose monitoring, but because this is a home therapy, there may not be compliance during the rest of the therapy interval. Another possible explanation for this clinical dilemma would be the effect normalization of Kt by a decreasing V in a malnourished patient has on Kt/V_{urea} calculation (described in the preceding section on discrepancy). Furthermore, if the dose of dialysis appears inadequate despite an adequate clinical assessment, these patients should be monitored very closely. The ADEMEX data provide scientific data to support this clinical approach. If the dose of dialysis is truly inadequate, subtle signs and symptoms of uremia should begin to develop and the prescription could be increased if necessary.

SUMMARY

The dose of dialysis delivered does influence outcome and does correlate with dietary protein intake. When considering adequacy of dialysis, one must monitor both of these parameters in addition to clinical assessment, blood pressure control, treatment of anemia, osteodystrophy, and other comorbid diseases. Periods of inadequate dialysis can result in subtle symptoms of uremia that are insidious in onset and may not be reversible. These can influence outcome in a negative way. To prevent this symptomatology and provide as close to optimal dialysis as possible, it is important to monitor dialysis dose so that changes in dialysis prescription can be made proactively rather than reactively. There does appear to be a "minimal" dose of dialysis measured in terms of small solute clearance that one should obtain to optimize outcomes. When tailoring peritoneal dialysis prescriptions, it is important that the prescribed dialysis dose be targeted to at least achieve these minimal doses. What is still unknown is if one was to achieve markedly higher small solute clearances would this result in an incremental improvement in outcome. Preliminary data would suggest no, but it is important to remember that these maneuvers did not concomitantly increase or improve other "adequacy" parameters such as middle molecular weight solute clearance or volume control. Further studies which specifically address these issues are needed.

ACKNOWLEDGMENT

The author thanks Sonya Ashburn for secretarial assistance.

REFERENCES

1. Lundin PA III. Prolonged survival on hemodialysis. In: Maher JF, ed. *Replacement of renal function,* 3rd ed. Dordrecht, the Netherlands: Kluwer Academic, 1989:1133–1140.
2. Held PJ, et al. Five-year survival for end-stage renal disease patients in the United States, Europe, and Japan 1982–1987. *Am J Kidney Dis* 1990;5:451–457.
3. Lamiere N, et al. Cardiovascular disease in peritoneal dialysis patients: the size of the problem. *Kidney Int* 1996;50(Suppl 56):S28–S36.
4. Sargent JA. Shortfalls in the delivery of dialysis. *Am J Kidney Dis* 1990;15:500–510.
5. Parker TF, et al. Delivering the prescribed dialysis. *Semin Dial* 1993; 6:13–15.
6. Moran J. Changes in the dose of peritoneal dialysis: have these independently improved outcomes? *Am J Kidney Dis* 1998;32(Suppl 4):S52–S57.
7. Wolfe RA. A critical examination of trends in outcomes over the past decade: presentation at special conference on strategies to improve outcomes in pre-ESRD and ESRD patients. Washington, DC, June 1998.
8. Peritoneal Dialysis Adequacy Work Group of the National Kidney Foundation. Dialysis Outcomes Quality Initiative (DOQI): clinical practice guidelines. *Am J Kidney Dis* 1997;30(Suppl 2):S67–S136.
9. National Kidney Foundation Dialysis Quality Initiative. NKF–K/DOQI clinical practice guidelines for peritoneal dialysis adequacy: update 2000. *Am J Kidney Dis* 2000;37(Suppl 1):S65–S136.
10. May RC, et al. Pathophysiology of uremia. In: Brenner BM, et al., eds. *The kidney.* Philadelphia: WB Saunders, 1991:1997–2018.
11. Luik AJ, et al. Hypertension in haemodialysis patients: is it only hypervolaemia? *Nephrol Dial Transplant* 1997;12:1557–1560.
12. Bagdade JD, et al. Hypertriglyceridemia: a metabolic consequence of chronic renal failure. *N Engl J Med* 1968;279:181–185.
13. Neilson VK. The peripheral nerve function in chronic renal failure. VII. Longitudinal course during terminal renal failure and regular hemodialysis. *Acta Med Scand* 1974;195:155.
14. Lowrie EG, et al. Effect of the hemodialysis prescription on patient morbidity. *N Engl J Med* 1981;305:1176–1181.
15. Churchill DN, et al. Adequacy of dialysis and nutrition in continuous peritoneal dialysis: association with clinical outcomes. *J Am Soc Nephrol* 1996;7:198–207.
16. Lindsay RM, et al. A hypothesis: the protein catabolic rate is dependent upon the type and amount of treatment in dialyzed uremic patients. *Am J Kidney Dis* 1989;13:382–389.
17. Churchill DN. Adequacy of peritoneal dialysis: how much do we need? *Kidney Int* 1994;46(Suppl 48):S2–S6.
18. Burkart JM, et al. Solute clearance approach to adequacy of peritoneal dialysis. *Perit Dial Int* 1996;16:457–470.
19. Popovich RP, et al. Kinetic modeling of peritoneal transport. *Contrib Nephrol* 1979;17:59–72.
20. Blake PG, et al. Urea kinetic modeling has limited relevance in assessing adequacy of dialysis in CAPD. In: Khanna R, et al., eds. *Advances in peritoneal dialysis.* Toronto: Peritoneal Dialysis Bulletin, 1992: 65–70.
21. De Alvaro F, et al. Adequacy of peritoneal dialysis: does Kt/V have the same predictive value as for HD? A multicenter study. In: Khanna R, et al., eds. *Advances in peritoneal dialysis.* Toronto: Peritoneal Dialysis Bulletin, 1992:93–97.
22. Lameire NH, et al. A longitudinal, five-year survey of urea kinetic parameters in CAPD patients. *Kidney Int* 1992;42:426–432.
23. Teehan BP, et al. Urea kinetic analysis and clinical outcome on CAPD: a five-year longitudinal study. In: Khanna R, et al., eds. *Advances in peritoneal dialysis.* Toronto: Peritoneal Dialysis Bulletin, 1990:181–185.
24. Maiorca R, et al. Predictive value of dialysis adequacy and nutritional indices for morbidity and mortality in CAPD and HD patients: a longitudinal study. *Nephrol Dial Transplant* 1995;10:2295–2305.
25. Churchill DN. Implications of the Canada–USA (CANUSA) study of the adequacy of dialysis on peritoneal dialysis schedule. *Nephrol Dial Transplant* 1998;13(Suppl 6):158–163.
26. Blake PG, et al. Guidelines for adequacy and nutrition in peritoneal dialysis. *J Am Soc Nephrol* 1999;10(Suppl 13):S311–S321.
27. Renal Association and Royal College of Physicians of London. Treatment of adult patients with renal failure: recommended standards and audit measures. London, 1997.
28. Szeto CC, et al. The impact of increasing the daytime dialysis exchange frequency on peritoneal dialysis adequacy and nutritional status of Chinese anuric patients. *Perit Dial Int* 2002;22:197–203.
29. Szeto CC, et al. Importance of dialysis adequacy in mortality and morbidity of Chinese CAPD patients. *Kidney Int* 2000;58:400–407.
30. Szeto CC, et al. Impact of dialysis adequacy on the mortality and morbidity of anuric Chinese patients receiving continuous ambulatory peritoneal dialysis. *J Am Soc Nephrol* 2001;12:355–360.
31. Davies SJ, et al. Analysis of the effects of increasing delivered dialysis treatment to malnourished peritoneal dialysis patients. *Kidney Int* 2000;57:1743–1754.
32. Davies SJ, et al. Peritoneal solute transport predicts survival on CAPD independently of residual renal function. *Nephrol Dial Transplant* 1998;13:962–968.
33. Bhaskaran S, et al. The effect of small solute clearance on survival of anuric peritoneal dialysis patients. *Perit Dial Int* 2000;20:181–187.
34. Agarwal M, et al. Survival outcomes in PD patients after DOQI guidelines: did we achieve the adequacy targets? *J Am Soc Nephrol* 2001;12:445a(abst).
35. Mak SK, et al. Randomized prospective study of the effect of increased dialytic dose on nutritional and clinical outcome in continuous ambulatory peritoneal dialysis patients. *Am J Kidney Dis* 2000; 36:105–114.
36. Paniagua R, et al. Effects of increased peritoneal clearances on mortality rates in peritoneal dialysis: Ademex, a prospective, randomized, controlled trial. *J Am Soc Nephrol* 2002;13:1307–1320.
37. Collins AJ, et al. Changing risk factor demographics endstage renal disease patients entering hemodialysis and the impact on long-term mortality. *Am J Kidney Dis* 1990;15:422–432.
38. Genestier S, et al. Prognostic factors in CAPD patients: a retrospective study of a 10-year period. *Nephrol Dial Transplant* 1995;10:1905–1911.
39. Churchill DN, et al. Increased peritoneal transport is associated with decreased CAPD technique and patient survival. *J Am Soc Nephrol* 1997;8:189A.
40. Davies SJ, et al. Peritoneal solute transfer is an independent predictor of survival on CAPD. *J Am Soc Nephrol* 1996;7:1443.
41. Heaf J. CAPD adequacy and dialysis morbidity: detrimental effect of a high peritoneal equilibrium rate. *Ren Fail* 1995;17:575–587.
42. Harty JC, et al. Is peritoneal permeability an adverse risk factor for malnutrition in CAPD patients? *Miner Electrolyte Metab* 1996;22: 97–101.

43. Blake P. What is the problem with high transporters? *Perit Dial Int* 1997;17:317–320.

44. Meyer KV, et al. Creatinine kinetics in peritoneal dialysis. *Semin Dial* 1998;11:88–94.

45. Shemin D, et al. Residual renal function and mortality risk in hemodialysis patients. *Am J Kidney Dis* 2001;38:85–90.

46. Bargman J, et al. Relative contribution of residual renal function and peritoneal clearance to adequacy of dialysis: a reanalysis of the CANUSA study. *J Am Soc Nephrol* 2001;12:2158–2162.

47. Diaz-Buxo JA, et al. Associate of mortality among peritoneal dialysis patients with special reference to peritoneal transport rates and solute clearance. *Am J Kidney Dis* 2000;33:523–534.

48. Rocco M, et al. Peritoneal dialysis adequacy and risk of death. *Kidney Int* 2000;58:446–457.

49. Jager KJ, et al. Mortality and technique failure in patients starting chronic peritoneal dialysis: results of the Netherlands Cooperative Study on the Adequacy of Dialysis. NECOSAD study group. *Kidney Int* 1999;55:1476–1485.

50. Merkus MP, et al. Physical symptoms and quality of life in patients on chronic dialysis: results of the Netherlands Cooperative Study on Adequacy of Dialysis (NECOSAD). *Nephrol Dial Transplant* 1999; 14:1163–1170.

51. Keshaviah P. Adequacy of CAPD: a quantitative approach. *Kidney Int* 1992;42(Suppl 38):S160–S164.

52. Kim DJ, et al. Dissociation between clearances of small and middle molecules in incremental peritoneal dialysis. *Perit Dial Int* 2001;21: 462–466.

53. Brophy DF, et al. Small and middle molecular weight solute clearance in nocturnal intermittent peritoneal dialysis. *Perit Dial Int* 1999;19: 534–539.

54. Leypoldt JK, et al. Small solute and middle molecule clearances during continuous flow peritoneal dialysis. *Adv in Perit Dial* 2002;18: 26–31.

55. Keshaviah PR, et al. The peak concentration hypothesis: a urea kinetic approach to comparing the adequacy of continuous ambulatory peritoneal dialysis (CAPD) and hemodialysis. *Perit Dial Int* 1989;9:257–260.

56. Fenton S, et al. Hemodialysis versus peritoneal dialysis: a comparison of adjusted mortality rates. *Am J Kidney Dis* 1997;30:334–342.

57. Collins AJ, et al. Mortality risks of peritoneal dialysis and hemodialysis. *Am J Kidney Dis* 1999;34:1065–1074.

58. Gotch FA, et al. Kinetic modeling in peritoneal dialysis. In: Nissenson AR, et al., eds. *Clinical dialysis*, 3rd ed. Norwalk, CT: Appleton & Lange, 1997:343–375.

59. Gokal R, et al. Are there limits on CAPD? Adequacy and nutritional considerations. *Perit Dial Int* 1996;16:437–441.

60. Blake PG. A review of the DOQI recommendations for peritoneal dialysis. *Perit Dial Int* 1998;18:247–251.

61. Satko SG, et al. Frequency and causes of discrepancy between Kt/V and creatinine. *Perit Dial Int* 1997;17:S23.

62. Gilbert R, et al. The gastrointestinal system. In: Eknoyan G, et al., eds. *The systemic consequences of renal failure*. New York: Grune and Stratton, 1984:133.

63. Ikizler TA, et al. Malnutrition in peritoneal dialysis patients: etiologic factors and treatment options. *Perit Dial Int* 1995;15:S63–S66.

64. Held PJ, et al. Survival probabilities and causes of death. In: Agadoa LYC, et al., eds. *USRDS annual data report 1991*, 2nd ed. Bethesda, MD: National Institutes of Health, NIDDKD, 1991:31–40.

65. Lowrie EG, et al. Death risk in hemodialysis patients: the predictive value of commonly measured variables and an evaluation of death rate differences between facilities. *Am J Kidney Dis* 1990;15:458–482.

66. Degoulet P, et al. Mortality risk factors in patients treated by chronic hemodialysis. *Nephron* 1982;31:103–110.

67. Kupin W, et al. Protein catabolic rate (PCR) as predictor of survival in chronic hemodialysis patients. *Council Ren Nutr QJ* 1986;10:15–17.

68. Acchiardo SR, et al. Malnutrition as main factor in morbidity and mortality of hemodialysis patients. *Kidney Int* 1983;24(Suppl 15): S199–S203.

69. Harris T, et al. Body mass index and mortality among nonsmoking older persons: the Framingham Heart Study. *JAMA* 1988;259:1520–1524.

70. Hylander B, et al. What contributes to poor appetite in CAPD patients? *Perit Dial Int* 1991;11(Suppl 1):117.

71. Hylander B, et al. Appetite and eating behavior: a comparison between CAPD patients, HD patients, and healthy controls. *Perit Dial Int* 1992;12(Suppl 1):137A.

72. Lindholm B, et al. Nutritional management of patients undergoing peritoneal dialysis. In: Nolph KD, ed. *Peritoneal dialysis*, 3rd ed. Boston: Kluwer Academic, 1989:230–260.

73. Bannister DK, et al. Nutritional effects of peritonitis in continuous ambulatory peritoneal dialysis (CAPD) patients. *J Am Diet Assn* 1987; 87:53–56.

74. Ates K, et al. Peritoneal protein losses do not have a significant impact on nutritional status in CAPD patients. *Perit Dial Int* 2001;21: 519–522.

75. Wang AY, et al. Independent effects of residual renal function and dialysis adequacy on actual dietary protein, calorie, and other nutrient intake in patients on continuous ambulatory peritoneal dialysis. *J Am Soc Nephrol* 2001;12:2450–2457.

76. Lo WK, et al. Relationship between adequacy of dialysis and nutritional status, and their impact on patient survival on CAPD in Hong Kong. *Perit Dial Int* 2001;5:441–447.

77. Lindsay RM, et al. A hypothesis: the protein catabolic rate is dependent upon the type and amount of treatment in dialyzed uremic patients. *Am J Kidney Dis* 1989;13:382.

78. Bergstrom J, et al. Nutrition and adequacy of dialysis: how do hemodialysis and CAPD compare? *Kidney Int* 1993;43(Suppl 40): S39.

79. Gotch FA. The application of urea kinetic modeling to CAPD. In: La Greca G, et al., eds. *Peritoneal dialysis: proceedings of the Fourth International Course on Peritoneal Dialysis*. Milan, Italy: Wichtig Editore, 1991:47.

80. Harty JC, et al. Is the correlation between normalized protein catabolic rate and Kt/V due to mathematic coupling? *J Am Soc Nephrol* 1993;4:407.

81. Davies SJ, et al. Analysis of the effects of increasing delivered dialysis treatment to malnourished peritoneal dialysis patients. *Kidney Int* 2000;57:1743–1754.

82. Ronco C, et al. Adequacy of continuous ambulatory peritoneal dialysis: comparison with other dialysis techniques. *Kidney Int* 1994;46 (Suppl 48):S18–S24.

83. Lindsay RM, et al. Which comes first, Kt/V or PCR—chicken or egg? *Kidney Int* 1992;42:S32.

84. Bergstrom J, et al. Elevated serum C-reactive protein is a strong predictor of increased mortality and low serum albumin in hemodialysis (HD) patients. *J Am Soc Nephrol* 1995;6:573.

85. Qureshi AR, et al. Predictors of malnutrition in maintenance hemodialysis (HD) patients (abst.). *J Am Soc Nephrol* 1995;6:586.

86. Han DS, et al. Factors affecting low values of serum albumin in CAPD patients. In: Khanna R, ed. *Advances in peritoneal dialysis*. Toronto: Peritoneal Dialysis Publications, 1996;12:288–292.

87. Yeun JY, et al. Active phase proteins and peritoneal dialysate albumin loss are the main determinants of serum albumin in peritoneal dialysis patients. *Am J Kidney Dis* 1997;30:923–927.

88. Kaysen GA, et al. Determinants of albumin concentration in hemodialysis patients. *Am J Kidney Dis* 1997;29:658–668.

89. Kaysen GA, et al. Mechanisms of hypoalbuminemia in hemodialysis patients. *Kidney Int* 1995;48:510–516.

90. Haubitz M, et al. C-reactive protein and chronic *Chlamydia pneumoniae* infection—long-term predictors for cardiovascular disease survival in patients on peritoneal dialysis. *Nephrol Dial Transplant* 2001; 16:809–815.

91. Noh H, et al. Serum C-reactive protein: a predictor of mortality in continuous ambulatory peritoneal dialysis patients. *Perit Dial Int* 1998;18:387–394.

92. Ducloux D, et al. C-reactive protein and cardiovascular disease in peritoneal disease in peritoneal dialysis patients. *Kidney Int* 2002;62: 1417–1422.

93. Kim SB, et al. Persistent elevation of C-reactive protein and ischemic heart disease in patients with continuous ambulatory peritoneal dialysis. *Am J Kidney Dis* 2002;39:342–346.

94. Herzig KA, et al. Is C-reactive protein a useful predictor of outcome in peritoneal dialysis patients? *J Am Soc Nephrol* 2001;12:814–821.

95. Marckmann P. Nutritional status of patients on hemodialysis and peritoneal dialysis. *Clin Nephrol* 1988;29:75–78.

96. Chung SH, et al. Influence of initial nutritional status on continuous ambulatory peritoneal dialysis patient survival. *Perit Dial Int* 2000; 20:19–26.

97. Young GA, et al. Nutritional assessment of CAPD patients: an international study. *Am J Kidney Dis* 1991;17:462–471.

98. Tan SH, et al. Protein nutrition status of adult patients starting chronic ambulatory peritoneal dialysis. *Adv Perit Dial* 2000;16:291–293.

99. Passadakis P, et al. Nutrition in diabetic patients undergoing continuous ambulatory peritoneal dialysis. *Perit Dial Int* 1999;19(Suppl 2):S248–S254.

100. Jager KJ, et al. Nutritional status over time in hemodialysis and peritoneal dialysis. *J Am Soc Nephrol* 2001;12:1272–1279.

101. McCusker FM, et al. How much peritoneal dialysis is required for the maintenance of a good nutritional state? *Kidney Int* 1996;50: S56–S61.

102. Blake PG, et al. Serum albumin in patients on continuous ambulatory peritoneal dialysis: predictors and correlations with outcomes. *J Am Soc Nephrol* 1993;3:1501–1507.

103. Spiegel DM, et al. Serum albumin: a marker for morbidity in peritoneal dialysis adequacy. *J Am Soc Nephrol* 1992;3:417.

104. Rocco MV, et al. Lack of correlation between efficacy number and traditional measures of peritoneal dialysis adequacy. *J Am Soc Nephrol* 1992;3:417.

105. Koomen GCM, et al. Comparison between dye binding methods and nephelometry for the measurement of albumin in plasma of dialysis patients. *Perit Dial Int* 1992;12(Suppl 1):S133.

106. Rocco MV, et al. Report from the 1995 core indicators for peritoneal dialysis study group. *Am J Kidney Dis* 1997;30:165–173.

107. Liberek T, et al. Peritoneal dialysis fluid inhibition of phagocyte function: effects of osmolality and glucose concentration. *J Am Soc Nephrol* 1993;3:1508–1515.

108. Dawnay A. Advanced glycation end products in peritoneal dialysis. *Perit Dial Int* 1996;16:S50–S53.

109. Beelen RHJ, et al. CAPD, a permanent state of peritonitis: a study on peroxidase activity. In: Maher JF, et al., eds. *Frontiers in peritoneal dialysis*. New York: Field & Rich, 1986:524–530.

110. Dobbie JW. Durability of the peritoneal membrane. *Perit Dial Int* 1995;15:S87–S92.

111. Dobbie JW. Morphology of the peritoneum in CAPD. *Blood Purif* 1989;7:74–85.

112. Slingeneyer A, et al. Permanent loss of ultrafiltration capacity of the peritoneum in long-term peritoneal dialysis: an epidemiological study. *Nephron* 1983;33:133–138.

113. Afthentopoulos IE, et al. Sclerosing peritonitis in continuous ambulatory peritoneal dialysis patients: one center's experience and review of the literature. *Adv Ren Replace Ther* 1998;5:157–167.

114. Kopple JD, et al. A proposed glossary for dialysis kinetics. *Am J Kidney Dis* 1995;26:963–981.

115. Keshaviah P, et al. Protein catabolic rate calculations in CAPD patients. *ASAIO Trans* 1991;37:M400–M402.

116. Randerson DH, et al. Amino acid and dietary status in CAPD patients. In: Atkins RC, et al., eds. *Peritoneal dialysis*. Edinburgh: Churchill Livingstone, 1981:171–191.

117. Harty JC, et al. The normalized protein catabolic rate is a flawed marker of nutrition in CAPD patients. *Kidney Int* 1994;45:103–109.

118. Nolph KD, et al. Cross-sectional assessment of weekly urea and creatinine clearances and indices of nutrition in continuous ambulatory peritoneal dialysis patients. *Perit Dial Int* 1993;13:178–183.

119. Health Care Financing Administration. *2000 Annual Report: end-stage renal disease clinical performance measures project*. Baltimore: Department of Health and Human Services, Health Care Financing Administration, Office of Clinical Standards and Quality, December 2000.

120. Blumenkrantz MJ, et al. Metabolic balance studies and dietary protein requirements in patients undergoing continuous ambulatory peritoneal dialysis. *Kidney Int* 1982;21:849–861.

121. Diamond SM, et al. Nutrition and peritoneal dialysis. In: Mitch WE, et al., eds. *Nutrition and the kidney*. Boston: Little, Brown, 1988: 198–233.

122. *NKF–KDOQI clinical practice guidelines for nutrition in chronic renal failure*. New York: National Kidney Foundation, 2001.

123. Nolph KD. What's new in peritoneal dialysis: an overview. *Kidney Int* 1992;42(Suppl 38):S148–S152.

124. Lim VS, et al. Protein intake in patients with renal failure: comments on the current NKF–DOQI guidelines for nutrition in chronic renal failure. *Semin Dial* 2001;14:150–152.

125. Uribarri J, et al. Association of acidosis and nutritional parameters in hemodialysis patients. *Am J Kidney Dis* 1999;34:493–539.

126. Lindholm B, et al. Nutritional requirements of peritoneal dialysis. In: Gokal R, et al., eds. *Textbook of peritoneal dialysis*. Dordrecht: Kluwer Academic, 1994:443–472.

127. Grzegorzewska AE, et al. Nutritional intake during continuous ambulatory peritoneal dialysis. *Adv Perit Dial* 1997;13:150–154.

128. Fernstorm A, et al. Energy intake in patients on continuous ambulatory peritoneal dialysis and haemodialysis. *J Intern Med* 1996;240: 211–218.

129. Kopple JD. Therapeutic approaches to malnutrition in chronic dialysis patients: the different modalities of nutritional support. *Am J Kidney Dis* 1999;33:180–185.

130. Pickering WP, et al. Nutrition in CAPD: serum bicarbonate and the ubiquitin-proteasome system in muscle. *Kidney Int* 2002;61: 1286–1292.

131. Detsky AS, et al. What is subjective global assessment global assessment of nutritional status. *J Parenter Enteral Nutr* 1987;11:8–13.

132. Enia G, et al. Subjective global assessment of nutrition in dialysis patients. *Nephrol Dial Transplant* 1993;8:1094–1098.

133. Lutes R, et al. Loss of residual renal function in patients on peritoneal dialysis. In: Khanna R, et al., eds. *Advances in peritoneal dialysis*. Toronto: Peritoneal Dialysis Publications, 1993;9:69–72.

134. Gotch FA, et al. CAPD prescription in current clinical practice. In: Khanna R, et al., eds. *Advances in peritoneal dialysis*. Toronto: Peritoneal Dialysis Publications, 1993;9:69–72.

135. Rottembourg J, et al. Evolution of residual renal functions in patients undergoing maintenance hemodialysis or continuous ambulatory peritoneal dialysis. *Proc EDTA* 1993;19:397–403.

136. Cancarini GC, et al. Renal function recovery and maintenance of residual diuresis in CAPD and hemodialysis. *Perit Dial Bull* 1986;5: 77–79.

137. Lysaght MJ, et al. The influence of dialysis treatment modality on the decline of remaining renal function. *Trans ASAIO* 1991;37:598–604.

138. Hallet M, et al. Maintenance of residual renal function: CAPD versus HD. *Perit Dial Int* 1992;12(Suppl 1):124 (abst).

139. Tattersall JE, et al. Maintaining adequacy in CAPD by individualizing the dialysis prescription. *Nephrol Dial Transplant* 1994;9:749–752.

140. Page DE, et al. Role still exists for cycler therapy in anuric patients with a low-transport membrane. *Adv Perit Dial* 2001;17:114–116.

141. Twardowski ZJ. Clinical value of standardized equilibration tests in CAPD patients. *Blood Purif* 1989;7:95–108.

142. Blake P, et al. Recommended clinical practices for maximizing peritoneal dialysis clearances. *Perit Dial Int* 1996;16:448–456.

143. Twardowski ZJ. Nightly peritoneal dialysis (why? who? how? and when?). *ASAIO Trans* 1990;36:8–16.

144. Garred LJ, et al. A simple kinetic model for assessing peritoneal mass transfer in chronic ambulatory peritoneal dialysis. *ASAIO J* 1983;3: 131–137.

145. Popovich RP, et al. Transport kinetics. In: Nolph KD, ed. *Peritoneal dialysis*, 2nd ed. Boston: Martinus Nijhoff, 1985:115–158.

146. Vonesh EF, et al. Kinetic modeling as a prescription aid in peritoneal dialysis. *Blood Purif* 1991;9:246–270.

147. Krediet RT, et al. Peritoneal fluid kinetics during CAPD measured with intraperitoneal dextran 70. *ASAIO Trans* 1991;37:662–667.

148. Pannekeet MM, et al. The standard peritoneal permeability analysis: a tool for the assessment of peritoneal permeability characteristics in CAPD patients. *Kidney Int* 1995;48:866–875.

149. Pride ET, et al. Comparison of a 2.5% and a 4.25% dextrose peritoneal equilibration test. *Perit Dial Int* 2002;22:365–370.

150. Rippe B, et al. Peritoneal physiology-transport of solutes. In: Gokal R, et al., eds. *The textbook of peritoneal dialysis.* Dordrecht: Kluwer Academic, 1994:69–113.
151. Faller B, et al. Evolution of clinical parameters and peritoneal function in a cohort of CAPD patients followed over 7 years. *Nephrol Dial Transplant* 1994;9:280–286.
152. Selgas R, et al. Functional longevity of the human peritoneum: how long is continuous peritoneal dialysis possible? Results of a prospective medium long-term study. *Am J Kidney Dis* 1994;23:64–73.
153. Selgas R, et al. Preserving the peritoneal dialysis membrane in long-term peritoneal dialysis patients. *Semin Dial* 1995;8:326–332.
154. Selgas R, et al. Stability of the peritoneal membrane in long-term peritoneal dialysis patients. *Adv Ren Replace Ther* 1998;5:168–178.
155. Heimburger O, et al. Peritoneal transport characteristics in CAPD patients with permanent loss of ultrafiltration. *Kidney* 1990;38:495–506.
156. Watson PE, et al. Total body water volumes for adult males and females estimated from simple anthropometric measurements. *Am J Clin Nutr* 1980;33:27–39.
157. Hume R, et al. Relationship between total body water and surface area in normal and obese subjects. *J Clin Pathol* 1971;24:234–238.
158. Dubois D, et al. A formula to estimate the approximate surface area if height and weight be known. *Arch Intern Med* 1916;17:863–871.
159. Blake PG. Targets in CAPD and APD prescription. *Perit Dial Int* 1996;16:S143–S146.
160. Jensen RA, et al. Weight limitations for adequate therapy using commonly performed CAPD and NIPD regimens. *Semin Dial* 1994;7:61–64.
161. Nolph KD. Has peritoneal dialysis peaked? The impact of the CANUSA study. *ASAIO Trans* 1996;42:136–138.
162. Rocco MV. Body surface area limitations in achieving adequate therapy in peritoneal dialysis patients. *Perit Dial* 1996;16:617–622.
163. Jones MR. Etiology of severe malnutrition: results of an international cross-sectional study in continuous ambulatory peritoneal dialysis patients. *Am J Kidney Dis* 1994;23:412–420.
164. Johnson DW, et al. Is obesity a favorable prognostic factor in peritoneal dialysis patients? *Perit Dial Int* 2000;20:715–721.
165. Nolph KD, et al. Continuous ambulatory peritoneal dialysis with a high flux membrane: a preliminary report. *ASAIO J* 1993;39:M566–M568.
166. Burkart JM. Effect of peritoneal dialysis prescription and peritoneal membrane transport characteristics on nutritional status. *Perit Dial Int* 1995;15:S20–S35.
167. Kagan A, et al. Heterogeneity in peritoneal transport during continuous ambulatory peritoneal dialysis and its impact on ultrafiltration, loss of macromolecules and plasma level of proteins, lipids and lipoproteins. *Nephron* 1993;63:32–42.
168. Struijk DG, et al. Functional characteristics of the peritoneal membrane in long term continuous ambulatory peritoneal dialysis. *Nephron* 1991;59:213–220.
169. Mamoun H, et al. Peritoneal dialysis solutions with glucose and amino acids suppress appetite in the rat. *J Am Soc Nephrol* 1994;5:498.
170. Balaskas EV, et al. Effect of intraperitoneal infusion of dextrose and amino acids on the appetite of rabbits. *Perit Dial Int* 1993;13:S490–S498.
171. Mamoun AH, et al. Influence of peritoneal dialysis solutions with glucose and amino acids on ingestive behavior in rats. *Kidney Int* 1996;49:1276–1282.
172. Davies S, et al. Impact of peritoneal absorption of glucose on appetite, protein catabolism and survival in CAPD patients. *Clin Nephrol* 1996;45:194–198.
173. Twardowski ZJ, et al. Daily clearances with CAPD and NIPD. *ASAIO Trans* 1986;32:575–580.
174. Feriani M. Adequacy of acid base correction in continuous ambulatory peritoneal dialysis patients. *Perit Dial Int* 1994;14:S133–S138.
175. Feriani M, et al. Acid-base balance with different CAPD solutions. *Perit Dial Int* 1996;16:S126–S129.
176. La Greca G, et al. Acid-base balance on peritoneal dialysis. *Clin Nephrol* 1981;16:1–7.
177. Uribarri J, et al. Acid-base balance in chronic peritoneal dialysis patients. *Kidney Int* 1995;47:269–273.
178. Graham KA, et al. Acid-base regulation in peritoneal dialysis. *Kidney Int* 1994;46(Suppl 48):S47–S50.
179. Walls J, et al. Does metabolic acidosis have clinically important consequences in dialysis patients? *Semin Dial* 1998;11:18–19.
180. Bailey JL, et al. Does metabolic acidosis have clinically important consequences in dialysis patients? *Semin Dial* 1998;11:23–24.
181. Graham KA, et al. Correction of acidosis in CAPD decreases whole body protein degradation. *Kidney Int* 1996;49:1396–1400.
182. Lowrie EG, et al. Commonly measured laboratory variables in hemodialysis patients: relationships among them and to death risk. *Semin Nephrol* 1992;12:276–283.
183. Bergstrom J. Why are dialysis patients malnourished? *Am J Kidney Dis* 1995;26:229–241.
184. Acchiardo SR, et al. Evaluation of CAPD prescription. In: Khanna R, et al., eds. *Advances in peritoneal dialysis.* Toronto: Peritoneal Dialysis Bulletin, 1991;7:47–50.
185. Chen HH, et al. Discrepancy between weekly Kt/V and weekly creatinine clearance in patients on CAPD. In: Khanna R, ed. *Advances in peritoneal dialysis.* Toronto: Peritoneal Dialysis Publications, 1995:83–87.
186. Vonesh EF, et al. Peritoneal dialysis kinetic modeling: validation in a multicenter clinical study. *Perit Dial Int* 1996;16:471–481.
187. Doolan PD, et al. A clinical appraisal of the plasma concentration and endogenous clearance of creatinine. *Am J Med* 1962;32:65–79.
188. Tzamaloukas AH. Effect of edema on urea kinetic studies in peritoneal dialysis. *Perit Dial Int* 1994;14:398–400.
189. Tzamaloukas AH, et al. Volume of distribution and fractional clearance of urea in amputees on continuous ambulatory peritoneal dialysis. *Perit Dial Int* 1994;14:356–361.
190. Twardowski ZJ. Relationships between creatinine clearances and Kt/V in peritoneal dialysis patients: a critique of the DOQI document. *Perit Dial Int* 1998;18:252–255.
191. Tzamaloukas AH, et al. Indicators of body size in peritoneal dialysis: their relation to urea and creatinine clearances. *Perit Dial Int* 1998;18:366–370.
192. Nolph KD. Is total creatinine clearance a poor index of adequacy in CAPD patients with residual renal function? *Perit Dial Int* 1997;17:232–233.
193. Foley RN, et al. Clinical and echocardiographic disease in patients starting end-stage renal disease therapy. *Kidney Int* 1995;47:186–192.
194. Ates K, et al. Effect of fluid and sodium removal on mortality in peritoneal dialysis patients. *Kidney Int* 2001;60:767–776.
195. Brown EA, et al. Ultrafiltration and not solute clearance or solute transport status predicts outcomes at 2 years for APD in anuric patients. *J Am Soc Nephrol* 2002;13:70.
196. Gunal AI, et al. Strict volume control normalizes hypertension in peritoneal dialysis patients. *Am J Kidney Dis* 2001;37:588–593.
197. Abu AL, et al. Approach to fluid management in peritoneal dialysis: a practical algorithm. *Kidney Int* 2002;62(Suppl 81):S8–S16.
198. Mujais S, et al. Evaluation and management of ultrafiltration problems in peritoneal dialysis. International Society for Peritoneal Dialysis Ad Hoc Committee on Ultrafiltration Management in Peritoneal Dialysis. *Perit Dial Int* 2000;20(Suppl 4):S5–S21.
199. Moberly JB, et al. Pharmacokinetics of icodextrin in peritoneal dialysis patients. *Kidney Int* 2002;62(Suppl 81):S23–S33.
200. Mujias S, et al. Profiling of peritoneal ultrafiltration. *Kidney Int* 2002;62(Suppl 81):S17–S22.
201. Mistry CD, et al. MIDA Study Group. A randomized multicenter clinical trial comparing isoosmolar icodextrin with hyperosmolar glucose solution in CAPD. *Kidney Int* 1994;46:496–503.
202. Gokal R, et al. United Kingdom multicenter study of icodextrin in continuous ambulatory peritoneal dialysis (MIDAS). *Perit Dial Int* 1994;14(Suppl 2):S22–S27.
203. Plum J, et al. Efficacy and safety of a 7.5% icodextrin peritoneal dialysis solution in patients treated with automated peritoneal dialysis. *Am J Kidney Dis* 2002;39:862–871.
204. Woodrow G, et al. Comparison of icodextrin and glucose solutions for the daytime dwell in automated peritoneal dialysis. *Nephrol Dial Transplant* 1999;14:1530–1535.

205. Burkart JM, et al. Assessment of dialysis dose by measured clearance versus extrapolated data. *Perit Dial Int* 1993;13:184–188.
206. Misra M, et al. Six-month prospective cross-over study to determine the effects of 1.1% amino acid dialysate on lipid metabolism in patients on continuous ambulatory peritoneal dialysis. *Perit Dial Int* 1997;17:279–286.
207. Frankenfield DL, et al. For the ESRD Core Indicators Workgroup. Trends in clinical indicators of care for adult peritoneal dialysis patients in the U.S. from 1995–1997. *Kidney Int* 1999;55:1998–2010.
208. Blake PG, et al. Changes in peritoneal membrane transport rates in patients on long term CAPD. In: Khanna R, et al., eds. *Advances in peritoneal dialysis*, Vol 15. Toronto: Peritoneal Dialysis International, 1989:3–7.
209. Rocco MV, et al. 24-hour dialysate collection for determination of peritoneal membrane transport characteristics: longitudinal follow-up data for the dialysis adequacy and transport test. *Perit Dial Int* 1996;16:590–593.
210. Rocco MV, et al. Prevalence of missed treatments and early signoffs in hemodialysis patients. *J Am Soc Nephrol* 1993;4:1178–1183.
211. Keen ML, et al. The measured creatinine generation rate in CAPD suggests that only 78% of prescribed dialysis is delivered. In: Khanna R, et al., eds. *Advances in peritoneal dialysis*. Toronto: Peritoneal Publications, 1993:73–75.
212. Warren PJ, et al. Compliance with the peritoneal dialysis prescription is poor. *J Am Soc Nephrol* 1994;4:1627–1629.
213. Nolph KD, et al. Predicted and measured daily creatinine production in CAPD: identifying noncompliance. *Perit Dial Int* 1995;15:22–25.
214. Burkart JM, et al. An elevated ration of measured to predicted creatinine production in CAPD patients is not a sensitive predictor of noncompliance with the dialysis prescription. *Perit Dial Int* 1996;16:142–146.
215. Blake PG, et al. Comparison of measured and predicted creatinine excretion is an unreliable index of compliance in PD patients. *Perit Dial Int* 1996;16:147–153.
216. Blake PG, et al. A multicenter study of noncompliance with continuous ambulatory peritoneal dialysis exchanges in U.S. and Canadian patients. *Am J Kidney Dis* 2000;35:506–514.
217. Bernardini J, et al. Measuring compliance with prescribed exchanges in CAPD and CCPD patients. *Perit Dial Int* 1997;17:338–342.
218. Obrador GT, et al. Pre–end-stage renal disease care in the United States: a state of disrepair. *J Am Soc Nephrol* 1998;9:S44–S54.
219. Nolph KD. Rationale for early incremental dialysis with continuous ambulatory peritoneal dialysis. *Nephrol Dial Transplant* 1998;13 (Suppl 6):117–119.
220. Obrador GT, et al. What is the level of GFR at the start of dialysis in the U.S. ESRD population? *J Am Soc Nephrol* 1998;9:156A.
221. Ikizler TA, et al. Spontaneous dietary protein intake during progression of chronic renal failure. *J Am Soc Nephrol* 1995;6:1386–1391.
222. Kopple JD, et al. Modification of Diet in Renal Disease Study Group. Nutritional status of patients with different levels of chronic renal insufficiency. *Kidney Int* 1989;26:S184–S194.
223. Pollock CA, et al. Protein intake in renal disease. *J Am Soc Nephrol* 1997;8:777–783.
224. Mehrotra R, et al. Towards targets for imitation of dialysis: the relationship of protein catabolic rate to Kt/V$_{urea}$ in chronic renal failure patients. *J Am Soc Nephrol* 1996;7:1521.
225. Bonomini V, et al. Benefits of early initiation of dialysis. *Kidney Int* 1985;28:S57–S59.
226. Tattersall J, et al. Urea kinetics and when to commence dialysis. *Am J Nephrol* 1995;15:283–289.
227. Ratcliffe PJ, et al. Late referral for maintenance dialysis. *Br Med J* 1984;288:441–443.
228. Schulman G, et al. Improving outcomes in chronic hemodialysis patients: should dialysis be initiated early? *Semin Dial* 1996;9:225–229.
229. Jungers P, et al. Detrimental effects of late referral in patients with chronic renal failure: a case control study. *Kidney Int* 1993;43:S170–S173.
230. Heaf JG, et al. Initial survival advantage of peritoneal dialysis relative to hemodialysis. *Nephrol Dial Transplant* 2002;17:112–117.
231. Mehrota R, et al. Early initiation of chronic dialysis: role of incremental dialysis. *Perit Dial Int* 1997;17:497–508.
232. Blake PG, et al. *Peritoneal dialysis prescription management decision tree: a need for change.* McGaw, IL: Baxter Healthcare Corporation, 1997.
233. Caruana RJ, et al. Dialysate dumping: a novel cause of inadequate dialysis in continuous ambulatory peritoneal dialysis patients. *Perit Dial Int* 1989;9:319–320.
234. Sevick MA, et al. Measurement of CAPD adherence using a novel approach. *Perit Dial Int* 1999;19:23–30.
235. Mistry CD, et al. Ultrafiltration with an isosmotic solution during long peritoneal dialysis exchanges. *Lancet* 1987;2:178–182.
236. Twardowski ZJ. Influence of different automated peritoneal dialysis schedules on solute and water removal. *Nephrol Dial Transplant* 1998;13(Suppl 6):103–111.
237. Nolph KD, et al. Weekly clearances of urea and creatinine on CAPD and NIPD. *Perit Dial Int* 1992;12:298–303.
238. Vonesh EF, et al. Applications in kinetic modeling using PD ADE-QUEST. *Perit Dial Int* 1997;17(Suppl 2):S119–S125.
239. Gotch FA, et al. A urea kinetic modeling computer program for peritoneal dialysis. *Perit Dial Int* 1997;17:S126–S130.
240. Twardowski ZJ. New approaches to intermittent peritoneal dialysis therapies. In: Nolph KD, ed. *Peritoneal dialysis,* 3rd ed. Boston: Kluwer Academic, 1990:133–151.
241. Twardowski Z, et al. Intra-abdominal pressures during natural activities in patients treated with continuous ambulatory peritoneal dialysis. *Nephron* 1986;44:129–135.
242. Digenis G, et al. Abdominal hernias in patients undergoing continuous ambulatory peritoneal dialysis. *Perit Dial Bull* 1982;2:115–117.
243. Rocco M, et al. Abdominal hernias in chronic peritoneal dialysis review: a review. *Perit Dial Bull* 1985;5:171–174.
244. Coles GA. Have we underestimated the importance of fluid balance for the survival of PD patients. *Perit Dial Int* 1997;17:321–326.

CAUSES, DIAGNOSIS, AND TREATMENT OF PERITONEAL MEMBRANE FAILURE

STEPHEN M. KORBET AND ROGER A. RODBY

The success of peritoneal dialysis (PD) as a long-term therapeutic option in the treatment of end-stage renal disease (ESRD) depends on the efficient removal of both solute and fluid. The ability to provide "adequate" dialysis (see Chapter 14) is a function of patient compliance, residual renal function, the transport characteristics of the peritoneal membrane, and the capacity to deliver a required dialysate flow rate in a manner that is tolerable to the patient. Thus alterations in any of these factors, and not only in the characteristics of the peritoneal membrane, can significantly influence the efficiency of peritoneal dialysis (Table 15.1) leading to "inadequate" dialysis and "failure" of peritoneal dialysis as a technique.

Fortunately, failure to achieve adequate dialysis from a solute or fluid removal standpoint represents only 4% to 12% of the total transfers from continuous ambulatory peritoneal dialysis (CAPD) to hemodialysis ("technique failure") (1–6). Because patients are on peritoneal dialysis for longer periods of time, however, they are at an increased risk of incurring problems attaining adequate solute and fluid removal. In part, this is the result of alterations in peritoneal membrane function. Typically, these changes have a disproportionately greater effect on fluid removal as compared with solute removal, and therefore ultrafiltration failure represents the overwhelming majority of cases of membrane failure, whereas the inability to achieve adequate solute removal is relatively uncommon.

In most patients maintained on peritoneal dialysis for 4 or more years, peritoneal clearance of small solutes is stable or increases, whereas net ultrafiltration has been shown to decrease by as much as 40% from baseline (7–10). This is evident clini-

cally by an increased requirement for the use of hypertonic exchanges in order to maintain an adequate extracellular volume status (11). Thus signs and symptoms of fluid overload resulting from net ultrafiltration failure constitute one of the most common problems encountered in patients chronically maintained on peritoneal dialysis. Over an 18-month period, Davies et al. (12) observed ultrafiltration failure in 14% of their patients. Defined by the presence of edema and the inability to maintain a patient's dry weight for a month or greater despite three or more hypertonic (4.25%) exchanges per day and fluid restriction, Heimburger et al. (5) demonstrated the cumulative risk for permanent loss of net ultrafiltration capacity to be 2.6% at 1 year, 9.5% at 3 years, and in excess of 30% for those patients on CAPD for 6 years or more!

Although the inability to achieve adequate solute and fluid removal is often attributed to a "failure" of the peritoneal membrane, it must be remembered that this is but one of several factors that impact on the efficiency of peritoneal dialysis (Table 15.1). It is therefore critical that nephrologists consider and understand these issues when evaluating patients with signs and symptoms of ultrafiltration failure. In this chapter we review the factors that influence ultrafiltration efficiency and present an approach to evaluating and treating these patients in clinical practice.

SOLUTE AND FLUID TRANSPORT IN PERITONEAL DIALYSIS

The Peritoneal Membrane

Solute and fluid transport in peritoneal dialysis result from the development of concentration and pressure (hydrostatic and osmotic) gradients between blood and dialysate across the semipermeable peritoneal "membrane." Thus the physical characteristics (surface area and permeability) of the peritoneal membrane become major determinants in solute and fluid transport. The physical features of hemodialysis membranes are known by design; however, these properties are unknown for the peritoneal membrane and have largely been determined indirectly based on conceptual models and mathematical analyses. From these efforts our concept of the transport physiology of the peritoneal membrane is evolving.

TABLE 15.1. FACTORS INFLUENCING PERITONEAL DIALYSIS EFFICIENCY

Residual renal function
Patient compliance
Peritoneal membrane characteristics
  Permeability
  Effective surface area
Lymphatic absorption
Dialysate volume/osmolarity/flow
Effective blood flow

Originally, peritoneal transport properties were based on a "membrane model" in which the peritoneum was simply viewed as a single "membrane" comprised of capillary wall, interstitium, and mesothelium. In this model, a concentration gradient exists from the capillary lumen on one side of the "membrane" to the peritoneal cavity on the other (13). More recently, the concept of a "distributed model" has been proposed to better explain the observed transport properties of the peritoneum. Here the capillaries are viewed as "distributed" throughout the interstitium, resulting in varying distances between capillary lumens and the peritoneal cavity (14).

The "anatomic" surface area of the peritoneal membrane correlates best with body surface area (BSA) and is estimated to range from 1.7 to 2.0 m² (15). However, it is the "effective" surface area of the peritoneal membrane that is important in determining solute and fluid transport in peritoneal dialysis. The "effective" peritoneal surface area is defined as that area of peritoneal membrane perfused by capillaries that comes into contact with dialysate and contributes to solute and fluid transport (16–18). The effective peritoneal surface area therefore depends not only on the volume of dialysate used, but also on the "effective" peritoneal blood flow (that portion of the peritoneal microcirculation that actually comes into contact with dialysate and thus participates in solute and fluid transport). Most (47%) of the overall small solute diffusive transport is across the peritoneal membrane associated with hollow viscera. However, as much as 43% of diffusive transport during peritoneal dialysis occurs across the peritoneum associated with the liver (abdominal wall 6% and diaphragm 4%) (19).

The permeability of the peritoneal membrane is determined by the resistances created by the capillary wall, interstitium, and mesothelium. Of these, the capillary wall is the most and the mesothelium the least important as barriers to transport. Transport across the capillary wall is best explained based on a three-pore model (14,20,21). In this model, the capillary wall is comprised of ultrasmall or transcellular pores (radius, ≤0.8 nm), small pores (radius, 4 to 5 nm) and large pores (radius, 20 to 30 nm).

The ultrasmall pores are permeable only to water, and it is across these pores that the greatest osmotic effect of glucose is achieved. Therefore, although these pores comprise only 1% to 2% of the total pore area, they contribute up to 40% of the ultrafiltrate. Since the ultrafiltrate generated by the ultrasmall pores is solute-free, they are largely responsible for the sieving coefficient of the peritoneal membrane.

Small pores account for more than 90% of total pore area and are the primary route for the diffusive and convective transport of small-molecular-weight solutes (e.g., urea, creatinine, and electrolytes). More than 50% of glucose-induced ultrafiltration occurs through small pores. It is through back-diffusion across these pores that glucose absorption from the peritoneal cavity also occurs. However, small pores are essentially impermeable to macromolecules such as proteins.

A small number of large pores are responsible for the transport of macromolecules (e.g., albumin), which occurs exclusively by unidirectional convection. They account for less than 1% of the effective pore area for small solute diffusion and are relatively unimportant in water transport.

Solute Transport

Diffusive Transport

In peritoneal dialysis, solute removal results from a combination of diffusive and convective transport. Diffusion, the primary mechanism for small solute removal, results from the concentration gradient between blood and dialysate created across the peritoneal membrane with the instillation of dialysate into the peritoneal cavity. The rate of diffusion for a solute (J_s) depends on the product of the peritoneal membrane solute permeability (P_s), effective peritoneal surface area *(A)*, and the magnitude of the plasma to dialysate concentration gradient (ΔC) for that solute.

$$J_s = P_s \times A \times \Delta C \qquad [1]$$

The intrinsic permeability of the peritoneal membrane for a given solute is relatively constant and is determined by its molecular weight. The peritoneal membrane is therefore highly permeable to low-molecular-weight solutes such as urea and creatinine but has a low permeability to high-molecular-weight solutes such as β_2-microglobulin and other large proteins.

Increasing the effective peritoneal surface area, by increasing the intraperitoneal volume of dialysate, can significantly improve the rate of diffusive transport for small solutes (Fig. 15.1) (8). Keshaviah et al. (22) demonstrated that transport rates for urea, creatinine, and glucose doubled as infused volumes of dialysate were increased from 0.5 to 2.5 L. The infused volume producing the maximal diffusive transport rate for a given patient increased with increasing BSA, being 2.5 L for an average-sized person (BSA 1.7 m²) and 3 to 3.5 L for a person with a BSA of more than 2 m². The improved transport with larger volumes is felt to result from an increase in contact between dialysate and peritoneum, thereby increasing the "effective" peritoneal surface area by recruiting more peritoneal membrane. Beyond these maximal volumes, little to no improvement in diffusive transport is attained as the effective peritoneal surface area is completely exposed to dialysate and any further increases in volume results in "pooling" of dialysate.

Maintaining a maximal concentration gradient also enhances the rate of diffusive transport. This is dependent on the effective peritoneal blood flow as well as dialysate flow. The concentration gradient (ΔC) across the peritoneum is maximal early in the dwell cycle but decreases over time as solute diffuses from blood to dialysate. As the gradient decreases, the rate of diffusion decreases. Increasing the dialysate flow rate (shorter dwell times) and/or volume (increased exchange volumes) enhances the gradient, and thus the rate of diffusion can be increased (Fig. 15.1). Diffusion ceases when the concentration gradient between blood and dialysate no longer exists. Smaller molecules cross the peritoneal membrane more easily, equilibrate faster, and are influenced more by dialysate flow rates than are larger molecules (23,24).

It has generally been accepted that effective peritoneal blood flow is not a rate-limiting factor for the diffusive transport of small-molecular-weight solutes, as estimates of peritoneal blood flows are more than two to three times that estimated for the transport rates of small solutes like urea (13,14,25,26). However, given the large contribution of the

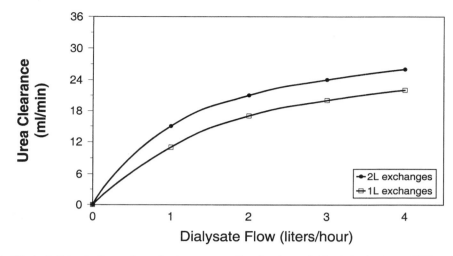

FIG. 15.1. Effect of dialysate flow rate and volume on small-molecular-weight solute clearance. With an increase in dialysate flow, clearances increase, but at a given flow rate the clearances are even better with the use of larger fill volumes. This results from an increase in diffusive transport due to the increase in effective peritoneal surface area with larger fill volumes. *Open circle,* 2-L volumes; *open square,* 1-L volumes. (Modified with permission from Robson M, et al. Influence of exchange volume and dialysate flow rate on solute clearance in peritoneal dialysis. *Kidney Int* 1978;14:486–490.)

liver-to-solute transport and the fact that the liver may be more permeable to small solutes than other vascular beds in the abdomen, the rate of transport across the sinusoids may be so rapid that blood flow could be a limiting factor for this vascular bed (19). The major contribution of the liver to small solute clearance may account, in part, for the increased solute transport observed in the supine position or with increased dwell volumes as these maneuvers increase the contact of dialysate with the liver (19,24,27,28).

Convective Transport

Solute removal also occurs through convection. As osmotic forces cause water to move across the peritoneal membrane and into the peritoneal cavity, frictional forces between the solvent (water) and solutes (e.g., Na$^+$, urea, etc.) result in these solutes being convectively carried along with water. This is referred to as "solvent drag." Since the peritoneal membrane provides greater resistance to solutes than to water (particularly by way of fluid transport across ultrasmall or transcellular pores), the concentration of solutes in the ultrafiltrate is less than that in plasma, and this is referred to as solute sieving. The sieving coefficient for a given solute is the ratio of the solute concentration in the ultrafiltrate to that in the plasma. The rate of solute transport by convection (J_s) is therefore related not only to the transcapillary ultrafiltrate rate or water flux (J_w), but also to the serum concentration (C_s) and sieving coefficient (*S*) for that solute.

$$J_s = J_w \times C_s \times S \qquad [2]$$

Since the rate of ultrafiltration decreases over the time course of a dwell (see the discussion of fluid transport later), the relative contribution of convective transport to overall solute removal also decreases during the same time period. The percent of total

solute transfer that is provided by convective as compared with diffusive transport increases significantly as the molecular size increases. It may be responsible for as little as 10% of total urea transport but may be responsible for more than 80% of protein transport (29,30).

Fluid Transport (Ultrafiltration)

Ultrafiltration occurs primarily through osmosis, resulting from the osmotic gradient created between the peritoneal blood compartment and the intraperitoneal dialysate compartment. This is achieved by utilizing hyperosmolar dialysate created by the addition of an osmotically active substance, usually dextrose, to the solution. The rate of transcapillary ultrafiltration or water flux (J_w) is dependent on the peritoneal membrane hydraulic permeability (L_p) and effective surface area (*A*), as well as the transmembrane osmotic ($\Delta\pi$) and hydrostatic pressure gradients (ΔP), where

$$J_w = L_p \times A \times (\Delta\pi + \Delta P) \qquad [3]$$

Transcapillary ultrafiltration is highest at the beginning of a peritoneal exchange when the osmotic gradient is greatest. As the osmotic gradient decreases over time, as a result of dilution of glucose by the ultrafiltrate and glucose absorption from the peritoneal cavity, the rate of ultrafiltration declines. The transcapillary ultrafiltration rate (and thus net ultrafiltration—see later) can be increased by either the use of larger dialysate volumes (which decrease the rate of dilution) or more hypertonic solutions (which increase the osmotic gradient) or both (Fig. 15.2). Factors that lead to an increase in peritoneal membrane permeability or effective surface area (e.g., peritonitis) increase solute transport (e.g., glucose absorption), resulting in a more rapid decline in the osmotic gradient and thus decrease the rate of ultrafiltration (31).

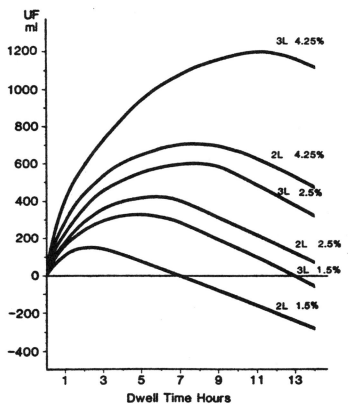

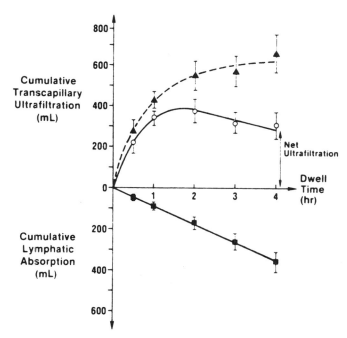

FIG. 15.2. Effect of osmolality and volume of dextrose dialysis solutions on net ultrafiltration. (Reproduced with permission from Twardowski Z, et al. Osmotic agents and ultrafiltration in peritoneal dialysis. *Nephron* 1986;42:93–101.)

FIG. 15.3. Net ultrafiltration *(open circle)* is a result of the additive effects of transcapillary ultrafiltration *(solid triangle)* and the negative effects of lymphatic absorption *(solid square)*. Net ultrafiltration actually decreases as lymphatic absorption rate exceeds transcapillary ultrafiltration. (Solution used is 2.5% dextrose.) (Reproduced with permission of the American Society for Clinical Investigation from Mactier RA, et al. Contribution of lymphatic absorption to loss of ultrafiltration and solute clearances in continuous ambulatory peritoneal dialysis. *J Clin Invest* 1987;80:1311–1316.)

Lymphatic absorption (LA) of fluid from the abdominal cavity opposes the effects of transcapillary ultrafiltration (UF). As shown in Fig. 15.3, the combined effects of these two forces determines the ultimate drain volume or net ultrafiltration (Net UF), where

$$\text{Net UF} = \text{UF} - \text{LA} \qquad [4]$$

Lymphatic absorption rates appear to be constant, irrespective of the initial volume or tonicity of the dialysate instilled, and have been estimated to average from 1 to 1.5 mL/min (18,32,33). As long as the rate of transcapillary ultrafiltration is greater than the rate of lymphatic absorption, intraabdominal fluid volume or net ultrafiltration increases above the initial fill volume (33,34). Peak intraperitoneal volume (Net UF) is reached when the rate of transcapillary ultrafiltration equals the rate of lymphatic absorption (Fig. 15.4). This actually precedes the point in time at which osmotic and glucose equilibration of dialysate and plasma occur. Thereafter the lymphatic absorption rate exceeds the rate of ultrafiltration resulting in a net absorption of fluid from the peritoneal cavity, causing a decline in the intraperitoneal volume (declining Net UF). Net ultrafiltration can be increased by measures that increase the transcapillary ultrafiltration rate (hypertonic dextrose solutions and/or increasing dialysate volume, as noted earlier), or by taking advantage of

the time of peak ultrafiltration (decrease the dwell time) (Figs. 15.2 and 15.3). In addition to affecting Net UF, absorption of peritoneal fluid by lymphatic uptake influences overall solute removal by partially negating the effects of both diffusive and convective transport.

EVALUATION OF PERITONEAL MEMBRANE FUNCTION

Unlike hemodialysis membranes, the solute and fluid transport characteristics (surface area and permeability) of the peritoneal membrane are unknown in a given patient. As a result, several indirect methods of evaluating the transport properties of the peritoneal membrane have been established. These protocols usually require that a peritoneal dialysis exchange be performed with a specified dialysate volume and dextrose concentration, assessing solute concentrations in serum and dialysate at specific points in time during a set dwell period, as well as determining the final drain volume. Through the information derived from these studies, a patient's transport characteristics can be established. This is most often done by determining either the dialysate-to-plasma (D/P) ratio—best standardized by the peritoneal equilibration test (PET) (35) or the peritoneal membrane mass transfer area coefficient (MTAC) (29,36,37) for various solutes. Since the D/P ratio of a given solute (the measure of

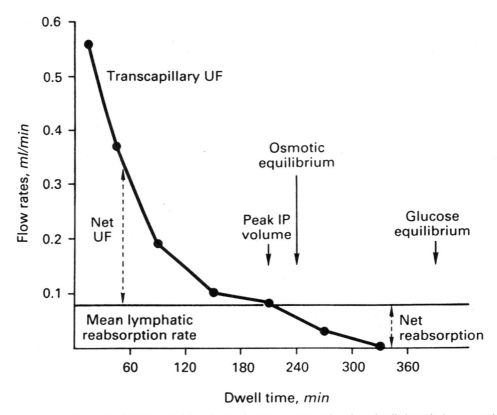

FIG. 15.4. Transcapillary ultrafiltration and lymphatic absorption rates related to dwell time during an exchange using 2 L of 1.5% dextrose. Peak intraperitoneal volume occurs when the rate of transcapillary ultrafiltration equals the rate of lymphatic absorption of fluid from the peritoneal cavity. This precedes osmotic equilibrium (there is still an osmolar gradient, although markedly attenuated because of the combined effects of dilution by ultrafiltrate and absorption of glucose from dialysate to blood) and glucose equilibration. (Reproduced with permission from Nolph KD, et al. The kinetics of UF during peritoneal dialysis: the role of lymphatics. *Kidney Int* 1987;32:219–226.)

transport utilized in the PET) depends upon both diffusive and convective transport, the MTAC was introduced to separate those influences on solute transfer from membrane function alone. From a practical perspective, information on peritoneal membrane function that is gained by the MTAC adds little to that of the PET alone (38).

Mass Transfer Area Coefficient

Mass transfer area coefficient represents the maximal diffusive clearance that could be obtained in the absence of both convection and solute build-up in the dialysate, and therefore is the most specific measure of peritoneal membrane transport. The MTAC (in mL/min) for a given solute is equal to the product of its peritoneal membrane solute permeability (P_s, in cm/min) and the effective peritoneal surface area (A, in cm^2) (see Eq. 1). The calculation of mass transport area coefficient (also referred to as diffusive mass transport) eliminates the effects of dialysate flow and convective clearance assessing only the diffusive properties of the peritoneum.

Some have considered MTAC the preferred method by which to measure and follow peritoneal membrane function (39). However, because of the variability of results, both among patients and between studies, and the complexity of the calcula-

tions for MTAC (36,37), this method of evaluation has not been widely accepted among clinical nephrologists. Furthermore, if one examines the equation for MTAC used by Vonesh et al. (40) (assuming isovolemia to occur between 2 and 4 hours following the infusion of 2.5% dextrose):

$$\text{MTAC} = -\frac{V_D}{t} \ln \frac{1-(C_D/C_B)}{1-(V^1_D C^1_D / V_D C_B)} \qquad [5]$$

where V_D is the dialysate volume drained at time t, t is time in minutes, C_D is the solute concentration in dialysate at time t, C_B is the average solute concentration in the plasma at time t, and superscript 1 represents the value immediately after infusion of fresh dialysate. It is evident that MTAC can be estimated from the dialysate to plasma (D/P) concentration ratio (e.g., C_D/C_B) for solutes such as urea and creatinine. If one assumes the concentration of a solute in the dialysate immediately after infusion C^1_D) is negligible or 0, Equation 5 can be further simplified to

$$\text{MTAC} = -V_D/t \times \ln[1 - (C_D/C_B)] \qquad [6]$$

From this relationship one can understand why an excellent correlation has been observed between the results of the MTAC and the D/P ratio established by the PET (41–43). The D/P ratio could overestimate the actual MTAC for low-transport patients (because of the larger contribution of convective transport to solute removal in these patients) and underestimate MTAC in the high-transport patients [because the relative contribution of lymphatic absorption has a greater negative effect on drain volume (V_D) in these patients]. As a result, this has led some researchers to recommend that the MTAC be the method of choice for assessing peritoneal membrane transport as it defines the maximal diffusive clearance without interference because of dialysate saturation with solute during the dwell and is not influenced by dialysate tonicity or volume (42). However, it has been shown that the contribution of convective transport to the overall removal of small-molecular-weight solutes, such as urea and creatinine, is negligible at 4 hours with the use of 2.5% dextrose solutions (the concentration used in the PET) (30). Furthermore, since the PET is standardized (performed with a specific dialysate tonicity and volume), it has been found to be highly reproducible. Thus, because of its simplicity, reliability, and reproducibility, the PET has become the accepted measure by which peritoneal membrane function is evaluated in clinical practice.

Peritoneal Equilibration Test

The peritoneal equilibration test as standardized and popularized by Twardowski et al. (35,38) has become the measure by which most clinicians initially assess and follow peritoneal membrane solute transport characteristics in their patients on peritoneal dialysis. This test semiquantitatively measures the peritoneal membrane transfer rates for solutes (usually urea and creatinine) based on the ratio of their concentration in dialysate and plasma (D/P ratio) at specific times *(t)* during the dialysate dwell; and for glucose, based on the ratio of dialysate glucose at dwell times *t* to dialysate glucose at 0 dwell time (D_t/D_0). Table 15.2 describes the standardized version of the PET.

TABLE 15.2. STANDARD PERITONEAL EQUILIBRATION TEST[a]

1. An 8- to 12-hour exchange with 4.25% dialysate precedes the test exchange.
2. Drain pretest exchange over 20 minutes in the vertical position (sending a sample for creatinine and glucose will allow for the determination of residual volume).
3. Infuse 2 L of 2.5%[a] dextrose dialysate over 10 minutes with patient supine.
4. After each volume of 400 mL is infused, have patient roll from side to side.
5. At the completion of the infusion, or 0 dwell time, and at 120 minutes dwell time, 200 mL of dialysate is drained, 10 mL is taken, and the remaining 190 mL is reinfused.
6. The patient is otherwise ambulatory during the dwell period.
7. At 120 minutes dwell time a serum sample is obtained.
8. At 240 minutes dwell time, with the patient in the vertical position, the dialysate is drained over 20 minutes, the volume is measured, and a final sample is obtained.
9. All samples are sent for glucose and creatinine concentrations.[b]

From Twardowski ZJ, et al. Peritoneal equilibration test. *Perit Dial Bull* 1987;7:138–147; Twardowski ZJ. Clinical value of standardized equilibration tests in CAPD patients. *Blood Purif* 1989;7:95–108.
[a]The Modified PET uses a 4.25% exchange.
[b]Sodium concentration may also be assessed when pursuing an abnormality in transcapillary ultrafiltration (type I ultrafiltration failure or an abnormality in transcellular pore function) vs an increase in lymphatic absorption rate. In this case an additional dialysate sample at 60 minutes may also be helpful.

In determining the D/P creatinine ratio it must be appreciated that high glucose levels will falsely elevate creatinine measurements when determined by the picric acid method. As a result, creatinine levels must be corrected for the glucose level using a correction factor, where

$$\text{Corrected Creatinine (mg/dL)} = \text{Creatinine (mg/dL)} - [\text{Glucose (mg/dL)} \times \text{correction factor}]$$

The correction factor in our laboratory is 0.00053, but this may differ from one lab to another, depending upon the analyzer used. Enzymatic methods of determining creatinine are not altered by glucose concentration and thus do not require the use of a correction factor.

From 103 PETs performed in 86 patients, on peritoneal dialysis from 0.1 to 84 months at the time of the PET, Twardowski et al. (35) categorized patients according to transport rates (based on the relationship of ±1 standard deviation from the mean) as low, low-average, high-average, and high (Figs. 15.5 and 15.6). The PET results have been found to be highly reproducible, varying by less than 3% in repeated studies (12,44). The PET provides a valuable tool for categorizing and monitoring changes in peritoneal membrane transport (solute transport), and while the standard PET is also useful in assessing ultrafiltration (water transport), it is limited by the fact that a maximal osmotic gradient is not created with the use of a 2.5% exchange (45). Nonetheless, information from the PET, in complement with clearance studies, aids in choosing an appropriate dialysis technique and developing a peritoneal dialysis prescription, as well as following peritoneal membrane function (46).

Because of the labor-intensive and time-consuming requirements of the standard PET, a "fast PET" was devised (47) (Table 15.3). The fast PET allows assessment of net ultrafiltration and categorization of solute transport status using only the 4-hour D/P creatinine ratio (Fig. 15.5) and glucose concentration (Table 15.4). The reproducibility of the fast PET results has also been shown to be quite good with coefficients of variation of less than 5% for the D/P creatinine and drain volumes (48). Transport category determinations obtained utilizing the results of the fast PET have been shown to correlate extremely well with those obtained by the standard PET method (49). One can therefore accurately follow patients using the more labor-efficient fast PET. One disadvantage of the fast PET is that intermediate evaluation points at 1-, 2-, or 3-hour dwell times cannot be obtained and may pose a problem when using this test for planning or altering dialysis prescriptions that use shorter dwell times such as continuous cyclic peritoneal dialysis (CCPD) regimens. Thus its primary value is as a tool for evaluating changes in membrane permeability over time.

Factors Influencing the Accuracy of PET

The accuracy and reproducibility of the PET depend on its being performed exactly as outlined in Table 15.2. Any alteration in the method (e.g., dialysate volume) could significantly alter the results. For example, a larger instilled volume of dialysate may delay equilibration and lead to a lower D/P ratio and vice versa. Although using a more hypertonic exchange (4.25%) has been shown to significantly change the D/D_0 glucose and drain volume, the effect on the D/P ratios for creatinine has been insignificant (50).

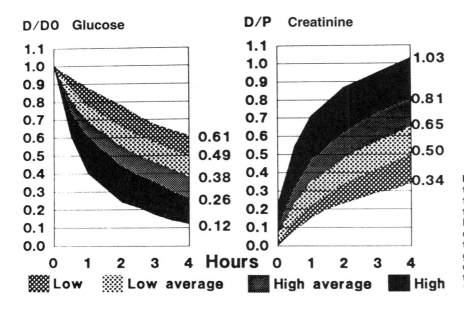

FIG. 15.5. Results of 103 peritoneal equilibration tests (PET) done in 86 patients. Areas shaded in different patterns portray results representing peritoneal transport rates that are high, high-average, low-average, and low. Creatinine concentrations in dialysate and plasma are corrected for glucose (see text). The numbers to the right separate the categories. (Reproduced with permission from Twardowski ZJ. Clinical value of standardized equilibration tests in CAPD patients. *Blood Purif* 1989;7:95–108.)

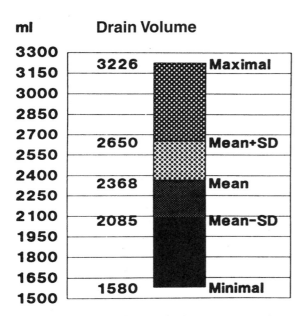

FIG. 15.6. Drain volumes after standardized 4-hour dwell time test exchanges (PET), *n* = 94. Patients with high solute transport rates usually have low drain volumes, and vice versa. (Reproduced with permission from Twardowski Z. Clinical value of standardized equilibration tests in CAPD patients. *Blood Purif* 1989;7:95–108.)

TABLE 15.3. FAST PERITONEAL EQUILIBRATION TEST

1. Steps 1, 2, and 3 of the standard PET are performed by the patient at home.
2. The exact time the infusion ended is noted by the patient.
3. The patient comes to the clinic at 240 minutes dwell time, in the vertical position, the dialysate is drained over 20 minutes.
4. The drained dialysate amount is measured and a sample is obtained.
5. A serum sample is obtained at 240 minutes dwell time.
6. All samples are sent for glucose and creatinine concentrations.

From Twardowski ZJ. The fast peritoneal equilibration test. *Semin Dial* 1990;3:141–142.

TABLE 15.4. DIALYSATE GLUCOSE CONCENTRATIONS AT 4 HOURS USING THE FAST PET

Permeability	Dialysate Glucose Concentration (mg/dL)
High	230–501
High average	502–723
Low average	724–944
Low	945–1,214

From Twardowski ZJ. The fast peritoneal equilibration test. *Semin Dial* 1990;3:141–142.

TABLE 15.5. COMMON ERRORS IN PERFORMING THE PET

1. Incomplete drainage of the overnight exchange
2. Incomplete final drainage of the PET exchange
3. Poor mixing of the dialysate during PET
4. Allowing fresh dialysate to flow into the drain bag
5. Errors in calculation

Table 15.5 outlines common errors in performing the PET. One additional note of caution is the use of the PET in patients with serum glucose concentrations of more than 300 mg/dL, as this can lead to unreliable results (47). Hyperglycemia decreases the dialysate-to-plasma glucose (osmotic) gradient, thereby reducing the transcapillary ultrafiltration rate as well as the rate of diffusion of glucose. This results in drain volumes that are less than expected and D/D_0 glucose concentrations that are higher than expected based on the patient's 4-hour D/P creatinine transport categorization.

Finally, peritoneal surface area is larger relative to body weight in infants and children as compared with adults, and correlates more closely to body surface area. Thus when performing the PET in infants and children, an exchange volume of 1,100 to 1,200 mL/m² BSA is recommended. This allows the use of the same transport categories defined for adults (35,38) to be applied to infants and children (51–53).

Modified Peritoneal Equilibration Test

Although standardized and highly reproducible, the standard PET is best suited to measure small solute clearance and categorize peritoneal membrane function. The use of the standard PET in determining ultrafiltration failure may not be optimal, since the osmotic gradient created by the use of a 2.5% exchange is modest and does not test maximal ultrafiltration, as would be seen using a 4.25% exchange. Thus it has been recommended that a modification of the standard PET be made and that a 4.25% exchange be used rather than a 2.5% exchange. Doing so, the presence of ultrafiltration failure is defined by a net ultrafiltration (drain volume) of less than 2,400 mL at 4 hours, allowing a more accurate diagnosis of ultrafiltration failure (54). The use of a 4.25% exchange does not result in any significant difference in MTAC or D/P creatinine transport group characterization compared with that determined using a 1.5% exchange (50). Thus the "Modified PET" (Table 15.2) is now considered the procedure of choice in the evaluation of ultrafiltration failure (water transport) and can be used to define peritoneal membrane function (solute transport) as well (45,50,54,55).

Alternative Methods of Evaluating Peritoneal Membrane Function

A number of authors have offered alternative approaches to evaluating and monitoring peritoneal transport. These are all variations on the principles of the PET but are felt to offer either greater accuracy or ease than the standard PET. Pannekeet et al. (42) have proposed the standardized peritoneal permeability analysis (SPA), a modification of the PET using 1.5% dextrose to which dextran 70 is added. The SPA results allow the determination of creatinine and urea MTAC, and lymphatic absorption and change in intraperitoneal volume for measurement of fluid kinetics and residual volume. There was a strong correlation between transport and ultrafiltration parameters defined by the PET when compared with those determined by the SPA. However, because of its complexity and the potential risk of anaphylaxis from the dextran, it is unlikely that the SPA will replace the PET in clinical practice.

The Dialysis Adequacy and Transport Test (DATT) described by Rocco et al. (56,57), utilizes the D/P creatinine and urea ratio established by the 24-hour dialysate collection available from clearance studies. The mean D/P creatinine for the 24-hour collection was 0.05 greater than that for the PET, and thus this amount is subtracted from the D/P creatinine determined by the DATT (no adjustment needed for urea). Correlation between the DATT and 4-hour PET results, and reproducibility of the DATT, has been demonstrated by these investigators, based on studies in more than 50 patients. Although simple, the evaluation is not standardized and the information gained for assessing and monitoring peritoneal transport and ultrafiltration is not only limited but potentially unreliable. Any changes in dialysis prescription (e.g., dialysate volume or tonicity, or dwell times) between DATT evaluations could significantly alter the results, making it impossible to compare one study with another. These issues, as well as the fact that the DATT is not recommended for patients on automated peritoneal dialysis, make it an inferior substitute for the PET.

The Peritoneal Permeability and Surface Area index (PSA) has been proposed by Sherman (58) to separate the contributions of diffusive and convective transport to the D/P ratio established by a PET, since the dialysate solute concentration is a result of both diffusive and convective transport. The PSA is based on the premise that the concentration of creatinine in ultrafiltrate (convective transport) is equal to that of plasma (giving a D/P ratio of 1 for the ultrafiltrate). Thus ultrafiltration increases the D/P creatinine through convection. The PSA index represents the D/P ratio achieved from diffusive transport alone and is determined by subtracting that portion of solute transport through convection from the "total" solute transport. The PSA index is calculated as follows:

$$PSA\ index = (D_V \times D_{Cr}/P_{Cr})/2 - (D_V - 2)/2 \quad [7]$$

where D_V is the drain volume at 4 hours in L, "2" is the instilled volume of dialysate in L, D_{Cr} is the dialysate concentration of creatinine (mg/dL) at 4 hours, and P_{Cr} is the plasma concentration of creatinine at 2 hours.

Comparison of the PET-determined D/P creatinine to the PSA index demonstrates the relative contribution of convective transport to solute removal (Table 15.6). Although the PSA

TABLE 15.6. THE PSA INDEX (DIFFUSIVE D/P)

PET D/PCr (4 h)	PET Drain Vol (L)	PSA Index	D/P Convection (% of Total)
0.81	2.1	0.8	1
0.65	2.4	0.58	10
0.5	2.7	0.33	35

appears to provide a simple way to define and follow the diffusive and convective transport properties of an individual, as well as among patients, its accuracy has been questioned (59).

THE COURSE OF PERITONEAL MEMBRANE FUNCTION

Peritoneal membrane characteristics can differ significantly among patients and may change significantly over time in a given patient. Establishing the baseline characteristics of a patient's peritoneal membrane is therefore critical not only in developing a dialysis prescription but in providing an important reference point with which to compare subsequent evaluations if problems arise.

The timing of the initial PET is important, as values for D/P creatinine obtained in the first few weeks on peritoneal dialysis are significantly lower when compared with repeat studies obtained after 4 weeks (60). It is speculated that the irritant effects of the hypertonic dialysate stimulate an initial increase in the local production of vasodilating prostaglandins by the "virgin" peritoneum, resulting in an increase in the peritoneal microcirculation volume and flow, and thus the effective surface area (8,60). It is therefore recommended that the initial PET not be done until after 1 month on dialysis (8,10,60).

Baseline PETs of patients initiating peritoneal dialysis demonstrate the majority to be high-average transporters (Table 15.7) followed by low-average transporters, both of whom can be managed effectively with standard CAPD or CCPD. Of the remaining patients, 17% are high transporters with excellent solute removal, but because of the rapid dissolution of the glucose gradient in these patients, an early ultrafiltration peak leads to reduced net ultrafiltration if placed on standard PD regimens. These patients benefit from PD regimens that take advantage of the early ultrafiltration peaks with shorter dwell times, such as nighttime intermittent peritoneal dialysis (NIPD) or daytime ambulatory peritoneal dialysis (DAPD). Fewer than 5% of patients are low-solute transporters with excellent ultrafiltration because of the ability to maintain the osmotic gradient for prolonged periods, but because of the reduced solute removal properties of the peritoneal membrane, these patients require "high-dose" CAPD/CCPD regimens to prevent uremic symptoms. Patients in the low-transport category are therefore subject to being inadequately dialyzed with PD and may require hemodialysis (38,61,62).

During the first several years on peritoneal dialysis, the transport properties of the peritoneum remain quite stable (63–65). Thereafter a significant increase in solute transport is observed in most patients, and this is often associated with a progressive decline in ultrafiltration capacity (7–10,66). What defines a "significant" change in peritoneal membrane transport varies among studies. Some investigators have defined this by a change in the 4-hour D/P creatinine or D/D$_0$ glucose of 15% to 22%, where most require a change of more than one standard deviation (SD; a change in essentially one transport category) from the patient's initial value (35,67,68).

Blake et al. (68) found a significant (>1 SD) increase in peritoneal transport rate by 18 months in 25% of patients, increasing to 42% by 24 months, with fewer than 10% having a decrease in transport status over the same time period. In a study by Lo et al. (44) of patients with repeat PETs performed when a change from baseline in peritoneal transport was actually suspected, an overall movement from the extremes of transport (high and low) toward the high-average and low-average categories, respectively, was observed (Table 15.8). Overall, 71% of patients had a change from their initial transport category, but in only 27% of patients was the change in D/P creatinine of more than 1 SD (44). The migration toward "high-average" transport was felt, in part, to explain the relatively infrequent dropout of patients from peritoneal dialysis due to poor solute clearance (low transporters) or ultrafiltration failure (high transporters).

The etiology(s) for the progressive increase in peritoneal transport is unclear. Even though patients who develop increased transport rates tend to have a higher incidence of peritonitis than patients with stable or decreased transport rates, no significant relationship has been firmly established (68–70). It has been suggested that it is the degree (PD leukocyte counts) and duration (total days of peritonitis) of inflammation to which the peritoneum has been exposed during episodes of peritonitis that best correlates with an increase in transport (7,10). Additionally, factors related to long-term exposure to dialysate alone, especially hypertonic solutions, may place a patient at risk for increased solute transport (66). Altered peritoneal function may result from the formation of advanced glycosylation endproducts (AGEs) in the peritoneum with prolonged exposure to high glucose concentrations such as those in dialysate. After years on dialysis, the peritoneal vessels are strongly positive for AGEs (71). Advanced glycosylation end-products are known to increase vascular permeability by altering the basement membrane structure and by causing cytokine release by macrophages (71). Thus the accumulation of AGEs in the vascular walls of the peritoneal vessels may contribute to the transport changes noted with increasing duration on peritoneal dialysis.

In addition to AGE-related biochemical changes in existing peritoneal blood vessels that may increase their permeability,

TABLE 15.7. PET CLASSIFICATION IN SOLUTE TRANSPORT

	Rodby et al. (139) (n = 153 pts[a])	Blake et al. (140) (n = 806 pts)
High	17%	10.4%
High average	51%	53.1%
Low average	30%	30.9%
Low	2%	5.6%

[a]Initial PETs done 1 month after initiation of PD.

TABLE 15.8. CHANGE IN SOLUTE TRANSPORT

	Initial PET	Follow-up PET
High	29%	14%
High average	31%	52%
Low average	27%	30%
Low	13%	4%

Fifty-five patients with two PETs or more performed over 22 ± 23 (m ± SD), Lo et al. (44).

an increase in the amount of microvasculature of the peritoneum would have the potential of increasing the effective peritoneal surface area, and thus solute clearance. Diabetic rats have been shown to have a much higher density of small blood vessels in their peritoneum than nondiabetic rats (72). This neovascularization resembles that seen in proliferative diabetic retinopathy. Since all patients receiving peritoneal dialysis (with the exclusion of some of the newer non–glucose-containing dialysis solutions) bathe their peritoneal membranes in a hyperglycemic milieu, the peritoneum of these patients has the potential of developing the neoangiogenesis described in diabetic rats. In accordance with this, biopsies from the Peritoneal Biopsy Registry of patients maintained on peritoneal dialysis for varying periods of time demonstrated a doubling of the density of the microvasculature as time increased on peritoneal dialysis (73). Despite all the above, it is of interest that baseline PET results among diabetics and nondiabetics are similar, and follow-up of more than 4 years has not found diabetics to be more prone to changes in peritoneal function than nondiabetics (10,35,68,74).

DIAGNOSTIC APPROACH, DIFFERENTIAL DIAGNOSIS, AND TREATMENT OF THE PATIENT WITH ULTRAFILTRATION FAILURE

Ultrafiltration failure is suspected clinically when patients cannot maintain an edema-free state or their target weight despite frequent use of hypertonic exchanges and dietary restriction. The observed increase in solute transport with time on dialysis explains, in part, the more frequent occurrence of signs and symptoms of ultrafiltration failure rather than that of inadequate solute removal (Table 15.9) (68–70,75). A change in peritoneal membrane function is, however, but one of a number of possible factors that must be considered in a patient with suspected evidence of ultrafiltration failure (Table 15.1). A diagnostic approach (Fig. 15.7) directed to the patient with possible ultrafiltration failure is therefore particularly germane.

When a patient presents with signs or symptoms of fluid overload, it is important to obtain a good medical history and to perform a thorough physical examination (Fig. 15.7A). Issues such as compliance with diet and dialysis are obviously critical, and a significant reduction in urine output may identify another potential reason for this problem. In addition, the time frame over which the fluid accumulation occurred can be extremely

TABLE 15.9. SIGNS AND SYMPTOMS OF INADEQUATE DIALYSIS

Ultrafiltration Failure
Increasing hypertension or edema
Increasing requirement for hypertonic exchanges
Solute Removal Failure
Increasing creatinine
Increasing or decreasing blood urea nitrogen
Worsening anemia or neuropathy
Anorexia, nausea, vomiting, lethargy, insomnia

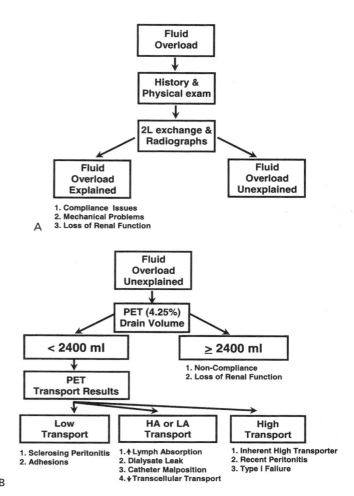

FIG. 15.7. Initial approach **(A)** to patients with fluid overload and **(B)** an algorithm incorporating the Modified (4.25%) PET to further evaluate those patients in whom the cause of fluid overload remains unexplained after the initial assessment.

helpful. Patients with membrane failure as well as those with increased lymphatic absorption usually develop ultrafiltration failure gradually, whereas those with mechanical problems (malpositioned catheter or dialysate leak) have a more acute presentation. When the dialysate flow is described as positional, this suggests a malpositioned catheter. Findings of edema localized to the abdomen or inguinal area can be important clinical clues to the presence of a peritoneal leak.

At the time of the initial office evaluation of a patient with fluid overload, we will often do a quick "fill and drain" with 2 L of dialysate to directly observe the nature and rate of in-flow and out-flow. The presence of fibrin clots may explain abnormalities with flow that reduce the efficiency of drainage and volume removal and can often be resolved with intraperitoneal heparin. If incomplete drainage or positional drainage are observed, a flat-plate radiograph of the abdomen will assess the possibility of a malpositioned catheter (Fig. 15.8). When a peritoneal leak is suspected by clinical examination, computerized tomography of the abdomen will often confirm its presence (Figs. 15.9 and

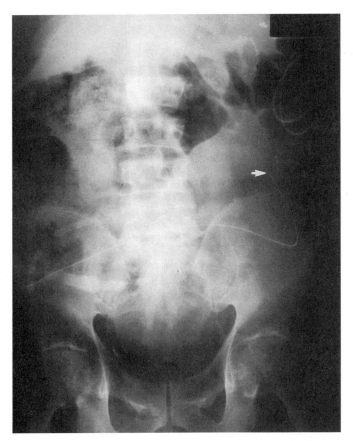

FIG. 15.8. Plain roentgenogram (flat-plate) of the abdomen demonstrating malpositioned catheter. Catheter tip can be seen in left upper abdomen *(arrow)*.

15.10). It is extremely important to communicate to the radiologist the purpose of any radiographic procedure used in assessing problems with peritoneal dialysis, as well as to review the radiograph(s) personally.

When the etiology of fluid overload is not apparent after the initial clinical assessment, the use of the Modified PET is now recommended as the best way to evaluate patients suspected of having ultrafiltration failure (45). The Modified PET allows one to construct a logical approach to the differential diagnosis and treatment of this common problem (Fig. 15.7B).

FLUID OVERLOAD WITHOUT ULTRAFILTRATION FAILURE

When a patient presents with unexplained fluid overload without ultrafiltration failure (drain volume ≥2,400 mL), the possibility of noncompliance with diet or dialysis prescription must be entertained (Fig. 15.7B). In addition, the unrecognized and thus uncompensated loss of residual renal function is a common cause for signs and symptoms of inadequate fluid removal, particularly in high-transport patients.

Patient Compliance

Noncompliance with dialysis prescription and/or diet is a common problem that is difficult to prove, as it is almost totally dependent on the patient's willingness to be honest. Estimates of the rate of noncompliance with the dialysis prescription alone have ranged from 13% to 78% (76–80). Unfortunately, the methods presently used in documenting dialysis noncompliance

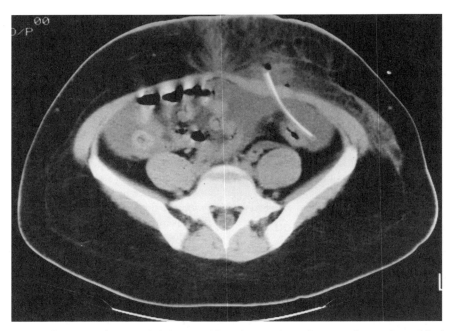

FIG. 15.9. Computed tomography scan of abdomen without intraperitoneal contrast in a patient with ultrafiltration failure and abdominal wall edema. Increased markings, representing fluid, can be seen within the anterior and left lateral subcutaneous tissues adjacent to the Tenckhoff catheter and indicate a dialysate leak.

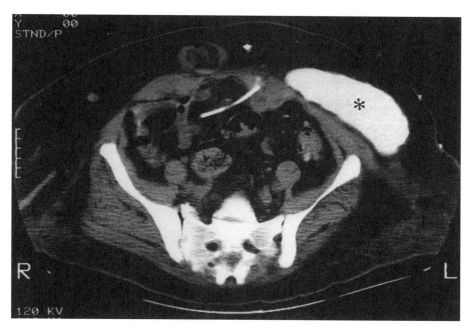

FIG. 15.10. Computed tomography scan of abdomen in patient with ultrafiltration failure and abdominal wall swelling. Radiocontrast material has been injected into dialysate to facilitate tracking. A large collection of contrast material can be seen in the anterior abdominal wall and subcutaneous tissues (*), indicating a dialysate leak.

such as comparing measured to calculated creatinine production are highly inaccurate (78). An estimate of dialysate use can be obtained through the shipping records of the dialysate supply company and thus may allow an objective parameter by which to judge a patient's compliance. Although difficult to resolve, education and positive reinforcement may help improve this problem in a motivated patient.

Residual Renal Function

At the initiation of chronic dialysis, most patients still have residual renal function that can contribute as much as 30% to the overall maintenance of solute and fluid balance (81). Nonetheless, residual renal function (creatinine clearance) continues to decline on dialysis (Table 15.10), albeit faster in patients maintained on hemodialysis (6% per month) than in those maintained on peritoneal dialysis (3% per month) (82,83). This decline in clearance is associated with a significant decrease in urine volume as well (Table 15.10). In our experience, the urine volume decreases by almost 30% at 1 year and

by more than 60% at 2 years. Since peritoneal membrane function changes little over the first several years on dialysis, most changes in peritoneal dialysis prescription during this time result from the progressive decrease in residual renal function. This is particularly true for patients at the extremes of peritoneal transport status. In high transporters, maneuvers to enhance net ultrafiltration (shorter dwells, more hypertonic exchanges, and when available, the use of glucose polymer solutions such as icodextrin) are required to compensate for the declining urine volume, whereas in low transporters, the loss in residual solute clearance must be compensated for by enhancing peritoneal clearances (larger fill volumes to maximize effective peritoneal surface area and thus clearances). To closely monitor for changes in renal function and thus minimize the potential for problems, it is recommended that 24-hour urine volumes and clearances be assessed every 6 months (16).

FLUID OVERLOAD WITH ULTRAFILTRATION FAILURE

A drain volume of less than 2,400 mL following a 4-hour 4.25% exchange defines a patient with ultrafiltration failure. Ultrafiltration failure occurs when the balance between the transcapillary ultrafiltration rate and lymphatic absorption rate has been altered, resulting in a decrease in drain volume (Fig. 15.7B). Clinically, this is identified by the need for more hypertonic exchanges to resolve signs of volume overload. These changes can be the result of (a) an increase in surface area/permeability leading to greater glucose absorption and a more rapid dissolution of the osmolar gradient (type I ultrafiltration failure), (b) a severe decrease in effective peritoneal surface area/permeability

TABLE 15.10. RESIDUAL RENAL FUNCTION[a]

Time	N	Creatinine Clearance (mL/min)		Urine Volume (mL/day)
Baseline	20	5.4	(3.8–7.9)	713 (509–948)
12 months	20	2.8	(2.4–4.9)	512 (420–743)
24 months	20	1.3	(0.9–2.6)	262 (189–527)

[a]Repeated measures in 20 patients on peritoneal dialysis at RUSH Medical Center with more than 1 mL/min residual creatinine clearance at baseline, medians, and 95% confidence intervals (unpublished data).

that significantly restricts the transport of both solute and fluid (type II ultrafiltration failure), (c) an increase in lymphatic absorption (type III ultrafiltration failure), and (d) an increase in residual volume that leads to a more rapid loss of osmotic gradient by dilution (8). Thus a number of factors, in addition to changes in the peritoneal membrane, must be considered in the differential diagnosis (Table 15.11). The PET allows an important assessment of both water and solute transport, which aids in the evaluation of ultrafiltration failure.

Patients with High-Average or Low-Average Solute Transport (D/P Creatinine 0.5 to 0.81)

When ultrafiltration failure is associated with high-average or low-average solute transport, conditions such as an increase in lymphatic absorption, mechanical problems (e.g., a peritoneal leak or malpositioned catheter), and a decrease in transcellular water transport should be considered (Fig. 15.7B).

Increased Lymphatic Flow (Type III Ultrafiltration Failure)

Lymphatic absorption of peritoneal fluid negatively influences the overall removal of water (decreases net ultrafiltration) and solute (partially negating the effect of diffusive and convective solute transport). Since the absorption of peritoneal fluid by lymphatics does not alter the concentration of solutes in the dialysate, the D/P ratio remains unchanged, with increased lymphatic flow even though net ultrafiltration can be significantly decreased. It has been estimated that an increase in the rate of lymphatic absorption may be a contributing factor in up to 60% of patients with permanent loss of ultrafiltration (42).

The rate of lymphatic absorption is estimated by measuring the disappearance of macromolecules, such as albumin or dextran 70 from the peritoneal cavity (molecules too large for transcapillary transfer by either diffusion or convection). Using 2 L of 2.5% dextrose solution, lymphatic absorption rates average 0.95 to 1.0 mL/min when studied with the patient upright (32,42), and 1.5 mL/min in the supine position, possibly due to a relative increase in intraperitoneal pressure in the subdiaphragmatic area, where a large proportion of the lymphatic stomata exist (33).

Intraperitoneal pressure is 10 to 20 cm H_2O 2 hours after a 2-L exchange utilizing a 4.25% dextrose solution but may vary from 5 to 25 cm H_2O. A correlation between intraperitoneal pressure and net ultrafiltration has been reported, with each increase of 1 cm H_2O pressure associated with a decrease in net ultrafiltration of 74 mL over a 2-hour dwell (84). Increased intraabdominal pressure causes a decline in net ultrafiltration primarily by the increase in lymphatic absorption rate (1.9 mL/min versus 1.0 mL/min), but also by a slight decrease in transcapillary ultrafiltration rate (1.73 mL/min versus 2.0 mL/min) (18). This problem may become more of an issue as larger dwell volumes are required for adequate solute clearance.

Measurement of lymphatic flow is uncommon in clinical practice because of the complexity of the procedure. Thus ultrafiltration failure secondary to increased lymphatic absorption becomes a diagnosis of exclusion. Since transcapillary ultrafiltration is normal in this situation, osmotically mediated water transport into the intraperitoneal cavity results in a dilution of the sodium concentration of the dialysate. (Because the sieving coefficient for sodium is 0.5, the sodium concentration in ultrafiltrate is 50% that of serum, leading to an increase in intraperitoneal free water that dilutes the initial dialysate sodium concentration.) A 2 to 4 mEq/L decrease in the dialysate sodium concentration will normally be observed within 2 hours of a 2-L 2.5% dextrose dialysate dwell (the decrease in dialysate sodium being even more pronounced with a 4.25% exchange) and has been used as indirect evidence of normal transcapillary ultrafiltration (Fig. 15.11) (70). In patients with reduced net ultrafiltration secondary to increased lymphatic absorption, the normal decline in sodium concentration is maintained. However, when transcapillary ultrafiltration rate is significantly reduced (e.g., due to a rapid decline in osmotic gradient in a high solute transporter), the initial decrease in sodium is markedly diminished. Profiling the change in sodium concentration as part of the PET requires no additional work and can be useful in defining the process primarily responsible for loss of ultrafiltration.

Patients with increased lymphatic absorption have demonstrated a deficiency in the dialysate content of phosphatidylcholine. Although oral administration of phosphatidylcholine alone (0.2 g qid) was not proven successful in one study (85), the oral administration of lecithin in another study (two 1.2-g capsules tid) improved ultrafiltration in patients with type III ultrafiltration failure (86). Lecithin preparations, available in health food stores are derived from soybeans and contain phos-

TABLE 15.11. FACTORS RESULTING IN ULTRAFILTRATION FAILURE

I. Peritoneal membrane function
  A. Increased effective surface area/permeability
    1. Peritonitis
    2. Type I ultrafiltration failure[a]
  B. Decreased effective surface area/permeability
    1. Type II ultrafiltration failure[b]
      a. Sclerosing peritonitis
      b. Adhesions
    2. Selective impairment in transcellular pore function
II. Lymphatic absorption
  A. Increased
    1. Primary increase (type III ultrafiltration failure[c])
    2. Secondary increase (dialysate leak)
III. Dialysate volume/osmolarity/flow
  A. Increased residual volume (diluting osmotic gradient)
    1. Malpositioned catheter
    2. Loculations from adhesions
IV. Peritoneal blood flow
  A. Decreased
    1. Vascular disease

[a]The term applied to ultrafiltration failure when unexplained changes in membrane properties result in high solute transport. This has also been referred to as type I membrane failure.
[b]The term applied to ultrafiltration failure when changes in membrane properties result in decreased water and (low) solute transport as seen with sclerosing peritonitis or severe abdominal adhesions. This has also been referred to as type II membrane failure.
[c]The term applied to ultrafiltration failure as a result of a primary increase in lymphatic absorption.

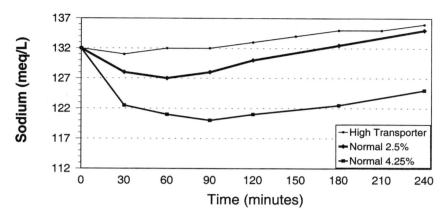

FIG. 15.11. Dialysate sodium concentration over 4 hours using 2-L dialysate volumes in normal patients with 2.5% and 4.25% glucose concentrations, and in high transporters (or patients with impaired transcellular pore transport) with ultrafiltration failure using 2 L of dialysate with 2.5% glucose concentration. The normal drop in sodium concentration is essentially lost in patients with markedly attenuated transcapillary ultrafiltration (high-transport patients or patients with impaired transcellular pore transport). (Adapted from refs. 5, 30, 99.)

phatidylcholine in addition to phosphatidylethanolamine, phosphatidylinositol, phytoglycolipids, other phospholipids, and soybean oil. It is unclear why differing results are obtained with these two preparations, since the daily amount of phosphatidylcholine was similar in both studies (0.8 g/d (85) versus 1.08 g/d (86), but this may relate to the other lipids found in the lecithin preparation. The addition of phosphatidylcholine directly to dialysate has also led to an increase in net ultrafiltration (87). This occurs without a change in solute transport, indicating that the increase in ultrafiltration is secondary to a decrease in lymphatic absorption. This later intraperitoneal approach is not clinically practical.

More recently, the oral administration of bethanechol chloride, 0.27 mg/kg/d up to 50 mg, in four divided doses before each exchange has demonstrated an 18% increase in net ultrafiltration in patients with type III ultrafiltration failure. Bethanechol chloride is similar to phosphatidylcholine in both having cholinergic properties. An increase in cholinergic tone appears to contract the subdiaphragmatic lymphatic stomata, thereby reducing lymph flow (88). Phosphatidylcholine also has a potential effect on the negative ionic charge of lymphatic endothelium. Because these anionic charges repel one another, they may play a role in keeping the subdiaphragmatic lymphatic stomata open. Phosphatidylcholine is cationic and may serve to neutralize these charges. This would result in a relative closure of the stomata and a decrease in lymphatic flow (89).

Experience with larger numbers of patients is necessary to confirm the benefits of these therapies. However, in the meantime, these oral preparations appear to be well tolerated and provide an option in the management of the patient, with ultrafiltration failure presumed to be secondary to high lymphatic absorption. Certainly this therapy, if successful, may obviate the need for an increased exposure to hypertonic dialysate exchanges and their potential long-term deleterious effects.

Dialysate Leak

Dialysate leaks from the intraabdominal cavity to extraabdominal tissues, usually the abdominal wall, result in a decrease in ultrafiltration drain volume. Although the reason drain volume is lowered is obvious, the interstitial leak of fluid is subsequently

removed by the lymphatic system and therefore falls into the category of ultrafiltration failure secondary to increased lymphatic flow. An extraperitoneal dialysate leak is frequently accompanied by an abdominal wall hernia or a history of multiple abdominal surgeries (90). Edema localized to the abdominal wall or a subcutaneous fluid collection is usually evident. Diagnosis may be confirmed by utilizing a radiographic technique that includes intraperitoneal infusion of radiographic contrast through the catheter followed by plain roentgenogram or computed tomography (Tables 15.12 and 15.13; Figs. 15.9 and 15.10) or through the intraperitoneal infusion of a radioisotope evaluated with peritoneal scintigraphy (91–96). Peritoneal membrane function is not compromised in patients with dialysate leaks. Therefore peritoneal transport as evaluated by the PET is not changed compared with a patient's baseline study.

Treatment of peritoneal leaks is aimed at repairing the defect in the peritoneum. Leaks associated with hernias usually require surgical repair of the hernia and a temporary transfer to hemodialysis for several weeks until adequate healing has occurred. Leaks that occur in the absence of a hernia usually represent a tear in the parietal peritoneum. These patients frequently have a history of multiple abdominal surgeries, pregnancies, recent corticosteroid usage, or abdominal straining (coughing, Valsalva maneuver). These leaks may respond to a several-week period of peritoneal rest on hemodialysis without the need for surgical repair. Response to this maneuver is more likely to be successful if the leak is considered small, although many of these will recur and eventually require surgical repair (90).

Catheter Malposition

Mechanical problems, such as a malpositioned catheter (Fig. 15.8), resulted in ultrafiltration failure in 7% of patients in

TABLE 15.12. PERITONEOGRAPHY

1. Take flat-plate radiogram of the abdomen.
2. Place 100 to 200 mL of nonionic contrast in dialysate (2-L bag).
3. Infuse 1 to 2 L of the dialysate into the supine patient.
4. Have the patient change positions for mixing.
5. Repeat flat-plate radiogram of the abdomen.

TABLE 15.13. PERITONEAL COMPUTERIZED TOMOGRAPHY

1. Take plain CT of abdomen.
2. Place 100 to 200 mL of nonionic contrast in dialysate (2-L bag).
3. Infuse 1 or 2 L of the dialysate into the supine patient.
4. Have the patient change positions for mixing.
5. Repeat CT of abdomen.

one center (12). Although this may occur because of improper initial catheter placement, it often results from the migration of catheters originally in good position (97). A malpositioned catheter does not drain the peritoneal cavity effectively and leads to an increase in residual volume. A normal residual volume *(R)* is approximately 200 to 250 mL (35) and can be measured from information obtained during the PET using the following equation:

$$R = V_{in} (S_3 - S_2)/(S_1 - S_3) \qquad [8]$$

where V_{in} = instillation volume, S_1 = solute concentration (urea or creatinine) in the pretest drain, S_2 = solute concentration of the instilled fluid (0 for urea or creatinine), and S_3 = solute concentration immediately following instillation (35). An increase in residual volume dilutes the glucose concentration in the freshly instilled dialysate. This decreases the osmotic gradient and thus reduces the rate of transcapillary ultrafiltration without any significant effect on solute transport. Net ultrafiltration is decreased and the D/P ratio remains essentially unchanged.

An increase in the calculated residual volume should raise the suspicion of a malpositioned catheter. However, the presence of this problem is often clinically apparent and the diagnosis is easily made with the aid of simple radiographic techniques (Fig. 15.8), as peritoneal dialysis catheters have radiopaque material imbedded within. Laparotomy or laparoscopy repositioning of the catheter tip can be done; however, recurrence is common and may require replacing or repositioning the straight Tenckhoff catheter through a new exit site, decreasing the angle (or bend) between the exit site and tunnel. This maneuver tends to force the path of the catheter caudad into the pelvis and may prevent recurrent migration. Success with nonsurgical manipulation of catheter position through the usage of a stiff guide wire and fluoroscopy has been reported (98). However, despite catheter repositioning with various procedures, recurrent malpositioning may occur in up to two-thirds of patients utilizing the straight Tenckhoff catheter. If this occurs the catheter may be replaced with either a column–disc catheter (98) or a swan neck catheter, as malposition recurrence with these catheters appears to be rare.

Decreased Transcellular Water Transport

A group of patients has recently been described with ultrafiltration failure in whom no associated increases in solute transport (for creatinine or glucose), residual volume, or lymphatic absorption rate could be identified (99,100). However, in all these patients, the normal drop in dialysate sodium concentration (Fig. 15.11) was lost (thus no sieving was noted) and felt to represent a loss of transcapillary ultrafiltration. Since the solute

transport properties had not changed (a function of the "small" pores), it was speculated that the loss of transcapillary ultrafiltration was best explained by a selective impairment in water transport by the "ultrasmall" or transcellular pores. The incidence and etiology of this selective defect in peritoneal membrane function is unknown but has been suggested to result from changes in permeability associated with the formation of AGEs within the peritoneal vasculature as the patients developing this problem had been on peritoneal dialysis for an average of 48 months (71,99). The likelihood of continuing peritoneal dialysis once this complication has occurred is poor, as essentially all cases have required transfer to hemodialysis for adequate volume control (99).

Patients with High Solute Transport (D/P Creatinine ≥0.81)

Solute transport typically increases with time on dialysis, and in some patients this results in a significant decrease in net ultrafiltration (Fig. 15.7B). This is attributed to an increase in effective surface area and permeability that increases the rate of glucose absorption, leading to a more rapid decline in osmolar gradient. Of those patients who develop a permanent loss of ultrafiltration capacity, high solute transport or type I ultrafiltration failure is felt to be at least partially if not totally responsible in up to 70% to 80% of cases (5,8,12,42,70,99). Since peritonitis leads to a similar but transient increase in transport, a diagnosis of type I ultrafiltration failure cannot be made in the presence of a recent episode. Finally, patients who are inherently high solute transporters may present with ultrafiltration failure when they lose residual renal function.

Type I Ultrafiltration Failure

The etiology of type I failure is unknown but peritonitis and the frequent use of hypertonic exchanges have been implicated, although it is unclear if the latter is a cause or a consequence of a hyperpermeable membrane (11,101). In most studies however, no significant correlation between these factors and the development of ultrafiltration failure has been found (5,70). Whatever the cause, the risk of type I ultrafiltration failure increases with time on peritoneal dialysis, implying that this alone is a major contributing factor (5,101).

The structural changes seen in these patients are similar to those described earlier in patients with recent peritonitis. Peritoneal biopsies demonstrate mesothelial desquamation, increased gaps between mesothelial cells and hypervascularization (102). The absence of mesothelium allows direct contact of dialysate with the connective tissue, which causes vasodilatation (recruiting more peritoneal capillary flow) and an increase in the effective peritoneal surface area. This increases solute transport for glucose, thus lowering net ultrafiltration. Discontinuing peritoneal dialysis and resting the peritoneum for at least 4 weeks by a temporary transfer to hemodialysis has been associated with significant improvement in ultrafiltration capacity and normalization of solute transport characteristics in more than 81% of patients (101–103). This discontinuation of peritoneal dialysis is felt to allow time for repair and remesothelialization of the damaged peritoneal membrane. A peritoneal biopsy performed in one patient after a period of peritoneal rest with the subsequent clinical recovery of ultrafiltration and transport properties demonstrated complete remesothelialization of the peritoneal membrane (102).

Cancer antigen 125 (CA125) is a high-molecular-weight glycoprotein that is secreted by mesothelial cells. The level in PD fluid is considered a marker of mesothelial cell mass (104). A decrease in CA125 levels in the absence of peritonitis has been seen before the development of type I membrane failure. Serial evaluations of CA125 may therefore provide a means by which to monitor mesothelial mass, allowing for peritoneal resting before the development of type I membrane failure. More research is required, however, to determine the best method for measuring CA125 and to establish normal values (104).

In most patients with type I ultrafiltration failure, especially those previously managed on standard CAPD, a change in the PD prescription to a regimen that takes advantage of shorter dwell times (e.g., NIPD and DAPD) may improve ultrafiltration. Recent experience with the glucose polymer solution icodextrin 7.5% (not yet available in the United States), has proven beneficial in enhancing ultrafiltration in patients with type I membrane failure, enabling them to remain on CAPD (105–107). Some patients cannot be maintained with these measures, fail peritoneal dialysis, and require a transfer to hemodialysis for better volume control. The peritoneal catheter may be left in place and the PET may be repeated after a peritoneal rest period of 1 to 2 months. If solute transfer and ultrafiltration normalize, peritoneal dialysis may be reinitiated. If the patient's peritoneal membrane remains hyperpermeable, the transfer should be considered permanent and the peritoneal dialysis catheter should be removed. An additional concern for patients with type I ultrafiltration failure is the fact that some patients have been reported to progress to type II ultrafiltration failure or sclerosing peritonitis (see later) (6,67).

Recent Peritonitis

During an episode of peritonitis, the PET demonstrates an increase in the D/P creatinine, a proportionate decrease in the D/D_0 glucose, and a significant reduction in net ultrafiltration as compared with baseline (108). As a result, patients frequently become fluid overloaded, requiring a change in their dialysis prescription to improve ultrafiltration: an increase in the hypertonicity or number of hypertonic exchanges, the use of icodextrin, or a regimen that utilizes shorter dwell times (e.g., NIPD and DAPD). Fortunately, these membrane permeability changes are generally transient and patients are usually able to resume their previous PD prescription within a month of the peritonitis episode.

In experimental peritonitis, increased transport rates are associated with denudation of the mesothelial surface, separation of the mesothelial cells, and an increase in mesenteric vascularity, all of which can contribute to an increase in effective peritoneal surface area and permeability (109). Similar structural changes have been seen in peritoneal biopsy specimens of patients with active or recent peritonitis (110–112). Recovery of peritonitis

may not be associated with significant remesothelialization of the peritoneum until 6 weeks or more have elapsed, even though clinical recovery of peritonitis may occur within days (111). Thus the PET should be delayed for at least 4 weeks after an episode of peritonitis, as it may otherwise not be representative of a patient's ultimate transport characteristics.

In some patients, however, remesothelialization fails to occur even long after the patient has clinically recovered from peritonitis (110). In these patients, the increase in transport persists, leading to type I ultrafiltration failure.

Inherent High Transporter

When patients originally defined as high transporters present with volume overload, it may be the result of a loss of residual renal function. When this occurs, a change in the dialysis regimen similar to that for type I membrane failure and strict dietary restriction are required. If there is no change from baseline in the residual renal function, an evaluation for mechanical problems as well as compliance issues must be pursued.

Patients with Low-Solute Transport (D/P Creatinine ≤0.5)

A much less common cause for ultrafiltration failure is that associated with a low-solute transport (Fig. 15.7B), which often stems from conditions leading to a severe reduction in effective peritoneal membrane surface area and permeability (type II ultrafiltration failure) (8,42,99). Thus signs and symptoms of both fluid overload and solute removal failure can be present (Table 15.9). This is observed in patients who have sclerosis of the peritoneal membrane (sclerosing peritonitis) as well as in patients with extensive intraabdominal adhesions.

Sclerosing Encapsulating Peritonitis

Sclerosing encapsulating peritonitis (SEP) is fortunately a rare but dire complication of chronic peritoneal dialysis. It affects less than 2% of patients and, except for a few reports of clusters of cases, it remains a sporadic finding (67,113). However, the prevalence of SEP increases over time and has been reported to exceed 10% for patients maintained on PD for more than 6 years (113). Characteristically, the PET demonstrates a decrease in both solute transport and ultrafiltration. The diagnosis of SEP is suggested clinically by nausea, vomiting, abdominal pain, or signs and symptoms of partial bowel obstruction but may need to be confirmed by surgical exploration and peritoneal biopsy. The radiographic findings of peritoneal thickening, peritoneal calcifications, or thickened bowel wall on computerized tomography (Fig. 15.12) or flat-plate radiograph of the abdomen have been found to be highly consistent with the presence of SEP and serve as a noninvasive method for the diagnosis of this disorder (114–117). Computerized tomography provides a valuable tool in screening patients in whom SEP has progressed to the point where there is radiographic evidence of the fibrosing process. However, early diagnosis, before the development of irreversible fibrosis and encapsulation, becomes critical in the prevention and treatment of SEP. Unfortunately,

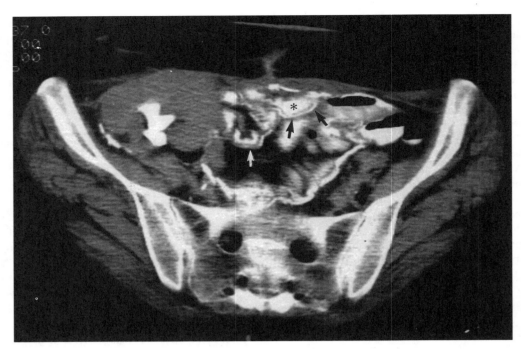

FIG. 15.12. Computed tomography scan of abdomen after oral contrast in a patient with sclerosing peritonitis demonstrating intestinal intraluminal coral contrast (*) and a diffusely thickened and calcified peritoneum *(arrows)*.

there is as yet no reliable noninvasive method by which to screen and thus diagnose patients during the preclinical and potentially "reversible" phase of this condition.

A number of risk factors have been implicated in the pathophysiology of this disorder (67). Because of the frequent association of this condition with bacterial peritonitis, various theories related to the production of pyrogens as a result of the peritoneal infection have been proposed. It is postulated that the pyrogens stimulate peritoneal macrophages to secrete lymphokines, which stimulate fibroblasts and result in proliferation and fibrosis (118–120). A number of other peritoneal irritants have been proposed to initiate this reaction (67) (Table 15.14). Because this condition is rare and often insidious, and therefore difficult to study, its exact etiology remains a mystery and may be multifactorial.

Serial PET testing has provided some added insight into the course and possible pathogenesis of this condition. In many cases of sclerosing peritonitis, the development of a markedly decreased solute transport rate and loss of ultrafiltration is actually preceded by a period of high solute transport (type I ultrafiltration failure). Verger et al. (121) postulate that this early high-permeability state may be related to mesothelial alterations that eventually lead to complete denudation of the peritoneum, with total loss of the mesothelial cells. This may be a reversible stage of this condition if the peritoneal membrane is put to rest. A temporary transfer to hemodialysis at this stage may allow "healing" of the peritoneal membrane and prevent the later progression to sclerosis. As the process continues, however, a reactive sclerosis of the peritoneal membrane may ensue associated with severely impaired irreversible solute. Since mesothelial cell injury and loss precedes the development of fibrosis, some suggest the routine assessment of peritoneal effluent markers of mesothelial cell mass, such as CA125, as a means to more closely monitor the status of the peritoneal membrane (122,123). A sudden and persistent decrease in the level of CA125 in the peritoneal effluent has been associated with the presence of peritoneal sclerosis (123,124). Although encouraging, the actual role of this test in the early diagnosis of sclerosing peritonitis has yet to be established (104).

Recently, a subset of patients diagnosed with sclerosing peritonitis has been described in whom the initial increase in small solute transport actually persists (17). It is speculated that stimulation of macrophages in sclerosing peritonitis leads to production of interleukin-1, which results in increased synthesis of collagen by fibroblasts (decreasing the effective surface area and permeability) and increased release of vasodilating prostaglandins by vascular endothelium. These vasodilating prostaglandins can lead to the development or recruitment of capillaries in poorly vascularized parts of the peritoneum, or in

TABLE 15.14. FACTORS ASSOCIATED WITH THE DEVELOPMENT OF SCLEROSING ENCAPSULATING PERITONITIS

Length of time on peritoneal dialysis (118, 141)[a]
Recurrent peritonitis (118, 141)
Acetate-containing dialysate (142, 143)
Bacterial filters (118, 144)
Chlorhexidine (145–152)
β-blocking agents (153–155)
Endotoxins (118, 119)
Hyperosmolar solutions (156, 157)
Intraperitoneal administration of drugs (17)

[a]See references for further information.

areas where new connective tissue is being formed and in doing so enhances solute transport by increasing the effective peritoneal surface area (17). Thus, depending on which process prevails, either a low- or a high-solute transport may develop. For the overwhelming majority of patients with sclerosing peritonitis, however, the fibrosing process predominates, leading to low-solute transport.

Progressive peritoneal sclerosis, with the formation of intraabdominal adhesions, leads to signs and symptoms of intestinal obstruction and strangulation (67). The transmural extension of the sclerosing process results in encapsulation of bowel, transforming the peritoneum into a "leathery cocoon." In patients with milder or earlier forms of sclerosis, treatment with a period of peritoneal resting may be of benefit. However, once this condition becomes encapsulating, improvement is unlikely to occur with this maneuver. The subsequent gastrointestinal manifestations of obstruction and poor motility lead to malnutrition, requiring aggressive intravenous hyperalimentation. In patients with bowel obstruction, intervention with surgical viscerolysis may be required; however, this is generally associated with a high mortality (>75%), often from sepsis (125,126).

Despite the historically abysmal prognosis of this condition, recent reports of improved survival after renal transplantation provide cause for optimism (127–129). It is unclear, however, if the improved prognosis is related to the discontinuation of peritoneal dialysis, immunosuppression, transplantation, or a combination of these factors. Some patients have improved with immunosuppression alone (130,131), suggesting that it is the inhibitory effects of these agents on lymphokine production, and thus fibroblast activity, that is responsible for the improvement in patients receiving renal transplantation.

Tamoxifen has also been reported to stabilize the process of peritoneal sclerosis (132). This antiestrogen agent acts by inhibiting protein kinase C, a mediator of cell proliferation (133). It has been used to treat retroperitoneal fibrosis, a condition that has some similarities to sclerosing peritonitis (134). Although data on the use of immunosuppression or tamoxifen are limited, the experience with these agents is encouraging and at least provides an option in the treatment of this highly fatal disease.

Abdominal Adhesions

Recurrent or severe peritonitis, catastrophic intraabdominal events, or complicated abdominal surgery may lead to the development of extensive intraabdominal adhesions (135). Adhesions limit dialysate flow throughout the abdominal cavity and decrease the effective surface area of the peritoneum, thereby compromising both solute transport and ultrafiltration. Diagnosis can be made by radiographic techniques that utilize the intraperitoneal infusion of a radiographic contrast material through the dialysis catheter with plain roentgenogram or computed tomography visualization, or with the intraperitoneal infusion of a radioisotope and peritoneal scintigraphy (91–96). If adhesions are present, peritoneal fluid will not distribute equally throughout the abdominal cavity despite changes in patient position or posture (Fig. 15.13). Surgical lysis of adhesions may result in an improvement of dialysate flow and distribution, but if adhesions are extensive, this procedure may not

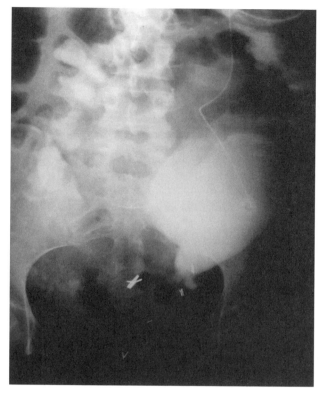

FIG. 15.13. Plain roentgenogram (flat-plate) of the abdomen in a patient with ultrafiltration failure. Before the radiographic examination, 2 L of dialysate containing 100 mL of nonionic radiocontrast were infused into the abdomen. Adhesions in the left lower quadrant of the abdomen result in a loculation of dialysate. This limits flow throughout the abdominal cavity and causes a decrease in the effective peritoneal surface area.

increase the peritoneal membrane surface area enough to allow adequate solute transport for peritoneal dialysis.

Compromised Peritoneal Blood Flow

Although a severe reduction in effective peritoneal blood flow or vascular permeability could theoretically compromise both fluid and solute removal, this must be an extremely rare cause for ultrafiltration failure, as we have seen no reports to date. A significant decrease in the peritoneal clearance of urea and creatinine has been observed in a few patients with systemic vascular disease (e.g., systemic lupus erythematosus, vasculitis, scleroderma, or malignant hypertension), but this was not associated with ultrafiltration failure (136–138).

CONCLUSION

As patients are successfully maintained on peritoneal dialysis for longer periods of time the potential for ultrafiltration failure increases. As a result, assessment of peritoneal membrane function (PET) and residual renal function should be done on an annual basis or more frequently if clinically indicated. Ultrafiltration failure is usually attributed to changes in the function of the peritoneal membrane that occur with increasing frequency as time on dialysis is prolonged. However, one must recognize that a number of other factors, including loss of residual renal function, can significantly impact on the efficiency of this therapy and must be considered when faced with a volume-overloaded (or inadequately dialyzed) patient. Although the initial office evaluation may identify the cause of this problem in many cases, the Modified PET (using a 4.25% exchange with ultrafiltration failure defined by a 4-hour drain volume of less than 2,400 mL) becomes an essential tool to further assist in the work-up of those patients in whom the etiology of volume overload remains unexplained. With the valuable information provided by the PET and the diagnostic algorithm we provide, a logical approach to the assessment of patients with ultrafiltration failure can be developed. Once the appropriate diagnosis is defined, a therapeutic approach can be devised.

REFERENCES

1. Termination of continuous peritoneal dialysis. In: Lindblad A, et al., eds. *Continuous ambulatory peritoneal dialysis in the USA: final report of the National CAPD Registry 1981–1988.* Boston: Kluwer Academic, 1989:43–60.
2. Nissenson A, et al. Morbidity and mortality of continuous ambulatory peritoneal dialysis: regional experience and long-term prospects. *Am J Kidney Dis* 1986;7:229–234.
3. Pollock C, et al. Continuous ambulatory peritoneal dialysis: eight years' experience in a single center. *Medicine* 1989;68:293–308.
4. Gokal R, et al. Outcome in patients on continuous ambulatory peritoneal dialysis and haemodialysis: 4-year analysis of a prospective multicenter study. *Lancet* 1987;2:1105–1109.
5. Heimburger O, et al. Peritoneal transport in CAPD patients with permanent loss of ultrafiltration capacity. *Kidney Int* 1990;38:495–506.
6. Huarte-Loza E, et al. Peritoneal membrane failure as a determinant of the CAPD future. *Contrib Nephrol* 1987;57:219–229.
7. Davies SJ, et al. Longitudinal changes in peritoneal kinetics: the effects of peritoneal dialysis and peritonitis. *Nephrol Dial Transplant* 1996;11:498–506.
8. Struijk DG, et al. A prospective study of peritoneal transport in CAPD patients. *Kidney Int* 1994;45:1739–1744.
9. Struijk DG, et al. Functional characteristics of the peritoneal dialysis membrane in long-term continuous ambulatory peritoneal dialysis. *Nephron* 1991;59:213–220.
10. Selgas R, et al. Functional longevity of the human peritoneum: how long is continuous peritoneal dialysis possible? Result of a prospective medium long-term study. *Am J Kidney Dis* 1994;23:64–73.
11. Ota K, et al. Functional deterioration of the peritoneum: does it occur in the absence of peritonitis? *Nephrol Dial Transplant* 1987;2:30–33.
12. Davies SJ, et al. Clinical evaluation of the peritoneal equilibration test: a population-based study. *Nephrol Dial Transplant* 1993;8:64–70.
13. Nolph K, et al. Determinants of low clearances of small solutes during peritoneal dialysis. *Kidney Int* 1978;13:117–123.
14. Flessner M. Peritoneal transport physiology: insights from basic research. *J Am Soc Nephrol* 1991;2:122–135.
15. Wegner G. Chirurgische bemerkingen uber die peritoneal hole, mit besonderer berucksichti der ovariotomie. *Arch Klin Chir* 1877;20:51–59.
16. Nolph KD. Clinical implications of membrane transport characteristics on the adequacy of fluid and solute removal. *Perit Dial Int* 1994;14(Suppl 3):S78–S82.
17. Krediet RT, et al. The time course of peritoneal transport kinetics in continuous ambulatory peritoneal dialysis patients who develop sclerosing peritonitis. *Am J Kidney Dis* 1989;13:299–307.
18. Imholz AL, et al. Effect of an increased intraperitoneal pressure on fluid and solute transport during CAPD. *Kidney Int* 1993;44:1078–1085.
19. Flessner MF, et al. Role of the liver in small-solute transport during peritoneal dialysis. *J Am Soc Nephrol* 1994;5:116–120.
20. Rippe B, et al. Simulations of peritoneal solute transport during CAPD: application of two-pore formalism. *Kidney Int* 1989;35:1234–1244.
21. Stelin G, et al. A phenomenological interpretation of the variation in dialysate volume with dwell time in CAPD. *Kidney Int* 1990;38:465–472.
22. Keshaviah P, et al. Relationship between body size, fill volume, and mass transfer are coefficient in peritoneal dialysis. *J Am Soc Nephrol* 1994;4:1820–1826.
23. Nolph K, et al. Equilibration of peritoneal dialysis solutions during long dwell exchanges. *J Lab Clin Med* 1979;93:246–256.
24. Robson M, et al. Influence of exchange volume and dialysate flow rate on solute clearance in peritoneal dialysis. *Kidney Int* 1978;14:486–490.
25. Ronco C, et al. Pathology of ultrafiltration in peritoneal dialysis. *Periton Dial Int* 1990;10:119–126.
26. Grzegorzewska A, et al. Ultrafiltration and effective peritoneal blood flow during peritoneal dialysis in the rat. *Kidney Int* 1991;39:608–617.
27. Mactier R, et al. Influence of dwell time, osmolality, and volume of exchanges on solute mass transfer and ultrafiltration in peritoneal dialysis. *Semin Dial* 1988;1:40–49.
28. Imholz AL, et al. Residual volume measurements with exogenous and endogenous solutes during CAPD. *Adv Perit Dial* 1992;8:33–38.
29. Pyle W. Mass transfer in peritoneal dialysis (PhD dissertation). University of Texas, 1981.
30. Heimburger O, et al. A quantitative description of solute and fluid transport during peritoneal dialysis. *Kidney Int* 1992;41:1320–1332.
31. Leypoldt JK. Evaluation of peritoneal membrane permeability, *Adv Ren Replace Ther* 1995;2:265–273.
32. Abensur H, et al. Use of dextran 70 to estimate peritoneal lymphatic absorption rate in CAPD. *Adv Perit Dial* 1992;8:3–6.
33. Mactier RA, et al. Contribution of lymphatic absorption to loss of ultrafiltration and solute clearances in continuous ambulatory peritoneal dialysis. *J Clin Invest* 1987;80:1311–1316.
34. Nolph KD, et al. The kinetics of ultrafiltration during peritoneal dialysis: the role of lymphatics. *Kidney Int* 1987;32:219–226.
35. Twardowski ZJ, et al. Peritoneal equilibration test. *Perit Dial Bull* 1987;7:138–147.
36. Garred L, et al. A simple kinetic model for assessing peritoneal mass transfer in continuous ambulatory peritoneal dialysis. *ASAIO J* 1983;6:131–137.
37. Hiatt M, et al. A comparison of the relative efficiency of CAPD and hemodialysis in the control of solute concentration. *Artif Organs* 1980;4:37–43.
38. Twardowski ZJ. Clinical value of standardized equilibration tests in CAPD patients. *Blood Purif* 1989;7:95–108.
39. Hallett M, et al. Adequacy of peritoneal dialysis. *Semin Dial* 1990;3:230–236.
40. Vonesh E, et al. Kinetic modeling as a prescription aid in peritoneal dialysis. *Blood Purif* 1991;9:246–270.
41. Tiexido J, et al. Peritoneal function tests: usefulness of simplified methods. *Adv Perit Dial* 1992;8:177–180.
42. Pannekeet MM, et al. The standard peritoneal permeability analysis: a tool for the assessment of peritoneal permeability characteristics in CAPD patients. *Kidney Int* 1995;48:866–875.
43. Heimburger O, et al. Dialysate to plasma solute concentration (D/P) versus transport parameters in CAPD. *Nephrol Dial Transplant* 1994;9:47–59.
44. Lo WK, et al. Changes in the peritoneal equilibration test in selected chronic peritoneal dialysis patients. *J Am Soc Nephrol* 1994;4:1466–1474.
45. Mujais S, et al. Evaluation and management of ultrafiltration problems in peritoneal dialysis. International Society for Peritoneal Dialysis Ad Hoc Committee on Ultrafiltration Management in Peritoneal Dialysis. *Perit Dial Int* 2000;20(Suppl 4):S5–S21.
46. Twardowski ZJ, et al. Limitations of the peritoneal equilibration test. *Nephrol Dial Transplant* 1995;10:2160–2161.

47. Twardowski ZJ. The fast peritoneal equilibration test. *Semin Dial* 1990;3:141–142.

48. Enia G, et al. The reproducibility of the fast peritoneal equilibration test. *Perit Dial Int* 1995;15:382–384.

49. Adcock A, et al. Clinical experience and comparative analysis of the standard and fast peritoneal equilibration test (PET). *Adv Perit Dial* 1992;8:59–61.

50. Smit W, et al. A comparison between 1.36% and 3.86% glucose dialysis solution for the assessment of peritoneal membrane function. *Perit Dial Int* 2000;20:734–741.

51. Warady BA, et al. Peritoneal membrane transport function in children receiving long-term dialysis. *J Am Soc Nephrol* 1996;7:2385–2391.

52. Kohaut EC, et al. The effect of changes in dialysate volume on glucose and urea equilibration. *Perit Dial Int* 1994;14:236–239.

53. Bouts AH, et al. Standard peritoneal permeability analysis in children. *J Am Soc Nephrol* 2000;11:943–950.

54. Ho-dac-Pannekeet MM, et al. Analysis of ultrafiltration failure in peritoneal dialysis patients by means of standard peritoneal permeability analysis. *Perit Dial Int* 1997;17:144–150.

55. Rippe B. How to measure ultrafiltration failure: 2.27% or 3.86% glucose? *Perit Dial Int* 1997;17:125–128.

56. Rocco MV, et al. Determination of peritoneal transport characteristics with 24-hour dialysate collections: dialysis adequacy and transport test. *J Am Soc Nephrol* 1994;5:1333–1338.

57. Rocco MV, et al. 24-hour dialysate collection for determination of peritoneal membrane transport characteristics: longitudinal follow-up data for the dialysis adequacy and transport test (DATT). *Perit Dial Int* 1996;16:590–593.

58. Sherman RA. The peritoneal permeability and surface area index. *Perit Dial Int* 1994;14:240–242.

59. Emerson PF, et al. The PSA index does not correct for ultrafiltration. *Perit Dial Int* 1995;15:185–186.

60. Rocco MV, et al. Changes in peritoneal transport during the first month of peritoneal dialysis. *Perit Dial Int* 1995;15:12–17.

61. Twardowski ZJ. Peritoneal dialysis glossary III. *Perit Dial Int* 1990;10:173–175.

62. Twardowski ZJ, et al. *Advances in continuous peritoneal dialysis.* Toronto: University of Toronto Press, 1987:171–178.

63. Kush R, et al. Long-term continuous ambulatory peritoneal dialysis: mass transfer and nutritional and metabolic stability. *Blood Purif* 1990;8:1–13.

64. Park M, et al. Peritoneal solute clearances after four years of continuous ambulatory peritoneal dialysis (CAPD). *Perit Dial Int* 1989;9:75–78.

65. Selgas R, et al. Peritoneal functional parameters after five years on CAPD: the effect of late peritonitis. *Perit Dial Int* 1989;9:329–332.

66. Davies SJ, et al. Peritoneal glucose exposure and changes in membrane solute transport with time on peritoneal dialysis. *J Am Soc Nephrol* 2001;12:1046–1051.

67. Diaz-Buxo J. Peritoneal sclerosis in a woman on continuous cyclic peritoneal dialysis. *Semin Dial* 1992;5:317–320.

68. Blake PG, et al. Changes in peritoneal membrane transport rates in patients on long-term CAPD. *Adv Perit Dial* 1989;5:3–7.

69. Passlick-Deetjen J, et al. Changes of peritoneal membrane function during long-term CAPD. *Adv Perit Dial* 1990;6:35–43.

70. Pollack C, et al. Loss of ultrafiltration in continuous ambulatory peritoneal dialysis (CAPD). *Perit Dial Int* 1989;9:107–110.

71. Nakayama M, et al. Immunohistochemical detection of advanced glycosylation end-products in the peritoneum and its possible pathophysiological role in CAPD. *Kidney Int* 1997;51:182–186.

72. De Vriese AS, et al. Diabetes-induced microvascular proliferation and hyperpermeability in the peritoneum: role of vascular endothelial growth factor. *J Am Soc Nephrol* 2001;12:1734–1741.

73. Williams JD, et al. Submesothelial fibrosis in the peritoneal membrane of patients on peritoneal dialysis correlates with the presence of vasculopathy. *J Am Soc Nephrol* 2000;11:314a(abst).

74. Coronel F, et al. Peritoneal clearances, protein losses and ultrafiltration in diabetic patients after four years on CAPD. *Adv Perit Dial* 1991;7:35–38.

75. Hallett M, et al. Is the peritoneal membrane durable indefinitely? *Adv Perit Dial* 1990;6:197–201.

76. Warren PJ, et al. Compliance with the peritoneal dialysis prescription is poor. *J Am Soc Nephrol* 1994;4:1627–1629.

77. Caruana R, et al. Dialysate dumping: a novel cause of inadequate dialysis in continuous ambulatory peritoneal dialysis (CAPD) patients. *Perit Dial Int* 1989;9:319–320.

78. Brandes JC. Do we have an objective method to determine compliance with the peritoneal dialysis prescription? *Perit Dial Int* 1996;16:114–115.

79. Tzamaloukas AH, et al. Symptomatic fluid retention in patients on continuous peritoneal dialysis. *J Am Soc Nephrol* 1995;6:198–206.

80. Blake PG, et al. A multicenter study of noncompliance with continuous ambulatory peritoneal dialysis exchanges in U.S. and Canadian patients. *Am J Kidney Dis* 2000;35:506–514.

81. Canada–USA (CANUSA) Peritoneal Dialysis Study Group. Adequacy of dialysis and nutrition in continuous peritoneal dialysis: associations with clinical outcomes. *J Am Soc Nephrol* 1996;7:198–207.

82. Lysaght M, et al. The influences of dialysis treatment modality on the decline of residual renal function. *ASAIO Trans* 1991;37:598–604.

83. Rottembourg J. Residual renal function and recovery of renal function in patients treated by CAPD. *Kidney Int* 1993;43(Suppl 40):106–110.

84. Durand P, et al. Intraperitoneal pressure, peritoneal permeability and ultrafiltration in CAPD. *Adv Perit Dial* 1992;8:22–25.

85. De Vecchi A, et al. Phosphatidylcholine administration in continuous ambulatory peritoneal dialysis (CAPD) with reduced ultrafiltration. *Perit Dial Int* 1989;9:207–210.

86. Chan H, et al. Oral lecithin improves ultrafiltration in patients on peritoneal dialysis. *Perit Dial Int* 1989;9:203–205.

87. Krack G, et al. Intraperitoneal administration of phosphatidylcholine improves ultrafiltration in continuous ambulatory peritoneal dialysis patients. *Perit Dial Int* 1992;12:359–364.

88. Baranowska-Daca E, et al. Use of bethanechol chloride to increase available ultrafiltration in CAPD. *Adv Perit Dial* 1995;11:69–72.

89. Khanna R, et al. Pharmacologic alterations of ultrafiltration. *Contrib Nephrol* 1990;85:150–158.

90. Tzamaloukas AH, et al. Early and late peritoneal leaks in patients on CAPD. *Adv Perit Dial* 1990;6:64–71.

91. Korzets Z, et al. Tear of the intraperitoneal segment of the Tenckoff catheter as an unusual cause of catheter malfunction. *Perit Dial Bull* 1986;6:107–108.

92. Twardowski ZJ, et al. Computerized tomography CT in the diagnosis of subcutaneous leak sites during continuous ambulatory peritoneal dialysis (CAPD). *Perit Dial Bull* 1984;4:163–166.

93. Schultz S, et al. Computerized tomographic scanning with intraperitoneal contrast enhancement in a CAPD patient with localized edema. *Perit Dial Bull* 1984;4:253–254.

94. Lupo A, et al. Abdominal hernias in CAPD patients: Incidence, risk factors and outcome. *Adv Perit Dial* 1988;4:107–109.

95. Wankowicz Z, et al. Colloid peritoneoscintigraphy in complications of CAPD. *Adv Perit Dial* 1988;4:138–143.

96. Kopecky R, et al. Prospective peritoneal scintigraphy in patients beginning continuous ambulatory peritoneal dialysis. *Am J Kidney Dis* 1990;15:228–236.

97. Schleifer C, et al. Migration of peritoneal catheters: personal experience and survey of 72 other units. *Perit Dial Bull* 1987;7:189–193.

98. Moss J, et al. Malpositioned peritoneal dialysis catheters: a critical reappraisal of correction by stiff-wire manipulation. *Am J Kidney Dis* 1990;15:305–308.

99. Monquil MCJ, et al. Does impaired transcellular water transport contribute to net ultrafiltration failure during CAPD? *Perit Dial Int* 1995;15:42–48.

100. Dobbie JW, et al. A 39-year-old man with loss of ultrafiltration. *Perit Dial Int* 1994;14:384–394.

101. Miranda B, et al. Peritoneal resting and heparinization as an effective treatment for ultrafiltration failure in patients on CAPD. *Contrib Nephrol* 1991;89:199–204.

102. Verger C, et al. *Frontiers in peritoneal dialysis.* New York: Field, Rich and Associates, 1986:88–93.

103. De Alvaro F, et al. Peritoneal resting is beneficial in peritoneal hypermeability and ultrafiltration failure. *Adv Perit Dial* 1993;9:56–61.

104. Krediet RT. Dialysate cancer antigen 125 concentration as marker of peritoneal membrane status in patients treated with chronic peritoneal dialysis. *Perit Dial Int* 2001;21:560–567.
105. Peers E, et al. Icodextrin: overview of clinical experience. *Perit Dial Int* 1997;17:22–26.
106. Krediet RT, et al. Augmenting solute clearance in peritoneal dialysis. *Kidney Int* 1998;54:2218–2225.
107. Krediet RT, et al. Pathophysiology of peritoneal membrane failure. *Perit Dial Int* 2000;20(Suppl 4):S22–S42.
108. Panasiuk E, et al. Characteristics of peritoneum after peritonitis in CAPD patients. *Adv Perit Dial* 1988;4:42–45.
109. Verger C, et al. Acute changes in peritoneal morphology and transport properties with infectious peritonitis and mechanical injury. *Kidney Int* 1983;23:823–831.
110. Dobbie J, et al. Categorization of ultrastructural changes in peritoneal mesothelium, stroma and blood vessels in uremia and CAPD patients. *Adv Perit Dial* 1990;8:3–12.
111. Dobbie J. Morphology of the peritoneum in CAPD. *Blood Purif* 1989;7:74–85.
112. Henderson I, et al. Structure of the peritoneum and changes brought about by infection. *Contrib Nephrol* 1987;57:30–40.
113. Kawaguchi Y, et al. Encapsulating peritoneal sclerosis: definition, etiology, diagnosis, and therapy. *Perit Dial Int* 2000;20(Suppl 4):S43–S55.
114. Krestin GP, et al. Imaging diagnosis of sclerosing peritonitis and relation of radiologic signs to the extent of the disease. *Abdom Imaging* 1995;20:414–420.
115. Campbell S, et al. Sclerosing peritonitis: identification of diagnostic, clinical, and radiological features. *Am J Kidney Dis* 1994;24:819–825.
116. Cox SV, et al. Sclerosing peritonitis with gross peritoneal calcification: a case report. *Am J Kidney Dis* 1992;20:637–642.
117. Korzets A, et al. Sclerosing peritonitis: possible early diagnosis by computerized tomography of the abdomen. *Am J Nephrol* 1988;8:143–146.
118. Shaldon S, et al. Pathogenesis of sclerosing peritonitis in CAPD. *ASAIO Trans* 1984;30:193–194.
119. Shaldon S. The interleukin hypothesis: a reappraisal after 6 years. *Semin Dial* 1989;2:172–175.
120. Dobbie JW. Pathogenesis of peritoneal fibrosing syndromes (sclerosing peritonitis) in peritoneal dialysis. *Perit Dial Int* 1992;12:14–27.
121. Verger C, et al. Peritoneal permeability and encapsulating peritonitis. *Lancet* 1985;1:986–987.
122. Ho-dac-Pannekeet MM, et al. Longitudinal follow-up of CA125 in peritoneal effluent. *Kidney Int* 1997;51:888–893.
123. Ho-dac-Pannekeet MM, et al. Inflammatory changes in vivo during CAPD: what can the effluent tell us? *Kidney Int* 1996;50(Suppl 56):S12–S16.
124. Krediet RT, et al. Markers of peritoneal tissue in stable CAPD patients and patients with sclerosing peritonitis. *Perit Dial Int* 1995;15(Suppl 2):S43(abst).
125. Pusateri R, et al. Sclerosing encapsulating peritonitis: report of a case with small bowel obstruction managed by long-term home parenteral hyperalimentation, and a review of the literature. *Am J Kidney Dis* 1986;8:56–60.
126. Carbonnel F, et al. Sclerosing peritonitis: a series of 10 cases and review of the literature. *Gastroenterol Clin Biol* 1995;19:876–882.
127. Bhandari S. Recovery of gastrointestinal function after renal transplantation in patients with sclerosing peritonitis secondary to continuous ambulatory peritoneal dialysis. *Am J Kidney Dis* 1996;27:604.
128. Hawley CM, et al. Recovery of gastrointestinal function after renal transplantation in a patient with sclerosing peritonitis secondary to continuous ambulatory peritoneal dialysis. *Am J Kidney Dis* 1995;26:658–661.
129. Bowers VD, et al. Sclerosing peritonitis. *Clin Transplant* 1994;8:369–372.
130. Junor BJ, et al. Immunosuppression in sclerosing peritonitis. *Adv Perit Dial* 1993;9:187–189.
131. Mori Y, et al. A case of a dialysis patient with sclerosing peritonitis successfully treated with corticosteroid therapy alone. *Am J Kidney Dis* 1997;30:275–278.
132. Turner M, et al. Successful therapy of sclerosing peritonitis. *Semin Dial* 1992;5:316.
133. Horgan K, et al. Inhibition of protein kinase C mediated signal transduction by tamoxifen: importance for antitumor activity. *Biochem Pharmacol* 1986;35:4463–4465.
134. Clark C, et al. The response of retroperitoneal fibrosis to tamoxifen. *Surgery* 1991;109:502–506.
135. Twardowski ZJ. *Contemporary issues in nephrology.* Vol 22, *Peritoneal dialysis.* New York: Churchill Livingstone, 1990:67–100.
136. Nolph K, et al. Altered peritoneal permeability in patients with systemic vasculitis. *Ann Intern Med* 1971;75:753–755.
137. Brown S, et al. Reduced peritoneal clearances in scleroderma increased by intraperitoneal isoproterenol. *Ann Intern Med* 1973;78:891–894.
138. Copley J, et al. Continuous ambulatory peritoneal dialysis and scleroderma. *Nephron* 1985;40:353–356.
139. Rodby RA, et al. Re-evaluation of solute transport groups using the peritoneal equilibration test. *Perit Dial Int* 1999;19:438–441.
140. Blake P, et al. Recommended clinical practices for maximizing peritoneal dialysis clearances. *Perit Dial Int* 1996;16:448–456.
141. Novello A, et al. Sclerosing encapsulating peritonitis. *Int J Artif Organs* 1986;9:393–396.
142. Slingeneyer A, et al. Progressive sclerosing peritonitis: a late and severe complication of maintenance peritoneal dialysis. *ASAIO Trans* 1983;29:633–640.
143. Rottembourg J, et al. Severe abdominal complication in patients undergoing continuous ambulatory peritoneal dialysis. *Proc Eur Dial Trans Assoc* 1983;20:236–242.
144. Mion C, et al. Reduction in incidence of peritonitis associated with CAPD. *Proc Clin Dial Trans Forum* 1979;9:63.
145. Buckle R, et al. The effect of chlorhexidine in peritoneal cavity. *Lancet* 1963;1:193.
146. Fabgri L, et al. Peritonitis in CAPD: treatment with chlorhexidine. *Dial Transplant* 1982;11:483.
147. Junor B, et al. Sclerosing peritonitis: the contribution of chlorhexidine in alcohol. *Perit Dial Bull* 1985;5:101–104.
148. Sobel J, et al. Nosocomial *Pseudomonas cepacia* infection associated with chlorhexidine contamination. *Am J Med* 1982;73:183–186.
149. Sommerville P, et al. Chlorhexidine is unsuitable for long-term use in patients on CAPD. *Perit Dial Bull* 1982;2:195.
150. Suessmuth R, et al. Mutagenic effect of 1,1'-hexamethylene-bis [5 p-chlorophenyl-biguanide]. *Chem Biol Interact* 1979;28:249.
151. Lo WK, et al. Sclerosing peritonitis complicating prolonged use of chlorhexidine in alcohol in the connection procedure for continuous ambulatory peritoneal dialysis. *Perit Dial Int* 1991;11:166–172.
152. Lo WK, et al. Sclerosing peritonitis complicating continuous ambulatory peritoneal dialysis with the use of chlorhexidine in alcohol. *Adv Perit Dial* 1990;6:79–84.
153. Greffberg N, et al. Sclerosing obstructive peritonitis, beta-blockers and continuous ambulatory peritoneal dialysis. *Lancet* 1983;2:733–734.
154. Ahmad S. Sclerosing peritonitis and propranolol. *Chest* 1981;79:361–362.
155. Bradley J, et al. Sclerosing obstructive peritonitis after continuous ambulatory peritoneal dialysis. *Lancet* 1983;2:113–114.
156. Fracasso A, et al. Peritoneal sclerosis: role of plasticizers. *ASAIO Trans* 1987;33:676–682.
157. Mion C, et al. Analysis of factors responsible for formation of adhesion during chronic peritoneal dialysis. *Am J Med Sci* 1965;250:675–679.

HYPERTENSION IN DIALYSIS PATIENTS

VITO M. CAMPESE AND ADINA TANASESCU

The association between hypertension and chronic renal disease has been recognized since the pioneering work of Richard Bright at Guy's Hospital in 1836. Renal disease is by far the commonest cause of secondary hypertension, and hypertension is an important presenting feature of renal disease and doubtless contributes to its progression (1). Hypertension occurs in approximately 80% of patients with end-stage renal disease (ESRD). The data collected by regional ESRD networks and summary statistics published annually by the Health Care Financing Administration (HCFA) and the National Forum of ESRD Networks indicate that hypertensive ESRD accounts for a progressively larger number of new Medicare program enrollees, whereas glomerulonephritis-induced ESRD is on the decline.

Cardiovascular disease (CVD) is the leading cause of death in patients receiving maintenance hemodialysis (HD), especially in the first year of treatment. A history of long-lasting arterial hypertension is associated with an increase in cardiovascular (CV) deaths in these patients (2). Controlled studies are not available on the beneficial effect of antihypertensive therapy on patients in HD. However, maintaining a controlled blood pressure (BP) is unanimously agreed to be of great importance for long-term survival (3,4). Hypertension is the single most important predictor of coronary artery disease in uremic patients, even more so than cigarette smoking and hypertriglyceridemia (5).

DETECTION

BP should be measured as recommended by the Seventh Report of the Joint National Committee on Prevention, Detection, Evaluation, and Treatment of High Blood Pressure (JNC VI). Patients should be seated in a chair with their backs supported and their arms bared and supported at heart level. Measurements should begin after at least 5 minutes of rest. Two or more readings separated by 2 minutes should be averaged. If the first two readings differ by more than 5 mm Hg, additional readings should be performed and averaged. In all dialysis patients, BP should also be measured after standing 2 minutes. BP measurements should be performed both before and after each dialysis or at every office visit.

The ankle-to-arm blood pressure index (AABI) has been recently found to be a strong predictor of CV and overall mortality (6). In a study of 142 patients on HD, Fishbane et al. (7) observed that patients with coronary artery disease, cerebrovascular disease, and peripheral vascular disease had significantly lower AABI index than patients without CVD. Thus, this simple index has been proposed as a powerful marker for the presence and intensity of systemic atherosclerotic vascular disease.

IMPORTANCE OF SYSTOLIC, DIASTOLIC, AND PULSE BLOOD PRESSURE

In the general population, the relationship between both systolic blood pressure (SBP) and diastolic blood pressure (DBP) and CV events appears to be linear. By contrast, in ESRD patients this relationship seems to be U-shaped. Low predialysis SBP (<110 mm Hg) is associated with decreased survival. Likewise, systolic BP greater that 180 mm Hg is associated with poor outcome (8–10). In a study of 649 HD patients, Salem and Bower (11) observed that hypertension was associated with improved 1-year survival. However, the effect of hypertension was mostly caused by the associated antihypertensive treatment, because untreated hypertensive patients have survival rates equal to normotensive patients.

Currently, there is increasing evidence that pulse pressure (PP), particularly in middle-aged and older subjects, is an independent predictor of risk of coronary heart disease, compared with mean arterial pressure (MAP). From age 30 to 50 years, SBP and DBP track together in a parallel manner; however, after age 60 years, DBP decreases, while SBP continues to rise. This accounts for the increase in PP after age 60 years (12). Recent evidence has shown that PP provides important predictive value for coronary events in normotensive and untreated hypertensive middle-aged and elderly adults (13).

An overview of seven trials (EWPHE, HEP, MRC1, MRC2, SHEP, Syst-Eur, and STOP), which included hypertensive patients with a wide range of ages and BP, indicates that PP is an independent risk factor for overall and CV mortality (14).

In a recent study of a large cohort of nondiabetic patients on chronic HD, PP was found to be an independent predictor of total mortality (15) and superior to systolic and diastolic BP in predicting total mortality. A recent prospective cohort study of 180 ESRD patients on maintenance HD, followed-up for a mean duration of 52 ±36 months, has shown that carotid pulse pressure and aortic pulse wave velocity (PWV) were strong independent predictors of all-cause (including CV) mortality. Brachial BP, including PP had no predictive value for mortality (16). In a cohort study of 432 ESRD patients (261 HD and 171 peritoneal dialysis) followed prospectively for an average of 41 months, each 10 mm Hg rise in mean arterial pressure increased the relative risk of left ventricular hypertrophy (LVH) by 48% on follow-up echocardiography, increased the risk of de novo congestive heart failure (CHF) by 44%, and the risk of de novo ischemic heart disease by 39%. Interestingly, in this study low mean arterial pressure was independently associated with mortality [relative risk (RR) 1.36 per 10 mm Hg fall, $p = 0.009$] (17).

IMPORTANCE OF 24-HOUR BLOOD PRESSURE RECORDING IN DIALYSIS PATIENTS

Ambulatory BP monitoring has improved the existing knowledge of the relationship between circadian variability of arterial BP and end-organ damage. Normally, BP tends to be the highest during the morning, gradually decreasing during the course of the day to reach the lowest levels at night (18–21). Some hypertensive patients (approximately 10% to 25% of patients with essential hypertension) fail to manifest this normal nocturnal dipping of BP, defined as a nighttime BP fall of more than 10%. These patients are called "nondippers" (22,23), whereas those with a normal circadian rhythm are called "dippers." Among patients with advanced renal disease (24) and those on maintenance HD (25–27), the lack of diurnal variation in BP and of the nocturnal dipping of BP can affect as many as 74% to 82% of patients. At times, in these patients, nocturnal BP can be greater than BP measured during the day. Because BP is usually measured during the day, this may lead to the erroneous impression of good antihypertensive control (28). Using ambulatory BP monitoring, Agarwal (29) observed that in HD patients BP decreased after dialysis and during the first night, but by the next morning reached predialysis levels and it did not decrease during the second night.

The mechanisms responsible for the abnormal circadian rhythm of BP in patients with renal failure remain elusive. Autonomic dysfunction (30), reduced physical activity (31), sleep-disordered breathing (32,33), and volume overload (34) has been implicated. Because the phenomenon of non-dipping is more prevalent among salt-sensitive patients with essential hypertension and because this disturbance improves with salt-restriction (35,36) and diuretic therapy (37), one would predict that volume expansion would play a major role in the phenomenon of BP non-dipping among HD patients. However, several observations do not support a primary role of volume expansion in HD patients. First, interdialytic weight gain does not correlate with the phenomenon of nondipping (38); second, slow and short, daily HD does not change nocturnal dipping despite reduced extracellular water and better BP control (39,40).

The correlation between BP measured in the physician's office and CV end-points is usually weak. A large body of evidence from subjects with essential hypertension has shown that average 24-hour ambulatory BP correlates with the incidence of CV complications (41–45) better than office BP. A relationship seems also to exist between the absence of the nocturnal dipping of arterial BP and severity of CV target organ damage. Verdecchia et al. (23) observed that left ventricular (LV) mass index was significantly greater in nondippers than in dippers. A statistically significant inverse correlation was present between LV mass index and percentage of nocturnal reduction in BP. In a large number of hypertensive patients, we observed a significant correlation between nighttime SBP and DBP and urinary albumin excretion (UAE) and between 24-hour SBP and UAE in all hypertensive patients; in addition, a significant correlation was present between 24-hour DBP and nighttime DBP and UAE in nondippers (46).

Among HD patients, equally compelling is the evidence that absence of normal dipping of BP may predict CV events. In a study of 57 treated hypertensive HD patients, Amar et al. (47) observed that after an average follow-up of 34.4 ±20.4 months and after adjusting for age, sex, and previous CV events, an elevated nocturnal and 24-hour PP and low office DBP predict CV mortality. However, one has to remember that among HD patients there is a substantial day-to-day variability in the day-night BP profile (26). Moreover, nocturnal BP measurements predict CV outcome only in patients with reproducible BP profile (48).

AORTIC STIFFNESS IN ESRD PATIENTS

Epidemiologic studies have shown that aortic stiffness is increased in ESRD patients and that this factor is an independent marker of CV risk in ESRD patients (49), as well as in the general population (50). Aortic stiffness, determined by the measurement of aortic PWV depends on the arterial wall structure and function, which can be influenced by BP and aging (51). PWV frequently improves when BP is reduced, particularly when angiotensin-converting enzyme (ACE) inhibitors (52) or calcium channel blockers (53) are used. In ESRD patients, failure of PWV to improve in response to decreased BP is associated with worse CV outcomes (54).

GOAL BLOOD PRESSURE IN THE DIALYSIS POPULATION

According to JNC VI recommendations, SBP less than 120 mm Hg and DBP less than 80 mm Hg are considered optimal. In patients with essential hypertension receiving antihypertensive therapy the recommended goal BP is 135 to 138/83 to 85 mm Hg. This recommendation is based on the HOT study (55). The same study, however, has shown that in diabetic patients the goal BP should be set at lower levels and probably in the range of less than 130/80 mm Hg.

In patients with renal disease, and particularly those with proteinuria greater than 1 g /24 hours, goal BP should be approximately 125/75 mm Hg (AASK and MDRD studies) (56,57).

Despite the obvious importance of this issue, the ideal goal BP for dialysis patients has not been ascertained. HCFA has suggested that BP of less than 150/90 mm Hg is a reasonable goal for most patients undergoing HD (58). The Working Group on chronic renal failure (CRF) and renovascular hypertension, however, recommended a goal BP of less than 130/85 mm Hg (59). In the only prospective study so far performed in the dialysis population, a BP of 140/90 mm Hg minimized the occurrence of LVH and death (17).

These different recommendations reflect the existing confusion in the literature on what levels of BP predict better outcomes in this patient population. Charra et al. (60) were able to achieve a better BP control and survival with longer and slow dialysis (average *Kt/V* of 1.67). This group showed a 2.2-fold increase in the risk of CV death in patients with a mean predialysis BP of 98 mm Hg (equivalent to a BP of 130/80 mm Hg), compared with patients with BP values of less than 98 mm Hg (61). Other investigators have also shown better regression of LVH with slow dialysis (62). Foley et al. (63) found that, after adjusting for age, diabetes, ischemic heart disease, hemoglobin, and serum albumin, each 10 mm Hg rise in mean arterial BP was independently associated with a progressive increase of concentric LVH, the development of de novo cardiac failure, and de novo ischemic heart disease. This means that, amongst the burden of CVD risk factors of the dialysis population, hypertension plays a significant and independent role in cardiac damage. Other studies, however, have not shown a consistent association between BP and subsequent mortality in the dialysis population. Zager et al. (64) observed a "U-shaped" relationship between BP and mortality, with excess mortality risk in patients with the lowest and with the highest levels of BP. Port et al. (65) using the U.S. Renal Data System database observed an 86% increase in mortality over a follow-up period of 2 to 3 years among patients with low (<110 mm Hg) predialysis SBP. Salem (66) has shown no adverse effect of hypertension on 2-year survival. However, the studies from Charra et al. suggest that observations longer than 5 years are required to see the beneficial effect of BP control. The reason for the controversies surrounding the relationship between hypertension and outcome may be mainly due to the fact that, after being exposed to hypertension for several years, many ESRD patients develop cardiac failure with consequent reduction of BP values (so-called reverse causality). Therefore, observational studies based on cross-sectional evaluation of risk patterns may reach misleading conclusions.

It is also unclear which BP reading should be used as the guide for therapy and control of CVD. Some data suggest that predialysis SBP correlates best with LVH (67). Another report suggests that postdialysis BP is the most representative of mean interdialytic BP measured by ambulatory BP monitoring (68). Others have suggested that an average of predialysis and postdialysis BP may be a better predictor of mean interdialysis BP (69). In reality, neither is a particularly good predictor of interdialytic BP (70). This issue is complicated by the known fall in BP during dialysis in a large number (40%–50%) of patients and by the fact that this fall is short lived (12 to 24 hours). Thus, perhaps ABPM (ambulatory blood pressure monitoring) or self-measured home BP are better markers of interdialytic BP load, but, for practical and financial reasons, these tools cannot be applied to all dialysis patients.

PARADOXICAL RISE OF BLOOD PRESSURE DURING DIALYSIS

Hypertension induced by HD is a topic that has received little attention. It occurs in a small number of patients during HD.

The causes of this phenomenon have not been well worked-out. Sometimes it is precipitated by removal of certain antihypertensive drugs with dialysis.

HD reduces blood levels of ACE inhibitors, minoxidil, and has a minimal effect on calcium channel blockers.

At times excessive volume depletion may result in hypertension rather than in hypotension. This has been attributed to excessive stimulation of the renin-angiotensin system precipitated by the decrease in blood volume (BV). An alternative possibility, which has not been properly investigated, is that this might be the result of excessive activation of the sympathetic nervous system (SNS). Activation of this system plays an important role in the pathogenesis of hypertension associated with kidney disease and it could result in dialysis-induced hypertension.

In a recent study of seven patients with this characteristic, all with marked cardiac dilation, intense ultrafiltration reduced BP and cardiac dilatation and eliminated the paradoxical elevation of BP during dialysis (71). The explanation of this phenomenon remains elusive.

PATHOGENESIS OF HYPERTENSION IN ESRD PATIENTS

The pathogenesis of hypertension in ESRD patients is complex and probably multifactorial (Table 16.1). It is our belief that the sodium and volume status and activation of the SNS play a key role (Fig. 16.1).

Role of Sodium and Volume Status

Excessive intravascular volume is a major pathogenic factor of hypertension in patients with CRF. However, the relationship between weight gain during two dialyses and hypertension are contradictory. Some studies have established that volume gain affects interdialytic BP, whereas other studies have not shown such a relationship (72). The strongest evidence supporting a role for extracellular volume expansion derives from observations by the group in Tassin that when excessive body fluids are removed with slow-dialysis (8 hours × 3 times weekly) and "dry weight" is achieved, BP normalizes in more than 90% of dialysis-dependent patients. Although at the time of initiation of maintenance HD 89% of patients were receiving antihypertensive drugs, less than 5% of them still required antihypertensive drugs 3 months later

TABLE 16.1. FACTORS IMPLICATED IN THE PATHOGENESIS OF HYPERTENSION IN END-STAGE RENAL DISEASE

Sodium and volume excess
The renin-angiotensin-aldosterone system
The adrenergic system and baroreceptor activity
Endothelium-derived vasodepressor substances
Endothelium-derived vasoconstrictor substances
Erythropoietin use
Divalent ions and parathyroid hormone
Atrial natriuretic peptide
Structural changes in the arteries
Preexistent essential hypertension
Miscellaneous: anemia, AV fistula, vasopressin, serotonin, thyroid function, calcitonin gene-related peptide

AV, arteriovenous.

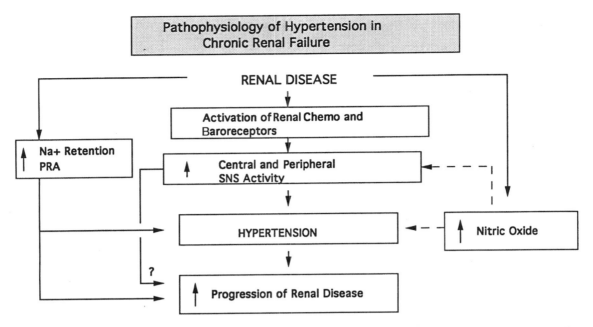

FIG. 16.1. Pathophysiology of hypertension in chronic renal failure: a schematic representation of how several processes combine to cause hypertension. As indicated in the left side of the figure, Na+ retention and enhanced renin activity may contribute to the elevation of blood pressure. As shown on the right side of the figure, renal disease may also stimulate increased nitric oxide synthesis and release, which tends to cause vasodilation and decrease blood pressure.

(73). It is of interest that, although the normalization of the extracellular volume was achieved in the first month of dialysis treatment, BP continued to decrease for another 8 months, despite the withdrawal of antihypertensive medication. It is also important to underscore that the long-slow dialysis performed in Tassin was associated with very low incidence of hypotensive episodes and muscular cramps during dialysis.

The reasons for long-slow dialysis achieving a more effective BP control may be due to more effective control of the ECV expansion with a low rate of hypotension episodes. Moreover, dry weight is probably more difficult to achieve with short than with long-slow HD.

The Tassin group has compared the fluid status and BP control in normotensive patients on long-slow dialysis in their center with that of normotensive and hypertensive HD patients on short HD (3 to 5 hours) at centers in Sweden (74). The fluid status was monitored by bioimpedance, ultrasonographic determination of the inferior vena cava diameter (IVCD), and on-line monitoring of changes in BV. Normotensive patients, either belonging to the Tassin or to the Swedish centers, did not differ significantly regarding ECV and IVCD before and after dialysis. Swedish hypertensive patients had significantly higher ECV and IVCD than normotensive patients. The fall in BV during dialysis was greater in the Swedish normotensive than in the Tassin patients, presumably resulting from higher ultrafiltration rates. The dialysis dose, as assessed by Kt/V_{urea}, was higher in the whole cohort of the Tassin patients (1.93 ±0.43), but it was not different between hypertensive and normotensive Swedish patients (1.58 ±0.34 vs. 1.55 ±0.43, respectively). On the whole, these data indicate that normotension in dialysis patients can be

achieved independently of the duration and dose of dialysis, provided that the control of the postdialysis ECV is adequate.

Several studies have shown that short daily HD treatment may be associated with a significant reduction of BP, antihypertensive medications, and LV mass index (40,75,76). Data collected from the Dialysis Morbidity and Mortality Study by the U.S. Renal Data System have shown that an interdialytic weight gain and noncompliance with the dialysis regimen were independent predictors of a higher BP (77). The normalization of patients' volume status appears also to improve the circadian BP rhythm that may be abnormal in the presence of volume expansion (78).

In patients who remain hypertensive despite intense ultrafiltration, the sodium and volume excess may play only a secondary role. The lack of correlation between exchangeable sodium and/or extracellular volume and BP in these patients supports this notion (79,80).

The mechanisms by which sodium excess may lead to arterial hypertension in the uremic patient are complex (Table 16.2). According to Guyton's hypothesis (81), sodium excess leads to volume expansion and increased cardiac output, which is followed by an increase in total peripheral vascular resistance (TPR) because of local autoregulation. In patients with terminal renal failure and normal BP, the tendency toward a high cardiac output is fully compensated by a decrease in peripheral vascular resistance, but this compensatory adaptation of peripheral vascular resistance does not occur in patients with hypertension (82). According to some investigators, this may be due to inappropriately elevated levels of angiotensin II or plasma catecholamines in relation to the body fluids and volume status or to increased sensitivity to endogenous pressor.

TABLE 16.2. MECHANISMS BY WHICH SODIUM EXCESS MAY LEAD TO HYPERTENSION

Increased extracellular volume
Increased vascular responsiveness to pressor hormones
Increased peripheral vascular resistance
Increased secretion of digitalis-like substances that reduce Na$^+$K$^+$ ATPase activity
Increased adrenergic activity
Structural changes in the vessel wall

An alternative explanation is that sodium overload may increase the secretion of digitalis-like inhibitors of vascular smooth muscle Na$^+$K$^+$ ATPase (83,84).

Boero et al. (85) measured erythrocyte Na$^+$K$^+$ ATPase activity in 38 uremic dialyzed patients and noted a lower pump activity in the hypertensive than in normotensive subjects. In the hypertensive group, an inverse correlation was present between Na$^+$K$^+$ ATPase activity and peripheral vascular resistance. As a consequence of the Na$^+$K$^+$ ATPase pump inhibition, intracellular sodium would increase, paralleled by an increase in cytosolic calcium, resulting in enhanced basal vascular tone and vascular responsiveness to vasoconstrictor agents. The increase in intracellular sodium may also cause swelling of arteriolar walls, narrowing of the lumen of arterioles, and increased peripheral vascular resistance (86).

Role of the Renin-Angiotensin System

The role of excessive renin secretion in relation to the state of sodium and volume has long been recognized as an important factor in the pathogenesis of hypertension in dialysis patients (87). Patients with the so-called dialysis-refractory hypertension are usually considered to have renin-dependent hypertension (88). Several factors support a role for the renin-angiotensin system in the pathogenesis of hypertension in dialysis patients. First, one can frequently find in these patients an abnormal relationship between exchangeable sodium or BV and plasma renin activity (PRA) or plasma levels of angiotensin II. This suggests that even "normal" plasma concentrations of renin may, in some instances, be inappropriately high in the face of sodium excess or increased BV. Second, a direct relationship between PRA and BP can be found in dialysis patients (although this finding has not been confirmed by all investigators). Third, BP can be effectively reduced in most of these patients by the administration of converting enzyme inhibitors (CEIs) or angiotensin II antagonists. Finally, bilateral nephrectomy results in normalization of BP in most of these patients (although this normalization could be also due to other factors, such as elimination of afferent inputs from the kidney to the central SNS).

Recent studies have shown that aldosterone contributes to hypertension and renal injury in the remnant kidney model in the rat. ACE inhibitors and angiotensin II receptor antagonists reduced the elevated aldosterone levels. In this model, the antihypertensive effect of these drugs appears to be in large part mediated by the suppressive effects on aldosterone (89).

Role of Increased Sympathetic Nervous System (SNS) Activity

Animal studies have shown that the kidney is not only an elaborate filtering device but also a sensory organ, richly innervated with sensory and afferent nerves. There are two main functional types of renal sensory receptors and afferent nerves: (a) renal baroreceptors, which increase their firing in response to changes in renal perfusion and intrarenal pressure and (b) renal chemoreceptors, which are stimulated by ischemic metabolites or uremic toxins (90,91).

In rats, these chemoceptive receptors are further classified into R1 and R2 based on their resting level of activity and the types of stimuli that elicit a response. The activation of these chemosensitive receptors may, through the renal afferent nerves, establish connections with integrative nuclei of the SNS in the central nervous system (CNS) (92,93). In experimental animals, stimulation of these afferent nerves by either ischemic metabolites such as adenosine or by uremic toxins such as urea evokes reflex increases in sympathetic nerve activity and BP (94). Chronic stimulation of these afferent nerves may lead to sympathetic overactivity and hypertension (Fig. 16.1).

Both direct and indirect evidence implicates increased SNS activity in the pathogenesis of hypertension in patients with CRF (95–99). Plasma norepinephrine (NE) levels are usually increased in HD patients (100,101), but these levels, whether measured predialysis or postdialysis, are poorly correlated with levels of BP (101,102). Direct recording of neuronal activity from postganglionic sympathetic fibers in the peroneal nerves of patients on chronic dialysis treatment have shown a greater rate of sympathetic nerve discharge than in control subjects (103). HD patients who had undergone bilateral nephrectomy had sympathetic nerve discharge similar to that of normal subjects and normal BP. However, the cross-sectional nature of these patient-oriented studies does not prove causality between the neurogenic signal from the failing kidney and the increasing SNS activity.

Our studies on 5/6 nephrectomized (CRF) rats have provided the most convincing evidence yet for a role of the SNS in the pathogenesis of hypertension associated with CRF. The turnover rate (104) and the secretion of NE (105) from the posterior hypothalamic (PH) nuclei were greater in CRF than in control rats. Bilateral dorsal rhizotomy at the level T-10 to L-3 prevented the increase in BP, the increase in NE turnover in the PH, and the progression of renal disease in CRF rats (106). These studies led us to postulate that increased renal sensory impulses generating in the affected kidney and then transmitted to the CNS activate regions in the CNS involved in the noradrenergic control of BP resulting in hypertension.

This possibility is supported by additional studies in animals as well as in humans. Ligtenberg et al. (107) reported an increase in muscle sympathetic nerve discharge in patients with CRF and renin-dependent hypertension, when compared with age- and weight-matched control. Klein et al. (108) have observed increased muscle sympathetic nerve activity in hypertensive patients with polycystic kidney disease regardless of kidney function. Activation of renal afferents appears also to be the primary mechanism for calcineurin inhibitors-induced hypertension in rats (109,110).

Other mechanisms potentially responsible for the increase in sympathetic nerve activity in uremic patients include reduced central dopaminergic tone (111). Hypertensive patients with CRF have a heightened DOPA and dopamine sulfoconjugating propensity, and dopamine sulfate attenuates the biologic action of free dopamine. The increase in sympathetic activity in CRF could also be due to reduced baroreceptors sensitivity (112), abnormal vagal function (113), increased intracellular calcium concentration (114), and increased plasma β-endorphin and β-lipotropin (115). Increased neuropeptide Y in response to fluid overload may also participate to hypertension in ESRD (116).

ACE inhibitors reduce peripheral sympathetic nerve activity in patients with CRF (107). Similarly, AT-1 receptor blockers reduced central SNS activity in a model of neurogenic hypertension caused by renal injury (117).

Role of the Vascular Endothelium

As the interface between the circulating blood and the vascular smooth muscle cells (VSMCs), the endothelial cells have several key functions (118) including (a) they serve as a first barrier to circulating antigens and actively participate in the defense reactions; (b) they play a cardinal role in both preventing and promoting clot formation through their interaction with platelets, the fibrinolytic system, and the clotting cascade; (c) they clear from the blood substances such as NE and serotonin; (d) they activate peptides such as angiotensin and inactivate others such as bradykinin; (e) they may play a key role in promoting thickening and fibrosis of blood vessels through mitogenic effects; and (f) the endothelium plays a crucial role in regulating regional blood flow and vascular resistance.

In 1977 Moncada et al. (119) demonstrated that the endothelium is the major source of prostacyclin. In 1980 Furchgott et al. (120) showed that acetylcholine-induced arterial relaxation is endothelium dependent and is caused by the generation of a diffusible and transferable substance that relaxes smooth muscle cells. This substance, initially called endothelium-derived relaxing factor (EDRF), is now characterized as nitric oxide (NO) (121–123).

Yanagisawa et al. (124) identified a 21-amino-acid peptide called endothelin (ET), the most potent vasoconstrictor isolated so far. Other endothelium-derived contracting factors (EDCFs) being studied include PGH_2 (125) and epidermal growth factor (EGF), which is a mitogen for smooth muscle cells in vitro and causes arterial strips to contract. Glomerular mesangial cells express EGF receptors, thus making it possible for EGF to regulate glomerular filtration rate (GFR) (126).

A number of investigators have speculated that these vasoactive peptides may play a role in disease states such as hypertension (127,128). The possibilities include the following:

1. Altered balance between EDRF and EDCF may result in a rise in renal and systemic vascular resistance and hypertension.
2. Hypertensive vascular endothelial damage may lead to abnormal production of endothelium-derived vasoactive factors (129).
3. The endothelium may affect systemic hemodynamics by secreting substances that have effects on other key regulators.

ET, for example, stimulates atrial natriuretic peptide (ANP) release.

Endothelium-Derived Vasoconstrictor Factors

The role of ET in dialysis-related hypertension has been the focus of active research and controversy. Three ET genes have been cloned from a human genomic library that encodes three distinct isopeptides: endothelin 1 (ET-1), endothelin 2 (ET-2), and endothelin 3 (ET-3) (130). They are all synthesized from a large precursor molecule, preproendothelin (prepro-ET). Prepro-ET-1 is a 203-amino-acid peptide, and pro-ET (big endothelin) is a peptide containing 92 amino acids. ET-1 is formed from big ET-1 by the action of endothelin-converting enzyme (ECE). Phosphoramidon, a metalloprotease inhibitor that blocks the action of ECE, when administered intravenously to conscious spontaneously hypertensive rats leads to a reduction of BP (131).

The three ETs are expressed differently in various tissues. Only ET-1 is expressed in vascular endothelial cells, but it is also expressed in various nonvascular cells within the brain, kidney, lung, and other tissues. ET-2 and ET-3 are expressed in the brain, kidney, adrenal glands, and intestine. Two distinct complementary deoxyribonucleic acids (DNAs) of ET receptors have been identified, one expressed in VSMCs (ET_A-receptor), and the other (ET_B-receptor) is probably present on endothelial cells and is responsible for the release of prostacyclin and NO.

The order of affinity for the ET_A receptor is ET-1 > ET-2 > ET-3 (ET-1 affinity is about 100 times greater than ET-3). ET_B receptors have equal affinity for all three isoforms. ET-2 is the most potent vasoconstrictor, followed by ET-1 and ET-3. Subpressor doses of ET-1 potentiate the vasoconstrictor effects of other hormones, such as NE. Calcium channel antagonists inhibit the pressor and the potentiating effects of ET-1.

In addition to its contractile actions on vascular smooth muscle, ET has mitogenic action on the vascular smooth muscle, mesangial cells, and fibroblasts. It potently contracts nonvascular smooth muscle (bronchial, uterine, intestinal, and urinary bladder), and it has prominent cardiac effects (positive isotropic, chronotropic, and stimulates ANP release). Cytokines, thrombin, and vasoactive hormones such as epinephrine, A-II (angiotensin II), and vasopressin stimulate ET release from endothelial cells. In addition, physical stimuli such as shear stress can enhance ET production (80). ET-1 also plays an important role as a locally procured vasoactive peptide in the regulation of renal hemodynamic and excretory function (132).

Compelling evidence that ET-1 might play a role in the pathophysiology of hypertension was reported by Yokokawa et al., who described two patients with hemangioendothelioma, a rare malignant vascular neoplasm, who had plasma levels of ET 10- to 15-fold greater than in normal and hypertensive patients. Surgical removal of the tumor led to resolution of hypertension in both cases. In one patient the tumor recurred along with a rise in plasma ET level and hypertension (133). Increased plasma ET-1 levels have been shown in patients with essential hypertension by some investigators (134) but not by others (135).

Hypertensive patients with CRF have higher plasma ET-1 levels than normotensive subjects (136,137). Suzuki et al. (138)

found elevated plasma ET-1 and ET-3 levels in HD patients, which could be either due to the uremic state or to exposure of the cells to an extracorporeal circuit during HD (139). Miyauchi et al. (140) found elevated ET-1 and ET-3 levels in hemodialyzed patients and a positive correlation between ET-1 levels and BP. Lebel et al. (141) observed higher ET-1 concentration and mean BP in HD patients than in continuous ambulatory peritoneal dialysis (CAPD) patients. Further studies using ET-1 receptor antagonists may be necessary to prove whether ET-1 plays a causal role in the hypertension of uremic patients.

Endothelium-Derived Vasodilator Factors

Endothelial cells cause vasodilatation in response to increases in flow, shear stress, and agonists through the release of several mediators. These include prostaglandin I_2 (PGI_2), endothelium-derived hyperpolarizing factor (EDHF), and NO.

PGI_2 is activated by bradykinin and it increases cyclic adenosine monophosphate (cAMP) levels in the VSMCs, leading to vasodilatation. It also inhibits platelet adhesion and has thrombolytic and cytoprotective actions. PGI_2 and NO potentiate each other's vascular and platelet antiaggregating effects even at subthreshold concentrations (142–144).

In 1988 Feketou and Vanhoutte (145) discovered an EDHF in the canine femoral artery. EDHF opens vascular smooth muscle calcium-activated potassium K_{Ca} channels, allowing potassium efflux, hyperpolarization, and relaxation. Depolarization of smooth muscle cells with high extracellular potassium or inhibitors of channels blocks this action of EDHF. The activity of EDHF is attenuated by ouabain, a sodium-potassium ATPase inhibitor and not by inhibitors of cyclooxygenase or NO synthase. The chemical identity of EDHF remains controversial. Hydrogen peroxide and potassium are possible candidates for EDHF. In diabetes and hypertension, impairment of EDHF contributes to endothelial dysfunction (146).

Of the various vasodilator substances so far identified, EDRF, an endogenous stimulator of the guanylate-cyclase, has attracted the most attention. The formation of NO by NO synthase in the vascular endothelium from the amino acid L-arginine has opened up a new area of biologic research. Several forms of NO synthase have been identified. The first is a constitutive form, cytosolic Ca^{2+}/calmodulin-dependent, that releases NO for short periods in response to receptor or physical stimulation and acts as a transduction mechanism underlying several physiologic responses. The second inducible form of NO synthase is cytosolic Ca^{2+} independent; its activation requires tetrahydrobiopterin, among other cofactors, and can be inhibited by glucocorticoids. This second form of NO synthase may be activated by cytokines in macrophages, endothelial cells, and a number of other cells; its only clearly established role is as a cytotoxic molecule for invading microorganisms and tumor cells, but a role in pathologic vasodilatation and tissue damage is also possible. Among the other forms of NO synthase that have been isolated, the one found in the brain, nNOS, appears to modulate the activity of the SNS.

In 5/6 nephrectomized rats, Vaziri et al. (147) have observed the presence of downregulation of e-NOS and iNOS and these

authors have suggested that this may contribute to the elevation of BP in these animals.

Chronic inhibition of NO synthesis by N^wL-nitro-L-arginine-methyl ester (L-NAME) has been recently used as a new model of arterial hypertension in animals. Administration of nitro-L-arginine to rats causes systemic hypertension, marked renal vasoconstriction, and hypoperfusion, as well as a fall in GFR and a rise in filtration fraction (FF) and in plasma renin levels (which could partly be responsible for the severe vasoconstrictor activity) (148,149). Renal histologic examination revealed widespread arteriolar narrowing, focal arteriolar obliteration, and segmental fibrinoid necrosis of the glomeruli, findings that have been confirmed by other investigators (150,151). Sakuma et al. (152) have shown that administration of N^G-methyl-L-arginine (NO synthase inhibitor) to male Wistar rats increases renal SNS activity and causes systemic hypertension. They have also shown that the increase in renal SNS activity and in BP could be reduced by spinal C-1 to C-2 transection, implying that NO may play a role in the central regulation of sympathetic tone.

Vallance et al. (153) have shown both in vitro and in vivo that NO synthesis can be inhibited by an endogenous compound, N^GN^G-dimethylarginine (asymmetrical dimethylarginine, ADMA). They have also found significantly higher plasma levels of ADMA and a significantly lower plasma arginine-to-dimethylarginine ratio in uremic patients on chronic HD, raising the intriguing possibility that hypertension in the uremic patient on maintenance dialysis might be due to NO synthesis inhibition caused by increased levels of this circulating endogenous inhibitor. ADMA may be significantly reduced by the dialysis procedure (154). ADMA levels are increased in salt-sensitive hypertensive patients (155) and Dahl rats (156). There is also a body of evidence that ADMA may be involved in the pathophysiology of atherosclerosis (157).

We have evaluated the effects of L-arginine and L-NAME on BP and SNS activity in Sprague Dawley 5/6 nephrectomized or sham-operated rats. SNS activity was determined by measuring NE turnover rate in several brain nuclei involved in the regulation of BP. In the same brain nuclei, we measured NO content and NOS gene expression using reverse transcription polymerase chain reaction.

In CRF rats, NE turnover rate was increased in the PH nuclei, locus ceruleus, paraventricular nuclei, and the rostral ventral medulla, whereas NOS mRNA gene expression and NO_2/NO_3 content were increased in all brain nuclei tested. L-NAME increased BP and NE turnover rate in several brain nuclei of both control and 5/6 nephrectomized rats. In CRF rats, a significant relationship was present between the percent increment in NOS mRNA gene expression related to the renal failure and the percent increase in NE turnover rate caused by L-NAME. This suggests that endogenous NO may partially inhibit the activity of the SNS in brain nuclei involved in the neurogenic regulation of BP, and this inhibition is enhanced in CRF rats (158).

These studies have demonstrated that the increase in SNS activity in the PH nuclei and in the locus ceruleus of CRF rats is partially mitigated by increased local expression of NOS mRNA (Fig. 16.1).

Adrenomedullin

When infused systemically, adrenomedullin significantly decreases BP in healthy subjects (159). In patients on maintenance HD, plasma adrenomedullin levels were greater than in control subjects even after fluid removal by ultrafiltration (160).

The increased levels of adrenomedullin may partially mitigate the rise in BP in HD patients.

Oxidative Stress and Hypertension (see Chapter 20)

Considerable attention has been given to the effects of short-lived reactive oxygen species (ROS) and reactive nitrogen species on BP and CV toxicity. ROS or oxygen free radicals are O_2 molecules with an unpaired electron, and include superoxide anion (O_2^-), hydrogen peroxide (H_2O_2), and hydroxyl ion (OH^-). Among reactive nitrogen species is peroxynitrate. These molecules are chemically unstable and highly reactive, and nicotinamide adenine dinucleotide phosphate (NADPH) oxidase, xanthine oxidase, and nitric oxide synthase (NOS) enzymes regulate their concentration. NADPH oxidase is a multimeric enzyme and is responsible for the reduction of oxygen and electron transport and superoxide production at the cell surface (161). The vascular isoform of NADPH is constitutively active and is a major source of vascular superoxide production (162). Although NOS is a major source of NO, under conditions of L-arginine deficiency, this enzyme may also generate the NO-scavenger superoxide. All three isoforms of NOS, the neuronal, inducible, and endothelial are capable of superoxide production (163).

The cytochrome b558 subunits, p22phox and gp91phox, of NAD(P)H oxidase are important for electron transport and the reduction of molecular oxygen to superoxide. Transfection of p22phox DNA in rats (164), or knockout of gp91phox in mice (161), have demonstrated these subunits to be functionally important for both NAD(P)H oxidase and angiotensin II-dependent superoxide production (165).

Oxygen radicals and endogenous scavenging systems, such as superoxide dismutase, modulate vascular tone and function. They stimulate proliferation and hypertrophy of VSMCs and fibroblasts (166) and influence vascular remodeling by increasing adhesion molecule expression, activation of matrix metalloproteinases, and induction of VSMC growth and migration (164,167). In addition, ROS may stimulate vascular contraction directly or through quenching of the vasodilator NO and production of peroxinitrite ($O_2^- + NOO^- \rightarrow ONOO^-$) (168). Peroxinitrite may induce oxidative damage to DNA, lipids, and proteins in vascular cells and result in endothelial dysfunction (169,170).

ROS production is increased in several experimental models of hypertension (171–175) including uremic hypertension (176). Vaziri et al. (177) have shown that ROS are increased in uremic rats and they react with NO producing cytotoxic reactive nitrogen species capable of nitrating proteins and damaging other molecules. Antioxidant therapy ameliorated the CRF-induced hypertension, improved vascular tissue NO production, and lowered tissue nitrotyrosine. Depletion of glutathione, an endogenous scavenger of ROS, by means of the GSH synthase inhibitor, butathionine sulfoximine (BSO), caused a marked elevation of nitrotyrosine, the footprint of peroxynitrite and marked elevation of BP in rats (178).

The exact mechanism through which oxidative stress may raise BP has not been fully elucidated.

One possibility is that ROS may play a role in the regulatory processes of noradrenergic transmission in the brain. Given that NO exerts a tonic inhibition on central SNS activity, increased production of ROS may enhance oxidation and inactivation of NO and result in activation of the SNS. NO actively reacts with superoxide (O_2^-) and other ROS to produce peroxynitrate ($ONOO^-$), a highly cytotoxic reactive nitrogen species. Peroxynitrate reacts with other proteins, such as tyrosine to produce nitrotyrosine, which can be detected in plasma and tissues. Nitrotyrosine is the footprint of the NO-ROS interaction and is used as an indicator of NO oxidation by ROS (179,180).

We have shown that tempol (4-hydroxy-2,2,6,6-tetramethyl piperidinoxyl), a superoxide dismutase mimetic, when injected in the lateral ventricle of rats, increases the abundance of interleukin-1β (IL-1β) and nNOS in the PH and paraventricular nuclei, and this is associated with reduced NE secretion from the PH and lower BP. In the phenol-renal injury model of hypertension in rat, we have shown that tempol prevents the activation of SNS and the rise in BP caused by renal injury (personal observations). These data support the hypothesis that oxygen radicals may modulate central SNS activation through regulation of local NO production and participate to hypertension in renal injury models.

Role of Erythropoietin

The advent of recombinant human erythropoietin (rhEPO) has substantially improved the management of anemia and the quality of life in patients with CRF. However, increasing the hematocrit (Hct) with rhEPO can lead to several adverse side effects, including worsening of hypertension. In patients with CRF, worsening of BP control may accelerate the progression of renal disease; in dialysis patients this may increase the requirement for antihypertensive drugs and potentially increase CV morbidity.

During studies in dialysis and prephase III multicenter trials of rhEPO in dialysis patients, an increase in DBP of more than 10 mm Hg and/or a need to increase antihypertensive therapy occurred in 88 of 251 (35%) of previously hypertensive patients. A similar increase in BP was noted in 31 of 71 (44%) of normotensive patients; in 32% of these patients, antihypertensive therapy had to be instituted (181,182). This adverse rise in BP has not been noted in patients receiving rhEPO for other reasons, suggesting that renal disease may confer a particular susceptibility (183) to the hypertensive action of rhEPO. The rise in BP during rhEPO administration usually occurs within 2 to 16 weeks, although some patients may experience a rise in BP several months after the initiation of therapy.

Patients who are at greater risk for developing hypertension during rhEPO therapy are those with severe anemia, those whose anemia is corrected too rapidly, those with preexisting hypertension, and perhaps those with their native kidneys.

Clinical and experimental studies have confirmed the importance of Hct in the regulation of both systemic and renal hemodynamics (184,185). Anemia causes a hyperdynamic state that is necessary to maintain an adequate oxygen supply to peripheral tissues. The hyperdynamic state is characterized by an increase in cardiac output and a decrease in TPR. LV mass and end-diastolic diameter also increase in response to the hyperdynamic state. Correction of the anemia with rhEPO leads to a decrease in cardiac output and a rise in TPR. Patients who become hypertensive or experience an exacerbation of their BP during rhEPO therapy either have an exaggerated rise of TPR in response to the increase in Hct or a cardiac output that does not decrease to the same extent as in patients who remain normotensive (Table 16.3). The failure of the myocardium to adapt to these changes could be the result of reduced compliance or of impaired baroreflex function. The increase in blood viscosity during rhEPO therapy correlates with the increase in TPR but not with BP changes (186). In patients with essential hypertension, elevated Hct leads to increased blood viscosity (187) and TPR. There is also reduced peripheral capillary dilation secondary to better tissue delivery of O_2 (188). Increased blood viscosity not only increases TPR and reduces blood flow but it also decreases plasma volume, further increasing the blood viscosity.

Hypertension induced by rhEPO cannot be due exclusively to increased blood viscosity, because studies in rats have shown that renal insufficiency is a prerequisite for the development of hypertension during rhEPO therapy (189). Thus, other mechanisms must participate (Table 16.3), such as enhanced pressor responsiveness to NE and A-II (190,191). Evidence of whether rhEPO has a direct vasoconstrictor action on smooth muscle cells is conflicting. After infusion of rhEPO, some studies have shown no vasoconstriction in the isolated rat kidney or isolated human resistance arterioles (192,193), whereas others have observed vasoconstriction in isolated renal and mesenteric resistance vessels of rats (110,194). This action was endothelium independent and was not affected by verapamil or phentolamine.

Some studies suggest that rhEPO may affect intracellular calcium homeostasis. An increase in platelet cytosolic free calcium has been shown in volunteers who received rhEPO (195). Others found no correlation between absolute BP levels and platelet

intracellular calcium in hemodialyzed patients treated with rhEPO (196).

Azzadin et al. (197) have shown that administration of rhEPO to normal and uremic rats caused a rise in blood and platelet serotonin and an increase in BP. These effects were abolished by ketanserin, an antagonist of 5-HT_2 receptors. The study suggests that serotonin may play a role in the development of hypertension caused by rhEPO.

Others have shown that HD patients on rhEPO therapy manifest increased ET-1 levels, suggesting a potential involvement in the pathogenesis of hypertension in these patients (198). There is no evidence that decreased NO activity is responsible for rhEPO-associated hypertension. In fact, NO production is stimulated by administration of rhEPO (199).

In humans as well as animals, anemia is associated with proportionately greater increase in renal plasma flow (RPF) than in GFR, so that FF tends to decrease. Micropuncture studies in the rat have shown that an acute decrease in Hct from 51% to 20% results in an acute increase in the glomerular capillary RPF, a less steep rise in single-nephron GFR, and, hence, a fall in FF. Both the afferent (RA) and efferent (RE) arteriolar resistances decrease, resulting in a fall in glomerular capillary pressure (PGC) (200). In addition to the direct effects on glomerular hemodynamics, a rise in Hct with a resultant increase in blood viscosity also modulates glomerular permselectivity to macromolecules and hence may increase proteinuria (201). In support of this is the massive glomerular enlargement, the proteinuria, and the progressive glomerulosclerosis observed in cyanotic patients with heart disease and marked polycythemia and hyperviscosity (202).

Role of Divalent Ions and Parathyroid Hormone (PTH)

A relationship between platelet or lymphocyte [Ca^{2+}]i and BP has been demonstrated in patients with essential hypertension (203,204) as well as in patients with ESRD (205). The mechanisms leading to the increase in [Ca^{2+}]i are not clear. This could be the result of increased circulating pressor hormones, such as NE or angiotensin II, or increased secretion of a ouabain-like factor in response to volume expansion. Finally, the increase in cytosolic calcium in VSMCs could be caused by secondary hyperparathyroidism. CRF is frequently associated with secondary hyperparathyroidism which leads to increased intracellular calcium [Ca^{2+}]i in almost any organ.

Recently, Raine et al. (206) studied 36 patients with CRF, 10 with normal serum PTH levels, 17 with elevated serum PTH, and 9 with elevated PTH but treated with nifedipine. Platelet [Ca^{2+}]i was significantly greater in the 17 patients with increased serum PTH than in patients with normal serum PTH. In addition, a significant relation was present between serum PTH and platelet [Ca^{2+}]i or between platelet [Ca^{2+}]i and mean BP and between PTH and mean BP. In patients with high serum PTH receiving nifedipine, platelet [Ca^{2+}]i was not increased. Nine patients with hyperparathyroidism were restudied during treatment with alfacalcidol, a vitamin D metabolite. In these patients, serum PTH, platelet [Ca^{2+}]i, and mean BP all decreased significantly. The changes in BP during treatment

TABLE 16.3. FACTORS IMPLICATED IN THE PATHOGENESIS OF HYPERTENSION IN ESRD PATIENTS ON ERYTHROPOIETIN

Increased blood viscosity
Increased blood volume
Increased total peripheral resistance
Loss of hypoxic vasodilation
Baroreceptor malfunction and/or impaired cardiac compliance
Enhanced sensitivity to circulating catecholamines and angiotensin II
Alterations in glomerular hemodynamics
Direct vasoconstrictor effect?
Increased cytosolic calcium?
Binding of local EDRF?
Stimulation of endothelin
Stimulation of serotonin

EDRF, endothelium-derived relaxing factor.

with alfacalcidol were linearly related with the changes in serum PTH and in $[Ca^{2+}]i$. These studies suggest that increased serum levels of PTH may be responsible for both the rise in $[Ca^{2+}]i$ and the increase in BP in these patients. Treatment of secondary hyperparathyroidism with oral calcium also may reduce BP in HD patients (207). However, parathyroidectomy failed to normalize BP in HD patients (208).

Dialysis patients may occasionally develop hypercalcemia as a result of exogenous administration of vitamin D analogs, oral calcium supplementation, granulomatous diseases, multiple myeloma, or severe secondary hyperparathyroidism. In these patients, hyperkalemia may either aggravate or cause hypertension. Hypercalcemia is more likely to raise BP in the presence of increased serum levels of PTH and it does so primarily by increasing systemic vascular resistance; cardiac output usually remains unchanged (209,210). We have observed that in rats with CRF the hypercalcemia-induced hypertension was more severe than in normal rats (210). This appeared to be secondary to the state of secondary hyperparathyroidism, because parathyroidectomy reduced the pressor response to acute hypercalcemia. These studies suggest that the presence of PTH plays an important role for the hypertensive action of hypercalcemia.

Natriuretic Factors in ESRD Patients

Plasma levels of α-ANP and pro-ANP are usually increased in patients with hypertension in an apparent attempt to offset volume retention and lower BP. In ESRD patients, predialysis plasma levels of α-ANP and pro-ANP are substantially greater than values in control subjects (211,212). Following HD, α-ANP levels were significantly reduced. No correlation was evident between predialysis levels of α-ANP and interdialytic weight gain or between these levels and volume removal with HD. Thus, plasma α-ANP is not a useful marker of volume status in HD patients.

Cardiac natriuretic peptides are related to LV mass and function in dialysis patients and predict CV mortality (213).

Cyclosporine A and Hypertension

Cyclosporine A (CyA) is a potent orally active immunosuppressive agent used in the management of patients with a variety of renal diseases and organ transplantation. CyA is known to be nephrotoxic and to raise BP.

CyA-induced hypertension appears to be dose-related, but the correlation between blood levels of CyA and BP is weak. The mechanisms of CyA-induced hypertension are complex. The increase in peripheral vascular resistance caused by CyA could be caused by direct vasoconstriction, because it can be shown in isolated vascular preparations. CyA causes marked vasoconstriction and decrease in renal blood flow; this action is not prevented by captopril. The renal vasoconstriction may depend on activation of the renal SNS because renal denervation and α-blocking agents prevent the decrease in renal blood flow. Direct measurements in conscious rats have shown that CyA increases the activity of afferent (214) and efferent sympathetic nerves and decreases fractional excretion of sodium.

The role of the SNS in CyA-induced hypertension in human subjects is less clear. Plasma and urinary catecholamines do not change during administration of CyA, but these levels are a poor marker of regional SNS activity.

The role of the renin-angiotensin system is also uncertain. Acute administration of CyA increases PRA, but after chronic treatment PRA levels are normal or suppressed.

CyA increases the production of thromboxane A_2 and inhibits the production of prostaglandin E_2. Administration of inhibitors of thromboxane improves the renal hemodynamic effects of CyA.

CyA increases the concentration of serotonin in the blood and platelets (215), but the role of serotonin in CyA-induced hypertension remains to be established.

CyA can cause magnesium deficiency, which may also cause increased peripheral vascular resistance.

MANAGEMENT OF HYPERTENSION IN DIALYSIS SUBJECTS

The management of hypertension in the dialysis patient is frequently challenging and it requires knowledge of the pharmacokinetic and pharmacodynamic properties of all the agents used. We propose an algorithm that may be useful in the management of hypertension in these patients (Fig. 16.2).

Lifestyle modifications should be an integral part of the management of every patient with hypertension, including those with ESRD. In dialysis patients, achievement of dry weight is essential for BP control.

If those measures are unsuccessful (and frequently they are), antihypertensive drugs should be initiated. We propose as the first line of treatment, one of three classes of antihypertensive

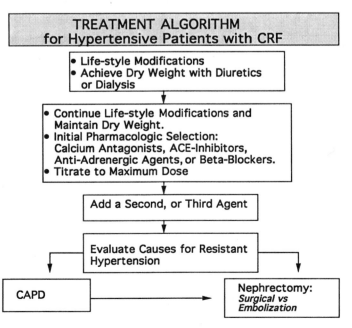

FIG. 16.2. Treatment of hypertension in chronic renal failure.

agents: calcium channel antagonists, ACE inhibitors, and β-blockers. The selection of one class of antihypertensive drugs over another must be dictated in large part by concomitant diseases or risk factors. If full doses of one agent are ineffective, a second or a third drug should be added. If BP is not controlled with dialysis and three antihypertensive agents of different classes, the patient should be evaluated for potential secondary causes of resistant hypertension. If no evident cause for resistant hypertension is found, one should consider treating the patient with CAPD. If CAPD proves ineffective, surgical or embolic nephrectomy should be considered.

Lifestyle Modifications

Lifestyle modification, such as weight reduction, dietary sodium restriction, moderation of alcohol intake, and increased physical activity, can be used effectively as adjunct therapy in the management of hypertension in dialysis patients as it is in patients with essential hypertension (Table 16.4) (216):

- *Salt and fluids.* Among the potential interventions, dietary salt and fluid restriction is the most important. Dietary sodium intake should be restricted to 1 to 1.5 g/day and fluid intake should match urine output plus insensible losses of 10 mL/kg/day. Admittedly, compliance with such severe fluid and salt restriction is very difficult to achieve and requires continued reinforcement and education.
- Studies mostly obtained in genetic strains of hypertensive rats, such as stroke-prone spontaneously hypertensive rats, and Dahl salt-sensitive rats have demonstrated that high salt intake may decrease carotid artery distensibility and compliance and increase wall thickness and extracellular matrix, independently of effects on BP. Salt restriction prevents these effects (217,218).
- *Calcium.* Some evidence suggests that calcium supplementation may have a beneficial effect on BP control in some patients with essential hypertension, provided it does not result in hypercalcemia. There are no data on the effects on BP of the calcium-containing compounds used to control hyperphosphatemia.
- *Exercise.* Regular physical exercise has been demonstrated to decrease BP in dialysis patients.

TABLE 16.4. LIFESTYLE MODIFICATIONS IN HYPERTENSIVE DIALYSIS PATIENTS

Of Proven Efficacy
    Moderate dietary sodium intake
    Achieve and maintain dry weight
    Increase physical activity
    Limit daily alcohol intake to ≤1 ounce of ethanol
    Avoid tobacco for CVD risk reduction
    Reduce dietary saturated fat and cholesterol for CVD risk reduction
    Eliminate the use of cocaine or amphetamines
Of Unproven Efficacy
    Reduction of caffeine intake
    Relaxation and biofeedback
    Calcium supplementations

CVD, cardiovascular disease.

- *Alcohol and substance abuse.* Moderation of alcoholic intake and avoidance of cocaine or amphetamines may also result in remarkable BP reduction among dialysis patients who abuse these substances. In some cases, a toxicology screening may be required to ascertain the diagnosis.
- *Tobacco use.* Tobacco use is a CV risk factor, and thus avoidance of tobacco is of extreme importance in dialysis patients.

Control of Fluid and Volume Status with Dialysis

In addition to sodium and fluid restrictions, an adequate dialysis strategy should be established to achieve and maintain dry weight. When beginning dialysis, optimal dry weight should be achieved gradually over 4 to 8 weeks and the negative fluid balance should not exceed 1 to 2 kg/week, because overzealous ultrafiltration may result in hypotension, rapid reduction of the residual renal function, and, in predisposed patients, in cerebral or coronary ischemic events. Dry weight is defined as that body weight at the end of dialysis below which further reduction results in hypotension. However, estimation of dry weight is a difficult problem. Several methods have been proposed but none of them is applicable to extensive clinical use. The gold standard for evaluation of total body water is the use of tracer dilution techniques, but this is not clinically applicable. Some have proposed the use of postdialytic echocardiographic measurement of IVCD (68), but this method is not without its critics (74). Probably the most promising method to assess fluid status during dialysis is by multifrequency electrical bioimpedance. More recently, Zucchelli et al. have proposed the use of continuous plasma volume measurement during dialysis and ultrafiltration stops to determine dry weight (78).

As previously discussed, the control of the fluid status is of paramount importance for BP control in most dialysis patients.

Occasionally, paradoxical hypertension can occur as a result of excessive ultrafiltration when the ultrafiltration leads to excessive activation of the renin-angiotensin system. More rapid ultrafiltration is necessary, however, in patients with signs of LV failure, malignant hypertension, hypertensive encephalopathy, acute pulmonary edema, pericardial effusion, or dissecting aneurysm of the aorta.

In a patient beginning dialysis, if BP is only moderately elevated (stage 1 or 2 according to the new JNC VI classification) (Table 16.5), antihypertensive therapy should not be instituted until dry weight is achieved. In patients already on antihypertensive agents, the dosage of medications should be gradually tapered when BP progressively decreases as a result of ultrafiltration. When dry weight is achieved, BP becomes normal in more than half of these patients. During the interdialytic period, BP may rise again in proportion to the amount of sodium and fluid retention. If during the interdialytic periods BP does not exceed 160/95 mm Hg, antihypertensive therapy may be withheld, because administration of antihypertensive agents before dialysis may result in frequent and severe intradialytic hypotensive episodes. Antihypertensive therapy should be instituted in patients with more severe hypertension or those with accelerated hypertension, severe retinopathy, CHF, cerebrovascular accidents, or aortic aneurysm.

Excessive ultrafiltration may cause dialysis-induced hypotension and a rapid decline of the residual renal function. In a

TABLE 16.5. CLASSIFICATION OF BLOOD PRESSURE FOR ADULTS AGE 18 YEARS AND OLDER

Category[a]	Systolic (mm Hg)	Diastolic (mm Hg)
Optimal	<120 and	<80
Normal	<130 and	<85
High normal	130–139 or	85–89
Hypertension[b]		
Stage 1 (mild)	140–159 or	90–99
Stage 2 (moderate)	160–179 or	100–109
Stage 3 (severe)	≥180 or	≥110

[a]When systolic and diastolic blood pressure fall into different categories, the higher category should be selected to classify the individual's blood pressure.
[b]Based on the average of two or more readings taken at each of two or more visits following an initial screening.
Adapted from Joint National Committee on Detection, Evaluation, and Treatment of High Blood Pressure. The Sixth Report of the Joint National Committee on Detection, Evaluation, and Treatment of High Blood Pressure JNC VI. *Arch Intern Med* 1997;153:154–183, with permission.

minority of patients, this may also result in angina pectoris or in transitory cerebral ischemia. Aggressive ultrafiltration should be instituted only in patients with signs of CHF, hypertensive emergencies, hypertensive encephalopathy, or pulmonary edema.

Therapy with Antihypertensive Drugs

The goal of antihypertensive therapy in dialysis patients is to achieve and maintain BP 140/90 mm Hg or lower by the least intrusive methods possible. This is not always easy to achieve in these patients because of the tendency for BP to increase in the interdialytic periods and to decrease during dialysis. The ultimate goal of antihypertensive therapy is to reduce CV morbidity and mortality related to hypertension.

At the initiation of dialysis treatment, in patients who have a DBP ranging between 90 and 114 mm Hg or SBP ranging between 140 and 179 mm Hg and no major CV complications, antihypertensive medications can be withheld until dry weight is achieved. In fact, once dry weight is achieved the BP will normalize in more than half of these patients, and it will remain normal as long as body weight remains close to dry weight.

During the interdialytic periods, BP frequently rises in proportion to the amount of sodium and fluid intake. If BP does not exceed 150/95 mm Hg during interdialytic periods, antihypertensive drugs should not be given to avoid the risk of intradialytic hypotension.

When hypertension persists despite achievement of dry weight, antihypertensive drugs should be initiated.

In patients already taking antihypertensive medications at the beginning of dialysis, the same drugs should be continued and the dose tapered as BP decreases with ultrafiltration. Antihypertensive drugs should be immediately instituted in patients with BP 180/115 mm Hg or in patients with significant end-organ damage, such as severe retinopathy, CHF, cerebrovascular accident, or aortic aneurysm.

Patients with poor compliance with sodium and fluid restrictions and frequent episodes of CHF and/or volume-dependent hypertension can be best managed with CAPD, because this treatment allows more steady maintenance of dry weight.

Choice of Antihypertensive Drugs

An extensive number of effective antihypertensive agents are currently available. With the exception of diuretics, which are not commonly used in dialysis patients because of their lack of efficacy, the criteria for drug selection do not substantially differ from those used in patients with essential hypertension.

In choosing among antihypertensive agents, consideration should be given to the coexisting diseases as well as the patient's demographic characteristics, risk profile, lifestyle, and financial situation (Table 16.6).

TABLE 16.6. ANTIHYPERTENSIVE DRUG THERAPY IN DIALYSIS: GUIDELINES FOR SELECTION

Clinical Situation	Preferred	Requires Special Monitoring	Relatively or Absolutely Contraindicated
Angina pectoris	β-Blockers, calcium antagonists,	—	Direct vasodilators
Post-myocardial infarction	Non-ISA β-blockers	—	Direct vasodilators
Hypertrophic cardiomyopathy with diastolic dysfunction	β-Blockers, diltiazem, verapamil	—	Direct vasodilators, α_1-blockers
Bradycardia, heart block, sick sinus syndrome		—	β-Blockers, labetalol, verapamil, diltiazem
Heart failure (decreased LV ejection fraction)	ACE inhibitors	—	β-Blockers, labetalol, calcium-antagonists (except amlodipine?)
Peripheral vascular disease		—	β-Blockers
Diabetes mellitus	ACE inhibitors, calcium antagonists	—	β-Blockers, labetalol
Asthma/COPD			β-Blockers, labetalol
Cyclosporine-induced hypertension	Nifedipine, labetalol	Nicadipine,[a] verapamil,[a] diltiazem[a]	
Liver disease		Labetalol	Methyldopa
Erythropoietin-induced hypertension	Calcium antagonists	ACE inhibitors	

[a]May increase serum levels of cyclosporine.
ACE, angiotensin-converting enzyme; COPD, chronic obstructive pulmonary disease; ISA, intrinsic sympathomimetic activity; LV, left ventricular.

Patient Demographics

Patients who are less likely to comply with the antihypertensive regimen, either because of their lifestyle or because of poor intellectual capacity to adhere to a therapeutic regimen, should be treated preferentially with long-acting agents that can be administered once daily or, even better, once weekly.

Certain antihypertensive agents, such as β-blockers and centrally acting antiadrenergic agents, may affect mental acuity and physical strength and should be avoided in patients who perform activities requiring alertness, mental acuity, or strenuous physical feats. In these instances, drugs such as ACE inhibitors or calcium channel blockers, which have little impact on mental or physical performance, are preferred.

Antiadrenergic drugs are more likely to cause sexual dysfunction, an important consideration when managing dialysis patients because 50% have significant impotence as a result of uremia.

Cost

The cost of therapy, not only of the drugs themselves, should be taken into consideration in choosing antihypertensive agents. ACE inhibitors and calcium antagonists are more expensive than β-blockers or some antiadrenergic agents. When a less expensive agent is efficacious and free of undesirable side effects, it should be preferred, particularly for financially deprived patients. The physician must remember that the excessive cost of drugs may limit the patient's compliance and thus affect the long-term control of the patient's hypertension.

Coexisting Disease

The presence of concomitant diseases should also guide the physician in the choice of antihypertensive drugs. For example, β-blockers should not be used in patients with asthma or with peripheral vascular disease, because these conditions can be aggravated by the administration of these drugs.

Patients with coronary artery disease, previous myocardial infarction, arrhythmias, hyperdynamic circulation, nervousness, and migraine headaches should be preferentially treated with β-blockers or calcium antagonists. However, these latter patients should avoid vasodilators such as hydralazine or minoxidil, which activate the SNS. Similarly, because of their vasodilator action on the coronary arteries, calcium antagonists are preferred in patients with coronary artery disease.

Patients with type-1 diabetes mellitus should not be treated with nonselective β-blockers, because they may aggravate the control of diabetes and may mask the usual signs of hypoglycemia in patients with diabetes and autonomic dysfunction. Antiadrenergic agents that are more likely to cause or aggravate orthostatic hypotension should be avoided.

Patients with dyslipidemia should be preferentially treated with agents that do not alter the lipid profile, such as calcium antagonists and ACE inhibitors, or with agents that may actually improve the lipid profile, such as the α_1-receptor blockers.

Dialysis in the Treatment of Hypertension in ESRD Patients

In patients with renal failure, the metabolism and disposition of antihypertensive drugs are abnormal and may result in accumulation of the intact drug or of its metabolites and in more frequent untoward effects. Furthermore, some drugs are more easily removed with dialysis than others. In general, water-soluble drugs are removed with dialysis more readily than are lipid-soluble agents. Postdialysis hypertension is more commonly observed in patients taking dialyzable drugs, because the removal of drugs with dialysis may result in sudden decrease in blood levels and in hypertensive rebounds. It is for these reasons that the choice of antihypertensive drugs in the dialysis patient requires knowledge of the pharmacodynamic and pharmacokinetic properties of these agents.

Use of Antihypertensive Drugs in ESRD Patients

We describe in this section some of the principal pharmacologic differences among the groups of antihypertensive agents and the usual doses of administration (Tables 16.7 to 16.9).

Calcium Antagonists

Intracellular calcium exerts critical functions in the regulation of the CV system. Calcium regulates the excitation-contraction coupling in smooth muscle cells, the activity of cardiac pacemaker cells, and atrioventricular (AV) conduction. In addition, intracellular calcium regulates the secretion of several pressor or depressor hormones, such as catecholamines, renin, aldosterone, and prostaglandins. Several membrane channels and pumps regulate the movement of calcium from the extracellular to the intracellular compartment or vice versa. The various calcium channels are structurally different and have different affinities for different calcium channel antagonists. Calcium channel antagonists primarily inhibit the voltage-dependent calcium channels. This results in reduced movement of calcium across vascular smooth muscle and cardiac cells and inhibition of the excitation-contraction process.

The chemical structure of these agents varies. Nifedipine is a dihydropyridine derivative, whereas verapamil is structurally similar to papaverine and diltiazem to the benzodiazepines. Several classifications for these agents have been proposed, but the division into type I and type II agents are the most often used. Type I refers to the dihydropyridines such as nifedipine, felodipine, amlodipine, nitrendipine, nimodipine, isradipine, nisoldipine, nilvadipine, and some others still under investigation. Type II agents include diltiazem, which is structurally related to the benzodiazepines, and verapamil, which is structurally similar to papaverine (Table 16.7).

Calcium antagonists lower BP by interfering with calcium-dependent contraction of VSMCs and reducing peripheral vascular resistance. As a result of their negative inotropic action, verapamil and diltiazem may lower BP in part by reducing cardiac output. The dihydropyridine derivatives have a more selective action on peripheral VSMCs and, thereby, are more likely

TABLE 16.7. PHARMACOKINETIC PROPERTIES OF ANTIHYPERTENSIVE AGENTS IN PATIENTS WITH END-STAGE RENAL FAILURE

Dialysis	Oral Bioavailability (%)	Protein Binding (%)	T½ (hours) Normal	T½ (hours) (ESRD)	Renal Excretion of Unchanged Drug (% dose)	Dose Change with ESRD	Removal with Dialysis Hemo	Removal with Dialysis Peritoneal	Active Hemo Metabolites
Antiadrenergic Agents									
Clonidine	75	20–40	5–13	17–40	50	↓ (50–75%)	5%	?	No
Guanabenz	40	40	50–100	83–323	Small	↓ (Yes)	None	None	No
Guanethidine	5–60	0	48–72	Prolonged	30–50	↓ (Yes)	None	None	Slight
Guanfacine	100	65	15–20	Slightly increased	30–50	↓ (Yes lowered dose)	None	None	No
Methyldopa	26–74	<20	1–2	1.7–3.6	50	12–24%	60%	30–40	Yes
Monoxidine	90	7–9	1.7–3.5	3.2–10.6	55–65	50%			
Rilmenidine	100	7–8	7–9	31–37	60–70	50%			
α-Adrenergic Blocking Agents									
Doxazosin	60–70	98–99	10–15	10–15	9	None	None	NA	Yes/None
Guanadrel	70–80	20	3–5	10–30	40–50	↓	?	NA	
Prazosin	48–68	97	2.5–4.0	2.5–4.0	<10		None	None	None
Terazosin	80–90	90–94	10–15	10–15	40	None	?	NA	None
Urapidil	70–75	79–82	2–5	5–8	10–15	None	None	None	Yes
β-Adrenergic Blocking Agents									
Acebutolol	50	30	3.5	3.5	40	↓ 70%	50%	?	Yes
Atenolol	50	<5	6–9	<120	85–100	↓ 75%	53%	48%	No
Betaxolol	89 ± 5	50	14–22	28–44	15	50%	None	None	No
Bisoprolol	80–90	30	10–12	20–25	45–55	50%	None	None	No
Carteolol	80–85	20–30	5–7	30–40	55–65	25%	NA	NA	Yes
Carvedilol	25	95	4–7	4–7	2	None	None	None	Yes
Cetamolol	—		6–8	10–12	30–40	33%	NA	NA	NA
Esmolol	—	55	7.2	7.1	2	None	None	None	Slight
Labetalol IV	NA	50	5.5	5.5	50–60	Smaller doses work	<1%	<1%	No
Labetalol PO	33	50	3–4	3–4	20–40	Slight ↓	<1%	<1%	No
La-propranolol	20	90	10	10	<1	Slight ↓	None	None	Yes
Metoprolol	40–50	12	3–4	3–4	13	None	High	?	Slight
Nadolol	30	30	14–24	45	70	50% ↓	High	?	Yes
Pindolol	90	57	2–3	2–3	40	Slight ↓	Probable	?	No
Propranolol	30	90	2–4	2–4	<1	Slight ↓	None	None	Yes
Timolol	75	10	4–6	4–6	20	Slight ↓	?	?	No
ACE Inhibitors									
Alacepril			4–6	15–20		↓			
Benazepril	37	97	10–11	Prolonged	1	Yes ↓[b]	None		
Captopril	75	30	2–3	20–30	30–40	Yes[b]	Yes	?	No
Cilazapril	77	2–3	4–6	65–85	25%	Yes			
Delapril	55	0.5		2	?				Yes
Enalapril	60	High	11	Prolonged	70	Yes[b]	35%	?	Yes
Fosinopril	36	95	12	Prolonged	Negligible	None	2	7	Yes
Lisinopril	25–30	3–10	12.7	54.3	29	↓ 75%	50%	?	No
Moexipril	13	2–9						Yes	
Pentopril	50	0.7–1.0	No change	20–25					
Pentoprilat		2–3	10–14	35–45		↓			
Perindopril	66			78	Yes				
Quinapril	60	97	2–3	Prolonged	5–6	NA	NA	NA	Yes
Ramipril	54–65	73	10.8	Prolonged	2	50%	Yes	?	Yes
Trandolapril	10	80	6	12	33	50%			Yes
Zofenopril	96	80–85	5–6	10	5	50%			
Vasodilators									
Diazoxide	Low	85	20–36	Prolonged	50	None	Yes	Yes	?
Hydralazine	10–30	90	2–4	Prolonged	10	Yes, slight ↓	NA	None	No
Minoxidil	95	Minimal	2.8–4.2	4.2	10	None	Yes	Yes	No
Nitroprusside	0	?	3–4 min	Prolonged	High	None	Yes	Yes	No
Calcium Channel Blockers									
Amlodipine	60–70	97	30–50	10%	<1	None	NA	NA	?
Diltiazem	20	80	α: 20 h (β: — 4 H)	Unchanged	35	None	?	?	No
Felodipine	15–20	97	10–20	<0.5%	<0.5	None			
Isradipine	15–20	96	8–12	Unchanged	<5				
Lercanidipine hydrochloride	6%	>98%	8–10	?	44%	NA	?	?	No
Nicardipine	6–30 (dose dependent)	98–99	3–6	Unchanged	<5	Decreased			No
Nifedipine	65	90	α: 2.5–3.0 h β: 5 h	Unchanged	70–80	None	Low	Low	No
Nilvadipine	15	85–90	10–13	<5					
Nimodipine	6–10	98	1–1.5	<1					No
Nisoldipine	8–10	98–99	1.0–1.5	<1	None				No
Nitrendipine	10–30	98	1.0–1.5	<1	None				No

TABLE 16.7. (CONTINUED)

Dialysis	Oral Bioavailability (%)	Protein Binding (%)	T½ (hours) Normal	T½ (hours) (ESRD)	Renal Excretion of Unchanged Drug (% dose)	Dose Change with ESRD	Removal with Dialysis Hemo	Removal with Dialysis Peritoneal	Active Hemo Metabolites
Verapamil	10–32	90	α: 15–30 h β: 3–7 hª	α: 4.5 (β: 2.3 h)ª3	3–4%	? (none)	None	Yes	Yes
Angiotensin II Inhibitor									
Candesartan Cilexetil	15	>99	9	?	26%	Yes ↓	None	?	No
Eprosartan	13	98	5–9	?	IV 37% Oral 7%	None	Poorly	No	No
Losartan	33	98.70	2	4	4	None	None	None	Yes
Olmesartan Medoxomil	26–28	?	10–15	?	35–50%	?	?	?	Olmesartan
Telmisartan	42–58	>99.5	24	?	0.49–0.91	None	None	?	No
Virsartan	10–35	95	6	?	13	?	None	None	No
Irbesartan	60–80	90	11–15	11–15	20	None	None	None	No

ACE, angiotensin-converting enzyme; NA, not applicable.
ªα, initial fast T½; β, late slow T½.
ᵇMaximum dose is same. Start with lower dose (50% ↓); it usually works.

TABLE 16.8. USUAL DOSAGE OF ANTIHYPERTENSIVE DRUGS IN DIALYSIS SUBJECTS

Drug	Dosage (mg/day)	Doses/Day	Mechanisms of Action	Special Considerations
ACE Inhibitors				
Benazepril	5–20	1	Block conversion of angiotensin I to angiotensin II. Decrease aldosterone. May increase bradykinin and vasodilatory prostaglandins. Decrease SVR. CO =.	When added to diuretics may cause hypotension. May cause hyperkalemia in patients with renal failure, those with hypoaldosteronism, in those receiving K-sparing diuretics or NSAIDs. Can cause acute renal failure in patients with bilateral renal artery stenosis, renal artery stenosis of a solitary kidney, creatinine >3 mg/dL, or severe CHF, contraindicated in pregnancy.
Captopril	12.5–50	2		
Cilazapril	1.25–2.5	1–2		
Enalapril	2.5–10	1–2		
Fosinopril	10–40	1–2		
Lisinopril	2.5–10	1		
Moexipril	7.5–30	1–2		
Perindopril	0.25–4	1–2		
Quinapril	2.5–20	1–2		
Ramipril	1.25–10	1–2		
Spirapril	6.25–25	1–2		
Trandolapril	1–4	1		
Angiotensin II Blockers				
Losartan	25–50	1	Block the vasoconstrictor and aldosterone secreting effects of angiotensin II by selectively blocking the binding of angiotensin II to the AT-1 receptor.	If severe renal impairment, and/or volume depletion, reduce dose.
Valsartan	80–320			
Irbesartan	150–300			
Calcium Antagonists				
Diltiazem	90–360	3	Block the entry of calcium into smooth muscle cells, causing vasodilation. Decrease SVR. CO =.	Inhibit slow calcium channels in the heart resulting in decreased heart rate. May cause heart block, particularly when combined with β-blockers.
Diltiazem SR	120–360	2		
Diltiazem (extended release)	180–360	1		
Verapamil	80–480	2		
Verapamil (long-acting)	120–480	1		
Dihydropiridines				
Amlodipine	2.5–10	1	Same as diltiazem and verapamil. May increase heart rate and CO.	More potent vasodilators than dilitiazem and verapamil. May cause dizziness, headache, tachycardia, flushing, edema.
Felodipine	5–20	2		
Isradipine	2.5–10	2		
Nicardipine	60–120	3		
Nifedipine	30–120	3		
Nifedipine (GITS)	30–120	1		

Continued on next page

TABLE 16.8. (CONTINUED)

Drug	Dosage (mg/day)	Doses/Day	Mechanisms of Action	Special Considerations
Adrenergic Inhibitors				
β-Blockers				
Cardioselective				
Atenolol	25–100	1	Inhibit β_1 receptors. Decrease CO; increase SVR; decrease PRA.	In higher doses will also inhibit β_2 receptors.
Betaxolol	10–20	1		
Carvedilol	12.5–50	1		
Metoprolol	50–200	1–2		
Noncardioselective				
Nadolol	20–120	1	Inhibit β_1 and β_2 receptors.	More likely to cause metabolic side effects.
Propranolol	40–240	1–2		
Timolol	20–40	2		
With Intrinsic Sympathomimetic Activity (ISA)				
Acebutolol	200–1,200	2	Have partial agonistic activity on β-adrenergic receptors. Decrease SVR; CO remains unchanged.	No clear advantage except for less bradycardia. Cause less metabolic side effects than other β-blockers.
Carteolol	2–10	1		
Penbutolol	20–80	1		
Pindolol	10–6	2		
α-β Blockers				
Labetalol	200–1,200	2	Same as blockers plus α-blockade. Decrease SVR; CO remains unchanged.	May cause postural hypotension. Causes less metabolic side effects.
Antiadrenergic Agents				
Centrally Acting				
Clonidine	0.1–0.6	2	Stimulate α_2-adrenergic receptors in the brainstem resulting in inhibitions of efferent sympathetic activity. Decrease SVR.	Sudden withdrawal may result in hypertensive crisis.
Clonidine TTS	0.1–0.3	once per week		
Guanabenz	4–64	2		
Guanfacine	1–3	1		
Methyldopa	250–2,500	2		
Peripherally Acting				
Guanadrel	10–75	2	Inhibit norepinephrine release from sympathetic nerve terminals. Decrease SVR.	Frequently cause orthostatic hypotension and sexual dysfunction.
Guanethidine	10–100	1		
Reserpine	0.05–0.25	1	Depletion of norepinephrine storages. Decrease SVR.	Causes frequent neurologic side effects.
α_1-Receptor Blockers				
Doxazosin	2–16	1	Inhibit α-adrenergic receptors. Decrease SVR. CO = or increases.	"First-dose" effect. Postural hypotension. Useful for prostatic hypertrophy.
Prazosin	2–20	1–2		
Terazosin	1–20	1		
Direct Vasodilators				
Hydralazine	50–200	2–4	Direct relaxation of smooth muscle cells, causing arteriolar vasodilation. Decrease SVR, increase CO.	Limited efficacy if given alone due to fluid retention and reflex tachycardia. Should be combined with a diuretic and a β-blocker.
Minoxidil	2.5–40	1		
Lecarnidipine				Contraindicated in patients with CrCl <10 mL/min.
Olmesartan Medoxomil	20–40 mg	1	Angiotensin type II blocker.	Pharmacokinetics in patients undergoing HD not studied.
Candesartan	max 8 mg	1	Angiotensin type II blocker.	Hemodynamic effects pronounced during HD due to volume.
Cilexetil				Contraction.
Eprosartan	200–300	2	Angiotensin type II blocker.	No initial dosage adjustment.
Telmisartan	40–80	1	Angiotensin type II blocker.	

The = sign indicates no changes.
CHF, congestive heart failure; CO, cardiac output; GITS, gastrointestinal therapeutic system; HD, hemodialysis; NSAIDs, nonsteroidal antiinflammatory drugs; PRA, plasma renin activity; SVR, systemic vascular resistance.

to cause reflex stimulation of the SNS and tachycardia (see later).

Dihydropyridine-derivative calcium channel blockers have usually been shown to raise SNS activity. However, studies have shown that N-type calcium channel blockers, such as cilnidipine may actually inhibit SNS activity. Cilnidipine inhibits the increase in BP and plasma NE levels in response to cold stress and to electrical sympathetic neurotransmission in pithed spontaneously hypertensive rats (SHR) (219). Cilnidipine also attenuated the decrease in renal blood flow and in urinary sodium excretion caused by renal nerve stimulation in anesthetized dogs (220).

TABLE 16.9. MOST COMMON SIDE EFFECTS AND PRECAUTIONS IN THE USE OF ANTIHYPERTENSIVE DRUGS IN DIALYSIS SUBJECTS

Drugs	Common Side Effects	Precautions and Special Considerations
ACE Inhibitors	Cough, skin rash, angioneurotic edema, hyperkalemia, dysgeusia. Rarely can cause neutropenia.	Hypotension may occur in patients receiving diuretics or with CHF.
Angiotensin II Blockers Losartan	Hyperkalemia in patients with renal failure.	Hypotension may occur in patients receiving diuretics or with CHF.
Calcium Antagonists Dihydropiridines Amlodipine Felodipine Isradipine Nicardipine Nifedipine	Headache, dizziness, peripheral edema, tachycardia, gingival hyperplasia, flushing, nausea.	Have mild negative inotropic action and should be used with caution in CHF. Amlodipine may improve exercise tolerance in patients with class 1–2 CHF treated with diuretics, digitalis, and ACE inhibitors.
Diltiazem and Verapamil	Headache, dizziness, gingival hyperplasia, constipation (particularly verapamil), bradycardia, AV block, peripheral edema (less common than with the dihydropiridines).	Should not be used in patients with sick sinus syndrome, second- or third-degree heart block, and low left ventricular ejection fraction. May be beneficial in patients with diastolic heart failure.
Direct Vasodilators Hydralazine Minoxidil	Headache, tachycardia, and angina. May cause positive antinuclear antibody test. Hypertrichosis, pericardial effusion, increased salt and water retention between dialysis.	May precipitate angina and myocardial infarction in patients with coronary artery disease. Should be combined with a β-blocker or ACE inhibitor.
Antiadrenergic Agents Centrally acting Clonidine Guanabenz Guanfacine	Drowsiness, sedation, dry mouth, fatigue, orthostatic hypotension.	Rebound hypertension may occur when these drugs are abruptly discontinued and especially when given in combination with β-blockers.
Clonidine TTS (patch)	Same as for clonidine. May cause skin rash at the site of the patch.	
Methyldopa	Same as for clonidine.	May cause liver damage, Coombs-positive hemolytic anemia, fever.
Peripherally Acting α₁-Receptor Blockers	"First-dose phenomenon." Orthostatic hypotension, syncope, palpitations, headache, nausea, diarrhea.	Use with caution in patients with autonomic dysfunction, and in elderly patients because of orthostatic hypotension. May decrease LDL and increase HDL.
Guanethidine Guanadrel	Orthostatic hypotension, impotence, diarrhea.	Can cause severe orthostatic hypotension.
Reserpine	Lethargy, depression, nasal congestion.	Contraindicated in patients with history of mental depression and peptic ulcer.
β-Blockers	Bronchospasm, fatigue, insomnia, Raynaud's phenomenon, may aggravate peripheral arterial insufficiency, may aggravate hypoglycemia and mask the symptoms of hypoglycemia in insulin-dependent diabetes (IDDM), sick sinus syndrome, peripheral vascular disease. If discontinued abruptly, may precipitate myocardial infarction.	Avoid in patients with asthma, CHF, chronic obstructive pulmonary disease (COPD), heart block greater than first-degree; increase triglycerides, decrease HDL.
α-β-Blockers Labetalol	Same as β-blockers. Orthostatic hypotension.	Same as β-blockers.

ACE, angiotensin-converting enzyme; AV, arteriovenous; CHF, congestive heart failure; HDL, high-density lipoprotein; LDL, low-density lipoprotein.

The dihydropyridines have a significant hepatic first-pass effect, and their bioavailability is between 6% and 30%. Less than 1% of felodipine, nisoldipine, nitrendipine, and nimodipine and approximately 10% of the other dihydropyridines is excreted unchanged in the urine. Therefore, these drugs may be used in dialysis patients without any change in dose or frequency of administration. Because of their poor water solubility, high protein binding, and large volume of distribution, the dihydropyridines are not significantly cleared by HD, eliminating the need for a supplementary postdialysis dose. The dihydropyridines form many metabolites, all of which are inactive. The type 2 calcium channel antagonists are also poorly excreted by the kidneys and require no dose adjustment in patients with renal failure on maintenance dialysis.

Some calcium channel antagonists may provide the advantage of treating comorbid conditions, in addition to their primary antihypertensive efficacy. For example, verapamil, and to a lesser extent diltiazem, may prolong AV conduction and are thereby useful in the treatment of supraventricular tachycardia. Verapamil is useful for the prophylaxis of migraine. Nicardipine and nimodipine appear to have more selective action on the cerebral circulation and to be useful in the setting of cerebrovascular accidents. Some studies have shown that these drugs may prevent ischemia-induced mitochondrial overload of calcium during reperfusion. As a result of peripheral vasodilation, dihydropyridines may reduce the incidence of Raynaud's phenomenon. Experimental evidence indicates that calcium channel antagonists may inhibit the progression of atherosclerosis; however, the clinical significance of these observations remains to be established.

Dihydropyridine-derivative calcium channel blockers have usually been shown to raise SNS activity. However, studies have shown that N-type calcium channel blockers, such as cilnidipine, may actually inhibit SNS activity. Cilnidipine inhibits the increase in BP and plasma NE levels in response to cold stress and to electrical sympathetic neurotransmission in pithed SHR (219). Cilnidipine also attenuated the decrease in renal blood flow and in urinary sodium excretion caused by renal nerve stimulation in anesthetized dogs (220).

Calcium channel blockers are usually well tolerated. The dihydropyridines are more likely to cause flushing, headache, tachycardia, ankle edema, and nausea. Verapamil is more likely to cause conduction disturbances, bradycardia, and constipation. Because verapamil and diltiazem have negative inotropic and chronotropic actions, caution should be used when combining these agents with β-blockers, because CHF and severe, life-threatening conduction defects may occur.

Nifedipine capsules should not be used for the management of hypertensive crisis or severe hypertension because of increased risk of myocardial infarction and stroke. The practice of using this agent in dialysis patients presenting with "higher than usual" BP or in patients whose BP rises during dialysis should be abandoned.

Calcium channel blockers do not increase PTH levels, and determination of vitamin D metabolites reveals no change in 1,25-dihydroxy vitamin D levels. Levels of 25-hydroxy vitamin D are significantly elevated, likely because of reduced cytosolic calcium stimulating α-hydroxylase activity in the hepatocyte.

Converting Enzyme Inhibitors

The CEI class of antihypertensive agents inhibits kininase II (ACE), thereby reducing the conversion of angiotensin I to angiotensin II.

The first ACE inhibitor was isolated from the venom of the Brazilian arrowhead viper, *Bothrops jararaca*. Since then, literally hundreds of ACE inhibitors have been isolated, and several of them have already reached the American market. CEIs can be classified into three main chemical categories: sulfhydryl-, carboxyl-, and phosphoryl-containing compounds (221):

Sulfhydryl Agents. The sulfhydryl agents are prodrugs, which in vivo are converted to captopril. Examples are alacepril, delapril, and moveltopril. These newer sulfhydryl-containing compounds have a slower onset and longer duration of action than captopril. Zofenopril has greater potency and is partially eliminated by the liver.

Carboxyl Agents. The carboxyl-containing CEIs (of which enalapril is an example) are prodrugs converted in vivo to the active metabolite. The kidney, with the exception of spirapril that is totally eliminated by the liver, principally excretes them. Benazepril has an earlier peak time and a slightly shorter terminal half-life than enalapril. Delapril, quinapril, trandolapril, and spirapril have an earlier peak time and shorter half-life, whereas perindopril has a peak time and half-life similar to enalapril. Lisinopril is an enalapril-like diacid, which is not a prodrug, and has poor oral bioavailability (30%).

Phosphoryl Agents. The last class of CEIs, the phosphoryl-containing group comprises fosinopril, a drug that is partially eliminated by the liver and does not require dose adjustment in patients with renal failure.

ACE inhibitors diminish the circulating levels of angiotensin II and aldosterone, and, as a result of reduction of the negative feedback of angiotensin II on renin secretion, they increase PRA. To the extent that the maintenance of BP depends on the renin angiotensin system, ACE inhibitors reduce BP. This explains the greater antihypertensive efficacy of these agents in patients with increased PRA, although they are also effective, but to a lesser extent, in patients with low PRA. The reason for their efficacy in patients with low PRA is less clear, but it may be due to tissue inhibition of angiotensin II formation. In addition, because kininase II also blocks the degradation of kinin, the antihypertensive action of these drugs may depend in part on increased levels of bradykinin at the tissue level.

CEIs decrease peripheral vascular resistance without increasing heart rate, cardiac output, pulmonary wedge pressure, and without reflex activation of the SNS. To the contrary, treatment with enalapril normalized BP and muscle sympathetic nerve activity in patients with CRF. By contrast, amlodipine treatment also lowered BP but increased muscle sympathetic nerve activity (107). Cerebral blood flow usually remains unchanged.

Side Effects

Captopril, the first ACE inhibitor to reach the market, was initially associated with a high incidence of side effects, in large part resulting from the high doses that were initially used. Also, captopril contains a sulfhydryl group, which increases the frequency of side effects that are not present in other ACE inhibitors. Side effects such as cough, skin rash, angioedema, dysgeusia, and leukopenia are still reported with most of these agents. Neutropenia and agranulocytosis may appear after 3 to 12 weeks of therapy, particularly in patients with autoimmune collagen vascular diseases.

Another notable side effect is the worsening of anemia in dialysis patients. In patients with CRF, CEIs may aggravate anemia. This is not associated with decreased levels of erythropoietin or increased hemolysis, but it appears to be related to a direct or indirect interference of angiotensin II with the signal transduction of erythropoietin at the cellular level.

Because angiotensin II may stimulate thirst, ACE inhibitors may reduce thirst, oral fluid intake, and interdialytic weight gain.

Of particular interest is the report of anaphylactic reactions in dialysis patients treated with ACE inhibitors. Specifically, this phenomenon has been observed in the setting of patients treated with CEIs while undergoing dialysis with a high-flux (AN 69) capillary dialyzer. Symptoms may range from mild edema of the mucosa of the eyes to nausea and vomiting, bronchospasm, hypotension, and angioedema (222).

Angiotensin II Receptor Antagonists

Saralasin was the first competitive antagonist of angiotensin II to be discovered and introduced in the market for the treatment of hypertensive emergencies. This agent has had limited clinical use in the management of hypertension because it can only be administered intravenously, has a very short half-life, and is a partial agonist.

Losartan (DuP 753), a derivative of imidazole, was the first orally active and highly specific antagonist of angiotensin II receptor with vasodilator and antihypertensive activity to be introduced into the market (223).

Subsequently, several other angiotensin II receptor blockers have been introduced in the U.S. market including valsartan, irbesartan, candesartan, telmisartan, eprosartan, and olmesartan (224).

The mechanism of antihypertensive action of these drugs appears to be due to inhibition of the renin-angiotensin system. We have recently shown that when injected in the lateral ventricle, losartan normalizes BP and SNS activity in CRF rats (117). These studies suggest that locally produced angiotensin II in the brain may mediate the central activation of the SNS caused by renal injury.

Because losartan does not affect the activity of kininase II, it does not appear to cause cough, a well-known adverse effect of ACE inhibitors. Losartan has a half-life of 1.5 hours; the active metabolite has a longer half-life of 9 hours. Losartan blocks angiotensin II-induced responses. The antihypertensive activity of losartan is comparable to that of ACE inhibitors when given in doses of 50 to 100 mg once daily. To date the drug appears to be well tolerated.

Molecular techniques have identified at least two angiotensin II receptor subtypes: AT_1 and AT_2 (225–227). Losartan and valsartan are selective AT_1 antagonists; AT_1 receptors mediate the vasoconstriction of resistance vessels. Stimulation of AT_2 receptors produces vasodilation, inhibits cell proliferation, increases apoptosis and cell differentiation, and regulates pressure-natriuresis (228–230). The AT_2 receptor is highly expressed during fetal life and to a lesser extent in a few selected organs in adults (heart, adrenal medulla, uterus, brain). Mice with AT_2 gene disruption that do not express the AT_2 receptor are hypersensitive to angiotensin II, suggesting that AT_2 stimulation opposes the vasoconstrictor effect of angiotensin II (231). Several types of nonpeptidergic AT-receptor antagonists are now being developed, including selective AT_2 antagonists (e.g., PD 123177). DuP 753 has approximately 10,000-fold selectivity for the AT_1 receptor, whereas PD 123177 is about 3,500 times more specific for the AT_2 receptor.

Potential Beneficial Effect of Drugs that Inhibit the Renin-Angiotensin-Aldosterone (RAA) System on Cardiovascular Diseases Independent of Blood Pressure

Angiotensin II stimulates the production of a variety of growth factors and of collagen (232,233). Conversely, drugs that inhibit the RAA system appear to prevent accumulation of collagen in the aorta and to reduce arterial stiffness (234). The effects of ACE inhibitors on arterial stiffness appear to be independent of effects on BP, because the nonspecific vasodilator hydralazine had no effects on arterial stiffness despite similar reduction in BP.

Large-scale clinical trials are needed to ascertain whether these pharmacologic effects will translate into clinical benefits. So far, the evidence that drugs that inhibit the renin angiotensin system may provide clinical advantages on the CV system independent of antihypertensive effects is inconclusive. The HOPE study in patients at high risk for CV events compared the effects of administration of an ACE inhibitor versus placebo on CV events. Patients who received ramipril manifested a 27% risk reduction of overall CV events compared with patients that received placebo. In this study, however, it is practically impossible to exclude the possibility that the observed benefits were due to BP reduction rather than to inhibition of the RAA (235).

By contrast, the LIFE study, which compared the effects of losartan and atenolol on CV morbidity and mortality, demonstrated that losartan was more effective than atenolol in reducing CV morbidity and mortality in patients with hypertension, diabetes, and LVH, and these effects appeared to be independent of BP (236).

Experimental studies have also shown that angiotensin II may influence atherosclerosis by actions on endothelial function, activation of adhesion molecule and cytokines, monocyte activation and binding, VSMC proliferation and migration, and oxidation of low-density lipoprotein (LDL) (237–242). Both ACE inhibitors and angiotensin receptor blockers may prevent atherosclerosis (243–246). The clinical relevance of these observations remains to be established.

A prospective study on a cohort of 150 ESRD patients followed for up to 136 months has demonstrated that survival in these patients was positively associated with ACE inhibitor use (53).

β-Adrenergic Blocking Agents

In the past, β-blockers in combination with vasodilators were extensively used in the management of hypertension in patients with CRF, based on the notion that these agents would, at least in part, reduce BP by inhibiting renin secretion. Since the advent of ACE inhibitors and calcium channel blockers, however, the use of these drugs in the management of hypertensive patients with renal failure has decreased. More recent studies have demonstrated that β-blockers may improve survival in patients with coronary artery disease as well as in patients with CHF (247). Based on these studies, and given the very high prevalence of coronary heart disease and CHF among dialysis patients, the use of these agents has received renewed interest.

The mechanisms of action of β-blockers are not well established. They reduce heart rate, myocardial contractility, AV conduction time, and automaticity, so their antihypertensive action may be, at least in part, due to reduction of cardiac output. Peripheral vascular resistances initially rise, presumably because of inhibition of β-receptors, which mediate vasodilatation and unopposed stimulation of α-receptors or to stimulation of the

SNS as a secondary adaptive response to a fall in cardiac output. After prolonged therapy, some studies found a persistent increase of peripheral vascular resistance; others found a decrease in peripheral vascular resistance in those patients in whom BP fell.

β-Blockers may reduce PRA, and some studies have shown a relationship between hypotensive action and pretreatment renin or degree of renin suppression (248,249). Other studies suggest that renin suppression is not a major mechanism of action, because patients with low renin also respond to β-blockers, and agents such as pindolol may effectively lower BP without decreasing PRA (250). Moreover, the hypotensive action of β-blockers reaches its peak after several days of treatment, whereas the decrease in plasma renin occurs more rapidly.

Some have postulated that after penetration in the CNS, β-blockers inhibit the sympathetic discharge from the CNS (251). Infusion of propranolol directly into the cerebral ventricle of dogs caused a fall in BP in direct proportion to the increase in NE in the cerebrospinal fluid. This mechanism, however, does not appear to be essential for the antihypertensive action of β-blockers; predominantly hydrosoluble agents such as atenolol, with little penetrance into the brain, exert equal antihypertensive action (252). In addition, β-blockers usually increase plasma levels of catecholamines, rather than decreasing them, as one would expect from a reduction of sympathetic outflow from the brain.

A large number of β-adrenergic blocking agents with differing pharmacodynamic and pharmacokinetic properties are available (Table 16.7). The most important pharmacologic differences among these agents are lipid solubility, intrinsic sympathomimetic activity (ISA), and selectivity for β₁-adrenergic receptors (cardioselectivity):

1. Lipid solubility. The degree of lipid solubility affects both CNS penetration and the extent of hepatic metabolism. High lipid solubility results in both more CNS side effects, as well as more extensive hepatic metabolism. For example, propranolol, acebutolol, and metoprolol are well absorbed from the small intestine, but, because of extensive first-pass metabolism by the liver, only 30% to 50% of these drugs reach the systemic circulation. The concomitant use of drugs that affect hepatic blood flow may further reduce the bioavailability of these β-blockers. Conversely, atenolol, acebutolol, and nadolol, agents with low degrees of lipid solubility, are primarily renally excreted. Accumulation of β-blockers with low lipid solubility may result in excessive bradycardia. Consequently, the dose of most liposoluble agents needs not be adjusted, and the dose of agents with low lipid solubility should be adjusted in patients with renal failure.
2. Cardioselectivity. The second important characteristic distinguishing these agents is cardioselectivity. Cardioselectivity is considered a property of limited clinical relevance with respect to the antihypertensive efficacy but is of considerable importance with respect to side effects. Cardioselective β-blockers are less likely to cause bronchospasm, Raynaud's phenomenon, or disturbances of lipid and carbohydrate metabolism. The β₁-selective β-blockers include atenolol, metoprolol, and acebutolol.

3. ISA. The third characteristic of β-blockers worthy of note is ISA. Pindolol, and to a lesser degree acebutolol, have ISA. These agents have a dual action of both blocking and directly stimulating β-adrenoreceptors. Hemodynamically, this results not only in decreased peripheral vascular resistance but also in less pronounced reductions in heart rate, cardiac output, and plasma renin secretion.

β-Blockers are particularly useful in the treatment of hypertension in patients with angina or arrhythmias and are the drugs of choice in patients with a history of a previous myocardial infarction. Studies have shown a 25% decrease in recurrence of myocardial infarction in patients treated with β-blockers. The DOPPS study has shown that the use of β-blockers in dialysis patients with hypertension and coronary heart disease reduces mortality by 9% and 13%, respectively (253).

β-Blockers, and particularly carvedilol, have been shown to reduce mortality in patients with heart failure (254), In ESRD patients with CHF and dilated cardiomyopathy, carvedilol reduced LV volumes and function and improved clinical status (255).

With the exception of β-blockers that are renally excreted (i.e., not highly lipid soluble), most β-blockers do not require dose adjustment in dialysis patients. Atenolol and nadolol are removed in significant amounts by HD and, thus, should be administered after dialysis.

Side Effects

Simultaneous administration of β-blockers and calcium channel blockers must be avoided in patients with CRF. This is to avoid an increase of the negative inotropic effect each of these agents exerts on the heart. Similarly, administration of cyclooxygenase inhibitors should be avoided because they may antagonize the antihypertensive effect of β-blockers. Hypotensive episodes during HD may occur more frequently with the use of β-blockers as a result of a blunting of reflex tachycardia.

The most frequent side effects of β-blockers are bradycardia, muscular fatigue, tiredness, AV blocks, sick-sinus syndrome, heart failure, cold extremities, and Raynaud's phenomenon. Bradycardia and heart failure are less likely to occur with β-blockers with ISA.

β-Blockers increase serum triglycerides and decrease high-density lipoproteins (HDL), but they do not significantly affect serum levels of LDL cholesterol. β-Blockers with ISA, however, cause little or no increase in triglycerides.

β-Blockers can cause several CNS symptoms, including insomnia, nightmares, hallucinations, and depression. Because β-blockers increase the number of receptor sites on VSMCs, caution must be exercised when these drugs are to be withdrawn, because of the possibility of coronary artery spasm or arrhythmias.

Simultaneous administration of β-blockers with calcium antagonists (particularly diltiazem and verapamil) must be avoided because of increased incidence of AV block and heart failure.

Labetalol

Labetalol is a nonselective β-blocker with little ISA but with α₁-blocking properties. The ratio of α- to β-blocking activity is between 1:3 and 1:7. It lowers BP by decreasing both peripheral vascular resistance and cardiac output. After prolonged therapy, the decrease in BP is sustained primarily by a fall in peripheral vascular resistance, whereas cardiac output returns to pretreatment levels. The drug acutely may cause slight reflex tachycardia, but chronic administration may actually decrease heart rate. Labetalol is particularly useful as adjunct therapy in patients with CRF and severe or refractory hypertension.

Labetalol can be used both orally and intravenously. The intravenous form has been used with some success in hypertensive emergencies, although its efficacy is not as predictable and immediate as that of sodium nitroprusside.

The most common side effect is orthostatic hypotension, which is related to the α-blocking properties. Labetalol is less likely to cause bronchospasm and has no deleterious effects on serum lipids. Occasionally it can increase the titer of antinuclear and antimitochondrial antibodies.

Centrally Acting Agents: Antiadrenergic Agents

α-Methyldopa

The antihypertensive action of α-methyldopa is primarily caused by activation of α_2-adrenergic receptors in the brainstem and partially by biotransformation into a false neurotransmitter. The drug also lowers PRA, but this is not considered to be of primary importance for the drug's antihypertensive action.

α-Methyldopa is biotransformed into pharmacologically active metabolites, which may accumulate in patients with renal failure. These metabolites may cause untoward side effects. Among the more common side effects of methyldopa are those involving the CNS, such as drowsiness and lethargy. Orthostatic hypotension and impotence are also well-known side effects. Occasionally the drug can cause hepatitis or Coombs-positive hemolytic anemia.

α-Methyldopa is easily removed by HD and should be administered after dialysis to avoid fluctuations in BP. The recommended initial dose is 250 mg twice daily. The dose for ESRD patients should not exceed 1,000 mg daily.

Clonidine

Clonidine is an imidazoline derivative that lowers BP primarily by activating presynaptic α_2-adrenergic receptors in the nucleus tractus solitarius and in the rostral ventrolateral medulla, thereby causing a decrease in SNS activity. Part of the antihypertensive effect of clonidine may be mediated by central I_1-imidazoline receptors localized in the rostral ventrolateral medulla (256). Inhibition of renin secretion contributes to the BP-lowering properties of clonidine but to a lesser extent. The drug is readily absorbed from the intestine and reaches peak plasma levels within 1 hour. The antihypertensive action appears within 30 minutes and it peaks within 2 to 4 hours.

Because the kidneys excrete 40% to 50% of the drug, the dosage should be reduced in patients with ESRD. The mean HD clearance of clonidine is 59 ± 7.8 mL/minute (257). The use of this drug has decreased substantially in recent years because of the high incidence of untoward side effects related to the CNS, including drowsiness, lethargy, dry mouth, impotence, and orthostatic hypotension. In addition, hypertensive crisis may

occur when the drug is discontinued abruptly. This rebound effect is more frequent and severe when the drug is given in doses exceeding 0.6 mg daily or in combination with β-adrenergic blocking agents. In this instance, the surge of catecholamines that occurs after withdrawal of the drug binds preferentially to unoccupied α-receptors rather than to the drug-bound β-receptors, resulting in greater vasoconstriction and more severe hypertension.

In recent years, in addition to the oral form clonidine has become available as a transdermal therapeutic system (TTS), which allows steady and continuous transdermal delivery of the drug for 1 week. This limits fluctuations in BP, which are commonly observed with oral dosing, and reduces the incidence of side effects. The TTS of clonidine is particularly useful for noncompliant dialysis patients; a dialysis nurse can apply the patient's patch once a week to ensure compliance. Despite some removal of clonidine with HD, the blood levels remained therapeutic beyond 1 week. The transdermal form of delivery can cause skin rash at the site of adherence of the patch. Clonidine has been reported to be useful in the treatment of restless leg syndrome of chronic dialysis and in the treatment of gastrointestinal autonomic dysfunction in diabetic patients.

Clonidine should be given at initial doses of 0.05 to 0.1 mg twice daily. The total daily dose should not exceed 0.3 mg twice daily. When given in conjunction with β-blockers the maximum dose should not exceed 0.4 mg daily.

Guanabenz

Guanabenz is an aminoguanidine with mechanisms of action similar to those of clonidine. The liver mainly excretes the drug and no dose adjustment is necessary in patients with renal failure. The dose is 4 to 16 mg given orally twice daily.

Guanfacine

Guanfacine is a clonidine-like drug that has a more prolonged duration of action than clonidine and may be given twice daily. This drug probably causes less CNS side effects than clonidine.

Rilmenidine and Monoxidine

Rilmenidine and monoxidine are antihypertensive agents that lower BP by binding to central I_1-imidazolone adrenoceptors in the rostral ventrolateral medulla. These drugs cause sedation less frequently and less intensively than clonidine.

Serotonergic 5-hydroxytryptamine (5HT)$_{1A}$-receptor Antagonists

The rostral ventrolateral medulla contains serotonergic receptors of the $5HT_{1A}$. Urapidil and ketanserin appear to exert their antihypertensive effect in part through this mechanism and in part through blockade of α_1-adrenoreceptors.

Peripherally Acting Agents α$_1$-Adrenergic Receptor Blocking Agents

Prazosin

Prazosin is a quinazoline derivative with a dual mechanism of antihypertensive activity: the agent has direct smooth muscle relaxant effects as well as peripheral α_1-adrenergic receptor inhibition. This latter property does not significantly affect the presynaptic α_2 receptors; therefore, epinephrine and NE occupy the presynaptic inhibitory α_2 receptors, thereby reducing further release of catecholamines from the sympathetic end-terminals. This may partially explain why this vasodilator stimulates neither heart rate nor plasma renin release.

The efficacy of the drug is similar to that of hydralazine, but prazosin is less likely to cause tolerance. Prazosin has a short half-life (2 to 3 hours) and must be administered twice daily. Primarily the liver metabolizes prazosin and no dose adjustment is necessary in renal failure.

The most troublesome side effect of prazosin is the "first-dose phenomenon." This consists of significant orthostatic hypotension occurring after administration of the first dose. This phenomenon is particularly common in patients receiving ultrafiltration with dialysis or those on sodium restriction. Other side effects include syncope, dizziness, diarrhea, and nausea, in addition to a postural hypotension that is independent of the first-dose effect. Prazosin has a favorable effect on the lipid profile in that it decreases LDL cholesterol and increases the cholesterol ratio.

Terazosin

Terazosin is a congener of prazosin with similar α_1-adrenergic inhibition. The oral absorption of this drug is more gradual than that of prazosin. This results in higher blood levels 8, 12, and 16 hours after administration of an oral dose. The half-life of terazosin is approximately 12 hours and is not altered by renal failure. This makes it possible to administer the drug once daily. The side effects are similar to those of prazosin.

Doxazosin

Like terazosin, doxazosin is a quinazoline derivative with a long half-life, making it suitable for once a day administration. The main route of elimination is the gut and it is poorly dialyzed.

This drug (as well as other drugs of the same group) should not be used as first-line therapy because of an increased risk of heart failure (ALL-HAT Trial).

Urapidil

Urapidil is a new antihypertensive agent derived from arylpiperazine uracil. Urapidil is a peripheral α_1-adrenergic receptor-blocking agent with an additional central component that is different from that of clonidine because it does not involve stimulation of central α_2-adrenoceptors. This compound stimulates serotonergic receptors in the $5HT_{1A}$ subtype located in the rostral ventrolateral medulla. Stimulation of these receptors lowers BP without causing sedation. The dose is not altered in renal failure, and it is poorly dialyzed.

Reserpine

Reserpine decreases BP by reducing NE storage at the adrenergic nerve terminals. The bioavailability of the drug is approximately 40%. Although the liver primarily metabolizes the drug, the dose is nonetheless reduced in cases of ESRD. The drug is not removed by dialysis.

This drug is of little use in patients with CRF or in transplant recipients because of its side effects, including high incidence of depression, psychosis, Parkinson-like syndrome, impaired ejaculation, and reactivation or induction of peptic ulcer disease.

Guanethidine

Guanethidine decreases BP by inducing depletion of NE storage at the sympathetic nerve terminals. The oral bioavailability is variable, and the urinary excretion of the unchanged drug is 50%. In humans, guanethidine also undergoes extensive hepatic metabolism. The antihypertensive effects of the metabolites are one tenth that of the intact compound. Renal failure results in the accumulation of the drug and its metabolites, so the dosage must be reduced accordingly. The drug is not removed by dialysis.

Guanethidine has virtually no role in the management of patients with renal failure because of the high incidence of severe side effects. Orthostatic hypotension, impotence, and retardation of ejaculation are extremely common. Diarrhea, bradycardia, and nasal stuffiness are also common and are due to uninhibited parasympathetic activity.

Guanadrel

Guanadrel is an analog of guanethidine with a shorter half-life and a shorter duration of action. Disposition of this drug is significantly altered by renal insufficiency. The dose is substantially reduced in dialysis patients to 25 mg every 5 days.

Vasodilators

Vasodilators exert their antihypertensive effect by a direct action on VSMCs. Some are given intravenously and others by the oral route. Those given intravenously, such as sodium nitroprusside and diazoxide, are more suitable for the treatment of hypertensive emergencies. The vasodilators for oral use are more suitable for chronic therapy.

Sodium Nitroprusside

Sodium nitroprusside is the most effective intravenous vasodilator available. It has the advantage of being both an arteriolar and venous vasodilator, thus reducing both preload and afterload of the heart so that no increase in cardiac output occurs (258). The antihypertensive activity ensues immediately, and it also terminates rapidly because the drug is quickly biotransformed into inactive metabolites such as thiocyanate and cyanogen.

In patients with renal failure the toxic metabolites can accumulate and cause delirium, seizures, coma, and hypothyroidism. To prevent these toxic effects the drug should not be administered for more than 2 to 3 days in these patients. If more prolonged administration is required, serum thiocyanate levels and cyanate levels should be monitored closely, and, if needed, HD or peritoneal dialysis should be instituted to remove the toxic metabolites. Recent studies have shown that hydroxocobalamin may prevent cyanide transfer from red blood cells and plasma into tissue, thereby preventing cyanide toxicity from large intravenous doses of the drug (259).

Nitrates

Nitrates are effective antihypertensive drugs, but they cause a selective decrease in SBP and in PP (260). Because of these characteristics, nitrates are particularly useful in patients with isolated systolic hypertension and wide PP (261). This selective action of nitrates on PP without affecting DBP suggests that these drugs act primarily on large muscular arteries (from the medium-sized arteries to the origin of arterioles), whereas they have little effect on small resistance vessels.

Nitrates increase arterial compliance of elastic and muscular arteries. The increase in compliance is mainly due to an increase in arterial diameter, whereas distensibility and PWV does not change (262).

Diazoxide

Diazoxide is another vasodilator suitable for intravenous administration in hypertensive emergencies. Diazoxide is a benzothiadiazine derivative, chemically related to the thiazide diuretics. It primarily dilates arterioles and has little effect on capacitance vessels. This results in decreased afterload, with an increase in venous return, heart rate, and cardiac output. The drug has a rapid onset of action, and the antihypertensive activity may last from 4 to 24 hours. It has been customary to administer 100 to 150 mg of the drug by rapid intravenous bolus injection to achieve high concentrations of the unbound form at the level of the VSMCs, thus yielding a more rapid and effective antihypertensive response. More recently, it has been shown that slow intravenous infusion of diazoxide can cause a slower but equally effective reduction of BP. A slower reduction allows prevention of complications from sudden reductions in BP such as angina, myocardial infarction, and cerebral ischemia.

The most common adverse reactions are sodium and water retention, hyperglycemia, electrocardiographic ischemic changes, angina pectoris, hypotension, nausea and vomiting, and hyperuricemia.

Hydralazine

Hydralazine is available in both oral and injectable forms. Hydralazine, like diazoxide, is predominantly an arteriolar vasodilator. The drug causes activation of the SNS and of the RAA system. This results in tachycardia, increased cardiac output, and sodium retention. Thus, it is of little therapeutic use when administered as monotherapy. Conversely, it is effective when used in conjunction with a β-blocker or an antiadrenergic agent. Also, it is of particular use when given in combination with nitrates in patients with CHF. Primarily the liver metabolizes hydralazine, but in dialysis patients dose adjustment is required. To prevent side effects a daily dose of 200 mg should not be exceeded. The most frequent side effects are headache, tachycardia, nausea, vomiting, palpitations, dizziness, fatigue, angina pectoris, sleep disturbances, nasal congestion, and a lupus-like syndrome.

Minoxidil

Minoxidil is an orally administered vasodilator that is more potent than hydralazine (263). It dilates primarily arterioles and has little effect on capacitance vessels. For patients with the most refractory forms of hypertension, it has been advocated as a valid alternative of bilateral nephrectomy. The drug is primarily metabolized by the liver and dose adjustments are not required in patients with renal failure. The drug induces reflex stimulation of the SNS as well as the RAA system producing tachycardia, increased cardiac output, and marked sodium and water retention. This combination of effects may result in pericardial effusion. Thus, minoxidil should be used in combination with a β-blocker or a CEI.

Patients receiving maintenance HD who are treated with minoxidil usually experience a greater increase in body weight during the interdialytic period. This is probably due to an increase in thirst and appetite for salt caused by reflex stimulation of the renin-angiotensin system. The most common adverse effects aside from fluid and sodium retention are tachycardia, angina pectoris, and ischemic electrocardiographic changes. Hypertrichosis is commonly seen, and this may limit use of the agents among females for cosmetic reasons. Pericardial effusion can develop in patients taking minoxidil, but its true incidence, particularly in patients with renal failure who are already predisposed to this particular complication of uremia, is difficult to establish.

The drug may be administered once or twice daily in doses of 5 to 40 mg.

RESISTANT HYPERTENSION

In dialysis patients, hypertension is considered resistant if BP in a compliant patient remains above 140/90 mm Hg after achieving dry weight and after an adequate and appropriate triple-drug regimen. In elderly patients with isolated systolic hypertension, resistant hypertension is defined as a failure of an adequate regimen to reduce SBP to less than 140 to 150 mm Hg. The regimen should include nearly maximal doses of at least three different pharmacologic agents selected from ACE inhibitors, calcium antagonists, β-blockers, antiadrenergic agents, or direct vasodilators.

Several factors can cause resistant hypertension, including patient noncompliance, inadequate regimen, drug-to-drug interactions, pseudoresistance, secondary hypertension, and unrecognized pressor mechanisms (Table 16.10).

TABLE 16.10. CAUSES OF RESISTANT HYPERTENSION IN DIALYSIS PATIENTS

Patient noncompliance
Dietary (excessive salt intake or alcohol consumption, inability to reduce excessive body weight)
Drug Regimen
  Inadequate regimen
  Drug-to-drug interaction
  Administration of epoetin
  Secondary hypertension (renovascular, pheochromocytoma, primary aldosteronism, hypothyroidism)
  Pseudoresistance
  Unrecognized pressor mechanisms
  Hemodynamic alterations
  Drug abuse (cocaine, amphetamines, Ritalin, etc.)
  Sleep apnea

Noncompliance or Inadequate Regimen

Noncompliance can be dietary (excessive sodium intake, inability to reduce weight, or excessive alcohol consumption) or pharmacologic (failure to take the prescribed drugs or to follow the prescribed dose regimen). Several clues may be useful to ascertain noncompliance, including the patient's failure to renew the prescribed drugs on time, to know the type and dose of the prescribed medications, or to recognize the prescribed drugs. Another clue can be a failure to observe the expected physiologic or laboratory evidence of drug ingestion; for example, one expects to observe bradycardia in a patient receiving a β-blocker or some types of calcium channel blockers. Frequently noncompliance is caused by inappropriate patient education about the importance and goals of the therapeutic regimen, drug prescriptions, and potential side effects or by the patient's lack of involvement in his or her own treatment plan.

Finally, probably the most common cause of noncompliance is the cost of the medications.

Drug-to-Drug Interactions

Before a patient can be defined as having resistant hypertension, he or she must have achieved and be maintaining dry weight and receive a triple-drug regimen that includes a calcium antagonist, an ACE inhibitor, and an antiadrenergic agent or a direct vasodilator, such as hydralazine or minoxidil:

- Nonsteroidal antiinflammatory drugs (NSAIDs), including aspirin and ibuprofen, can reduce the efficacy of most antihypertensive agents by inhibiting the production of renal prostaglandins. Selective COX-2 inhibitors are not immune from this problem.
- Oral contraceptives containing estrogens can also elevate BP.
- Sympathomimetic amines such as phenylpropanolamine (which can be obtained in over-the-counter cold and diet preparations), pseudoephedrine, ephedrine, and epinephrine can increase BP and cause resistance to other antihypertensive agents.
- Our experiences in a large inner-city community hospital have found that many patients with resistant hypertension abuse amphetamines or cocaine.

A detailed drug history is essential to rule out these possibilities. Occasionally, toxicology screening tests may be necessary to exclude the ingestion of drugs such as amphetamines, cocaine, or methylphenidate (Ritalin).

Pseudoresistance

Some patients may manifest pseudohypertension. This is particularly frequent in elderly patients with significant hardening of their brachial or radial arteries; they may manifest spuriously elevated BP measured by the cuff method but normal intraarterial pressure. Hardening of the arterial walls is not uncommon even in younger dialysis patients with hypertension. In these situations, measurements of BP by cuff can overestimate DBP by 20 mm Hg—and occasionally even by as much as 40 to 50 mm Hg.

The Osler maneuver may help to diagnose pseudohypertension. The cuff is inflated well above the measured SBP; if the brachial or radial arteries remain palpable, the maneuver is considered positive: the cuff method may be overestimating the true intraarterial pressure. Skepticism, however, remains about the practical validity of this maneuver.

Pseudohypertension characterized by a false elevation of DBP may also be diagnosed in obese patients when an inappropriately small cuff is used. In these patients, the use of a thigh cuff (19 cm wide) will minimize the risk of falsely high readings.

Pseudoresistance should be suspected in patients with high indirect BP but little or no end-organ damage. Occasionally, home BP monitoring or direct intraarterial BP recording may be necessary to rule out this possibility.

Secondary Hypertension

Secondary causes of hypertension such as renovascular hypertension, renal cyst formation, primary aldosteronism, pheochromocytoma, hypothyroidism, or sleep apnea should be considered in dialysis patients who have resistant hypertension with no other possible cause for the resistance:

- Renovascular hypertension. Renovascular hypertension should be suspected in patients with resistant hypertension, particularly those with a history of heavy cigarette smoking, clinical evidence of diffuse atherosclerotic vascular disease, and abdominal bruits.
- Cyst formation. Occasionally, cyst formation may cause constriction of renal arterioles and increase renin secretion.
- Pheochromocytoma. Pheochromocytoma should be suspected in patients with palpitations, headaches, diaphoresis, and orthostatic hypotension. It is important, however, to recognize that the presentation of pheochromocytoma can be deceiving. Patients may be totally asymptomatic, or may present with signs and symptoms consistent with diabetes mellitus, hyperthyroidism, hypercalcemia, CHF, myocardial infarction, shock, transient ischemic attacks, or stroke. Every patient with resistant hypertension should be screened for pheochromocytoma by measurement of plasma catecholamines. Levels in excess of 2,000 pg/mL are unusual in patients with CRF and should lead to further tests to determine the diagnosis (264).
- Primary aldosteronism. Primary aldosteronism is another possible cause of resistant hypertension. In dialysis patients with this condition, hypokalemia is not a common finding and, therefore, is not a useful screening test, like in patients with normal renal function. Plasma aldosterone levels may be indicated.
- Hypothyroidism. Dialysis patients with resistant hypertension should also be screened for hypothyroidism.
- Sleep apnea. Sleep apnea has recently been recognized as a cause of hypertension and possibly of resistant hypertension. Patients with resistant hypertension and a typical history of excessive snoring, interrupted sleep, daytime somnolence, obesity, polycythemia, and elevated carbon dioxide should receive a sleep study.

Pressor Mechanisms

Occasionally, resistance may be caused by hemodynamic (such as an unrecognized increase in plasma volume or in cardiac output) or neurohumoral aberrations (an increase in plasma catecholamines, PRA, or aldosterone). Recognition of these pressor mechanisms may be necessary in occasional patients with truly resistant hypertension to establish appropriate therapeutic interventions.

For example, in patients treated with direct vasodilators such as hydralazine or minoxidil, hypertension may be sustained by an increase in cardiac output or by retention of sodium and water. In this instance, the addition of a β-blocker or verapamil may reduce cardiac output and improve BP control. On the other hand, the increase in BV may benefit from more aggressive ultrafiltration. Similarly, specific antagonists of catecholamines or angiotensin II may be used when the activity of these hormones appears to be increased as a result of peripheral vasodilatation or exaggerated response to volume contraction.

REFERENCES

1. Klag MJ, et al. Blood pressure and end-stage renal disease in men. *N Engl J Med* 1996;334:13–18.
2. Ritz E, et al. Morbidity and mortality due to hypertension in patients with renal failure. *Am J Kidney Dis* 1993;21[Suppl 2]:113–118.
3. Schupak E, et al. Chronic hemodialysis in unselected patients. *Ann Intern Med* 1967;67:708–717.
4. Klooker P, et al. Treatment of hypertension in dialysis patients. *Blood Purif* 1985;3:15–26.
5. Curtis JR, et al. Maintenance hemodialysis. *Q J Med* 1969;38:49–89.
6. Newman AB, et al. Morbidity and mortality in hypertensive adults with a low ankle/arm blood pressure index. *JAMA* 1993;270:487–489.
7. Fishbane S, et al. Ankle-arm blood pressure index as a marker for atherosclerotic vascular diseases in hemodialysis patients. *Am J Kidney Dis* 1995;25:34–39.
8. Duranti E, et al. Is hypertension a mortality risk factor in dialysis? *Kidney Int* 1996;55:S173–S174.
9. United States Renal Data System. USRDS 1998 Annual Data Report. U.S. Department of Health and Human Services. Bethesda, MD: National Institutes of Health, National Institute of Diabetes and Digestive and Kidney Diseases, April 1998.
10. Lowrie EG, et al. Death risk in hemodialysis patients: the predictive value of commonly measured variables and an evaluation of death rate differences between facilities. *Am J Kidney Dis* 1990;15:458–482.
11. Salem MM, et al. Hypertension in the hemodialysis population: any relation to one-year survival? *Am J Kidney Dis* 1996;28:737–740.
12. Franklin SS, et al. Hemodynamic patterns of age-related changes I blood pressure: the Framingham Heart Study. *Circulation* 1997;96:308–315.
13. Franklin SS, et al. Is pulse pressure useful in predicting risk for coronary heart disease? The Framingham Heart Study. *Circulation* 1999;100:354–360.
14. Gasowski J, et al. Pulsatile blood pressure component as predictor of mortality in hypertension: a meta-analysis of clinical trial control. *J Hypertens* 2002;20:145–151.
15. Tozawa M, et al. Pulse pressure and risk of total mortality and cardiovascular events in patients on chronic hemodialysis. *Kidney Int* 2002;61:717–726.
16. Safar ME, et al. Central pulse pressure and mortality in end-stage renal disease. *Hypertension* 2002;39:735–738.
17. Foley RN, et al. Impact of hypertension on cardiomyopathy, morbidity and mortality in end-stage renal disease. *Kidney Int* 1996;49:1379–1385.
18. Millar-Craig MW, et al. Diurnal variation of blood pressure. *Lancet* 1979;1:795–797.
19. National High Blood Pressure Education Program Coordinating Committee. National High Blood Pressure Education Program working group report on ambulatory blood pressure monitoring. *Arch Intern Med* 1990;150:2270–2280.
20. Mancia G, et al. Blood pressure and hearth rate variabilities in normotensive and hypertensive human beings. *Circ Res* 1983;53:96–104.
21. Shimada K, et al. Diurnal blood pressure variations and silent cerebrovascular damage in elderly patients with hypertension. *J Hypertens* 1992;10:875–878.
22. O'Brien E, et al. Dippers and non dippers. *Lancet* 1988;2:397.
23. Verdecchia P, et al. Diurnal blood pressure changes and left ventricular hypertrophy in essential hypertension. *Circulation* 1990;81:528–536.
24. Farmer CK, et al. An investigation of the effect of advancing uraemia, renal replacement therapy and renal transplantation on blood pressure diurnal variability. *Nephrol Dial Transplant* 1997;12:2301–2307.
25. Baumgart P, et al. Blood pressure elevation in the night in chronic renal failure, hemodialysis and renal transplantation. *Nephron* 1991;57:293–298.
26. Peixoto AJ, et al. Ambulatory blood pressure monitoring in chronic renal disease: technical aspects and clinical relevance. *Curr Opin Nephrol Hypertens* 2002;11:507–516.
27. Ritz E, et al. Ambulatory blood pressure monitoring: fancy gadgetry or clinically useful exercise? *Nephrol Dial Transplant* 2001;16:1550–1554.
28. Sokolow M, et al. Relationship between level of blood pressure measured casually and by portable recorders and severity of complications in essential hypertension. *Circulation* 1966;34:279–298.
29. Agarwal R. Role of home blood pressure monitoring in hemodialysis patients. *Am J Kidney Dis* 1999;33:682–687.
30. Perin PC, et al. Sympathetic nervous system, diabetes, and hypertension. *Clin Exp Hypertens* 2001;23:45–55.
31. O'Shea JC, et al. Nocturnal blood pressure dipping: a consequence of diurnal physical activity blipping? *Am J Hypertens* 2000;13:601–606.
32. Hanly PJ, et al. Improvement of sleep apnea in patients with chronic renal failure who undergo nocturnal hemodialysis. *N Engl J Med* 2001;344:102–107.
33. Zoccali C, et al. Nocturnal hypoxemia, night-day arterial pressure changes and left ventricular geometry in dialysis patients. *Kidney Int* 1998;53:1078–1084.
34. Sorof JM, et al. Ambulatory blood pressure monitoring and interdialytic weight gain in children receiving chronic hemodialysis. *Am J Kidney Dis* 1999;33:667–674.
35. Uzu T, et al. Sodium restriction shifts circadian rhythm of blood pressure from nondipper to dipper in essential hypertension. *Circulation* 1997;96:1859–1862.
36. Higashi Y, et al. Nocturnal decline in blood pressure is attenuated by NaCl loading in salt-sensitive patients with essential hypertension: noninvasive 24-hour ambulatory blood pressure monitoring. *Hypertension* 1997;30:163–167.
37. Uzu T, et al. Diuretics shift circadian rhythm of blood pressure from nondipper to dipper in essential hypertension. *Circulation* 1999;100:1635–1638.
38. Toth L, et al. Diurnal blood pressure variations in incipient and end-stage diabetic renal disease. *Diabetes Res Clin Pract* 2000;49:1–6.
39. McGregor DO, et al. Ambulatory blood pressure monitoring in patients receiving long, slow home haemodialysis. *Nephrol Dial Transplant* 1999;14:2676–2679.
40. Fagugli RM, et al. Short daily hemodialysis: blood pressure control and left ventricular mass reduction in hypertensive hemodialysis patients. *Am J Kidney Dis* 2001;38:371–376.
41. Perloff D, et al. The prognostic value of ambulatory blood pressure. *JAMA* 1983;249:2792–2798.
42. Devereux RB, et al. Left ventricular hypertrophy in patients with hypertension: importance of blood pressure responses to regularly recurring stress. *Circulation* 1983;68:470–476.
43. White WB, et al. Average daily blood pressure, not office blood pressure, determines cardiac function in patients with hypertension. *JAMA* 1989;261:873–877.

44. Parati G, et al. Relationship of 24-hour blood pressure mean and variability to severity of target organ damage in hypertension. *J Hypertens* 1987;5:93–98.

45. Sluniade K, et al. Silent cerebrovascular disease in the elderly: correlation with ambulatory pressure. *Hypertension* 1990;16:692–699.

46. Bianchi S, et al. Diurnal variation of blood pressure and microalbuminuria in essential hypertension. *Am J Hypertens* 1994;7:23–29.

47. Amar J, et al. Nocturnal blood pressure and 24-hour pulse pressure are potent indicators of mortality in hemodialysis patients. *Kidney Int* 2000;57:2485–2491.

48. Omboni S, et al. Reproducibility and clinical value of nocturnal hypotension: prospective evidence from the SAMPLE study. Study on Ambulatory Monitoring of Pressure and Lisinopril Evaluation. *J Hypertens* 1998;16:733–738.

49. Blacher J, et al. Impact of aortic stiffness on survival in end-stage renal disease. *Circulation* 1999;99:2434–2439.

50. Blacher J, et al. Aortic pulse wave velocity as a marker of cardiovascular risk in hypertensive patients. *Hypertension* 1999;33:1111–1117.

51. Avolio AP, et al. Effects of aging on changing arterial compliance and left ventricular load in a northern Chinese urban community. *Circulation* 1983;68:50–58.

52. Asmar RG, et al. Reversion of cardiac hypertrophy and reduced arterial compliance after converting enzyme inhibition in essential hypertension. *Circulation* 1988;78:941–950.

53. London GM, et al. Salt and water and calcium blockade in uremia. *Circulation* 1990;2:105–113.

54. Guerin AP, et al. Impact of aortic stiffness attenuation on survival of patients in end-stage renal failure. *Circulation* 2001;103:987–992.

55. Hansson L, et al. For the HOT Study Group. Effects of intensive blood pressure lowering and low-dose aspirin in patients with hypertension: principal results of the Hypertension Optimal Treatment (HOT) randomized trial. HOT Study Group. *Lancet* 1998;351:1755–1762.

56. Klahr S, et al. The effects of dietary protein restriction and blood pressure control on the progression of chronic renal disease. *N Engl J Med* 1994;330:877–884.

57. Agodoa LY, et al. Effect of ramipril vs amlodipine on renal outcomes in hypertensive nephrosclerosis: a randomized controlled trial. *JAMA* 2001;285:2719–2728.

58. Highlights from the 1996 Core Indicators Project for hemodialysis patients. HCFA. *Dial Transplant* 1997;April:188–191.

59. National High Blood Pressure Education Program Working Group, 1995. Update of the working group reports on chronic renal failure and renovascular hypertension. *Arch Int Med* 1996;156:1938–1947.

60. Charra B, et al. Survival as an index of adequacy of dialysis. *Kidney Int* 1992;41:1286–1291.

61. Charra B. Control of blood pressure in long slow hemodialysis. *Blood Purif* 1994;12:252–258.

62. Ozkahya M, et al. Treatment of hypertension in dialysis patients by ultrafiltration: the role of cardiac dilation and "time factor." *Am J Kidney Dis* 1999;34:218–221.

63. Foley RN, et al. Cardiovascular disease and mortality in ESRD. *J Nephrol* 1998;11:239–245.

64. Zager PG, et al. "U" curve association of blood pressure and mortality in hemodialysis patients. Medical Directors of Dialysis Clinic, Inc. *Kidney Int* 1998;54:561–517.

65. Port FK, et al. Predialysis blood pressure and mortality risk in a national sample of maintenance hemodialysis patients. *Am J Kidney Dis* 1999;33:507–517.

66. Salem MM. Hypertension in the haemodialysis population: any relationship to 2-years survival? *Nephrol Dial Transplant* 1999;14:125–128.

67. Conlon PJ, et al. Predialysis systolic blood pressure correlates strongly with mean 24-hour systolic blood pressure and left ventricular mass in stable hemodialysis patients. *J Am Soc Nephrol* 1996;7:2658–2663.

68. Kooman JP, et al. Blood pressure during the interdialytic period in hemodialysis patients: estimation of representative blood pressure values. *Nephrol Dial Transplant* 1992;7:917–923.

69. Coomer RW, et al. Ambulatory blood pressure monitoring in dialysis patients and estimation of mean interdialytic blood pressure. *Am J Kidney Dis* 1997;29:678–684.

70. Agarwal R, et al. Prediction of hypertension in chronic hemodialysis patients. *Kidney Int* 2001;60:1982–1989.

71. Cirit M, et al. Paradoxical rise in blood pressure during ultrafiltration in dialysis patients. *Nephrol Dial Transplant* 1995;10:1417–1420.

72. Horl MP, et al. Hemodialysis-associated hypertension: pathophysiology and therapy. *Am J Kidney Dis* 2002;39:227–244.

73. Chazot C, et al. Interdialysis blood pressure control by long haemodialysis sessions. *Nephrol Dial Transplant* 1995;10:831–837.

74. Katzarski KS, et al. Fluid state and blood pressure control in patients treated with long and short haemodialysis. *Nephrol Dial Transplant* 1999;14:369–375.

75. Kooistra MP, et al. Daily home hemodialysis in the Netherlands: effects on metabolic control, haemodynamics, and quality of life. *Nephrol Dial Transplant* 1998;13:2853–2860.

76. Taeger J, et al. Daily versus standard hemodialysis: one year experience. *Artif Organs* 1998;22:558–563.

77. Rahman M, et al. Interdialytic weight gain, compliance with dialysis regimen, and age independent predictors of blood pressure in hemodialysis patients. *Am J Kidney Dis* 2000;35:257–265.

78. Zucchelli P, et al. Dry weight in hemodialysis: volume control. *Semin Nephrol* 2001;21:286–290.

79. Schalekamp MADH, et al. Interrelationships between blood pressure, renin, renin substrate and blood volume in terminal renal failure. *Clin Sci Mol Med* 1973;45:417–428.

80. Schultze G, et al. Blood pressure in terminal renal failure: fluid spaces and renin-angiotensin system. *Nephron* 1980;25:15–24.

81. Coleman TG, et al. Hypertension caused by salt loading in the dog: III. Onset transients of cardiac output and other variables. *Circ Res* 1969;25:153–160.

82. Weidman P. Pathogenesis of hypertension associated with chronic renal failure. *Contr Nephrol* 1984;41:47–65.

83. DeWardener HE, et al. Dahl's hypothesis that a saluretic substance may be responsible for a sustained rise in arterial pressure: its possible role in essential hypertension. *Kidney Int* 1980;18:1–9.

84. Graves SW, et al. Volume expansion in renal failure patients: a paradigm for a clinically relevant [Na,K]ATPase inhibitor. *J Cardiovasc Pharmacol* 1993;22[Suppl 2]:S54–S57.

85. Boero R, et al. Pathogenesis of arterial hypertension in chronic uremia: the role of reduced Na+K+ATPase activity. *J Hypertension* 1988;6 [Suppl 14]:S363–S365.

86. Tobian L Jr, et al. Tissue cations and water in arterial hypertension. *Circulation* 1952;5:754–758.

87. Lazarus JM, et al. Hypertension in chronic renal failure: treatment with hemodialysis and nephrectomy. *Arch Intern Med* 1974;133:1059–1065.

88. Weidman P, et al. Plasma renin activity and blood pressure in terminal renal failure. *N Engl J Med* 1971;285:757–762.

89. Greene EL, et al. Role of aldosterone in the remnant kidney model in the rat. *J Clin Invest* 1996;98:1063–1068.

90. Recordati G, et al. Renal chemoreceptors. *J Auton Nerv Syst* 1981;3:237–251.

91. Katholi RE. Renal nerves and hypertension: an update. *Fed Proc* 1985;44:2846–2850.

92. Faber JE, et al. Afferent renal nerve-dependent hypertension following acute renal artery stenosis in the conscious rat. *Circ Res* 1985;57:676–688.

93. Calaresu FR, et al. Renal afferent nerves affect discharge rate of medullary and hypothalamic single units in cat. *J Auton Nerv Syst* 1981;3:311–320.

94. Katholi RE, et al. Intrarenal adenosine produces hypertension by activating the sympathetic nervous system via the renal nerves. *J Hypertension* 1984;2:349–352.

95. Atuk NO, et al. Red blood cell catechol-o-methyl transferase, plasma catecholamines and renin in renal failure. *Trans Am Soc Artif Intern Organs* 1976;22:195–200.

96. Lake CR, et al. Plasma levels of norepinephrine and dopamine-beta-hydroxylase in CRF patients treated with dialysis. *Cardiovasc Med* 1979;1:1099–1111.

97. Henrich WL, et al. Competitive effects of hypokalemia and depletion on plasma renin activity, aldosterone, and catecholamine concentrations in hemodialysis patients. *Kidney Int* 1977;12:279–284.

98. Izzo JL, et al. Sympathetic nervous system hyperactivity in maintenance hemodialysis patients. *Trans Am Soc Artif Organs* 1982;28:604–607.

99. Ishii M, et al. Elevated catecholamines in hypertensives with primary glomerular diseases. *Hypertension* 1983;5:545–551.

100. Cuche JL, et al. Plasma free, sulfo- and glucuro-conjugated catecholamines in uremic patients. *Kidney Int* 1986;30:566–572.

101. Campese VM, et al. Mechanisms of autonomic nervous system dysfunction in uremia. *Kidney Int* 1981;20:246–253.

102. Grekas D, et al. Effects of sympathetic and plasma renin activity on hemodialysis hypertension. *Clin Nephrol* 2001;55:115–120.

103. Converse RL, et al. Sympathetic overactivity in patients with CRF. *N Engl J Med* 1992;327:1912–1918.

104. Bigazzi R, et al. Altered norepinephrine turnover in the brain of rats with chronic renal failure. *J Am Soc Nephrol* 1994;4:1901–1907.

105. Ye S, et al. Renal afferent impulses, the posterior hypothalamus, and hypertension in rats with chronic renal failure. *Kidney Int* 1997;51:722–727.

106. Campese VM, et al. Renal afferent denervation prevents the progression of renal disease in the renal ablation model of chronic renal failure in the rat. *Am J Kidney Dis* 1995;26:861–865.

107. Ligtenberg G, et al. Reduction of sympathetic hyperactivity by enalapril in patients with chronic renal failure. *N Engl J Med* 1999;340:1321–1328.

108. Klein IHHT, et al. Sympathetic activity is increased in polycystic kidney disease and is associated with hypertension. *J Am Soc Nephrol* 2001;12:2427–2433.

109. Moss NG, et al. Intravenous cyclosporine activates afferent and efferent renal nerves and causes sodium retention in innervated kidneys in rats. *Proc Natl Acad Sci* 1985;82:8222–8226.

110. Zhang W, et al. Calcineurin inhibitors cause renal afferent activation in rats: a novel mechanism of cyclosporine-induced hypertension. *Am J Hypertens* 2000;13:999–1004.

111. Kuchel OG, et al. Dopaminergic abnormalities in hypertension associated with moderate renal insufficiency. *Hypertension* 1994;23[Suppl 1]:I240–I245.

112. Pickering TG, et al. Baroreflex sensitivity in patients on long-term hemodialysis. *Clin Sci* 1972;43:645–647.

113. Zucchelli P, et al. Influence of ultrafiltration on plasma renin activity and adrenergic system. *Nephron* 1978;21:317–324.

114. Zimlichman RR, et al. Vascular hypersensitivity to noradrenaline: a possible mechanism of hypertension in rats with chronic uremia. *Clin Sci* 1984;67:161–166.

115. Elias AN, et al. Plasma catecholamines in chronic renal disease. *Int J Artif Org* 1985;8:243–244.

116. Odar-Cederlof I, et al. Is neuropeptide Y a contributor to volume induced hypertension? *Am J Kidney Dis* 1998;31:803–808.

117. Ye S, et al. Losartan reduces central and peripheral sympathetic nerve activity in a rat model of neurogenic hypertension. *Hypertension* 2002;39:1101–1106.

118. Henrich WL. The endothelium: a key regulator of vascular tone. *Am J Med Sci* 1991;302:319–328.

119. Moncada S, et al. Differential formation of prostacyclin (PGX or PGI2) by layers of the arterial wall: an explanation for the anti-thrombotic properties of vascular endothelium. *Thromb Res* 1977;11:323–344.

120. Furchgott RF, et al. The obligatory role of endothelial cells in the relaxation of arterial smooth muscle by acetylcholine. *Nature* 1980;299:373–376.

121. Palmer RMJ, et al. Nitric oxide release accounts for the biological activity of endothelium-derived relaxation factor. *Nature* 1987;327:524–526.

122. Amezuca JL, et al. Acetylcholine induces vasodilation in the rabbit isolated heart through release of nitric oxide, the endogenous vasodilator. *Br J Pharmacol* 1988;95:830–834.

123. Palmer RMJ, et al. Vascular endothelial cells synthesize nitric oxide from L-arginine. *Nature* 1988;333:664–666.

124. Yanagisawa M, et al. A novel vasoconstrictor peptide produced by vascular endothelial cells. *Nature* 1988;332:411–415.

125. Kato T, et al. Prostaglandin H2 may be the EDCF released by acetylcholine in the aorta of the rat. *Hypertension* 1990;15:475–481.

126. Harris RC, et al. Mediation of renal vascular effects of epidermal growth factor by arachidonate metabolites. *FASEB* 1990;4:1654–1660.

127. Luscher TF. The endothelium—target and promoter of hypertension? *Hypertension* 1990;15:482–485.

128. Shultz PJ, et al. Endothelial-derived vasoactive substances and the kidney. *Kidney* 1990;23:1–7.

129. McGuire PG, et al. Increased deposition of basement membrane macromolecules in specific vessels of the spontaneously hypertensive rat. *Am J Pathol* 1989;135:291–299.

130. Luscher TF, et al. Molecular and cellular biology of endothelin and its receptors. *J Hypertens* 1993;11:7–11.

131. McMahon EG, et al. Phosphoramidon blocks the pressor activity of big endothelin (1-39) and lowers blood pressure in spontaneously hypertensive rats. *J Cardiovasc Pharmacol* 1991;17[Suppl 7]:529–533.

132. Clavell AL, et al. Physiologic and pathophysiologic roles of endothelin in the kidney. *Curr Opinion in Nephrol and Hypertens* 1994;3:66–72.

133. Yokokawa K, et al. Hypertension associated with endothelin-secreting malignant hemangioendothelioma. *Ann Int Med* 1991;114:213–215.

134. Saito Y, et al. Increased plasma endothelin level in patients with essential hypertension. *N Engl J Med* 1990;322:205.

135. Schiffrin EL, et al. Plasma endothelin in human essential hypertension. *Am J Hypertens* 1991;4:303–308.

136. Shichiri M, et al. Plasma endothelin levels in hypertension and chronic renal failure. *Hypertension* 1990;15:493–496.

137. Koyama H, et al. Plasma endothelin levels in patients with uremia. *Lancet* 1989;i:991–992.

138. Suzuki N, et al. Endothelin-3 concentrations in human plasma: the increased concentrations in patients undergoing hemodialysis. *Biochem Biophys Res Commun* 1990;169:809–815.

139. Warrens AN, et al. Endothelin in renal failure. *Nephrol Dial Transplant* 1990;5:418–422.

140. Miyauchi T, et al. Plasma concentrations of endothelin-1 and endothelin-3 are altered differently in various pathophysiological conditions in humans. *J Cardiovasc Pharmacol* 1991;17[Suppl 7]:S394–S397.

141. Lebel M, et al. Plasma endothelin levels and blood pressure in hemodialysis and in CAPD patients: effect of subcutaneous erythropoietin replacement therapy. *Clin Exp Hypertens* 1994;16:565–575.

142. Radomski MW, et al. The anti-aggregating properties of vascular endothelium. Interaction between nitric oxide and prostacyclin. *Br J Pharmacol* 1987;92:639–646.

143. Shimokawa H, et al. Prostacyclin releases EDRF and potentiates its action in the coronary arteries of the pig. *Br J Pharmacol* 1988;95:1197–1203.

144. Kloog Y, et al. Sarfatoxin, a novel vasoconstrictor peptide: phosphoinositide hydrolysis in rat heart and brain. *Science* 1988;242:268–270.

145. Feketou M, et al. Endothelium-dependent hyperpolarization of canine coronary smooth muscle. *Br J Pharmacol* 1988;93:515–524.

146. Campbell WB, et al. What is new in endothelium-derived hyperpolarizing factors. *Curr Opin Nephrol Hypertens* 2002;11:177–183.

147. Vaziri ND, et al. Downregulation of nitric oxide synthase in chronic kidney insufficiency: role of excess PTH. *Am J Physiol Ren Physiol* 1998;274:F642–F649.

148. Hu LR, et al. Long-term cardiovascular role of nitric oxide in conscious rats. *Hypertension* 1994;23:185–194.

149. Johnson RA, et al. Sustained hypertension in the rat induced by chronic blockade of nitric oxide production. *Am J Hypertens* 1992;5[part 1]:919–922.

150. Baylis C, et al. Chronic blockade of nitric oxide synthesis in the rat produces systemic hypertension and glomerular damage. *J Clin Invest* 1992;90:278–281.

151. Chen PY, et al. L-arginine abrogates salt-sensitive hypertension in Dahl/Rapp rats. *J Clin Invest* 1991;88:1559–1567.

152. Sakuma I, et al. NG-methyl-L-arginine, an inhibitor of L-arginine-derived nitric oxide synthesis, stimulates renal sympathetic nerve activity. *Circ Res* 1992;70:607–611.

153. Vallance P, et al. Accumulation of an endogenous inhibitor of nitric oxide synthesis in chronic renal failure. *Lancet* 1992;339:572–575.

154. Kielstein JT, et al. Asymmetric dimethylarginine plasma concentrations differ in patients with end-stage renal disease: relationship to treatment method and atherosclerotic disease. *J Am Soc Nephrol* 1999; 10:594–600.

155. Fujiwara N, et al. Study on the relationship between plasma nitrite and nitrate level and salt sensitivity in human hypertension: modulation of nitric oxide synthesis by salt intake. *Circulation* 2000;101: 859–861.

156. Matsuoka H, et al. Asymmetrical imethylarginine, an endogenous nitric oxide synthase inhibitor, in experimental hypertension. *Hypertension* 1997;29:242–247.

157. Cooke JP. Does ADMA cause endothelial dysfunction? *Arterioscler Thromb Vasc Biol* 2000;20:2032–2037.

158. Ye S, et al. Nitric oxide (NO) modulates the neurogenic control of blood pressure in rats with chronic renal failure. *J Clin Invest* 1997; 99:540–548.

159. Lainchbury JG, et al. Adrenomedullin: a hypotensive hormone in man. *Clin Sci* 1997;92:467–472.

160. Mallamaci F, et al. Plasma adrenomedullin during acute changes in intravascular volume in hemodialysis patients. *Kidney Int* 1998;54: 1697–1703.

161. Gorlach A, et al. Oxidative stress and expression of P22^{phox} are involved in the up-regulation of tissue factor in vascular smooth muscle cells in response to activated platelets. *FASEB J* 2000;14: 1518–1528.

162. Cross AR, et al. Enzymatic mechanisms of superoxide production. *Biochem Biophys Acta* 1991;1057:281–298.

163. Berry C, et al. Oxidative stress and vascular damage in hypertension. *Curr Opin Nephrol Hypertens* 2001;10:247–255.

164. Ushio Fukai M, et al. P22(phox) is a critical component of the superoxide-generating NADH/NADPH oxidase system and regulates angiotensin II-induced hypertrophy in vascular smooth muscle cells. *J Biol Chem* 1996;271:23317–23321.

165. Pagano PJ, et al. Localization of a constitutively active, phagocyte-like NADPH oxidase in rabbit aortic adventitia: enhancement by angiotensin II. *Proc Natl Acad Sci U S A* 1997;94:14483–14488.

166. Rao GN, et al. Active oxygen species stimulate vascular smooth muscle cell growth and proto-oncogene expression. *Circ Res* 1992;70: 593–599.

167. Rajagopalan S, et al. Reactive oxygen species produced by macrophage-derived foam cells regulate the activity of vascular matrix metalloproteinases in vitro. *J Clin Invest* 1996;98:2572–2579.

168. Hu Q, et al. Hydrogen peroxide induces intracellular calcium oscillations in human aortic endothelial cells. *Circulation* 1998;97: 268–275.

169. Ballinger SW, et al. Hydrogen peroxide- and peroxynitrate induced mitochondrial DNA damage and dysfunction in vascular endothelial and smooth muscle cells. *Circ Res* 2000;86:960–966.

170. Mihm MJ, et al. Nitrotyrosine causes selective vascular endothelial dysfunction and DNA damage. *J Cardiovasc Pharmacol* 2000;36: 182–187.

171. Vaziri ND, et al. Increased nitric oxide inactivation by reactive oxygen species in lead-induced hypertension. *Kidney Int* 1999;56: 1492–1498.

172. Kerr S, et al. Superoxide anion production is increased in a model of genetic hypertension: role of the endothelium. *Hypertension* 1999; 33:1353–1358.

173. Lerman LO, et al. Increased oxidative stress in experimental renovascular hypertension. *Hypertension* 2001;27[part 2]:541–546.

174. Somers MJ, et al. Vascular superoxide production and vasomotor function in hypertension induced by deoxycorticosterone acetate-salt. *Circulation* 2000;101:1722–1728.

175. Swei A, et al. A mechanism of oxygen free radicals production in the Dahl hypertensive rat. *Microcirculation* 1999;6:179–187.

176. Vaziri ND, et al. Role of increased oxygen free radical activity in the pathogenesis of uremia hypertension. *Kidney Int* 1998;53: 1748–1754.

177. Vaziri ND, et al. Enhanced nitric oxide inactivation and protein nitration by reactive oxygen species in renal insufficiency. *Hypertension* 2002;39:135–141.

178. Vaziri ND, et al. Induction of oxidative stress by glutathione depletion causes hypertension in normal rats. *Hypertension* 2000;36: 142–146.

179. Eiserich JP, et al. Nitric oxide rapidly scavenges tyrosine and tryptophan radicals. *Biochem J* 1995;310:745–749.

180. Eiserich JP, et al. Formation of nitric oxide-derived inflammatory oxidants by myeloperoxidase in neutrophils. *Nature* 1998;391:393–397.

181. Eschbach JW, et al. Treatment of anemia of progressive renal failure with recombinant human erythropoietin. *N Engl J Med* 1989;321: 158–163.

182. Eschbach JW, et al. Recombinant human erythropoietin in anemic patients with end-stage renal disease: results of a Phase III multicenter clinical trial. *Ann Int Med* 1989;111:992–1000.

183. Adamson JW, et al. Treatment of anemia of chronic renal failure with recombinant human erythropoietin. *Ann Rev Med* 1990;41:349–360.

184. Raine AEG. Hypertension, blood viscosity, and cardiovascular morbidity in renal failure: Implications of erythropoietin therapy. *Lancet* 1988;1:97–100.

185. Garcia DL, et al. Anemia lessens and its prevention worsens glomerular injury and hypertension in rats with reduced renal mass. *Proc Natl Acad Sci U S A* 1988;85:6142–6146.

186. Steffen HM, et al. Peripheral hemodynamics, blood viscosity, and the renin-angiotensin system in hemodialysis patients under therapy with recombinant human erythropoietin. *Contrib Nephrol* 1989;76: 292–298.

187. Letcher RL, et al. Direct relationship between blood pressure and blood viscosity in normal and hypertensive subjects: role of fibrinogen and concentration. *Am J Med* 1981;70:1195–1202.

188. Coleman TG. Hemodynamics of uremic anemia. *Circulation* 1972; 45:510–511.

189. Poux JM, et al. Uraemia is necessary for erythropoietin-induced hypertension in rats. *Clin Exp Pharmacol Physiol* 1995;22:769–771.

190. Vasiri ND. Mechanism of erythropoietin-induced hypertension. *Am J Kidney Dis* 1999;33:821–828.

191. Yamakado M, et al. Mechanisms of hypertension induced by erythropoietin in patients on hemodialysis. *Clin Invest Med* 1991;14: 623–629.

192. Hand MF, et al. Erythropoietin enhances vascular responsiveness to norepinephrine in renal failure. *Kidney Int* 1995;48:806–813.

193. Vaziri ND, et al. In vivo and in vitro pressor effects of erythropoietin in rats. *Am J Physiol* 1995;269:F838–F845.

194. Eggena P, et al. Influence of recombinant human erythropoietin on blood pressure and tissue renin-angiotensin systems. *Am J Physiol* 1991;261:E642–E646.

195. van Geet C, et al. Recombinant human erythropoietin increases blood pressure, platelet aggregability and platelet free calcium mobilization in uremic children: a possible link? *Throm Haemost* 1990;64: 7–10.

196. Neusser M, et al. Erythropoietin increases cytosolic free calcium concentration in vascular smooth muscle cells. *Cardiovasc Res* 1993;27: 1233–1236.

197. Azzadin A, et al. Serotonin is involved in the pathogenesis of hypertension developing during erythropoietin treatment in uremic rats. *Thrombosis Res* 1995;77:217–224.

198. Carlini R, et al. Intravenous erythropoietin administration increases plasma endothelin and blood pressure in hemodialysis. *Am J Hypertens* 1993;6:103–107.

199. del-Castillo D, et al. The pressor effect of recombinant human erythropoietin is not due to decreased activity of the endogenous nitric oxide system. *Nephrol Dial Transplant* 1995;10:505–508.

200. Myers BD, et al. Dynamics of glomerular ultrafiltration in the rat. VIII. Effects of hematocrit. *Circ Res* 1975;36:425–435.

201. Simpson LO. Blood viscosity induced proteinuria. *Nephron* 1984;36:280–281.

202. Spear GS. The glomerulus in cyanotic congenital heart disease and primary pulmonary hypertension: a review. *Nephron* 1964;1: 238–248.

203. Erne P, et al. Correlation of platelet calcium with blood pressure. *N Engl J Med* 1984;310:1084–1088.

204. Alexiewicz JM, et al. Effect of dietary sodium intake on intracellular

calcium in lymphocytes of salt-sensitive hypertensive patients. *Am J Hypertens* 1992;5:536–541.

205. Schiffl H. Correlation of blood pressure in end-stage renal disease with platelet cytosolic free calcium concentration. *Klin Wochenschr* 1990;68:718–722.

206. Raine AEG, et al. Hyperparathyroidism, platelet intracellular free calcium and hypertension in chronic renal failure. *Kidney Int* 1993;43 :700–705.

207. Peterson LJ, et al. Long-term oral calcium supplementation reduces diastolic blood pressure in end-stage renal disease: a randomized, double-blind, placebo controlled study. *Int J Artif Organs* 1994;17:37–40.

208. Ifudu O, et al. Parathyroidectomy does not correct hypertension in patients on maintenance hemodialysis. *Am J Nephrol* 1998;18:28–34.

209. Marone C, et al. Acute hypercalcemic hypertension in man: role of hemodynamics, catecholamines and renin. *Kidney Int* 1980;20: 92–96.

210. Iseki K, et al. Effects of hypercalcemia and PTH on blood pressure in normal and renal failure rats. *Am J Physiol* 1986;250:F924–F929.

211. Winters CJ, et al. Change in plasma immunoreactive N-terminus, C-terminus, and 4,000-dalton midportion of atrial natriuretic factor prohormone with hemodialysis. *Nephron* 1991;58:17–22.

212. Franz M, et al. N-terminal fragments of the proatrial natriuretic peptide in patients before and after hemodialysis treatment. *Kidney Int* 2000;58:374–383.

213. Zoccali C, et al. Cardiac natriuretic peptides are related to left ventricular mass and function and predict mortality in dialysis patients. *J Am Soc Nephrol* 2001;12:1508–1515.

214. Zhang W, et al. Cyclosporine A-induced hypertension involves synapsin in renal sensory nerve endings. *PNAS* 2000;97:9765–9770.

215. Mysliwiec J, et al. The effect of tacrolimus (FK506) and cyclosporin A (Cya) on peripheral serotonergic mechanisms in uremic rats. *Thromb Res* 1996;83:175–181.

216. Joint National Committee on Detection, Evaluation, and Treatment of High Blood Pressure. The Sixth Report of the Joint National Committee on Detection, Evaluation, and Treatment of High Blood Pressure JNC VI. *Arch Intern Med* 1997;153:154–183.

217. Limas C, et al. Effect of salt on the vascular lesions of spontaneously hypertensive rats. *Hypertension* 1980;2:477–489.

218. Levy BI, et al. Sodium, survival and the mechanical properties of the carotid artery in stroke-prone hypertensive rats. *J Hypertens* 1997;15: 251–258.

219. Hosono M, et al. Inhibitory effect of cilnidipine on vascular sympathetic neurotransmission and subsequent vasoconstriction in spontaneously hypertensive rats. *Jpn J Pharmacol* 1995;69:127–134.

220. Takahara A, et al. Cilnidipine attenuates renal nerve stimulation-induced renal vasoconstriction and antinatriuresis in anesthetized dogs. *Jpn J Pharmacol* 1997;75:27–32.

221. Hoyer J, et al. Clinical pharmacokinetics of angiotensin converting enzyme (ACE) inhibitors in renal failure. *Clin Pharmacokinet* 1993; 24:230–254.

222. Tielemans C, et al. Anaphylactoid reactions during hemodialysis on AN69 membranes in patients receiving ACE inhibitors. *Kidney Int* 1990;38:982–984.

223. Chiu AT, et al. [3H]Dup 753, a highly potent and specific radioligand for the angiotensin-II receptor subtype. *Biochem Biophys Res Comm* 1990;172:1195–1202.

224. Criscione L, et al. Pharmacological profile of valsartan: a potent, orally active, nonpeptide antagonist of the angiotensin II AT1-receptor subtype. *Br J Pharmacol* 1993;110:761–771.

225. Whitebread S, et al. Preliminary biochemical characterization of two angiotensin II receptor subtypes. *Biochem Biophys Res Commun* 1989; 163:284–291.

226. Chang RSL, et al. Two distinct angiotensin II receptor binding sites in rat adrenal revealed by new selective non-peptide ligands. *Mol Pharmacol* 1990;29:347–351.

227. Inagami T, et al. Cloning, expression and regulation of angiotensin II receptor. *J Hypertens* 1992;10:713–716.

228. Stoll M, et al. The angiotensin AT2-receptor mediates inhibition of cell proliferation in coronary endothelial cells. *J Clin Invest* 1995; 95:651–657.

229. Yamada T, et al. Angiotensin II type 2 receptor mediates programmed cell death. *Proc Natl Acad Sci* 1996;93:156–160.

230. Lo M, et al. Subtype 2 of angiotensin II receptors controls pressure-natriuresis in rat. *J Clin Invest* 1995;95:1394–1397.

231. Ichiki T, et al. Effects on blood pressure and exploratory behaviour of mice lacking angiotensin II type-2 receptor. *Nature* 1995;271: 2729–2735.

232. Kato H, et al. Angiotensin II stimulates collagen synthesis in cultured vascular smooth muscle cells. *J Hypertens* 1991;9:17–22.

233. Gibbson GH, et al. Vascular smooth muscle cell hypertrophy vs hyperplasia: autocrine transforming growth factor-b1 expression determines growth response to angiotensin II. *J Clin Invest* 1992;90: 456–461.

234. Albaladejo P, et al. Angiotensin converting enzyme inhibition prevents the increase in aortic collagen in rats. *Hypertension* 1994;23: 74–82.

235. Yusuf S, et al. Effects of an angiotensin-converting-enzyme inhibitor, ramipril, on cardiovascular events in high-risk patients: the Heart Outcomes Prevention Evaluation Study Investigators. *N Engl J Med* 2000;342:145–153.

236. Dahlöf B, et al. Cardiovascular morbidity and mortality in the Losartan Intervention For Endpoint reduction in Hypertension Study (LIFE): a randomized trial against atenolol. *Lancet* 2002;359: 995–1003.

237. Ferrario CM, et al. Hypertension and atherosclerosis: a mechanistic understanding of disease progression. *Cardiovasc Risk Factors* 1996;6: 299–310.

238. Kubo A, et al. Inhibitory effect of an angiotensin II type 1 receptor antagonist on growth of vascular smooth muscle cells from spontaneously hypertensive rats. *J Cardiovasc Pharmacol* 1996;27:58–63.

239. Yanagitani Y, et al. Angiotensin II type 1 receptor-mediated peroxide production in human macrophages. *Hypertension* 1999;33[part II]:II-335–II-339.

240. Kim JA, et al. Angiotensin II increases monocyte binding to endothelial cells. *Biochem Biophys Res Commun* 1996;226:862–868.

241. Clozel M, et al. Endothelial dysfunction and subendothelial monocyte macrophages in hypertension. *Hypertension* 1991;18:132–141.

242. Keidar S, et al. Angiotensin II-modified LDL is taken up by macrophages via the scavenger receptor, leading to cellular cholesterol accumulation. *Arterioscler Thromb Vasc Biol* 1996;16:97–105.

243. Strawn WB, et al. Inhibition of early atherogenesis by losartan in monkeys with diet-induced hypercholesterolemia. *Circulation* 2000; 101:1586–1593.

244. Song K, et al. Induction of angiotensin converting enzyme and angiotensin II receptors in the atherosclerotic aorta of high cholesterol fed Cynomolgus monkeys. *Atherosclerosis* 1998;138:171–182.

245. Chobanian AV, et al. Antiatherogenic effect of captopril in the Watanabe heritable hyperlipidemic rabbit. *Hypertension* 1990;15:327–331.

246. Hernandez A, et al. Delapril slows the progression of atherosclerosis and maintains endothelial function in cholesterol-fed rabbits. *Atherosclerosis* 1998;137:71–76.

247. Packer M, et al. Effect of carvedilol on survival in severe chronic heart failure. *N Engl J Med* 2001;344:1651–1658.

248. Buhler FR, et al. Propanolol inhibition of renin secretion: a specific approach to diagnosis and treatment of renin-dependent hypertensive disease. *N Engl J Med* 1972;287:1209–1214.

249. Hollifield JW, et al. Proposed mechanisms of propranolol's antihypertensive effect in essential hypertension. *N Engl J Med* 1976;295:68–73.

250. Stokes GS, et al. β-blockers and plasma renin activity in hypertension. *Br Med J* 1974;1:60–62.

251. Frishman WH. Atenolol and timolol, two new systemic β-adrenoceptor antagonists. *N Engl J Med* 1982;306:1456–1462.

252. Myers MG, et al. Brain concentration of propranolol in relation to hypotensive effect in the rabbit with observations on brain propranolol levels in man. *J Pharmacol Exp Ther* 1975;192:327–335.

253. Bragg JL, et al. Beta adrenergic antagonist utilization among hemodialysis patients. *J Am Soc Nephrol* 2001;12:A1652.

254. Packer M, et al. for the Carvedilol Heart Failure Study Group. The effect of carvedilol on morbidity and mortality in patients with chronic heart failure. *N Engl J Med* 1966;334:1349–1355.

255. Cice G, et al. Dilated cardiomyopathy in dialysis patients: beneficial effects of carvedilol—a double-blind placebo-controlled trial. *J Am Coll Cardiol* 2001;37:407–411.

256. van Zwieten PA. Centrally acting antihypertensives: a renaissance of interest mechanisms and haemodynamics. *J Hypertens* 1997;15[Suppl 1]:S3–S8.

257. Rosansky SJ, et al. Use of transdermal clonidine in chronic hemodialysis patients. *Clin Nephrol* 1993;39:32–36.

258. Palmer RF, et al. Drug therapy: sodium nitroprusside. *N Engl J Med* 1975;292:294–297.

259. Cottrell JE, et al. Prevention of nitroprusside induced cyanide toxicity with hydroxycobalamin. *N Engl J Med* 1978;298:808–811.

260. Safar ME. Antihypertensive effects of nitrates in chronic human hypertension. *J Appl Cardiol* 1990;5:69–81.

261. Duchier J, et al. Antihypertensive effect of sustained-release isosorbide dinitrate for isolated systolic hypertension in the elderly. *Am J Cardiol* 1987;60:99–102.

262. Van Bortel LMAB, et al. Pulse pressure, arterial stiffness, and drug treatment of hypertension. *Hypertension* 2001;38:914–921.

263. Campese VM. Minoxidil: a review of its pharmacological properties and therapeutic use. *Drugs* 1981;22:257–278.

264. DeQuattro V, et al. Pheochromocytoma: diagnosis and therapy. In: DeGroot LJ, ed. *Endocrinology.* Philadelphia: WB Saunders, 1989:1780–1797.

LEFT VENTRICULAR DYSFUNCTION IN DIALYSIS PATIENTS

SEAN W. MURPHY AND PATRICK S. PARFREY

Cardiovascular (CV) disease is the leading cause of mortality in patients with end-stage renal disease (ESRD) and accounts for approximately one half of all deaths (1–3). The prevalence of left ventricular (LV) disorders or ischemic heart disease (IHD) is extremely high in this population. Roughly 80% of patients starting maintenance dialysis therapy already have established left ventricular hypertrophy (LVH) or systolic dysfunction, disorders that are predictive of heart failure (HF), IHD, and death (4). The annual incidence of myocardial infarction (MI) or acute coronary syndrome requiring hospitalization among hemodialysis patients is 8%; the per annum risk of developing HF requiring hospitalization or treatment with ultrafiltration is 10% (5).

The high burden of cardiac disease associated with chronic kidney disease (CKD) is likely the end result of many etiologic factors. The prevalence of many "traditional" risk factors for heart disease, for example, diabetes and hypertension, is clearly higher among patients with renal disease than in the general population. These same risk factors may be responsible for the development of CKD in many patients. This confounds analyses of CKD itself as an independent risk factor for CV disease, and currently there is some debate as to whether or not this is the case. Regardless, several metabolic and hemodynamic disturbances that occur and progress in relation to declining renal function do increase CV risk.

This chapter focuses on the pathogenesis, risk factors, and treatment of disorders of LV geometry and function in dialysis patients. The cardiomyopathy associated with uremia may manifest itself in many ways, including arrhythmia and dialysis-associated hypotension (Fig. 17.1). These disorders, therefore, also are considered in this section. IHD is discussed in detail elsewhere in this book, but it should be recognized that myocardial dysfunction and ischemic disease are closely associated and coexist in many patients.

LEFT VENTRICULAR HYPERTROPHY AND HEART FAILURE

Pathogenesis of Left Ventricular Disorders

Ventricular growth occurs in response to mechanical stresses, primarily volume or pressure overload (6). Volume overload results in addition of new sarcomeres in series, leading to increased cavity diameter (7). Larger diameter results in increased wall tension, a direct consequence of Laplace's law (Fig. 17.2). This increase in wall tension stimulates the addition of new sarcomeres in parallel. Such remodeling thickens the ventricular wall, distributing the tension over a larger cross-sectional area of muscle and returning the tension in each individual fiber back toward normal. This combination of cavity enlargement and wall thickening is called *eccentric hypertrophy.* Pressure overload, on the other hand, increases wall tension by increasing intraventricular pressure, resulting directly in the parallel addition of new sarcomeres. Because sarcomeres are not added in series, isolated pressure overload leads to *concentric hypertrophy,* that is, wall thickening without cavity enlargement.

Both eccentric and concentric hypertrophy are initially compensatory and therefore beneficial. Dilatation permits an increase in stroke volume without an increase in the inotropic state of the myocardium and as such is an efficient adaptation to volume overload (8). It also permits the maintenance of a normal stroke volume and cardiac output in the presence of *decreased* contractility. Muscular hypertrophy returns the tension per unit muscle fiber back to normal, decreasing ventricular stress.

If the stimuli for ventricular remodeling persist, however, LVH eventually becomes maladaptive. Hypertrophy is associated with progressive, deleterious changes in myocardial cells. Early in the evolution of LVH, abnormalities of cellular calcium handling leads to abnormal ventricular relaxation; combined with decreased passive compliance of a thickened ventricular wall, these changes may precipitate diastolic dysfunction (9). Decreased capillary density, impaired coronary reserves, and abnormal relaxation may decrease subendocardial perfusion, promoting ischemia (10). Frequent coexistence of coronary artery disease (CAD) may exacerbate the situation. Fibrosis of the cardiac interstitium also occurs and appears to be more marked in pressure than volume overload (11). In the late phases of chronic overload, oxidative stress is prominent and contributes to cellular dysfunction and demise (12). Together, these various processes lead to progressive cellular attrition, fibrosis, HF, and death.

Many factors unique to patients with CKD appear to contribute to cardiac dysfunction. Anemia, salt and water overload, and arteriovenous (AV) fistulas in hemodialysis patients are

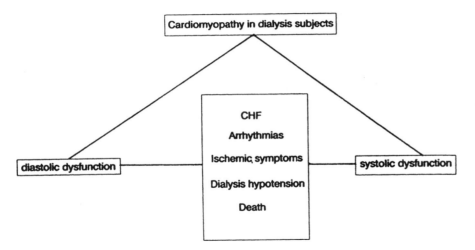

FIG. 17.1. Manifestations of cardiomyopathy in dialysis patients.

common causes of volume overload. Hypertension is highly prevalent in ESRD patients and is a major cause of pressure overload. These same factors promote arterial remodeling in the large and resistance arteries, characterized by diffuse arterial thickening and stiffening (arteriosclerosis), which can increase the effective load on the left ventricle independently of mean arterial pressure (12,13).

Aside from hemodynamic factors, the uremic milieu may also lead to myocyte death. Although CAD is the major factor promoting ischemia and infarction, hyperparathyroidism increases susceptibility to ischemia via dysregulation of cellular energy metabolism (14). Poor nutrition, oxidative stress, and inadequate dialysis may all additionally promote myocyte death (6,15,16).

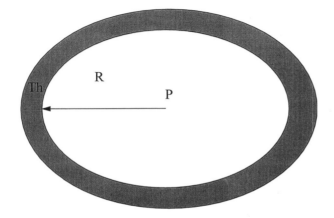

FIG. 17.2. The law of Laplace.

Diagnosis of Left Ventricular Disorders in Dialysis Patients

LV disorders can be asymptomatic, or they may be manifested clinically as HF, arrhythmias, dialysis-associated hypotension, or ischemic symptoms. The diagnosis of HF is based on clinical symptoms and signs and can usually be made with an appropriate history and physical examination. HF typically presents as progressive fatigue and decline in exercise tolerance or, alternatively, as a syndrome characterized by dyspnea and evidence of volume expansion.

Echocardiography is probably the single most useful method for the assessment of LV structure and function (17–19). It is widely available and noninvasive. Although LV mass measurement using echocardiography is highly reproducible between observers, its measurement varies over the course of a hemodialysis session by as much as 25 g/m^2 (19). This occurs because LV internal diastolic diameter decreases as the patient's blood volume decreases, as a result of fluid withdrawal. A concomitant decrease in LV wall thickness is not observed. Consequently the LV mass index measured predialysis is higher than the postdialysis measurement, although the actual LV mass has not changed. Therefore, when possible, imaging should be carried out when the patient has achieved "dry weight," the weight below which hypotension or symptoms such as muscle cramps occur.

Echocardiography provides relatively accurate measures of LV mass, cavity size, geometry, systolic function, and diastolic function. Systolic dysfunction is defined as an ejection fraction of less than 40%. It is often associated with LV dilatation (LV end-diastolic diameter ≥5.6 cm), defined as LV cavity volume index of greater than 90 mL/m^2 on echocardiogram (17). Concentric LVH is characterized by a thickened LV wall (≥1.2 cm during diastole) with normal cavity volume. Left ventricular mass index (LVMI) is a calculated parameter that reflects the degree of hypertrophy. In non-CKD patients the upper limits of normal are LVMI 130 g/m^2 for men and 102 g/m^2 for women (20). Echocardiograms have the additional benefit of allowing detection of valve disease or a pericardial effusion, conditions that can potentially precipitate HF.

Other imaging techniques, such as nuclear medicine imaging of the left ventricle using technetium-labeled red blood cells may be particularly useful in diagnosing areas of focal hypokinesis (usually resulting from ischemia). This method allows a more accurate estimate of global ejection fraction than does echocardiography alone.

Because most dialysis patients have echocardiographic abnormalities at the beginning of ESRD treatment, it is our routine practice to perform M-mode and two-dimensional echocardiography on all of our patients at or before the start of ESRD therapy. In addition to providing baseline information for future comparisons, the detection of LV disease at an earlier stage may allow more specific therapy to be employed in affected patients

Outcome of LV Disorders and Heart Failure

The presence of concentric LVH, LV dilation with normal contractility, and systolic dysfunction at baseline has been asso-

ciated with progressively worse survival, independent of age, gender, diabetes, and IHD (21). All three abnormalities are also associated with increased risk for the development of HF (Figs. 17.3 and 17.4). This relationship between LV mass and CV events in dialysis patients was confirmed recently, as was the prognostic impact of the different types of hypertrophy (22).

Symptomatic HF confers a poor prognosis for dialysis patients. In one cohort, the median survival of patients who had HF at or before initiation of ESRD therapy was 36 months, compared with 62 months in subjects without baseline HF. This adverse prognosis was independent of age, diabetes, and IHD. Among patients who had HF at baseline, 56% developed recurrent HF and 44% remained failure-free during follow-up. Median survival in those with recurrent HF was 29 months, significantly less than in those without recurrence (45 months) (23). It is interesting to note that HF has been consistently shown to be a strong independent risk factor for death, whereas the adverse impact of IHD is not a significant risk factor for

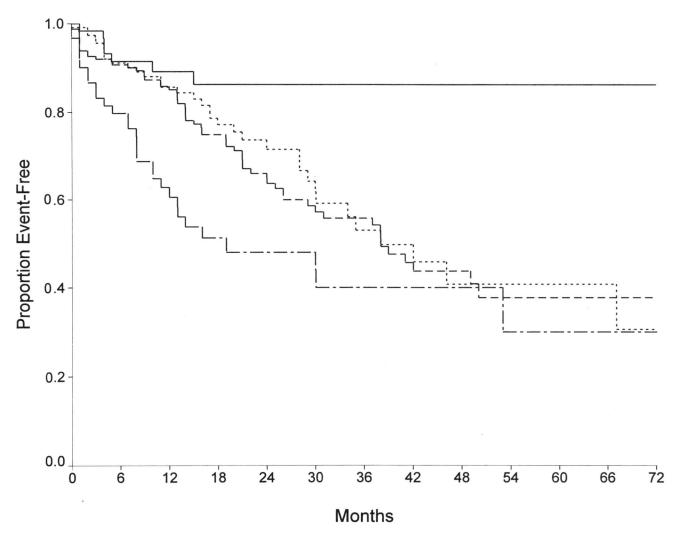

FIG. 17.3. Time to cardiac failure for patients with normal left ventricle (–), concentric left ventricular hypertrophy (———, left ventricular dilation (— -), and systolic dysfunction (— - —) at inception of dialysis therapy. (Slightly modified from Parfrey PS, et al. Outcome and risk factors for left ventricular disorders in chronic uraemia. *Nephrol Dial Transplant* 1996;11:1277–1285, with permission.)

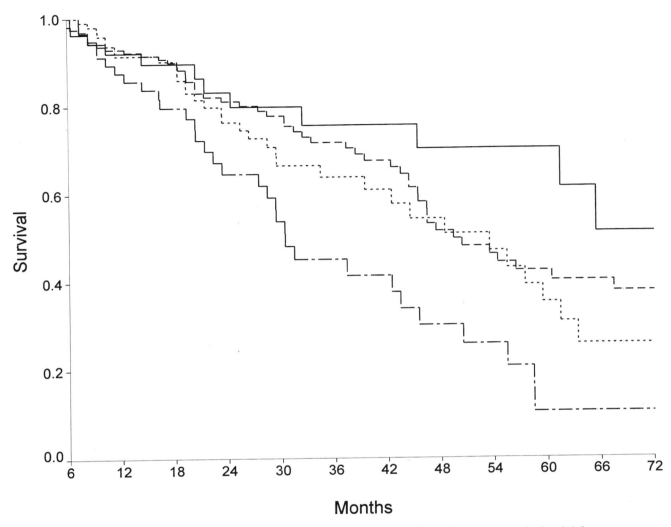

FIG. 17.4. Survival for patients with normal left ventricle (—), concentric left ventricular hypertrophy (——), left ventricular dilation (— -), and systolic dysfunction (— - —) at inception of dialysis therapy. (Slightly modified from Parfrey PS, et al. Outcome and risk factors for left ventricular disorders in chronic uraemia. *Nephrol Dial Transplant* 1996;11:1277–1285, with permission.)

death independent of age, diabetes, and presence of HF (23). This suggests that the adverse impact of IHD exerts its effect through compromising LV pump function.

Risk Factors for LV Disorders and Heart Failure

Independent predictors of HF at or before the time of ESRD therapy initiation include systolic dysfunction, older age, diabetes mellitus, and IHD. For patients without HF at baseline, predictors of the development of de novo HF include older age, systolic dysfunction, anemia, hypoalbuminemia, hypertension, and LVH (5,23). Numerous other risk factors, some unique to the dialysis patient, are known or suspected contributors to LV disorders. These include AV fistulas, disorders of divalent ion metabolism, chronic salt and water overload, altered oxidative stress, and chronic inflammation. The relative contribution of

each of these risk factors in the pathogenesis of LVH has not been fully elucidated.

Nonmodifiable Risk Factors

Diabetes Mellitus
Diabetic patients without ESRD appear to be subject to a specific type of cardiomyopathy (24,25). Glycation of collagen may induce cross-linking of collagen fibers (26), and this may be a reason for large and small vessel disease as well as myocardial dysfunction. In addition, LVH is more prevalent in hypertensive diabetic patients than in hypertensive nondiabetic patients (25,27).

In both the general and the dialysis population, diabetes is an independent risk factor for the development of HF and CAD (16,28,29). Some diabetic patients with ESRD have impairment of LV function despite normal coronary arteries, possibly resulting from the development of a diabetic cardiomyopathy as discussed previously. Having said this, any analysis of the contribution of diabetes to the development of LV dysfunction in uremic patients is confounded by the very high prevalence of other risk factors, particularly hypertension.

The impact of diabetes was examined in a cohort study of dialysis patients who survived at least 6 months following the initiation of dialysis; 15% of these patients had insulin-dependent diabetes and 12% non–insulin-dependent diabetes. On starting dialysis therapy the prevalence of clinical manifestations of cardiac disease was significantly higher in diabetic patients compared with nondiabetic patients. Only 11% of diabetic patients had normal echocardiographic dimensions compared with 25% of nondiabetic patients, predominantly because of the prevalence of severe LVH (34% vs. 18%) (30). Older age, LVH, history of smoking, IHD, cardiac failure, and hypoalbuminemia were independently associated with mortality. Diabetes was a strong risk factor for the development of IHD but not for cardiac failure (30), suggesting that the excessive cardiac morbidity and mortality of diabetic patients may be mediated via ischemic disease rather than progression of cardiomyopathy while patients are on dialysis. Echocardiographic determination of LV size and function was a good predictor of survival. Diabetic patients receiving dialysis therapy with abnormal LV wall motion and abnormal LV internal diameter had the lowest mean survival (8 months), a mortality rate not matched by any subgroup defined by coronary anatomy, ventricular function, or clinical manifestation (31).

Ischemic Heart Disease

The risk factors and outcome for IHD are discussed elsewhere in this book (see Chapter 18). CAD is an important cause of systolic and diastolic dysfunction in the general population and in dialysis patients (16,32).

Modifiable Risk Factors

Hypertension

The prevalence of hypertension is about 80% in hemodialysis patients, but it is closer to 50% in peritoneal dialysis patients (33). The 1996 Core Indicators project reported that 53% of prevalent adult hemodialysis patients had predialysis systolic blood pressures (BPs) in excess of 150 mm Hg, and 17% had predialysis diastolic BPs of 90 mm Hg or more. The comparable rates in peritoneal dialysis patients were 29% and 18%, respectively (34).

The impact of hypertension was assessed in a cohort of 261 hemodialysis and 171 peritoneal dialysis patients. These patients were followed prospectively for an average of 41 months per patient, and echocardiographic assessments were performed annually. The mean arterial BP level during dialysis therapy was 101 ±11 mm Hg. When adjustments were made for age, diabetes, and IHD and hemoglobin and serum albumin levels were measured serially, each 10 mm Hg rise in mean arterial BP was independently associated with the development of concentric LVH (OR 1.48, $p = 0.02$), IHD (OR 1.39, $p = 0.05$), and de novo HF (OR 1.44, $p = 0.007$) (35).

In the non-renal failure population, reductions in BP are associated with regression of LVH. Although a similar effect in ESRD patients seems highly likely, there is considerably less direct evidence that this is the case. In an attempt to determine the effect of BP lowering on LV size, while partially correcting anemia with erythropoietin, London et al. (36) enrolled 153 hemodialysis patients in a longitudinal study and followed them for a mean of 54 months. The first step to control BP was achievement of dry weight. If this failed to achieve the target BP, an angiotensin-converting enzyme (ACE) inhibitor, calcium channel blocker, and then α-blocker was added as required. Predialysis BP decreased from 169/90 to 147/78 mm Hg, and hemoglobin increased from 8.7 to 10.5 g/L. LV mass index decreased from 174 to 162 g/m². The hazard ratio associated with a 10% LV mass decrease was 0.78 for all cause mortality and 0.72 for CV mortality. The authors concluded that alteration of hemodynamic overload favorably influenced the natural history of LVH in hemodialysis by reducing LVH, an outcome that had a beneficial effect on survival.

Current guidelines for the treatment of hypertension in the general population do not recommend different target BP for patients with and without LVH (37,38). The optimal target BP for patients requiring dialysis is not at all clear. In this group, low BP has been repeatedly associated with increased mortality (39,40). It is likely that low BP is a marker for the presence of cardiac failure (and/or other comorbidity), confounding analyses of BP and death. This hypothesis is supported by recent analysis in the general population (41). In the absence of specific trial data, a conservative target is a predialysis BP of 140/90 mm Hg or less, unless the patient develops symptomatic hypotension during or after dialysis. This should be achieved primarily by maintenance of an accurate dry weight, with antihypertensive therapy added if satisfactory results are not achieved.

Anemia

There is considerable epidemiologic evidence that persistent anemia in patients with chronic renal failure is a risk factor for cardiac disease; it has been associated with LV dilatation and LVH in both CKD and ESRD patients [relative risk (RR) for LVH progression, per 10 g/L drop, is 1.74 in CKD and 1.48 in dialysis] (16,42–46). It is also a risk factor for the development of de novo HF and death but is not associated with de novo IHD (46).

Partial correction of anemia with recombinant erythropoietin has been shown by many investigators to lead to a decrease in elevated LV mass and improved hemodynamics (47,48). The optimal treatment target hemoglobin for anemia correction is currently the subject of intense debate. The largest trial to date addressing this question was performed by Besarab et al. (49) who compared normalization of hemoglobin versus partial correction in hemodialysis patients with preexisting IHD or HF. The primary outcome was death or MI. This trial was stopped early and increased mortality and a trend toward increased dialysis access loss was observed among the higher hemoglobin group. Another multicenter randomized controlled trial was undertaken in Canada in which hemodialysis patients without symptomatic cardiac disease were allocated to normalization of hemoglobin with erythropoietin or to partial correction of anemia. Two groups were studied, patients with preexisting LV dilatation and patients with concentric hypertrophy. In the former group mean LV volume was high at baseline (around 120 mg/m²) and a substantial minority had systolic dysfunction. Normalization of hemoglobin failed to induce regression of LV dilatation. In the latter group, normalization of hemoglobin failed to induce regression of LVH but it did prevent progressive LV dilatation (50).

These two studies suggest that (a) full correction of anemia is not beneficial in patients with established cardiac disease and (b) normalization of hemoglobin will not be effective when cardiac disease progresses to severe LV dilatation or to symptomatic presentation. The argument could be made that neither of these trials was sufficiently long to allow for significant improvements in cardiac status, and the number of dialysis patients entered in studies of the effect of erythropoietin on cardiac structure and function to date has been small. It seems likely that correction of anemia will induce regression of hypertrophy, but whether it will normalize mass is not clear. Irreversible myocardial fibrosis is probably responsible for some increase in LV mass and is likely to persist despite amelioration of anemia. If so, correction of anemia may not prevent all the clinical consequences of LVH. Furthermore, the impact of erythropoietin on various subsets of dialysis patients with other cardiac disease is not clear, and whether hemoglobin normalization at an earlier stage of renal disease may be beneficial is similarly unknown.

The optimal target hemoglobin for prevention of cardiac disease is thus currently not established. Although some authors have advocated individualized targets for ESRD patients, there has yet to be any outcome-based studies to demonstrate either the safety or efficacy of this approach. Until further data becomes available, it is reasonable to follow the current National Kidney Foundation-Dialysis Outcomes Quality Initiative (NKF-DOQI) guidelines for treatment of anemia for all patients, including those with cardiac disease. These guidelines recommend a target hematocrit of 33% to 36%, based on studies demonstrating improvement in quality of life and exercise tolerance at this level (51).

Hypoalbuminemia

Low albumin is a powerful predictor of poor outcome in dialysis patients and has been associated with LV dilatation, de novo HF, and IHD (52). The mechanisms underlying this association are unclear. It may be a marker for malnutrition, inadequate dialysis, vitamin deficiency, or a chronic inflammatory state. To date there is no real evidence as to the impact of the correction of any these factors on cardiac function.

Volume Overload

Sodium and water overload causes plasma volume expansion. Blood volume correlates directly with LV diameter in hemodialysis patients, as does the magnitude of weight changes between sessions (53,54). Despite these associations, it is difficult to clearly discern cause and effect. It is possible that salt and water retention is induced by preexisting systolic or diastolic dysfunction in some patients rather than predisposing to it.

Keeping the patient's dry weight optimal may minimize the degree of enlargement of the LV. It is interesting to note that LVH is more severe in long-term continuous ambulatory peritoneal dialysis (CAPD) patients than in hemodialysis patients (55). This finding is associated with evidence of more pronounced volume expansion, hypertension, and hypoalbuminemia.

Abnormal Divalent Ion Metabolism

There is considerable experimental and clinical evidence that the hyperparathyroid state associated with uremia contributes to cardiomyopathy, LVH, LV fibrosis, atherosclerosis, myocardial ischemia, and vascular and cardiac calcification (56). Registry data indicate that hyperphosphatemia and raised calcium × phosphate product are independent predictors of mortality (57), especially death from CAD and sudden death (58).

The appropriate use of vitamin D analogs and phosphate binders are recommended to achieve target levels for serum calcium of 9.2 to 9.6 mg/dL, for serum phosphorus of 2.5 to 5.5 mg/dL, for calcium × phosphate product of 55 mg/dL, and for intact parathyroid hormone (PTH) 100 to 200 pg/mL (59). The recent availability of aluminum and calcium-free phosphorus binders has significantly improved the management of ESRD patients. Sevelamer hydrochloride (Renagel) is an effective, although costly, phosphorus binder that is not associated with hypercalcemia. Calcimimetic agents are currently being developed and will likely further improve the treatment of hyperparathyroidism.

Valve Disease

Acquired aortic stenosis may occur in a few patients and may induce concentric LVH (60). Calcification of the aortic valve has been observed in 28% to 55% of dialysis patients in various series, whereas hemodynamically important stenosis has been reported in 3% to 13%. Progression at times may be extremely rapid. The major factors predisposing to aortic valve calcification appear to be hyperparathyroidism, duration of dialysis, and degree of elevation of calcium × phosphate product.

Mode and Quantity of ESRD Therapy

Although declining renal function has been associated with LV growth in patients with chronic renal failure, once patients reach ESRD the impact of quantity of dialysis on LVH is not definitively known. The question as to whether higher dosing targets for dialysis than those currently recommended will result in improvements in cardiac outcomes has been addressed by the recent HEMO study. In this study, 1,846 patients on three-times weekly hemodialysis were randomized to either "standard" dose (target equilibrated *Kt/V* = 1.05) or "high" dose (target equilibrated *Kt/V* = 1.45). No difference in the primary outcome of all-cause mortality or any of the prespecified secondary outcomes was observed between the groups (61).

Although some patients who are unable to tolerate the intradialytic volume expansion associated with intermittent hemodialysis may be more easily managed with peritoneal dialysis, there is no good evidence that either modality is associated with improved outcomes for patients with heart disease. Nocturnal hemodialysis has been associated with an improvement in many clinical parameters, including BP and regression of LVH (62,63). Whether the observed cardiac benefits are due to amelioration of hypertension, improvement in anemia, or higher dialysis dose is not yet clear.

Renal transplantation is undoubtedly the best treatment for ESRD and a good model of what happens to cardiac function when uremia is optimally treated. Following renal transplantation, concentric LVH and LV dilatation improves, but the most striking observation is the improvement in systolic dysfunction (64). It is not known which adverse risk factors characteristic of the uremic state have been corrected to produce the improvement in LV contractility, but hypertension and AV fistulas usually persist posttransplantation.

Management of LV Disorders and Heart Failure

Asymptomatic LV disease is usually detected with screening echocardiography. Aggressive treatment of risk factors, particularly hypertension, anemia, and IHD, is critical to prevent further myocardial dysfunction. Periodic echocardiography to assess the efficacy of such measures is prudent, and careful observation for clinical evidence of HF is required.

The initial step in the treatment of any patient with symptoms of HF should be a careful assessment for reversible precipitating or aggravating factors. Arrhythmias, uncontrolled hypertension, and use of drugs that may adversely affect cardiac performance (e.g., most calcium channel blockers, most antiarrhythmic agents, or nonsteroidal antiinflammatory drugs) are examples. IHD may be associated with HF. This diagnosis is not always obvious, especially in diabetic patients who may not have typical symptoms.

For some patients with CKD the appearance of HF symptoms refractory to standard treatment heralds the need for dialysis initiation. ESRD patients with severe HF will usually require hemofiltration for relief of their acute symptoms, and those on maintenance dialysis will require careful assessment of their target weights.

Distinguishing systolic from diastolic dysfunction on clinical grounds is difficult, although the presence of hypertension with signs of HF is suggestive of hypertrophic disease with diastolic dysfunction. Systolic and diastolic dysfunction may coexist, and the relative contribution of each process may change with the evolution of LV disease in a given patient. Nonetheless, the clinical management of HF differs according to whether systolic or diastolic dysfunction predominates. An echocardiographic diagnosis of mainly diastolic disease could lead to changes in therapy as discussed later. Consequently, an echocardiogram is an integral part of the evaluation of patients with HF.

A suggested approach to the treatment of LV disorders and HF is shown in Fig. 17.5.

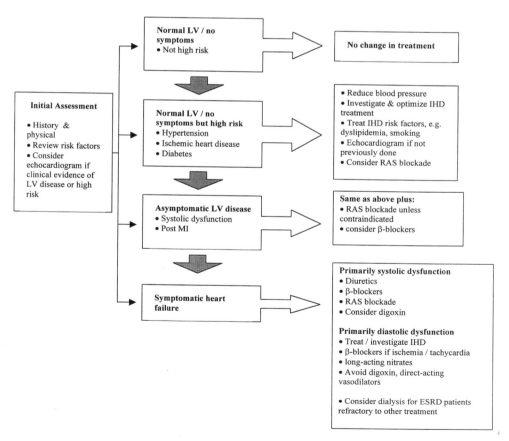

FIG. 17.5. Approach to the treatment of heart failure in dialysis patients. (From Murphy SW, et al. The management of heart failure and coronary artery disease in patients with chronic kidney disease. *Semin Dial* 2003;16:165–172, with permission).

Pharmacotherapy

Patients who have LVH without HF benefit from control of hypertension. Although many classes of drugs have been shown to improve LVH, ACE inhibitors reduce LVH beyond their BP lowering effect (65). Current guidelines recommend ACE inhibitors for patients who are either post-MI with a LV ejection fraction of less than 40% or who are asymptomatic with a LV ejection fraction of less than 35% (66,67). Although these drugs have not been as well studied in the ESRD population, it is reasonable to consider using them when there is no contraindication. Aggravation of hyperkalemia in hemodialysis patients is possible and patients should be monitored after starting treatment. Angiotensin-1 (AT_1) receptor antagonists are probably as effective as ACE inhibitors for this indication, but there is no evidence that risk of serious side effects is any lower.

β-Receptor antagonists improve the prognosis of persons with asymptomatic systolic dysfunction, regardless of whether or not the patient has had an MI (67). Comparable mortality-based trials have not been conducted in the dialysis population, but improvement in LV dimensions and fractional shortening have been demonstrated (68). For now one should consider the use of β-receptor antagonists in ESRD patients without contraindications (e.g., reactive airway disease, sinus-node dysfunction, and cardiac conduction abnormalities). As in any patient, these drugs should be started in low doses and titrated carefully. The dose of some drugs, such as atenolol, must be reduced for patients with renal impairment, and agents with intrinsic sympathomimetic activity appear to be detrimental and should not be used in patients with HF.

Non-renal failure patients with symptomatic HF resulting from systolic dysfunction are usually managed with a combination of renin-angiotensin system (RAS) blockade, β-receptor antagonists, diuretics, and/or digoxin. There have been many well-designed trials indicating that ACE inhibitors and β-receptor antagonists improve outcomes for patients with HF (67). Improvements in mortality and/or hospitalization have been shown in patients with mild to moderate symptomatic HF treated with carvedilol, bisoprolol, or controlled-release metoprolol (69–71). Individuals with significant renal impairment have almost always been excluded from these studies, however, and there is very little trial data specific to the CKD or ESRD populations. Despite this, the magnitude of the effect of both drug classes suggests that uremic patients are also very likely to benefit.

Loop diuretics are widely used to maintain euvolemia in most patients with HF, but their effect may be negligible in patients requiring dialysis. Thiazide diuretics usually become ineffective with a glomerular filtration rate (GFR) less than 30 mL/minute and are therefore not useful in patients with severe renal impairment. Aldosterone antagonists are similarly ineffective in patients with ESRD, but hyperkalemia can result when these drugs are combined with RAS blockade and β-receptor antagonists. They should be avoided in such patients.

Digoxin is useful in patients with atrial fibrillation and HF, and it improves exercise tolerance in nonuremic patients with symptomatic LV systolic dysfunction (72). Digoxin should be considered for similar patients with ESRD, provided that the dose is reduced appropriately. Low dialysate potassium levels should be avoided for hemodialysis patients, because hypokalemia may predispose to arrhythmias in the presence of digoxin. Peritoneal dialysis patients will frequently require potassium supplementation to maintain normal levels.

The treatment of diastolic dysfunction is less well defined. Attempts to eliminate the cause are generally the focus of therapy. This includes aggressive control of hypertension and IHD. Long-acting nitrates may be advantageous in some patients, and β-receptor antagonists are useful for treating IHD and tachycardia. Digoxin and direct vasodilators, such as prazosin, hydralazine, or minoxidil, are generally contraindicated in this setting (67).

CARDIAC ARRHYTHMIAS

In the general population, LVH and CAD appear to be associated with an increased risk of arrhythmias. These cardiac diseases are highly prevalent in dialysis patients. In addition, serum electrolyte levels that can affect cardiac conduction, including potassium, calcium, magnesium, and hydrogen, are often abnormal or undergo rapid fluctuations during hemodialysis. For all these reasons, cardiac arrhythmias should be common in these patients.

CAD has been associated with a higher frequency of arrhythmias in some (73,74) but not all studies on patients receiving hemodialysis (75,76). Also, the association with LVH has not been well documented in ESRD, and whether or not LVH is a cause of fatal arrhythmias (sudden death) in dialysis patients is not known. There are also conflicting data about the effect of dialysis and various dialysis compositions and dialysis protocols on the occurrence of rhythm disturbances. Some studies show higher incidence of premature ventricular contractions (PVCs) during dialysis or immediately after dialysis (76,77), whereas in others no differences could be observed (75).

In cross-sectional studies of patients with ESRD, the prevalence of atrial arrhythmias was between 68% and 88%, ventricular arrhythmias were present in 56% to 76% of patients, and PVCs were found in 14% to 21% (75–77). Older age, preexisting heart disease, LVH, and use of digitalis therapy were associated with higher prevalence and greater severity of cardiac arrhythmias (75).

Most PVCs observed are unifocal and below 30 per hour, but high-grade ventricular arrhythmias like multiple PVCs, ventricular couplets, and ventricular tachycardia have been found in 27% of 92 patients with 24-hour Holter monitoring (78). The finding of high-grade ventricular arrhythmias in the presence of IHD was associated with increased risk of cardiac mortality and sudden death (74,79). Whereas the dialysis method, membrane, and buffer used do not seem to have a direct effect on the incidence of arrhythmias (80), dialysis-associated hypotension seems to be an important factor in precipitating high-grade ventricular arrhythmias, irrespective of the type of dialysis (80,81).

Holter monitoring of cardiac rhythm of 21 peritoneal dialysis patients revealed a high frequency of atrial and/or ventricular premature beats (82). There were no differences in the type and frequency of the extrasystoles between the day on peritoneal dialysis and the day on which dialysis was deliberately withheld. It seems that, in contrast with hemodialysis, peritoneal dialysis is by itself not responsible for provoking or aggravating arrhythmias. The arrhythmias are more a reflection of the patient's age, underlying IHD, or an association with LVH (83,84).

A study in which 27 peritoneal dialysis patients were compared with 27 hemodialysis patients revealed that severe cardiac arrhythmias occurred in only 4% of CAPD and in 33% of the hemodialysis group (85). Patients in both groups were matched for age, sex, duration of treatment, and cause of chronic renal failure. The lower frequency of LVH, the maintenance of a relatively stable BP, the absence of sudden hypotensive events, and the significantly lower incidence of severe hyperkalemia in patients on peritoneal dialysis may explain the lower incidence of severe arrhythmias in CAPD patients (86).

Digoxin use in hemodialysis patients has raised concern regarding precipitation of arrhythmias, especially in the immediate postdialysis period, when both hypokalemia and relative hypercalcemia may occur (73,74,87). Keller et al. (88) studied 55 patients in a crossover study of "on-and-off" digoxin and found no increase in incidence of arrhythmias when patients were on the drug.

Currently, the treatment of arrhythmias with pharmacologic agents is controversial, regardless of the patient population. Certain antiarrhythmics may increase the likelihood of sudden death (89). In renal failure, pharmacokinetics are altered, and hemodialysis per se may have a major effect on antiarrhythmic drug levels. In general, management should first be directed at the underlying cardiac disease and the amelioration of any aspects of the dialysis procedure or uremic state that may be aggravating the situation. Only then should drug therapy be considered. It is our policy to be conservative in initiating treatment with antiarrhythmic drugs in dialysis patients.

DIALYSIS-ASSOCIATED HYPOTENSION

The hemodynamic response to hemodialysis depends on the amount and rate of fluid removal and the presence and nature of any underlying ventricular dysfunction. Fluid removal during hemodialysis leads to a decrease in plasma volume and a reduction in end-diastolic volume and diameter. Arterial hypotension may also result. The normal defense against such hypotension is mediated by the sympathetic nervous system that causes peripheral vasoconstriction, increasing systemic vascular resistance and heart rate with a resultant rise in cardiac output. In dialysis patients this compensatory response may be defective if autonomic dysfunction is present.

The influence of the nature of the underlying cardiac disease on the occurrence of dialysis hypotension has not been well studied. Theoretically, hypotension also may occur if LV dysfunction does not allow a compensatory rise in cardiac output. In patients with diastolic dysfunction there is a shift of the normal end-diastolic volume and pressure relationship (Fig. 17.6). These individuals are more likely to develop decreased cardiac output and hypotension with smaller decreases in intravascular volume. Conversely, they are also more likely to develop HF with smaller increments in intravascular volume.

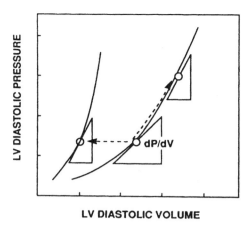

FIG. 17.6. Compliance characteristics of the left ventricle during diastolic filling. In uremia, compliance is decreased, with a leftward shift of the pressure-volume curve. (From Palmer BF, et al. The effect of dialysis on left ventricular contractility. In: Parfrey PS, et al., eds. *Cardiac dysfunction in chronic uremia.* Boston: Kluwer Academic, 1992, with permission.)

If the amount and rate of volume removal is too high, hypotension may result even in the presence of an intact autonomic nervous system and the absence of cardiac disease. Dialysis-associated hypotension is therefore often multifactorial. Indeed, it cannot entirely be explained by changes in volume status, because hypotension occurs more readily with conventional hemodialysis than with ultrafiltration, given identical fluid removal. The stability of plasma osmolality during ultrafiltration may be an important factor (90,91).

The most important means of preventing hypotensive episodes is the prescription of an accurate dry weight. Stepwise reduction of weight with clinical assessment at each stage is still the most common method of achieving this, but newer methods such as ultrasonic inferior vena cava measurement and bioelectric impedance determination are becoming more widely used. Cooling of the dialysate or sympathicomimetic agents such as midodrine are useful in selected patients. Sodium modelling during dialysis and reduction in ultrafiltration rates are also useful strategies to try. Overall the prevention and treatment of hypotension are no different in patients with underlying cardiac disease than in those with normal hearts. The existence of underlying ventricular dysfunction should, however, alert the clinician that hypotension is more likely, particularly for patients with severe LVH.

CONCLUSION

LV dysfunction and HF is a common problem in ESRD patients. Such disease may be asymptomatic and may contribute to arrhythmias or dialysis-associated hypotension. Our understanding of the optimal treatment of ESRD patients is still evolving. In the absence of specific trial data, it is wise to consider treating this patient group in much the same way as the general population. Management is aimed at treating any reversible causes, optimizing salt and water balance, and ameliorating uremic anemia. RAS blockade is a cornerstone of treatment, and β-receptor antagonists should be considered. Digoxin may be useful in patients with systolic dysfunction even in the absence of atrial fibrillation, but it should be avoided in those patients with predominantly diastolic dysfunction. Prevention of LV disease through early and aggressive treatment of risk factors is likely the best way to reduce morbidity and mortality.

REFERENCES

1. Foley RN, et al. Epidemiology of cardiovascular disease in chronic renal disease. *J Am Soc Nephrol* 1998;9[Suppl 12]:S16–S23.
2. United States Renal Data Systems: USRDS 1998 annual data report. U.S. Department of Health and Human Services. Bethesda, MD: The National Institute of Health, National Institute of Diabetes and Digestive and Kidney Diseases, August 1998.
3. 1999 report, volume 1: dialysis and renal transplantation. Ottawa, Canada: Canadian Organ Replacement Register, Canadian Institute for Health Information, June 1999.
4. Foley RN, et al. The prognostic importance of left ventricular geometry in uremic cardiomyopathy. *J Am Soc Nephrol* 1995;5:2024–2031.
5. Churchill D, et al. Canadian Hemodialysis Morbidity Study. *Am J Kidney Dis* 1992;19:214–234.
6. London GM, et al. Cardiac disease in chronic uremia: pathogenesis. *Adv Ren Replace Ther* 1997;4:194–211.
7. Grossman W, et al. Wall stress and patterns of hypertrophy in the human left ventricle. *J Clin Invest* 1975;56:56–64.
8. Grossman W. Cardiac hypertrophy: useful adaptation or pathological process? *Am J Med* 1980;69:576–584.
9. Rozich JD, et al. Dialysis induced alterations in left ventricular filling: mechanisms and clinical significance. *Am J Kidney Dis* 1991;3:277–285.
10. Hofman JI. Transmural myocardial perfusion. *Prog Cardiovasc Dis* 1987;29:429–464.
11. Amann K, et al. Cardiac disease in chronic uremia: pathophysiology. *Adv Ren Replace Ther* 1997;4:212–216.
12. London GM, et al. Cardiac and arterial interactions in end-stage renal disease. *Kidney Int* 1996;50:600–608.
13. London GM, et al. Atherosclerosis and arteriosclerosis in chronic renal failure. *Kidney Int* 1997;51:1678–1695.
14. Massry SG, et al. Mechanisms through which parathyroid hormone mediates its deleterious effects on organ function in uremia. *Semin Nephrol* 1994;14:219–231.
15. Rigatto C, et al. Oxidative stress in uremia: impact on cardiac disease in dialysis patients. *Semin Dial* 1999;12:91–96.
16. Parfrey PS, et al. Outcome and risk factors for left ventricular disorders in chronic uremia. *Nephrol Dial Transplant* 1996;11:1277–1285.
17. Pombo JF, et al. Left ventricular volumes and ejection fractions by echocardiography. *Circulation* 1971;43:480–490.
18. Devereux R, et al. Ultrasonic techniques for the evaluation of hypertension. *Curr Opin Nephrol Hypertens* 1994;3:644.
19. Harnett JD, et al. The reliability and validity of echocardiographic measurement of left ventricular mass in hemodialysis patients. *Nephron* 1993;65:212–214.
20. Levy D, et al. Echocardiographic criteria for left ventricular hypertrophy: the Framingham Study. *Am J Cardiol* 1987;59:956–960.
21. Foley R, et al. Clinical and echocardiographic disease in end-stage renal disease: prevalence, associations, and risk factors. *Kidney Int* 1995;47:186–192.
22. Zoccali C, et al. Prognostic impact of the indexation of left ventricular mass in patients undergoing dialysis. *J Am Soc Nephrol* 2001;12:2768–2774.
23. Harnett JD, et al. Congestive heart failure in dialysis patients: prevalence, incidence, prognosis and risk factors. *Kidney Int* 1995;47:884–890.
24. Galdeisi M, et al. Echocardiographic evidence for a distinct diabetic cardiomyopathy (The Framingham Heart Study). *Am J Cardiol* 1991;68:85–89.
25. Grossman E, et al. Diabetic and hypertensive heart disease. *Ann Intern Med* 1996;125:304–310.
26. Bromlee M, et al. Advanced glycosylation end products in tissue and biochemical basis of diabetic complications. *N Engl J Med* 1988;318:1315.
27. Van Hoeven K, et al. A comparison of the pathological spectrum of hypertensive, diabetic, and hypertensive-diabetic heart disease. *Circulation* 1990;82:848–855.
28. Greaves S, et al. Determinants of left-ventricular hypertrophy and systolic dysfunction in chronic renal failure. *Am J Kidney Dis* 1994;24:768–776.
29. Kannel WB, et al. Diabetes and cardiovascular disease. The Framingham Study. *JAMA* 1979;241:2035.
30. Foley RN, et al. Cardiac disease in diabetic end-stage renal disease. *Diabetologia* 1997;40:1307–1312.
31. Weinrauch LA, et al. Usefulness of left ventricular size and function in predicting survival in chronic dialysis patients with diabetes mellitus. *Am J Cardiol* 1992;70:300–303.
32. Saxon L, et al. Predicting death from progressive heart failure secondary to ischemic or idiopathic dilated cardiomyopathy. *Am J Cardiol* 1993;72:62–65.
33. Mailloux LU, et al. Hypertension in patients with chronic renal disease. *Am J Kid Dis* 1998;32[5 Suppl 3]:S120–S141.
34. Rocco MV, et al. Report from the 1995 core indicators for peritoneal dialysis study group. *Am J Kid Dis* 1997;30:165–173.
35. Foley RN, et al. Impact of hypertension on cardiomyopathy, morbidity and mortality in end-stage renal disease. *Kidney Int* 1996;49:1379–1385.
36. London GM, et al. Alterations of left ventricular hypertrophy in and survival of patients receiving hemodialysis: follow-up of an interventional study. *J Am Soc Nephrol* 2001;12:2759–2767.
37. The sixth report of the Joint National Committee on prevention, detection, evaluation and treatment of high blood pressure. *Arch Intern Med* 1997;157:2413–2446.
38. Canadian Hypertension Recommendations Working Group. The 2001 Canadian recommendations for the management of hypertension: part one—assessment for diagnosis, cardiovascular risk, causes and lifestyle modification. *Can J Cardiol* 2002;18:604–624.
39. Zager PG, et al. "U" curve association of blood pressure and mortality in hemodialysis patients. *Kidney Int* 1998;54:561–569.
40. Lowrie EG, et al. Commonly measured laboratory values in hemodialysis patients: relationships among them and to death risk. *Semin Nephrol* 1992;12:276–283.
41. Boutitie F, et al. J-shaped relationship between blood pressure and mortality in hypertensive patients: new insights from a meta-analysis of individual-patient data. *Ann Intern Med* 2002;136:438–448.
42. Levin A, et al. Left ventricular mass index increase in early renal disease: impact of decline in hemoglobin. *Am J Kidney Dis* 1999;34:125–134.
43. Foley RN, et al. The long-term evolution of cardiomyopathy in dialysis patients. *Kidney Int* 1998;54:1720–1725.
44. Huting J, et al. Analysis of left ventricular changes associated with chronic hemodialysis: a non-invasive follow-up study. *Nephron* 1988;49:284–290.
45. Parfrey P, et al. The clinical course of left ventricular hypertrophy in dialysis patients. Nephron 1990;55:114-120.
46. Foley RN, et al. The impact of anemia on cardiomyopathy, morbidity, and mortality in end-stage renal disease. *Am J Kidney Dis* 1996;28:53–61.
47. Martinez-Vea A, et al. Long-term myocardial effects of correction of anemia with recombinant human erythropoietin in aged dialysis patients. *Am J Kidney Dis* 1992;14:353–357.
48. Fellner S, et al. Cardiovascular consequences of the correction of anemia of renal failure with erythropoietin. *Kidney Int* 1993;44:1309–1315.
49. Besarab A, et al. The effects of normal as compared with low hematocrit values in patients with cardiac disease who are receiving hemodialysis and epoietin. *N Engl J Med* 1998;339:584–590.
50. Foley RN, et al. Effect of hemoglobin levels in hemodialysis patients with asymptomatic cardiomyopathy. *Kidney Int* 2000;58:1325–1335.

51. NKF-DOQI clinical practice guidelines for the treatment of anemia of chronic renal failure. National Kidney Foundation-Dialysis Outcomes Quality Initiative. *Am J Kidney Dis* 1997;30[4 Suppl 3]:S192–S240.

52. Foley RN, et al. Hypoalbuminemia, cardiac morbidity and mortality in end-stage renal disease. *J Am Soc Nephrol* 1996;7:728–736.

53. Chaignon M, et al. Effect of hemodialysis on blood volume distribution and cardiac output. *Hypertension* 1981;13:327–332.

54. London GM, et al. Cardiovascular function in hemodialysis patients. In: Grunfeld JP, et al., eds. *Advances in nephrology,* vol 20. St. Louis: Mosby Year Book, 1991.

55. Enia G, et al. Long-term CAPD patients are volume expanded and display more severe left ventricular hypertrophy than hemodialysis patients. *Nephrol Dial Transplant* 2001;16:1459–1464.

56. Rostand SG, et al. Parathyroid hormone, vitamin D, and cardiovascular disease in chronic renal failure. *Kidney Int* 1999;56:383–392.

57. Block GA, et al. Association of serum phosphorus and calcium × phosphate product with mortality risk on chronic hemodialysis: a national study. *Am J Kidney Dis* 1998;31:607–617.

58. Ganesh SK, et al. Association of elevated serum PO_4, Ca × PO_4 product, and parathyroid hormone with cardiac mortality risk in chronic hemodialysis patients. *J Am Soc Nephrol* 2001;12:2131–2138.

59. Block GA, et al. Re-evaluation of risks associated with hyperphosphatemia and hyperparathyroidism in dialysis patients: recommendations for a change in management. *Am J Kidney Dis* 2000;35:1226–1237.

60. Raine AEG. Acquired aortic stenosis in dialysis patients. *Nephron* 1994;68:159–168.

61. Eknoyan G, et al. Primary results from the HEMO study. *J Am Soc Neph* 2002;13:421A.

62. Chan CT, et al. Regression of left ventricular hypertrophy after conversion to nocturnal hemodialysis. *Kidney Int* 2002;61:2235–2239.

63. Chan CT, et al. Improvement in ejection fraction by nocturnal haemodialysis in end-stage renal failure patients with coexisting heart failure. *Nephrol Dial Transplant* 2002;17:1518–1521.

64. Parfrey PS, et al. Impact of renal transplantation on uremic cardiomyopathy. *Transplantation* 1995;60:908–914.

65. Cruikshank JM, et al. Reversibility of left ventricular hypertrophy by differing types of antihypertensive therapy. *J Hum Hypertens* 1992;6:85–90.

66. Steering Committee and Membership of the Advisory Council to Improve Outcomes Nationwide in Heart Failure: Consensus recommendations for the management of chronic heart failure. *Am J Cardiol* 1999;83:2A–38A.

67. Hunt SA, et al. ACC/AHA guidelines for the evaluation and management of chronic heart failure in the adult: A report to the ACC/AHA task force on practice guidelines (committee to revise the 1995 guidelines for the evaluation and management of heart failure), 2001, available at ACC web site (www.acc.org).

68. Hara Y, et al. Beneficial effect of β-adrenergic blockade on left ventricular function in hemodialysis patients. *Clin Sci* 2001;101:219–225.

69. Packer M, et al. The effect of carvedilol on morbidity and mortality in patients with chronic heart failure. *N Engl J Med* 1996;334:1349–1355.

70. CIBIS Investigators and Committees. The Cardiac Insufficiency Bisoprolol Study II (CIBIS II): a randomized trial of beta-blockade in heart failure. *Lancet* 1999;353:9–13.

71. MERIT-HF Study Group. Effect of metoprolol CR/XL in chronic heart failure. Metoprolol CR/XL randomized intervention trial in congestive heart failure (MERIT-HF). *Lancet* 1999;353:2001–2007.

72. Young JB, et al. Superiority of "triple" drug therapy in heart failure. Insights from the PROVED and RADIANCE trials. *J Am Coll Cardiol* 1998;32:686–692.

73. Blumberg A, et al. Cardiac arrhythmias in patients on maintenance hemodialysis. *Nephron* 1983;33:91–95.

74. D'Elia JA, et al. Application of the ambulatory 24-hour electrocardiogram in the prediction of cardiac death in dialysis patients. *Arch Intern Med* 1988;148:2381–2385.

75. Wizemann V, et al. Cardiac arrhythmias in patients on maintenance hemodialysis: causes and management. *Contrib Nephrol* 1986;52:42–53.

76. Gruppo Emodialisi e Pathologia Cardiovasculari. Multicentre cross-sectional study of ventricular arrhythmias in chronically hemodialysed patients. *Lancet* 1988;6:305–309.

77. Kimura K, et al. Cardiac arrhythmias in hemodialysis patients: a study of incidence and contributory factors. *Nephron* 1989;53:201–207.

78. Niwa A, et al. Echocardiographic and Holter findings in 321 uremic patients on maintenance hemodialysis. *Jpn Heart J* 1985;26:403–411.

79. Sforzini S, et al. Ventricular arrhythmias and four-year mortality in hemodialysis patients. *Lancet* 1992;339:212–213.

80. Wizemann V, et al. Dialysis-induced cardiac arrhythmias: fact or fiction? *Nephron* 1985;39:356–360.

81. Qellhorst E, et al. Hemofiltration: an improved method of treatment for chronic renal failure. *Contrib Nephrol* 1985;4:194–211.

82. Peer G, et al. Cardiac arrhythmia during chronic ambulatory peritoneal dialysis. *Nephron* 1987;45:192–195.

83. McLenachan JM, et al. Ventricular arrhythmias in hypertensive left ventricular hypertrophy. *Am J Hypertens* 1990;3:735–740.

84. Canziani ME, et al. Risk factors for the occurrence of cardiac arrhythmias in patients on continuous ambulatory peritoneal dialysis. *Perit Dial Int* 1993;13[Suppl 2]:S409–S411.

85. Canziani ME, et al. Hemodialysis versus continuous ambulatory peritoneal dialysis: effects on the heart. *Artif Organs* 1995;19:241–244.

86. Tzamaloukas A, et al. Temporal profile of serum potassium concentration in nondiabetic and diabetic outpatients on chronic dialysis. *Am J Nephrol* 1987;7:101–109.

87. Morrison G, et al. Mechanism and prevention of cardiac arrhythmias in chronic hemodialysis patients. *Kidney Int* 1980;17:811–819.

88. Keller F, et al. Effect of digitoxin on cardiac arrhythmia in hemodialysis patients. *Klin Wschr* 1987;65:1081–1086.

89. The Cardiac Arrhythmia Suppression Trial (CAST) Investigators. The Cardiac Arrhythmia Suppression Trial investigations: increased mortality due to Encainide or Flecainide in a randomized trial of arrhythmia suppression after myocardial infarction. *N Engl J Med* 1989;321:406–412.

90. Henrich WL. Hemodynamic instability during hemodialysis. *Kidney Int* 1986;30:605–612.

91. Keshaviah P, et al. A critical examination of dialysis-induced hypotension. *Am J Kidney Dis* 1982;2:290–301.

CORONARY ARTERY DISEASE IN END-STAGE RENAL DISEASE PATIENTS

L. DAVID HILLIS AND WILLIAM L. HENRICH

Coronary artery disease with or without left ventricular systolic dysfunction occurs commonly in subjects with end-stage renal disease (ESRD). In this patient population, in fact, it accounts for almost half of all deaths (1–3). In the 5 years following a myocardial infarction, ESRD patients have a very high mortality (about 70%) (4). Subjects with ESRD have a high prevalence of atherosclerotic coronary artery disease for several reasons. First, the average age of patients in whom dialysis is initiated has increased steadily over the past 10 to 20 years, so that nowadays it is not unusual to have patients older than 70 years on maintenance dialysis. At the same time, even young hemodialysis patients have a high prevalence of cardiovascular death; among ESRD subjects aged 20 to 44 years, the incidence of cardiovascular death is roughly 40 per 1,000 patient-years (5). The percentage of deaths that are cardiovascular in cause is similar in all age groups with ESRD (Fig. 18.1), suggesting that atherosclerosis may be accelerated in this patient population (6). Second, diabetes mellitus is the leading cause of ESRD in the United States (7). In many patients with diabetes mellitus and resultant ESRD, atherosclerosis is well established by the time dialysis is initiated. Many patients have manifestations of previous myocardial infarction, peripheral vascular disease, ischemic bowel disease, or cerebrovascular events at the time that dialysis is begun (8).

RISK FACTORS FOR ATHEROSCLEROSIS IN PATIENTS WITH ESRD

Is Atherosclerosis Accelerated in Patients with ESRD?

More than 25 years ago, Lindner et al. (6) hypothesized that atherogenesis is accelerated in patients with ESRD on maintenance hemodialysis. Of 39 subjects undergoing hemodialysis for an average of 6.5 years, 23 (59%) died; 14 of these deaths were attributed to complications of atherosclerosis (myocardial infarction in 8, cerebrovascular accident in 3, refractory congestive heart failure in 3). The incidence of these complications was many times higher than that noted in normal and hypertensive patients of similar age but without ESRD. Subsequent postmortem (9) and angiographic (10–13) studies confirmed that

the prevalence of atherosclerotic coronary artery disease is increased in dialysis patients when compared with patients of similar age without renal impairment. For example, in a postmortem examination of dialysis patients, Ansari et al. (9) found more than 50% luminal diameter narrowing of at least one epicardial coronary artery in 60% and at least some degree of atherosclerotic coronary artery disease in 86%.

The high prevalence of coronary artery disease among patients on maintenance dialysis appears to result from a multiplicity of risk factors for atherosclerosis rather than from dialysis per se. Rostand et al. (14) reported that most patients who developed symptomatic coronary artery disease during the 5 to 6 years after the initiation of dialysis had known coronary artery disease beforehand or developed it within a year of dialysis initiation, suggesting that coronary arterial atherosclerosis was already present when dialysis was begun. A recently completed cross-sectional comparison of 1,041 dialysis patients and the general population (via the National Health and Nutrition Examination database) found a high prevalence of diabetes mellitus (54%), hypertension (96%), electrocardiographic evidence of left ventricular hypertrophy (22%), limited physical activity (80%), and hypertriglyceridemia (36%) in those with ESRD (15). Even after adjusting for race, gender, and atherosclerotic vascular disease, the factors enumerated above remained more common in ESRD patients (15). In keeping with the observation that atherosclerosis often is advanced in patients with ESRD, other studies have demonstrated an increased carotid arterial intima-media thickness ratio and increased stiffness of these vessels in ESRD subjects when compared with patients of similar age without ESRD (16,17). In fact, even patients with only a modestly elevated serum creatinine (1.5 to 3.0 mg/dL) appear to have an increased morbidity and mortality in association with a variety of general surgical procedures, which may be caused, at least in part, by underlying vascular disease (18). Long-term studies (19–21) have failed to show a clear correlation between the duration of dialysis and the occurrence of cardiac events, a relation that might be expected if dialysis, in fact, promoted atherogenesis. In short, ESRD per se does not appear to cause accelerated atherosclerosis. Instead, the presence of numerous risk factors for atherosclerosis in these patients appears to be responsible for the increased prevalence of atherosclerotic vascular disease among them. Those factors that cause

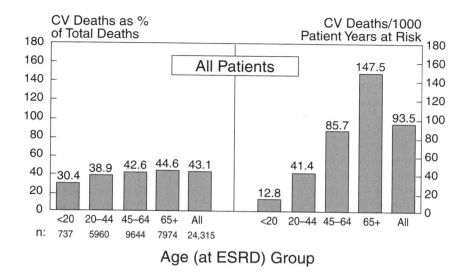

FIG. 18.1. Cardiovascular deaths, expressed as a percentage of total death *(left panel)* and per 1,000 patients at risk *(right panel)*. (From Held PJ, et al. Cardiac disease in chronic uremia. In: Parfrey PS, et al., eds. *Cardiac dysfunction in chronic uremia.* Boston: Kluwer Academic, 1992:3–17, with permission.)

oxidation of low-density lipoprotein (LDL), endothelial dysfunction, and the enhanced inflammatory state contribute to the vascular disease so often seen in ESRD patients (see Chapters 20 and 28 for a detailed discussion).

Risk Factors for Atherosclerosis in Patients with ESRD

The dramatically increased prevalence of atherosclerotic cardiovascular disease in patients with ESRD is influenced by numerous risk factors for atherosclerosis, most often systemic arterial hypertension, diabetes mellitus, hypercholesterolemia, and hyperhomocystinemia (22–27). Systemic arterial hypertension, which is extremely common in patients with ESRD, is believed to be the predominant risk factor for atherosclerosis in this patient population (26,28). Despite aggressive dialysis and antihypertensive therapy, hypertension is not optimally controlled in about half the patients with ESRD (see Chapter 16 for details). Aside from its role as a major risk factor for atherosclerosis, poorly controlled hypertension is associated with an increased likelihood of complex ventricular arrhythmias (29,30). Furthermore, the hypertension-induced increase in left ventricular mass enhances the morbidity and mortality of such arrhythmias, should they occur (31–33). Not surprisingly, a reduction of left ventricular mass (e.g., brought about by an increase in hematocrit, effective antihypertensive therapy, sympathetic nervous system blockade, or improved control of intravascular volume) is associated with a reduced morbidity and mortality in ESRD patients (34–37).

Diabetes mellitus is present in almost half the patients with ESRD, and diabetics with ESRD have a cardiovascular mortality twice that of age-matched nondiabetics (see Chapter 36). Furthermore, subjects with diabetes mellitus and associated nephropathy are at a particularly increased risk of such disease. The incidence of coronary artery disease in diabetics with nephropathy is 8 to 15 times higher than in diabetics without nephropathy (23,25). In patients with diabetes mellitus in whom coronary angiography is performed routinely as a prelude

to renal transplantation, significant coronary artery disease is noted in 25% to 50% (10–12,22). The prevalence of coronary artery disease in diabetics awaiting renal transplantation is particularly high in those older than 45 years (38).

Although virtually all studies of coronary artery disease have defined "significant" coronary atherosclerosis as a luminal diameter narrowing greater than 50% to 70%, the extent of luminal diameter narrowing and the occurrence of acute coronary events (unstable angina pectoris, myocardial infarction, or sudden cardiac death) are not tightly coupled. Ambrose et al. (39) and Little et al. (40) showed that the extent of atherosclerotic coronary arterial narrowing often does not predict the risk of thrombotic occlusion, in that many acute ischemic events are caused by thrombotic occlusion of a coronary artery without a significant stenosis.

Patients with ESRD often have serum lipid abnormalities (Table 18.1 and Chapter 28) (41–44). The cause of renal failure does not appear to influence the specific abnormalities that are seen. The most common pattern, seen in 50% to 75% of patients on hemodialysis, is an elevated serum triglyceride concentration in conjunction with a normal LDL concentration (41–44). This pattern is caused by diminished removal of triglyceride from the serum resulting from an acquired deficiency of lipoprotein lipase and hepatic triglyceride lipase (42,43). Apoprotein CII, an activator of lipoprotein lipase, is reduced in ESRD patients, whereas apoprotein CIII, an inhibitor of lipoprotein lipase, is increased (21,44). In addition, the serum concentration of high-density lipoprotein (HDL) is reduced substantially, probably because of a reduction in its synthesis and turnover (Table 18.1) (43–46). Rapoport et al. (45), for example, reported that dialysis patients had an average HDL concentration of only 26 mg/dL, substantially lower than the average of 52 mg/dL in normal individuals.

Because hypertriglyceridemia is only weakly associated with coronary artery disease in patients with ESRD, it appears likely that other more complex lipid abnormalities are important in promoting atherogenesis in these patients (44,47–49). Deficiencies of lipoprotein lipase and hepatic triglyceride lipase delay

TABLE 18.1. LIPID ABNORMALITIES IN PATIENTS WITH END-STAGE RENAL DISEASE

Increased serum concentrations of triglycerides and triglyceride remnants
Decreased serum concentrations and cholesterol content of high-density lipoprotein
Increased triglyceride content of very low density, intermediate density, low-density, and high-density lipoproteins
Cholesterol enrichment of very low density lipoprotein
Increased apo(E) content of very low density, low-density, and high-density lipoproteins
Increased serum concentrations of lipoprotein(a)

hydrolysis of triglycerides, allowing intestinal and hepatic triglyceride remnants to accumulate, thereby enriching the triglyceride content of very low density lipoprotein (VLDL), intermediate-density lipoprotein, and LDL (Table 18.1) (49). Apoproteins A-IV and B-48, absent in the serum of normal individuals during fasting, are present in patients with ESRD (49). Prolonged exposure of vascular endothelium to these remnant lipoproteins may promote atherogenesis (48,49). The cholesterol content of VLDL is increased and that of HDL is decreased in patients with ESRD (44). This cholesterol-enriched form of VLDL, termed beta-VLDL (because of its electrophoretic properties), may be more atherogenic than VLDL (Table 18.1). In addition, the apo E content of VLDL is increased in patients with ESRD, and this may allow VLDL to interact with LDL at apo B and apo E receptors (Table 18.1) (44). Finally, lipoprotein(a) [Lp(a)] concentrations are increased in patients with ESRD, independent of the cause of renal failure (50). All these factors, combined with the decreased antiatherogenic defense mechanisms that accompany a decreased HDL, likely contribute to the development of atherosclerosis.

Homocysteine is a sulfur-containing amino acid produced when methionine is demethylated. It can be oxidized to disulfide homocysteine or a mixed disulfide, homocysteine-homocysteine (6). Several recently published studies have shown a strong association between hyperhomocystinemia and advanced atherosclerotic disease (51,52). The most convincing of these, a 5-year prospective study involving almost 15,000 male physicians, showed a 3.4-fold greater risk of myocardial infarction in those with an elevated serum homocysteine concentration (53). The increased risk of myocardial infarction associated with hyperhomocystinemia was independent of other known risk factors for atherosclerosis. Numerous reports have described an increased serum level of free or protein-bound homocysteine in ESRD patients (54), and some of these reports have shown that hyperhomocystinemia persists following renal transplantation (50). This increase in the homocysteine concentration translates into a greater than 100-fold increase in the risk of atherosclerosis in comparison with controls (Fig. 18.2) (50).

The cause of hyperhomocystinemia in ESRD patients is not well understood (55). Possibly the loss of normal renal metabolism contributes to vitamin B-refractory hyperhomocystinemia in these patients (50). Studies in rats have shown that the kidney extracts homocysteine (56). With a loss of renal function, therefore, serum homocysteine concentrations rise. In fact, the

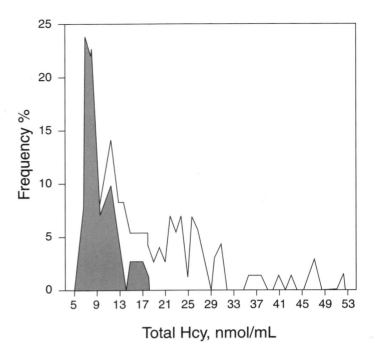

FIG. 18.2. Distribution of total fasting homocysteine (tHcy) levels in dialysis-dependent ESRD patients (*n* = 71), and age-, sex-, and race-matched controls free of renal disease (*n* = 71). *Shaded area* denotes ESRD. (From Bostom AG, et al. Hyperhomocystinemia, hyperfibrinogenemia, and lipoprotein(a) excess in maintenance dialysis patients: a matched case-control study. *Atherosclerosis* 1996;125:91–101, with permission.)

average elimination half-life of homocysteine is increased from 3.5 hours in patients with normal renal function to 11 hours in those with ESRD (56). Finally, successful renal transplantation lowers homocysteine concentrations by 23% to 33% (57).

An elevated serum homocysteine concentration is associated with an increased risk of atherosclerotic coronary artery disease and resultant events in patients with and without ESRD (58,59). Each 5 µmol/L incremental increase in serum homocysteine concentration above 10 µmol/L is associated with a 60% to 80% increased risk of coronary artery disease (58). Massy et al. (59) followed 73 dialysis patients for an average of 17 months, during which 16 of them had a cardiovascular event. The fasting serum homocysteine concentrations of those having an event were substantially higher than the concentrations in those who were event-free. Elevated homocysteine levels increased the risk of a fatal cardiovascular event 7-fold and a nonfatal event 3.5-fold.

The therapy of hyperhomocystinemia in patients with ESRD should consist of (a) folate 5 to 15 mg/day and possibly (b) N-acetylcysteine 1.2 g/day (60–68). It is unknown if it is necessary to give more than 5 mg/day of folate to achieve a maximal reduction in homocysteine concentrations. Distressingly, about two thirds of dialysis patients with serum homocysteine concentrations greater than 15 µmol/L will continue to have high homocysteine concentrations despite 15 mg/day of folic acid. Neither vitamin B$_6$ 3 to 4 g/day nor betaine 6 g/day influences homocysteine concentrations.

Oxidant Stress (See Chapter 20 for a Full Discussion)

Several reports have highlighted the importance of oxidative stress in subjects with uremia (69–73). Although some studies have shown a decrease in fatal cardiac events in non-renal failure patients who consume large amounts of β-carotene or vitamin E (74,75), prospective and randomized trials in patients with ESRD have not observed a reduction in the incidence of fatal cardiac events with antioxidant dietary supplementation (76). Nonetheless, vitamin E may slow the progression of coronary arterial atherosclerosis in ESRD patients (77), and endothelium-dependent vasoreactivity may be improved by the combination of antioxidant and lipid-lowering therapy (78,79). Patients with uremia may have an imbalance between the magnitude of oxidizing activity and the availability of antioxidants, with a resultant increase in oxidative stress. In this regard, a reduced concentration of endogenous antioxidants, such as vitamin C and vitamin E, has been noted (80,81).

Exogenous factors may contribute to the increased oxidant activity noted in ESRD patients. The use of incompatible dialysis membranes (cellulosic) may dramatically increase H_2O_2 release from activated granulocytes (82). This increase in reactive oxygen species and activated neutrophils in close proximity to endothelial cells may contribute to endothelial cell injury. The chronic, cumulative exposure to cellulosic membranes may augment lipid peroxidation, thereby contributing to the generation of oxidized LDL (see Chapter 28) (83,84). The use of cellulosic membranes may lead to an increased production of reactive oxygen species by complement-dependent and complement-independent processes (82,85). Nagasi et al. (85) have shown that antioxidant activity is significantly improved with hemodialysis to a level comparable to that of healthy controls (Fig. 18.3). In short, ESRD patients manifest diminished oxygen-scavenging activity, which is improved with dialysis.

Advanced Glycosylation End Products (See Chapter 20 for a Full Discussion)

Advanced glycosylation end products (AGEs) accumulate in ESRD patients and are not removed by dialysis (86,87). By contributing to the increased oxidative stress that exists in patients with ESRD, AGEs may contribute to the excessive cardiovascular disease seen in this patient population (88,89). In addition, AGEs may consume nitric oxide, thereby diminishing vasodilatation. Based on data from experimental animals, Palinski et al. (90) have suggested that AGEs are present in atherosclerotic lesions. Through all these mechanisms, it seems feasible that AGEs may potentiate atherosclerosis in ESRD patients (91).

Oxidized Low-Density Lipoproteins

The dyslipidemias associated with renal failure are discussed in detail in Chapter 28. In the setting of increased oxidative stress, the in vivo oxygenation of LDL may promote atherosclerotic disease by causing endothelial injury. Cellular lipoxygenase and reactive oxygen species are believed to inaugurate LDL oxidation (92,93), which leads to a chemical rearrangement of fatty

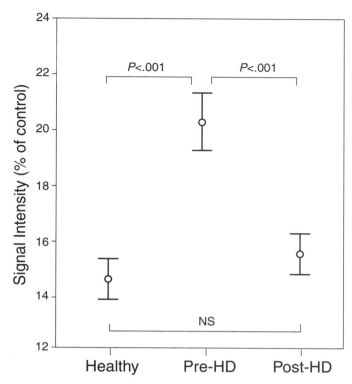

FIG. 18.3. Comparison of electron spin resonance (ESR) signal intensity among the reaction mixtures containing healthy, prehemodialysis (pre-HD), and post-HD sera. *Open circles* indicate the mean, and *bars* indicate the standard deviation of signal intensities. The ESR signals of the reaction mixture containing pre-HD sera are significantly stronger than those containing healthy sera (unpaired *t* test, *p* <0.001, *n* = 19 and 23) or those containing post-HD sera (paired *t* test, *p* <0.001, *n* = 19), and there is no significant difference in the signal intensities between the reaction mixtures containing post-HD sera and healthy sera. (From Nagasi S, et al. Favorable effect of hemodialysis on decreased serum antioxidant activity in hemodialysis patients demonstrated by electron spin resonance. *J Am Soc Nephrol* 1997;8: 1157–1163, with permission.)

acid structure and subsequent fragmentation, resulting in aldehyde and ketone formation. These alterations favor the recognition of oxidized LDL by monocytes, which act as scavengers in the subendothelial space. Scavenger cells that take up oxidized LDL gradually become cholesterol enriched and form foam cells, the initial "building block" of atherosclerosis (93).

Leukocyte-endothelial cell interaction further promotes the process of atherosclerosis by potentiating monocyte chemotaxis. In addition, oxidized LDL directly damages endothelial cells (94). One intriguing new observation is that LDL oxidation can occur in vivo and generate antigenic epitopes (95), leading Salonen et al. (96) to propose that autoantibody formation against oxidized LDL may contribute to the progression of atherosclerosis. Other reactions, such as the carbamylation of LDL, may contribute to altered LDL clearance and influence the scavenger pathway in ESRD patients. An elevated urea nitrogen concentration can trigger condensation of cyanate with lipoprotein lysine residues, leading to reduced clearance and increased pathogenicity (97).

Oxidized LDL is present in chronic dialysis patients, and several studies have demonstrated an increase in lipid peroxidation products in the plasma and the lipoprotein fractions of ESRD patients (84–96,98–100). Finally, Itabe et al. (101) showed that oxidized LDL was increased more than eightfold in chronic dialysis patients when compared with controls. In short, ESRD patients on dialysis clearly have increased levels of oxidized LDL, which play an important role in accelerated atherogenesis.

Lipoprotein(a)

Lp(a) has been linked to atherogenesis in the general population and in ESRD patients (see Chapter 28). Its atherogenicity may be related to its binding of apolipoprotein B and subsequent uptake by macrophages, forming foam cells. Lp(a) accumulates in atherosclerotic plaque, after which it undergoes further alterations, including oxidation, which may contribute to its atherogenicity (102). In addition, Lp(a) inhibits plasminogen activation and may stimulate vascular smooth muscle proliferation, each of which may further enhance atherosclerotic plaque formation (103). Lp(a) serum concentrations are typically two to three times higher in ESRD patients than in healthy controls (104), resulting largely from a decreased renal catabolism of Lp(a). Certain Lp(a) phenotypes may be particularly atherogenic; for example, the low-molecular-weight phenotype of Lp(a) may increase the risk of atherosclerosis in ESRD patients.

Other Factors

Malnutrition may contribute to atherosclerosis, in that there is an inverse relation between a low serum albumin concentration and an elevated Lp(a) level in chronic dialysis patients (105). Whether vascular reactivity is altered by poor nutrition is unknown, but Ritz et al. (106) have suggested that malnour-ished patients may have diminished nitric oxide production. Hypoalbuminemia is associated with an increased risk of ischemic heart disease (107) and cardiovascular death in ESRD patients. The precise mechanisms underlying this observation are unclear, but it is possible that albumin may act as an oxidative product scavenger so that hypoalbuminemia renders the patient more vulnerable to atherogenesis. In diabetic subjects with ESRD, Koch et al. (108) demonstrated an association between lower skin fold thickness and mortality.

Recent attention has centered on the association of a high calcium-phosphorus product and both vascular calcifications and decreased arterial compliance in ESRD patients. One such study documented a dramatic increase in arterial stiffness in subjects with a high calcium-phosphorous product; in addition, it suggested that calcium-containing phosphate binders may contribute to the appearance of vascular disease (109). Arterial calcification in ESRD subjects most often involves the vessel media; a recently published study has postulated that the deposition of calcium and phosphorus in the arterial media may follow the deposition of bone matrix proteins, such as osteopontin (110). A randomized comparison of 12 months duration of the non–calcium-containing binder, sevelamer, versus calcium-containing binders demonstrated diminished coronary arterial calcification (as measured by electron beam tomography) in those receiving sevelamer (*p* <0.01) (111) (Fig. 18.4). Whether a diminution of vessel calcification will be associated with a reduction in adverse cardiovascular events is unknown (112). In addition, it is unknown if other agents, such as vitamin E, will reduce the magnitude of arterial calcification (111). Finally, it should be remembered that a low calcium-phosphorus product—and particularly a low phosphate concentration—is associated with a higher mortality in ESRD patients (113).

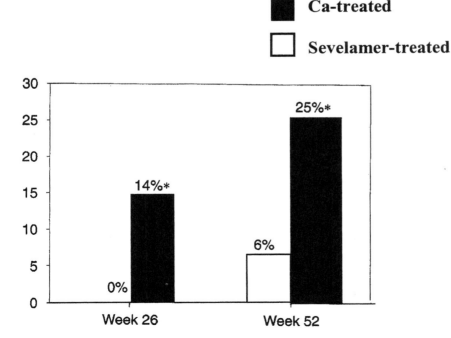

Ca-treated

Sevelamer-treated

FIG. 18.4. Median percent change in coronary artery calcification scores from baseline to weeks 26 and 52 in patients with calcification scores ≥30 at baseline. Calcium-treated patients have significantly greater increases than sevelamer-treated patients at weeks 26 and 52. (From Chertow GM, et al. Sevelamer attenuates the progression of coronary and aortic calcification in hemodialysis patients. *Kidney Int* 2002;62:245–252, with permission.)

CLINICAL PRESENTATIONS OF CORONARY ARTERY DISEASE IN PATIENTS WITH ESRD

Myocardial ischemia is caused by a relative imbalance of myocardial oxygen supply and demand. Most often, it occurs during transient increases in oxygen demand in the presence of atherosclerotic narrowing of one or more coronary arteries. Less often, it may be caused by (a) a transient primary fall in myocardial oxygen supply, such as that caused by coronary arterial vasospasm, or (b) an excessive augmentation of myocardial oxygen demand without a limitation of supply, such as that which may occur with severe aortic stenosis, a sustained supraventricular or ventricular tachyarrhythmia, or severe sustained systemic arterial hypertension.

Myocardial ischemia is usually diagnosed when typical angina pectoris occurs during exertion, emotional excitement, or hemodialysis. Physical exertion or emotional excitement often cause an increase in the three major determinants of myocardial oxygen demand (heart rate, left ventricular wall tension, and cardiac contractility). Hemodialysis may induce myocardial ischemia by producing hypotension, thereby diminishing myocardial oxygen supply, or by provoking tachycardia and/or increased cardiac contractility, thereby increasing myocardial oxygen demand. It is not surprising, therefore, that angina pectoris often is provoked during hemodialysis.

The clinical significance of "silent" (painless) myocardial ischemia is controversial. It is considered to be present when, in the absence of chest pain, (a) ST segment alterations of ischemia are noted during provocative testing or ambulatory electrocardiographic monitoring, (b) reversible myocardial perfusion defects appear with thallium imaging, or (c) reversible segmental wall motion abnormalities are noted by echocardiography. Although the pathogenesis of silent ischemia has not been resolved, three mechanisms have been proposed. First, some patients may have altered neural pathways, so they cannot sense the pain of myocardial ischemia. Cardiac transplant recipients, in whom the heart is surgically denervated, and diabetic patients with generalized neuropathy are particularly likely to have such episodes. Second, patients with silent myocardial ischemia may have unusually high thresholds for pain and thus do not sense painful stimuli as other individuals do. Third, differences in the duration and severity of ischemic episodes may explain why some of them occur without pain. Because chest pain is a relatively late manifestation of myocardial ischemia, short-lived episodes of ischemia may interfere with myocardial relaxation and contraction, inducing electrocardiographic and perfusion abnormalities but resolving before chest pain appears.

Silent myocardial ischemia provides valuable prognostic information. In asymptomatic patients without a cardiac history, silent ischemia identifies those at increased risk of a subsequent cardiac event, such as the onset of angina pectoris, myocardial infarction, or sudden cardiac death. Patients with silent as well as painful ischemia or a previous myocardial infarction are more likely to have an adverse outcome (such as subsequent myocardial infarction, the need for coronary revascularization, or the occurrence of cardiac death) in comparison to those without silent ischemia. However, no difference in prognosis is apparent between patients with silent ischemia and those with symptomatic ischemia. As a result, although agents that are useful in treating angina pectoris are effective in treating silent ischemia, the overall impact of therapy (medical or nonmedical) on prognosis is unknown.

DIAGNOSIS OF CORONARY ARTERY DISEASE IN ESRD PATIENTS

In stable ESRD patients, the development of angina pectoris, pulmonary edema without major changes in intravascular volume, unexplained hypotension, or a marked change in exercise capacity may trigger an investigation into the presence of coronary artery disease.

In the patient with ESRD who is being considered for renal transplantation, atherosclerotic coronary artery disease, symptomatic or asymptomatic, is associated with an increased incidence of allograft failure and mortality (11–13,22,114,115). For example, Philipson et al. (114) performed coronary angiography in 53 diabetic transplant candidates, detecting significant coronary artery disease in 20 (38%). During an average follow-up of 1 year, mortality was 44% in those with and only 5% in those without coronary artery disease. Because of data such as these, transplant candidates with angina or evidence of previous myocardial infarction typically undergo coronary angiography as a part of their pretransplant evaluation, and subsequent transplantation may be denied if coronary artery disease is extensive and not amenable to revascularization (13,114,115).

Patients with ESRD without angina or with atypical symptoms of coronary artery disease pose a difficult management problem, because many of them, particularly if they are diabetic, have coronary artery disease. For example, Weinrauch et al. (12) reported that 41% of asymptomatic diabetic patients with ESRD awaiting transplantation had significant coronary artery disease, and their 2-year survival was only 22%, compared with 88% in those without coronary artery disease. Similarly, Bennett et al. (13) reported that 11 consecutive diabetics without symptoms of coronary artery disease who were awaiting renal transplantation had angiographic evidence of multivessel coronary artery disease, even though only 4 had positive exercise tests. Over the subsequent 20 months, 8 of the 11 died. Similar findings were reported by Braun et al. (116), who noted in addition that depressed left ventricular systolic performance was associated with a particularly guarded cardiovascular outcome (22,116–118).

Perhaps the most exciting recent development in the identification and risk stratification of ESRD patients with possible coronary artery disease is the so-called cardiac biomarkers, such as troponin T. Data from Zoccali et al. (119) and deFilippi et al. (120) suggest that ESRD patients with a troponin T ≥0.07 to 0.10 ng/mL are at a particularly high risk for underlying coronary artery disease and its associated adverse events. Other studies have found that cardiac troponin T concentrations are useful in predicting short-term prognosis in patients with a wide range of renal function (121–124). In addition to the relationship between cardiac troponin T concentrations and atherosclerotic coronary artery disease (119–121), elevated troponin T levels have been linked to increased left ventricular mass in dialysis

TABLE 18.2. SENSITIVITY/SPECIFICITY OF NONINVASIVE TESTING FOR CAD

	No Renal Disease (%)		Renal Disease (%)	
	Sensitivity	Specificity	Sensitivity	Specificity
Exercise ECG	50–85	85	QNS	QNS
Exercise thallium-201	82	91	67	62
Dipyridamole	79	76	37–86	73–79
Adenosine thallium	83	76	QNS	QNS
Exercise echocardiogram	76–84	95	QNS	QNS
Dobutamine echocardiogram	72–89	85–95	69–96	95
Dipyridamole echocardiogram	52–60	95	QNS	QNS

CAD, coronary artery disease; ECG, electrocardiogram; QNS, quantity not sufficient.
Murphy SW, Parfrey PS. Screening for cardiovascular disease in dialysis patients. *Curr Opin Nephrol* 1996;5:539.

patients (124,125). In this regard, the measurement of brain natriuretic peptide (BNP) also appears to correlate with prognosis in this patient population (126,127). Cardiac troponin I appears to have limited value in cardiovascular risk stratification in ESRD patients, perhaps because its half life is relatively short (120,128). In addition to cardiac troponin T, markers of inflammation, such as C-reactive protein, appear to be associated with a poor prognosis (129,130).

How then should the cardiovascular evaluation of a candidate for renal transplantation proceed? Because coronary angiography is costly, invasive, and not risk-free, it is not an ideal screening procedure for all patients with ESRD under consideration for transplantation. Among its potential deleterious effects, contrast-induced nephrotoxicity may cause further deterioration in patients with some degree of residual renal function.

Therefore, coronary angiography should be reserved for those who are likely to have significant coronary artery disease or those who may benefit from revascularization. Patients with typical angina, evidence of previous myocardial infarction (by history or electrocardiogram), or congestive heart failure should be considered to be at high risk, and cardiac catheterization should be performed to assess left ventricular systolic function as well as the presence and magnitude of coronary artery disease. Other noninvasive studies for the diagnosis of coronary artery disease are provided in Table 18.2.

Patients with congestive heart failure are considered to be high risk, because those with impaired left ventricular systolic performance and coronary artery disease have a particularly guarded prognosis and may derive an improved survival with surgical revascularization. The reader is directed to Fig. 18.5 for

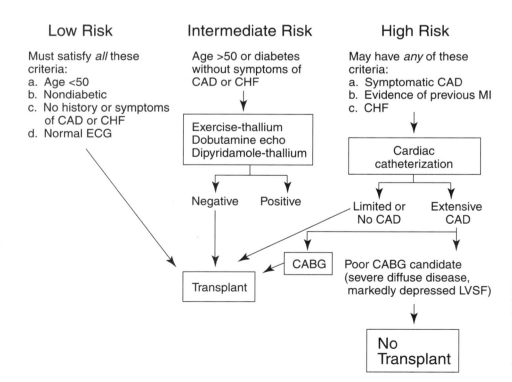

FIG. 18.5. Proposed management strategy for end-stage renal disease patients who are candidates for renal transplantation. (From DeLemos JA, et al. Diagnosis and management of coronary artery disease in patients with end-stage renal disease on hemodialysis. *J Am Soc Nephrol* 1996; 7:2044–2054, with permission.)

a suggested approach to the management of patients with ESRD and possible coronary artery disease.

Several investigators have attempted to devise a strategy whereby low risk patients, who can safely undergo renal transplantation without a preoperative cardiovascular evaluation, can be identified quickly, inexpensively, and noninvasively. Le et al. (131) prospectively enrolled 196 consecutive candidates for renal transplantation in a risk stratification program based on the presence of five risk variables: insulin-dependent diabetes mellitus, age older than 50 years, a history of angina, a history of congestive heart failure, and an abnormal electrocardiogram. Patients were considered to be low risk if they had none of these variables and high risk if any was present. Over a follow-up period averaging almost 4 years, cardiac mortality was 17% in the 95 high-risk patients and only 1% in the 94 low-risk patients.

Other investigators have used a similar approach in diabetics with ESRD. Manske et al. (132) retrospectively identified several clinical variables that were associated with coronary artery disease in diabetic transplant candidates: age older than 45 years, a greater than 5 pack-year history of cigarette smoking, more than 25 years of diabetes mellitus, and nonspecific ST-T wave abnormalities on a resting electrocardiogram. In a small group of patients studied prospectively, they showed that these variables provided a sensitivity of 97% and a negative predictive value of 96% for detecting angiographically significant coronary artery disease. Furthermore, they concluded that diabetics younger than 45 years with none of these predictors could safely undergo renal transplantation without a preoperative cardiovascular assessment.

If transplant candidates are not clearly high or low risk, they are considered to be at intermediate risk. This intermediate risk group includes older patients without symptoms of coronary artery disease, previous myocardial infarction, or congestive heart failure, as well as most diabetics with no symptoms or atypical symptoms of coronary artery disease. This intermediate risk group constitutes most patients who are considered for renal transplantation. Noninvasive testing may be particularly useful in the pretransplant cardiac evaluation of these subjects (133–136).

Many patients with ESRD have electrocardiographic abnormalities at rest that make the electrocardiogram difficult or impossible to interpret during provocation (often because of left ventricular hypertrophy), and many patients, particularly those who are diabetic, fail to attain a sufficient heart rate during exercise to provide a reasonable predictive accuracy (10,52,137). As a result, provocative pharmacologic testing with concomitant cardiac imaging (using nuclear scintigraphy or echocardiography) has been used in an attempt to identify patients with underlying coronary artery disease.

There are conflicting reports in the literature concerning the utility of thallium imaging with dipyridamole to identify coronary artery disease in patients with ESRD awaiting transplantation. On the one hand, Marwick et al. (138) and Boudreau et al. (139) concluded that such imaging was of little use in identifying angiographically significant coronary artery disease or in predicting cardiac prognosis in this patient population. Of Marwick's 45 transplant candidates (138), thallium imaging with dipyridamole offered only fair specificity and poor sensitivity in identifying coronary artery disease. Importantly, five of the six individuals who died of cardiac causes over a mean follow-up of 2 years had normal thallium imaging studies. Of the 80 patients reported by Boudreau et al. (139), 36 had negative dipyridamole thallium studies, 6 (17%) of whom had significant angiographic coronary artery disease, giving a negative predictive value of only 83% (Table 18.2).

On the other hand, several reports have concluded that thallium imaging with dipyridamole provides an effective noninvasive means of identifying transplant candidates with no chest pain or atypical chest pain who are at increased risk of having a subsequent cardiac event. Camp et al. (133) showed that six of nine patients with dipyridamole-induced reversible thallium defects had a subsequent cardiovascular event, whereas none of 31 patients without reversible defects had a subsequent event. Other studies (117,140) have supported the contention that thallium imaging with dipyridamole can identify the patients at increased risk of an adverse cardiovascular outcome. In addition, a normal thallium imaging study appears to predict a very low likelihood of a subsequent cardiovascular event (117,131,133).

Why are these dipyridamole-thallium data disparate? The reasons are not entirely clear but may include differences in study design, definition of end points, interpretation of "positive" thallium images, and patient selection. Most of these studies used only patients referred for noninvasive evaluation, and the differences in referral patterns between centers may explain some of the variability in results (141).

Two-dimensional echocardiography during the intravenous infusion of dobutamine (so-called dobutamine stress echocardiography) was recently evaluated in 97 patients (both diabetic and nondiabetic) with ESRD awaiting renal transplantation (134). In these patients, this technique had a sensitivity of 95% and a specificity of 86% for predicting death or cardiovascular complications during the subsequent year. Although the positive predictive value was poor (only 14%), the negative predictive value was excellent (97%). These promising results await confirmation by others (Table 18.2). In a recent assessment of symptoms, electrocardiographic findings, thallium dipyridamole scintigraphic results, and echocardiographic results in 42 ESRD patients and 42 patients after renal transplantation indicated that the presence of angina offered the best prognostic information by far (142), whereas the other methods lacked sensitivity and/or specificity in the identification of those with coronary artery disease.

In summary, all high-risk transplant candidates—those with symptoms of coronary artery disease, electrocardiographic evidence of previous myocardial infarction, or congestive heart failure—should have coronary angiography before renal transplantation. At the opposite extreme, young, nondiabetic patients without symptoms of coronary artery disease or electrocardiographic evidence of previous myocardial infarction comprise a low-risk group, and they do not require cardiac evaluation before transplantation. In addition, young diabetics, particularly nonsmokers who have had diabetes for less than 25 years and whose electrocardiograms are normal, may not require cardiac evaluation before renal transplantation. Patients are considered to be at intermediate risk if they are neither high nor low risk;

this group includes older patients without symptomatic coronary artery disease as well as most diabetics with no symptoms or atypical symptoms of coronary artery disease. In preparation for transplantation, these patients should undergo noninvasive evaluation (with dobutamine stress echocardiography or dipyridamole-thallium imaging), recognizing that neither procedure is perfect. Because most insulin-dependent diabetics younger than 45 years have underlying coronary artery disease, we recommend that these individuals routinely undergo coronary angiography, even in the absence of angina or electrocardiographic evidence of previous myocardial infarction (Fig. 18.4) (135).

MANAGEMENT OF ESRD PATIENTS WITH CORONARY ARTERY DISEASE

Medical Management

Several initial steps should be taken in the medical management of patients with ESRD and coronary artery disease. First, correction of the hematocrit to between 33% and 35% to improve oxygen-carrying capacity should be pursued with erythropoietin therapy (see Chapter 32) (143,144). Such an improvement in hematocrit may allow the patient to participate in exercise training, which by itself offers additional benefits (145). Second, control of blood pressure (see Chapter 16) is important in reducing the magnitude of left ventricular hypertrophy and myocardial oxygen demand, resulting in reduced anginal frequency, ventricular irritability, and perhaps even mortality (7,146–148). Obviously, careful control of intravascular volume is implicit in this strategy; in addition, measures to reduce left ventricular mass are important (Chapter 17). The use of high sodium dialysate, sodium-modeling regimens, cool temperature dialysis, and other strategies to protect blood pressure during ultrafiltration dialysis are discussed in Chapter 19. One or more of these strategies may be necessary to achieve an ideal dry weight.

Several antianginal medications may be useful in patients with stable angina on dialysis. Long-acting nitrates are effective orally or cutaneously in reducing anginal frequency and severity, but their influence on survival is unknown (7). Twice daily dosing with a long nitrate-free period is recommended so that nitrate tolerance is minimized. The use of sublingual nitroglyc-

erin may induce hypotension, particularly if the patient uses it during dialysis.

Other drugs that are often prescribed in patients with ESRD and angina include β-blockers, which reduce heart rate, contractility, and left ventricular wall tension, and calcium channel blockers, which induce coronary arterial vasodilation and simultaneously reduce the determinants of myocardial oxygen demand. These agents reduce anginal frequency and the number of cardiovascular events that occur in patients with silent myocardial ischemia (149). Caution should be used in administering these agents to patients with ESRD, because some of them depend on normal renal function for their metabolism. For example, the β-blocker, atenolol, is excreted unchanged in the urine, and its half-life is increased fourfold in patients with ESRD. As a result, the dose of atenolol should be reduced by 50% to 75% and its dosing frequency increased to avoid β-blocker intoxication in patients with ESRD. Because propranolol and metoprolol are largely metabolized by the liver, their dosage and frequency are not altered in patients with ESRD. Similarly, the calcium channel blockers—diltiazem, verapamil, and the dihydropyridines—are metabolized by the liver; as a result, dosing adjustments are unnecessary in patients with ESRD. For patients with known coronary artery disease, low-dose aspirin is recommended.

Nonmedical Management

Table 18.3, adapted from the work of Fellner et al. (150), summarizes recommendations for coronary artery bypass grafting in patients with ESRD. In general, the indications for bypass grafting in ESRD patients are similar to those in subjects with normal renal function. First, individuals with limiting angina despite adequate medical therapy should be considered for bypass grafting to eliminate or to improve symptoms. Second, certain patient subgroups should be considered for bypass grafting to improve long-term survival. This includes patients with (a) greater than 50% luminal diameter narrowing of the left main coronary artery; (b) greater than 70% luminal diameter narrowing of two or three major epicardial coronary arteries, in whom the proximal portion of the left anterior descending coronary artery is significantly narrowed; and (c) greater than 70% luminal diameter narrowing of all three major epicardial coronary arteries in association with left ventricular systolic dysfunc-

TABLE 18.3. GENERAL RECOMMENDATIONS FOR AORTOCORONARY BYPASS SURGERY

Generally Indicated	Intermediate Indications	Not Indicated
Left main disease of greater than 50%	Stable, 2-vessel disease with mild to moderate to severe LV dysfunction	Asymptomatic[a] and 1- or 2-vessel disease
Severe 3-vessel disease (greater than 70% narrowing) or symptomatic	Symptomatic 2-vessel disease with a normal left ventricle	Stable angina with 1-vessel disease
Severe 2- or 3-vessel disease with moderate to severe left ventricular dysfunction or symptomatic	Symptomatic[a] 1-vessel disease	Angina with no significant coronary artery disease
Severe 2-vessel disease including a proximal left anterior descending artery	Stable 1-vessel disease with severe LV dysfunction	Unstable 1-vessel disease

LV, left ventricular.
[a]*Symptomatic* can refer to clinical symptoms or an abnormal exercise stress test result. *Asymptomatic* refers to no symptoms or a negative stress test result.

tion (ejection fraction <0.50) (151). It should be emphasized that no data from prospectively performed, randomized trials have shown that bypass grafting is superior to antianginal medical therapy in improving survival in subjects with ESRD and any of these three coronary arterial anatomic patterns. Subjects with no or mild symptoms obviously do not require bypass grafting for symptom relief. Those with less extensive coronary artery disease (involving one, two, or all three coronary arteries without involvement of the proximal portion of the left anterior descending coronary artery) do not manifest a better survival with bypass grafting than with antianginal medical therapy.

Numerous reports have emphasized the high perioperative mortality and morbidity in patients with ESRD who undergo coronary artery bypass grafting (152–163). In all these reports, the perioperative mortality of ESRD subjects is 5% to 10% (in contrast to the 1% to 2% perioperative mortality in patients with normal renal function). In addition, perioperative morbidity, such as stroke, mediastinitis, and excessive bleeding, occurs in as many as 20% of ESRD patients (Fig. 18.6). Recently developed "off-pump" bypass grafting, with which surgical revascularization is accomplished on the beating heart without cardiopulmonary bypass, may be associated with less morbidity and mortality than the classic "on-pump" procedure (164), but adequately sized, randomized comparisons of on-pump and off-pump bypass grafting have not yet been reported.

The 5-year survival of ESRD patients undergoing bypass grafting is only 50%; as noted previously, it is unknown if this is superior, similar, or inferior to antianginal medical therapy in this patient population (165,166).

As experience with percutaneous coronary interventional procedures has grown, it has become clear that subjects with renal insufficiency, particularly ESRD patients on maintenance dialysis, have a substantially increased risk of periprocedural and postprocedural morbidity and mortality. Furthermore, the likelihood of adverse periprocedural and postprocedural events is related directly to the magnitude of preprocedural renal dysfunction. Best et al. (167) reviewed all adverse events that occurred in-hospital and within 1 year of percutaneous coronary intervention in 5,327 subjects undergoing balloon angioplasty alone (in 25%–30%) or intracoronary stenting (in 65%–70%) at the Mayo Clinic between January, 1994, and August, 1999, after which they related these events to the estimated preprocedural creatinine clearance. Periprocedural in-hospital death occurred in 0.5% of those with a creatinine clearance greater than 70 mL/minute, 0.7% of those with a clearance of 50 to 69 mL/minute, 2.3% of those with a creatinine clearance of 30 to 49 mL/minute, 7.1% of those with a clearance less than 30 mL/minute, and 6.0% of those on dialysis. Similarly, death between hospital discharge and 1 year later occurred in 1.5% of those with a creatinine clearance greater than 70 mL/minute, 3.6% of those with a clearance of 50 to 69 mL/minute, 7.8% of those with a clearance of 30 to 49 mL/minute, 18.3% of those with a clearance less than 30 mL/minute, and 19.9% of those on dialysis. Rubenstein et al. (168) reviewed the experience at the Massachusetts General Hospital from 1994 to 1997 in 3,334 patients undergoing a variety of percutaneous coronary interventional procedures. Of these, 362 had a preprocedural serum creatinine greater than 1.5 mg/dL, whereas the other 2,972 had

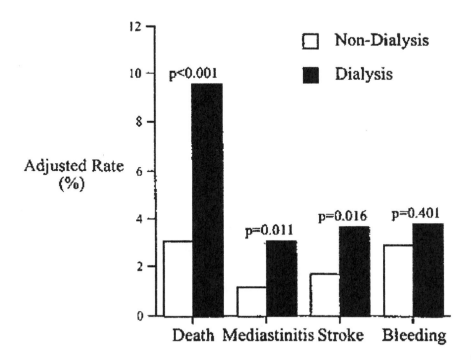

FIG. 18.6. Adjusted adverse outcome rates after bypass surgery according to the presence or absence of dialysis-dependent renal failure. Note the significantly higher adverse rates in end-stage renal disease patients. (From Liu JY, et al. Risks of morbidity and mortality in dialysis patients undergoing coronary artery bypass surgery. *Circulation* 2000;102:2973–2977, with permission.)

a creatinine less than 1.5 mg/dL. In comparison to those with a serum creatinine less than 1.5 mg/dL, those with a creatinine greater than 1.5 mg/dL had a somewhat lower rate of procedural success (90% vs. 93%, $p = 0.007$), and they had a markedly increased periprocedural mortality (10.8% vs. 1.1%, $p <0.0001$). Similar data most recently have been reported by Gruberg et al. (169). In summary, percutaneous coronary interventions of all types (balloon angioplasty, intracoronary stenting, or atherectomy) are associated with substantial periprocedural and short-term postprocedural morbidity and mortality, and this is particularly true in subjects with severely compromised renal function, such as those with ESRD.

During the 1 to 12 months after a successful percutaneous coronary intervention, a minority of patients develop so-called restenosis, a process by which smooth muscle cells migrate to the area of mechanical endothelial injury and then proliferate. If the magnitude of smooth muscle cell proliferation is large, the patient complains of recurrent angina resulting from severely limited flow in the involved coronary artery. In subjects with normal renal function, the likelihood of symptomatic restenosis following balloon angioplasty is about 35% and following intracoronary stenting, 20% to 25%. Through mechanisms that are not understood, the incidence of restenosis after balloon angioplasty in subjects with ESRD is considerably higher, namely 65% to 80% (170,171). Few data are available concerning the incidence of restenosis following intracoronary stenting, although some reports have suggested that its incidence in subjects with ESRD is similar to that of individuals with normal renal function (172).

REFERENCES

1. United States Renal Data System. 1991 annual report. Bethesda, MD: National Institute of Health, National Institute of Diabetes and Digestive and Kidney Diseases, August 1991.
2. Held PJ, et al. Cardiac disease in chronic uremia. In: Parfrey PS, et al., eds. *Cardiac dysfunction in chronic uremia.* Boston: Kluwer Academic, 1992:3–17.
3. Tyroler HA. Nutrition and coronary heart disease epidemiology. *Adv Exp Med Biol* 1995;369:7–19.
4. Herzog CA, et al. Poor long-term survival after acute myocardial infarction among patients on long-term dialysis. *N Engl J Med* 1998;339:799–805.
5. Becker BN, et al. Reassessing the cardiac risk profile in chronic hemodialysis patients: a hypothesis on the role of oxidant stress and other non-traditional cardiac risk factors. *J Am Soc Nephrol* 1996; 8:475–486.
6. Lindner A, et al. Accelerated atherosclerosis in prolonged maintenance hemodialysis. *N Engl J Med* 1974;290:697–701.
7. Rostand SG, et al. Coronary artery disease in end-stage renal disease. In: Henrich WL, ed. *Principles and practice of dialysis.* Baltimore: Williams & Wilkins, 1994:181–195.
8. Rostand SG, et al. Cardiovascular complications in renal failure. *J Am Soc Nephrol* 1991;2:1053–1062.
9. Ansari A, et al. Cardiac pathology in patients with end-stage renal disease maintained on hemodialysis. *Int J Artif Organs* 1993;16:31–36.
10. Rostand S, et al. The epidemiology of coronary artery disease in patients on maintenance hemodialysis: implications for management. *Contrib Nephrol* 1986;52:34–41.
11. Weinrauch L, et al. Asymptomatic coronary artery disease: angiographic assessment of diabetics evaluated for renal transplantation. *Circulation* 1978;58:1184–1189.
12. Weinrauch L, et al. Asymptomatic coronary artery disease: angiography in diabetic patients before renal transplantation. *Ann Intern Med* 1978;88:346–348.
13. Bennett W, et al. Natural history of asymptomatic coronary arteriographic lesions in diabetic patients with end-stage renal disease. *Am J Med* 1978;65:779–784.
14. Rostand S, et al. Ischemic heart disease in patients with uremia undergoing maintenance hemodialysis. *Kidney Int* 1979;16:600–611.
15. Longenecker JC, et al. Traditional cardiovascular disease risk factors in dialysis patients compared with the general population: the CHOICE study. *J Am Soc Nephrol* 2002;13:1918–1927.
16. Shoji T, et al. Advanced atherosclerosis in predialysis patients with chronic renal failure. *Kidney Int* 2002;61:2187–2192.
17. Konings C, et al. Arterial wall properties in patients with renal failure. *Am J Kid Dis* 2002;39:1206–1212.
18. O'Brien MM, et al. Modest serum creatinine elevation affects outcome after general surgery. *Kidney Int* 2002;62:585–592.
19. Nicholls A, et al. Accelerated atherosclerosis in long-term dialysis and renal-transplant patients: fact or fiction? *Lancet* 1980;1:276–278.
20. Burke J, et al. Accelerated atherosclerosis in chronic dialysis patients—another look. *Nephron* 1978;21:181–185.
21. Ritz E, et al. Is atherogenesis accelerated in uremia? *Contrib Nephrol* 1986;52:1–9.
22. Braun W, et al. Coronary artery disease in 100 diabetics with end-stage renal failure. *Transplant Proc* 1984;16:603–607.
23. Krolewski A, et al. Magnitude and determinants of coronary artery disease in juvenile-onset, insulin-dependent diabetes mellitus. *Am J Cardiol* 1987;59:750–755.
24. Manske C, et al. Prevalence of, and risk factors for, angiographically determined coronary artery disease in type 1-diabetic patients with nephropathy. *Arch Intern Med* 1992;152:2450–2455.
25. Jensen T, et al. Coronary heart disease in young type 1 (insulin-dependent) diabetic patients with and without diabetic nephropathy: incidence and risk factors. *Diabetologia* 1987;30:144–148.
26. Rostand S, et al. Relationship of coronary risk factors to hemodialysis-associated ischemic heart disease. *Kidney Int* 1982;22:304–308.
27. Bachmann J, et al. Hyperhomocystinemia and the risk for vascular disease in hemodialysis patients. *J Am Soc Nephrol* 1995;6:121–125.
28. Vincenti F, et al. The role of hypertension in hemodialysis-associated atherosclerosis. *Am J Med* 1980;68:363–369.
29. DeLima JJG, et al. Blood pressure influences the occurrence of complex ventricular arrhythmia in hemodialysis patients. *Hypertension* 1995;26:1200–1203.
30. Morales MA, et al. Signal-averaged ECG abnormalities in hemodialysis patients. *Nephrol Dial Transplant* 1998;13:668–673.
31. Meier P, et al. Ventricular arrhythmias and sudden cardiac death in end-stage renal disease patients on chronic hemodialysis. *Nephron* 2001;87:199–214.
32. Verdeccia P, et al. Left ventricular mass and cardiovascular morbidity in essential hypertension: the MAVI study. *J Am Coll Cardiol* 2001; 38:1829–1835.
33. Foley RN, et al. Serial change in echocardiographic parameters and cardiac failure in end-stage renal disease. *J Am Soc Nephrol* 2000;11: 912–916.
34. Harnett JD, et al. Cardiac function and hematocrit level. *Am J Kidney Dis* 1995;25:S3–S7.
35. Kestenbaum B, et al. Calcium channel blocker use and mortality among patients with end-stage renal disease. *Kidney Int* 2002;61: 2157–2164.
36. Cice G, et al. Dilated cardiomyopathy in dialysis patients—beneficial effects of carvedilol: a double-blind, placebo-controlled trial. *J Am Coll Cardiol* 2001;37:407–411.
37. Chan CT, et al. Regression of left ventricular hypertrophy after conversion to nocturnal hemodialysis. *Kidney Int* 2002;61:2235–2239.
38. Manske C. Coronary artery disease in diabetic patients with nephropathy. *Am J Hypertens* 1993;6[Suppl]:S367–S374.
39. Ambrose J, et al. Angiographic progression of coronary artery disease and the development of myocardial infarction. *J Am Coll Cardiol* 1988;12:56–62.
40. Little W, et al. Can coronary angiography predict the site of a subse-

quent myocardial infarction in patients with mild-to-moderate coronary artery disease? *Circulation* 1988;78:1157–1166.

41. Goldberg I. Lipoprotein metabolism in normal and uremic patients. *Am J Kidney Dis* 1993;21:87–90.

42. Bagdade J. Uremic lipemia: an unrecognized abnormality in triglyceride production and removal. *Arch Intern Med* 1970;126:875–881.

43. Appel G. Lipid abnormalities in renal disease. *Kidney Int* 1991;39:169–183.

44. Drueke T, et al. Recent advances in factors that alter lipid metabolism in chronic renal failure. *Kidney Int* 1983;24[Suppl]:S134–S138.

45. Rapoport J, et al. Defective high-density lipoprotein composition in patients on chronic hemodialysis. *N Engl J Med* 1978;299:1326–1329.

46. Fuh M, et al. Effect of chronic renal failure on high-density lipoprotein kinetics. *Kidney Int* 1990;37:1295–1300.

47. Hahn R, et al. Analysis of cardiovascular risk factors in chronic hemodialysis patients with special attention to the hyperlipoproteinemias. *Atherosclerosis* 1983;48:279–288.

48. Nestel P, et al. Increased lipoprotein-remnant formation in chronic renal failure. *N Engl J Med* 1982;307:329–333.

49. Weintraub M, et al. Severe defect in clearing postprandial chylomicron remnants in dialysis patients. *Kidney Int* 1992;42:1247–1252.

50. Bostom AG, et al. Hyperhomocystinemia, hyperfibrinogenemia, and lipoprotein(a) excess in maintenance dialysis patients: a matched case-control study. *Atherosclerosis* 1996;125:91–101.

51. Fermo I, et al. Prevalence of moderate hyperhomocystinemia in patients with early-onset venous and arterial occlusive disease. *Ann Intern Med* 1995;123:747–753.

52. Glueck CJ, et al. Evidence that homocysteine is an independent risk factor for atherosclerosis in hyperlipidemic patients. *Am J Cardiol* 1995;75:132–136.

53. Stampfer MJ, et al. A prospective study of plasma homocysteine and risk of myocardial infarction in U.S. physicians. *JAMA* 1992;268:877–881.

54. Bostom AG, et al. Hyperhomocystinemia in end-stage renal disease: prevalence, etiology, and potential relationship to arteriosclerotic outcomes. *Kidney Int* 1997;52:10–20.

55. Dennis VW, et al. Homocystinemia and vascular disease in end-stage renal disease. *Kidney Int* 1996;50[Suppl 57]:S11–S17.

56. Bostom AG, et al. Net uptake of plasma homocysteine by the rat kidney in vivo. *Atherosclerosis* 1995;116:59–62.

57. Van Guldener C, et al. Short-term effect of kidney transplantation on plasma homocysteine in dialysis patients. *Irish J Med Sci* 1995;164:22(abst).

58. Boushey CJ, et al. A quantitative assessment of plasma homocysteine as a risk factor for vascular disease. *JAMA* 1995;274:1049–1057.

59. Massy ZA, et al. Hyperhomocystinemia: a significant risk factor for cardiovascular disease in renal transplant recipients. *Nephrol Dial Transplant* 1994;9:1103–1108.

60. Bostom AG, et al. High dose B-vitamin treatment of hyperhomocystinemia in dialysis patients. *Kidney Int* 1996;49:147–152.

61. Bostom AG, et al. Hyperhomocystinemia and traditional cardiovascular disease risk factors in end-stage renal disease patients on dialysis: a case control study. *Atherosclerosis* 1995;114:93–103.

62. Janssen MJFM, et al. Folic acid treatment of hyperhomocystinemia in dialysis patients. *Miner Electrol Metab* 1996;22:110–114.

63. Bostom AG, et al. Brief report: lack of effect of oral N-acetylcysteine on the acute dialysis-related lowering of total plasma homocysteine in hemodialysis patients. *Atherosclerosis* 1996;120:242–244.

64. Wilcken DEL, et al. Folic acid lowers elevated plasma homocysteine in chronic renal insufficiency: possible implications for prevention of vascular disease. *Metabolism* 1988;37:697–701.

65. Arnadottir M, et al. The effect of high dose pyridoxine and folic acid supplementation on serum lipid and plasma homocysteine concentrations in dialysis patients. *Clin Nephrol* 1993;40:236–240.

66. Chauveau P, et al. Long-term folic acid (by not pyridoxine) supplementation lowers elevated plasma homocysteine level in chronic renal failure. *Miner Electrol Metab* 1996;22:106–109.

67. Bostom AG, et al. Short-term betaine therapy fails to lower elevated fasting total plasma homocysteine levels in hemodialysis patients maintained on chronic folic acid supplementation. *Atherosclerosis* 1995;113:129–142.

68. Robinson K, et al. Hyperhomocystinemia confers an independent increased risk of atherosclerosis in end-stage renal disease and is closely linked to plasma folate and pyridoxine concentrations. *Circulation* 1996;94:2743–2748.

69. Giardini O, et al. Evidence of red blood cell membrane lipid peroxidation in hemodialysis patients. *Nephron* 1984;36:235–237.

70. Kuroda M, et al. Serum antioxidant activity in uremic patients. *Nephron* 1985;41:293–298.

71. Lucchi L, et al. Oxidative metabolism of polymorphonuclear leukocytes and serum opsonic activity in chronic renal failure. *Nephron* 1989;51:44–50.

72. Shainkin-Kestenbaum R, et al. Reduced superoxide dismutase activity in erythrocytes of dialysis patients: a possible factor in the etiology of uremic anemia. *Nephron* 1990;55:251–253.

73. Toborek M, et al. Effect of hemodialysis on lipid peroxidation and antioxidant system in patients with chronic renal failure. *Metabolism* 1992;41:1229–1232.

74. Gey KF, et al. Plasma levels of antioxidant vitamins in relation to ischemic heart disease and cancer. *Clin Nutr* 1987;45:1368–1377.

75. Rimm EB, et al. Dietary intake and risk of coronary heart disease among men. *N Engl J Med* 1993;328:1450–1456.

76. Jha P, et al. The antioxidant vitamins and cardiovascular disease: a critical review of epidemiologic and clinical trial data. *Ann Intern Med* 1995;123:860–872.

77. Hodis HN, et al. Serial coronary angiographic evidence that antioxidant vitamin intake reduces progression of coronary artery atherosclerosis. *JAMA* 1995;273:1849–1854.

78. Anderson TJ, et al. The effect of cholesterol-lowering and antioxidant therapy on endothelium-dependent coronary vasomotion. *N Engl J Med* 1995;332:488–493.

79. Levine GN, et al. Ascorbic acid reverses endothelial vasomotor dysfunction in patients with coronary artery disease. *Circulation* 1996;93:1107–1113.

80. Ponka A, et al. Serum ascorbic acid in patients undergoing chronic hemodialysis. *Acta Med Scand* 1983;213:305–307.

81. Cohen JD, et al. Plasma vitamin E levels in a chronically hemolyzing group of dialysis patients. *Clin Nephrol* 1986;25:42–47.

82. Himmelfarb J, et al. Intradialytic granulocyte reactive oxygen species production: a prospective crossover trial. *J Am Soc Nephrol* 1993;4:178–186.

83. Loughrey CM, et al. Oxidative stress in hemodialysis. *QJM* 1994;87:679–683.

84. Toborek M, et al. Effect of hemodialysis on lipid peroxidation and antioxidant system in patients with chronic renal failure. *Metabolism* 1992;41:1229–1232.

85. Nagasi S, et al. Favorable effect of hemodialysis on decreased serum antioxidant activity in hemodialysis patients demonstrated by electron spin resonance. *J Am Soc Nephrol* 1997;8:1157–1163.

86. Bucala R, et al. Lipid advanced glycosylation: pathway for lipid oxidation in vivo. *Proc Natl Acad Sci U S A* 1993;90:6434–6438.

87. Vlassara H. Serum advanced glycosylation end products: a new class of uremic toxins. *Blood Purif* 1994;12:54–59.

88. Mullarkey C, et al. Free radical generation by early glycation products: a mechanism for accelerated atherogenesis in diabetes. *Biochem Biophys Res Commun* 1990;173:932–939.

89. Schmidt AM, et al. Cellular receptors for advanced glycation end products. *Arterioscler Thromb* 1994;14:1521–1528.

90. Palinski W, et al. Immunological evidence for the presence of advanced glycosylation end products in atherosclerotic lesions of euglycemic rabbits. *Arterioscler Thromb Biol* 1995;15:571–582.

91. Hou FF, et al. Receptor for advanced glycation end products on human synovial fibroblasts: role in the pathogenesis of dialysis-related amyloidosis. *J Am Soc Nephrol* 2002;13:1296–1306.

92. Parthasarathy S, et al. A role for endothelial cell lipoxygenase in the oxidative modification of low density lipoprotein. *Proc Natl Acad Sci U S A* 1988;86:1046–1050.

93. Bjorkhem I, et al. The antioxidant butylated hydroxytoluene protects against atherosclerosis. *Arterioscler Thromb* 1991;11:15–22.

94. Thomas JP, et al. Lethal damage to endothelial cells by oxidized low density lipoprotein: role of selenoperoxidases in cytoprotection against lipid hydroperoxide-mediated and iron-mediated reactions. *J Lipid Res* 1993;332:218–220.

95. Palinski W, et al. Antisera and monoclonal antibodies specific for epitopes generated during oxidative modification of low density lipoproteins. *Arteriosclerosis* 1990;10:325–335.

96. Salonen JT, et al. Autoantibody against oxidized LDL and progression of carotid atherosclerosis. *Lancet* 1992;339:883–887.

97. Horkko S, et al. Decreased clearance of uremic and mildly carbamylated low-density lipoprotein. *Eur J Clin Invest* 1994;24:105–113.

98. Maggi E, et al. Enhanced LDL oxidation in uremic patients: an additional mechanism for accelerated atherosclerosis? *Kidney Int* 1994;45:876–883.

99. Jackson P, et al. Effect of hemodialysis on total antioxidant capacity and serum antioxidants in patients with chronic renal failure. *Clin Chem* 1995;41:1135–1138.

100. Jain SK, et al. Lipofuscin products, lipid peroxides and aluminum accumulation in red blood cells of hemodialyzed patients. *Am J Nephrol* 1995;15:305–311.

101. Itabe H, et al. Sensitive detection of oxidatively modified low density lipoprotein using a monoclonal antibody. *J Lipid Res* 1996;37:45–53.

102. Cressmann MD, et al. Lipoprotein(a) is an independent risk factor for cardiovascular disease in hemodialysis patients. *Circulation* 1992;86:475–482.

103. Grainger DJ, et al. Proliferation of human smooth muscle cells promoted by lipoprotein(a). *Science* 1993;260:1655–1658.

104. Kronenburg F, et al. Multicenter study of lipoprotein(a) and apolipoprotein(a) phenotypes in patients with end-stage renal disease treated by hemodialysis or continuous ambulatory peritoneal dialysis. *J Am Soc Nephrol* 1995;6:110–120.

105. Churchill DN, et al. Canadian hemodialysis morbidity study. *Am J Kidney Dis* 1992;19:214–234.

106. Ritz E, et al. The effect of malnutrition on cardiovascular mortality in dialysis patients: is L-arginine the answer? *Nephrol Dial Transplant* 1994;9:129–130.

107. Foley RN, et al. Risk factors for cardiac morbidity and mortality in dialysis patients. *Curr Opin Nephrol Hypertens* 1994;3:608–614.

108. Koch M, et al. Apolipoprotein A, fibrinogen, age, and history of stroke are predictors of death in dialysed diabetic patients: a prospective study in 412 subjects. *Nephrol Dial Transplant* 1997;12:2603–2611.

109. Guerin AP, et al. Arterial stiffening and vascular calcifications in end-stage renal disease. *Nephrol Dial Transplant* 2000;15:1014–1021.

110. Moe SM, et al. Medial artery calcification in ESRD patients is associated with deposition of bone matrix proteins. *Kidney Int* 2002;61:638–647.

111. Yukawa S, et al. Prevention of aortic calcification in patients on hemodialysis by long-term administration of vitamin E. *J Nutr Sci Vitam* 1992;S-5-2:187–190.

112. Chertow GM, et al. Sevelamer attenuates the progression of coronary and aortic calcification in hemodialysis patients. *Kidney Int* 2002;62:245–252.

113. Ganesh SK, et al. Association of elevated serum PO4, Ca × PO4 product, and parathyroid hormone with cardiac mortality risk in chronic hemodialysis patients. *J Am Soc Nephrol* 2001;12:2131–2138.

114. Philipson J, et al. Evaluation of cardiovascular risk for renal transplantation in diabetic patients. *Am J Med* 1986;81:630–634.

115. Ramos E, et al. The evaluation of candidates for renal transplantation. *Transplantation* 1994;57:490–497.

116. Braun W, et al. Coronary arteriography and coronary artery disease in 99 diabetic and nondiabetic patients on chronic hemodialysis or renal transplantation programs. *Transplant Proc* 1981;13:128–135.

117. Brown K, et al. Noninvasive cardiac risk stratification of diabetic and nondiabetic uremic renal allograft candidates using dipyridamole-thallium-201 imaging and radionuclide ventriculography. *Am J Cardiol* 1989;64:1017–1021.

118. Weinrauch L, et al. Preoperative evaluation for diabetic renal transplantation: impact of clinical, laboratory, and echocardiographic parameters on patient and allograft survival. *Am J Med* 1992;93:19–28.

119. Zoccali C, et al. Cardiac natriuretic peptides are related to left ventricular mass and function and predict mortality in dialysis patients. *J Am Soc Nephrol* 2001;12:1508–1515.

120. deFilippi C, et al. Troponin T predicts adverse cardiac events and multi-vessel coronary artery disease in end-stage renal disease: an angiographic and outcomes study. *J Am Soc Nephrol* 2001;12:376A.

121. Aviles RJ, et al. Troponin T levels in patients with acute coronary syndromes, with or without renal dysfunction. *N Engl J Med* 2002;346:2047–2052.

122. Antman EM. Decision making with cardiac troponin tests. *N Engl J Med* 2002;346:2079–2082.

123. Porter GA, et al. Long-term follow p of the utility of troponin T to assess cardiac risk in stable chronic hemodialysis patients. *Clin Lab* 2000;46:469–476.

124. Iliou MC, et al. Factors associated with increased serum levels of cardiac troponins T and I in chronic haemodialysis patients: chronic haemodialysis and new cardiac markers evaluation (CHANCE) study. *Nephrol Dial Transplant* 2001;16:1452–1458.

125. Mallamaci F, et al. Troponin is related to left ventricular mass and predicts all-cause and cardiovascular mortality in hemodialysis patients. *Am J Kidney Dis* 2002;40:68–75.

126. Maisel AS, et al. Rapid measurement of B-type natriuretic peptide in the emergency diagnosis of heart failure. *N Engl J Med* 2002;347:161–167.

127. Peacock WF. The B-type natriuretic peptide assay: a rapid test for heart failure. *Cleve Clin J Med* 2002;69:243–251.

128. Khan IA, et al. Prognostic value of serum cardiac troponin I in ambulatory patients with chronic renal failure undergoing long-term hemodialysis: a two-year outcome analysis. *J Am Coll Cardiol* 2001;38:991–998.

129. Chang JW, et al. Effects of simvastatin on high-sensitivity C-reactive protein and serum albumin in hemodialysis patients. *Am J Kidney Dis* 2002;39:1213–1217.

130. Memoli B, et al. Changes of serum albumin and C-reactive protein are related to changes of interleukin-6 release of peripheral blood mononuclear cells in hemodialysis patients treated with different membranes. *Am J Kid Dis* 2002;39:266–273.

131. Le A, et al. Prospective risk stratification in renal transplant candidates for cardiac death. *Am J Kid Dis* 1994;24:65–71.

132. Manske C, et al. Screening diabetic transplant candidates for coronary artery disease: identification of a low risk subgroup. *Kidney Int* 1993;44:617–621.

133. Camp A, et al. Prognostic value of intravenous dipyridamole thallium imaging in patients with diabetes mellitus considered for renal transplantation. *Am J Cardiol* 1990;65:1459–1463.

134. Reis G, et al. Usefulness of dobutamine stress echocardiography in detecting coronary artery disease in end-stage renal disease. *Am J Cardiol* 1995;75:707–710.

135. Braun W, et al. Coronary artery disease in renal transplant recipients. *Cleve Clin J Med* 1994;61:370–385.

136. Williams M. Management of the diabetic renal transplant recipient. *Kidney Int* 1995;48:1660–1674.

137. Morrow C, et al. Predictive value of thallium stress testing for coronary and cardiovascular events in uremic diabetic patients before renal transplantation. *Am J Surg* 1983;146:331–335.

138. Marwick TH, et al. Ineffectiveness of dipyridamole SPECT thallium imaging as a screening technique for coronary artery disease in patients with end-stage renal failure. *Transplant* 1990;49:100–103.

139. Boudreau RJ, et al. Perfusion thallium imaging of type I diabetes patients with ESRD: comparison of oral and intravenous dipyridamole administration. *Radiology* 1990;175:103–105.

140. Derfler K, et al. Predictive value of thallium-201-dipyridamole myocardial stress scintigraphy in chronic hemodialysis patients and transplant recipients. *Clin Nephrol* 1991;36:192–202.

141. Kasiske B, et al. The evaluation of renal transplant candidates: clinical practice guidelines. *J Am Soc Nephrol* 1995;6:1–34.

142. Schmidt A, et al. Informational contribution of noninvasive screening tests for coronary artery disease in patients on chronic renal replacement therapy. *Am J Kidney Dis* 2001;37:56–63.

143. Foley RN, et al. Cardiac disease in chronic uremia: clinical outcome and risk factors. *Adv Ren Replace Ther* 1997;4:235–248.

144. London GM, et al. Cardiac disease in chronic uremia: pathogenesis. *Adv Ren Replace Ther* 1997;4:194–211.
145. Painter P, et al. Effects of exercise training plus normalization of hematocrit on exercise capacity and health-related quality of life. *Am J Kidney Dis* 2002;39:257–265.
146. Silverberg JS, et al. Impact of left ventricular hypertrophy on survival in end-stage renal disease. *Kidney Int* 1989;36:286–290.
147. Sargoca MA, et al. Left ventricular hypertrophy as a risk factor for arrhythmias in hemodialysis patients. *J Cardiovasc Pharmacol* 1991;17 [Suppl 2]:S136–S138.
148. Zoccali C, et al. Left ventricular hypertrophy, cardiac remodeling and asymmetric dimethylarginine (ADMA) in hemodialysis patients. *Kidney Int* 2002;62:339–345.
149. Gottlieb SO. Asymptomatic or silent myocardial ischemia in angina pectoris: pathophysiology and clinical implications. *Cardiol Clin* 1991;9:49–61.
150. Fellner SK, et al. Ischemic heart disease in patients with end-stage renal disease. *Adv Ren Replace Ther* 1996;3:240–249.
151. Hillis LD. Coronary artery bypass surgery: risks and benefits, realistic and unrealistic expectations. *J Invest Med* 1995;43:17–27.
152. DeMeyer M, et al. Myocardial revascularization in patients on renal replacement therapy. *Clin Nephrol* 1991;36:147–151.
153. Manske CL, et al. Coronary revascularization in insulin-dependent diabetic patients with chronic renal failure. *Lancet* 1992;340:998–1002.
154. Deutsch E, et al. Coronary artery bypass surgery in patients on chronic hemodialysis. *Ann Intern Med* 1989;110:369–372.
155. Batiuk TD, et al. Coronary artery bypass operation in dialysis patients. *Mayo Clin Proc* 1991;66:45–53.
156. Liu JY, et al. Risks of morbidity and mortality in dialysis patients undergoing coronary artery bypass surgery. *Circulation* 2000;102:2973–2977.
157. Franga DL, et al. Early and long-term results of coronary artery bypass grafting in dialysis patients. *Ann Thorac Surg* 2000;70:813–819.
158. Castelli P, et al. Immediate and long-term results of coronary revascularization in patients undergoing chronic hemodialysis. *Eur J Cardiothorac Surg* 1999;15:51–54.
159. Osake S, et al. Immediate and long-term results of coronary artery bypass operation in hemodialysis patients. *Artif Organs* 2001;25:252–255.
160. Okamura Y, et al. Coronary artery bypass in dialysis patients. *Artif Organs* 2001;25:256–259.
161. Naruse Y, et al. Coronary artery bypass grafting in patients with dialysis-dependent renal failure. *Artif Organs* 2001;25:260–262.
162. Higashiue S, et al. Coronary artery bypass grafting in patients with dialysis-dependent renal failure. *Artif Organs* 2001;25:263–267.
163. Nishida H, et al. Coronary artery bypass grafting in 105 patients with hemodialysis-dependent renal failure. *Artif Organs* 2001;25:268–272.
164. Hirose H, et al. Efficacy of off-pump coronary bypass grafting for the patients on chronic hemodialysis. *Jpn J Thorac Cardiovasc Surg* 2001;49:693–699.
165. DeLemos JA, et al. Diagnosis and management of coronary artery disease in patients with end-stage renal disease on hemodialysis. *J Am Soc Nephrol* 1996;7:2044–2054.
166. Opsahl J, et al. Coronary artery bypass surgery in patients on maintenance dialysis: long-term survival. *Am J Kidney Dis* 1988;12:271–274.
167. Best PJM, et al. The impact of renal insufficiency on clinical outcomes in patients undergoing percutaneous coronary interventions. *J Am Coll Cardiol* 2002;39:1113–1119.
168. Rubenstein MH, et al. Are patients with renal failure good candidates for percutaneous coronary revascularization in the new device era? *Circulation* 2000;102:2966–2972.
169. Gruberg L, et al. Comparison of outcomes after percutaneous coronary revascularization with stents in patients with and without mild chronic renal insufficiency. *Am J Cardiol* 2002;89:54–57.
170. Kahn JK, et al. Short- and long-term outcome of percutaneous transluminal coronary angioplasty in chronic dialysis patients. *Am Heart J* 1990;119:484–489.
171. Ahmed WA, et al. Outcome of coronary artery angioplasty in hemodialysis patients. *Semin Dial* 1994;7:96–99.
172. Le Feuvre C, et al. Comparison of clinical outcome following coronary stenting or balloon angioplasty in dialysis versus non-dialysis patients. *Am J Cardiol* 2000;85:1365–1368.

AUTONOMIC NEUROPATHY AND HEMODYNAMIC STABILITY IN END-STAGE RENAL DISEASE PATIENTS

BIFF F. PALMER AND WILLIAM L. HENRICH

The usual manifestation of hemodynamic instability during ultrafiltration dialysis (in which fluid removal is the primary goal) is hypotension. The incidence of a symptomatic reduction in blood pressure during or immediately following dialysis ranges from 15% to 50% of dialysis sessions (1,2). In some patients, the development of hypotension necessitates intravenous fluid replacement before the patient leaves the dialysis unit, which results in volume overload. In addition, symptomatic hypotension may necessitate a premature discontinuation of the treatment, which if repetitive can lead to inadequate clearance. As a result, the occurrence of episodes of hypotension during dialysis treatments contributes substantially to the morbidity of the therapy (Table 19.1).

A second type of dialysis-related hypotension is a chronic, persistent form of hypotension that occurs in approximately 5% of dialysis patients (3). This second form of hypotension is usually observed in patients who have been on hemodialysis (HD) for a long period (usually ≥5 years). Such patients often come to the dialysis unit with a systolic blood pressure of less than 90 mm Hg (3). Epidemiologic studies show that patients with this form of hypotension have an increased mortality (4,5). Low blood pressure may be a manifestation of malnutrition and/or cardiovascular disease in chronic HD patients (6). This chapter emphasizes the problem of episodic hypotension, which is the most frequent form of HD-related hemodynamic instability.

OVERVIEW OF THE PROBLEM

A normal individual subjected to volume loss is able to maintain blood pressure by employing mechanisms that involve the autonomic and cardiovascular systems. One compensatory response to volume loss is vasoconstriction of the venous side of the circulation and in particular the splanchnic and dermal beds. Venoconstriction redistributes volume to the central circulation where it then becomes available for cardiac refilling. Cardiac refilling is also maintained by refilling of the intravascular space by fluid transfer from the extracellular and intracellular compartments. This transfer of fluid ensures that the decline in intravascular volume is less than the amount of fluid removed

from the body. Refilling of the heart in the setting of normal systolic and diastolic function allows for an adequate cardiac output to be maintained. If the cardiac output begins to decline, blood pressure is further stabilized by sympathetic nervous system-induced increases in peripheral vascular resistance.

The chronic dialysis patient often demonstrates disturbances in either one or several of these compensatory steps and is thus prone to develop hypotension in the setting of fluid removal. Such disturbances are the result of the chronic uremic state as well as accompanying comorbid conditions. The following sections review the various abnormalities in the autonomic and cardiovascular systems that contribute to the development of episodic dialysis hypotension (Table 19.2). The chapter concludes with a discussion of the prevention and management of dialysis-related hypotension.

CARDIAC SYSTEM

Normal systolic and diastolic function of the heart are required to generate an adequate cardiac output in the face of volume removal. Myocardial dysfunction is commonly present in patients with end-stage renal disease (ESRD) and can be an important cofactor in dialysis-induced hypotension (7–10).

Diastolic Dysfunction

The frequent occurrence of hypertension and on occasion aortic stenosis contributes to pressure overload of the left ventricle and accounts for the frequent occurrence of concentric left ventricular hypertrophy (LVH) (11). In addition, the presence of an arteriovenous fistula, anemia, and hypervolemia contribute to left ventricular (LV) volume overload ultimately causing LV dilation with hypertrophy (8,9,11,12).

As a result of these structural abnormalities, ventricular performance in most patients with ESRD differs strikingly from that seen in the normal heart. A high incidence of LVH and abnormal diastolic function lead to diminished diastolic distensibility, such that the volume-pressure relationship during diastolic filling is steeper and shifted to the left (Fig. 19.1). When

TABLE 19.1. COMPLICATIONS OF INTRADIALYTIC HYPOTENSION

Myocardial ischemia
Stroke
Mesenteric ischemia
Clotted access
Ischemic atrophy of the optic nerve with loss of vision
Inadequate clearance secondary to shortened treatment time
Persistent posttreatment volume overload

LV compliance is diminished, a small rise in left ventricular end-diastolic volume (LVEDV) may cause a disproportionately large increase in left ventricular end-diastolic pressure (LVEDP) with consequent pulmonary venous congestion but little or no increase in stroke volume. Even in the presence of well-preserved systolic function, the preload reserve of the left ventricle can be exceeded by abrupt or large increases in plasma volume or because decreased ventricular compliance leads to inappropriately high filling pressure and pulmonary congestion. Furthermore, decreases in plasma volume, as during ultrafiltration in the setting of a steep volume-pressure relationship, can critically decrease the filling pressure of the heart and result in hypotension. In short, many patients with ESRD operate within a narrow LV volume-pressure relationship such that changes in plasma volume are often not well tolerated.

The contribution of LVH to hemodynamic instability during dialysis is highlighted by a number of studies that have shown LVH to be more common in dialysis patients who experience episodic dialysis hypotension (13,14). Ritz et al. (15) observed that the LV mass-to-volume ratio was 37% greater in 27 patients with recurrent intradialytic hypotension than in 27 patients without this complication. Similarly, Wizemann et al. (16) noted that the incidence of dialysis hypotension was several times greater in patients with echocardiographic LVH than in those with normal ventricular mass. In fact, a recent study of

TABLE 19.2. FACTORS THAT PREDISPOSE TO INTRADIALYTIC HYPOTENSION

Myocardial dysfunction
  Diastolic dysfunction
  Systolic dysfunction
Impaired vascular refilling
  Declining plasma osmolality
  Decreased volume of interstitial fluid
  Local Starling forces
Impaired cardiac refilling
  Venous dysfunction
  Splanchnic vasodilation
  Arterial dysfunction
  Increased core body temperature
Vasoactive mediators
  Nitric oxide
  Adenosine
Autonomic neuropathy
High ultrafiltration rates, volume depletion
Antihypertensive medicines

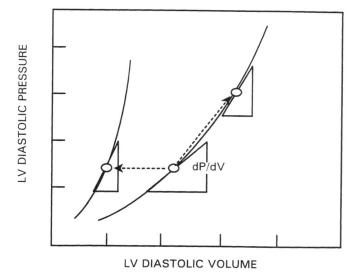

FIG. 19.1. Compliance characteristics (left ventricular end-diastolic volume/left ventricular end-diastolic pressure) of the left ventricle during diastolic filling. Patients with end-stage renal disease often have the pressure-volume relationship of the left ventricle shifted to the left such that myocardial compliance is decreased.

patients with recurrent intradialytic hypotension showed that they had a lower predialysis blood pressure, more severe concentric LVH, and lower LV compliance (17).

Patients with diastolic dysfunction are particularly difficult to treat. The problem is that of impaired ventricular relaxation; a small amount of volume replacement can potentially trigger pulmonary edema. Furthermore, therapy with inotropic agents exacerbates the problem by further impairing ventricular relaxation. One intriguing therapeutic possibility for this group of subjects is the use of calcium channel blockers, agents that lead to improved LV relaxation. In one small study, the use of calcium channel blockers produced a functional improvement in cardiac performance and a reduction in the frequency of hypotension (18). However, it must be emphasized that the use of vasodilator calcium channel blockers has the potential disadvantage of lowering blood pressure. Hence the trade-off of improving LV relaxation may not be tolerated in all patients because of the effect of the drugs to lower blood pressure.

On a more chronic basis, therapy can be instituted with the goal of reducing LV mass toward normal and presumably improve ventricular diastolic function. Partial or complete regression can be achieved by control of hypertension and by correction of anemia with erythropoietin (19,20). Studies in nonuremic hypertensive subjects suggest that, at equivalent blood pressure control, angiotensin-converting enzyme inhibitors, angiotensin receptor blockers, and calcium channel blockers reduce LV mass more rapidly and perhaps more effectively than most other antihypertensive drugs. It is not clear if these observations apply to the patient with renal failure (21). Correction of anemia with erythropoietin presumably acts by improving tissue oxygen delivery, thereby allowing the cardiac output (which is increased in anemia) and, therefore, cardiac work to fall toward normal. These changes have been associated with a 10% to 30% reduction in LV mass index (20). However, attention must also be paid to the frequent elevation in blood pressure following erythropoietin, an effect that may partially counteract the benefit associated with the elevation in hematocrit.

Systolic Dysfunction

Impaired systolic function of the heart is common in dialysis patients. Depressed systolic function may be the result of a prior myocardial infarction, ischemic or hypertensive cardiomyopathy, or ischemic injury resulting from microvascular disease as in diabetes mellitus. Some patients with this disorder manifest the chronic persistent form of hypotension. More commonly impaired systolic function contributes to an increased frequency of dialysis-associated hemodynamic instability. Decreased myocardial contractility leads to poor LV performance and, importantly, a diminished cardiac reserve in the context of a hemodynamic challenge. Support for the importance of diminished cardiac reserve is provided by the results of dobutamine stress echocardiography among 18 patients with dialysis instability and 18 without such instability (22). The baseline cardiac index was similar in the two groups. However, cardiac reserve, as determined by the increase in cardiac index with dobutamine, was significantly lower among the patients who were prone to hypotension during dialysis. An inability to generate a sufficient cardiac output despite adequate cardiac filling can contribute to intradialytic hypotension and pulmonary edema.

CARDIAC AND VASCULAR REFILLING DURING ULTRAFILTRATION DIALYSIS

Vascular Refilling

In a typical dialysis procedure an ultrafiltrate volume that is equal to or greater than the entire plasma volume is often removed. Despite the large ultrafiltrate volume, plasma volume typically decreases by only approximately 10% to 20% (23,24). This ability to maintain plasma volume requires mobilization of fluid from the extravascular and intravascular space. The success of vascular refilling is influenced by the stability of plasma osmolality, the rate of fluid removal, and other patient characteristics that dictate the distribution of fluid between the body fluid compartments.

Stable Plasma Osmolality

The importance of a stable plasma osmolality as a key element in preventing dialysis hypotension is discussed in detail in Chapter 3. The main mechanism by which a stable plasma osmolality contributes to hemodynamic stability appears to be through the maintenance of a more stable extracellular fluid volume and plasma volume (25). The rapid fall in plasma osmolality that results from solute removal leads to the movement of water to intracellular loci (Fig. 19.2). This movement of water will decrease the amount of fluid accessible for vascular refilling (25). The use of a higher dialysate sodium (Na) concentration limits the decline in plasma osmolality and therefore leads to the removal of volume during ultrafiltration from both intracellular and extracellular compartments. This limits the compromise in the plasma volume that normally occurs during rapid falls in plasma osmolality coupled with a very large ultrafiltration rate. Another potential mechanism by which a decline in plasma osmolality may contribute to dialysis hypotensive episodes is that of impairing peripheral vasoconstriction during volume removal (26–28). A decline in plasma osmolality may also have an adverse effect on baroreceptor function (27), as inhibitory effects on afferent sensing mechanisms may exacerbate autonomic dysfunction.

In dialysis practice today, the usual dialysate Na concentration is maintained at 140 mEq/L or higher. There has been recent attention given to the possibility that a changing dialysate Na concentration during dialysis (termed "Na modeling") may allow for improved ultrafiltration at either the beginning or the end of the dialysis procedure (29–31). Although most of these Na modeling studies have failed to show a clear advantage of a variable dialysate Na during the course of dialysis (29,30), this approach may be useful in hypotensive-prone patients.

Local Starling Forces

Several patient characteristics that affect Starling forces operating at the capillary level influence the process of vascular refill-

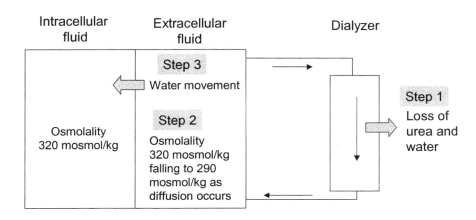

FIG. 19.2. A decline in extracellular osmolality can contribute to hemodynamic instability. The first step is a reduction in osmolality as urea and other solutes are removed from the body across the dialyzer. This solute removal results in a decline in extracellular osmolality relative to the intracellular space. The third step is the osmotic movement of water from the extracellular to intracellular space.

ing. One such characteristic is the amount of interstitial fluid present, a parameter clinically reflected by the dry weight of the patient. When the volume of interstitial fluid is small, any ultra-filtrate volume will more likely be associated with hemodynamic instability. This explains the development of hypotension when patients are dialyzed below their true dry weight. By contrast increased amounts of interstitial fluid will expand the volume of fluid accessible for refilling of the intravascular space and, therefore, decrease the likelihood of hypotension. In most patients a dry weight is selected that minimizes the amount of interstitial fluid present because chronic volume overload has long-term deleterious effects on the cardiovascular system. However, in patients with recurrent intradialytic hypotension or chronic persistent hypotension that is not amenable to other interventions it may be necessary to purposely maintain the patient in a hypervolemic state so that the dialysis procedure can be employed with a lower likelihood of hemodynamic instability.

Patient characteristics that influence oncotic and hydrostatic pressure at the tissue level will affect vascular refilling. For example, well-nourished patients with a higher serum albumin concentration are likely to have better preserved vascular refilling. The administration of vasodilators may impair vascular refilling by allowing excessive transmission of arterial pressure into the capillary bed resulting in increased hydrostatic pressure.

Cardiac Refilling

Through the process of vascular refilling most episodes of intradialytic hypotension are not associated with a sudden decrease in intravascular volume. However, hemodynamic analysis often demonstrates evidence of decreased cardiac filling (32,33). Reduced cardiac filling in the setting of a preserved vascular volume implies a failure to redistribute intravascular volume into the central circulation. This failure can be traced to abnormalities in both the functional and structural characteristics of the venous system, abnormalities in arterial structure and tone, vasoactive mediators, and abnormalities in autonomic function.

Venous Dysfunction

Because most plasma volume is located on the venous side of the circulation, even a small decrease in tone of the venous system can potentially limit cardiac filling because of a decrease in central blood volume. Abrupt splanchnic vasodilation can be the cause of intradialytic hypotension. Such vasodilation may result from ingestion of food during the dialysis procedure or withdrawal of sympathetic tone resulting from an increase in core body temperature. Increased production of vasodilators such as adenosine or nitric oxide may also play a role in this complication.

Decreased venous compliance has also been demonstrated in hypertensive HD patients (34,35). Such a disturbance in venous compliance can lead to hemodynamic instability in at least two ways. First, decreased venous compliance leads to a steep volume-to-pressure relationship such that a major drop in cardiac filling pressure can occur with only a small decrease in plasma volume. In this regard, an inverse relationship has been observed between venous compliance and the fall in central venous pressure in dialysis patients during isolated ultrafiltration (34). Second, impaired venous compliance can reduce vascular refilling from the interstitium because of an altered capillary Starling equilibrium. A greater decrease in plasma volume during ultrafiltration has been observed in patients with decreased venous compliance (34,35). The basis for altered venous function in chronic uremia may relate to structural abnormalities of the venous wall. Morphologic studies of the ileac and inferior caval veins of hypertensive patients with ESRD have shown increased thickness of the media in the venous wall (36). Structural and functional abnormalities of the venous system may also impair the ability to mobilize erythrocytes from the splanchnic or splenic circulation into the systemic circulation during ultrafiltration (37). This mechanism may be particularly important in patients with impaired autonomic function.

Arterial Dysfunction

Disturbances in arterial function may contribute to impaired mobilization of fluid into the central circulation. A decrease in arterial tone resulting from impaired autonomic function or increases in core body temperature can result in more direct transmission of systemic pressure into the venous circulation. A sudden increase in venous pressure will increase the holding capacity of the venous compartment potentially leading to the sequestration of fluid and, therefore, limiting cardiac refilling (23).

Structural abnormalities of the arterial circulation are also common in the chronic renal failure patient. Such changes lead to increased wall stiffness and importantly contribute to the development of LVH (38,39). The vascular lesion in arteries of uremic patients is characterized by intimal fibrosis and medial calcifications with little to no deposition of lipid droplets (40). These changes tend to be more reminiscent of accelerated aging or diabetic macroangiopathy rather than typical atherosclerosis. The causes of these pathologic changes are presumably related to age, effects of hypertension, and abnormalities of calcium and phosphorus metabolism (41).

Vasoactive Mediators

Adenosine

In the setting of hypotension, no matter what the cause, tissue ischemia will result in net negative balance between the synthesis and degradation of adenosine triphosphate (ATP). As a consequence, ATP metabolites will begin to accumulate and be released into the extracellular fluid. One such metabolite of ATP is adenosine. It has been suggested that this metabolite may play a role in dialysis-induced hypotension (42,43) (Fig. 19.3). Adenosine has vasodilatory properties and increased levels have been reported just before hypotensive episodes during dialysis (42). In an attempt to demonstrate that accumulation of adenosine during dialysis-induced hypotension is more than just a marker of the ischemic event, Shinzato et al. (43) measured the metabolites of ATP before, during, and after dialysis-induced hypotension in a group of hypotensive-prone chronic dialysis patients. In this study, plasma levels of inosine, hypoxanthine, and xanthine rose sharply with the development of sudden

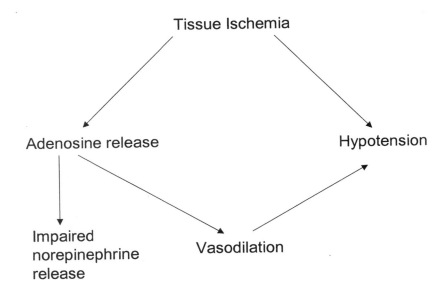

FIG. 19.3. A cycle in which tissue ischemia can lead to intradialytic hypotension via the generation of adenosine. Adenosine can potentially exacerbate hypotension by its direct vasodilatory effects and secondarily by inhibiting norepinephrine.

intradialytic hypotension and quickly decreased as the blood pressure was restored. By contrast, there was no significant variation in the plasma levels of the metabolites when hypotension developed more gradually during the course of the procedure. Adenosine levels were not measured because of the short half-life of the metabolite. These patients were then treated with caffeine, an adenosine-receptor blocker, and the frequency of hypotensive episodes was examined. A 250-mg capsule of caffeine administered 2 hours into the procedure resulted in a significant decrease in the development of hypotensive episodes. These results support the idea that tissue ischemia can contribute to intradialytic hypotension through the release of vasodilatory metabolites of ATP such as adenosine.

Nitric Oxide

Another intriguing and as yet ill-defined contributor to the development of HD hypotension is that of nitric oxide (44). It has been proposed that blood bioincompatibility with dialysis membranes leads to the activation of monocytes in the peripheral circulation (see Chapter 1). This is thought to produce a variety of cytokines including interleukin-1 (IL-1) and tumor necrosis factor (TNF). These cytokines in turn induce the synthesis of nitric oxide by endothelial cells (45). The support for this hypothesis is derived from several sources. First, plasma levels of IL-1 and TNF are elevated in ESRD patients on dialysis (46). Furthermore, IL-1 and TNF induce hypotension when administered in vivo, predominantly as a result of a decline in systemic vascular resistance (47). In vitro studies have also shown that IL-1 and TNF promote nitric oxide synthesis in endothelial cells. Nitric oxide has a direct effect as a smooth muscle vasodilator, working via intracellular cyclic guanylyl monophosphate (GMP) as a second messenger. In addition, IL-1 is also capable of inducing the synthesis of vasodilator prostaglandins (PGs), including PGE_2 and PGI_2 in human vascular smooth muscle cells and endothelial cells (48). These arachidonic acid metabolites are direct smooth muscle vasodila-

tors as well and could thereby contribute to a decline in peripheral vascular resistance.

The concentration of the stable end products of endogenously released nitric oxide, nitrite and nitrate, are increased in chronic renal failure patients undergoing HD as compared with normal controls (49–51). Normally, these levels decrease significantly during a dialysis treatment in otherwise hemodynamically stable patients. By contrast, at least two studies have shown that these metabolites actually increase in patients who develop intradialytic hypotension (49,50). A higher predialysis fractional exhaled nitric oxide concentration has also been found in patients with intradialytic hypotension as compared with those with stable hemodynamics (51). These findings suggest that increased synthesis of nitric oxide may be contributing to hemodynamic instability in hypotensive-prone subjects. The basis for increased nitric oxide activity is unknown but may be related to the dialytic removal of the nitric oxide inhibitor, asymmetric dimethylarginine (ADMA) (52). If further studies confirm an important role for increased synthesis of nitric oxide in dialysis-associated hemodynamic instability, administration of an antagonist to nitric oxide production such as N(G)-monomethyl-L-arginine acetate (L-NMMA) may ultimately prove useful in the treatment of hypotensive-prone patients.

AUTONOMIC NEUROPATHY

Autonomic Dysfunction in Uremia

The importance of autonomic dysfunction as a contributing factor to dialysis hypotension has been the subject of vigorous investigation for the past 15 years. One of the first clinical associations between impaired autonomic nervous system control and hypotension was described by Bradbury and Eggelston in 1925 (53). They observed that the autonomic nervous system was essential in the orthostatic regulation of arterial pressure through baroreflex mechanisms. Subsequently, the central and peripheral neuronal pathways that control vasomotor tone, heart rate, myocardial contractility, and venous capacitance have been described in greater detail (54–56).

An autonomic reflex arc is composed of an afferent limb that consists of sensory nerve fibers originating from the vascular tree, visceral organs, and the skin. These afferent fibers travel to the central nervous system mainly via the spinal cord and vagus nerves. Arterial baroreceptors are located in the aortic arch and carotid sinus and sense changes in blood pressure; cardiopulmonary baroreceptors are located in the atrium, ventricles, great veins, and pulmonary vessels and sense changes in cardiac filling pressures. Information about these pressure changes is integrated in the central nervous system at several different levels including the brainstem, cerebellum, hypothalamus, and cerebral hemispheres. The efferent limb of the system consists of both sympathetic and parasympathetic pathways that exit the brainstem to the spinal cord and travel to the heart and circulation (57,58).

Abnormalities in autonomic function are commonly present in patients with chronic renal failure (58–60). The presence of these abnormalities can potentially impair the patient's ability to maintain systemic blood pressure following a large degree of fluid removal by ultrafiltration. Under normal conditions, sympathetic neural outflow is under tonic restraint by baroreceptors in the aortic arch and carotid sinus and by baroreceptors in the cardiopulmonary region. With the volume removal that accompanies HD, reductions in central venous pressure and arterial blood pressure would be expected to unload these baroreceptors and thus reduce their tonic restraint on the vasomotor center, resulting in reflex increases in sympathetic outflow to the heart and peripheral circulation to help maintain blood pressure. Defects in this homeostatic response may play an important role in the development of hypotension during the dialytic procedure.

Numerous tests have been employed to assess the autonomic nervous system in patients with chronic renal failure. These tests may be used to try to localize the defect in the autonomic nervous system. For example, the Valsalva test probes the integrity of the entire autonomic nervous system: low- and high-pressure baroreceptors in the cardiopulmonary circulation, the afferent and efferent limbs of these pathways, and both sympathetic and parasympathetic function (61). This test is, therefore, useful in detecting a defect but not in identifying the site of the abnormality. The amyl nitrate inhalation test may be used to test low-pressure baroreceptors and the resultant efferent sympathetic outflow expected when blood pressure declines (62). The cold pressor test (performed by placing a cold cloth on the patient's forehead or by submerging a hand in ice slush) predominantly reflects efferent sympathetic function activated by cold-induced peripheral vasoconstriction (58). The precise role of the autonomic nervous system in dialysis patients has been difficult to assess in part because tests of autonomic function have not been routinely included in large surveys of dialysis subjects (63). For this reason, the natural history of changes in the autonomic nervous system in ESRD subjects is not presently clear.

The initial study that suggested that a defect in the autonomic nervous system could be related to HD hypotension was published in 1976 by Lilley et al. (64). These investigators performed a variety of autonomic tests and concluded that the defect in the autonomic nervous system in ESRD patients was on the afferent side of the autonomic loop. More specifically, they concluded that the defect resided in the baroreceptors. The finding of autonomic dysfunction at the levels of the afferent branch of the baroreflex arc is consistent with numerous other studies published in the literature in which selective testing of the vasomotor center and the efferent sympathetic tract (cold pressor test, handgrip test, mental stress) showed normal function (59,64–69), whereas tests of the complete baroreflex arc showed a diminished response (59,63,64–68,70–74).

The precise mechanism of the autonomic dysfunction remains unclear but, because efferent sympathetic function appears to be normal, the most likely sites of primary damage are the baroreceptors or their afferent fibers or central nervous system connections. Chronic fluid overload leading to persistent overstretching has been suggested as one cause of baroreceptor dysfunction (75). In addition, there has been some sentiment that uremic "poisoning" of baroreceptors is involved in dialysis hypotension (63,64,76–80). Chronic exposure to uremic toxins has been thought to poison the baroreceptors, leading in some patients to almost complete removal of their tonic inhibitory effects on sympathetic vasomotor outflow (63,64,76–78). According to this hypothesis, uremia-induced sinoaortic baroreceptor deafferentation would cause central sympathetic outflow to be nearly maximal under basal conditions so that it could not possibly increase much further during the hypotensive stress of HD. However, the experimental support for this hypothesis is indirect, relying mainly on plasma catecholamines and semiquantitative bedside tests to assess sympathetic neural function, and a definitive relation between impaired baroreflexes and dialysis-induced hypotension has not been established (68,78,79, 81,82).

Paradoxical Withdrawal of Sympathic Tone in Dialysis-Induced Hypotension

To better characterize the role of autonomic dysfunction in the genesis of intradialytic hypotension, Converse et al. (83) examined baroreflex control of heart rate, efferent sympathetic nerve activity, and vascular resistance in 16 hypotension-resistant and 7 hypotension-prone HD patients. Hypotension-prone patients were defined as those in whom a sudden, symptomatic decrease in mean arterial pressure of greater than 30 mm Hg occurred during at least one third of maintenance HD sessions. Patients with diabetes were excluded from the study because autonomic neuropathy is a well-known complication of diabetes mellitus (84). Direct measurements of sympathetic nerve activity and several quantifiable reflex maneuvers were employed to test the effects of chronic uremia on a number of specific reflexes, including arterial baroreflex control of heart rate and cardiopulmonary baroreflex control of vascular resistance. By studying the same patients both during the interdialytic period and during actual sessions of maintenance HD, these investigators were able to separate the autonomic effects of chronic uremia from the acute autonomic effects of the HD procedure.

To assess whether a chronic abnormality was present in either arterial or cardiopulmonary baroreceptors, both groups of patients were first studied during the interdialytic period. Measurement of heart rate and sympathetic nerve activity during the intravenous infusion of nitroprusside and measurement of fore-arm vascular resistance during the application of negative pressure to the lower body disclosed no abnormalities in either group of patients. These results suggested that there was no baseline autonomic defect chronically present to account for dialysis-induced hypotension in this select group of nondiabetic patients. It should be pointed out that in other groups of dialysis patients, such as those with diabetic autonomic neuropathy, impaired baroreflexes indeed may contribute more to hypotension during HD.

Studies were then undertaken to examine autonomic function during the dialytic procedure. In a subgroup of patients who developed severe hypotension on dialysis, baroreceptor function was again normal, that is, a small initial decrease in blood pressure was accompanied by the appropriate reflex increases in sympathetic nerve activity, heart rate, and peripheral vascular resistance. As the hypotensive episode became severe, however, normal baroreflex function was replaced by the sudden appearance of an inappropriate vasodepressor reaction. With the additional fall in blood pressure, sympathetic activity, heart rate, and vascular resistance did not increase further but rather fell paradoxically back to or below baseline levels. Shortly after the onset of the hypotension and loss of sympathetic activation, classic signs and symptoms of vasovagal syncope developed in the patients, including nausea, abdominal discomfort, diaphoresis, and giddiness.

To further examine the mechanism triggering this vasodepressor reaction, additional experiments were performed in which the normal HD procedure was separated into its component parts, ultrafiltration alone and dialysis alone. Using measurements of calf vascular resistance it was found that ultrafiltration reproduced both the increases and decreases in vascular resistance (including vasodilation and hypotension), whereas dialysis alone had no effect on calf vascular resistance in either group of patients. These results suggested that withdrawal of volume appears to be the key stimulus triggering this vasodepressor reaction, which in turn exacerbates the volume-dependent fall in blood pressure.

An inhibitory reflex arising in the heart is the most likely mechanism causing this paradoxical bradycardia and vasodilation during hypovolemic hypotension (85–93). In addition to being a pump, the heart is also a sensory organ, being richly innervated with sensory (or afferent) nerves (92). Many of these sensory nerves function as mechanoreceptors and thus signal the brain of changes in loading conditions and contractility of the ventricles (93). Their function is to inhibit sympathetic outflow. During euvolemia, these sensory nerves normally exert a tonic inhibitory influence on sympathetic vasomotor outflow. During mild hypovolemia, this inhibitory influence is reduced. During severe hypovolemia, however, this inhibitory influence is not reduced further but instead increases paradoxically. The theory is that the receptive fields of these endings are deformed as the adrenergically stimulated heart contracts forcefully around an almost empty ventricular chamber.

It was hypothesized that mild hypovolemia might simulate nonhypotensive HD: unloading of inhibitory ventricular afferents causing reflex sympathetic activation. In contrast, severe hypovolemia might simulate HD-induced hypotension: paradoxical activation of inhibitory ventricular afferents causing

reflex inhibition of sympathetic outflow resulting in bradycardia and peripheral vasodilation. Echocardiographic measurements of LV volumes before the onset of severe hypotension showed near obliteration of the LV cavity possibly accounting for the paradoxical activation of inhibitory LV afferents.

Thus, in a subset of hypotensive-prone dialysis patients, a form of acute autonomic neuropathy plays an etiologic role. For this paradoxical sympathetic failure to occur, severe volume depletion must occur. To determine the prevalence of this type of hypotension (bradycardic hypotension) in the dialysis population, Zoccali et al. (94) identified 20 patients out of a total population of 106 who suffered from intradialytic hypotension. In 60 hypotensive episodes recorded in the 20 patients, heart rate increased in 35 episodes, remained unchanged in 19 episodes, and decreased in 6 episodes. The five patients who developed bradycardic hypotension were characterized by high ultrafiltration rates and smaller LV end-diastolic diameters as compared with those with tachycardic or fixed heart rate.

Autonomic Dysfunction and Chronic Hypotension

As mentioned previously, a small fraction of HD patients have difficulty maintaining a normal blood pressure and are chronically hypotensive between dialysis treatments. The role of autonomic dysfunction in this condition was examined in one study that compared numerous measures of autonomic function among hypotensive HD patients, normotensive HD patients, and control patients (all groups consisted of 17 individuals) (95). Chronically hypotensive individuals exhibited a significant downregulation of α- and β-adrenergic receptors, suggesting an inability to produce an adequate sympathetic response.

Autonomic Dysfunction and Arrhythmias

The presence of myocardial dysfunction, fluid and electrolyte shifts, poor oxygen saturation, and other factors, either alone or in combination, favor the development of cardiac arrhythmias in ESRD. A previously unrecognized predisposing factor may be autonomic dysfunction. One study of 41 dialysis patients evaluated the correlation between arrhythmia (as determined by 24-hour Holter examination) and autonomic dysfunction (as determined by blood pressure and heart rate responses) (96). Compared with patients with normal autonomic function, a significantly increased incidence of atrial and/or ventricular arrhythmia was found among those with one or more autonomic abnormalities (41 abnormal rhythms in 26 patients with autonomic dysfunction vs. 1 in 15 with normal autonomic responses).

Sympathetic Nervous System and Hypertension in the Uremic State

Despite the frequent presence of autonomic dysfunction, baseline plasma catecholamine levels are often elevated in chronic renal failure (66). Increased sympathetic tone, decreased degradation, and diminished neuronal reuptake all may contribute to this finding. The physiologic significance of this finding is uncertain but sympathetic overactivity could contribute to the common development of hypertension in ESRD. The signal for this increased sympathetic tone may in part originate with stimulation of renal afferent nerves.

Chemosensitive renal afferent nerves have been implicated in the pathogenesis of hypertension by causing reflex activation of sympathetic outflow to the heart and peripheral circulation (97–99). Stimulation of these afferent nerves by either ischemic metabolites, such as adenosine, or by uremic toxins, such as urea, evokes reflex increases in sympathetic nerve activity and blood pressure in experimental animals (99,100). Reduced sympathetic activity may be one important mechanism by which bilateral nephrectomy lowers blood pressure in some HD patients (101).

THERAPIES FOR HEMODYNAMIC INSTABILITY DURING HEMODIALYSIS

General

In patients in whom dialysis hypotension has not been a problem but in whom it develops suddenly, the differential diagnoses must be expanded to include occult septicemia and unrecognized cardiac or pericardial disease. In this regard, the exclusion of a pericardial effusion and tamponade and/or a significant segmental wall motion abnormality are important in the assessment in any patient with hypotensive episodes occurring frequently. Other serious underlying conditions that can give rise to new onset hypotension include intestinal ischemia with impending bowel infarction and occult hemorrhage. Hypotension during the early part of the procedure should make one consider exaggerated cytokine release resulting from a reaction with the dialysis membrane. After excluding these processes, there are several options available for the treatment and prevention of episodic dialysis hypotension (Table 19.3).

TABLE 19.3. TREATMENT OF HEMODYNAMIC INSTABILITY

Exclude nondialysis related causes (cardiac ischemia, pericardial effusion, infection)
Individualize the dialysis prescription
  Accurate setting of the dry weight
  Optimize dialysate composition
    Na concentration greater than or equal to 140 mEq/L
    Na modeling
    HCO_3 buffer
    Avoid low Mg dialysate
    Avoid low Ca dialysate
  Optimize method of ultrafiltration (Uf)
    Volume controlled Uf
    Uf modeling
    Sequential Uf and isovolemic dialysis
  Cool temperature dialysate
Maximize cardiac performance
Avoidance of food
Avoid antihypertensive medicines on dialysis day
Pharmacologic prevention
  Erythropoietin therapy to keep hematocrit >33%
  Midodrine
  Sertraline
  Others: ephedrine, phenylephrine, carnitine

Individualizing the Dialysis Prescription

Accurate Setting of the "Dry Weight"

At present, the determination of dry weight is largely assessed empirically by trial and error. The dry weight is set at the weight below which unacceptable symptoms, such as cramping, nausea and vomiting, or hypotension occur. The dry weight is highly variable in many patients and can fluctuate with intercurrent illnesses (such as diarrhea or infection) and with changes in hematocrit (as with erythropoietin). Other modalities have been evaluated in an effort to more objectively estimate dry weight. Plasma atrial natriuretic peptide levels, which vary with cardiac filling pressures, do not appear to predict the state of hydration (102). It has been suggested that a noninvasive assessment of conductivity, which is measured with electrodes around the lower leg, is an accurate estimate of the extracellular volume and can detect underhydration after dialysis (102). However, conductivity measurement is not widely available and needs further testing. Other ways that have been suggested to noninvasively assess dry weight include determination of inferior caval vein diameter by echocardiography, plasma levels of cyclic guanosine 3'5'-monophosphate, and plasma levels of calcitonin gene-related peptide (103).

Dialysate Composition

A detailed discussion is provided in Chapter 3 on how the composition of the dialysate can be adjusted to maximize hemodynamic stability. Summary statements regarding these components are provided in the following sections.

Dialysate Sodium Concentration and Sodium Modeling

The use of a higher dialysate Na concentration (>140 mEq/L) has been among the most efficacious and best tolerated therapies for episodic hypotension. The high Na concentration prevents a marked decline in the plasma osmolality during dialysis, thereby protecting the extracellular volume by minimizing osmotic fluid loss into the cells. Na modeling is a technique in which the dialysate Na concentration is varied during the course of the procedure. Most commonly, a high dialysate Na concentration is used initially with a progressive reduction toward isotonic or even hypotonic levels by the end of the procedure. This method of Na control allows for a diffusive Na influx early in the session to prevent the rapid decline in plasma osmolality resulting from the efflux of urea and other small molecular weight solutes. During the remainder of the procedure, when the reduction in osmolality accompanying urea removal is less abrupt, the dialysate Na level is set at a lower level, thereby minimizing the development of hypertonicity and any resultant excessive thirst, fluid gain, and hypertension in the interdialytic period. The precise role of Na modeling has not been fully defined as yet; studies with positive and negative findings have been performed. It is a procedure associated with low morbidity and is, therefore, worthy of a trial in individual problem dialysis patients.

Dialysate Buffer

In prior years the use of acetate as a dialysis buffer had been a potential cofactor in causing dialysis hypotension by leading to peripheral vasodilatation. The current use of high-efficiency and high-flux dialysis procedures prohibits the use of acetate as a dialysis buffer. Bicarbonate is now widely available and adaptable to all new dialysis machines. In general, blood pressure is generally better maintained with bicarbonate. The cost differential between bicarbonate dialysate and acetate dialysate has decreased sufficiently to make this issue of dialysate buffer moot.

Dialysate Magnesium Concentration

Low magnesium in the dialysate may also contribute to intradialytic hypotension. One study, for example, randomized 78 clinically stable patients on HD to treatment with dialysate containing low (0.38 mmol/L) or high (0.75 mmol/L) concentrations of magnesium in combination with either bicarbonate or acetate buffer (104). For both bicarbonate and acetate solutions, patients dialyzed with the low magnesium concentration solution experienced a significant increase in the number of episodes of hypotension and a lower absolute decrease in mean arterial pressure compared with those dialyzed with the higher concentration.

Dialysate Calcium Concentration

Cardiac contractility can be enhanced in many dialysis patients by increasing the dialysate calcium concentration. A limitation of this approach is the development of hypercalcemia particularly in patients being treated with calcium-containing phosphate binders and vitamin D. In patients prone to intradialytic hypotension who are at risk for hypercalcemia, dialysate calcium profiling can be used as a strategy to improve hemodynamic stability and yet minimize the potential for hypercalcemia (105). In one study of patients dialyzed for 4 hours, the dialysate calcium concentration was set low (1.25 mmol/L) for the first 2 hours and then increased to 1.75 mmol/L for the last 2 hours (105). Use of the varying dialysate calcium concentration was associated with greater hemodynamic stability as compared with a fixed dialysate calcium concentration of either 1.25 or 1.5 mmol/L. This hemodynamic benefit was accomplished via an increase in cardiac output. At the end of 3 weeks there was no difference in the predialysis ionized calcium concentration between the three groups.

Optimized Method of Ultrafiltration

Volumetrically Controlled Ultrafiltration

Modern dialysis machines have helped in the avoidance of dialysis hypotension by allowing clinicians to program the volume removal pattern from patients during dialysis. These machines use an accurate volumetric device to evenly program ultrafiltration. Hence, a steady and even ultrafiltration rate throughout the course of dialysis is achievable. In the absence of an ultrafiltration control device, the rate of ultrafiltration can fluctuate considerably as the pressure across the membrane tends to vary. In addition, high venous pressures can lead to exaggerated rates of fluid removal. To minimize the risk for excessive fluid removal when such a device is not available, membranes with a low water permeability (KUf) should be used.

Ultrafiltration Modeling

Clinicians may desire to ultrafilter more volume at the beginning of the procedure and less toward the conclusion of the procedure. In this manner, dialysis ultrafiltration may be tailored to the individual dialysis subject. This approach may prove particularly effective when combined with a Na modeling program that has also been individually tailored (106).

Sequential Ultrafiltration and Isovolemic Dialysis

A similar goal of maintenance of the plasma osmolality can be attained by initial ultrafiltration alone (without dialysis) followed by isovolemic dialysis in which little or no further fluid removal occurs because of reduced transmembrane pressures. This sequential procedure often allows a large volume of fluid to be removed without inducing hemodynamic instability. The downside to this approach is that adequacy can be impaired unless the period of dialysis is prolonged.

Cool Temperature Dialysate

In response to ultrafiltration, increased activity of the sympathetic nervous system leads to vasoconstriction of the dermal circulation. As a result heat dissipation is impaired and core body temperature tends to increase. Indirect evidence suggests that the increase in body temperature is directly related to the amount of ultrafiltration (107). In addition to impaired heat dissipation there is also increased central heat production that accompanies the dialysis procedure. At some point, the increase in core body temperature can overcome peripheral vasoconstriction and precipitate acute hypotension (Fig. 19.4).

Recently, the simple maneuver of lowering the dialysis temperature 2°C from 37°C to 35°C has been associated with improvement in both symptoms and blood pressure (108–111). Use of cooler temperature dialysate results in increased myocardial contractility in stable dialysis patients (112,113). In patients selected for frequent episodic hypotension or predialysis hypotension use of the 35°C dialysate has also been shown to increase peripheral vasoconstriction (113). The peripheral vasoconstrictive response was measured directly by venous occlusion plethysmography in these studies. The increase in peripheral vasoconstriction resulted in an improvement in both supine and standing blood pressure following ultrafiltration HD in both groups of hypotensive-prone patients. No episodes of hypotension were recorded during the 35°C procedure, whereas many were noted when the patients were on the 37°C procedures. Also, the 35°C procedure was associated with an increase in plasma norepinephrine levels. In addition to increased myocardial contractility and peripheral vasoconstriction, lowering the dialysate temperature is also associated with better preservation of central blood volume through enhanced mobilization of pooled venous blood (114). Taken together, these findings suggest that the combination of an improvement in myocardial

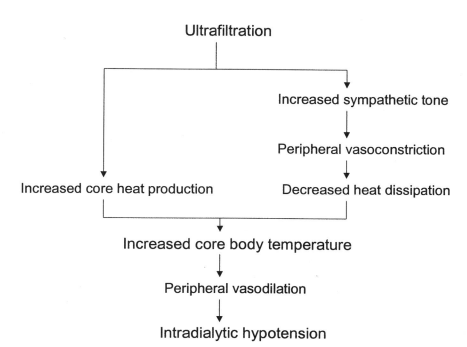

FIG. 19.4. There is an increase in core body temperature that typically occurs during the dialysis procedure. The degree to which core body temperature rises is related to the amount of ultrafiltration. At some point the increased body temperature overcomes peripheral vasoconstriction and leads to the sudden onset of hypotension.

contractility, increased peripheral vasoconstriction, and less venous pooling add to providing improved support for blood pressure in patients undergoing ultrafiltration dialysis.

This hemodynamic protection is present even in those patients with the highest proclivity to develop dialysis hypotension. When applied to a more general dialysis population, those patients with subnormal predialysis temperatures (present in up to 23% of patients) may derive the greatest hemodynamic benefit from this procedure (115). The mechanism of the protection would appear to be an increase in efferent autonomic outflow, as deduced from the increase in plasma norepinephrine levels seen on exposure to 35°C dialysis. The improved hemodynamic stability observed with convective dialysis treatments such as hemofiltration may, in part, be related to the lower extracorporeal blood temperature typical of this procedure (116).

Despite the potential for cool temperature dialysis to increase the degree of urea compartmentalization as a result of peripheral vasoconstriction, the procedure has been shown to have no significant effect on dialysis efficiency (117). Although tolerated well in most patients, it should be noted that 35°C dialysis may not be tolerated in all patients. This may be particularly true of patients who are sensitive to temperature changes and in patients who develop excessive vasoconstriction and symptoms and signs of either coronary insufficiency or peripheral vascular insufficiency.

A recent refinement in the implementation of cool temperature dialysate is the use of what has been termed isothermic dialysis. This technique employs a blood temperature monitor that senses temperature changes in the arterial and venous catheters of the extracorporeal circuit. This information is used to then adjust the dialysate temperature on an ongoing basis such that body temperature remains unchanged. Use of isothermic dialysis allows for dialysate temperature to be individualized and adjusted throughout the procedure rather than subjecting every patient to the same cold stress. The procedure takes into account patient-to-patient variability in predialysis body temperature and the increase in body temperature as ultrafiltration volume varies. The effectiveness of this technique was recently verified in a large group of patients selected because of the frequent occurrence of intradialytic hypotension (118).

Maximize Cardiac Performance

The frequency of dialysis-associated hemodynamic instability is greatly increased in patients with a prior history of congestive heart failure, cardiomegaly, or ischemic heart disease. These conditions lead to poor LV performance and, importantly, a diminished cardiac reserve in the context of a hemodynamic challenge. As discussed previously, cardiac contractility can be enhanced in many dialysis patients by increasing the dialysate calcium concentration, using cool temperature HD, and correcting anemia with erythropoietin.

Avoidance of Food

Food ingestion during dialysis leads to a significant decline in systemic vascular resistance that can contribute to a fall in blood pressure (119). In addition, increased splanchnic pooling of blood will impair maintenance of central blood volume and thereby limit cardiac refilling. This effect is not corrected by the concurrent intake of caffeine.

Pharmacologic Prevention of Hypotension

Erythropoietin Therapy

Correction of anemia can potentially improve hemodynamic stability in several ways. An increase in the hematocrit is associated with an exponential rise in blood viscosity that in turn is an important component of peripheral vascular resistance (120). For this reason maintenance of a hematocrit higher than 33% may help maintain vascular resistance in the face of volume removal. Use of erythropoietin to treat anemia may further increase vascular tone through effects that are independent of the hematocrit (120,121). Correction of the hematocrit has been shown to be beneficial in causing regression of LVH (122). Finally, an increased hematocrit may result in less tissue ischemia, thus minimizing the release of the vasodilatory metabolite, adenosine.

Caffeine

Adenosine is an endogenous vasodilator that has been related to hypotensive episodes in a subset of patients on HD (39). This response can be blunted in some patients by the administration of caffeine, which may act as an adenosine receptor antagonist in this setting (39). This therapy may be limited by the fact that caffeine is rapidly removed by dialysis and chronic use may be associated with considerable tolerance to the hemodynamic effects (123).

Midodrine

Midodrine is a selective α-1 adrenergic pressor agent that has been used to treat patients with frequent intradialytic hypotension (124,125). In addition to increasing peripheral vascular resistance, midodrine has been shown to limit venous pooling and effectively restore central blood volume and maximize cardiac refilling (114).

A recent pilot study examined 21 patients with severe hypotension during dialysis and reported a significant beneficial effect on hemodynamic stability (124). The dose was initiated at 2.5 mg given before the procedure and then titrated in 2.5-mg increments to maintain the systolic pressure above 100 mm Hg. The mean dose was 8 mg, and the drug was well tolerated. Studies examining the chronic efficacy of the drug also demonstrated a significant hemodynamic benefit in patients suffering from intradialytic hypotension (126,127). It is noteworthy that many of the patients enrolled in these studies were elderly and had several comorbid conditions including diabetes mellitus, coronary artery disease, and peripheral vascular disease. Despite the high-risk nature of the patients studied, the drug was well tolerated and safe to use. The dose should be individually titrated according to blood pressure and symptoms; most patients require 10 to 20 mg administered 30 minutes predialysis.

Sertraline

Preliminary evidence suggests that sertraline, a central nervous system serotonin reuptake inhibitor, may also be beneficial in dialysis-induced hypotension (128). A retrospective study of nine patients placed on sertraline (50 to 100 mg/day) for depression compared the blood pressure response during dialysis for the 6-week period before drug initiation to the response during an equivalent period immediately after the drug was begun. Sertraline was associated with an increase in the lowest mean blood pressure measured during dialysis (68 vs. 55 mm Hg), a lower frequency of hypotensive episodes (0.6 vs. 1.4 episodes per ses-

sion), and fewer required therapeutic interventions for hypotension during the study period (1.7 vs. 11.0). This benefit may be due to an attenuation of sympathetic withdrawal. Although more data are needed, sertraline is considered a safe drug and, therefore, should be considered as a reasonable agent to administer in hypotension-prone patients.

Other Drugs

Other drugs that have been used to treat patients with intradialytic hypotension include ephedrine (129) and phenylephrine (130). In a study of 6 patients with refractory HD-induced hypotension, intranasal lysine vasopressin administered 1 hour before a dialysis treatment and again 12 hours later resulted in a significant decline in the number of hypotensive episodes and in the volume of intravenous fluids used in the treatment of hypotension (131). Finally, in a multicenter study of otherwise stable chronic dialysis patients, intravenous infusion of carnitine was found to significantly decrease the incidence of intradialytic hypotension and cramps as compared with a control group (132).

Comparative Studies

All of the measures delineated previously provide some degree of prophylactic benefit. However, their relative efficacy in the same patient is unclear and comparative studies are limited.

In one study the efficacy and tolerability of midodrine, cool temperature dialysate, or the combination were compared in a study of 11 patients with intradialytic hypotension (133). All three therapies were found to be equally effective in improving hemodynamic stability. There was a trend for the combined group to have superior improvement in hemodynamic stability; however, this did not reach statistical significance.

A second study compared five different procedures in a single-blinded cross-over study of 10 patients with a history of intradialytic hypotension (134). After 1 week of standard dialysis, all patients underwent 1 week of each of the following four strategies: high Na dialysate, Na modeling, sequential ultrafiltration and isovolemic dialysis, and cool temperature dialysis. The following results were reported: high Na dialysate, Na modeling, and cool temperature dialysis resulted in significantly fewer hypotensive events than that observed with standard dialysis. Compared with the other test strategies, sequential ultrafiltration and isovolemic dialysis had a significantly greater number of hypotensive episodes. Postdialysis upright blood pressure was best with Na modeling and cool temperature dialysis, compared with that measured with standard and isolated ultrafiltration dialysis. Weight loss was virtually identical with all protocols. In general, the best tolerated and most effective strategy was Na modeling. High Na and cool temperature dialysis were also effective, whereas sequential ultrafiltration and isovolemic dialysis was significantly less useful.

ACUTE TREATMENT OF HYPOTENSION

Although occasionally asymptomatic, patients with hypotension may suffer from light-headedness, muscle cramps, nausea, vom-

TABLE 19.4. ACUTE TREATMENT OF INTRADIALYTIC HYPOTENSION

Stop or slow rate of ultrafiltration
Place patient in Trendelenburg position
Decrease blood-flow rate
Restore intravascular volume (hypertonic saline)
Assess for ischemic injury
Check patency of vascular access

iting, and dyspnea. The acute management of low blood pressure associated with HD includes stopping or slowing the rate of ultrafiltration, placing the patient in the Trendelenburg position, decreasing the blood flow rate, and restoring intravascular volume (Table 19.4).

The use of hypertonic saline solutions appears to be particularly effective; it allows Na to be administered in a small volume of water, and the rapid rise in plasma osmolality may have a positive effect on cardiac inotropy (135). One study found that three different regimens safely and effectively raised the blood pressure: 10 mL of 23% saturated hypertonic saline; 30 mL of 7.5% hypertonic saline; and the latter solution with 6% dextran-70 (135). The addition of dextran appeared to prolong the duration of the blood pressure response.

Further treatment is based on the cause of the hypotension; the prompt recognition of life-threatening causes of low blood pressure is essential. Particular concerns should include occult sepsis, previously unrecognized cardiac and/or pericardial disease, and gastrointestinal bleeding.

REFERENCES

1. Rosa AA, et al. Dialysis symptoms and stabilization in long-term dialysis—practical applications of the CUSUM plot. *Arch Intern Med* 1980;140:804–880.
2. Kjellstrand CM. Can hypotension during dialysis be avoided? In: Schriner GE, et al., eds. *Controversies in nephrology,* vol II. Basel: S. Karger AG, 1980;12–28.
3. Moore TJ, et al. Reduced angiotensin receptors and pressor responses in hypotensive hemodialysis patients. *Kidney Int* 1989;36:696–701.
4. Zager PG, et al. "U" curve association of blood pressure and mortality in hemodialysis patients. Medical Directors of Dialysis Clinic, Inc. *Kidney Int* 1998;54:561–569.
5. Port FK, et al. Predialysis blood pressure and mortality risk in a national sample of maintenance hemodialysis patients. *Am J Kidney Dis* 1999;33:507–517.
6. Iseki K, et al. Low diastolic blood pressure, hypoalbuminemia, and risk of death in a cohort of chronic hemodialysis patients. *Kidney Int* 1997;51:1212–1217.
7. Foley RN, et al. Left-ventricular hypertrophy in dialysis patients. *Semin Dial* 1992;5:34–41.
8. Harnett JD, et al. Risk factors for the development of left ventricular hypertrophy in a prospectively followed cohort of dialysis patients. *J Am Soc Nephrol* 1994;4:1486–1490.
9. Levin A, et al. Prevalent left ventricular hypertrophy in the predialysis population: identifying opportunities for intervention. *Am J Kidney Dis* 1996;27:347–354.
10. Foley RN, et al. The prognostic importance of left ventricular geometry in uremic cardiomyopathy. *J Am Soc Nephrol* 1995;5:2024–2031.
11. Parfrey PS, et al. Risk factors for cardiac dysfunction in dialysis patients: implications for patient care. *Semin Dial* 1997;10:137–141.
12. Coomer RW, et al. Ambulatory blood pressure monitoring in dialysis patients and estimation of mean interdialytic blood pressure. *Am J Kidney Dis* 1997;29:678–684.
13. Ritz E, et al. Dialysis hypotension: is it related to diastolic left ventricular malfunction? *Nephrol Dial Transplant* 1987;2:293–297.
14. Klein J, et al. Hypertrophic cardiomyopathy: an acquired disorder of end-stage renal disease. *ASAIO Trans* 1983;29:120.
15. Ritz E, et al. Cardiac changes in uraemia and their possible relationship to cardiovascular instability on dialysis. *Nephrol Dial Transplant* 1990;5[Suppl 1]:93–97.
16. Wizemann V, et al. Options in dialysis: significance of cardiovascular findings. *Kidney Int* 1993;43:S85–S91.
17. Ruffmann K, et al. Doppler echocardiographic findings in dialysis patients. *Nephrol Dial Transplant* 1990;5:426–431.
18. Whelton PK, et al. Calcium channel blockers in dialysis patients with left ventricular hypertrophy and well-preserved systolic function. *J Cardiovasc Pharmacol* 1987;5:185–186.
19. Silberberg, J, et al. Regression of left ventricular hypertrophy in dialysis patients following correction of anemia with recombinant human erythropoietin. *Can J Cardiol* 1990;6:1.
20. Harnett JD, et al. Cardiac function and hematocrit level. *Am J Kidney Dis* 1995;25[Suppl 1]:S3.
21. Roithinger FX, et al. The influence of ACE-inhibition on myocardial mass and diastolic function in chronic hemodialysis patients with adequate control of blood pressure. *Clin Nephrol* 1994;42:309–314.
22. Poldermans D, et al. Cardiac evaluation in hypotension-prone and hypotension-resistant hemodialysis patients. *Kidney Int* 1999;56:1905–1911.
23. Daugirdas JT. Pathophysiology of dialysis hypotension: an update. *Am J Kidney Dis* 2001;38[4 Suppl 4]:S11–S17.
24. Krepel HP, et al. Variability of relative blood volume during haemodialysis. *Nephrol Dial Transplant* 2000;15:673–679.
25. Van Stone JC, et al. The effect of dialysate sodium concentration on body fluid distribution during hemodialysis. *Trans Am Soc Artif Intern Organs* 1980;26:383–386.
26. Palmer BF. The effect of dialysate composition on systemic hemodynamics. *Semin Dial* 1992;5:54–60.
27. Kunze DL, et al. Sodium sensitivity of baroreceptors-reflux effects on blood pressure and fluid volume in the cat. *Circ Res* 1978;42:714–720.
28. Schultze G, et al. Prostaglandin E$_2$ promotes hypotension on low-sodium hemodialysis. *Nephron* 1984;37:250–256.
29. Daugirdas JT, et al. A double-blind evaluation of sodium gradient hemodialysis. *Am J Nephrol* 1985;5:163–168.
30. Raja R, et al. Sequential changes in dialysate sodium (D$_{Na}$) during hemodialysis. *Trans Am Soc Artif Intern Organs* 1983;24:649–651.
31. Bedichek E, et al. Comparison of the hemodynamic and hormonal effects of hemodialysis using programmable vs. constant sodium dialysate. *J Am Soc Nephrol* 1992;3:354.
32. Cavalcanti S, et al. Role of short-term regulatory mechanisms on pressure response to hemodialysis-induced hypovolemia. *Kidney Int* 2002;61:228–238.
33. Nakamura Y, et al. The role of peripheral capacitance and resistance vessels in hypotension following hemodialysis. *Am Heart J* 1991;121:1170–1177.
34. Kooman JP, et al. Role of the venous system in hemodynamics during ultrafiltration and bicarbonate dialysis. *Kidney Int* 1992;42:718–726.
35. Kooman JP, et al. Compliance and reactivity of the peripheral venous system in chronic intermittent hemodialysis. *Kidney Int* 1992;41:1041–1048.
36. Kooman JP, et al. Morphological changes of the venous system in uremic patients. *Nephron* 1995;69:454–458.
37. Yu AW, et al. Splanchnic erythrocyte content decreases during hemodialysis: a new compensatory mechanism for hypovolemia. *Kidney Int* 1997;51:1986–1990.
38. London GM, et al. Aortic and large artery compliance in end-stage renal failure. *Kidney Int* 1990;37:137–142.
39. Marchais SJ, et al. Wave reflections and cardiac hypertrophy in chronic uremia. *Hypertension* 1993;22:876–883.
40. Ibels LS, et al. Arterial calcification and pathology in uremic patients undergoing dialysis. *Am J Med* 1979;66:790–796.

41. Raine AEG. The susceptible patient. *Nephrol Dial Transplant* 1996; 11:6–10.

42. Shinzato T, et al. Relationship between dialysis-induced hypotension and adenosine released by ischemic tissue. *Trans Am Soc Artif Organs* 1992;38:M286–M290.

43. Shinzato T, et al. Role of adenosine in dialysis-induced hypotension. *J Am Soc Nephrol* 1994;4:1987–1994.

44. Beasley D, et al. Role of nitric oxide in hemodialysis hypotension. *Kidney Int* 1992;42(38):S96–S100.

45. Shaldon S, et al. Hemodialysis hypotension: the interleukin hypothesis restated. *Proc Eur Dial Transplant Assoc* 1985;22:229–243.

46. Herbelin A, et al. Influence of uremia and hemodialysis on circulating interleukin-1 and tumor necrosis factor α. *Kidney Int* 1990; 37:116–125.

47. Weinberg JR, et al. Interleukin-1 and tumor necrosis factor cause hypotension in the conscious rabbit. *Clin Sci* 1988;75:251–255.

48. Rossi V, et al. Prostacyclin synthesis induced in vascular cells by interleukin-1. *Science* 1985;229:174–176.

49. Noris M, et al. Enhanced nitric oxide synthesis in uremia: implications for platelet dysfunction and dialysis hypotension. *Kidney Int* 1993;44:445–450.

50. Yokokawa K, et al. Increased nitric oxide production in patients with hypotension during hemodialysis. *Ann Intern Med* 1995;123:35–37.

51. Raj DS, et al. Hemodynamic changes during hemodialysis: role of nitric oxide and endothelin. *Kidney Int* 2002;61:697–704.

52. Kang ES, et al. Hypotension during hemodialysis: role for nitric oxide. *Am J Med Sci* 1997;313:138–146.

53. Bradbury S, et al. Postural hypotension: report of three cases. *Am Heart J* 1925;1:73–86.

54. Rowell LB. Reflex control of regional circulation in humans. *J Autonom Nerv Sys* 1984;11:101–114.

55. Damprey RAL, et al. Role of ventrolateral medulla in vasomotor regulation, correlative, anatomical and physiological study. *Brain Res* 1982;249:223–235.

56. Bannister R. *Autonomic failure.* Oxford: Oxford University Press, 1983.

57. Travis M, et al. Autonomic nervous system and hemodialysis hypotension. *Semin Dial* 1989;2:158–162.

58. Henrich WL. Autonomic insufficiency. *Arch Intern Med* 1982;142: 339–344.

59. Ewing DJ, et al. Autonomic function in patients with chronic renal failure on intermittent haemodialysis. *Nephron* 1975;15:424–429.

60. Malik S, et al. Chronic renal failure and cardiovascular autonomic function. *Nephron* 1986;43:191–195.

61. Sharpey-Schafer EP. Effect of Valsalva's maneuver on the normal and failing circulation. *Br Med J* 1955;1:693.

62. Lazarus JM, et al. Baroreceptor activity in normotensive and hypertensive uremic patients. *Circulation* 1973;47:1015.

63. Campese VM, et al. Mechanisms of autonomic nervous system dysfunction in uremia. *Kidney Int* 1981;20:246–253.

64. Lilley JJ, et al. Adrenergic regulation of blood pressure in chronic renal failure. *J Clin Invest* 1976;57:1190–1200.

65. Friess U, et al. Failure of arginine-vasopressin and other pressor hormones to increase in severe recurrent dialysis hypotension. *Nephrol Dial Transplant* 1995;10:1421–1427.

66. Daul AE, et al. Arterial hypotension in chronic hemodialyzed patients. *Kidney Int* 1987;32:728–735.

67. Tajiri M, et al. Autonomic nervous dysfunction in patients on long-term hemodialysis. *Nephron* 1979;23:10–13.

68. Nies AS, et al. Hemodialysis hypotension is not the result of uremic peripheral autonomic neuropathy. *J Lab Clin Med* 1979;94:395–402.

69. Koch KM, et al. Autonome Kreislaufregulation in der Uramie. *Klin Wochenschr* 1980;58:1037–1042.

70. Pickering TG, et al. Baroreflex sensitivity in patients on long-term haemodialysis. *Clin Sci* 1972;43:645–657.

71. Kersh ES, et al. Autonomic insufficiency in uremia as a cause of hemodialysis-induced hypotension. *N Engl J Med* 1974;290:650–653.

72. Stojceva-Taneva O, et al. Autonomic nervous system dysfunction and volume nonresponsive hypotension in hemodialysis patients. *Am J Nephrol* 1991;11:123–126.

73. Cavalcanti S, et al. Autonomic nervous function during haemodialysis assessed by spectral analysis of heart-rate variability. *Clin Sci* 1997;92:351–359.

74. Enzmann G, et al. Autonomic nervous function and blood volume monitoring during hemodialysis. *Int J Artif Organs* 1995;18: 504–508.

75. Heber ME, et al. Baroreceptor, not left ventricular, dysfunction is the cause of hemodialysis hypotension. *Clin Nephrol* 1989;32:79–86.

76. McLeod JG. Autonomic dysfunction in peripheral nerve disease. In: Bannister R, ed. *Autonomic failure.* Oxford: Oxford University Press, 1988:615–616.

77. Lazarus JM, et al. Baroreceptor activity in normotensive and hypertensive uremic patients. *Circulation* 1973;82:1015–1021.

78. Zoccali C, et al. Defective reflex control of heart rate in dialysis patients: evidence for an afferent autonomic lesion. *Clin Sci* 1982; 63:285–292.

79. Nakashima Y, et al. Localization of autonomic nervous system dysfunction in dialysis patients. *Am J Nephrol* 1987;7:375–381.

80. Mallamaci F, et al. Autonomic function in uremic patients treated by hemodialysis or CAPD and in transplant patients. *Clin Nephrol* 1986; 25:175–180.

81. Naik RB, et al. Cardiovascular and autonomic reflexes in haemodialysis patients. *Clin Sci* 1981;60:165–170.

82. Ligtenberg G, et al. No change in autonomic function tests during uncomplicated haemodialysis. *Nephrol Dial Transplant* 1996;11: 651–656.

83. Converse RL, et al. Paradoxical withdrawal of reflex vasoconstriction as a cause of hemodialysis-induced hypotension. *J Clin Invest* 1992; 90:1657–1665.

84. Ewing DJ, et al. Assessment of cardiovascular effects in diabetic autonomic neuropathy and prognostic implications. *Ann Intern Med* 1980;92(Part 2):308–311.

85. Henrich WL, et al. Role of osmolality in blood pressure stability after dialysis and ultrafiltration. *Kidney Int* 1980;18:480–488.

86. Morita H, et al. Opiate receptor-mediated decrease in renal nerve activity during hypotensive hemorrhage in conscious rabbits. *Circ Res* 1988;63:165–172.

87. Smith ML, et al. Naloxone does not prevent vasovagal syncope during simulated orthostasis in humans. *Physiologist* 1991;27:2.

88. Morgan DA, et al. Serotonergic mechanisms mediate renal sympathoinhibition during severe hemorrhage in rats. *Am J Physiol* 1988;255:H496–H502.

89. Peuler JD, et al. Inhibition of renal sympathetic activity and heart rate by vasopressin in hemorrhaged diabetes insipidus rats. *Am J Physiol* 1990;258:H706–H712.

90. Landgren S. On the excitation mechanism of the carotid baroreceptors. *Acta Physiol Scand* 1952;26:1–34.

91. Bishop VS, et al. Cardiac mechanoreceptors. In: Shepherd JT, et al., ed. *Handbook of physiology,* section 2: The cardiovascular system, vol III. Bethesda, MD: American Physiological Society, 1983:497–555.

92. Abboud FM. Ventricular syncope: is the heart a sensory organ? *N Engl J Med* 1989;320:390–392.

93. Sander-Jensen R, et al. Vagal slowing of the heart during hemorrhage: observation from 20 consecutive hypotensive patients. *Br Med J (Clin Res)* 1986;292:365–366.

94. Zoccali C, et al. The heart rate response pattern to dialysis hypotension in haemodialysis patients. *Nephrol Dial Transplant* 1997;12:519–523.

95. Armengol NE, et al. Vasoactive hormones in uraemic patients with chronic hypotension. *Nephrol Dial Transplant* 1997;12:321–324.

96. Jassal SV, et al. Autonomic neuropathy predisposing to arrhythmias in hemodialysis patients. *Am J Kidney Dis* 1997;30:219–223.

97. Faber JE. Afferent renal nerve-dependent hypertension following acute renal artery stenosis in the conscious rat. *Circ Res* 1985;57: 676–688.

98. Katholi RE, et al. Intrarenal adenosine produces hypertension by activating the sympathetic nervous system via the renal nerves. *J Hypertension* 1984;2:349–359.

99. Siggaard-Andersen J. Venous occlusion plethysmography on the calf: evaluation of diagnosis and results in vascular surgery. *Dan Med Bull* 1970;17[Suppl 1]:1–68.

100. Recordati G, et al. Renal chemoreceptor. *J Autonomic Nerv Sys* 1981; 3:237–251.
101. Converse RL, et al. Sympathetic overactivity in patients with chronic renal failure. *N Engl J Med* 1992;327:1912–1918.
102. Kouw PM, et al. Assessment of postdialysis dry weight: a comparison of techniques. *JASN* 1993;4:98–104.
103. Franz M, et al. Living on chronic hemodialysis between dryness and fluid overload. *Kidney Int* 1997;51:39–42.
104. Rakash NR, et al. Dialysate magnesium concentration predicts the occurrence of intradialytic hypotension. *J Am Soc Nephrol* 1996;7: 1496(abst).
105. Kyriazis J, et al. Dialysate calcium profiling during hemodialysis: use and clinical implications. *Kidney Int* 2002;61:276–287
106. Levin A, et al. The benefits and side effects of ramped hypertonic sodium dialysis. *JASN* 1996;7:242–246.
107. Rosales LM, et al. Isothermic hemodialysis and ultrafiltration. *Am J Kidney Dis* 2000;36:353–361
108. Maggiore Q, et al. Blood temperature and vascular stability during hemodialysis and hemofiltration. *Trans Am Soc Artif Intern Organs* 1982;28:523–527.
109. Sherman RA, et al. Amelioration of hemodialysis-associated hypotension by the use of cool dialysate. *Am J Kidney Dis* 1985;5:124–127.
110. Mahida BH, et al. Effect of cooled dialysate on serum catecholamines and blood pressure stability. *Trans Am Soc Artif Intern Organs* 1993; 29:384–389.
111. Schneditz D, et al. Effect of controlled extracorporeal blood cooling on ultrafiltration-induced blood volume changes during hemodialysis. *JASN* 1997;8:956–964.
112. Levy FL, et al. Improved left ventricular contractility with cool temperature hemodialysis. *Kidney Int* 1992;41:961–965.
113. Jost CMT, et al. Effects of cooler temperature dialysate on hemodynamic stability in "problem" dialysis patients. *Kidney Int* 1993;44: 606–612.
114. Hoeben H, et al. Hemodynamics in patients with intradialytic hypotension treated with cool dialysate or midodrine. *Am J Kidney Dis* 2002;39:102–107
115. Fine A, et al. The protective effect of cool dialysate is dependent on patients predialysis temperature. *Am J Kidney Dis* 1996;28:262–265.
116. van Kuijk WHM, et al. Critical role of the extracorporeal blood temperature in the hemodynamic response during hemofiltration. *JASN* 1997;8:949–955.
117. Yu AW, et al. Effect of dialysate temperature on central hemodynamics and urea kinetics. *Kidney Int* 1995;48:237–243.
118. Maggiore Q, et al. Study group of thermal balance and vascular stability: the effects of control of thermal balance on vascular stability in hemodialysis patients: results of the European randomized clinical trial. *Am J Kidney Dis* 2002;40:280–290.
119. Barakat MM, et al. Hemodynamic effects of intradialytic food ingestion and the effects of caffeine. *JASN* 1993;3:1813–1818.
120. Radermacher J, et al. Treatment of renal anemia by erythropoietin substitution: the effects on the cardiovascular system. *Clin Nephrol* 1995;44[Suppl 1]:S56–S60.
121. Bode-Boger SM, et al. Recombinant human erythropoietin enhances vasoconstrictor tone via endothelin-1 and constrictor prostanoids. *Kidney Int* 1996;50:1255–1261.
122. Portoles J, et al. Cardiovascular effects of recombinant human erythropoietin in predialysis patients. *Am J Kidney Dis* 1997;29: 541–548.
123. Daugirdas JT. Preventing and managing hypotension. *Semin Dial* 1994;7:276–283.
124. Flynn JJ III, et al. Midodrine treatment for patients with hemodialysis hypotension. *Clin Nephrol* 1996;45:261–267.
125. Blowey DL, et al. Midodrine efficacy and pharmacokinetics in a patient with recurrent intradialytic hypotension. *Am J Kidney Dis* 1996;28:132–136.
126. Cruz DN, et al. Midodrine is effective and safe therapy for intradialytic hypotension over 8 months of follow-up. *Clin Nephrol* 1998;50: 101–107.
127. Perazella MA. Pharmacologic options available to treat symptomatic intradialytic hypotension. *Am J Kidney Dis* 2001;38[4 Suppl 4]: S26–S36.
128. Dheenan S, et al. Effect of sertraline hydrochloride on dialysis hypotension. *Am J Kidney Dis* 1998;31:624–630.
129. Hirszel IP, et al. Uremic autonomic neuropathy: evaluation of ephedrine sulphate therapy for hemodialysis-induced hypotension. *Int Urol Nephrol* 1976;8:313–321.
130. Warren SE, et al. Use of phenylephrine HCL for treatment of refractory dialysis- aggravated hypotension. *Dial Transplant* 1980;9:492–496.
131. Lindberg JS, et al. Lysine vasopressin in the treatment of refractory hemodialysis-induced hypotension. *Am J Nephrol* 1990;10:269–275.
132. Ahmad S, et al. Multicenter trial of L-carnitine in maintenance hemodialysis patients. II: clinical and biochemical effects. *Kidney Int* 1990;38:912–918.
133. Cruz DN, et al. Midodrine and cool dialysate are effective therapies for symptomatic intradialytic hypotension. *Am J Kidney Dis* 1999;33:920–926.
134. Dheenan S, et al. Preventing dialysis hypotension: a comparison of usual protective maneuvers. *Kidney Int* 2001;59:1175–1181
135. Gong R, et al. Comparison of hypertonic saline solutions and dextran in dialysis-induced hypotension. *JASN* 1993;3:1808–1812.

OXIDANT STRESS IN END-STAGE RENAL DISEASE

RAVINDER K. WALI

DEFINITION OF OXIDANT STRESS

Oxidative stress is a pathologic state in which reactive oxygen intermediates (ROI) or reactive oxygen species (ROS) can cause oxidation of cellular and matrix macromolecules including sugars, proteins, deoxyribonucleic acid (DNA) bases, and lipids (1). During the past several years, the role of increased oxidant stress in the pathogenesis of inflammation, end-organ complications of diabetes mellitus, normal aging, and atherosclerosis has been gradually evolving (2,3). Increasing evidence suggests that oxidative stress may have a significant role in the development of complications in patients with renal failure requiring dialysis. Understanding the role of oxidant stress in the pathogenesis of dialysis-associated pathology will ultimately help to develop the strategies for the prevention and the treatment of increased oxidant stress in renal failure.

GENERATION OF ROS IN THE BIOLOGIC SYSTEM

In biologic systems, cells generate energy aerobically to generate adenosine triphosphate (ATP) by reducing molecular oxygen (O_2) to water. The cytochrome-C oxidase-catalyzed reactions involve transfer of four electrons (e^-) to oxygen; the consumption of oxygen at the mitochondrial level is associated with production of oxygen intermediates. One percent to 2% of total oxygen consumption may, in fact, be converted to superoxide anion radical (O_2^-).

Formation of O_2^- anion radical leads to a cascade of other ROS (4) (Fig. 20.1). Superoxide dismutase (SOD) rapidly converts O_2^- to hydrogen peroxide (H_2O_2) and oxygen. Because O_2^- is more toxic than H_2O_2, its rapid removal is of paramount importance for the proper function of the microenvironment (5). H_2O_2 is a versatile ROS because it can cross plasma membranes, increase intracellular hydroxyl radicals and trigger peroxidation of cell membrane lipids, promote protein aggregation, and damage and/or cleave to DNA (6). H_2O_2 is reduced by several general mechanisms:

1. It is the substrate for two enzymes, catalase (CAT) and the GSH form of glutathione peroxidase (GPx), that catalyze the conversion of H_2O_2 to $H_2O + O_2$. This presumably is a detoxification mechanism.
2. H_2O_2 is converted by the abundant myeloperoxidase (MPO) enzyme in neutrophils to hypochlorous acid (HOCl) (6). This appears to be a mechanism for the generation of a physiologic but toxic agent, because HOCl is a strong oxidant that acts as a bactericidal agent in phagocytic cells. Reaction of HOCl with H_2O_2 yields singlet oxygen ($^1O_2$) and water.
3. H_2O_2 also reacts spontaneously with intracellular iron to form highly reactive hydroxy radical (OH^-) (7) by the Haber-Weiss cycle or Fenton reaction (8). The hydroxyl radical reacts instantaneously with any biologic molecule to produce reactive amines (RH) from which it can abstract a hydrogen atom with the production of longer lived ROS than the hydroxyl radical (9).
4. O_2^- anion also regulates the bioavailability of nitric oxide (NO), because superoxide anion can react with NO and result in the formation of peroxynitrite ($ONOO^-$) (9). $ONOO^-$ is a strong oxidant with vasoconstrictor activities as compared with the vasodilator potential of NO (10). In addition, $ONOO^-$ reacts nonenzymatically with arachidonic acid components of phospholipids resulting in the formation of isoprostanes (8-iso-PGF2α), a potent vasoconstrictor with prolonged half-life (11).

ROS have a very short life and excessive production and prolonged exposure of cell constituents to these evanescent radicals can result in oxidative modification of cellular macromolecules. In vivo measurements of ROS modified cellular macromolecules serve as indirect markers of prevailing oxidative stress. These include carbohydrate and protein oxidation (12,13), lipid peroxidation (14), and nucleic acid breaks leading to DNA fragmentation with instability and mutation (15,16).

PHYSIOLOGIC ANTIOXIDANT SYSTEM

An imbalance between the production of ROS and the available antioxidants results in the excessive exposure of the tissue macromolecules to ROS, resulting in the production of biomarkers of oxidant stress (17). Under physiologic conditions, protection against oxidant stress is offered by the presence of different types of antioxidants, enzymatic and nonenzymatic antioxidants (1).

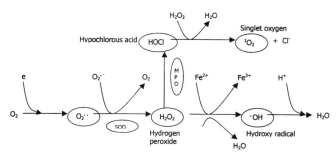

FIG. 20.1. Generation of reactive oxygen species, where MPO is myeloperoxidase and SOD is superoxide dismutase. The biologically active oxygen-free radicals are the radical ion superoxide O_2^-, hydroxide ion HO^-, and peroxide ion $O^2_2^-$. These radicals are intermediates in the respiratory process at the mitochondrial level, in which dioxygen (O^2_2) is reduced to water in a stepwise six-electron process in the presence of glutathione(s) and catalases. H_2O_2 rapidly diffuses across the lipid membranes and is converted into strong oxidants. H_2O_2 in the presence of cytoplasmic MPO produces HOCl, a free radical ion with toxic effects.

Enzymatic antioxidants include glutathione dismutase (GPx), glutathione reductase (GR) and glutathione transferase (GT), speroxide dismutase (SOD), and catalase (CAT). GPx is a selenium-dependent enzyme present in the plasma and red blood cell (RBC) and is mainly produced in the kidneys. GPx exists in three different forms (GST, GSSG, and GSH). GR uses nicotinamide adenine dinucleotide phosphate (NADPH) to convert oxidized glutathione (GSSG) to its reduced form (GSH).

The major nonenzymatic antioxidants include α-tocopherol (vitamin E); vitamin C (ascorbic acid); albumin; and others such as transferrin, ceruloplasmin, and microamounts of extracellular superoxide dismutases (ecSOD) (18). α-Tocopherol (vitamin E) is perhaps the major lipid-soluble chain-breaking antioxidant (reacting with chain-propagating radicals such as peroxyl radicals) (19). This antioxidant is particularly important because it prevents lipid peroxidation. Ascorbic acid on the other hand has mostly scavenging properties and other minor antioxidant properties. It scavenges the singlet oxygen ($^1O_2$), O_2^- and H_2O at a constant rate at optimal pH (7.4). It is a powerful scavenger of HOCl and also can be a substrate for the enzyme MPO to prevent the generation of HOCl (20). However, ascorbic acid at occasions can also be a prooxidant (21).

Acute-phase reactive proteins such as ferritin, transferrin, ceruloplasmin, haptoglobin, and others also function as effective antioxidants by binding to transitional metals such as iron, copper, and bromide to prevent the formation of halides, hemes, and chloramines (22).

PATHOPHYSIOLOGY OF OXIDATIVE STRESS IN DIALYSIS PATIENTS

Patients with progressive renal failure and those who subsequently require dialysis therapy have increased risk of exposure to oxidant stress because of qualitative and quantitative changes in the physiologic antioxidants. This is further complicated by the increased production or decreased removal of ROS and related oxidation products. These sequences of events culminate in excessive tissue damage from the ROS and its end products.

Increased Generation of Oxidant Radicals (ROS) in Dialysis Patients

Advanced renal failure is associated with increased production of ROS and this oxidant stress is further aggravated with the initiation of dialysis therapy. There are several pathways involved in the excessive generation of ROS in renal failure. The increased oxidative stress in renal failure and in dialysis patients could be due to activation of monocyte-macrophage cells by the uremic milieu and further aggravated by exposure of blood to extracorporeal circulation (see Chapter 2).

Activation of phagocytes is associated with oxidative activity that results in phagocytic function along with respiratory burst activity with the production of ROS necessary for host defenses, cell activation, and cell signaling (23). The respiratory burst activity is associated with activation of mitochondrial NADPH-oxidases that catalyzes the single electron transfer and generates superoxide anion (O_2^-) at the electron transfer chain level (24). The NADPH-oxidases are a very highly regulated group of homologous proteins comprised of cytoplasmic (p47, p67, p40) and membrane bound proteins (gp91 and p22) (25). Deficiency or dysfunction of NADPH-oxidases are associated with increased risk of bacterial infections and result in the development of chronic granulomatous disease (CGD).

In addition phagocytic cells have abundant MPO in the azurophilic granules, which is released on stimulation. The MPO enzyme system in phagocytic cells catalyzes the oxidation of halides like chloride, bromide, and iodide. MPO in the presence of chloride (Cl^-) ions converts H_2O_2 to HOCl. In addition to its primary function of bactericidal killing, HOCl is a potent oxidant by oxidation of thiol groups of membrane proteins and intracellular enzymes, and it inhibits the mitochondrial cytochrome system, perpetuating the production of ROS. HOCl can react with endogenous amines (R-NHI) to result in the production of long-lasting oxidants called chloramines (RNH-Cl) (5).

Himmelfarb et al. (26) studied phagocytic function in patients on hemodialysis and peritoneal dialysis (PD) and demonstrated an exaggerated respiratory burst activity of phagocytes after in vitro stimulation. This respiratory burst production of ROS coincides with the peak of complement activation during dialysis treatment (27).

With the advent of biocompatible membranes, it was hoped that the generation of ROS and the activation of complement cascade could be prevented. However, cross-over studies have demonstrated that a primed state of phagocytes and production of ROS persist with so-called biocompatible membranes (28). Furthermore, Tepel et al. (29) showed increased ROS production from peripheral lymphocytes both spontaneously and after phorbol-myristate-acetate (PMA)-induced stimulation in patients on maintenance dialysis and remained unchanged before and after dialysis using biocompatible membranes.

Increased levels of plasma oxidant activity measured by electron spin resonance spectroscopy were reported in dialysis

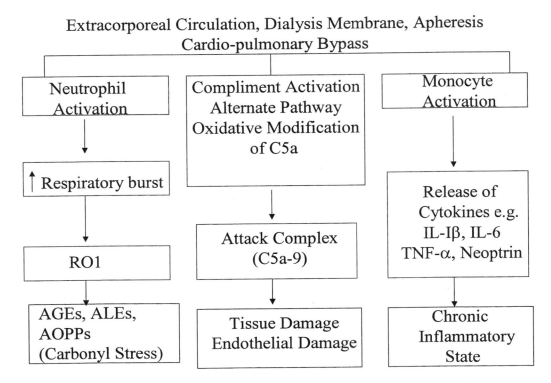

FIG. 20.2. Different pathways of ROS production on exposure to extracorporeal circulation.

patients by Roselaar et al. (30); these levels remained unchanged after dialysis treatment. 8-Hydroxy 2'-deoxygaunosine (8-OHdG) is a novel marker for the assessment of oxidative DNA damage, and increased 8-OHdG levels in peripheral mononuclear cells have been demonstrated in dialysis patients as compared with healthy controls (31).

These observational studies provide compelling evidence that patients on maintenance dialysis (hemodialysis or PD) have an increased burden of oxidative stress. This excessive burden of ROS in dialysis patients could also be due, in part, to the presence of factors other than the biocompatibility of dialysis membranes (32): the inability to remove all uremic toxins by dialysis, increased production and decreased removal of cytokines [interleukin-6 (IL-6), IL-1β, tumor necrosis factor-α (TNF-α), transforming growth factor-β (TGF-β)] on repeated exposure to extracorporeal circulation (33), back leak of microamounts of bacteria (34,35), and recurrent endotoxemia resulting from increased endotoxin levels in the water used for regular dialysis (36) (Fig. 20.2).

Qualitative or Quantitative Changes in Physiologic Antioxidants

The effect of increased production of ROS in dialysis patients is further aggravated by decreased levels or impaired function of both enzymatic and nonenzymatic antioxidants. Thus, imbalance between the increased ROS production and reduced availability of antioxidants aggravates the prevailing oxidative stress.

GPx converts H_2O_2 to 2 H_2O. It is mainly produced in the kidney and both serum and RBC levels decrease in proportion to the decreasing glomerular filtration rate (GFR). All three forms of glutathione (GST, GSSG, and GSH) decrease in patients with advanced renal failure and in patients on renal replacement therapy (hemodialysis or PD). Ross at al. (37) and Mimic-Oka et al. (38) demonstrated that whole blood and RBC glutathione and CAT levels (CATs also convert H_2O_2 to H_2O and O_2) were significantly decreased in patients with renal failure of different causes and in dialysis-dependent patients.

The levels of nonenzymatic antioxidants like vitamin C and vitamin E have been demonstrated to be low normal or below normal in dialysis patients as compared with healthy controls. The reasons for decreased levels of antioxidants in patients with renal disease are multifactorial: increased consumption resulting from increased burden of ROS, relative deficiency of vitamin C and vitamin E (possibly related to a decreased intake and dietary restriction of fresh fruits and vegetables to avoid hyperkalemia), and the excessive losses of nutrients of different molecular weights with dialysis (39,40).

It is also possible that uremic toxins that persist despite an adequate dialysis dose may cause functional deficiency of these physiologic antioxidants. Hypoalbuminemia is often present in dialysis-dependent patients and results in decreased antioxidant stores in blood (41).

High doses of oral vitamin E at 800 U per day (SPACE trial) (42) and the use of vitamin E-modified dialysis membranes has been shown to decrease the degree of oxidant stress, perhaps by replenishing the antioxidant factors (43).

BIOMARKERS OF OXIDATIVE STRESS

Because ROS have a very short half-life, their in vivo presence is extremely transient. Therefore, to understand the consequences of the presence of excessive amounts of ROS, one has to study the downstream effects of excessive ROS, called "footprints" of increased oxidative stress. Wolff and Dean (1987) introduced the concept of the Maillard reaction to describe the role of reducing sugars as catalysts in the oxidative modification and cross-linking of proteins, defined as reactive carbonyls (RCO): autoxidative glycosylation leading to production of reactive dicarbonyls such as methylglyoxal, 3-deoxyglucosone and glyoxal. These Schiff bases undergo spontaneous rearrangements (Amadori products) resulting in the formation of advanced glycation end products (AGEs) (2).

ADVANCED GLYCATION END PRODUCTS (AGEs)

Baynes et al. (44) demonstrated almost a decade ago that hyperglycemia is associated with increased production of ROS resulting in the modification of long-lived extracellular proteins such as collagen, elastin, laminin, and myelin sheath proteins. This is associated with structural changes in tissues rich in these proteins (lens, vascular wall, basement membranes) resulting in the development of complications associated with diabetes mellitus. Similar changes in collagen, elastin, and basement membranes, both physical and chemical, develop gradually during the process of normal aging, and these processes appear to be accelerated in diabetes (45) and chronic renal failure (CRF), depending on the severity and duration of disease. However, increased levels of fructosamine (a marker of hyperglycemia) have not been demonstrated in aging and nondiabetic renal failure. This supports the hypothesis that increased AGE in aging and renal failure are not due to glycemic stress but related to increased levels of oxidant stress (46).

Three different carbohydrate-derived oxidation products are identified as N^ε-(carboxymethyl)lysine (CML), N^ε-(carboxymethyl)hydroxylysine (CMhL), and pentosidine (47). Intravenous administration to animals of experimentally prepared AGE-modified albumin or enzymatically prepared AGE-peptides results in widespread vascular leakage, increased macrophage chemotactic activity, impaired NO-induced vasodilatation, and glomerulosclerosis (48,49).

Sell and Monnier (50) reported increased tissue levels of the AGE-specific moiety pentosidine in collagen tissues of patients with end-stage renal disease (ESRD) and aging patients. Makita et al. (51) with the use of radioreceptor assays demonstrated significantly higher levels of AGEs in medium-sized arteries of diabetics and nondiabetics. Diabetics with ESRD had twice the levels of tissue AGEs as compared with diabetic patients without renal failure. Dialysis-dependent diabetic patients had mean AGE levels five times higher than those diabetics without renal

failure. Although serum creatinine decreased by 75% with each dialysis session, AGE levels decreased by less than 25%. Successful kidney transplantation, however, is associated with a decrease in the plasma levels of AGEs commensurate with the decrease in creatinine, but levels of AGEs remain higher than in healthy controls.

Different sizes of AGEs have been noted in the blood of diabetic and uremic patients: those with AGEs less than 10 kDa versus greater than 10 kDa. Makita et al. measured peptide-linked degradation products of AGEs, labeled as low molecular weight AGE-modified molecules (LMW-AGEs), with a molecular weight of 2,000 to 6,000. Serum levels of LMW-AGE remain five- to sixfold higher in patients undergoing dialysis therapy with cuprophane or high flux membranes and in PD patients than in healthy controls (52).

The use of high-flux membranes was associated with at least a 50% decrease in LMW-AGE in both diabetic and nondiabetic dialysis patients. However, these levels returned to baseline values within the first 4 hours at the end of dialysis. In vitro experiments demonstrated that LMW-AGEs retain strong chemical activity against tissue collagen and vascular endothelium; this interaction was abrogated with the use of inhibitors of AGE-cross-linking, such as aminoguanidine. These results suggest that LMW-AGEs are refractory to removal by current modes of dialysis therapy and may be a component of the "middle molecule" uremic toxin (53).

ADVANCED LIPID PEROXIDATION (ALEs)

Nonenzymatic oxidation of polyunsaturated fatty acids either in the plasma or cell membranes by H_2O_2 and HOCl results in the formation of lipid hydroperoxides and reactive aldehydes (54,55). These lipid hydroperoxides and reactive aldehydes are unstable and undergo spontaneous rearrangements or break down into different smaller and stable compounds such as malondialdehyde (MDA), 4-hydroxynonenal, glyoxal, and acrolein (55).

Isoprostanes (8-iso-PGF2α) are generated by peroxidation of arachidonic acid of cell membrane lipids. The peroxidation occurs in situ in membrane phospholipids; these are then cleaved by endogenous phospholipases and circulate as isoprostanes. These new classes of oxidative stress byproducts are strong vasoconstrictors (56). Elevated levels of urinary isoprostanes decrease with antioxidant treatment in healthy volunteers (57).

Serum MDA is the breakdown product of oxidized polyunsaturated fatty acids such as linoleic acid and linolenic acid. Diaz et al. (58) validated the methods of measuring plasma MDA as an indirect marker of cumulative end-product of lipid peroxidation in plasma and RBCs. Toborek et al. (59) demonstrated increased lipid peroxidation and decreased levels of SOD after each session of hemodialysis. Zima et al. (60) measured thiobarbituric acid reactive substances (TBRS) by spectroscopy as an indirect marker of MDA and found that hemodialysis is associated with intensification of lipid peroxidation. Boaz et al. (61) found that patients with highest levels of posthemodialysis MDA were almost four times more likely to have accelerated atherosclerosis.

ADVANCED OXIDIZED PROTEIN PRODUCTS (AOPPs)

ROS can alter the primary, secondary, or tertiary structure of proteins resulting initially in denaturation and fragmentation and finally cross-linking (12). Such cross-linked proteins are less susceptible to proteolytic digestion, resulting in long-term accumulation (12). Witko-Sarsat et al. (62) developed a novel spectrophotometric assay for the detection of oxidatively modified proteins called AOPP. The plasma levels of AOPP were significantly increased in patients on dialysis (hemodialysis or PD), and in patients with advanced renal failure but not on dialysis when compared with healthy controls.

The plasma levels of AOPP in dialysis patients correlated well with increased levels of methylgaunidine (a marker of oxidant-induced protein cross-linking and aggregation), TBARS and pentosidine as markers of ALE and AGE, respectively. Similarly, the levels of AOPP were closely related to soluble markers of monocyte activation such as neopterin and TNF-α (63).

In vitro exposure of control plasma samples and human serum albumin (HSA) to HOCl (a strong oxidizing agent) results in the dose-dependent formation of AOPP. In vitro exposure of HSA-AOPP aggregate is capable of triggering the respiratory burst of isolated neutrophils in a dose-dependent manner. In view of these findings, it is postulated that neutrophils generate HOCl leading to the formation of AOPP, and these molecules will in turn stimulate phagocytes and release more HOCl (62). The molecular mechanisms that allow AOPP to stimulate monocytes may be dependent on ligand-receptor type interaction. These in vitro experiments demonstrate that AOPPs per se can perpetuate the oxidative stress (63).

CONSEQUENCES OF INCREASED OXIDATIVE STRESS

Increased markers of oxidant stress (especially in patients with diabetes mellitus) correlate with the severity of diabetic complications. In patients with renal failure, oxidant stress-related processes are more diverse and intense, with an attendant alteration of a variety of cellular components irrespective of the level of blood glucose. These oxidized products play a prominent role in a variety of complications and may contribute a significant degree of morbidity and mortality in dialysis patients (Figs. 20.3 and 20.4).

OXIDANT STRESS AND ACCELERATED ATHEROSCLEROSIS

Patients with CRF and patients on long-term dialysis are characterized by a vasculopathic state because about 50% patients die of cardiovascular disease (see Chapter 18). This vasculopathic state is not completely explained by the presence of traditional risk factors for the development of atherosclerosis (64,65). Increased production of ROS can potentiate the atherosclerotic process by several different mechanisms, such as increased production of oxidized low density lipoprotein (LDL) and ROS-associated endothelial dysfunction.

Minor modifications in the lipid or protein components of LDL prevent its uptake by the LDL-receptor pathways. LDL is susceptible to modifications in dialysis patients by different pathways such as oxidation as a result of increased generation of ROS or modifications by increased levels of AGE, ALE (MDA), and AOPP (66).

Perhaps the most common modification is the oxidation of LDL, resulting in the formation of ox-LDL. As LDL becomes oxidized, the lipoprotein loses its ability to be recognized by the LDL receptor, and it becomes easily available to be phagocytosed by other scavenger cells such as macrophages. The macrophages become lipid loaded with decreased degradation and decreased mobility, and these changes result in the conversion of such macrophages into foam cells. The accumulation of foam cells in the intima of blood vessels is an initial step in the development of the fatty streak of the atherosclerotic lesion. Steinberg and others demonstrated the role of early fatty streak (the precursor lesion) that subsequently leads to the development of an intermediate lesion and finally the complicated lesion of atherosclerotic plaques (67,68).

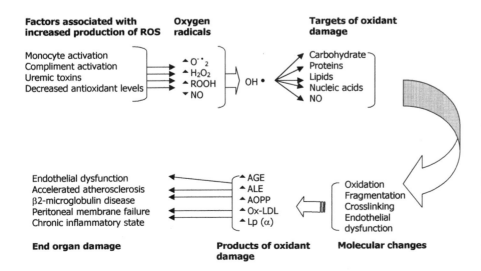

FIG. 20.3. General pathway by which increased production of reactive oxygen species may contribute to the development of complications in patients with end-stage renal disease. Intermediate oxygen radicals such as a (O·⁻₂) superoxide, (H₂O₂) hydrogen peroxide, and (ROOH) lipid peroxides are precursors to toxic reactive species, such as (OH•) hydroxyl radicals. These radicals can cause chemical modifications of biologic molecules. These include advanced glycation end products (AGEs), advanced lipid oxidation products (ALEs), advanced oxidized protein products (AOPPs), oxidized low-density lipoprotein LDL (ox-LDL), and increased lipoprotein (a) with decreased availability of nitric oxide.

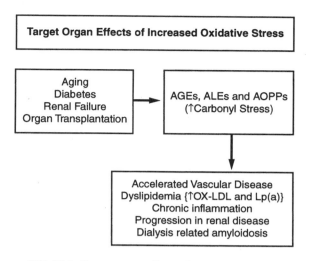

Target Organ Effects of Increased Oxidative Stress

Aging
Diabetes
Renal Failure
Organ Transplantation

→

AGEs, ALEs and AOPPs
(↑Carbonyl Stress)

↓

Accelerated Vascular Disease
Dyslipidemia {↑OX-LDL and Lp(a)}
Chronic inflammation
Progression in renal disease
Dialysis related amyloidosis

FIG. 20.4. Target organ effects of increased oxidative stress.

Increased levels of autoantibodies against the epitopes of ox-LDL and MDA-LDL have been demonstrated in the atherosclerotic plaques of coronary arteries and in the blood of dialysis patients with and without coronary artery disease. Several longitudinal studies in subjects with normal renal function have shown that the titers of circulating antibodies against ox-LDL are independent cardiovascular risk factors for progression in atherosclerosis (69). Maggi et al. (70) showed that LDL from uremic and dialysis-dependent patients is easily susceptible to in vitro oxidation. Increased ratio of plasma antioxidized LDL antibodies to anti-native LDL was present in patients with advanced uremia and in patients on maintenance dialysis compared with healthy controls (Fig. 20.4).

Treatment with an antioxidant drug such as probucol without lipid lowering potential has been reported to reduce the extent and the progression of atherosclerotic lesions in Watanabe heritable hyperlipidemic rabbits (WHHL) (71). Based on these data it is reasonable to speculate that, in addition to the usual lipid abnormalities, enhanced in vivo LDL oxidation seen in dialysis patients plays an important role in the process of accelerated atherosclerosis. Therefore, pharmacologic interventions that can decrease LDL oxidation should provide an important tool to ameliorate the accelerated progression in atherosclerosis in dialysis-dependent patients.

Recent introduction of vitamin E-bonded dialysis membranes may have the potential to reduce the overall oxidant stress, decrease lipid peroxidation, and LDL oxidation by providing site-specific high-dose vitamin E to prevent the release of ROS in the extracorporeal circulation (72).

ROLE OF ROS IN THE PATHOGENESIS OF β_2-MICROGLOBULIN (β_2-M) DISEASE (SEE CHAPTER 23)

Progression in renal failure and subsequently the need for dialysis is associated with accumulation of middle molecular weight proteins (11.8 kD) called β_2-M (levels in dialysis patients are usually 30-fold higher than normal healthy controls) (73,74).

Gejyo et al. (73,75) described increased serum levels of β_2-M in patients on maintenance hemodialysis that did not correlate with the joint or bone disease as seen in dialysis-related amyloidosis (DRA). This questioned the concept of simple deposition disease of dialysis amyloidosis. It is postulated that unknown amyloid-enhancing factors result in the qualitative or conformational changes in the β_2-molecule that plays an important role in the pathogenesis of amyloid disease. Subsequently, Miyata et al. (76) demonstrated that β_2-M produces tissue injury after it is modified by products of oxidant stress such as AGE, ALE, or AOPP.

AGE-modified β_2-M stimulates monocyte-macrophage cells, releases cytokines TNF-α and IL-1β and induces collagenase gene expression in rabbit synovial cells (77). In addition β_2-M increases the expression of IL-8 and profibrogenic cytokine TGF-β (78) with increased recruitment of polymorphonuclear neutrophils (PMNs) (79) and increased expression of fibroblasts in the synovial membranes of DRA-affected joints. These markers of neutrophil activation and tissue damage were absent in the presence of β_2-M deposition but without accompanying joint damage.

Further insights about the AGE and ALE modification of β_2-M were demonstrated by the use of anti-AGE monoclonal antibodies for the epitopes of imidazoline and N$^\varepsilon$-carboxymethyl-lysine adducts of β_2-M in the synovial tissues of patients with dialysis-related arthropathy along with increased serum levels of both imidazolone and CML-modified β_2-M (76).

These studies support the evidence that excessive generation of ROS in dialysis patients results in β_2-M modification by AGEs, AOPPs, and ALEs; such a modification could be an important factor in the pathogenesis of tissue injury at the site of deposition of β_2-M and subsequent development of DRA (77). The combined use of hemoperfusion and hemodialysis devices are being developed to increase the rate of removal of β_2-M and to prevent the development of DRA (80). The use of adsorbent columns to increase the removal of β_2-M is being evaluated in a multicenter trial by the National Institutes of Health (NIH).

ROS AND THEIR ROLE IN PERITONEAL MEMBRANE FAILURE IN PERITONEAL DIALYSIS PATIENTS

Progressive loss of ultrafiltration is the most common cause of the PD failure. The morphologic changes associated with ultrafiltration failure include mesothelial denudation, interstitial fibrosis, and increase in extracellular matrix proteins; the end result is peritoneal membrane thickening (81). Electron microscopy reveals a characteristic replication of the basement membrane of the peritoneal capillaries and hyalinization of vascular media. These structural changes are well described in diabetic nephropathy (82). AGEs and pentosidine have been demonstrated in the peritoneal tissues and peritoneal blood vessel walls. Increased levels of AGEs and pentosidine have been correlated with the degree of peritoneal fibrosis and have been linked to the cumulative peritoneal glucose load (83,84).

Whether the use of low glucose or nonglucose dialysate solutions will prevent the production of local AGEs remains to be studied and could provide new therapeutic strategies for the preservation of peritoneal function in long-term continuous ambulatory peritoneal dialysis (CAPD) patients.

ROS AND THEIR ROLE IN THE PATHOGENESIS OF INFLAMMATION AND CARDIOVASCULAR DISEASE

There is growing evidence that strongly suggests a link between increased oxidant stress, inflammation, and endothelial dysfunction. Several observational studies have demonstrated increased levels of markers of chronic microinflammatory state in patients with renal failure and on dialysis. The production of increased amounts of ROS with accumulation of the products of glycation, lipid peroxidation, and protein adducts could play a significant role in the initiation and progression of the chronic inflammatory state.

It has been demonstrated that AGEs can react with corresponding receptors called receptors for AGE (RAGE) (85) and other scavenger receptors on macrophages, vascular endothelial cells, and smooth muscle cells. Such a receptor/ligand interaction leads to the activation of endothelial cells and release of vascular cell adhesion molecules (VCAM-1) and further attracts monocytes to the vessel wall (86). AGE interaction with binding sites on monocyte-macrophages activates a host of intracellular signaling pathways. Activation of these signaling pathways results in the release of IL-1β, IL-6, TNFα, and stimulation of NADPH oxidases with release of superoxide (O_2^-), thus aggravating the already existent oxidative state (87).

IL-6 is one of the mediators of increased production of acute phase proteins of acute inflammatory response. IL-6 acts directly on the hepatocytes and increases the synthesis of C-reactive protein (CRP), fibrinogen, and serum amyloid A (88,89). Whether AGE can act directly on the hepatocytes and increase the synthesis and/or release of CRP remains to be determined.

Increased levels of CRP and other acute-phase proteins in apparently healthy people (90) and in dialysis patients have been demonstrated to be the potential markers of predicting cardiovascular and overall mortality independent of other well-defined risk factors for cardiovascular disease (91).

ENDOTHELIAL DYSFUNCTION

CRF has been associated with impaired NO bioavailability and endothelial dysfunction in the absence of other associated risk factors, even in children with renal failure. The reduced NO bioavailability in renal failure and in dialysis patients is perhaps multifactorial such as decreased NO production (92), increased NO degradation, or both. Also decreased NO production could be related to low levels of NO synthase (NOS) activity, which in turn can be the result of a decreased clearance of the endogenous NOS inhibitor such as asymmetric dimethylarginine (ADMA) by dialysis (93,94) or decreased bioavailability of the NOS substrate L-arginine because of poor intake, accompa-

nying malnutrition or increased losses via dialysis. However, the important mechanism involved with NO dysfunction is the ability of the AGEs to quench NO resulting in vasomotor dysfunction in the absence of underlying atherosclerosis (95). The use of vitamin E-bonded dialyzers have been demonstrated to reduce the level of oxidant stress and to improve the endothelial function (96).

The combination of increased production of ox-LDL, decreased availability of endogenous NO, and increased levels of CRP could be hypothesized as important elements of nontraditional risk factors, thus establishing the link between traditional and nontraditional risk factors for the development of accelerated atherosclerosis in dialysis-dependent patients.

CAN DIALYSIS-ASSOCIATED INCREASED OXIDATIVE STRESS BE PREVENTED?

Therapeutic approaches to prevent or to decrease the oxidant stress are aimed at minimizing inflammatory cell activation, removing inflammatory cytokines or mediators, maintaining host antioxidant defenses, and using strategies to adsorb or to chelate the ROS.

Minimizing Inflammatory Cell Activation and Release of ROS

The use of biocompatible membranes (to some extent) prevents complement activation, neutrophil sequestration and activation (24), although it does not completely abrogate the production of ROS. Hence ROS continue to have a significant effect on the generation and maintenance of oxidative stress and lipid peroxidation as measured by serum levels of MDA and ox-LDL (97).

Other investigators have demonstrated that use of ultrapure water and sterile dialysate (98) could possibly decrease the inflammatory responses. These steps (combined use of biocompatible membranes, ultrapure water, and sterile dialysate) can decrease the production of ROS and also abolish the inflammatory responses.

Measures to Improve the Removal of Inflammatory Cytokines

Hemolipodialysis (HLD) improves oxidant stress by decreasing inflammatory cell activation, removing inflammatory mediators, and maintaining antioxidant levels (99). HLD uses liposomes with vitamin E added in the liposomal bilayer and vitamin C added directly in the dialysate. Liposomes have a high affinity for proteins, drugs, and cytokines. Use of liposomes can increase the removal of inflammatory mediators, whereas vitamin E in the liposomal bilayer and vitamin C in the dialysate will act synergistically to replenish the antioxidant levels ordinarily lost via diffusion during dialysis (100).

Role of Vitamin E-modified Hemodialysis Filters

Improved bioreactivity and biocompatibility of vitamin E-modified multilayer hemodialysis filters can reduce the production of

TABLE 20.1. EFFECT OF VITAMIN E-MODIFIED DIALYSIS MEMBRANE ON OXIDIZED LOW DENSITY LIPOPROTEIN (OX-LDL) AND MALODIALDEHYDE (MDA) LEVELS AFTER 9 MONTHS OF TREATMENT

	Oxidized LDL ng/ μg LDL Protein	MDA nmol/ mg LDL Protein
Normal range	0.257 ± 0.132	1.9 ± 0.5
Hemodialysis group		
Month		
0	1.653 ± 0.76	4.329 ± 0.955
1	1.623 ± 0.966	4.091 ± 0.891
3	1.592 ± 1.064	3.997 ± 1.045
6	1.406 ± 0.568	3.656 ± 0.788
9	1.357 ± 0.852	3.459 ± 0.658[a]

Results are expressed as mean ± SD. Plasma oxidized LDL and MDA levels were significantly higher in hemodialysis (HD) patients compared to controls. These values slowly decreased and were significantly lower after 9 months of treatment using vitamin E-modified dialyzer.
[a]$p <0.05$ vs. 0 month (prior to using the vitamin E-modified dialyzer). Modified from Shimazu T, et al. Antioxidant effects of the vitamin E-modified dialyzer, *Kidney Int* 2001;59:S137–S143, with permission.

ROS. Galli et al. showed that vitamin E-modified hemodialysis filters (CL-E) as compared with cuproammonium rayon (CL-S) filters provides site-specific and time-dependent protection against ROS at the site of their generation by activated PMNs in the extracorporeal circulation. Such membranes have the potential to replenish antioxidant stores in plasma and RBCs, significantly inhibit the leukocyte respiratory burst and ROS production (72,101).

Vitamin E-coated membrane filters have been shown to prevent dialysis-induced endothelial dysfunction by maintaining the bioreactivity of endothelium-derived NO and also decreasing the levels of ox-LDL as compared with dialysis treatment with cellulose or other synthetic membranes (96). Hemodialysis using vitamin E-modified membranes has also been shown to increase plasma and erythrocyte vitamin E content, increase plasma levels of reduced glutathione, improve leukocyte function, and decrease mononuclear cell apoptosis and complement activation (102) (Table 20.1).

Taken together, these recent studies show that vitamin E-modified dialysis membranes can reduce the release of ROS and could reduce the oxidant stress. Prospective randomized studies to compare the patient outcomes with new techniques of dialysis like HLD, high-flux polysulfones, and vitamin E-modified filters are clearly needed.

Restoring the Host Antioxidant Defenses

Role of Vitamin E and Vitamin C Supplements

Several observational and epidemiologic studies in the general population have demonstrated conflicting evidence about the efficacy of various antioxidants such as vitamins A, E, and C and beta-carotene in reducing the incidence of secondary cardiovascular outcomes or death from any cause (103,104). The secondary Prevention with Antioxidants of Cardiovascular Disease (SPACE) trial used vitamin E 800 IU (as naturally occurring α-tocopherol) and demonstrated significantly lower primary and

secondary cardiovascular events in the treatment group as compared with the placebo group (42). However, the results of this study have not been reproduced to date.

Use of Angiotensin-Converting Enzyme Inhibitors

The use of angiotensin-converting enzyme inhibitors is associated with decreased incidence of cardiovascular events in high-risk populations, and this effect is remarkable even without significant changes in blood pressure (HOPE study).

De Cavanagh et al. (105) and Boaz et al. (61) demonstrated that treatment of dialysis patients with enalapril at 10 mg per day for 6 months resulted in higher levels of antioxidants and reduced levels of ROS. Therefore, enalapril treatment may have the potential of enhancing the endogenous antioxidant defenses and, hence, protect the cells from the oxidant-related injury.

Value and Efficacy of Chelators of ROS

Use of BetaSorb in Dialysis

BetaSorb hemodialysis is an accessory device for hemodialysis, placed upstream from the dialyzer in the hemodialysis circuit. Its intended use is to improve the removal of middle molecular weight uremic toxins like β_2-M, ROS, and proinflammatory cytokines such as complement factors, TNF-α, IL-1, and interleukin-8 (106,107). Hence, BetaSorb polymers remove size-selective toxins by adsorption. The BetaSorb device has been approved for human clinical testing by the Food and Drug Administration (FDA), and clinical trials are underway to assess the efficacy of BetaSorb devices to remove β_2-M in hemodialysis patients using the combination of high-flux dialyzer and BetaSorb as compared with the use of high-flux membrane dialyzers.

Use of Compounds that Inhibit the Action of ROS, AGE, and ALE

Aminoguanidine (AGN) and second-generation AGN-like compounds [± 2-isopropylictenehydrazono-4-oxo-thiazolindin-5 acetanilide (OPB-9195)] are small nucleophilic compounds that inhibit the formation of AGEs and also inhibit the action of ROS at the molecular level. Both AGN and OPB-9195 inhibit glycoxidation and lipidoxidation reactions at the cellular level, thereby preventing the formation of AGE, ALE, and AOPP (108). These agents prevent diabetes-induced glycation protein cross-linking in blood vessels and, hence, decrease the rate of atherosclerosis. These substances have been shown to decrease the levels of AGEs in PD fluid and in the blood of rodents with diabetes mellitus (109). After balloon dilatation of carotid arteries (which results in the local accumulation of AGEs, ALEs, and neointimal proliferation), all these metabolites were significantly reduced by oral administration of OPB-9195 (108,109).

However, the development of less toxic and more specific inhibitors of glycoxidation and lipidoxidation (that are effective not only in decreasing the production of such products but also in protecting the tissues from their toxic effects after their generation) is urgently needed.

SUMMARY

Patients with chronic kidney disease receiving different types of dialysis are at risk for increased oxidative stress as measured by the biomarkers of oxidant stress such as ROS, AGEs, ALEs, AOPP, and ox-LDL. Increased oxidative stress may contribute directly or indirectly in the pathogenesis of accelerated atherosclerosis, the chronic inflammatory state, and the development of DRA. In light of these findings, clinical trials are needed to assess the efficacy and safety of different interventions that can abrogate the production of ROS and/or restore the function of antioxidants in the early stages of development of renal failure and after the initiation of dialysis therapy. Similarly, dialysis modalities using high-flux polysulfones in combination with other evolving modalities of dialysis, such as the use of BetaSorb cartridges or vitamin E-modified hemodialysis filters, can be used to reduce the burden of oxidative stress and, hopefully, the associated complications in dialysis patients and those with chronic kidney disease.

REFERENCES

1. Halliwell B, et al. Free radicals, antioxidants, and human disease: where are we now? *J Lab Clin Med* 1992;119:598–620.
2. Brownlee M, et al. Advanced glycosylation end products in tissue and the biochemical basis of diabetic complications. *N Engl J Med* 1988; 318:1315–1321.
3. Cross CE, et al. Oxygen radicals and human disease. *Ann Intern Med* 1987;107:526–545.
4. Malech HL, et al. Current concepts: immunology—neutrophils in human diseases. *N Engl J Med* 1987;317:687–694.
5. Weiss SJ, et al. Long-lived oxidants generated by human neutrophils: characterization and bioactivity. *Science* 1983;222:625–628.
6. Weiss SJ. Tissue destruction by neutrophils. *N Engl J Med* 1989;320:365–376.
7. Nemoto S, et al. Role for mitochondrial oxidants as regulators of cellular metabolism. *Mol Cell Biol* 2000;20:7311–7318.
8. Britigan BE, et al. Hydroxyl radical formation in neutrophils. *N Engl J Med* 1988;318:858–859.
9. Radi R, et al. Peroxynitrite-induced membrane lipid peroxidation: the cytotoxic potential of superoxide and nitric oxide. *Arch Biochem Biophys* 1991;288:481–487.
10. Nathan C. Nitric oxide as a secretory product of mammalian cells. *FASEB J* 1992;6:3051–3064.
11. Morrow JD, et al. Free radical-induced generation of isoprostanes in vivo: evidence for the formation of D-ring and E-ring isoprostanes. *J Biol Chem* 1994;269:4317–4326.
12. Dean RT, et al. Biochemistry and pathology of radical-mediated protein oxidation. *Biochem J* 1997;324:1–18.
13. Davies KJ, et al. Protein damage and degradation by oxygen radicals. IV. Degradation of denatured protein. *J Biol Chem* 1987;262:9914–9920.
14. Peuchant E, et al. Lipoperoxidation in plasma and red blood cells of patients undergoing haemodialysis: vitamins A, E, and iron status. *Free Radic Biol Med* 1994;16:339–346.
15. Imlay JA, et al. DNA damage and oxygen radical toxicity. *Science* 1988;240:1302–1309.
16. Imlay JA, et al. Toxic DNA damage by hydrogen peroxide through the Fenton reaction in vivo and in vitro. *Science* 1988;240:640–642.
17. Gosslau A, et al. [Oxidative stress, age-related cell damage and antioxidative mechanisms.] *Z Gerontol Geriatr* 2002;35:139–150.
18. Fang X, et al. Overexpression of human superoxide dismutase inhibits oxidation of low- density lipoprotein by endothelial cells. *Circ Res* 1998;82:1289–1297.
19. Ingold KU, et al. Vitamin E remains the major lipid-soluble, chain-breaking antioxidant in human plasma even in individuals suffering severe vitamin E deficiency. *Arch Biochem Biophys* 1987;259:224–225.
20. Frei B, et al. Ascorbate is an outstanding antioxidant in human blood plasma. *Proc Natl Acad Sci U S A* 1989;86:6377–6381.
21. Levine M, et al. Does vitamin C have a pro-oxidant effect? *Nature* 1998;395:231, discussion 232.
22. Halliwell B, et al. The antioxidants of human extracellular fluids. *Arch Biochem Biophys* 1990;280:1–8.
23. Henson PM, et al. Tissue injury in inflammation: oxidants, proteinases, and cationic proteins. *J Clin Invest* 1987;79:669–674.
24. Himmelfarb J, et al. Intradialytic granulocyte reactive oxygen species production: a prospective, crossover trial. *J Am Soc Nephrol* 1993;4:178–186.
25. Griendling KK, et al. NAD(P)H oxidase: role in cardiovascular biology and disease. *Circ Res* 2000;86:494–501.
26. Himmelfarb J, et al. Reactive oxygen species production by monocytes and polymorphonuclear leukocytes during dialysis. *Am J Kidney Dis* 1991;17:271–276.
27. Descamps-Latscha B, et al. Establishing the relationship between complement activation and stimulation of phagocyte oxidative metabolism in hemodialyzed patients: a randomized prospective study. *Nephron* 1991;59:279–285.
28. Vanholder R, et al. Phagocytosis in uremic and hemodialysis patients: a prospective and cross sectional study. *Kidney Int* 1991;39:320–327.
29. Tepel M, et al. Increased intracellular reactive oxygen species in patients with end- stage renal failure: effect of hemodialysis. *Kidney Int* 2000;58:867–872.
30. Roselaar SE, et al. Detection of oxidants in uremic plasma by electron spin resonance spectroscopy. *Kidney Int* 1995;48:199–206.
31. Tarng DC, et al. 8-hydroxy-2′-deoxyguanosine of leukocyte DNA as a marker of oxidative stress in chronic hemodialysis patients. *Am J Kidney Dis* 2000;36:934–944.
32. Markert M, et al. Dialyzed polymorphonuclear neutrophil oxidative metabolism during dialysis: a comparative study with 5 new and reused membranes. *Clin Nephrol* 1988;29:129–136.
33. Pereira BJ, et al. Cytokine production during in vitro hemodialysis with new and formaldehyde- or Renalin-reprocessed cellulose dialyzers. *J Am Soc Nephrol* 1995;6:1304–1308.
34. Pereira BJ, et al. Diffusive and convective transfer of cytokine-inducing bacterial products across hemodialysis membranes. *Kidney Int* 1995;47:603–610.
35. Panichi V, et al. Cytokine production in haemodiafiltration: a multicentre study. *Nephrol Dial Transplant* 1998;13:1737–1744.
36. Sundaram S, et al. Transmembrane passage of cytokine-inducing bacterial products across new and reprocessed polysulfone dialyzers. *J Am Soc Nephrol* 1996;7:2183–2191.
37. Ross EA, et al. Low whole blood and erythrocyte levels of glutathione in hemodialysis and peritoneal dialysis patients. *Am J Kidney Dis* 1997;30:489–494.
38. Mimic-Oka J, et al. Alteration in plasma antioxidant capacity in various degrees of chronic renal failure. *Clin Nephrol* 1999;51:233–241.
39. Lim VS, et al. The effect of hemodialysis on protein metabolism: a leucine kinetic study. *J Clin Invest* 1993;91:2429–2436.
40. Ikizler TA, et al. Amino acid and albumin losses during hemodialysis. *Kidney Int* 1994;46:830–837.
41. Stenvinkel P, et al. Strong association between malnutrition, inflammation, and atherosclerosis in chronic renal failure. *Kidney Int* 1999;55:1899–1911.
42. Boaz M, et al. Secondary prevention with antioxidants of cardiovascular disease in endstage renal disease (SPACE): randomised placebo-controlled trial. *Lancet* 2000;356:1213–1218.
43. Galli F, et al. Bioreactivity and biocompatibility of a vitamin E-modified multi-layer hemodialysis filter. *Kidney Int* 1998;54:580–589.

44. Baynes JW, et al. The Amadori product on protein: structure and reactions. *Prog Clin Biol Res* 1989;304:43–67.

45. Baynes JW. Role of oxidative stress in development of complications in diabetes. *Diabetes* 1991;40:405–412.

46. Miyata T, et al. Autoxidation products of both carbohydrates and lipids are increased in uremic plasma: is there oxidative stress in uremia? *Kidney Int* 1998;54:1290–1295.

47. Miyata T, et al. Alterations in nonenzymatic biochemistry in uremia: origin and significance of "carbonyl stress" in long-term uremic complications. *Kidney Int* 1999;55:389–399.

48. Vlassara H, et al. Exogenous advanced glycosylation end products induce complex vascular dysfunction in normal animals: a model for diabetic and aging complications. *Proc Natl Acad Sci U S A* 1992;89:12043–12047.

49. Fu MX, et al. Role of oxygen in cross-linking and chemical modification of collagen by glucose. *Diabetes* 1992;41[Suppl 2]:42–48.

50. Sell DR, et al. End-stage renal disease and diabetes catalyze the formation of a pentose-derived crosslink from aging human collagen. *J Clin Invest* 1990;85:380–384.

51. Makita Z, et al. Advanced glycosylation end products in patients with diabetic nephropathy. *N Engl J Med* 1991;325:836–842.

52. Miyata T, et al. Clearance of pentosidine, an advanced glycation end product, by different modalities of renal replacement therapy. *Kidney Int* 1997;51:880–887.

53. Miyata T, et al. Advanced glycation and lipidoxidation of the peritoneal membrane: respective roles of serum and peritoneal fluid reactive carbonyl compounds. *Kidney Int* 2000;58:425–435.

54. Stocker R. Lipoprotein oxidation: mechanistic aspects, methodological approaches and clinical relevance. *Curr Opin Lipidol* 1994;5:422–433.

55. Esterbauer H, et al. Chemistry and biochemistry of 4-hydroxynonenal, malonaldehyde and related aldehydes. *Free Radic Biol Med* 1991;11:81–128.

56. Morrow JD, et al. Non-cyclooxygenase-derived prostanoids (F2-isoprostanes) are formed in situ on phospholipids. *Proc Natl Acad Sci U S A* 1992;89:10721–10725.

57. Meagher EA, et al. Effects of vitamin E on lipid peroxidation in healthy persons. *JAMA* 2001;285:1178–1182.

58. Diaz J, et al. Reference intervals for four biochemistry analytes in plasma for evaluating oxidative stress and lipid peroxidation in human plasma. *Clin Chem* 1998;44:2215–2217.

59. Toborek M, et al. Effect of hemodialysis on lipid peroxidation and antioxidant system in patients with chronic renal failure. *Metabolism* 1992;41:1229–1232.

60. Zima T, et al. Lipid peroxidation on dialysis membranes. *Biochem Mol Biol Int* 1993;29:531–537.

61. Boaz M, et al. Serum malondialdehyde and prevalent cardiovascular disease in hemodialysis. *Kidney Int* 1999;56:1078–1083.

62. Witko-Sarsat V, et al. Advanced oxidation protein products as novel mediators of inflammation and monocyte activation in chronic renal failure. *J Immunol* 1998;161:2524–2532.

63. Descamps-Latscha B, et al. Importance of oxidatively modified proteins in chronic renal failure. *Kidney Int* 2001;59[Suppl 78]:S108–S113.

64. London GM, et al. Atherosclerosis and arteriosclerosis in chronic renal failure. *Kidney Int* 1997;51:1678–1695.

65. Luke RG. Chronic renal failure—a vasculopathic state. *N Engl J Med* 1998;339:841–843.

66. Sutherland WH, et al. Oxidation of low density lipoproteins from patients with renal failure or renal transplants. *Kidney Int* 1995;48:227–236.

67. Steinberg D, et al. Beyond cholesterol. Modifications of low-density lipoprotein that increase its atherogenicity. *N Engl J Med* 1989;320:915–924.

68. Witztum JL, et al. Role of oxidized low density lipoprotein in atherogenesis. *J Clin Invest* 1991;88:1785–1792.

69. Salonen JT, et al. Autoantibody against oxidised LDL and progression of carotid atherosclerosis. *Lancet* 1992;339:883–887.

70. Maggi E, et al. Enhanced LDL oxidation in uremic patients: an additional mechanism for accelerated atherosclerosis? *Kidney Int* 1994;45:876–883.

71. Carew TE, et al. Antiatherogenic effect of probucol unrelated to its hypocholesterolemic effect: evidence that antioxidants in vivo can selectively inhibit low density lipoprotein degradation in macrophage-rich fatty streaks and slow the progression of atherosclerosis in the Watanabe heritable hyperlipidemic rabbit. *Proc Natl Acad Sci U S A* 1987;84:7725–7729.

72. Galli F, et al. Vitamin E, lipid profile, and peroxidation in hemodialysis patients. *Kidney Int* 2001;59[Suppl 78]:S148–S154.

73. Gejyo F, et al. Serum levels of beta 2-microglobulin as a new form of amyloid protein in patients undergoing long-term hemodialysis. *N Engl J Med* 1986;314:585–586.

74. Capeillere-Blandin C, et al. Structural modifications of human beta 2 microglobulin treated with oxygen-derived radicals. *Biochem J* 1991;277:175–182.

75. Gejyo F, et al. A new form of amyloid protein associated with chronic hemodialysis was identified as beta 2-microglobulin. *Biochem Biophys Res Commun* 1985;129:701–706.

76. Miyata T, et al. beta 2-Microglobulin modified with advanced glycation end products is a major component of hemodialysis-associated amyloidosis. *J Clin Invest* 1993;92:1243–1252.

77. Miyata T, et al. Involvement of beta 2-microglobulin modified with advanced glycation end products in the pathogenesis of hemodialysis-associated amyloidosis: induction of human monocyte chemotaxis and macrophage secretion of tumor necrosis factor-alpha and interleukin-1. *J Clin Invest* 1994;93:521–528.

78. Matsuo K, et al. Transforming growth factor-beta is involved in the pathogenesis of dialysis-related amyloidosis. *Kidney Int* 2000;57:697–708.

79. Takayama F, et al. Involvement of interleukin-8 in dialysis-related arthritis. *Kidney Int* 1998;53:1007–1013.

80. Schwalbe S, et al. Beta 2-microglobulin associated amyloidosis: a vanishing complication of long-term hemodialysis? *Kidney Int* 1997;52:1077–1083.

81. Churchill DN. Implications of the Canada-USA (CANUSA) study of the adequacy of dialysis on peritoneal dialysis schedule. *Nephrol Dial Transplant* 1998;13:158–163.

82. Dobbie JW, et al. Categorization of ultrastructural changes in peritoneal mesothelium, stroma and blood vessels in uremia and CAPD patients. *Adv Perit Dial* 1990;6:3–12.

83. Nakayama M, et al. Immunohistochemical detection of advanced glycosylation end-products in the peritoneum and its possible pathophysiological role in CAPD. *Kidney Int* 1997;51:182–186.

84. Honda K, et al. Accumulation of advanced glycation end products in the peritoneal vasculature of continuous ambulatory peritoneal dialysis patients with low ultra-filtration. *Nephrol Dial Transplant* 1999;14:1541–1549.

85. Neeper M, et al. Cloning and expression of a cell surface receptor for advanced glycosylation end products of proteins. *J Biol Chem* 1992;267:14998–15004.

86. Schmidt AM, et al. Advanced glycation endproducts interacting with their endothelial receptor induce expression of vascular cell adhesion molecule-1 (VCAM- 1) in cultured human endothelial cells and in mice: a potential mechanism for the accelerated vasculopathy of diabetes. *J Clin Invest* 1995;96:1395–1403.

87. Abo A, et al. Activation of the NADPH oxidase involves the small GTP-binding protein p21rac1. *Nature* 1991;353:668–670.

88. Herbelin A, et al. Elevated circulating levels of interleukin-6 in patients with chronic renal failure. *Kidney Int* 1991;39:954–960.

89. Herbelin A, et al. Influence of uremia and hemodialysis on circulating interleukin-1 and tumor necrosis factor alpha. *Kidney Int* 1990;37:116–125.

90. Ridker PM, et al. Inflammation, aspirin, and the risk of cardiovascular disease in apparently healthy men. *N Engl J Med* 1997;336:973–979.

91. Zimmermann J, et al. Inflammation enhances cardiovascular risk and mortality in hemodialysis patients. *Kidney Int* 1999;55:648–658.

92. Lau T, et al. Arginine, citrulline, and nitric oxide metabolism in end-stage renal disease patients. *J Clin Invest* 2000;105:1217–1225.

93. Vallance P, et al. Endogenous dimethylarginine as an inhibitor of nitric oxide synthesis. *J Cardiovasc Pharmacol* 1992;20:S60–S62.

94. Vallance P, et al. Accumulation of an endogenous inhibitor of nitric oxide synthesis in chronic renal failure. *Lancet* 1992;339:572–575.

95. Bucala R, et al. Advanced glycosylation products quench nitric oxide and mediate defective endothelium-dependent vasodilatation in experimental diabetes. *J Clin Invest* 1991;87:432–438.

96. Miyazaki H, et al. Hemodialysis impairs endothelial function via oxidative stress: effects of vitamin E-coated dialyzer. *Circulation* 2000; 101:1002–1006.

97. Panichi V, et al. The link of biocompatibility to cytokine production. *Kidney Int* 2000;[Suppl 76]:S96–S103.

98. Baz M, et al. Using ultrapure water in hemodialysis delays carpal tunnel syndrome. *Int J Artif Organs* 1991;14:681–685.

99. Wratten ML, et al. Haemolipodialysis. *Blood Purif* 1999;17:127–133.

100. Ziouzenkova O, et al. Oxidative stress during ex vivo hemodialysis of blood is decreased by a novel hemolipodialysis procedure utilizing antioxidants. *Free Radic Biol Med* 2002;33:248–258.

101. Mydlik M, et al. A modified dialyzer with vitamin E and antioxidant defense parameters. *Kidney Int* 2001;59[Suppl 78]:S144–S147.

102. Shimazu T, et al. Effects of a vitamin E-modified dialysis membrane on neutrophil superoxide anion radical production. *Kidney Int* 2001; 59[Suppl 78]:S137–S143.

103. Davey PJ, et al. Cost-effectiveness of vitamin E therapy in the treatment of patients with angiographically proven coronary narrowing (CHAOS trial). Cambridge Heart Antioxidant Study. *Am J Cardiol* 1998;82:414–417.

104. Virtamo J, et al. Effect of vitamin E and beta carotene on the incidence of primary nonfatal myocardial infarction and fatal coronary heart disease. *Arch Intern Med* 1998;158:668–675.

105. de Cavanagh EM, et al. Higher levels of antioxidant defenses in enalapril-treated versus non-enalapril-treated hemodialysis patients. *Am J Kidney Dis* 1999;34:445–455.

106. Tetta C, et al. Removal of cytokines and activated complement components in an experimental model of continuous plasma filtration coupled with sorbent adsorption. *Nephrol Dial Transplant* 1998;13: 1458–1464.

107. Dhondt A, et al. The removal of uremic toxins. *Kidney Int* 2000; [Suppl 76]:S47–S59.

108. Brownlee M, et al. Aminoguanidine prevents diabetes-induced arterial wall protein cross-linking. *Science* 1986;232:1629–1632.

109. Yamauchi A, et al. Effects of aminoguanidine on serum advanced glycation endproducts, urinary albumin excretion, mesangial expansion, and glomerular basement membrane thickening in Otsuka Long-Evans Tokushima fatty rats. *Diabetes Res Clin Pract* 1997;34: 127–133.

INFECTION AND IMMUNITY IN END-STAGE RENAL DISEASE

BÉATRICE DESCAMPS-LATSCHA, VÉRONIQUE WITKO-SARSAT, AND PAUL JUNGERS

Infection is still a major cause of morbidity and mortality in patients with end-stage renal disease (ESRD) treated with hemodialysis (HD) or peritoneal dialysis (PD). Infection is second only to cardiovascular disease as a cause of death in ESRD patients, although the proportion of deaths by infection among dialysis patients markedly decreased in recent years, going from more than 40% in the early 1970s (1) to about 15% in the 1990s in U.S. (2,3), European (4), and Japanese (5) centers.

This high susceptibility of ESRD patients reflects their state of immunodeficiency, which has been considered a hallmark of chronic uremia for many years. Indeed, almost 50 years ago, Dammin et al. (6) reported abnormally long survival of skin allografts in ESRD patients and first suggested that it was due to impaired immunity. Subsequently, profound alterations in both humoral and cellular immunity were described. Clinically, in addition to bacterial and viral infections, ESRD patients exhibit an abnormally high incidence of autoimmune diseases and neoplasia (7), show cutaneous anergy in delayed-type hypersensitivity reactions to common antigens (8), and respond poorly to vaccination implying T-cell dependent antigens, for example, influenza virus (9) and hepatitis B virus (HBV) (10,11).

Several hypotheses have been put forward to elucidate the mechanisms of such an immune system dysregulation in dialysis patients. A number of factors acting along both the humoral and the cellular axes of the immune system have been incriminated.

One puzzling observation, emerging in particular from studies by our group (reviewed in reference 12), is that clinical and biologic immune deficiency paradoxically coexists with activation of most immunocompetent cells. This state of activation also has its clinical impact in the most serious complications linked to long-term dialysis such as β_2-microglobulin amyloid arthropathy and atherosclerosis-related cardiovascular complications.

Another interesting observation was that the immune dysregulation is present in chronic renal failure (CRF) patients long before the start of dialysis therapy, which itself further triggers phagocytic cell activation inducing a chronic inflammation state dominated by oxidative stress and its related pathology (13). The dialysis procedure per se brings additional risk factors for inflammation such as bioincompatible membranes and impure dialysate. A syndrome whereby raised levels of proinflammatory cytokines [interleukin-1β (IL-1β), tumor necrosis factor-α (TNF-α), and interleukin-6 (IL-6)] are a common link between inflammation, malnutrition, and atherosclerosis has been recently identified by Stenvinkel et al. (14).

On the side of immunodeficiency, malnutrition (15), zinc deficiency, and especially iron overload known to enhance bacterial growth and virulence (16) and to alter cell-mediated immune responses (17,18) also contribute to amplify the immunodeficiency state of HD patients. In addition to these factors, circulating uremic toxins appear more and more to be critical (19).

After a review of the current knowledge on the ESRD-associated immune dysregulation and chronic inflammation state, this chapter presents a comprehensive review of the clinical aspects of infections in ESRD patients and ends with a survey of the preventive strategies that could be relevant for the uremic patient.

IMMUNE SYSTEM DYSREGULATION IN ESRD

Despite extensive studies, the origin of the immune system dysregulation observed in the uremic patient still remains unclear. Signs of functional deficiency coexist with phenotypic and functional signs of activation (12). This dual aspect will serve hereafter as a pattern for describing the cellular actors of ESRD-associated immune system dysregulation.

T Lymphocytes

T-Lymphocyte Deficiency

Immunologists have long sought in T cells the origin of the immunodeficiency state associated with uremia. A decreased T-cell number combined with a shortened lifespan might play a role in the T-cell impairment associated with ESRD inasmuch as it would affect preferentially one of the CD4+ (helper T cells) or CD8+ (cytotoxic suppressive T cells) subsets. However, evaluation of the CD4 to CD8 ratio showed no significant changes (20).

Precise evaluation of T-cell functions has clearly established that uremic T cells exhibit impaired responses to most mitogens and allogeneic lymphocytes (reviewed in reference 21). Defective T-cell proliferative responses to anti-CD3 monoclonal antibodies have also been reported (22–24). Incubation for 24 hours with uremic serum lowered TCR/CD3 receptor density on normal and uremic CD4 T cells, thus supporting the hypothesis that blunted T-cell response to antigens in uremia is due to downregulation of the TCR/CD3 receptor complex by the uremic milieu (23).

The expression of T-cell receptor (TCR) variable (V) beta chain, which holds a place in tolerance, autoimmunity, and response to external agents, has also been studied in HD patients. An impressive increase of TCR Vβ6.7 positive T cells and a massive deletion of TCR V β8 have been reported (25).

Among the other cell types that could contribute to T-cell dysfunction the monocyte is a good candidate. This effect could be mediated either directly via an impaired antigen processing by monocytes and subsequently altered presentation to the T cell and/or indirectly following their defective delivery of costimulatory signals (e.g., monocyte-derived cytokines to the T-cell responses). The demonstration that T-cell activation blockade was observed in monocyte-dependent stimulation (which is the case for all antigens, most mitogens and anti-CD3 antibody) but not in monocyte-independent stimulation (by anti-CD2 antibody) strongly supports the possibility that monocytes largely contribute to the T-cell deficiency (22). The subsequent observation that the T-cell proliferation was restored to normal by adding normal monocytes and/or anti-CD28 antibody confirmed a prominent role for monocytes in the T-cell defect (26). This was corroborated by the findings that although the expression of B7-2 (CD86, mainly monocytic) is markedly reduced, the expression of B7-1 (CD80, mainly lymphocytic) and of the primary signaling molecule (antigen class II) is not affected in HD patients.

The observation that T-cell alterations were more marked in the presence of autologous serum and that uremic plasma markedly reduced the proliferative response of normal T cells suggests that circulating uremic toxins could play a significant role in the T-cell defect (reviewed in reference 27). Finally, an immunosuppressive effect of blood transfusions and iron had also been suggested (28,29) and is in keeping with later reports showing that administration of recombinant erythropoietin partially corrects defective T-cell responses (30,31).

Impaired Production of Interferon Gamma (IFNγ) and Interleukin-2 (IL-2)

Whatever its underlying mechanisms, the defective proliferation of T cells is associated with abnormally low IL-2 and IFNγ production. The regulation of IL-2 and IFNγ gene expression has also been recently investigated in T-cell culture conditions that measure the transient, phytohemagglutinin-induced expression of IL-2 and IFNγ messenger ribonucleic acid (mRNA), as well as the intactness of posttranscriptional and suppressor T cell–dependent mechanisms that control this expression (32). A complete loss of inducibility of the IL-2 gene, concomitant with decreased inducibility of IFNγ mRNA was found in patients on maintenance HD.

The possibility of an increased IL-2 consumption by its own receptor leading to its decreased bioavailability for inducing the T-cell response has been suggested (33) and was at the origin of IL-2 boosting immunomodulating strategies in uremic patients who were nonresponders to HBV vaccination.

T-Lymphocyte Activation

Evidence for a state of activation of T cells in dialysis patients relies on both increased numbers of cells expressing the Tac antigen or IL-2 receptor (IL-2R) CD25 and higher density of IL-2R at the T-cell surface (34), and elevated serum levels of the soluble form of IL2R in the circulation (35,36) (Fig. 21.1). Both the number of CD25+ T cells and the level of soluble IL2R are increased from the incipient stage of CRF, further rise with progression of CRF, and culminate in dialysis patients (36). The role of dialysis-membrane bioincompatibility in this accentuation of T-cell activation has also been reported (37).

More recent reports have shown that the expression of early T-cell activation markers (CD69) is also increased in ESRD patients and highly correlates with apoptosis markers (38).

Imbalance Between Th-1 and Th-2 Type Cytokines

A major concept emerged in the mid-1980s from the work of Mosmann et al. (39) who proposed that CD4+ T lymphocytes, which provide help for humoral or cellular responses, were distinct and could be differentiated according to the cytokines that they produced (Fig. 21.2). As reviewed elsewhere (21), two types of cytokine-producing cells termed Th1 and Th2 were characterized first in mice and subsequently in humans. Th1 subsets produce IL-2 and IFNγ and preferentially participate in cell-mediated immune responses such as delayed-type hypersensitivity reactions. Th2 clones synthesize IL-4, IL-5, IL-6, IL-10, and IL-13 and provide efficient help for B-cell proliferation and differentiation and for antibody production. Importantly, Th1 and Th2-type cells have profound cytokine-mediated counterregulatory effects on each other, which explains that humoral and cellular responses to a given antigen often alternate in reciprocal dominance. Thus, IFNγ produced by Th1 cells inhibits Th2 cell proliferation and IL-10 produced by Th2 cells inhibits Th1 cell function. IL-12 produced by monocyte/macrophages was shown to be important for driving the response toward Th2 (reviewed in reference 40). Moreover, the presence of IL-4 at the time of antigen triggering may be essential to shift the balance toward Th2. Polarization of specific responses toward a preferential Th1 or Th2 phenotype has been associated with a number of pathologic situations that include T-cell mediated organ-specific autoimmune diseases and organ allograft rejection for Th1 and parasitic infections, atopic diseases, infection with human immunodeficiency virus (HIV), and systemic non-organ-specific autoimmunity for Th2.

Based on the study of the balance between Th1- and Th2-type cytokines, Sester et al. (41) first reported that T-cell activation follows a Th1 pattern in HD patients, and they showed that the skewed helper cell responses correlate with a higher percentage of monocytes capable of secreting the Th1-promoting cytokine IL-12, thus providing a link between overproduction of proinflammatory cytokines and imbalanced T-cell activation. Our own study also concluded in an imbalance of Th1 over Th2

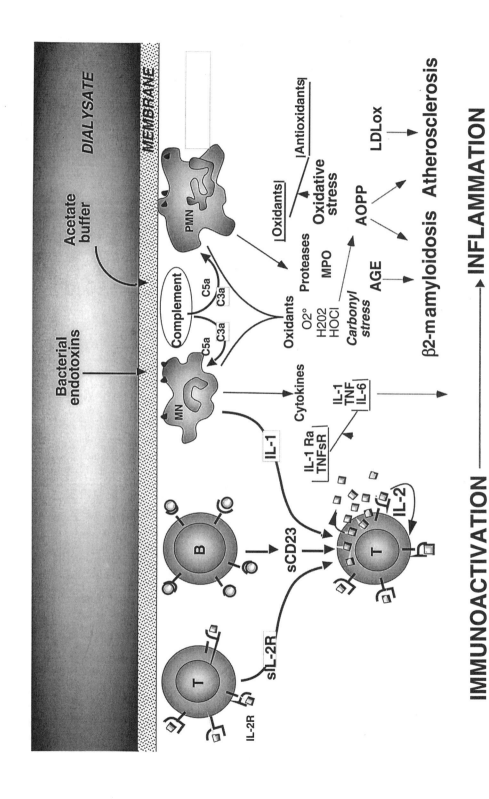

FIG. 21.1. Hemodialysis-induced immunoactivation: mechanisms and consequences.

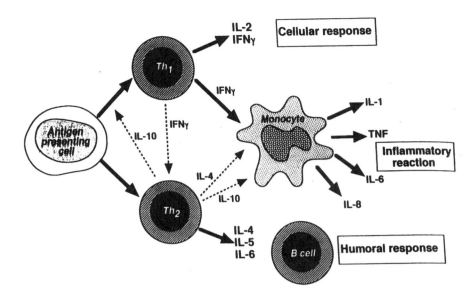

FIG. 21.2. The Th-1 and Th-2 type cytokines and their respective effects in cell-mediated and humoral immunity. *Solid arrows* indicate stimulatory effects. *Dotted arrows* indicate inhibitory effects.

cytokines in patients who were nonresponders to HBV vaccine as opposed to the responders (unpublished data). However, other authors (42,43) observed a polarization of T cells toward Th2 type, which is in keeping with the increased IL-10 basal production observed in hemodialyzed patients (44).

B Lymphocytes

B-Lymphocyte Deficiency

Although plasma levels of IgG, IgM, and IgA are usually in the normal range in ESRD patients, specific antibody responses of B cells, both in vivo and in vitro, are abnormally depressed (reviewed in reference 38). This is particularly well illustrated in vivo by the impaired antibody responses of ESRD patients to vaccines.

B-Lymphocyte Activation

An increased incidence of autoantibodies has been reported in dialysis patients (45) and in patients on PD (46). Likewise, the presence of IgE antibodies to the ethylene oxide used for sterilizing dialysis equipment (47) is also suggestive of abnormal sensitization in these patients, although this varies greatly among centers.

Our finding of elevated plasma levels of the soluble form of the low-affinity Fc receptor of IgE (CD23), which is predominantly expressed on activated B cells, is also suggestive of a B-cell activation state (48) (Fig. 21.1). With regard to the biologic significance of soluble CD23, its gradual accumulation during the progression of CRF along with the demonstration that it can be a cofactor in T-cell activation led to proposing this novel cytokine as "the missing link" in the T-cell activation associated with uremia.

Impaired Response to Vaccines

Most studies of responses to vaccines against T cell-independent antigens have indicated that antibody titers in uremic patients are lower than those achieved in the normal host and decline

more quickly (49). The impairment is even more evident for vaccines against T cell-dependent antigens such as *Pneumococcus* (50), tetanus toxoid (51), and *Haemophilus influenzae* (9,52) or, as mentioned previously, HBV (10,11,53,54).

Several factors, such as age, renal failure, immunosuppression, and route of administration are known to be associated with a decreased antibody responsiveness to vaccination. Genes within the major histocompatibility complex (MHC), which play a major role in the presentation of antigenic peptides to immunocompetent cells (see previous), have also been shown to modulate immune responses to HBV in healthy subjects.

An increased frequency of various DR alleles among nonresponders to hepatitis B surface (HBs) antigen has been reported (55), and special attention has been focused on a recessive A1 B8 DR3 haplotype involved in a defective humoral response related to the absence of T-cell help (56–59). Subsequently, the human leukocyte antigen (HLA) genetic heterogeneity of HBs vaccine response was reevaluated in a large series of hemodialyzed patients by using a deoxyribonucleic acid (DNA) class II oligotyping technique (60). A significantly decreased DR2 frequency in nonresponders to HBV was observed, whereas contrary to previous reports (61), the frequency of DR3 was not higher than in responders.

Interestingly, administration of erythropoietin has been reported to improve B-cell function (62,63) and antibody titers after HBV vaccination (64).

Monocytes

Monocyte Deficiency

Evidence for monocyte deficiency was first suggested by Ruiz et al. (65) who first showed that monocyte Fc receptor-dependent function is markedly impaired in HD patients. Although not specifically studied, impairment of phagocytic and bactericidal activities of monocytes is highly probable, given that it is the case with their phagocyte counterparts, the neutrophils.

As mentioned previously, the defective capacity of uremic monocytes for providing the costimulatory signal necessary for antigen presentation to T cell via B7/CD28 is further evidence for monocyte deficiency. However, whether this results from an intrinsic defect of the uremic monocyte or from toxins specifically targeted toward monocytes remains to be determined (19).

Monocyte Activation

The concept that uremic patients present a state of activation mainly originated from the first studies showing increased circulating levels of monocyte-derived cytokines (IL-1, TNF-α, and IL-6) (Fig. 21.1). This was further confirmed by the demonstration of the concomitant presence of elevated levels of neopterin, a specific marker of monocyte activation (36).

Further evidence of monocyte activation in ESRD patients comes by studies showing that the phenotypic expression of the lipopolysaccharide (LPS) ligand CD14 and of adhesion molecules including CD18, CD49, and CD54 is upregulated in dialysis patients (66,67). More recently, CD14+ and CD16+ monocytes, a potent phagocytosing and antigen-presenting subpopulation, have been reported to be expanded in HD patients (68) and closely related to dialysis membrane bioincompatibility.

Finally, of special interest are recent reports indicating that monocytes of ESRD patients exhibit an increased rate of apoptosis directly related to the degree of biocompatibility of the dialysis membrane (67). As stressed by these authors, this senescent profile may also generate a defective cellular response in acute stress situations, explaining (at least in part) the altered immune response observed in dialysis patients.

Imbalance Between Proinflammatory Cytokines and Their Inhibitors

In 1983, the "IL-1 hypothesis" was proposed (69), based on the observation that (a) both the clinical symptoms, for example, hypotension, fever, and other acute-phase responses observed during dialysis sessions and the sites of complications in long-term hemodialyzed patients closely reflect the systemic effects and the target organs of IL-1 and (b) numerous dialysis-related factors can trigger the production of IL-1 by monocytes. This hypothesis was soon verified by several studies showing elevated levels of IL-1β in the plasma of dialysis patients (reviewed in reference 70), and has been extended to TNF-α and IL-6, which share with IL-1β most of its biologic activities (reviewed in reference 13).

The IFNγ-inducing cytokine IL-18 (71), a proinflammtory cytokine capable of inducing gene expression and synthesis of TNF-α, could be involved in host defense against pathogens (72) but remains to be investigated in uremic patients.

At the cellular level, increased cell-associated IL-1 activity has also been reported (73), together with constitutively increased production of proinflammatory cytokines by cultured monocytes (74) from dialysis patients. Further evidence for a monocyte activation has been provided by several studies showing that dialysis induces the gene expression of IL-1β, TNF-α (75), and IL-6 (76) in circulating monocytes. Lastly, studies showing that cell-associated levels of IL-1β (74) and plasma levels of both TNF-α (77) and IL-6 (78) are elevated in predialysis patients, suggested that such monocyte activation is associated with uremia and further aggravated by dialysis.

It is now established that the potentially harmful effects of monocyte-derived proinflammatory cytokines are counteracted by specific inhibitors concomitantly synthesized in response to infectious or inflammatory challenge (Fig. 21.3). Among these, TNF-soluble receptors (TNF-sR55 and TNF-sR75), which bind to TNF-α and neutralize its effects, and the IL-1 receptor antagonist (IL-1Ra), which competitively binds to the IL-1 receptor without triggering an activation signal, deserved special attention in dialysis patients (79). Increased plasma levels of TNF-soluble receptors have been reported in ESRD patients (36,80,81). In our study (36), both TNF-sR55 and TNF-sR75 were elevated from the incipient stage of CRF, increased in parallel with the progression of renal failure, and further rose dur-

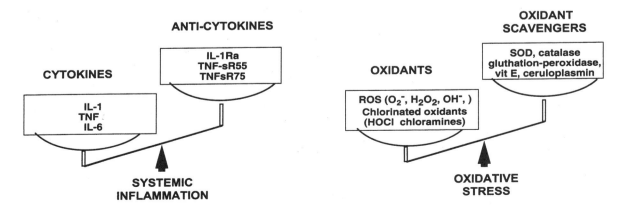

FIG. 21.3. The balance between cytokines and anticytokines and between oxidants and antioxidants involved in the inflammatory state of uremic patients.

ing the course of dialysis sessions. IL-1Ra levels were also elevated from the incipient stage of chronic uremia but were only moderately increased in the course of renal failure and, contrary to TNF soluble receptors, tended to decrease during dialysis sessions.

Neutrophils

Neutrophil Deficiency

In 1977, Craddock et al. (82) first reported that the dialysis session induces a profound but transient neutropenia, which was attributed to the sequestration of neutrophils into the lung by activated complement components themselves induced by the contact of blood with cellulosic membranes (83). The development of non-complement activating membranes has now decayed this phenomenon.

Most studies of neutrophil functions in ESRD patients, motivated by the increased susceptibility of these patients to infections, have concluded in an overall depression in their expected responses to pathogens, for example, chemotaxis, phagocytosis, and bactericidal activities (84–86).

With regard to the underlying mechanisms, the downregulation of opsonin receptors (CR1 and CR3) and C5a receptors following activation by complement components could easily explain neutrophil defective responses (87). Malnutrition and iron overload also largely contribute to neutrophil defectiveness (17,88,89), which is partly restored by recombinant human erythropoietin (31).

The role of uremic toxins in such an impairment of neutrophil responses has also been well documented. During the past years, a number of compounds that accumulate in the blood of uremic patients have been shown to inhibit neutrophil functions (reviewed in reference 19). Among these, p-cresol impairs neutrophil production of reactive oxygen species (85); the granulocyte inhibitory protein GIP I with homology to free immunoglobulin light chains inhibits several functions, for example, chemotaxis, glucose uptake, oxidative metabolism, and phagocytosis (90); GIP II, which shares a great homology with β_2-microglobulin, inhibits deoxyglucose uptake and neutrophil oxidative metabolism (91); a degranulation inhibitory protein (DPI 1 or angiogenin) selectively inhibits the release of collagenase, gelatinase, and lactoferrin without affecting other neutrophil functions (92).

Neutrophil Activation

Neutrophil activation triggered by activated complement components has been well documented in dialysis patients. It is evidenced by a massive generation of highly reactive oxygen species (ROS) (93,94) and granular enzymes (95) and results in the overexpression of the adhesion molecules CD11b, CD11a, CD54, and CD45 (96–98). A common finding is that it closely reflects the complement activating potential of dialysis membranes up to C5-B9 and may be used as an index of bioincompatibility.

Evidence of an imbalance between prooxidants and antioxidants (Fig. 21.3) has been abundantly documented in patients on maintenance HD (reviewed in reference 99). The salient observations are that (a) blood interaction with complement-activating dialysis membranes triggers circulating phagocytes to produce ROS and chlorinated oxidants via activation of NADPH oxidase and myeloperoxidase, respectively (Fig. 21.4); (b) the potential of plasma components to scavenge ROS, especially the glutathione system, is likely to be overwhelmed, and

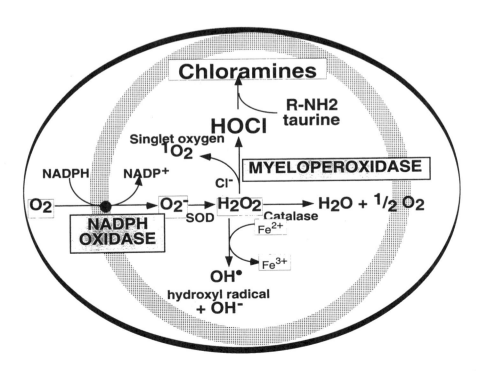

FIG. 21.4. Oxidant generation pathways in phagocytes.

(c) there is a severe defect in antioxidant enzyme cofactors such as zinc or manganese (for superoxide dismutase) and selenium (for glutathione peroxidase), and antioxidant vitamins. Interestingly, our own study showed that glutathione abnormalities are observed from the early stage of CRF; progress with renal failure; and culminate in dialysis, which induces a profound loss of reduced glutathione (100).

Until recently, evidence for in vivo oxidative stress almost solely relied on increased concentrations of lipid peroxidation byproducts such as malondialdehyde, thiobarbituric acid-reactive substances, or conjugated diene fatty acids, the relevance of which is still debated (101).

Advanced Oxidation Protein Products (AOPPs) as Novel Mediators of Inflammation

In the search for the presence of oxidatively modified proteins in uremic patients we recently characterized a novel protein oxidation marker referred to as advanced oxidation protein products (AOPPs) in reference with advanced glycation end products (AGEs) with which AOPPs were found to share several homologies (102).

In more recent studies (reviewed in reference 103), we showed that AOPP plasma levels are (a) already elevated from the early stage of CRF and increase with the progression of renal failure, (b) are correlated with AGE pentosidine and protein oxidation markers such as dityrosine and carbonyls but not with lipid peroxidation markers, (c) are also closely related to monocyte activation markers (neopterin, TNF-α and its soluble

receptors) but not to markers of T-cell activation (soluble IL-2 receptor) or B-cell activation (soluble CD23), and (d) in vitro human serum albumin-AOPP (HSA-AOPP) preparations trigger monocyte activation in a dose-dependent manner along with the degree of HSA-AOPP oxidation.

Taken together, these findings led us to propose AOPP as potential mediators of inflammation notably involved in monocyte activation (Fig. 21.5). Several recent reports, mainly from the group of Himmelfarb et al. (104), have also stressed the importance of oxidatively modified proteins in the chronic inflammatory state associated with uremia.

As another pathway the hypothesis that oxidation acts together with glycation in the formation of AGE (105) has also been proposed and has led to the concept of carbonyl stress (106).

Accelerated Rate of Apoptosis

In recent years, several indices of an increased rate of apoptosis of T cells (38), monocytes, and neutrophils (107,108) have been reported in HD patients and ascribed to both bioincompatibility and the retention of uremic toxins. However, a recent study of the Fas/Fas ligand system, a key regulatory apoptotic pathway, showed that the serum level of the soluble Fas (CD95) was increased in patients with various degrees of CRF and suggested that this could minimize mediation of cellular apoptosis.

In conclusion, immune system dysregulation combines a deficiency and an activation state in all cell types, as summarized in Table 21.1. Clinically, this dual process is involved in both the susceptibility of ESRD patients to infection and in the chronic

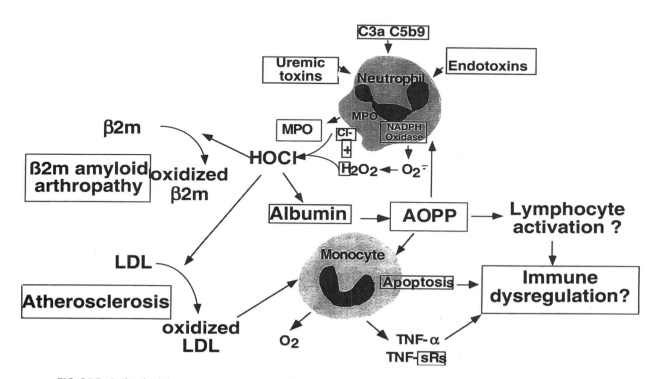

FIG. 21.5. Pathophysiologic role of advanced oxidation protein products (AOPP) in uremia. (From Descamps-Latscha B, et al. Importance of oxidatively modified proteins in chronic renal failure. *Kidney Int* 2001;78[Suppl]:S108–S113, with permission.)

TABLE 21.1. THE DUAL ASPECT OF IMMUNE DYSREGULATION IN UREMIC PATIENTS

	Immune Deficiency	Immunoactivation
T cells	Poor delayed type hypersensitivity response	Increased IL-2 R expression and release
	Defective proliferation and cytotoxic potential	Increased expression of early activation markers
	Impaired production of IL-2 and IFNγ	Increased rate of apoptosis
	Imbalance between Th_1/Th_2 cytokines	
B cells	Defective production of opsonins (IgG and IgM)	Increased incidence of autoantibodies
	Poor antibody response to vaccines	Increased CD23 expression and release
Monocytes	Downregulation of opsonin receptors	Increased level of neopterin
	Defective antigen presentation	Increased expression of CD14
	Poor antibody response to vaccines	Imbalance between CD14/CD16 monocyte subsets
	Impaired chemotaxis, adhesion, migration,	Overexpression of adhesion molecules
	phagocytosis, and bactericidal activities	Increased production of IL-1, TNF and IL-6
		Increased generation of reactive oxygen species and chlorinated oxidants
Neutrophils	Downregulation of opsonin receptors	Overexpression of adhesion molecules
	Impaired chemotaxis, adhesion, migration,	Increased generation of reactive oxygen species and chlorinated
	phagocytosis, and bactericidal activities	oxidants
		Increased liberation of proteases

INFγ, interferon gamma; IL-2, interleukin-2.

inflammatory state responsible for malnutrition, β2-microglobulin amyloidosis, and accelerated atherosclerosis. With regard to infections, immune deficiency is primarily involved in the defective response to bacterial pathogens but immunostimulation also contributes to the risk of infection, by inducing a priming state of neutrophils and a subsequent downregulation of opsonin receptors involved in bacteria recognition.

INFECTIONS IN ESRD

Epidemiologic Data

Mortality from Infection in Dialysis Patients

The proportion of deaths secondary to infection has decreased substantially from the early period of maintenance dialysis until more recent years. This evolution is clearly apparent from the survey by Mailloux et al. (1) in the United States. Among 532 consecutive patients who started dialysis between 1970 and 1985, the role of infection as the cause of death was 44.4% in 1970 to 1973, 42.9% in 1974 to 1977, 36.2% in 1978 to 1981, and 21.6% in 1982 to 1985. The proportion of deaths related to infections further decreased to 14.8% in patients on dialysis therapy in the United States during years 1995 to 1997 (2,3). Infection, in the form of septicemia in most cases, accounted for an incidence of deaths of 34.2 per 1,000 patient-years on dialysis, that is, 14.8% of an overall death rate of 231 per 1,000 patient-years (2,3). In Europe, during the period 1991 to 1999, infection was the cause of death in 16% of patients treated with HD, and 18% of those treated with PD (Fig. 21.6) (4).

Sarnak et al. (109) examined annual mortality rates caused by sepsis in ESRD patients compared with the general population, using data from the U.S. Renal Data System 1994 to 1996. Overall, the annual percentage of mortality secondary to sepsis, adjusted for age and diabetes was at least 50-fold higher in dialysis patients compared with the general population. These findings clearly highlight the susceptibility of dialysis patients to septic accidents and their vulnerability to sepsis.

Incidence of Septicemia

Septicemia accounts for at least half of deaths secondary to septic causes in ESRD patients. Incidence of septicemia in dialysis patients appears to have decreased from the early times of dialysis therapy but has remained virtually at the same level over the past two decades (110). In 1978, Dobkin et al. (111) reported an incidence of 15 septicemic episodes per 100 patient-years among HD patients. In a retrospective longitudinal cohort study based on 4,918 patients who started maintenance dialysis in the United States in 1986 to 1987, 11.7% of HD and 9.4% of PD patients experienced at least one septicemic episode at some time during a follow-up period of 7 years (112). A subsequent study based on the same cohort reported a comparable incidence of septicemia in diabetic and nondiabetic patients, 11.1% and 12.5%, respectively (113). A prospective study in

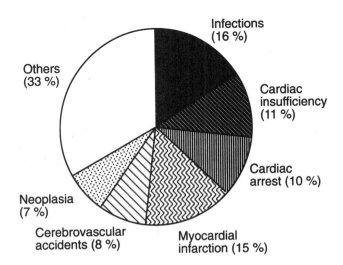

FIG. 21.6. Distribution of causes of death in hemodialysis patients. (From USRDS. VI. Causes of death in ESRD. *Am J Kidney Dis* 1999;34:S87–S94, with permission.)

the United States in 1994 to 1996 identified 65 episodes of *Staphylococcus aureus* bacteremia among 445 patients, an incidence of 14.4 episodes per 100 patient-years (114). In France, the prospective EPIBACDIAL study conducted by Kessler's group recorded an incidence of 11.1 bacteremic episodes per 100 patient-years (115). In a previous multicentric study conducted some years earlier (116), the same authors reported a comparable incidence of septicemic episodes of 8.4 per 100 patient-years, which indicates that incidence of septicemia did not decrease over the past decade despite all preventive efforts. A nationwide retrospective epidemiologic study was performed recently in the United States by Abbott et al. (117), based on 327,993 patients who initiated maintenance dialysis between January 1992 and June 1997. Of them, 13.2% had been hospitalized at least once for septicemia, with an estimated incidence of 6.8 episodes per 100 patient-years.

Bacterial Infections

Gram-Positive Agents

Gram-positive microorganisms are the most frequently identified pathogens in patients with bacteremia or local infections, the proportion being 40% to 70% among patients with septicemic episodes (111,115–117). *S. aureus* is the most commonly encountered gram-positive agent, but coagulase-negative staphylococci are nearly as often responsible for bacteremia such as *S. aureus* in HD patients mainly in the form of *Staphylococcus epidermidis* (115); *Staphylococcus lugdunensis* was also responsible for several cases of valvular endocarditis (118). Other gram-positive agents such as streptococci, or less often pneumococci, may be isolated from blood culture in septicemic patients (117).

The most frequent portal of entry of *S. aureus* is angioaccess infection in HD patients (115) because of the frequent *S. aureus* carriage in the nose, throat, and skin and the required repetitive punctures of the vascular access in these patients (117, 119–121). *S. aureus* or coagulase-negative staphylococci bacteremia may result in multiple secondary septic foci, such as septic pulmonary emboli (111,115), metastatic infection in bones or joints (122), or endocarditis (114,115,123). Strategies aimed at eradication of *S. aureus* carriage, in particular nasal application of mupirocin (124) or regular oral administration of rifampicin (120), may have contributed to reduce incidence of bacteremias in HD patients, although Hoen et al. (115) did not observe a significantly different incidence of bacteremias whether or not patients were *S. aureus* carriers. In a recent study by Perl et al. (125), prophylactic nasal application of mupirocin did not reduce the rate of *S. aureus* postoperative local infection at the surgical site, thus suggesting a major role for nosocomial transmission of staphylococci by health care staff. A *S. aureus* vaccine has been reported to elicit antibody production in a small cohort of dialysis patients, but its clinical applicability still remains to be evaluated on a larger scale (126).

In PD patients, formation of a bacterial biofilm on the walls of the peritoneal catheter is often the cause of repeat peritonitis episodes with the same *S. aureus* or *S. epidermidis* strain, thus requiring catheter change to prevent reinfection (127).

Gram-Negative Organisms

Gram-negative organisms were the cause of bacteremic episodes in 25% of vascular access site-related septicemic episodes reported by Dobkin (111) and in 25% of septicemic episodes observed by Hoen et al. (115). Among gram-negative organisms, *Escherichia coli* is the most often encountered (115,117), although *Pseudomonas* or *Serratia* may be responsible for septicemic episodes. *E. coli* bacteremia usually originates in the gastrointestinal or the genitourinary tract (121,128). Indeed, significant bacteriuria was found in 27% of 182 patients with CRF and clinical urinary tract infection in 19%, in the study by Saitoh et al. (128). Urinary tract infection was especially frequent in oliguric HD patients and in those with polycystic kidney disease or chronic pyelonephritis as underlying disease. Likewise, defects in the mechanisms for the concentration of antibiotics at sites of infection explain the abnormal durability of *E. coli* bacteriuria and the development of perinephritic abscesses that are refractory to systemic antibiotic therapy and that may necessitate nephrectomy.

More recently, attention has focused on latent chronic *Chlamydia pneumoniae* infection in dialysis and predialysis patients, associated with elevated C-reactive protein (CRP) plasma level and increased risk of atherosclerosis (14,129), as already observed in the general population (130). Indeed, IgG and IgA antibodies (the latter being indicative of a chronic and still active infectious process) were found in a high proportion of uremic patients treated by PD, and a strong correlation was found between IgA antibody titer and CRP level (129). Although a causative link between *C. pneumoniae* infection and atherosclerotic complications in dialysis patients remains to be demonstrated, ongoing trials using macrolide antibiotherapy will allow assessment of whether eradication of these inapparent infections results in reduced atherosclerotic morbidity (131).

Nonbacteremic Infections

Even if septicemia is the most severe form of infectious complication in ESRD patients, nonbacteremic infections are more frequent and may also be life threatening.

Angioaccess local infection was a very frequent event in the early times of dialysis therapy, when Scribner's external shunt was used. The generalized use of internal radiocephalic fistula led to a significant decrease in vascular access-related infections, but the increasing use of polytetrafluoroethylene (PTFE) prosthetic devices in recent years, especially in the United States, is responsible for a dramatically increasing incidence of thrombotic and infectious complications (132–134). In particular, late occult infections can arise from old prosthetic vascular grafts several months or years after implantation, resulting from the production of a biofilm by coagulase-negative staphylococci. Such focal infection induces an inflammatory state that may be revealed by a resistance to recombinant erythropoietin (135). The diagnosis may be helped by evidencing presence of antibodies against staphylococcal slime antigens, as recently proposed by Selan et al. (136). Gram-positive organisms are responsible for more than 80% of access-related infections, with a nearly equal frequency of *S. aureus* and *S. epidermidis* (137).

Also, the increased use of central catheters, either for temporary or long-standing use, is associated with a high incidence of exit-site infections that, in turn, may result in bacteremia (138,139). Angioaccess infections represented 20% of nonbacteremic infections in the study of Kessler et al. (116).

Respiratory tract infections are also frequent. They accounted for 35% of nonbacteremic infections in the study of Kessler et al. (116), with an incidence of 6.2 episodes per 1,000 patient-months. A similar incidence of pulmonary infection episodes was reported by others, at 5.7 per 1,000 patient-months (140) or 6.9 per 1,000 patient-months (141).

Urinary tract infections are favored by the reduced urinary output that results from progressive loss of residual renal function, especially in HD patients. Patients with polycystic kidney disease or with a history of chronic pyelonephritis are especially prone to this complication. Urinary tract infection episodes accounted for 23% of nonbacteremic infection episodes in the prospective study of Kessler et al. (116), an incidence of 5.2 per 1,000 patient-months. *E. coli* was identified as the causative microorganism in two thirds of cases. The treatment of urinary tract infections is often difficult because of the low concentration of antibacterial agents in urine and in kidney parenchyma in patients with advanced renal failure, thus requiring long-duration antibacterial therapy with agents having a high tissular penetration.

Tuberculosis

An abnormally high incidence of tuberculosis has been consistently reported in dialysis patients, when compared with its incidence in the general population in the same countries (recently reviewed in reference 142), with an incidence of tuberculosis 5 to 15 times higher than in the normal population (143–149). However, incidence of active tuberculosis is markedly higher in developing countries than in industrial ones (150).

Recent epidemiologic studies confirm this previous observation. Simon et al. (151) recorded all cases of incident tuberculosis in patients treated with maintenance dialysis in New Jersey in 1994 and 1995. In this statewide study, they recorded three cases among 4,550 dialysis patients in 1994 (an incidence of 66 per 1,000 patient-years) and four cases among 4,831 patients in 1995 (an incidence of 83 per 1,000 patient-years), that is, seven times higher than in the general population of this state (10.7 to 10.8 per 1,000 person-years). By contrast, in a countrywide study during year 1997 by Chou et al. (152) in Taiwan, the annual incidence of tuberculosis in dialysis patients was 493 per 1,000 patient-years (i.e., 6.9 times higher than in the Taiwanese population) and also six times higher than in U.S. dialysis patients. Mortality rates among their tuberculous patients was 3.3 times higher than in people affected with tuberculosis in the general population.

Tuberculosis in uremic patients is often extrapulmonary, which rends the diagnosis difficult and delayed. In the survey of Rutsky et al. (147) in the United States, 56 of 885 dialyzed patients had predominantly extrapulmonary disease, and in the study by Taskapan in Turkey (153), 7 of 18 (38%) patients diagnosed between 1980 to 1998 had extrapulmonary tuberculosis, mainly peritoneal. Tuberculous peritonitis was observed in 33% of 24

HD patients in an Indian study (154), and more than 50 cases of tuberculous peritonitis have been reported in PD patients (155).

Diagnosis is often difficult because skin reactions are frequently negative for tuberculosis, as are routine direct examination or culture of sputum. Thus, diagnosis is often delayed, which results in increased mortality because of late treatment (147,153–155). The recently developed molecular detection by polymerase chain reaction (PCR) technology is expected to be of considerable help in rapidly identifying the presence of *Mycobacterium tuberculosis* in sputum samples (156) or in pleural fluid (157) in patients with persisting cough or fever of unknown origin, and the same is probably true of ascitic fluid. In such cases, chest computed tomography (CT) scan may be of help to identify lung or pleuritic tuberculous involvement, as shown by Coskun et al. (158). Finally, thanks to more rapid diagnosis, pulmonary or extrapulmonary tuberculosis should be treated earlier, thus resulting in lesser mortality, because the response to specific antibiotics is usually good.

Unusual Pathogens

Other intracellular bacteria may be occasionally responsible for local or systemic infections in a dialysis patient treated with immunosuppressive drugs. *Legionella pneumophila* (the agent of legionnaire's disease) caused fistula infection in hemodialyzed patients (159) and pneumonia in a dialysis patient on immunosuppression for systemic vasculitis (160), thus evidencing the favoring effect of immunosuppression. The same is true of *Listeria monocytogenes,* which was responsible for bacteremia and endocarditis in some patients (115,123,160,161). In the two cases reported by Goldman et al. (160), affected patients had recently received immunosuppression for graft failure that required return to dialysis. Iron overload was considered the favoring factor in a patient who had received multiple blood transfusions (162).

Dialysis patients are susceptible to mucormycosis (*Rhizopus* infection). In observations reported in the literature, patients presented with dissemination or rhinocerebritis in most cases, and the fatality rate was very high despite amphotericin B therapy. The major risk factor was administration of deferoxamine, chiefly given because of aluminium overload. Indeed, the deferoxamine-iron chelate acts as a siderophore to *Rhizopus,* thus stimulating its growth and pathogenicity, as shown experimentally by Van Cutsem et al. (163).

Clostridium difficile is a cause of colitis and diarrhea in dialysis patients, especially in those treated with broad-spectrum antibiotics (164,165), but impaired host defenses in malnourished patients have been implicated (166).

Of note, opportunistic infections are infrequent in ESRD patients, because the degree of immunodeficiency secondary to the uremic state per se is much lesser than that induced by HIV infection or immunosuppressive agents.

Viral Infections

The HD patient is at an increased risk of viral hepatitis (especially type B and C) because of the frequent need for blood transfusions (see Chapter 22 for a detailed discussion). Unlike healthy subjects, uremic patients infected with HBV usually have mild (almost asymptomatic) infections. However, because of their deficient immune status, a high proportion of patients are unable to produce antibodies to HBV surface antigens and, therefore, become chronic carriers able to transmit the infection to other patients, dialysis unit staff, other categories of hospital personnel, and their own families (167).

Various immunomodulating strategies have been tried in an attempt to overcome the poor response of ESRD patients to HBV vaccine, by enhancing antibody production through concomitant administration of various agents. Zinc supplementation was proposed as an adjuvant (168), but its efficacy was not confirmed by others (169,170). Thymopentin injected by subcutaneous route was reported to improve the antibody response of dialysis patients previously unresponsive to vaccination (171), but its beneficial effect was not confirmed in subsequent prospective controlled studies (172,173). IFNγ failed to enhance the response rate or increase antibody titers in a prospective controlled study (174). Concomitant local administration of HBV vaccine and a preparation of purified IL-2 was reported to induce an antibody response in patients who previously were nonresponders to a standard vaccination protocol (175). However, in a prospective placebo-controlled trial, we did not find a significant enhancement of antibody response in previously unresponsive patients with the concomitant use of recombinant IL-2, as compared with patients who received the recombinant vaccine alone (176).

More recently, Anandh et al. (177) reported a beneficial effect of a subcutaneous injection of 4 to 5 μg/kg of granulocyte macrophage-stimulating factor (GM-CSF) 24 hours before the first injection of HBV vaccine, in HD patients naive to vaccination or nonresponders to prior vaccination receiving a booster dose of vaccine. However, the number of patients was very limited and these encouraging results must be confirmed.

In view of the deleterious effects of HBV infection in dialyzed and transplanted patients, achieving immunization before starting dialysis therapy and kidney transplantation should be considered an important goal. Ideally, vaccination should be initiated early in the predialysis phase, at a time when immunodeficiency still is of moderate degree, as part of the optimal predialysis management of patients (178,179).

Whereas HBV infection could be virtually eradicated from dialysis units thanks to the generalized practice of HBV vaccine, at least in industrialized countries, hepatitis C virus (HCV) infection still remains an important problem in dialysis units. Fortunately, testing of blood products with sensitive techniques (180,181) virtually eliminated the risk of bloodborne transmission of HCV, inasmuch as widespread use of recombinant erythropoietin therapy has dramatically reduced the need for blood transfusion in dialysis patients. However, patients may be seropositive for HCV before referral, and nosocomial transmission in the absence of any blood transfusion is possible (182). Presently, HCV infection is the most common cause of morbidity and mortality from chronic liver disease in HD (183) and transplant patients (184). In the absence of a vaccine against HCV, the only means of preventing nosocomial HVC transmission is scrupulous respect of the universal precautions for patients undergoing dialysis, which are also mandatory to prevent nosocomial transmission of bacterial pathogens or other viruses such as HIV.

Risk Factors and Prevention of Infection

Risk Factors for Bacterial Infections in ESRD Patients

Even if depressed immunity is the main factor for the abnormally high incidence of bacterial infections (either bacteremic or local) in dialysis patients, risk factors associated with the dialysis procedure may also contribute (Fig. 21.7). These risk factors are important to identify because most of them are amenable by specific measures.

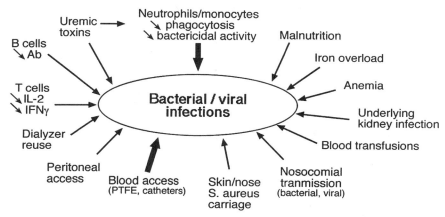

FIG. 21.7. Endogenous and exogenous factors involved in the pathogenesis of bacterial and viral infections in dialysis patients.

Vascular Access and Dialysis Technique

Infection of vascular access is well established as the leading cause of bacteremia, especially infection resulting from *S. aureus* or coagulase-negative staphylococci.

The type of vascular access has a prominent influence on the occurrence of local infections and bacteremic episodes. Churchill et al. (132) reported that prosthetic grafts were associated with a much higher incidence of bacteremia than were native arteriovenous fistulas, with a 12-month incidence of 19.7% versus 4.5%, respectively. In the French EPIBACDIAL prospective study (115), PTFE grafts entailed a 29% higher risk of bacteremia than native arteriovenous fistulas. A similarly higher risk of infections with prosthetic grafts was also found by others, both in nondiabetic patients with a relative risk of 1.34 (112) and in diabetics with a relative risk of 1.41 (113). Marr et al. (114) observed a high rate of bacteremia recurrence in patients dialyzed through PTFE grafts. Such increased risk of infection with prosthetic devices is an argument to favor creation of a native arteriovenous fistula, rather than implantation of a PTFE graft in patients starting HD, as recommended by the National Kidney Foundation-Dialysis Outcomes Quality Initiative (NKF/DOQI) (185).

In fact, use of central vein catheters entails the highest risk of infection. In the EPIBACDIAL study (115), the relative risk of bacteremia associated with use of permanent central catheters, relative to native arteriovenous fistulas, was 7.64, whereas the temporary use of a central catheter was not associated with a significantly higher risk. In a 1-year prospective study on 67 long-term catheters inserted in 43 HD patients, Nielsen et al. (139) observed an incidence of septicemia as high as 49 per 100 patient-years; presence of *S. aureus* at the cutaneous catheter insertion site, rather than nasal carriage, was the most significant predictive factor of the risk of subsequent septicemia. In the longitudinal retrospective study of Powe et al. (112) the temporary short-term use of a central catheter was associated with a relative risk of 1.48, whereas use of a permanent catheter entailed a relative risk of 2.0. Similar findings were observed in diabetic patients by Jaar et al. (113).

Influence of dialysis modality (either HD or PD) was evaluated in two recent studies. The conclusion from both studies was that there was a marginally higher infectious risk with HD than PD (112,117).

Comorbidity

A poor nutritional status of the patient as reflected by a serum albumin level <35g/L was associated with an increased frequency of infection with a relative risk of 1.66 in HD patients (112).

Influence of diabetes is variably estimated. Some authors did not find a significant difference between diabetics and nondiabetics (115,186), whereas others reported a higher risk of bacterial infections in diabetics (112,113,117,187). However, peripheral arteriopathy in diabetics was shown to be a strong risk factor for infection (113) because of the presence of infected foot ulcers secondary to diabetic neuropathy and distal arteriopathy.

Iron Overload

The intricate influence of iron overload, anemia, and erythropoietin therapy is worthy to consider. In the pre-erythropoi-etin era, Goldman et al. (160) observed that multiple transfusions in HD patients were a risk factor for *E. coli* sepsis. The average number of blood transfusions per month was 2.60 ±0.93 in 10 patients who suffered bacteremia, compared with 1.15 ±0.22 (*p* <0.001) in 13 patients without bacteremia. This observation was confirmed in the first study of Kessler et al. (116) who observed that a high ferritin plasma level (>1,000 µg/L) resulting from multiple previous transfusions was observed four times more frequently among patients who experienced bacteremia than in those who did not. In a subsequent study (186), these authors confirmed high plasma ferritin level as an independent, significant risk factor for bacterial infections, either bacteremic or not, the relative risk of infection being 1.79 in patients with a plasma ferritin level greater than 500 µg/L. In their most recent study (115), iron overload was no longer a risk factor for bacteremia, because most patients were treated with epoetin at that time, and the proportion of patients with a high ferritin level had declined to less than 5%. However, they found anemia to be a risk factor for infection, with each decrease by 1 g/dL of hemoglobin level being associated with a 30% higher risk of infection. Accordingly, it has been shown that recombinant erythropoietin helps to reverse the neutrophil dysfunction in iron-overloaded anemic dialysis patients (31,188). Abbott et al. (117) also reported that a hematocrit level less than 25% was associated with an increased risk of infection.

Iron overload increases the risk of bacterial infections in dialysis patients through several mechanisms (188). Iron is essential for growth of microorganisms and excess iron availability enhances bacterial growth and virulence. In addition, iron overload impairs chemotactic and phagocytic activities of neutrophils (189). Thanks to epoetin therapy since the early 1990s, the need for blood transfusions has been dramatically reduced, thus lowering the risk of iron accumulation. Moreover, erythropoiesis stimulated by epoetin therapy results in mobilization of ferrous hepatic stores without inducing high circulating iron levels in patients with previous hemosiderosis. By contrast, mobilization of iron stores by means of deferoxamine may rapidly increase plasma iron concentration, thus resulting in the increased risk of sudden growth of iron-dependent microorganisms.

It is noteworthy that infection is mostly confined to ESRD patients treated with HD or PD, whereas infectious complications are much less frequent in predialysis patients even at the advanced stage of renal failure, although immune deficiency and activation still are present. There are several reasons for the increased incidence of bacteremic and nonbacteremic infections in dialysis patients: (a) dialysis does not restore a state of normal renal function (at variance with kidney transplantation) but maintains a state of chronic uremia corresponding to a glomerular filtration rate (GFR) reduced at 15 to 20 mL/minute; (b) the dialysis procedure by itself, especially HD, further increases lymphocyte, monocyte, and polymorphonuclear neutrophil (PMN) dysfunction (through complement activation by poorly biocompatible membranes and/or bacterial endotoxins issued from dialysis fluid); (c) malnutrition, anemia, and iron overload are frequent and favor infection or depress host defenses; (d) the dialysis technique and environment entails a number of situations that may predispose to bacteremic or local infection (e.g., nasal or skin staphylococcus portage; multiple, repetitive access punctures for dialysis; skin break at the cutaneous exits of central vein or peritoneal catheters; nosocomial transmission of bacteria or viruses in center-treated patients; and decreased urine output favoring development of severe renal infection especially in patients with underlying polycystic kidney disease or chronic pyelonephritis). None of these factors is present at the predialysis phase of CRF.

Thus, increased incidence of bacterial infections results from the combined effects of underlying endogenous uremia-associated immune deficiency and triggering external factors associated with the dialysis procedure.

Preventive Measures

Measures aimed at preventing, or at least limiting, morbidity and mortality from infection in ESRD patients derive from the previously mentioned considerations. They are summarized in Table 21.2.

Of note, uremia-associated immune dysfunction will never be suppressed even with optimal dialysis efficacy, and it constitutes an incompressible part of the risk. By contrast, factors linked to dialysis technique and environment are amenable through careful respect of hygienic precautions, avoidance of prosthetic blood access devices, and correction of anemia. In this respect, improvements in practice already achieved in the United States thanks to the NKF/DOQI recommendations, namely better correction of anemia by recombinant human erythropoietin (rHuEPO) and more generalized use of native fistulas is encouraging and will hopefully result in a decreased incidence of morbidity and mortality from infection in ESRD patients.

TABLE 21.2. PREVENTIVE MEASURES AIMED AT LIMITING BACTERIAL VIRAL INFECTION IN ESRD PATIENTS

Risk Factors	Therapeutic Intervention
Uremia-associated immune dysfunction	Optimal dialysis efficacy
	Optimal nutritional status
	Correction of anemia
Complement activation	Use of biocompatible membranes
	Avoiding of reuse
Dialysate endotoxins	Use of ultrapure dialysate fluid
Nasal staphylococci carriage	Nasal mupirocin ointment
Blood viruses transmission	Avoidance of blood transfusions
Nosocomial transmission	Respect of the universal precautions
	Careful disinfection of dialysis equipment
Iron overload	Avoidance of blood transfusions
	rHuEPO
Iron mobilization	Avoidance of deferoxamine
Vascular access	Preferred use of native fistulae
Peritoneal access, central vein catheters	Close surveillance of cutaneous issues of catheters

rHuEPO, recombinant human erythropoietin.

REFERENCES

1. Mailloux LU, et al. Mortality in dialysis patients: analysis of the causes of death. *Am J Kidney Dis* 1991;18:326–335.
2. The USRDS annual data report. *Am J Kidney Dis* 1997;30[Suppl 1]: S107–S117.
3. USRDS. VI. Causes of death in ESRD. *Am J Kidney Dis* 1999;34:S87–S94.
4. van Dijk PC, et al. Renal replacement therapy in Europe: the results of a collaborative effort by the ERA-EDTA registry and six national or regional registries. *Nephrol Dial Transplant* 2001;16:1120–1129.
5. Shinzato T, et al. Report of the annual statistical survey of the Japanese Society for Dialysis Therapy in 1996. *Kidney Int* 1999;55: 700–712.
6. Dammin GJ, et al. Prolonged survival of skin homografts in uremic patients. *Ann N Y Acad Sci* 1957;94:967–976.
7. Lindner A, et al. High incidence of neoplasia in uremic patients receiving long-term dialysis: cancer and long-term dialysis. *Nephron* 1981;27:292–296.
8. Kirkpatrick CH, et al. Immunologic studies in human organ transplantation: observation and characterization of suppressed cutaneous reactivity in uremia. *J Exp Med* 1964;119:727–742.
9. Cappel R, et al. Impaired humoral and cell-mediated immune responses in dialyzed patients after influenza vaccination. *Nephron* 1983;33:21–25.
10. Crosnier J, et al. Randomised placebo-controlled trial of hepatitis B surface antigen vaccine in french haemodialysis units. II: haemodialysis patients. *Lancet* 1981;i:797–800.
11. Benhamou E, et al. Long-term results of hepatitis B vaccination in patients on dialysis. *N Engl J Med* 1986;314:1710–1711.
12. Descamps-Latscha B. The immune system in end-stage renal disease. *Curr Opin Nephrol Hypertens* 1993;2:883–891.
13. Descamps-Latscha B, et al. Immunological and chronic inflammatory abnormalities in end-stage renal disease. In: Jacobs CMKC, et al., eds. *Replacement of renal function by dialysis,* 4th ed. Boston: Kluwer Academic, 1996.
14. Stenvinkel P, et al. Strong association between malnutrition, inflammation, and atherosclerosis in chronic renal failure. *Kidney Int* 1999;55:1899–1911.
15. Lawson JA, et al. Prevalence and prognostic significance of malnutrition in chronic renal insufficiency. *J Ren Nutr* 2001;11:16–22.
16. Sunder-Plassmann G, et al. Pathobiology of the role of iron in infection. *Am J Kidney Dis* 1999;34:S25–S29.
17. Mattern WD, et al. Malnutrition, altered immune function, and the risk of infection in maintenance hemodialysis patients. *Am J Kidney Dis* 1982;1:206–218.
18. Keown PA, et al. Ferroproteins and the immune response. *Lancet* 1984;i:44.
19. Vanholder R, et al. Uremic toxicity: present state of the art. *Int J Artif Organs* 2001;24:695–725.
20. Deenitchina SS, et al. Cellular immunity in hemodialysis patients: a quantitative analysis of immune cell subsets by flow cytometry. *Am J Nephrol* 1995;15:57–65.
21. Descamps-Latscha B, et al. T cells and B cells in chronic renal failure. *Semin Nephrol* 1996;16:183–191.
22. Meuer SC, et al. Selective blockade of the antigen-receptor-mediated pathway of T cell activation in patients with impaired primary immune responses. *J Clin Invest* 1987;80:743–749.
23. Stachowski J, et al. Does uremic environment down-regulate T cell activation via TCR/CD3 antigen receptor complex? *J Clin Lab Immunol* 1991;36:15–21.
24. Ankersmit HJ, et al. Impaired T cell proliferation, increased soluble death-inducing receptors and activation-induced T cell death in patients undergoing haemodialysis. *Clin Exp Immunol* 2001;125:142–148.
25. Sunder-Plassmann G, et al. T-cell selection and T-cell receptor variable beta-chain usage in chronic hemodialysis patients. *Clin Nephrol* 1992;37:252–259.
26. Girndt M, et al. T cell activation defect in hemodialysis patients: evidence for a role of the B7/CD28 pathway. *Kidney Int* 1993;44: 359–365.

27. Vanholder R, et al. Protein-bound uremic solutes: the forgotten toxins. *Kidney Int* 2001;78[Suppl]:S266–S270.
28. Keown PA, et al. Improved renal allograft survival after blood transfusion: a nonspecific, erythrocyte-mediated immunoregulatory process? *Lancet* 1979;i:20–22.
29. Keown P, et al. In vitro suppression of cell-mediated immunity by ferroproteins and ferric salts. *Cell Immunol* 1983;80:257–266.
30. Pfaffl W, et al. Lymphocyte subsets and delayed cutaneous hypersensitivity in hemodialysis patients receiving recombinant human erythropoietin. *Contrib Nephrol* 1988;66:195–204.
31. Veys N, et al. Correction of deficient phagocytosis during erythropoietin treatment in maintenance hemodialysis patients. *Am J Kidney Dis* 1992;19:358–363.
32. Gerez L, et al. Regulation of interleukin-2 and interferon-gamma gene expression in renal failure. *Kidney Int* 1991;40:266–272.
33. Chatenoud L, et al. Immune deficiency of the uremic patient. *Adv Nephrol Necker Hosp* 1990;19:259–274.
34. Chatenoud L, et al. Presence of preactivated T cells in hemodialyzed patients: their possible role in altered immunity. *Proc Natl Acad Sci U S A* 1986;83:7457–7461.
35. Walz G, et al. Soluble interleukin 2 receptor and tissue polypeptide antigen serum concentrations in end-stage renal failure. *Nephron* 1990;56:157–161.
36. Descamps-Latscha B, et al. Balance between IL-1 beta, TNF-alpha, and their specific inhibitors in chronic renal failure and maintenance dialysis: relationships with activation markers of T cells, B cells, and monocytes. *J Immunol* 1995;154:882–892.
37. Zaoui P, et al. Hemodialysis with cuprophane membrane modulates interleukin-2 receptor expression. *Kidney Int* 1991;39:1020–1026.
38. Meier P, et al. Early T cell activation correlates with expression of apoptosis markers in patients with end-stage renal disease. *J Am Soc Nephrol* 2002;13:204–212.
39. Mosmann TR, et al. Two types of murine helper T cell clone. I. Definition according to profiles of lymphokine activities and secreted proteins. *J Immunol* 1986;136:2348–2357.
40. Colombo MP, et al. Interleukin-12 in anti-tumor immunity and immunotherapy. *Cytokine Growth Factor Rev* 2002;13:155–168.
41. Sester U, et al. T-cell activation follows Th1 rather than Th2 pattern in haemodialysis patients. *Nephrol Dial Transplant* 2000;15:1217–1223.
42. Libetta C, et al. Polarization of T-helper lymphocytes toward the Th2 phenotype in uremic patients. *Am J Kidney Dis* 2001;38:286–295.
43. Yokoyama T, et al. Identification of T helper cell subsets in continuous ambulatory peritoneal dialysis patients. *Nephron* 2001;89:215–218.
44. Brunet P, et al. IL-10 synthesis and secretion by peripheral blood mononuclear cells in haemodialysis patients. *Nephrol Dial Transplant* 1998;13:1745–1751.
45. Nolph KD, et al. Antibodies to nuclear antigens in patients undergoing long-term hemodialysis. *Am J Med* 1976;60:673–676.
46. Gagnon RF, et al. Auto-immunity in patients with end-stage renal disease maintained on hemodialysis and continuous ambulatory peritoneal dialysis. *J Clin Lab Immunol* 1983;11:155–158.
47. Rumpf KW, et al. Association of ethylene-oxide-induced IgE antibodies with symptoms in dialysis patients. *Lancet* 1985;ii:1385–1387.
48. Descamps-Latscha B, et al. Soluble CD23 as an effector of immune dysregulation in chronic uremia and dialysis. *Kidney Int* 1993;43:878–884.
49. Girndt M, et al. Tetanus immunization and its association to hepatitis B vaccination in patients with chronic renal failure. *Am J Kidney Dis* 1995;26:454–460.
50. Rytel MW, et al. Pneumococcal vaccine immunization of patients with renal impairment. *Proc Soc Exp Biol Med* 1986;182:468–473.
51. Guerin A, et al. Response to vaccination against tetanus in chronic haemodialysed patients. *Nephrol Dial Transplant* 1992;7:323–326.
52. Rautenberg P, et al. Influenza subtype-specific IgA, IgM and IgG responses in patients on hemodialysis after influenza vaccination. *Infection* 1988;16:323–328.
53. Kohler H, et al. Active hepatitis B vaccination of dialysis patients and medical staff. *Kidney Int* 1984;25:124–128.
54. Stevens CE, et al. Hepatitis B vaccine in patients receiving hemodialysis: immunogenicity and efficacy. *N Engl J Med* 1984;311:496–501.
55. Desombere I, et al. Response to hepatitis B vaccine: multiple HLA genes are involved. *Tissue Antigens* 1998;51:593–604.
56. Bach JF, et al. Letter: HL-A 1,8 phenotype and HBs antigenaemia in haemodialysis patients. *Lancet* 1975;ii:707.
57. Descamps B, et al. HLA-A1, B8-phenotype association and HBs antigenemia evolution in 440 hemodialyzed patients. *Digestion* 1977;15:271–277.
58. Alper CA, et al. Genetic prediction of nonresponse to hepatitis B vaccine. *N Engl J Med* 1989;321:708–712.
59. Varla-Leftherioti M, et al. HLA-associated non-responsiveness to hepatitis B vaccine. *Tissue Antigens* 1990;35:60–63.
60. Caillat-Zucman S, et al. HLA genetic heterogeneity of hepatitis B vaccine response in hemodialyzed patients. *Kidney Int* 1993;41[Suppl]:S157–S160.
61. Pol S, et al. Genetic basis of nonresponse to hepatitis B vaccine in hemodialyzed patients. *J Hepatol* 1990;11:385–387.
62. Grimm PC, et al. Effects of recombinant human erythropoietin on HLA sensitization and cell mediated immunity. *Kidney Int* 1990;38:12–18.
63. Paczek L, et al. Suppression of immunoglobulin and interleukin-6 production from peripheral blood mononuclear cells by dialysis membranes. *ASAIO Trans* 1990;36:459–461.
64. Sennesael JJ, et al. Treatment with recombinant human erythropoietin increases antibody titers after hepatitis B vaccination in dialysis patients. *Kidney Int* 1991;40:121–128.
65. Ruiz P, et al. Impaired function of macrophage Fc gamma receptors in end-stage renal disease. *N Engl J Med* 1990;322:717–722.
66. Carracedo J, et al. Role of adhesion molecules in mononuclear cell apoptosis induced by cuprophan hemodialysis membranes. *Nephron* 2001;89:186–193.
67. Carracedo J, et al. Cell apoptosis and hemodialysis-induced inflammation. *Kidney Int* 2002;61[Suppl 80]:89–93.
68. Kawanaka N, et al. Expression of Fc gamma receptor III (CD16) on monocytes during hemodialysis in patients with chronic renal failure. *Nephron* 2002;90:64–71.
69. Henderson LW, et al. Hemodialysis hypotension: the interleukin hypothesis. *Blood Purif* 1983;1:3–8.
70. Dinarello CA. Cytokines: agents provocateurs in hemodialysis? *Kidney Int* 1992;41:683–694.
71. Dinarello CA. Interleukin-18, a proinflammatory cytokine. *Eur Cytokine Netw* 2000;11:483–486.
72. Stuyt RJ, et al. Differential roles of interleukin-18 (IL-18) and IL12 for induction of gamma interferon by staphylococcal cell wall components and superantigens. *Infect Immunol* 2001;69:5025–5030.
73. Haeffner-Cavaillon N, et al. In vivo induction of interleukin-1 during hemodialysis. *Kidney Int* 1989;35:1212–1218.
74. Herbelin A, et al. Influence of first and long-term dialysis on uraemia-associated increased basal production of interleukin-1 and tumour necrosis factor alpha by circulating monocytes. *Nephrol Dial Transplant* 1991;6:349–357.
75. Roccatello D, et al. Induction of mRNA for tumor necrosis factor alpha in hemodialysis. *Kidney Int* 1993;39[Suppl]:S144–S148.
76. Pertosa G, et al. Influence of hemodialysis on interleukin-6 production and gene expression by peripheral blood mononuclear cells. *Kidney Int* 1993;39[Suppl]:S149–S153.
77. Herbelin A, et al. Influence of uremia and hemodialysis on circulating interleukin-1 and tumor necrosis factor alpha. *Kidney Int* 1990;37:116–125.
78. Herbelin A, et al. Elevated circulating levels of interleukin-6 in patients with chronic renal failure. *Kidney Int* 1991;39:954–960.
79. Dinarello CA. Interleukin-1 and tumor necrosis factor and their naturally occurring antagonists during hemodialysis. *Kidney Int* 1992;38[Suppl]:S68–S77.
80. Brockhaus M, et al. Plasma tumor necrosis factor soluble receptors in chronic renal failure. *Kidney Int* 1992;42:663–667.
81. Pereira BJ, et al. Plasma levels of IL-1 beta, TNF alpha and their specific inhibitors in undialyzed chronic renal failure, CAPD and hemodialysis patients. *Kidney Int* 1994;45:890–896.

82. Craddock PR, et al. Hemodialysis leukopenia: pulmonary vascular leukostasis resulting from complement activation by dialyzer cellophane membranes. *J Clin Invest* 1977;59:879–888.

83. Hakim RM, et al. Complement activation and hypersensitivity reactions to dialysis membranes. *N Engl J Med* 1984;311:878–882.

84. Vanholder R, et al. Phagocytosis in uremic and hemodialysis patients: a prospective and cross sectional study. *Kidney Int* 1991;39:320–327.

85. Vanholder R, et al. Contributing factors to the inhibition of phagocytosis in hemodialyzed patients. *Kidney Int* 1993;44:208–214.

86. Haag-Weber M, et al. Uremia and infection: mechanisms of impaired cellular host defense. *Nephron* 1993;63:125–131.

87. Lewis SL, et al. Alterations in chemotactic factor-induced responses of neutrophils and monocytes from chronic dialysis patients. *Clin Nephrol* 1988;30:63–72.

88. Haag-Weber M, et al. Effect of malnutrition and uremia on impaired cellular host defence. *Miner Electrolyte Metab* 1992;18:174–185.

89. Kalantar-Zadeh K, et al. Relative contributions of nutrition and inflammation to clinical outcome in dialysis patients. *Am J Kidney Dis* 2001;38:1343–1350.

90. Horl WH, et al. Physicochemical characterization of a polypeptide present in uremic serum that inhibits the biological activity of polymorphonuclear cells. *Proc Natl Acad Sci U S A* 1990;87:6353–6357.

91. Haag-Weber M, et al. Isolation of a granulocyte inhibitory protein from uraemic patients with homology of beta 2-microglobulin. *Nephrol Dial Transplant* 1994;9:382–388.

92. Tschesche H, et al. Inhibition of degranulation of polymorphonuclear leukocytes by angiogenin and its tryptic fragment. *J Biol Chem* 1994;269:30274–30280.

93. Nguyen AT, et al. Hemodialysis membrane-induced activation of phagocyte oxidative metabolism detected in vivo and in vitro within microamounts of whole blood. *Kidney Int* 1985;28:158–167.

94. Ritchey EE, et al. Chemiluminescence and superoxide anion production by leukocytes from chronic hemodialysis patients. *Kidney Int* 1981;19:349–358.

95. Horl WH, et al. Plasma levels of main granulocyte components in patients dialyzed with polycarbonate and cuprophan membranes. *Nephron* 1987;45:272–276.

96. Arnaout MA, et al. Increased expression of an adhesion-promoting surface glycoprotein in the granulocytopenia of hemodialysis. *N Engl J Med* 1985;312:457–462.

97. Himmelfarb J, et al. Modulation of granulocyte LAM-1 and MAC-1 during dialysis—a prospective, randomized controlled trial. *Kidney Int* 1992;41:388–395.

98. Tielemans CL, et al. Adhesion molecules and leukocyte common antigen on monocytes and granulocytes during hemodialysis. *Clin Nephrol* 1993;39:158–165.

99. Canaud B, et al. Imbalance of oxidants and antioxidants in haemodialysis patients. *Blood Purif* 1999;17:99–106.

100. Ceballos-Picot I, et al. Glutathione antioxidant system as a marker of oxidative stress in chronic renal failure. *Free Radic Biol Med* 1996;21:845–853.

101. Cristol JP, et al. Impairment of antioxidant defense mechanisms in elderly women without increase in oxidative stress markers: "a weak equilibrium." *Lipids* 1999;34[Suppl]:S289.

102. Witko-Sarsat V, et al. Advanced oxidation protein products as a novel marker of oxidative stress in uremia. *Kidney Int* 1996;49:1304–1313.

103. Descamps-Latscha B, et al. Importance of oxidatively modified proteins in chronic renal failure. *Kidney Int* 2001;78[Suppl]:S108–S113.

104. Himmelfarb J, et al. Albumin is the major plasma protein target of oxidant stress in uremia. *Kidney Int* 2001;60:358–363.

105. Miyata T, et al. Oxidation conspires with glycation to generate noxious advanced glycation end products in renal failure. *Nephrol Dial Transplant* 1997;12:255–258.

106. Miyata T, et al. Alterations in nonenzymatic biochemistry in uremia: origin and significance of "carbonyl stress" in long-term uremic complications. *Kidney Int* 1999;55:389–399.

107. Jaber BL, et al. Apoptosis of leukocytes: basic concepts and implications in uremia. *Kidney Int* 2001;78[Suppl]:S197–S205.

108. Nahar N, et al. Dialysis membrane-induced neutrophil apoptosis is mediated through free radicals. *Clin Nephrol* 2001;56:52–59.

109. Sarnak MJ, et al. Mortality caused by sepsis in patients with end-stage renal disease compared with the general population. *Kidney Int* 2000;58:1758–1764.

110. Marr KA. *Staphylococcus aureus* bacteremia in patients undergoing hemodialysis. *Semin Dial* 2000;13:23–29.

111. Dobkin JF, et al. Septicemia in patients on chronic hemodialysis. *Ann Intern Med* 1978;88:28–33.

112. Powe NR, et al. Septicemia in dialysis patients: incidence, risk factors, and prognosis. *Kidney Int* 1999;55:1081–1090.

113. Jaar BG, et al. Septicemia in diabetic hemodialysis patients: comparison of incidence, risk factors, and mortality with nondiabetic hemodialysis patients. *Am J Kidney Dis* 2000;35:282–292.

114. Marr KA, et al. Incidence and outcome of *Staphylococcus aureus* bacteremia in hemodialysis patients. *Kidney Int* 1998;54:1684–1689.

115. Hoen B, et al. EPIBACDIAL: a multicenter prospective study of risk factors for bacteremia in chronic hemodialysis patients. *J Am Soc Nephrol* 1998;9:869–876.

116. Kessler M, et al. Bacteremia in patients on chronic hemodialysis: a multicenter prospective survey. *Nephron* 1993;64:95–100.

117. Abbott KC, et al. Etiology of bacterial septicemia in chronic dialysis patients in the United States. *Clin Nephrol* 2001;56:124–31.

118. Kamaraju S, et al. *Staphylococcus lugdunensis* pulmonary valve endocarditis in a patient on chronic hemodialysis. *Am J Nephrol* 1999;19:605–608.

119. Kirmani N, et al. *Staphylococcus aureus* carriage rate of patients receiving long-term hemodialysis. *Arch Intern Med* 1978;138:1657–1659.

120. Yu VL, et al. *Staphylococcus aureus* nasal carriage and infection in patients on hemodialysis: efficacy of antibiotic prophylaxis. *N Engl J Med* 1986;315:91–96.

121. Khan IH, et al. Long-term complications of dialysis: infection. *Kidney Int* 1993;41[Suppl]:S143–S148.

122. Mathews M, et al. Septic arthritis in hemodialyzed patients. *Nephron* 1980;25:87–91.

123. Leonard A, et al. Bacterial endocarditis in regularly dialyzed patients. *Kidney Int* 1973;4:407–422.

124. Boelaert JR, et al. *Staphylococcus aureus* infections in haemodialysis patients: pathophysiology and use of nasal mupirocin for prevention. *J Chemother* 1995;7[Suppl 3]:49–53.

125. Perl TM, et al. Intranasal mupirocin to prevent postoperative *Staphylococcus aureus* infections. *N Engl J Med* 2002;346:1871–1877.

126. Welch PG, et al. Safety and immunogenicity of *Staphylococcus aureus* type 5 capsular polysaccharide-Pseudomonas aeruginosa recombinant exoprotein A conjugate vaccine in patients on hemodialysis. *J Am Soc Nephrol* 1996;7:247–253.

127. Finkelstein ES, et al. Patterns of infection in patients maintained on long-term peritoneal dialysis therapy with multiple episodes of peritonitis. *Am J Kidney Dis* 2002;39:1278–1286.

128. Saitoh H, et al. Urinary tract infection in oliguric patients with chronic renal failure. *J Urol* 1985;133:990–993.

129. Haubitz M, et al. C-reactive protein and chronic *Chlamydia pneumoniae* infection—long-term predictors for cardiovascular disease and survival in patients on peritoneal dialysis. *Nephrol Dial Transplant* 2001;16:809–815.

130. Danesh J, et al. Chronic infections and coronary heart disease: is there a link? *Lancet* 1997;350:430–436.

131. Zoccali C, et al. Atherosclerosis in dialysis patients: does *Chlamydia pneumoniae* infection contribute to cardiovascular damage? *Nephrol Dial Transplant* 2002;17:25–28.

132. Churchill DN, et al. Canadian Hemodialysis Morbidity Study. *Am J Kidney Dis* 1992;19:214–234.

133. Schwab SJ, et al. The hemodialysis catheter conundrum: hate living with them, but can't live without them. *Kidney Int* 1999;56:1–17.

134. Schwab SJ, et al. Vascular access for hemodialysis. *Kidney Int* 1999;55:2078–2090.

135. Nassar GM, et al. Occult infection of old nonfunctioning arteriovenous grafts: a novel cause of erythropoietin resistance and chronic inflammation in hemodialysis patients. *Kidney Int* 2002;61[Suppl 80]:49–54.

136. Selan L, et al. Diagnosis of vascular graft infections with antibodies against staphylococcal slime antigens. *Lancet* 2002;359:2166–2168.

137. Rinehart A, et al. Host defenses and infectious complications in maintenance hemodialysis patients. In: Jacobs CMKC, et al., eds. *Replacement of renal function by dialysis,* 4th ed. Boston: Kluwer Academic, 1996.

138. Marr KA, et al. Catheter-related bacteremia and outcome of attempted catheter salvage in patients undergoing hemodialysis. *Ann Intern Med* 1997;127:275–280.

139. Nielsen J, et al. Dialysis catheter-related septicaemia—focus on *Staphylococcus aureus* septicaemia. *Nephrol Dial Transplant* 1998;13:2847–2852.

140. Keane WF, et al. Incidence and type of infections occurring in 445 chronic hemodialysis patients. *Trans Am Soc Artif Intern Organs* 1977;23:41–47.

141. Kaplowitz LG, et al. A prospective study of infections in hemodialysis patients: patient hygiene and other risk factors for infection. *Infect Control Hosp Epidemiol* 1988;9:534–541.

142. Hussein M, et al. Tuberculosis and chronic renal disease. *Saudi J Kidney Dis Transplant* 2002;13:320–330.

143. Pradhan RP, et al. Tuberculosis in dialyzed patients. *JAMA* 1974;229:798–800.

144. Lundin AP, et al. Tuberculosis in patients undergoing maintenance hemodialysis. *Am J Med* 1979;67:597–602.

145. Papadimitriou M, et al. Tuberculosis in patients on regular haemodialysis. *Nephron* 1979;24:53–57.

146. Sasaki S, et al. Ten years' survey of dialysis-associated tuberculosis. *Nephron* 1979;24:141–145.

147. Rutsky EA, et al. Mycobacteriosis in patients with chronic renal failure. *Arch Intern Med* 1980;140:57–61.

148. Andrew OT, et al. Tuberculosis in patients with end-stage renal disease. *Am J Med* 1980;68:59–65.

149. Belcon MC, et al. Tuberculosis in dialysis patients. *Clin Nephrol* 1982;17:14–18.

150. Hachicha J, et al. High incidence of tuberculosis in chronic dialysis patients in developing countries. *Nephron* 1989;52:189.

151. Simon TA, et al. Tuberculosis in hemodialysis patients in New Jersey: a statewide study. *Infect Control Hosp Epidemiol* 1999;20:607–609.

152. Chou KJ, et al. Tuberculosis in maintenance dialysis patients. *Nephron* 2001;88:138–143.

153. Taskapan H, et al. The outcome of tuberculosis in patients on chronic hemodialysis. *Clin Nephrol* 2000;54:134–137.

154. Vachharajani T, et al. Diagnosis and treatment of tuberculosis in hemodialysis and renal transplant patients. *Am J Nephrol* 2000;20:273–277.

155. Talwani R, et al. Tuberculous peritonitis in patients undergoing continuous ambulatory peritoneal dialysis: case report and review. *Clin Infect Dis* 2000;31:70–75.

156. Kaul KL. Molecular detection of *Mycobacterium tuberculosis*: impact on patient care. *Clin Chem* 2001;47:1553–1558.

157. Nagesh BS, et al. Evaluation of polymerase chain reaction for detection of *Mycobacterium tuberculosis* in pleural fluid. *Chest* 2001;119:1737–1741.

158. Coskun M, et al. Thoracic CT findings in long-term hemodialysis patients. *Acta Radiol* 1999;40:181–186.

159. Kalweit WH, et al. Hemodialysis fistula infections caused by *Legionella pneumophila. Ann Intern Med* 1982;96:173–175.

160. Goldman M, et al. Bacterial infections in chronic hemodialysis patients: epidemiologic and pathophysiologic aspects. *Adv Nephrol Necker Hosp* 1990;19:315–332.

161. Zeitlin J, et al. Graft infection and bacteremia with *Listeria monocytogenes* in a patient receiving hemodialysis. *Arch Intern Med* 1982;142:2191–2192.

162. Mossey RT, et al. Listeriosis in patients with long-term hemodialysis and transfusional iron overload. *Am J Med* 1985;79:397–400.

163. Van Cutsem J, et al. Effects of deferoxamine, feroxamine and iron on experimental mucormycosis (zygomycosis). *Kidney Int* 1989;36:1061–1068.

164. Leung AC, et al. *Clostridium difficile*-associated colitis in uremic patients. *Clin Nephrol* 1985;24:242–248.

165. Aronsson B, et al. *Clostridium difficile*-associated diarrhoea in uremic patients. *Eur J Clin Microbiol* 1987;6:352–356.

166. Barany P, et al. *Clostridium difficile* infection—a poor prognostic sign in uremic patients? *Clin Nephrol* 1992;38:53–57.

167. Degos F, et al. Viral infections in dialysis patients: dialysis-associated hepatitis. In: Jacobs CMKC, et al., eds. *Replacement of renal function by dialysis,* 4th ed. Boston: Kluwer Academic, 1996.

168. Rawer P, et al. Seroconversion rate, hepatitis B vaccination, hemodialysis, and zinc supplementation. *Kidney Int* 1987;22[Suppl]:149–152.

169. Migneco G, et al. [Serum zinc concentration and antibody response to hepatitis B vaccine in hemodialysis patients.] *Minerva Med* 1990;81:19–21.

170. Kouw PM, et al. Effects of zinc supplementation on zinc status and immunity in haemodialysis patients. *J Trace Elem Electrolytes Health Dis* 1991;5:115–119.

171. Donati D, et al. Controlled trial of thymopentin in hemodialysis patients who fail to respond to hepatitis B vaccination. *Nephron* 1988;50:133–136.

172. Dumann H, et al. Influence of thymopentin on antibody response, and monocyte and T cell function in hemodialysis patients who fail to respond to hepatitis B vaccination. *Nephron* 1990;55:136–140.

173. Palestini M, et al. [Brief treatment with thymopentin as adjuvant in vaccination for hepatitis B: controlled study in patients on periodic hemodialysis.] *Riv Eur Sci Med Farmacol* 1990;12:135–139.

174. Quiroga JA, et al. Recombinant gamma-interferon as adjuvant to hepatitis B vaccine in hemodialysis patients. *Hepatology* 1990;12:661–663.

175. Meuer SC, et al. Low-dose interleukin-2 induces systemic immune responses against HBsAg in immunodeficient non-responders to hepatitis B vaccination. *Lancet* 1989;i:15–18.

176. Jungers P, et al. Randomised placebo-controlled trial of recombinant interleukin-2 in chronic uraemic patients who are non-responders to hepatitis B vaccine. *Lancet* 1994;344:856–857.

177. Anandh U, et al. Granulocyte-macrophage colony-stimulating factor as an adjuvant to hepatitis B vaccination in maintenance hemodialysis patients. *Am J Nephrol* 2000;20:53–56.

178. Jungers P, et al. Detrimental effects of late referral in patients with chronic renal failure: a case-control study. *Kidney Int* 1993;41[Suppl]:S170–S173.

179. Pereira BJ. Optimization of pre-ESRD care: the key to improved dialysis outcomes. *Kidney Int* 2000;57:351–365.

180. Garson JA, et al. Detection of hepatitis C viral sequences in blood donations by "nested" polymerase chain reaction and prediction of infectivity. *Lancet* 1990;335:1419–1422.

181. Van der Poel CL, et al. Confirmation of hepatitis C virus infection by new four-antigen recombinant immunoblot assay. *Lancet* 1991;337:317–319.

182. Jadoul M, et al. Incidence and risk factors for hepatitis C seroconversion in hemodialysis: a prospective study. The UCL Collaborative Group. *Kidney Int* 1993;44:1322–1326.

183. Espinosa M, et al. Risk of death and liver cirrhosis in anti-HCV-positive long-term haemodialysis patients. *Nephrol Dial Transplant* 2001;16:1669–1674.

184. Pereira BJ, et al. Effects of hepatitis C infection and renal transplantation on survival in end-stage renal disease. The New England Organ Bank Hepatitis C Study Group. *Kidney Int* 1998;53:1374–1381.

185. Collins AJ, et al. United States Renal Data System assessment of the impact of the National Kidney Foundation-Dialysis Outcomes Quality Initiative guidelines. *Am J Kidney Dis* 2002;39:784–795.

186. Hoen B, et al. Risk factors for bacterial infections in chronic haemodialysis adult patients: a multicentre prospective survey. *Nephrol Dial Transplant* 1995;10:377–381.

187. Quarles LD, et al. *Staphylococcus aureus* bacteremia in patients on chronic hemodialysis. *Am J Kidney Dis* 1985;6:412–419.

188. Boelaert JR, et al. Iron overload in haemodialysis patients increases the risk of bacteraemia: a prospective study. *Nephrol Dial Transplant* 1990;5:130–134.

189. Tielemans CL, et al. Critical role of iron overload in the increased susceptibility of haemodialysis patients to bacterial infections: beneficial effects of desferrioxamine. *Nephrol Dial Transplant* 1989;4:883–887.

HEPATITIS AND HUMAN IMMUNODEFICIENCY VIRUS INFECTIONS IN END-STAGE RENAL DISEASE PATIENTS

SVETLOZAR N. NATOV, B.V.R. MURTHY, AND BRIAN J.G. PEREIRA

Patients on chronic dialysis are at increased risk of acquiring parenterally transmitted viruses such as hepatitis viruses and human immunodeficiency virus (HIV) infection from blood product transfusions or nosocomial transmission in hemodialysis units (1,2). Liver function abnormalities are seen in 10% to 44% of patients on chronic hemodialysis (1). In the past, hepatitis B virus (HBV) was the major cause of parenterally transmitted viral hepatitis in dialysis patients, and the remaining cases were attributed to non-A, non-B hepatitis (NANBH). The discovery of new parenterally transmitted hepatitis viruses such as hepatitis C virus (HCV) and GB virus (GBV)/hepatitis G virus (HGV) has shed light on the cause and clinical course of NANBH in patients on dialysis. Among dialysis patients, serum markers of HBV, HCV, and GBV/HGV have been reported in 0.3% to 25.9%, 3.3% to 59%, and 3.1% to 55%, respectively (3–5).

The clinical consequences of parenterally transmitted viral hepatitides acquired during dialysis are especially manifest after renal transplantation (6). Liver disease has been reported in 7% to 24% of transplant recipients, and liver failure is the cause of death in 8% to 28% of long-term survivors after renal transplantation (1). Patients with pretransplantation HBV or HCV infection are at increased risk of liver disease and death after transplantation. The advent of blood product screening for hepatitis B surface antigen (HBsAg) and anti-HCV has virtually eliminated the transmission of HBV and HCV infection by blood product transfusions (7). Consequently, the current debate is focused on other strategies to reduce the transmission of viral hepatitis among dialysis patients and to lessen the consequences of liver disease among patients already infected (1).

The prevalence of HIV infection among dialysis patients is also high. HIV infection has been reported in 0.3% to 38% of dialysis patients, but for a number of reasons, which will be discussed later, the reported prevalence underestimates the true prevalence (8). As in the case of viral hepatitides, strategies to reduce the transmission of HIV infection among dialysis patients and postexposure prophylaxis (PEP) among staff and patients accidentally exposed to the virus are a major cause for concern.

The modes of transmission of HBV in dialysis units and strategies for control have been extensively reviewed (9). On the other hand, information on the transmission and clinical consequences of GBV/HGV is as yet incomplete. Therefore, this review primarily focuses on prevention and treatment of HCV infection and strategies to control transmission of HIV infection in dialysis units.

HEPATITIS C VIRUS (HCV)

In 1989, HCV was cloned and identified as the major cause of parenterally transmitted NANBH (10,11). At present, HCV is the most common chronic bloodborne infection in the United States. The transmission of HCV by transfusion of blood products and by sharing of needles among intravenous drug abusers has been unequivocally demonstrated (12–14). Other modes of transmission are also possible. Horizontal transmission by sexual and/or household exposure and vertical transmission from mother to fetus have been implicated (1,15,16). HCV can also be transmitted with organ and tissue transplantation (17,18).

Since the cloning of the virus, numerous tests have been developed to detect antibodies to multiple HCV antigens (anti-HCV), to detect the presence of HCV ribonucleic acid (RNA), and to quantitate viral titers (11,19,20). These advances in the development of diagnostic tools for HCV enabled the study of the prevalence, transmission, and natural course of HCV infection in patients with end-stage renal disease (ESRD) (1).

HCV Genome

The HCV genome is illustrated in Fig. 22.1. HCV is a small (40 to 60 nm) spherical virus, which belongs to the Flaviviridae family (10,21). It has a lipid envelope and a single-stranded RNA viral genome of approximately 9,400 nucleotides. The N-termi-

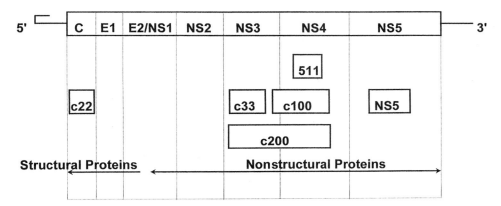

FIG. 22.1. Schematic representation of hepatitis C virus (HCV) genome. Boxes represent antigens used in anti-HCV test systems. C, core; E, envelope; NS, nonstructural. (From Pereira BJG, et al. Hepatitis C virus infection in dialysis and renal transplantation. *Kidney Int* 1997;51:981–999, with permission.)

nus encodes the basic nucleocapsid (C), followed by two glyco-protein domains, the envelope (E1), and second envelope/non-structural-1 (E2/NS1) regions (21).

Downstream to this region are the nonstructural genes NS2, NS3, NS4, and NS5. Significant genetic heterogeneity is present over the entire viral genome (22–24). The regions encoding the E1 and E2/NS1 are the most variable sequences, and the 5′ noncoding region (5′NCR) represents the most conserved one (1). Sequence analysis of the viral genome has identified a number of distinct HCV variants. The universal system for the classification and nomenclature of hepatitis C viral genotypes recognizes six major groups, designated as HCV *types* 1 through 6 with mean sequence homology of 65% (range from 55% to 72%) (25). Each major type consists of one or more closely related variants with mean sequence homology of 80% (range from 75% to 86%), which are designated as *subtypes* and named *a, b, c,* and so on, in order of discovery. Furthermore, each subtype may consist of individual isolates sharing sequence homology of 88%.

Tests for HCV RNA

Polymerase Chain Reaction and Branched-chain DNA Technology

The detection of HCV RNA by reverse transcriptase polymerase chain reaction (PCR) has been the gold standard to identify current HCV infection (1). Because the nucleotide sequence of the highly conserved 5′ end is shared by most HCV strains, "universal" primers directed to this region are used to identify the presence or absence of the virus. In patients with posttransfusion NANBH, high levels of HCV RNA are detected in the circulation within a week and before the appearance of anti-HCV or elevations in serum alanine aminotransferase (ALT) levels (12,19). There are two types of test for HCV RNA presently available–qualitative and quantitative assays:

- Qualitative PCR assays–The qualitative PCR assays report the results as presence or absence of HCV RNA. These assays

are considered the most sensitive tests for the diagnosis of HCV infection. However, they are not intended to be used as screening tests for detection of HCV infection (26). The reliability of these tests might be limited by false-positive and negative results. Because PCR can detect very low levels of HCV RNA (27,28), even minor contamination can give false-positive results (29). On the other hand, false-negative results may be due to imperfect handling and/or storage of blood samples causing a failure to detect HCV RNA in up to 40% of samples (30). Whole blood anticoagulated with eth-ylenediaminetetraacetic acid (EDTA) or with mixed anticoagulants [citrate phosphate dextrose adenine (CPDA-1) and EDTA] may be stored at up to 25°C (room temperature) for up to 5 days without any significant loss in plasma HCV RNA (31).

- Quantitative assays for HCV RNA–These tests measure HCV RNA titers. The results are usually expressed in number of HCV RNA copies per milliliter of serum. Two different types of tests have been developed: quantitative reverse transcriptase PCR (RT-PCR) assays and branched-chain deoxyribonucleic acid (bDNA) assays. Several commercial quantitative HCV RNA assays are presently available. The lower limit of detection for currently used bDNA assays is 200,000 RNA genome equivalents/mL, and the lower limit of detection for the RT-PCR method is fewer than 100 RNA genome equivalents/mL. Thus, theoretically, the quantitative RT-PCR assay is three orders of magnitude more sensitive than the bDNA assay (28).

Significant shortcomings of the PCR assays are their labor-intensive performance, lack of standardization, and wide variations in sensitivity and specificity. By comparison, the bDNA assays are automated, simpler to perform, and more reproducible but less sensitive than the quantitative PCR tests. In clinical practice, quantitative tests for HCV RNA should not be used as an initial diagnostic tool for HCV infection but should be reserved for pretreatment evaluation and monitoring patient response to antiviral therapies. Because of the great variability in sensitivity and lack of standardization across assays and laboratories, when a patient is tested repeatedly, particularly during monitoring the response to antiviral treatment, it is critical to use the same test and the same laboratory where previous testing was performed.

Tests for Genotypes

The universal system for classification and nomenclature of HCV genotypes is based on nucleotide sequence comparisons of the NS5 region (25). Although numerous tests can be used for HCV genotyping, the nucleic acid sequencing of the NS5 region is generally considered to be the gold standard for HCV genotyping. Other practical methods that can be used to identify HCV genotypes include PCR using subtype specific primers, restriction fragment length polymorphism (RFLP) analysis, cleavage fragment length polymorphism (CFLP) technology, and line probe assay (28). In addition, an enzyme-linked immunosorbent assay (ELISA) that detects antibodies to serotype-specific immunodominant epitopes from the NS4 region of the HCV genome and novel recombinant immunoblot assays (RIBAs) have been developed (32–34). HCV genotyping is mostly used as a tool for research or epidemiologic investigations tracing the source of infection. HCV genotype testing is unnecessary for the diagnosis of HCV infection but may potentially be useful in clinical practice to assist in tailoring antiviral therapy to the individual patient's HCV genotype.

Tests for Antibody to HCV (Anti-HCV)

Tests for anti-HCV are the mainstay of the diagnosis of HCV infection (1). ELISA and RIBA have been used to detect nonneutralizing antibodies. ELISA detects antibodies to specific HCV antigens in a standard ELISA plate; RIBA detects antibodies to HCV antigens on a strip that is read visually. ELISAs have been used as screening tests, whereas RIBAs have been considered confirmatory tests by virtue of their increased specificity.

The first-generation tests (ELISA1, RIBA1, which are now obsolete) detected nonneutralizing antibody to the C100-3 (and 5-1-1) protein(s) encoded by the NS3/NS4 region of the HCV prototype isolate (i.e., HCV genotype 1a) (Fig. 22.1). Because there is a substantial heterogeneity in C100-3 sequences of different genotypes, the performance of these anti-HCV tests was compromised by marked genotype dependence (32). In addition, there is a significant delay in antibody production to C100-3 antigen in response to HCV infection. This early stage in HCV infection, when HCV RNA is present but antibody response is not yet manifest, is defined as the "window" period (12) and, with the use of these tests, was reported to have a mean duration of 16 weeks but in some cases could be as long as 1 year (1).

The second-generation tests (ELISA1, RIBA1) incorporate c22 antigen from the nucleocapsid region and c200, which is a composite of c33 and c100-3 antigens from the NS3/NS4 region. RIBA2 uses four recombinant HCV antigens (c22, c33, c100, and 5-1-1). The use of an increased number of incorporated antigens with highly conserved protein sequences (negating any genotype dependence of the assay) coupled with a faster antibody response to c22 or c33 proteins, which can occur as

early as 4 weeks after exposure (35) and precedes the production of antibodies to c100-3 by at least 1 month (36), has contributed to the improved performance of these tests.

The third-generation anti-HCV tests are currently largely in use. They have demonstrated further improvement in sensitivity as a result of an additional recombinant antigen from the NS5 region of the HCV genome incorporated uniquely in these assays, an improved c33 antigen corresponding to the NS3 region, and even shorter window period (estimated at a mean of 70 days) (37,38,39).

Tests for Hepatitis C Core Antigen

Recently, new tests have been developed to detect the presence of viral antigenemia using a monoclonal antibody to the HCV core antigen (HCVcAg) (40–43). A commercial ELISA test for "free" HCVcAg is now available in some countries (43). Other tests that detect "total" HCVcAg, both free and complexed with anti-HCV antibody, are presently undergoing evaluation (42,43). Preliminary results have shown that assays for HCVcAg demonstrate excellent correlation with virologic tests for HCV RNA and make it possible to detect HCV infection before anti-HCV seroconversion, confirm anti-HCV positive status, assess patient infectivity, depict those anti-HCV patients who are most likely to be viremic, and monitor the dynamics of the infection and the therapeutic response in individuals receiving antiviral treatments (41–43). In addition, HCVcAg is a stable substance in contrast to HCV RNA, and extra precautions for handling and storage of blood specimens are expected to prove unnecessary (40). Overall, these tests seem to be a viable alternative to HCV RNA testing and are promising to find a large clinical application.

Difficulties in Interpreting Tests for HCV Infection

Anti-HCV-positive, but HCV RNA-negative Patients

The anti-HCV tests that are currently licensed for clinical use detect nonneutralizing antibodies to recombinant HCV antigens (1). Thus, the presence of anti-HCV does not necessarily imply the presence of HCV RNA in the serum. Indeed, HCV RNA has been detected in only 52% to 93% of dialysis patients with anti-HCV (44,45). However, there is some evidence to suggest that the presence of IgM anti-HCV may serve as a complementary marker of viral replication (46).

Several possibilities could account for the presence of anti-HCV in the absence of HCV RNA:

1. HCV may be sequestered at sites other than the bloodstream, such as the liver or peripheral blood mononuclear cells (PBMCs) (44,47).
2. Viremia could be intermittent and, therefore, HCV RNA may not be present in the plasma at the time of testing (12). Fluctuating viremia with virus-free intervals has been observed in 35% of HCV-infected dialysis patients (48).
3. The number of copies of HCV RNA may be below the limit of detection (49).

4. Antibodies to HCV may persist even after the viral RNA has disappeared. In this situation, anti-HCV-positive but HCV RNA-negative patients might represent a group that had been infected with the virus but no longer harbors it, and for this reason is no longer infective.

5. Anti-HCV may have been passively acquired from blood transfusions. In this situation, anti-HCV would disappear over the next few weeks in keeping with the half-life of IgG.

6. False-positive results can occur from nonspecific reactions, a problem that has been largely overcome with the current tests.

Anti-HCV-negative, but HCV RNA-positive Patients

More than 90% of nonimmunosuppressed individuals with HCV infection test positive for anti-HCV (50). Possible explanations for the presence of HCV RNA in the absence of anti-HCV include the following (1):

1. The anti-HCV test may not be sensitive enough to detect existing anti-HCV antibodies, either because of the low titer of antibody or because the antigen used in the assay system cannot detect the serum antibody response to the particular genotype. As an example, the first-generation anti-HCV tests demonstrated major genotype dependence, which significantly limited their performance (32).

2. Various diseases or pharmacologic immunosuppression could suppress or modify the anti-HCV response. Indeed, only 83% of HCV RNA-positive dialysis patients test positive for anti-HCV, and 2.5% to 12% of anti-HCV-negative dialysis patients test positive for HCV RNA (1). Of note, in an area endemic of HCV infection (Saudi Arabia), as high as 28% of the hemodialysis patients who were anti-HCV negative by third-generation ELISA tested positive for HCV RNA (51).

3. The patient may be in the window period between the time of acquiring the infection and the time of anti-HCV seroconversion.

4. After anti-HCV antibody has persisted for a certain period of time, it can disappear, despite the persistence of HCV RNA.

In addition to the previous possibilities, HCV RNA has been detected in the PBMCs from hemodialysis patients without anti-HCV or HCV RNA in the serum (52). The HCV RNA in these PBMC could serve as a viral reservoir and further frustrate efforts to identify HCV infection in hemodialysis patients.

Clinical Features of HCV Infection

Clinical Course

The incubation period of HCV is 15 to 150 days (mean 50 days). Acute infection typically remains asymptomatic or presents with only mild clinical symptoms. However, although rare, fatal cases of fulminant and subacute liver failure have been reported. Among patients with posttransfusion hepatitis C, HCV RNA is detected in the serum within 1 to 3 weeks after exposure, followed by elevated serum ALT levels several weeks later (12). Seroconversion for anti-HCV begins at 4 weeks but can take as long as 1 year (35). Anti-HCV antibodies usually persist indefinitely or at least over a long period (50, 53–56). Among patients with posttransfusion HCV infection, 50% have self-limited disease. The other 50% demonstrate persistently elevated serum ALT levels and develop chronic hepatitis C. If a chronic HCV carrier state is established, HCV RNA levels are usually sustained in serum over the time (57). Of those who undergo liver biopsy, 60% have chronic active hepatitis, and 10% to 20% have cirrhosis (58). Some of these patients progress to develop hepatocellular carcinoma (59).

The progression of liver disease is slow, and mortality among patients with posttransfusion NANBH followed for almost two decades was not significantly higher than that among patients without posttransfusion NANBH (60). However, a longer follow-up period might reveal a difference in the mortality between these two groups. Indeed, Kiyosawa et al. (59) have reported that the interval between the initial presentation and the onset of chronic hepatitis, cirrhosis, and hepatocellular carcinoma in patients with posttransfusion NANBH is 10, 21, and 29 years, respectively.

The natural history of acute HCV infection in patients on maintenance dialysis has not been well described. A recent prospective study of 19 dialysis patients with acute infection found that after a median follow-up of 3 years, nearly 80% of the patients remained viremic; 60% had increased transaminase levels and positive HCV RNA tests, with five patients exhibiting chronic active hepatitis on liver biopsy; and only four patients (21%) cleared the viral infection (61).

Relationship among Serum ALT Levels, HCV Infection, and Liver Disease

Serum ALT levels are a poor predictor of HCV-induced liver disease among patients on chronic hemodialysis. Indeed, among hemodialysis patients, serum ALT levels are elevated in only 4% to 67% of patients with anti-HCV, only 12% to 31% of patients with HCV RNA, and only one third of those with biopsy-proven hepatitis (1). There are several reasons for the discrepancy between serum ALT levels and the presence of anti-HCV (1):

1. Chronic hepatitis C characteristically has a fluctuating course with multiple peaks and troughs in ALT levels, which are usually within normal range. Consequently, patients with normal ALT levels may have advanced liver disease with severe histologic lesions.

2. HCV infection is not always associated with chronic liver disease. In fact, only 69% of anti-HCV-positive symptom-free blood donors who underwent liver biopsy had histologic evidence of chronic hepatitis, all of whom had HCV RNA in the serum (62). Therefore, it is likely that a healthy carrier state with no apparent liver damage can exist. In these cases, viral replication probably occurs at extrahepatic sites.

3. As discussed earlier, some anti-HCV-positive patients may have cleared the infection and anti-HCV may be the remnant of past infection.

4. Baseline ALT levels are depressed in patients on dialysis (63). Interestingly, elevated ALT levels have also been observed in 4% to 23% of anti-HCV-negative dialysis patients (1).

These patients could be carriers of HCV infection in whom anti-HCV production is absent, or the liver disease might be due to a non-A, non-B virus other than HCV or nonviral causes. Consequently, liver biopsy remains the only reliable method of confirming the presence and assessing the severity of liver disease in patients with HCV infection. This is particularly true for patients who are being considered for renal transplantation, because liver histology at the time of initial presentation has been shown to be a good predictor of intermediate and long-term outcomes after renal transplantation (64). Over a mean follow-up of 6 years, progression to liver failure and death was rare in transplant recipients with mild histologic abnormalities such as fat metamorphosis or chronic persistent hepatitis (64). In contrast, 35% of recipients with early chronic active hepatitis and 60% of recipients with advanced chronic active hepatitis progressed to liver failure and death (64).

Immunity

Humans exposed to HCV respond with production of antibodies targeted at multiple regions of the HCV genome. The majority of these antibodies are nonneutralizing and hence do not provide protective immunity. Although neutralizing antibodies to the envelope regions of HCV have recently been characterized, their role in protective immunity has not been demonstrated (65). Thus, in most cases of HCV infection, the immune responses fail to control the infection, which results in the development of a chronic carrier state. Indeed, studies in humans and animals with HCV infection have well documented lack of protective immunity and development of reinfection (new infection after the previous infection has cleared) with the same or different genotype (66,67) or superinfection (infection with a new genotype in the presence of preexisting infection) (68). The newly introduced HCV genotype may either replace ("take over" phenomenon), be eliminated, or coexist with the predecessor HCV genotype (68–71). The clinical implications of each of these virologic outcomes are currently unclear.

Prevalence of HCV Infection and Risk Factors for Infection in Dialysis Patients

Prevalence

The prevalence of anti-HCV among patients on dialysis is consistently higher than in healthy populations. Using ELISA1, the prevalence of anti-HCV among dialysis patients ranged from 8% to 36% in North America, 39% in South America, 1% to 54% in Europe, 17% to 51% in Asia, and 1.2% to 10% in New Zealand and Australia (1). The advent of second-generation tests has revealed an even higher prevalence of anti-HCV in dialysis patients (1). Pooled data from studies in which dialysis patients were tested by both ELISA1 and ELISA2 revealed that ELISA2 identified more than twice the number of patients who had tested positive by ELISA1 (72). The prevalence of anti-HCV antibodies among dialysis patients with the use of the second-generation anti-HCV tests has been reported to range between 10% to 36% in the United States, 2% to 63% in Europe, and 22% to 55.5% in Asia (1,73,74).

The third-generation anti-HCV tests have shown better sensitivity and specificity in patients receiving renal replacement therapy than the previous two generations of anti-HCV tests (38,39). In different studies, the prevalence of anti-HCV antibodies among dialysis patients by third-generation anti-HCV tests runs between 13.5% to 28% in Italy (39,75), 19% in the United States (76,77), 42% in France (53), 49% in Syria (78), and as high as 75% in Moldavia (79).

In addition to the wide range in the prevalence of HCV infection among different countries, there is also a wide variation in the prevalence of HCV infection among dialysis units within a single country. As an example, in the United States, the prevalence of anti-HCV by ELISA2 among the 61,400 patients from dialysis centers participating in the National Surveillance of Dialysis Associated Diseases in the United States in 1995 was 10.4%, with a range of 0% to 64% among centers with at least 40 patients (74). In 2000, the prevalence of anti-HCV among the 135,599 tested hemodialysis patients was 8.4% and ranged from 4.7% to 11.9% among the 12 ESRD networks in the United States, each of which represents different geographic areas of the country (80). Likewise, the prevalence of HCV infection among hemodialysis units in Portugal ranged from 0% to 75.5%, being lowest in the northern regions of the country and particularly high in the south and central regions (81). Within Saudi Arabia, the prevalence of anti-HCV among hemodialysis units varied between 15.4% to 94.7% (82).

Trends

The incidence and prevalence of HCV infection among patients on dialysis is steadily declining. Among member nations in the European Dialysis and Transplant Association, the prevalence of anti-HCV declined from 21% in 1992 to 17.7% in 1993 (4,83). Likewise, among hemodialysis units in Portugal, the incidence of HCV infection declined from 11.2% in 1991, to 7.2% in 1992, and to 6.5% in 1993 (81). Among hemodialysis patients in the United States, the incidence of NANBH (mainly caused by HCV) declined from 1.7% in 1982 to 0.2% in 1997 (84). The incidence rate of anti-HCV in 2000 was 0.27% (80).

The initial decline in the incidence of HCV infection among dialysis patients could be attributed to a reduction in posttransfusion HCV infection following the implementation of routine anti-HCV screening of blood donors and the introduction of erythropoietin therapy, which significantly decreased the blood transfusion requirements of ESRD patients. However, as discussed later, the subsequent decline in the incidence of HCV infection probably resulted from the implementation of infection-control measures to prevent nosocomial transmission of bloodborne infections within dialysis units.

In contrast to the decrease in the incidence, the prevalence of anti-HCV among hemodialysis patients in the United States has remained relatively stable over the last few years. Indeed, for the years 1992 through 2000, the prevalence of anti-HCV among tested patients varied only slightly between 8.1% and 8.4% (with a peak at 10.5% in 1994) (80). This fact, together with the reported incidence of anti-HCV as high as 15% in some hemodialysis units, testifies that HCV infection among dialysis patients remains an unresolved problem (1).

Risk Factors

The high incidence and prevalence of anti-HCV among patients on dialysis can be attributed to several risk factors.

Number of Blood Transfusions

Several studies in patients on dialysis before the advent of blood product screening for anti-HCV have shown that anti-HCV-positive hemodialysis patients had received significantly more units of blood products than anti-HCV-negative patients (1,85). Further, the prevalence of anti-HCV among hemodialysis patients is directly related to the number of blood transfusions received (Fig. 22.2).

Since the advent of screening of blood products for anti-HCV, the risk of acquiring posttransfusion HCV infection has declined to less than 1 per 103,000 units of blood products transfused (7), so future studies may not show the same association between anti-HCV and the number of blood products transfused.

Duration of ESRD

Several studies have shown that the interval since beginning dialysis was significantly longer among anti-HCV-positive patients compared with anti-HCV-negative patients (1). The risk of acquiring HCV infection increases significantly after a decade of hemodialysis treatment (86) and has been estimated at 10% per year on hemodialysis (87). In addition, the prevalence of anti-HCV has shown a stronger correlation with the duration of hemodialysis than with the number of units of blood transfused. Thus, duration of dialysis has emerged as an independent risk factor for HCV infection (88,89). Consequently, the risk of HCV infection is directly related to the interval since beginning dialysis (Fig. 22.3).

Mode of Dialysis

Centers that compared the prevalence of anti-HCV in peritoneal dialysis (PD) and hemodialysis patients have observed a consistently lower prevalence of anti-HCV among PD patients (Fig. 22.4) (90–100). In a group of 129 anti-HCV-negative patients on chronic dialysis, the rate of seroconversion was 0.15 per patient year on hemodialysis, compared with 0.03 per patient-year on continuous ambulatory peritoneal dialysis (CAPD) (99). Furthermore, most anti-HCV-positive CAPD patients may have acquired HCV infection while on hemodialysis. Huang et al. (93) reported a 15.4% prevalence of anti-HCV among PD patients, but when patients with prior hemodialysis treatment were excluded the prevalence decreased to 5.9%. This difference between hemodialysis and PD patients in the prevalence of HCV infection continues to be supported by current data. As an example, a recent study from Israel reported that the prevalence of HCV infection was 18% among hemodialysis patients but only 7% among PD patients (101).

Factors that can account for the lower risk of HCV infection among PD patients include the following:

1. PD patients have a lower requirement for blood transfusion than hemodialysis patients (94).
2. The absence of access site and extracorporeal blood circuit reduces the risk for parenteral exposure to the virus.
3. Because PD is primarily a home procedure, it offers a more isolated environment. Indeed, the prevalence of anti-HCV in patients receiving home hemodialysis is also lower than in patients receiving center hemodialysis (Fig. 22.5) (98, 102–104).

Prevalence of HCV Infection in the Dialysis Unit

Patients treated in hemodialysis units with a high prevalence of HCV infection are at increased risk of acquiring infection

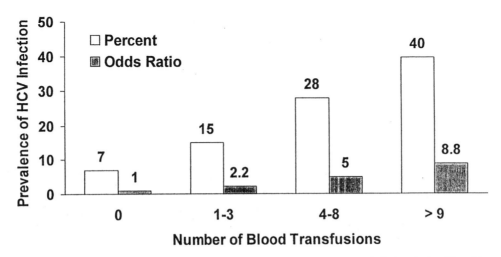

FIG. 22.2. Prevalence of hepatitis C virus (HCV) infection among patients on hemodialysis–relationship with number of blood transfusions received. HCV infection detected by second-generation anti-HCV test. (Adapted from Dussol B, et al. Hepatitis C virus infection among chronic dialysis patients in the south of France: a collaborative study. *Am J Kidney Dis* 1995;25:399–404, with permission.)

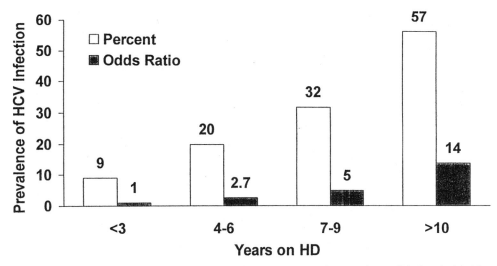

FIG. 22.3. Prevalence of hepatitis C virus (HCV) infection among patients on hemodialysis–relationship with duration of dialysis. HCV infection detected by second-generation anti-HCV test. (Adapted from Dussol B, et al. Hepatitis C virus infection among chronic dialysis patients in the south of France: a collaborative study. *Am J Kidney Dis* 1995;25:399–404, with permission.)

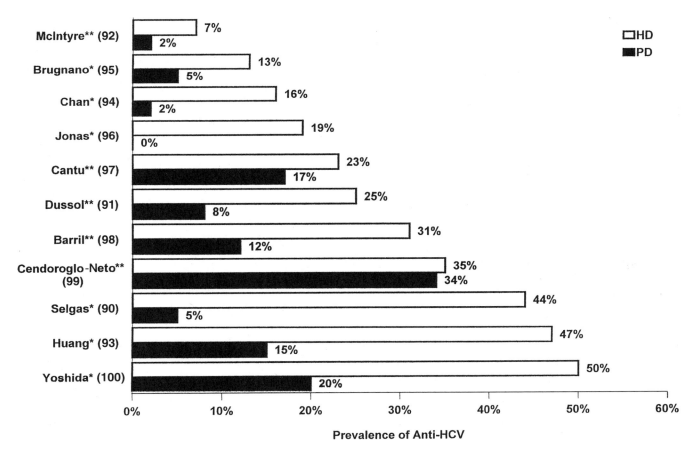

FIG. 22.4. Prevalence of antibodies to hepatitis C virus (anti-HCV) among patients on hemodialysis *(open bars)* and peritoneal dialysis *(filled bars)* in the same dialysis programs. Reference numbers are in parentheses. *First-generation anti-HCV; **second-generation anti-HCV. (From Pereira BJG, et al. Hepatitis C virus infection in dialysis and renal transplantation. *Kidney Int* 1997;51:981–999, with permission.)

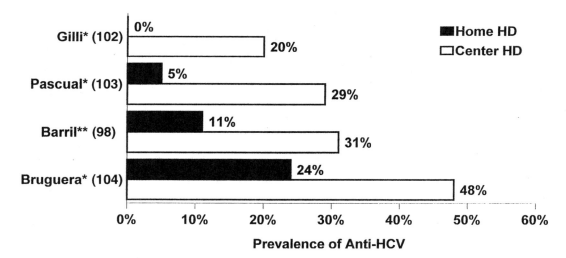

FIG. 22.5. Prevalence of antibodies to hepatitis C virus (anti-HCV) among patients on home hemodialysis *(filled bars)* and in-center hemodialysis *(open bars)* in the same dialysis programs. Reference numbers are in brackets. *First-generation anti-HCV; **second-generation anti-HCV. (From Pereira BJG, et al. Hepatitis C virus infection in dialysis and renal transplantation. *Kidney Int* 1997;51:981–999, with permission.)

(81,105). A survey by the Portuguese Society of Nephrology showed that the incidence of HCV correlated directly with the prevalence of the infection in the hemodialysis units (Fig. 22.6) (81). Among units with a prevalence of less than 19%, the annual incidence of seroconversion for anti-HCV was 2.5%, compared with 35.3% among units with a prevalence greater than 60%. In addition, a relative homogeneity of HCV variants has been reported among patients receiving hemodialysis treatment in the same unit (106).

Other Factors

- A history of previous organ transplantation is a risk factor for HCV infection in dialysis patients, possibly reflecting transmission from the organ donor (1).
- Intravenous drug use (IVDU) has been identified as another important risk factor for HCV infection in hemodialysis patients. History of IVDU was present in 30% of anti-HCV-positive patients receiving hemodialysis

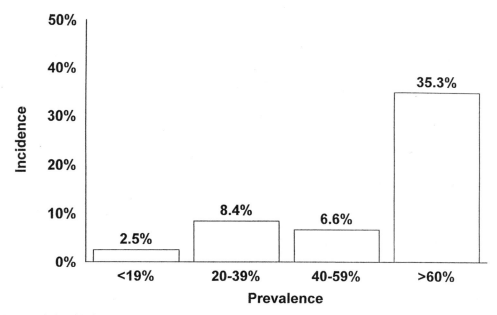

FIG. 22.6. Relationship between incidence and prevalence of hepatitis C virus (HCV) infection in hemodialysis units. The odds ratio of acquiring HCV infection was 1.05, 1.25, and 1.56 for 1%, 5%, and 10% increase in the prevalence in the hemodialysis unit, respectively. The number of patients in the analysis was 2,471, 2,320, 816, and 167, respectively, for units with anti-HCV prevalence of less than 19%, 20% to 39%, 40% to 59%, and more than 60%. (From Pinto dos Santos J, et al. Impact of dialysis room and reuse strategies on the incidence of HCV infection in HD units. *Nephrol Dial Transplant* 1996;11:2017–2022, with permission.)

at the Northwest Kidney Center, Seattle (49), and 73% in two urban hemodialysis units in Miami (107). Furthermore, in another study, multivariate logistic regression analysis identified a history of IVDU as an independent risk factor for anti-HCV positive status among the patients receiving hemodialysis treatment in an urban dialysis center in New York (89).

■ Males have been reported to have a higher prevalence of HCV infection than females (50,89). In addition, male hemodialysis patients infected with HCV have been found to have a significantly higher concentration of serum HCV RNA than females (49). However, there are currently no other data available regarding gender-related differences in the natural history of HCV infection.

Nosocomial Transmission of HCV in Hemodialysis Units

Modes of Transmission of HCV in Hemodialysis Units

The lower prevalence of HCV infection among PD and home hemodialysis patients, the correlation between interval since beginning hemodialysis and prevalence of anti-HCV, the relationship between prevalence and incidence of anti-HCV in hemodialysis units, and relative homogeneity of HCV variants in patients receiving treatment in the same hemodialysis unit strongly suggest patient-to-patient transmission of HCV in hemodialysis units (1). Furthermore, several studies have implicated a variety of potential modes of transmission.

Current molecular biologic techniques provide evidence for nosocomial transmission of HCV within hemodialysis units. In a Belgian hemodialysis unit, HCV genotyping by PCR and nucleotide sequencing of 23 seroconverters revealed that 20 of them were infected with exactly the same HCV strain (108). Similarly, in two studies, phylogenetic analysis of the nucleotide sequences of the hypervariable region 1 of the viral genome supported nosocomial transmission including possible patient-to-patient cross-infection (109,110). Comparison of the sequences in the E1 variable region of the viral genome also provided epidemiologic evidence of nosocomial transmission within a dialysis unit in southern France and permitted the reconstitution of the ways in which the dissemination of one specific HCV strain had occurred (111). Other investigators have used a technique called heteroduplex tracking analysis to screen for HCV genetic relatedness in a group of HCV-infected hemodialysis patients attending hemodialysis centers in one geographic area (112). Nucleotide sequencing and phylogenetic analysis of the apparently related HCV isolates were further used as the gold standard method to detect the truly related infections, which demonstrated that 10% of HCV-infected patients had genetically related HCV infections and enabled the authors to identify successfully the source of the infections. These findings strongly supported the probability that HCV transmission had occurred within the dialysis centers. In contrast, another study also using molecular biologic techniques found that patient-to-patient transmission of HCV was uncommon within a single dialysis facility (113).

Transmission of Infection to Dialysis Staff by Needlestick Injury

The prevalence of anti-HCV among dialysis staff ranges from 0% to 6% and is comparable to that in blood donors (1). In 2000, 40% of U.S. dialysis centers tested staff members for anti-HCV. Among the 20,091 staff members tested, the prevalence of anti-HCV was 1.7% (80). The risk of transmission of HCV from infected patients to medical staff via needlestick injury ranges from 2.7% to 10% (114,115). Genotype analysis has been used to document that the viral strain acquired by the medical staff following accidental needle exposure was identical to that in the index patient (23).

Breakdown in Standard Infection Control Practices

The implementation of universal precautions and measures to reduce the spread of HBV in dialysis units has resulted in a decline in the incidence of NANBH in dialysis units (116). Consequently, strict adherence to standard infection-control practices would also be expected to prevent the transmission of HCV. Several outbreaks of hepatitis C in hemodialysis units have been associated with a failure to rigidly enforce universal precautions and standard infection-control measures, such as sharing of a multidose heparin vial between patients with and without HCV infection and failure to change gloves between patients while performing hemodialysis treatments (1). In support of the importance of strict adherence to standard infection-control practices in controlling HCV infection, it has been well documented that rigorous infection-control measures, cleaning and disinfection of all instruments and environmental surfaces that are routinely touched, and a ban on sharing of articles among patients could decrease the incidence of HCV infection (117,118). Furthermore, in a multicenter prospective study from Belgium, enforcement of universal precautions alone fully prevented transmission of HCV in hemodialysis units (119). However, it has been reported that despite adherence to standard precautions, HCV RNA could still be detected on the hands of some dialysis nurses, suggesting that dialysis personnel should always be considered a potential vector for HCV transmission between hemodialysis patients (120).

A multicenter study conducted in 58 hemodialysis units in Italy has provided more indirect evidence to support the role of breaks in infection control practices in the dialysis unit for the nosocomial spread of HCV. This study demonstrated that understaffing (i.e., a low personnel-to-patient ratio) and a high prevalence of HCV-infected dialysis patients, a combination that indeed increases the probability of breakdowns in infection-control measures, was associated with an increased risk for nosocomial transmission of HCV infection in the dialysis setting (121).

Physical Proximity to an Infected Patient

In a multicenter study in Belgium, 38% of the hemodialysis patients who seroconverted had never been transfused and had no apparent risk factor for HCV infection (105). Interestingly, clustering of seroconversion occurred only in dialysis units in which anti-HCV-positive patients were being treated. Likewise, Da Porto et al. (122) have found that anti-HCV-positive hemodialysis patients were clustered in a group of patients who had never been transfused but who had been dialyzed in the same section of the unit. A Portuguese Society of Nephrology survey also found the lowest incidence of HCV infection among hemodialysis units that used isolated rooms to treat anti-HCV-positive patients (81). These data suggest that transmission of HCV may be enhanced by physical proximity.

Dialysis Machines

Some studies suggest that cross-infection through dialysis machines could account for nosocomial transmission of HCV in the dialysis setting (95,123–125). In one report, documented episodes of contamination of the transducer protectors in the external pressure tubing sets with patient blood reflux were suspected to have resulted in a potential contamination by blood of the pressure-sensing port of the machine, which is not accessible to routine disinfection. The use of a second transducer protector in combination with strict reinforcement of routine infection control measures prevented further cases of HCV infection (125).

A high incidence of HCV infection has been documented among dialysis patients who shared the same dialysis machines (95) and in dialysis centers that did not assign patients to receive hemodialysis treatment always on a particular dialysis machine (124). These findings are further supported by a survey of hemodialysis units conducted by the Portuguese Society of Nephrology, which found a significantly lower incidence of HCV infection among units that used dedicated machines for anti-HCV-positive patients (81). Other studies have also reported that the use of dedicated machines and isolated areas for anti-HCV-positive patients along with strict enforcement of universal precautions resulted in decreased incidence of seroconversion in hemodialysis centers (1).

The value of some of these practices has been challenged. As an example, in one study the use of dedicated dialysis machines for anti-HCV positive patients could not prevent nosocomial transmission of HCV in the dialysis unit. On the contrary, the rate of nosocomial HCV transmission was found to be lower in a hemodialysis unit in which treatment was provided only for anti-HCV-negative patients than in another hemodialysis unit where anti-HCV-positive and anti-HCV-negative patients were treated together. Therefore, separating anti-HCV-positive from anti-HCV-negative patients was considered to be effective and was strongly advocated (126).

In a recent survey on the spread of HCV infection in Italian dialysis centers conducted by the Italian branch of EDTNA-ERCA, the use of dedicated dialysis machines was felt to be useful in preventing nosocomial transmission of HCV and therefore was strongly recommended, at least for centers with a high prevalence of HCV infection. Isolation of anti-HCV-positive patients, although practiced by 25% of the dialysis centers that responded to the questionnaire, was found to be of uncertain benefit and associated with a high cost, and, therefore, it was considered unwise (127). This position was also supported by another recent study that demonstrated that the incidence of

HCV infection in a dialysis unit decreased in the absence of isolation of anti-HCV-positive patients but with strict adherence to universal precautions and infection control measures (128). Furthermore, a multicenter study from Belgium did not detect any new cases of HCV transmission over a 54-month study period, despite the fact that none of the participating hemodialysis centers used dedicated machines for anti-HCV positive patients, and more than 70% of the patients were dialyzed in units in which monitors were not disinfected after each session (119).

Regardless of the controversies about the role of dialysis machines in the nosocomial transmission of HCV infection, systematic monitor disinfection seems to be a simple and effective tool in preventing nosocomial transmission of HCV (129). In an experimental study, autoclaving of dialysate circuits was shown to eliminate HCV particles from artificially contaminated hemodialysis monitors (130). Therefore, systematic monitor disinfection, as simple as it could be, emerges as a valuable means in controlling HCV transmission in the hemodialysis unit and, in the opinion of some authors, its use should be mandatory (129). If this practice were implemented in conjunction with strict adherence to universal precautions, the use of dedicated machines for anti-HCV positive patients would appear to be unnecessary.

Overall, in our view, current data cannot provide enough evidence to support any significant role of hemodialysis machines in the nosocomial transmission of HCV infection. Therefore, it is likely that HCV transmission in hemodialysis settings results primarily from environmental contamination and horizontal, patient-to-patient, transmission.

Dialyzer Membranes and Hemodialysis Ultrafiltrate

Theoretically, the passage of HCV through intact dialyzer membranes seems improbable, because the viral particles have an estimated diameter of 35 nm, much higher than the pores of even the most permeable dialysis membrane (131). However, any alteration in pore size or disruption of the membrane integrity associated with the process of filter assembly, the dialysis session itself, or dialyzer reuse could hypothetically permit the passage of the virus into the dialysate compartment.

Several studies have reported that neither low-flux (cellulose) nor high-flux (cellulose-diacetate, polysulfone, and polyacrylonitrile) dialyzers permit contamination of the dialysis ultrafiltrate with HCV RNA (132,133). Likewise, in another study, HCV RNA could not be detected in ultrafiltrated spent dialysate when dialysis was performed with single use high-flux polysulfone membrane dialyzers and low transmembrane pressure (less than 18.72 mm Hg), despite the finding that serum HCV RNA levels decreased significantly postdialysis as compared with predialysis (134). Although the mechanism for this reduction of HCV copies in serum remained unclear, the authors have suggested that lower transmembrane pressure should be used in anti-HCV-positive patients to minimize the risk for HCV transmission by extravasation of HCV to the dialysate (134).

Reproducible decrease in serum HCV RNA titers has been observed in hemodialysis patients treated with polysulfone and hemophane membranes and only in a subgroup of hemodialysis patients treated with AN69 but has not occurred in patients dialyzed with a cuprophane membrane. In both in vitro and in vivo experiments, HCV RNA could be recovered from a polysulfone membrane following dialysis sessions but could not be detected in the ultrafiltrate. These findings indicate that the transient reduction in HCV RNA serum levels observed during or immediately after dialysis most likely results from membrane-dependent adsorption of HCV, which occurs during hemodialysis, and not from a transit of the virus to the ultrafiltrate (135).

In contrast, others have detected HCV RNA by PCR in the dialysate of apparently intact polyacrylonitrile membranes but not cellulose membranes (136).

The detection of HCV RNA in the dialysate by PCR may only imply the presence of fragments of viral RNA not necessarily the infective virus itself, a situation that may not lead to transmission of the infection. On the other hand, a negative result on a PCR test does not absolutely rule out the presence of viral RNA in the dialysis ultrafiltrate, because minimal amounts of HCV, below the detection threshold of the PCR assay, may have passed through the dialysis membrane. However, such a low viral load in the dialysis ultrafiltrate may represent only a negligible risk of transmission of HCV infection. To date, a higher prevalence of anti-HCV among hemodialysis patients has not been associated with any particular dialysis membrane (1).

Reprocessing of Dialyzers

In a prospective study in 15 hemodialysis units in Belgium, Jadoul et al. (105) did not find a higher incidence of HCV infection among patients treated in units that reprocessed dialyzers compared with those that did not. Likewise, a survey of the Portuguese Society of Nephrology also reported that the incidence of HCV infection among patients in hemodialysis units that reprocessed dialyzers was not significantly different from that among patients in units that did not reprocess dialyzers (81). However, among units that did reprocess dialyzers, the lowest incidence of HCV infection was observed among patients in units that used separate rooms to reprocess dialyzers from anti-HCV-positive and anti-HCV-negative patients or had a ban on reprocessing dialyzers from anti-HCV-positive patients (81).

In the United States, among hemodialysis units that reused dialyzers, the prevalence of anti-HCV was higher at centers that reused dialyzers on anti-HCV-positive patients (8.7%) than at those that did not (7.6%). However, the prevalence of anti-HCV among patients in hemodialysis units that reused dialyzers on anti-HCV-positive patients (8.3%) was not different from the prevalence among units that did not reprocess dialyzers on any patients (8.9%). The incidence rate of anti-HCV among hemodialysis patients was also similar at centers that reused dialyzers and at those that did not practice reuse of dialyzers (0.25% vs. 0.27%). However, among centers that reused dialyzers, the incidence of anti-HCV was marginally higher at centers that reused dialyzers on anti-HCV-positive patients (0.16% vs. 0.27%) (80). In another study, a decline in the prevalence of HCV seropositivity among hemodialysis patients occurred despite routine dialyzer reuse (137).

Overall, it appears that dialyzer reuse is not directly implicated in the nosocomial transmission of HCV. In fact, because reprocessed dialyzers are reused on the same patient, it is expected that reuse would not be associated with higher rates of HCV infection among hemodialysis patients. If such association occurs, the epidemiologic investigation should look for unmeasured confounding factors or episodes of environmental contamination resulting from improper handling (i.e., transport of used dialyzers to a reprocessing area without placing them in a leakproof container or contamination within the reprocessing room) that may become a vector for HCV transmission in hemodialysis units (80,81).

Strategies to Control the Transmission of HCV Infection in Hemodialysis Units

The high prevalence of HCV infection among patients on hemodialysis, the limitations of current tests in identifying these patients, and uncertainty regarding the modes of transmission within dialysis units have led to difficulty in formulating policies regarding HCV infection in hemodialysis units. The debate continues on the need for routine testing for anti-HCV and the controversies regarding the efficacy of patient isolation, dedicated machines, and banning reuse of dialyzers for controlling transmission of HCV infection in hemodialysis units have not been resolved. Arguments in favor of such strategies in hemodialysis units include the following:

1. HCV is parenterally transmitted, and hemodialysis patients are at risk of nosocomial transmission.
2. Other parenterally transmitted viruses such as HBV have been shown to be transmitted within hemodialysis units.
3. Similar strategies to reduce the transmission of HBV have resulted in a decrease in the incidence of HBV infection in hemodialysis units (80).

There are, however, strong arguments against a policy of isolating anti-HCV-positive patients and use of dedicated machines (1):

1. HCV is not as infective as HBV, circulates in low titers in infected serum, and is rapidly degraded at room temperature. Indeed, chimpanzee transmission studies have shown that the viral titer of human NANBH sera is generally less than 10^2 chimpanzee-infective units compared with 10^8 chimpanzee-infective units for HBeAg-positive sera and 10^{11} chimpanzee-infective units for hepatitis D virus-infected sera.
2. Currently licensed anti-HCV tests detect nonneutralizing antibodies and, therefore, do not distinguish between current and past infection. Also, a negative test result does not exclude HCV infection. Consequently, isolation of anti-HCV-positive patients does not eliminate the risk of transmission. Although the previous problem could potentially be circumvented by testing for HCV RNA by PCR, this test is expensive, requires a specialized laboratory, and has technical limitations that can lead to false-positive and false-negative results.
3. Although isolation may protect uninfected patients, it might also increase the risk of superinfection in patients originally

infected with a single strain (66). Indeed, infection with two or more different HCV genotypes has been observed in hemodialysis patients and in 13% of patients referred for renal transplantation (76). The clinical impact of such polygenotype infections is currently undefined.

In view of the previously mentioned debate, the U.S. Centers for Disease Control and Prevention (CDC) does not recommend dedicated machines, patient isolation, or a ban on dialyzer reuse in hemodialysis patients with HCV infection (138,139). Meanwhile, strict adherence to universal precautions, careful attention to hygiene, and strict sterilization of dialysis machines is recommended (1). Conventional cleansing and sterilization appear to be adequate to inactivate the virus (102,105).

Although these recommendations may suffice for developed countries, which have succeeded in implementing strict universal precautions, additional measures such as isolation, dedicated machines, and a ban on reuse of dialyzers for anti-HCV-positive patients may be required in underdeveloped countries where enforcement of universal precautions lags behind developed countries. Ironically, these measures are important in the very countries that can least afford them.

In 2001, the CDC released new recommendations for preventing transmission of infections among chronic hemodialysis patients (140). In this document, the CDC provides schedules for routine serologic testing for HCV infection. The CDC recommends that all hemodialysis patients should be tested for anti-HCV on admission to the dialysis unit to establish their baseline status. Subsequently, anti-HCV negative patients should be tested for anti-HCV semiannually. Undoubtedly, serologic surveillance for HCV will allow early detection of nosocomial transmission, which in turn should prompt a thorough epidemiologic investigation to identify the source of the infection and the mechanism of transmission. This will ultimately lead to corrective measures preventing further spread and outbreaks of HCV infection in the hemodialysis unit.

Finally eliminating the spread of HCV infection in hemodialysis units may require the development of treatments to eradicate the virus or vaccines to prevent infection.

Survival among Chronic Dialysis Patients with HCV Infection

Data on survival among chronic dialysis patients infected with HCV are limited. Among 200 chronic dialysis patients screened for HCV infection using enzyme immunoblot assay and PCR, the risk of death was increased in anti-HCV-positive and HCV RNA-positive patients–1.8 ($p = 0.04$) and 2.0 ($p = 0.01$), respectively–as compared with those who were not infected with HCV (141). Similarly, in a multicenter prospective cohort study of 1,470 chronic hemodialysis patients in Japan, after a 6-year follow-up, anti-HCV-positive patients had a significantly higher mortality rate than those who were anti-HCV-negative–33.0% versus 23.2% ($p < 0.01$). The relative risk of death associated with anti-HCV-positive status was 1.57 (95% confidence interval (CI), 1.23 to 2.00). As a cause of death, hepatocellular carcinoma and liver cirrhosis were significantly more frequent among anti-HCV-positive patients than among anti-HCV-neg-

ative patients (5.5% vs 0.0%, $p < 0.001$; 8.8% vs. 0.4%, $p < 0.001$, respectively) (142). In addition, a study from the New England Organ Bank found that, among patients referred for renal transplantation, the relative risk of death for those with HCV infection was increased (relative risk of 1.41), independent of whether they remained on dialysis or underwent transplantation (143). These data suggest that HCV infection adversely affects survival among patients with ESRD.

ROLE OF INTERFERON ALFA (IFNα) IN THE TREATMENT OF HCV INFECTION IN DIALYSIS PATIENTS

A number of randomized controlled trials have demonstrated the therapeutic efficacy of IFNα against HCV. Consequently, IFNα has become the mainstay of hepatitis C therapy and its use is currently recommended for the treatment of anti-HCV-positive patients with abnormal serum aminotransferase and well-compensated chronic hepatitis on liver biopsy (144,145). Four different forms of IFNα have been evaluated for clinical use in large trials: IFNα-2b (most commonly used), IFNα-2a, IFNα-n1, and IFN alfacon (or consensus interferon, CIFN) (144). They are similarly effective but differ in approved dosing and duration of therapy. Recently, a new modified form of IFNα, pegylated IFNα or also called peginterferon alfa, was developed by covalent attachment of a 40-kd branched-chain polyethylene glycol (PEG) moiety to recombinant IFNα. Compared with unmodified IFNα, this new compound is remarkable for its unique properties including better sustained absorption, a slower rate of clearance, and a longer half-life (146,147), all of which contribute to its improved therapeutic efficacy. Two formulations of pegylated IFNα have been developed based on IFNα-2a and IFNα-2b: pegylated IFNα-2a (Pegasys, Roche Pharmaceuticals), and pegylated IFNα-2b (Peg-Intron, Schering-Plough Corporation) (148–150).

The efficacy of INFα therapy is determined by the rates of biochemical, virologic, and histologic response. Biochemical response to IFNα treatment is defined as normalization of serum ALT and virologic response as clearance of HCV RNA from the serum. There is no uniform definition of histologic response, but most studies define histologic response as a two point or greater reduction in the histology activity index score (Knodell histologic score for inflammatory components only) (151). A complete biochemical and virologic response by the end of the treatment is defined as end-of-treatment response (ETR) and at 6 or 12 months following discontinuation of interferon therapy as a sustained response (SR) (145). Currently, the best indicator of effective treatment is a sustained virologic response, defined by the absence of detectable HCV RNA in the serum as shown by a qualitative HCV RNA assay with lower limit of detection of 50 IU/mL or less at 24 weeks after the end of treatment (152). Two therapeutic regimens using identical dosing (3 million units of IFNα administered subcutaneously three times weekly) but different duration of treatment (either 6 or 12 months) have been studied (144,145). Six-month treatment courses have resulted in biochemical and virologic ETR rates of 40% to 50% and 30% to 40%, respectively, and biochemical and virologic SR of 15% to 20% and 10% to 20%, respectively (145). The biochemical and virologic responses have been usually accompanied by histologic improvement. A twelve-month treatment regimen has not produced higher biochemical or virologic ETR but has increased SR rates to 20% to 30% (145). Therefore, treatment for at least 12 months is now considered to be the standard of care for patients who respond to interferon within the first 12 weeks of therapy. The benefit of treatment of longer duration (18 to 24 months) and/or with higher doses is currently under evaluation. Overall, although IFNα treatment has demonstrated favorable biochemical and virologic results, its effects on paramount clinical outcomes such as quality of life and disease progression have not been ascertained (145).

Recent clinical trials have demonstrated that an oral antiviral drug, called ribavirin, which is a synthetic guanosine analogue with activity against a broad spectrum of DNA and RNA viruses, can improve the response rates to IFNα therapy and, therefore, should be made a part of the therapeutic regimen for hepatitis C. Indeed, currently, the combination of IFNα and ribavirin is considered to be the best treatment option for chronic HCV infection (152). However, ribavirin clearance is impaired in patients with renal dysfunction. In addition, the drug is not removed by dialysis. Consequently, ribavirin metabolites may accumulate in erythrocytes of patients with advanced renal insufficiency or ESRD leading to the development of hemolytic anemia. For this reason, ribavirin is not recommended for patients with a creatinine clearance below 50 mL/minute.

Monotherapy with IFNα is the only currently accepted treatment option for HCV infection in ESRD patients. Most hemodialysis patients with HCV infection who receive IFNα therapy demonstrate good biochemical and virologic response and an improvement in liver histology (48,153–165). However, as in the case with nonrenal patients, despite frequently observed initial disappearance of HCV RNA from the serum, relapses are common after treatment is discontinued and long-term outcomes are not yet adequately defined (48,154,155). Furthermore, recurrence of viremia from extravascular sites remains a distinct possibility (52,155).

Antiviral therapy with IFNα is recommended for selected categories of HCV-infected hemodialysis patients based on pretreatment clinical, biochemical, viral, and histologic characteristics that have been found to predict, at least to some extent, the response to interferon therapy (145,152). Among these, liver histology, viral load, and HCV serologic type have been extensively studied.

Liver histology has been closely correlated to the success of IFNα therapy and, therefore, plays a major role in the selection of patients that are likely to benefit from antiviral treatment. Patients with moderate or severe chronic hepatitis with or without fibrosis should be offered IFNα treatment, unless they have a contraindication such as major depression. Treatment with IFNα should be considered on an individual basis in patients who have mild histologic activity because these patients usually have a relatively good long-term prognosis even without antiviral treatment and in patients with cirrhosis because they have a poor response rate to IFNα therapy. Patients with advanced liver cirrhosis and ESRD should not be treated with IFNα but considered for combined liver-kidney transplantation.

Viral load and serologic type of HCV infection have both been used to predict response to IFNα therapy. A low pretreatment viral load has been correlated with a SR to IFNα therapy, whereas relatively high HCV RNA levels have been associated with a nonsustained response or no response at all. However, in the individual patient, pretreatment HCV RNA levels correlate poorly with response to IFNα (48,166). The value of HCV genotype as a predictor of response to IFN therapy is debatable. In the general population, infections with HCV genotype 1 have been associated with a lower response rate to IFN therapy than infections with other HCV genotypes (167). In hemodialysis patients, however, some studies have failed to find any correlation between HCV genotype and response to IFN therapy (48,168). By comparison, in one study that included nonrenal and hemodialysis patients with HCV infection, HCV genotype 1b was associated with a better response to interferon treatment, as compared with HCV genotypes 1a and 2a, which seemed to predict a low response rate (48). In addition, in the general population, age younger than 40 years, pretreatment ALT levels less than three times the upper limit of normal, and posttransfusion rather sporadic infection have been associated with high response rates (169).

Although there is not enough evidence to allow firm recommendations concerning dose and treatment duration in patients on chronic dialysis, a regimen of 3 million units of IFNα-2b three times per week for 6 to 12 months (if tolerated) appears to be safe and effective in inducing biochemical, virologic, and histologic responses. However, in some studies, higher doses of IFNα (5 to 10 MU), daily administration (vs. three times per week) and longer duration of treatment (12 to 18 months vs. 6 months) have been associated with higher rates of biochemical, virologic, and histologic response in hemodialysis patients (168,170–172). Even more, among patients who relapsed after 1-year treatment with usual dose (3 MU three times a week), an additional year of IFNα resulted in sustained biochemical and virologic response (173). However, because of the particular pharmacokinetics of IFNα in patients with impaired renal function (hemodialysis patients have a 50% decrease in IFNα clearance, significantly longer half-lives of IFN-alpha2b, and markedly larger areas under the serum IFNα concentration curve than nonuremic patients) such regimens in hemodialysis patients may result in more frequent and more serious adverse effects than in the general population (162). Consequently, the safety of using daily and high-dose IFNα regimens in hemodialysis patients has been questioned.

Treatment with IFNα is frequently associated with significant side effects (a flulike syndrome with asthenia, myalgia, headache, neutropenia, thrombocytopenia, and depression), which are partially dose related (174) and are the reason for the high dropout rates (as high as 54%) among patients on renal replacement therapy (153–157,174). Importantly, in addition to its antiviral activity, IFNα exerts antiproliferative and immunomodulatory properties that can induce or facilitate acute steroid-resistant rejection in allograft recipients (175). An increased risk of acute rejection (40%–100%) among transplant recipients treated with IFNα for HCV-related chronic liver disease has been reported in most studies (155,159,161,176). Therefore, the National Institute of Health Consensus Statement on Management of Hepatitis C has listed renal transplant as a contraindication to interferon treatment (145).

In a number of studies, high rates of sustained biochemical and virologic response and no increased risk of rejection after subsequent renal transplantation have been reported among ESRD patients with chronic hepatitis C who were treated with IFNα while on dialysis (Table 22.1) (170,172,177,178). Furthermore, IFNα treatment of HCV-infected hemodialysis patients appears to exert a beneficial effect on the course of liver disease following renal transplantation, regardless of the virologic response (177). These data suggest that IFNα treatment before transplantation of HCV-infected dialysis patients, who are considered transplant candidates, seems to be a safer and particularly advisable, although probably less cost-effective, strategy (156,158,177). In contrast, other investigators have reported a high rate of relapse of HCV infection after renal transplantation (164) and have questioned the benefit from this strategy. Because current data appear limited and controversial, controlled studies are needed to evaluate the long-term effects of IFNα therapy in renal transplant candidates on the posttransplant course of liver disease, rates of transplantation, and graft and patient survival.

The introduction of pegylated interferons in clinical practice has raised great expectations. As mentioned previously, the specific pharmacokinetics of pegylated IFNα with enhanced half-life and more uniform interferon concentrations even though they are administered only once weekly provide certain therapeutic advantages. Indeed, in large randomized trials, pegylated interferons alfa-2a and alfa-2b have been found to be superior to their standard counterparts (IFNα-2a and IFNα-2b) with respect to sustained virologic response and tolerability and for the treatment of HCV-infected patients with cirrhosis or bridging fibrosis that typically have a poor response to standard IFNα monotherapy (148–150). However, there is still no information about the use of pegylated interferons in patients on renal replacement therapy.

Combination therapy with IFNα plus ribavirin in HCV-infected dialysis patients has been recently evaluated by a small pilot study. This trial has demonstrated that, despite the impaired clearance of ribavirin in patients with renal dysfunction, the drug could still be used safely if its dose is reduced and if its plasma concentrations and hemoglobin levels are closely monitored (179). More data are needed on the safety and efficacy of ribavirin use in reduced dose and with close monitoring

of ribavirin plasma concentrations and hemoglobin levels in patients with advanced impairment of renal function, including dialysis patients, before ribavirin can be recommended as a part of the therapeutic regimens for the treatment of HCV infection in this patient population.

Because pegylated interferons are likely to replace standard IFNα preparations in clinical practice, ongoing studies are evaluating combination therapy with pegylated interferon plus ribavirin. Preliminary results have demonstrated that peginterferon alfa-2a (or alfa-2b) plus ribavirin was associated with a higher sustained virologic response rate than therapy with standard IFNα-2b plus ribavirin (180,181). There is still no information about the use of this regimen in patients on renal replacement therapy.

Given the absence of data, we currently do not recommend the use of pegylated interferons and/or ribavirin in patients on renal replacement therapy

HEPATITIS G VIRUS (HGV)

Despite the development of reliable antibody assays and molecular probes for the detection of human hepatitis viruses A through E, the causative agents in about 10% to 20% of human hepatitis remain unexplained (182), suggesting the presence of other etiologic agents. In the United States, 25% of cases of presumed acute viral hepatitis are due to NANBH, of which only 82% (or 20.5% of the total) are caused by HCV (183). Consequently, in about 4.5% of patients with presumed acute viral hepatitis, the cause remains unexplained. Furthermore, most cases of non-A, non-B fulminant hepatic failure test negative for markers of HCV (184). The search for these elusive etiologic agents of hepatitis has been aided by the recent discovery of the GB group of viruses (GBV)/hepatitis G.

GBV/HGV

GB viruses are RNA viruses belonging to the Flavivirus family (185). In the late 1960s, Deinhardt et al. (186) demonstrated that an infective agent in plasma from a 34-year-old surgeon with acute hepatitis could be transmitted to marmosets and described the histology of the liver lesions caused by this agent in animals. Subsequent cross-challenge studies from this plasma suggested that the infective agent was distinct from hepatitis A, B, C, D, and E. More recently, using a subtractive PCR methodology known as representational difference analysis (RDA),

TABLE 22.1. INTERFERON-ALFA THERAPY IN RENAL TRANSPLANT CANDIDATES WITH HCV INFECTION

Author	No. of Patients	Follow-up (months)	Deaths/Ac. Rejection	Biochemical SR	Virologic SR
Huraib, et al.[170]	2	17; 28	0	2/2 (100%)	2/2 (100%)
Campistol, et al.[177]	10	3–24	0	10/10 (100%)	2/3 (66%)
Espinosa, et al.[172]	2	72	0	2/2 (100%)	2/2 (100%)
Casanovas-Taltavull, et al.[178]	14	41 ± 28	1/1	12/12 (100%)	8/12 (66%)

HCV, hepatis C virus; SR, sustained response.
From Natov SN, et al. Management of hepatitis C infection in renal transplant recipients. *Am J Transpl* 2002;2:483–490, with permission.

Simons et al. (187) cloned two specific nucleotide sequences from the plasma of a tamarin that had been infected with pooled sera derived from the serial passage in tamarins of the infective agent from the aforementioned surgeon. These two agents were named GB virus-A (GBV-A) and GBV-B, after the initials of the surgeon from whom the infected serum was obtained.

Subsequent studies on serum from a West African patient with antibody to GBV-A and B, revealed the presence of a nucleotide sequence with a nucleotide homology of 59% with GBV-A, 47.9% with GBV-B, and 53.7% with HCV-1 (188). The same unique sequence was also identified in sera of some patients with non-A-E hepatitis (188). The nucleotide sequence of this virus, named GBV-C, has since been cloned and shown to contain the highly conserved RNA helicase domain characteristic of other members of the Flaviviridae family, including GBV-A, GBV-B, and HCV-1 (189).

Concurrently, Linnen et al. (190) have identified an RNA virus from the plasma of a patient with chronic hepatitis and designated it as hepatitis G virus (HGV). HGV shows 95% amino acid sequence identity to GBV-C (85% at nucleotide level), suggesting that HGV and GBV-C are independent isolates of the same virus (191); therefore, the term *HGV* will be used hereafter.

Epidemiology of GBV-C

HGV has worldwide distribution. In individuals infected with HGV by blood transfusion, the humoral immune response usually triggers production of antibody (HGV E2 Ab) targeted to a protein located in the viral envelope 2 (E2) region (192). This results in HGV RNA clearance from the blood within several weeks, whereas HGV E2 Ab remains indefinitely. However, in some individuals infected with HGV, HGV E2 Ab production does not occur, either because of failure of the immune system to recognize the virus or the capability of the virus to escape effectively the immune defense mechanisms, leading to inability to clear HGV RNA from the blood and eventually to the establishment of persistent viremia. The presence of HGV RNA (with or without HGV E2 Ab) is interpreted as *current infection,* whereas the presence of HGV E2 Ab alone signifies *past infection. HGV exposure* (a positive test for HGV RNA and/or HGV E2 Ab) refers to all patients with current or past infection and is the best way to assess the actual prevalence of HGV infection.

Transmission of HGV

The prevalence of HGV infection among volunteer blood donors, as ascertained by the presence of HGV RNA, varies from 0.8% to 11% (193–199). The overall rate of exposure to HGV among them is even higher: 5% to 17% (198,200–202). Several lines of evidence suggest that HGV is a parenterally transmitted virus:

1. In animal experiments, transmission of HGV by inoculation of infected serum has been unequivocally demonstrated (203). In addition, the appearance of serum HGV RNA has been shown to coincide with transfusion-associated non-A-E hepatitis (190).

2. The prevalence of HGV infection (HGV RNA present in the bloodstream) is higher among populations at high risk of acquiring parentally transmitted infections such as hemophiliacs (1% to 24%) (190,195,204,205), multiply transfused individuals and commercial plasma donors (43% to 47%) (200,206), hemodialysis patients (3% to 55%) (195,197,199,207–215), renal transplant recipients (14% to 43%) (195,216–219), and intravenous drug users (16% to 33%) (190,200,220,221). The HGV exposure rate in these populations is even higher: 55% among hemophiliacs (201), 71% among multiply transfused individuals and commercial plasma donors (200), 11% to 44% among hemodialysis patients (197,199,202,211–215,222–224), 28% to 53% among renal transplant recipients (216,219,225), and 74% to 100 % among intravenous drug users (200,201).

3. The prevalence of HGV infection among cadaver organ donors is high especially among those with serum markers of other parenterally transmitted viral infections. Indeed, the prevalence of HGV infection among anti-HCV-positive donors (27.6%) was four times higher than that among anti-HCV-negative donors (7.3%) (226). Furthermore, the prevalence of serum markers of HBV such as anti-HBs and anti-HBc antibodies was higher among donors with HGV infection than without infection.

4. Dialysis patients with HGV infection had received a higher number of blood transfusions and had a trend toward a longer duration of dialysis compared with patients without HGV infection (227). These are both known risk factors for parenterally transmitted viral infections among dialysis patients (1).

These data suggest that HGV shares common modes of transmission with HBV and HCV and, hence, is also a parenterally transmitted virus.

Nonparenteral transmission of HGV is also possible. There is evidence to suggest that vertical (mother-to-baby) (228,229) and horizontal (sexual or household) transmission can occur (230,231).

Prevalence and Risk Factors for HGV Infection among Hemodialysis Patients

The prevalence of HGV RNA among patients on chronic hemodialysis ranges between 3% to 55% in Asia (199,207, 208,213,232), 18% to 34% in the United States (227,233), 12% to 21% in South America (234), and 13% to 38% in Europe (77,197,209,212,235–242). As in the general population, the rate of HGV exposure among hemodialysis patients is higher than the prevalence of HGV RNA and varies widely between 11% and 44% across geographic areas and dialysis units (197,202,211–214,222,223,243).

The risk factors for HGV infection and the potential modes of transmission among hemodialysis patients are as yet incompletely defined. In some studies, increasing time on dialysis, higher number of blood product transfusions, and glomerulonephritides-related renal failure have all been associated with an increased risk of HGV infection (227,236). In another report, although more than five blood transfusions increased significantly the risk of HGV infection, there was no association between HGV infection and the length of time on hemodialysis (242). In addition, others have observed that the rate of HGV infection seemed to increase only during the first 6 years of hemodialysis, whereas the overall risk of HGV infection did not correlate strictly with the duration of dialysis (202).

In contrast to cadaver organ donors, the prevalence of HGV infection is not increased among anti-HCV-positive dialysis patients compared with anti-HCV-negative patients. Indeed, the 23% prevalence of HGV infection among anti-HCV-positive dialysis patients in the New England region of the United States was not significantly different from the 17% prevalence among anti-HCV-negative patients (227). Likewise, the 45% prevalence of HGV infection among anti-HCV-positive dialysis patients in Miami, Florida, was not significantly different from the 32% prevalence among anti-HCV-negative patients (233). In accordance, another study from Argentina also found that HGV infection in hemodialysis patients was independent of HCV prevalence (234). These data suggest that dialysis patients probably acquire HCV and HGV infection from different sources.

The reason for the wide variation in the prevalence of HGV infection in different parts of the world is still not clearly understood. Possible explanations include variations in the prevalence of HGV infection among blood donors (190,207), difference in the primers used for the detection of virus, and geographic differences in the prevalence of HGV because of differences in host susceptibility or virulence of different strains of HGV. In addition, the high prevalence of HGV infection among hemodialysis patients seems to be correlated to a high prevalence of anti-HCV and in most cases probably reflects nosocomial transmission because of suboptimal infection control strategies.

Despite a high prevalence of HGV among healthy blood donors and in various disease states, HGV has not been uniformly associated with liver disease. Earlier studies that have favored the role of HGV in causing hepatitis based on a higher prevalence of HGV RNA among volunteer blood donors with elevated ALT levels (220), patients with hepatitis of unknown etiology (244), chronic non-A through E hepatitis (220), and fulminant hepatitis (245–247) have been challenged by more recent data suggesting lack of association between HGV and liver disease. In fact, there has been a growing consensus that HGV might not be a "hepatitis" virus based on the following data:

- Among patients with acute hepatitis resulting from community-acquired hepatitis A, B, or C infection, biochemical markers of liver disease were similar among patients with and without HGV infection (248). Furthermore, the prevalence of chronic hepatitis among patients with both HCV and HGV infections was similar to that among patients with HCV infection alone (248).
- Among blood transfusion recipients, the prevalence of HGV RNA was not significantly different between groups with hepatitis C, non-A, non-B, non-C hepatitis, or no hepatitis (249).
- Among patients with fulminant hepatic failure, serum HGV RNA was uniformly absent in blood samples at the time of admission before any blood transfusion (250).

- The prevalence of abnormal liver function tests was not significantly different between HGV RNA-positive and RNA-negative cadaver organ donors (226).
- Among patients who underwent liver transplantation for cryptogenic cirrhosis or for nonviral causes of end-stage liver disease, despite a high acquisition rate of HGV at the time of transplantation, the development of HGV infection did not predispose them to viral hepatitis and had no adverse effect on graft or patient survival (251,252).
- The prevalence of abnormal liver function tests among chronic hemodialysis patients was similar among patients with and without serum HGV RNA (207,209). HGV could not be implicated in the cause of posttransplantation hepatitis among liver transplant recipients (253) or posttransplant liver disease among renal transplant recipients (227).
- Coinfection with HGV did not affect the severity of liver disease or response to interferon therapy among patients with chronic HCV-induced liver disease (254).
- A study from the New England Organ Bank in Massachusetts reported that the prevalence of elevated serum ALT levels among HGV RNA-positive patients (7%) was not different from that among HGV RNA-negative patients (7%) (255).
- To date, HGV has not been shown to adversely affect the outcome of dialysis patients or renal transplant recipients. Results from the New England Organ Bank in the United States have shown that patient and graft survival among renal transplant recipients with HGV RNA in the pretransplant serum (76% and 59%, respectively) was not significantly different from that among recipients without HGV RNA in the pretransplant serum (76% and 55%, respectively) (5). Likewise, the presence of serum HGV RNA did not influence the survival among patients referred for renal transplantation, whether they underwent transplantation or remained on dialysis (256). Finally, among those with serum HGV RNA at the time of referral for transplantation, the survival among patients who underwent transplantation was not significantly different from that among those who remained on dialysis (256). Taken together, these data suggest that, at the present time, HGV is not associated with adverse outcomes among ESRD patients.

These studies suggest that HGV is unlikely to be associated with either acute or chronic liver disease. Even more, a feeling that HGV might not be a pathogen at all has been expressed. Until recently, except for sporadic case reports that linked the presence of serum HGV RNA to aplastic anemia (257,258), there had been no other data to suggest any HGV disease association. However, this might have reflected only our limited knowledge of HGV pathogenicity at that time (259) because more recently, new studies have emerged to demonstrate that HGV replicates in human liver (260,261) and is involved with some cases of acute and chronic hepatitis (244). An association between HGV and hepatitis C viremia and portal and periportal inflammation has been also reported (262). In addition, HGV has been found to replicate in the kidney and consequently has been considered a risk factor for developing glomerulonephritis (263). A case of de novo membranoproliferative glomerulonephritis (type 1) occurring in a renal transplant recipient was associated with HGV infection (264). However, the debate whether HGV is a true pathogen or just an innocent bystander has not been resolved. More data are needed before the clinical significance of HGV infection can be determined.

HIV INFECTION AMONG DIALYSIS PATIENTS

HIV infection has established itself as a global pandemic, with approximately 40 million people living with HIV and acquired immunodeficiency syndrome (AIDS) as of December 31, 2001 (265). The distribution of these patients across the globe is uneven with 29 million of these in sub-Saharan Africa alone, and 5.6 million in south and southeast Asia (265). Five million new cases of HIV and AIDS (about 14,000 per day) were added in the year 2001, with sub-Saharan Africa accounting for 3.5 million and Asia and Eastern Europe for another million. HIV and AIDS accounted for approximately 3 million deaths in the year 2001 with 2.2 million of these from sub-Saharan Africa and another 400,000 from southeast Asia. More than 95% of deaths are in developing countries. This infection affects people in the prime years of their life, with almost all the infections among adults occurring between ages 15 and 49 years. In sub-Saharan Africa, the prevalence of HIV and AIDS is 20% to 39% of the adult population. Although in the United States, the incidence and prevalence of HIV/AIDS has shown a downward trend, it still is a major health issue. Currently, about one-half million people are known to be living with HIV and AIDS in the United States, as of December 31, 2000 (266).

Renal manifestations from HIV infection occur in 6% to 10% of HIV-infected patients, and 40% of these require renal replacement therapy (RRT) (267,268). HIV-infected patients could also develop renal failure from causes unrelated to HIV.

Prevalence of HIV Infection among Dialysis Patients

The true prevalence of HIV infection among dialysis patients in the United States is unknown, because universal screening is not practiced. In addition, patient confidentiality issues result in incomplete reporting of HIV cases. For these reasons, the reported prevalence is an underestimate of the true prevalence. In the year 2000, 1.5% (range among networks 0.3% to 3.4%) of dialysis patients were reported to have HIV infection, and 0.4% (range among networks 0% to 1%) were reported to have AIDS in the United States. (80). However, the prevalence in different geographical regions of the United States ranges from 0.3% to 38% (8). The wide range in the prevalence of HIV infection among dialysis patients is related to large differences in the prevalence of HIV infection in the population served by these dialysis units. Dialysis units located in the inner cities report a higher prevalence of HIV infection compared with suburban dialysis units, reflecting the higher prevalence of HIV infection in the general population of the inner cities. Finally, there has been a steady increase in the number of HIV-positive patients receiving dialysis in the United States, from 244 (0.3% of the total) in 1985 to 3,447 (1.5% of the total) in 2000. Like-

wise, the proportion of dialysis centers treating HIV-infected patients increased from 11% in 1985 to 37% in 2000 (80).

Limited information is available on the prevalence of HIV infection among CAPD patients. Two single-center studies from the United States observed a prevalence of HIV infection of 7.5% and 8.5%, respectively, among CAPD patients (269,270). Interestingly, the prevalence of HIV infection among hemodialysis patients in those centers was also high (and similar to that among CAPD patients). The high prevalence of HIV infection among both CAPD and hemodialysis patients in those centers may be due to the fact that the centers were located in the inner city. Nonetheless, there could be a physician bias in selecting CAPD for HIV-positive patients to reduce the risk of occupational exposure to dialysis staff, thus resulting in increased prevalence among these patients.

Incident Dialysis Patients with HIV Infection

Again, because of a lack of policy for routine testing for HIV at entry to ESRD therapy, the annual incidence rate for HIV infection and ESRD (rate at which new patients with ESRD and HIV infection enter chronic dialysis therapy) in the United States is not available. Nevertheless, the incidence of ESRD resulting from HIV-associated nephropathy (HIVAN) appears to be increasing. Based on the data from the United States Renal Data System (USRDS), between the years 1987 and 1990, 297 patients with ESRD resulting from HIVAN started dialysis in the United States (average 74 per year) (271). In contrast, between the years 1991 and 1995, 2,738 patients (average 547 per year) (272), and between 1995 and 1999, 4,271 patients (average 854 per year), with ESRD resulting from HIVAN started dialysis (273). In the latter block years (1995 to 1999), HIVAN accounted for 1.1% of the incident ESRD population. The true incidence of HIVAN may be even higher, because HIVAN is not easy to distinguish from some other causes of progressive renal failure, without a renal biopsy. Furthermore, HIV infection is often underreported because of patient confidentiality issues. The single-center reports that have higher or lower incidence are subject to bias from several factors such as referral bias, reporting bias, and under- or overrepresentation of the susceptible population (such as the African-American race) in that community.

Survival Among HIV Infected Patients with Renal Disease

The effect of ESRD on the progression of HIV infection and the effect of HIV infection on survival among ESRD patients on dialysis continue to be debated. ESRD is associated with abnormalities of several immune functions including dysfunction of polymorphonuclear leukocytes, monocytes, and lymphocytes (274). Consequently, the course of HIV infection among ESRD patients would be expected to be accelerated. There is a paucity of information on the effect of ESRD on the course of HIV infection at the current time. In a study by Reiser et al. (275) over a 42-month period, it was observed that 11% of asymptomatic HIV-positive ESRD patients progressed to AIDS; the rate of progression was similar to that among non-ESRD HIV-positive patients over the same duration (10%). CD4 counts and viral load at initiation of dialysis therapy among those who progressed versus those who did not were not available. From this study, it appears that the course of HIV infection among ESRD patients is not significantly different from that among non-ESRD patients, if the patients start ESRD therapy in an asymptomatic state (from the HIV standpoint). Obviously further work must be done in this area.

Survival of HIV-positive patients on dialysis is significantly worse compared with HIV-negative patients on dialysis. Among HIV-positive patients, the determinants of survival include the stage of the disease, HIVAN as the cause of ESRD, CD4 counts, and use of antiretroviral therapy. Early reports suggested an extremely poor prognosis for HIV patients with renal disease. Rao et al. (276) reported a median survival of 1.4 months (range 1 to 9 months) for patients with AIDS starting hemodialysis, all of whom had AIDS-associated nephropathy (276). Similarly, the median survival of patients who developed AIDS while on maintenance hemodialysis was 1 month (range 1 to 3 months) from the time that the diagnosis of AIDS was established (276). However, subsequent studies reported a better survival (1.9 to 33 months) (269–277). Survival of HIV-positive patients on dialysis is critically dependent on the stage of HIV disease. Ortiz et al. (278) observed that the mean survival among hemodialysis patients with AIDS was approximately 3 months, compared with 9.5 months among asymptomatic HIV-positive patients. Likewise, among HIV-positive patients treated with CAPD, asymptomatic patients had a significantly better survival compared with patients with advanced disease (279). In another study by Ifudu et al. (280), among 34 ESRD patients with HIV infection from four dialysis centers (one hospital-based and three community-based), the median duration of ESRD was observed to be 57 months. Twenty-three of the 34 patients (68%) had AIDS before the diagnosis of ESRD, and the cause of ESRD was thought to be HIVAN in these patients. Thirty-one of the 34 (91%) patients were African American and the other three (9%) were Hispanic. These studies suggest that the survival of HIV-positive dialysis patients in the current era has significantly improved compared with the 1980s. This improvement may be the result of improved dialysis techniques, effective use of antiretroviral drugs, and advances in the diagnosis and therapy of opportunistic infections associated with HIV infection and AIDS. Use of antiretroviral therapy significantly improves survival among HIV-positive ESRD patients. In one of the earlier studies, use of antiretroviral therapy was associated with a mean survival of 15 months compared with 6 months among patients who did not receive any antiretroviral therapy (281). In the current era of aggressive and combination therapy, the survival is even better. Indeed, in a recent study, Ahuja et al. (282) observed that with highly active antiretroviral therapy (HAART) only 20% of dialysis patients with HIV infection died after a mean survival of 28 months, whereas 57% of HIV-positive dialysis patients on suboptimal therapy died after a mean survival of only 13 months.

HIVAN also appears to have an independent adverse effect on survival. Indeed, patients with HIVAN have a significantly poor survival (median 9.5 months from diagnosis of HIVAN) compared with patients with AIDS but without HIVAN (median 12.3 months from diagnosis of AIDS) (283). Survival among patients with HIVAN is also determined by the stage of HIV infection. Carbone et al. (277) observed that the median survival of patients with HIVAN who were asymptomatic at diagnosis was approximately 9.7 months, with HIVAN and AIDS-related complex (ARC) it was 3.6 months, and with HIVAN and AIDS it was 1.9 months. Despite the improved survival in the current era, HIVAN patients who undergo dialysis continue to have a shorter survival time compared with patients with ESRD from other causes (282). In a recent analysis using the USRDS database, Abbott et al. (284) observed that the 2-year all-cause unadjusted survival was 36% for ESRD patients with HIVAN compared with 64% for all other patients with ESRD.

As in the case of HIV patients in general, CD4 counts predict survival among HIV-infected ESRD patients. At the San Francisco General Hospital, Schoenfeld et al. (285) observed that dialysis patients with CD4 counts greater than 200 cells/μL (measured at the start of dialysis therapy) had a mean survival of 26 months compared with a mean survival of 8.4 months for patients with CD4 counts less than 200 cells/μL. In a Cox proportional model, among factors such as dialysis modality, weight loss, opportunistic infections, CD4 counts, albumin concentration, and cognitive motor dysfunction, only CD4 counts and neurologic disease correlated with survival (285). In addition to CD4 counts, other investigators have observed that survival was positively correlated with blood pressure (both systolic and diastolic) and negatively correlated with infection rate and degree of urine protein excretion (281).

Studies on the plasma viral load in the current era are still emerging. In the initial study by Ahuja et al. (282), the plasma viral load was significantly less in patients on HAART than on suboptimal therapy (3.35 vs. 4.63 $\log_{10}$ copies/mL). In addition, 7 of the 15 patients on HAART had undetectable viral load at the end of follow-up. Other studies did not show a significant decrease in viral loads with antiretroviral treatment among HIV patients on dialysis (286). The response of ESRD patients to HAART and the response of viral load to this treatment among these patients is still being investigated.

It is not clear whether any survival difference exists between patients undergoing hemodialysis and CAPD. Schoenfeld et al. (287) at the San Francisco General Hospital observed a better survival among HIV-positive patients who were able to do CAPD compared with patients treated with hemodialysis. However, most of these patients were in the earlier stages of HIV disease, and the results were not adjusted for the stage of HIV infection. In another study, Kimmel et al. (269) observed that the modality of dialysis was not a predictor of survival among ESRD patients with HIV infection. Tebben et al. (279) observed a cumulative patient survival of 58% and 54% in the first and second year, respectively, among patients on CAPD; asymptomatic (from the HIV standpoint) patients survived longer than symptomatic patients. Although these studies were conducted in the era when effective therapy for HIV was not available, no studies are available from the current era using HAART.

HIV-positive patients, particularly those with advanced HIV disease, are at increased risk of inadequate dialysis. Patients whose renal failure occurs during their hospital stay or who are admitted to the hospital for initiating hemodialysis are often dialyzed with temporary vascular accesses that do not permit high blood flows for an effective dialysis. Furthermore, HIV-positive patients who continue to abuse intravenous drugs have been observed to have an increased incidence of vascular access infections or clotting of the vascular accesses (276). Infection rate of synthetic grafts, but not native arteriovenous (AV) fistulas, is increased among HIV-positive patients (288). The resulting removal of these grafts tends to increase the use of temporary vascular accesses. These factors may contribute to inadequate dialysis and probably contribute to the decreased survival observed among HIV patients treated with hemodialysis. There may be a possibility of increased viral load with use of nonbiocompatible membranes, particularly if the patient is not receiving antiretroviral therapy (289). Whether use of nonbiocompatible dialysis membranes is associated with any difference in survival compared with use of biocompatible membranes is still unclear. In addition, other factors that are known to influence the survival among non-ESRD patients with HIV infection, such as demographic features, mode of infection, and opportunistic infections may also influence the survival among HIV patients with renal disease.

Choice of Dialysis Therapy

The choice of therapy among HIV-positive patients should be individualized. Because of lower risk of hospital-acquired infections, CAPD offers an advantage to patients. However, CAPD in HIV-positive patients is not without disadvantages. Some investigators have observed an increased incidence of peritonitis, often with opportunistic organisms (279). Also, loss of proteins through the dialysate in an already asthenic patient may result in malnutrition. Furthermore, CAPD is not a suitable option for patients with advanced disease and cognitive motor dysfunction and is often unsuccessful in patients with poor compliance (287). For staff, occupational exposure to HIV with CAPD is less than that of hemodialysis because the PD effluent is less contagious than blood. However, in dialysis units, transmission of HIV from a patient to a health care worker is extremely uncommon if adequate infection-control measures are followed. Indeed, over a 15-year period, only one documented case of transmission of HIV from a patient to a dialysis technician (through a needlestick injury) has been reported in the United States. (3). Hence, the risk to health care workers should not form the basis for a physician's decision on the modality of ESRD therapy. Every effort should be made to construct and preserve native AV fistulas among these patients.

Transmission of HIV Infection in Dialysis Units

Patient-to-Patient Transmission

Transmission of HIV infection from one patient to another is extremely unlikely in dialysis units that conform to the practice guidelines recommended by the CDC (290). Annual surveillance data collected by the CDC from individual dialysis units

in the United States revealed no instances of nosocomial transmission of HIV among patients on maintenance dialysis (290). Similarly, in a large multicenter prospective study of 667 patients from 12 dialysis centers across the United States followed for 48 weeks, no incidence of HIV seroconversion was observed (291). Likewise, Cendoroglo et al. (292) did not observe a single HIV seroconversion among 351 patients on chronic dialysis in Brazil, followed for a period of 3 years. Because the risk of patient-to-patient transmission of HIV is negligible, neither dedicated machines nor isolation from other patients is required for HIV-positive patients on hemodialysis or CAPD (3). The transmission of HIV through contaminated dialysis machines has not been shown so far. One of the reasons is likely from the fact that the average pore size of the dialyzer membrane is approximately 1 to 7 nm, whereas the HIV virion is 105 nm, making it difficult for it to pass through the dialysis membrane (293). Use of the same dialysis machine for HIV-positive and HIV-negative patients has not been shown to be associated with transmission of HIV. Although most dialysis units do not reuse dialyzers for HIV-infected patients, disinfection procedures for reprocessing of dialyzers and dialysis machines that are currently recommended for non-HIV patients should be followed for HIV-infected patients too, because these procedures are adequate to kill HIV (294).

A breach in infection-control measures can result in HIV transmission in dialysis units. Indeed, transmission of HIV in dialysis units has been reported from Colombia, Argentina, and Egypt (295–297). In all these instances, adequate precautions were not followed either for disinfection of dialyzers or vascular access needles. In the Colombian outbreak, an investigation by the CDC revealed that transmission of HIV in the dialysis center was probably due to cross-contamination of dialysis access needles or from inadvertent sharing of inadequately disinfected access needles between HIV infected and uninfected patients. In the Argentinean outbreak, either a multidose heparin vial or cross-use of filter or both may have been the reason for HIV transmission among many patients in the same dialysis facility (295). In the Egyptian outbreak, use of syringes for more than one patient was believed to be the reason for transmission of HIV (297). These outbreaks underline the importance of observing adequate procedures for disinfection of dialyzers and dialysis access devices and standard precautions for prevention of cross contamination.

Patient-to-Staff Transmission

Needlestick injuries and skin and mucous membrane exposures to blood or body fluids are not uncommon in dialysis units. In a study among Italian dialysis units, Ippolito et al. (298) reported an incidence of 5 needlestick exposures and 28 skin and mucous membrane exposures for every 10,000 dialyses. When such an exposure involves HIV-infected material, it is of considerable concern to the health care worker. However, transmission of HIV from a patient to a dialysis staff member is exceedingly rare with only one reported instance in the United States so far through a needlestick injury (293). Not necessarily in a dialysis setting, as of June 2001, the CDC received voluntary reports of 57 U.S. heath care workers with documented

HIV seroconversion associated with occupational exposure, with another 137 cases with exposure but without seroconversion (299). The actual rate of transmission may be higher because there is often a significant underreporting of HIV infection. Notwithstanding this low rate of transmission, it is worthwhile reviewing studies on occupational exposure to HIV to a health care worker.

Pooled analysis from 25 prospective studies suggests that the risk of acquiring HIV infection following occupational exposure resulting from needle punctures and similar percutaneous injuries is approximately 0.3% (95%, CI 0.2% to 0.5%) or 21 infections after 6,498 exposures (300,301). The risk following a mucous membrane exposure is even less (0.09%, CI 0.006 to 0.5%) (302). The risk following exposure through a nonintact skin is not well studied, although the risk appears to be less than that of mucous membrane exposure. In a multinational case-control study of health care workers with percutaneous occupational exposure to HIV-infected blood, the factors that were independently associated with a seroconversion were deep injury (odds ratio 15, 95% confidence interval 6–41), visible blood on sharp device (odds ratio 6.2, 95% confidence interval 2.2–21), needle used to enter blood vessel (odds ratio 4.3, 95% confidence interval 1.7–12), and a source patient who died within 60 days of the incident (odds ratio 5.6, 95% confidence interval 2–16). Zidovudine (AZT) prophylaxis was associated with a lower risk of acquiring HIV infection (odds ratio 0.19, 95% confidence interval 0.06–0.52) (303,304). These suggest that the risk is associated with exposure to a greater volume of infected blood, as supported by another study that demonstrated that needle (bore) size and depth of penetration were significantly associated with transfer volume (305). In addition, in the same study, the case patients were less likely to have taken AZT prophylaxis, suggesting thereby that AZT may have a protective value. Further evidence as to the protection by AZT is suggested by another study in which AZT prophylaxis after a percutaneous exposure to HIV was associated with a blunted in vitro response of cytotoxic T-lymphocyte (CTL) response to exposure to HIV-specific antigens (306). The source patient's viral titer for assessing the transmission risk has not yet been established. The plasma viral load reflects only the level of cell-free virus, and transmission by latent viruses in the peripheral mononuclear cells in the presence of an undetectable or low viral titer has not been ruled out (307). Alternately, some authors speculate that phenotypic and genotypic differences in the virus in terminally ill patients with AIDS may also account for the increased risk of transmission (308).

Transmission of HIV from a dialysis patient to a health care worker could also occur from improper handling or disposal of infected PD effluent. Indeed, HIV has been recovered from PD effluent (309). The effluent forms a good culture medium for HIV. The virus is not only known to survive but also to replicate for up to 7 days in the effluent (310). Furthermore, HIV has been shown to survive for up to 48 hours in PD exchange tubings (311). Because the effluent dialysate is also infectious, it is important that HIV-positive patients treated with CAPD are taught proper disposal of effluent dialysate at home. The Task Force on HIV and Kidney Disease has issued detailed recommendations for disinfection, at home and in the hospital, of PD effluent in HIV-infected patients (312). In view of some studies showing HIV multiplication in PD fluid effluent, some authors recommend additional disinfection measures (313). Chemicals known to inactivate HIV include Amukin, household bleach, and povidone-iodine mixture, and these are recommended to be added to the PD dialysis effluent before disposal.

Staff-to-Patient Transmission

To date, there have been no reports of transmission of HIV from a health care worker to a patient in a dialysis setting.

There are other important issues in dialysis units that accept patients with HIV infection. Patients with HIV infection are prone to infection with *Mycobacterium tuberculosis*. In contrast to HIV, *M. tuberculosis* infection is an aerosol-transmitted infection, and, therefore, precautions to prevent the spread of this infection to other patients should be taken. Importantly, *M. tuberculosis* infections among HIV-infected patients are often multidrug resistant. Nosocomial transmission of multidrug tuberculosis has been described (314). In addition to tuberculosis, HIV-infected patients are at increased risk of other communicable infections. Appropriate precautions should be observed to protect other patients in the dialysis facility and the staff caring for these patients.

Postexposure Prophylaxis (PEP)

Even if PEP is not provided, seroconversion following an occupational exposure to HIV is only 0.3% (304). Given such a low incidence of seroconversion, a prospective randomized trial to assess the value of PEP for occupational exposure to HIV requires recruiting several thousand health care workers. Because such a study is difficult to perform, we rely on animal studies and nonrandomized human studies to assess the effectiveness of PEP. In a study with inoculation of simian immunodeficiency virus (SIV) into macaque monkeys, a 4-week course of tenofovir starting before or within 24 hours of inoculation uniformly prevented seroconversion compared with untreated monkeys (315). Incomplete protection was observed if the prophylaxis was delayed up to 48 hours or later or the duration was curtailed to 3 or 10 days (316). Although there are other studies in the recent past confirming the efficacy of PEP in animals (317,318), these data have been difficult to extrapolate to humans because of differences in the controlled situation in the laboratory and in real-life situations. Furthermore, adverse effects of antiretroviral drugs are a matter of concern. In a study of 200 persons treated with AZT 200 mg five times a day for 4 weeks following an occupational exposure to HIV, one third of patients stopped the drug because of side effects (319). Two other studies have also reported a high dropout rate because of side effects (320,321). In the most quoted study by Cardo et al. (304), use of AZT was associated with an 81% reduction in the seroconversion. This study is limited by the fact that the number of cases were few and cases and controls were from different cohorts. In a different clinical setting of perinatal transmission of HIV, administration of AZT alone or in combination with lamivudine was associated with a significant reduction in perinatal transmission (322–326). Despite these evidences, skeptics argue that the situation of maternal-fetal transmission and that of occupational exposure are not similar in terms of transmission, that there are several reports of seroconversion following occupational exposure despite prophylaxis (327,328), and that concerns regarding delayed mutagenicity and carcinogenicity with AZT therapy cannot be ignored (329). Finally, none of the studies have examined the long-term effects of AZT in an otherwise healthy person.

Despite the limitations discussed previously, PEP for HIV can be recommended for several reasons. Early antiretroviral therapy may minimize the effective viral inoculum and thus abrogate or diminish the probability of acquiring the infection. There clearly exists a rationale for prophylaxis after an accidental occupational HIV exposure, because it takes several days for uptake, processing, and presentation of the viral particle before it starts to propagate (308). Extrapolation of the results from animal studies to humans may not also be appropriate, because the viral titer in most primate studies was substantially higher than in human occupational exposure (308). Furthermore, in these studies, animals were inoculated by the intravenous route, bypassing the cutaneous route whose defenses are important in viral elimination (308). The limited human experience with PEP shows a high dropout rate of approximately 33% because of side effects, more so with a three-drug regimen (308,330,331). The psychologic effects of an occupational exposure to HIV in an otherwise healthy person should also be considered.

To date, there are no published randomized trials of AZT for PEP to health care workers exposed to HIV. The updated guidelines for prophylaxis of occupational parenteral exposures to HIV have been recently released by the CDC (307). The CDC acknowledges that the recommendations are based on limited data regarding efficacy and toxicity of PEP. These recommendations are given in Tables 22.2 and 22.3, for percutaneous and mucous membrane and nonintact skin exposures, respectively. Chemoprophylaxis is recommended for workers after occupational exposures associated with known HIV-positive status. PEP is generally not recommended for exposures from a source patient with unknown HIV status or unknown source, unless there are concerns that there may be HIV risk factors in the source or exposure to HIV-infected person is likely. If the source patient is known to be HIV-negative, no PEP is recommended. These decisions should be based on a discussion between the exposed person and the treating physician and, if necessary, with consultation of a physician who has experience in using these medications. These decisions should take into consideration the risk of infection and potential toxicity of the drugs. Single-drug therapy for PEP should be avoided, because of potential resistance of HIV to this regimen. Typically, the two-drug regimens consist of one of the three combinations, AZT + lamivudine (3TC), 3TC + stavudine (d4T), or didanosine (ddI) + d4T. The expanded three-drug regimen consists of one of the previous combinations with addition of indinavir, nelfinavir, efavirenz, or abacavir.

Although animal experiments suggest that PEP probably is not effective when started later than 24 to 36 hours after the exposure, the interval after which there is no benefit from PEP for humans is undefined (332). Therefore, if appropriate for the exposure, PEP should be initiated even if the interval is longer than 36 hours (307). Although the optimal duration of PEP is unknown, the CDC recommends therapy for 4 weeks based on the results of earlier human and animal studies (304,316). The exposed person should be reevaluated within 72 hours, whenever possible, as more information is available about the exposure or the source person.

TABLE 22.2. RECOMMENDED HIV POSTEXPOSURE PROPHYLAXIS (PEP) FOR PERCUTANEOUS INJURIES

	Infection Status of Source				
Exposure Type	HIV-Positive Class 1[a]	HIV-Positive Class 2[a]	Source of Unknown HIV Status[b]	Unknown Source[c]	HIV-Negative
Less severe[d]	Recommend basic 2-drug PEP	Recommend expanded 3-drug PEP	Generally no PEP required; consider 2-drug PEP[e] for source with HIV risk factors[f]	Generally no PEP required; consider 2-drug PEP[e] in settings where exposure to HIV-infected person likely	No PEP warranted
More severe[g]	Recommend expanded 3-drug PEP	Recommend expanded 3-drug PEP	Generally no PEP required; consider 2-drug PEP[e] for source with HIV risk factors[f]	Generally no PEP required; consider 2-drug PEP[e] in settings where exposure to HIV-infected person likely	No PEP warranted

[a]HIV-positive, Class 1—asymptomatic HIV infection or known low viral load (<1,500 copies/mL). HIV-positive, Class 2—symptomatic HIV infection, AIDS, acute seroconversion, or known high viral load. If drug resistance is a concern, obtain expert consultation. Initiation of PEP should not be delayed pending expert consultation, and, because expert consultation alone cannot substitute for face-to-face counseling, resources should be available to provide immediate evaluation and follow-up care for all exposures.
[b]Source of unknown HIV status (e.g., deceased source person with no samples available for HIV testing).
[c]Unknown source (e.g., a needle from a sharp disposal container).
[d]Less severe (e.g., solid needle and superficial injury).
[e]The designation "consider PEP" indicates that PEP is optional and should be based on an individualized decision between the exposed person and the treating clinician.
[f]If PEP is offered and taken and the source is later determined to be HIV-negative, PEP should be discontinued.
[g]More severe (e.g., large-bore hollow needle, deep puncture, visible blood on device, or needle used in patient's artery or vein).
From D'Amico R, et al. Effect of zidovudine postexposure prophylaxis on the development of HIV-specific cytotoxic T-lymphocyte responses in HIV-exposed healthcare workers. *Infect Control Hosp Epidemiol* 1999;20:428–430, with permission.

TABLE 22.3. RECOMMENDED HIV POSTEXPOSURE PROPHYLAXIS (PEP) FOR MUCOUS MEMBRANE EXPOSURES AND NONINTACT SKIN[a] EXPOSURES

Exposure Type	HIV-Positive Class 1[b]	HIV-Positive Class 2[b]	Source of Unknown HIV Status[c]	Unknown Source[d]	HIV-Negative
			Infection Status of Source		
Small volume[e]	Recommend basic 2-drug PEP	Recommend expanded 3-drug PEP	Generally no PEP required; consider 2-drug PEP[f] for source with HIV risk factors[g]	Generally no PEP required; consider 2-drug PEP[f] in settings where exposure to HIV-infected person likely	No PEP warranted
Large volume[h]	Recommend expanded 3-drug PEP	Recommend expanded 3-drug PEP	Generally no PEP required; consider 2-drug PEP[f] for source with HIV risk factors[g]	Generally no PEP required; consider 2-drug PEP[f] in settings where exposure to HIV-infected person likely	No PEP warranted

[a]For skin exposures, follow-up is indicated only if there is evidence of compromised skin integrity (e.g., dermatitis, abrasion, or open wound).
[b]HIV-positive, Class 1—asymptomatic HIV infection or known low viral load (<1,500 copies/mL). HIV-positive, Class 2—symptomatic HIV infection, AIDS, acute seroconversion, or known high viral load. If drug resistance is a concern, obtain expert consultation. Initiation of PEP should not be delayed pending expert consultation, and, because expert consultation alone cannot substitute for face-to-face counseling, resources should be available to provide immediate evaluation and follow-up care for all exposures.
[c]Source of unknown HIV status (e.g., deceased source person with no samples available for HIV testing).
[d]Unknown source (e.g., splash from inappropriately disposed blood).
[e]Small volume (i.e., a few drops).
[f]The designation "consider PEP" indicates that PEP is optional and should be based on an individualized decision between the exposed person and the treating clinician.
[g]If PEP is offered and taken and the source is later determined to be HIV-negative, PEP should be discontinued.
[h]Large volume (i.e., major blood splash).
From D'Amico R, et al. Effect of zidovudine postexposure prophylaxis on the development of HIV-specific cytotoxic T-lymphocyte responses in HIV-exposed healthcare workers. *Infect Control Hosp Epidemiol* 1999;20:428–430, with permission.

Workers with occupational exposures to HIV should receive follow-up medical evaluation, including HIV-antibody tests at baseline and periodically for at least 6 months postexposure regardless of PEP. Extended follow-up to 12 months is recommended for exposures to a source coinfected with HIV and HCV. Monitoring should be done using the enzyme immunoassay (EIA) rather than direct viral assays (such as P24 antigen or HIV RNA), which only increase the false-positive results causing unnecessary anxiety (307). Drug-toxicity monitoring should include a complete blood count and renal and hepatic function tests at baseline and 2 weeks after starting PEP, in addition to the specific adverse effects of the corresponding drug(s).

Counseling is an integral part of the PEP, because the emotional effect of exposure is enormous although the risk of transmission is low. For the first 6 to 12 weeks after exposure when highest chance of seroconversion exists, some important pieces of advice include sexual abstinence or use of condoms; avoidance of pregnancy; discontinuation of breast feeding; and refraining from donating blood, tissue or organs. For detailed procedures and guidelines, the reader is referred to other resources available at the CDC Web site (www.cdc.gov).

REFERENCES

1. Pereira BJG, et al. Hepatitis C virus infection in dialysis and renal transplantation. *Kidney Int* 1997;51:981–999.
2. Dyer E. Argentinian doctors accused of spreading AIDS (news). *BMJ* 1993;307:584.
3. Tokars JI, et al. National surveillance of dialysis associated diseases in the United States—1994. *ASAIO J* 1997;43:108–119.
4. Valderrabano F, et al. Report on management of renal failure in Europe, XXIV, 1993. *Nephrol Dial Transplant* 1995;10[Suppl 5]:1–25.
5. Murthy BVR, et al. Impact of pre-transplantation GB virus C (GBV-C) infection on the outcome of renal transplantation. *J Am Soc Nephrol* 1997;8:1164–1173.
6. Pereira BJG, et al. The impact of pretransplantation hepatitis C infection on the outcome of renal transplantation. *Transplantation* 1995;60:799–805.
7. Schreiber GB, et al. The risk of transfusion-transmitted viral infections: the Retrovirus Epidemiology Donor Study [see comments]. *N Engl J Med* 1996;334:1685–1690.
8. Murthy BVR, et al. A 1990s perspective of hepatitis C, human immunodeficiency virus and tuberculosis infections in dialysis patients. *Semin Nephrol* 1997;17:346–363.
9. Alter MJ, et al. The changing epidemiology of hepatitis B in the United States: need for alternative vaccination strategies. *JAMA* 1990;263:1218–1222.
10. Choo Q, et al. Isolation of a cDNA clone derived from a blood-borne non-A, non-B viral hepatitis genome. *Science* 1989;244:358–362.
11. Kuo G, et al. An assay for circulating antibodies to a major etiologic virus of human non-A, non-B hepatitis. *Science* 1989;244:362–364.
12. Farci P, et al. A long-term study of hepatitis C virus replication in non-A, non-B hepatitis. *N Engl J Med* 1991;325:98–104.
13. Alter HJ, et al. Detection of antibody to hepatitis C virus in prospectively followed transfusion recipients with acute and chronic non-A, non-B hepatitis. *N Engl J Med* 1989;321:1494–1500.
14. Esteban JI, et al. Evaluation of antibodies to hepatitis C virus in a study of transfusion-associated hepatitis. *N Engl J Med* 1990;323:1107–1112.
15. Kassem AS, et al. Prevalence of hepatitis C virus (HCV) infection and its vertical transmission in Egyptian pregnant women and their newborns. *J Trop Pediatr* 2000;46:231–233.

16. Gibb DM, et al. Mother-to-child transmission of hepatitis C virus: evidence from preventable peripartum transmission. *Lancet* 2000; 356:904–907.

17. Pereira BJG, et al. Transmission of hepatitis C virus by organ transplantation. *N Engl J Med* 1991;325:454–460.

18. Pereira BJG, et al. Prevalence of HCV RNA in hepatitis C antibody positive cadaver organ donors and their recipients. *N Engl J Med* 1992;327:910–915.

19. Weiner AJ, et al. Detection of hepatitis C viral sequences in non-A, non-B hepatitis. *Lancet* 1990;335:1–3.

20. Okamoto H, et al. Detection of hepatitis C virus RNA by a two-stage polymerase chain reaction with two pairs of primers deduced from the 5′-noncoding region. *Jpn J Exp Med* 1990;60:215–222.

21. Houghton M, et al. Molecular biology of the hepatitis C viruses: implications for diagnosis, development and control of viral disease. *Hepatology* 1991;14:381–388.

22. Okamoto H, et al. Nucleotide sequence of the genomic RNA of hepatitis C virus isolated from a human carrier: comparison with reported isolates for conserved and divergent regions. *J Gen Virol* 1991;72:2697–2704.

23. Okamoto H, et al. Typing hepatitis C virus by polymerase chain reaction with type-specific primers: application to clinical surveys and tracing infectious sources. *J Gen Virol* 1992;73:673–679.

24. Simmonds P, et al. Classification of hepatitis C virus into six major region genotypes and a series of subtypes by phylogenetic analysis of the NS5 region. *J Gen Virol* 1993;74:2391–2399.

25. Simmonds P, et al. A proposed system for the nomenclature of hepatitis C virus genotypes. *Hepatology* 1994;19:1321–1324.

26. Podzorski R. Molecular testing in the diagnosis and management of hepatitis C virus infection. *Arch Pathol Lab Med* 2002;126:285–290.

27. Lau JYN, et al. Significance of antibody to the host cellular gene derived epitope GOR in chronic hepatitis C virus infection. *J Hepatol* 1993;17:253–257.

28. Hofgartner WT, et al. Hepatitis C virus quantitation: optimization of strategies for detecting low-level viremia. *J Clin Microbiol* 2000; 38:888–891.

29. Kwok S, et al. Avoiding false positives with PCR. *Nature* 1989;339: 237–238.

30. Busch MP, et al. Impact of specimen handling and storage on detection of hepatitis C virus RNA. *Transfusion* 1992;32:420–425.

31. Grant PR, et al. Effects of handling and storage of blood on the stability of hepatitis C virus RNA: implications for NAT testing in transfusion practice. *Vox Sang* 2000;78:137–142.

32. Nagayama R, et al. Genotype dependence of hepatitis C virus antibodies detectable by the first generation enzyme-linked immunosorbent assay with C100-3 protein. *J Clin Invest* 1993;92:1529–1533.

33. Stuyver L, et al. Typing of hepatitis C virus isolates and characterization of new. *J Gen Virol* 1993;74:1093–1102.

34. Fabrizi F, et al. Serotyping strip immunoblot assay for assessing hepatitis C virus strains in dialysis patients. *Am J Kidney Dis* 2000; 35:832–838.

35. Aach RD, et al. Hepatitis C virus infection in post-transfusion hepatitis. *N Engl J Med* 1991;325:1325–1329.

36. Nasoff MS, et al. Identification of an immunodominant epitope within the capsid protein of hepatitis C virus. *Proc Natl Acad Sci U S A* 1991;88:5462–5466.

37. Busch MP, et al. Declining value of alanine aminotransferase in screening of blood donors to prevent posttransfusion hepatitis B and C virus infection. *Transfusion* 1995;35:903–910.

38. Soffredini R, et al. Increased detection of antibody to hepatitis C virus in renal transplant patients by third-generation assays. *Am J Kidney Dis* 1996;28:437–440.

39. Fabrizi F, et al. Serologic survey for control of hepatitis C in haemodialysis patients: third-generation assays and analysis of cost. *Nephrol Dial Transplant* 1997;12:298.

40. Tanaka T, et al. Simple fluorescent enzyme immunoassay for detection and quantification of hepatitis C viremia. *J Hepatol* 1995;23: 742–745.

41. Tanaka E, et al. Evaluation of a new enzyme immunoassay for hepatitis C virus (HCV) core antigen with clinical sensitivity approximating that of genomic amplification of HCV RNA. *Hepatology* 2000;32: 388–393.

42. Aoyagi K, et al. Development of a simple and highly sensitive enzyme immunoassay for hepatitis C virus core antigen. *Vox Sang* 1999;37: 1802–1808.

43. Kurtz JB, et al. The diagnostic significance of an assay for 'total' hepatitis C core antigen. *J Virol Methods* 2001;96:127–132.

44. Dussol B, et al. Detection of hepatitis C infection by polymerase chain reaction among hemodialysis patients. *Am J Kidney Dis* 1993; 22:574–580.

45. Pol S, et al. Hepatitis C virus RNA in anti-HCV positive hemodialyzed patients: significance and therapeutic implications. *Kidney Int* 1993;44:1097–1100.

46. Dentico P, et al. Hepatitis C virus-RNA, immunoglobulin M anti-HCV and risk factors in haemodialysis patients. *Microbios* 1999;99: 55–62.

47. Williams M, et al. Hepatitis C virus-RNA in plasma and in peripheral blood mononuclear cells of hemophiliacs with chronic hepatitis C: evidence for viral replication in peripheral blood mononuclear cells. *J Med Virol* 1994;42:272–278.

48. Umlauft F, et al. Patterns of hepatitis C viremia in patients receiving hemodialysis. *Am J Gastroenterol* 1997;92:73–78.

49. DuBois DB, et al. Quantitation of hepatitis C viral RNA in sera of hemodialysis patients: gender-related differences in viral load. *Am J Kidney Dis* 1994;24:795–801.

50. Alter MJ, et al. The natural history of community-acquired hepatitis C in the United States: the Sentinel Countries Chronic non-A, non-B Hepatitis Study Team. *N Engl J Med* 1992;327:1899–1905.

51. al Meshari K, et al. New insights into hepatitis C virus infection of hemodialysis patients: the implications. *Am J Kidney Dis* 1995;25: 572–578.

52. Oesterreicher C, et al. HBV and HCV genome in peripheral blood mononuclear cells in patients undergoing hemodialysis. *Kidney Int* 1995;48:1967–1971.

53. Courouce A-M, et al. Hepatitis C (HCV) infection in haemodialysed patients: HCV-RNA and anti-HCV antibodies (third-generation assays). *Nephrol Dial Transplant* 1995;10:234–239.

54. Courouce AM, et al. A comparative evaluation of the sensitivity of seven anti-hepatitis C virus screening tests. *Vox Sang* 1995;69: 213–216.

55. Carrera F, et al. Persistence of antibodies to hepatitis C virus in a chronic hemodialysis population. *Nephron* 1994;68:38–40.

56. Simon N, et al. A twelve-year natural history of hepatitis C virus infection in hemodialyzed patients. *Kidney Int* 1994;46:504–511.

57. Yoshimura E, et al. No significant changes in levels of hepatitis C virus (HCV) RNA by competitive polymerase chain reaction in blood samples from patients with chronic HCV infection. *Dig Dis Sci* 1997;42:772–777.

58. Alter HJ. Chronic consequences of non-A, non-B hepatitis. In: Seeff LB, et al., eds. *Current perspectives in hepatology.* New York: Plenum, 1989:83–97.

59. Kiyosawa K, et al. Interrelationship of blood transfusion, non-A, non-B hepatitis and hepatocellular carcinoma: analysis by detection of antibody to hepatitis C virus. *Hepatology* 1990;12:671–675.

60. Seeff LB, et al. Long-term mortality after transfusion-associated non-A, non-B hepatitis. *N Engl J Med* 1992;327:1906–1911.

61. Espinosa M, et al. Natural history of acute HCV infection in hemodialysis patients. *Clin Nephrol* 2002;58:143–150.

62. Alberti A, et al. Hepatitis C viraemia and liver disease in symptom-free individuals with anti-HCV. *Lancet* 1992;340:697–698.

63. Wolf PL, et al. Low aspartate transaminase activity in serum of patients undergoing chronic hemodialysis. *Clin Chem* 1972;18:567–573.

64. Rao KV, et al. Value of liver biopsy in the evaluation and management of chronic liver disease in renal transplant recipients. *Am J Med* 1993;94:241–250.

65. Zibert A, et al. Antibodies in human sera to hypervariable region 1 of hepatitis C virus can block viral attachment. *Virology* 1995;208: 653–661.

66. Farci P, et al. Lack of protective immunity against reinfection with hepatitis C virus. *Science* 1992;258:135–140.

67. Lai ME, et al. Hepatitis C virus in multiple episodes of acute hepatitis in polytransfused thalassaemic children. *Lancet* 1994;343: 388–390.

68. Kao JH, et al. Superinfection of heterologous hepatitis C virus in a patient with chronic type C hepatitis. *Gastroenterology* 1993;105: 583–587.

69. Oldach D, et al. Clinical and virological outcomes in hepatitis C virus (HCV)-infected renal transplant recipients, 14th annual meeting of the American Society of Transplant Physicians, Chicago, May 14–17, 1995.

70. Widell A, et al. Hepatitis C superinfection in hepatitis C virus (HCV)-infected patients transplanted with an HCV-infected kidney. *Transplantation* 1995;60:642–647.

71. Qian KP, et al. Hepatitis C virus mixed genotype infection in patients on hemodialysis. *J Viral Hepatitis* 2000;7:153–160.

72. Natov SN, et al. Hepatitis C infection in patients on dialysis. *Semin Dial* 1994;7:360–368.

73. Natov SN, et al. Hepatitis C in dialysis patients. *Adv Ren Replace Ther* 1996;3:275–283.

74. Tokars JI, et al. National surveillance of dialysis associated diseases in the United States, 1995. *ASAIO J* 1998;44:98–107.

75. Biamino E, et al. Prevalence of anti-HCV antibody positivity and seroconversion incidence in hemodialysis patients. *Minerva Urol Nefrol* 1999;51:53–55.

76. Natov SN, et al. Serological and virological profiles of hepatitis C infection in renal transplant candidates. *Am J Kidney Dis* 1998;31: 920–927.

77. de Medina M, et al. Prevalence of hepatitis C and G virus infection in chronic hemodialysis patients. *Am J Kidney Dis* 1998;31:224–226.

78. Othman B, et al. Prevalence of antibodies to hepatitis C virus among hemodialysis patients in Damascus, Syria. *Infection* 2001;29:262.

79. Covic A, et al. Hepatitis virus infection in haemodialysis patients from Moldavia. *Dial Nephrol Transplant* 1999;14:40–45.

80. Tokars JI, et al. National surveillance of dialysis-associated diseases in the United States, 2000. *Semin Dial* 2002;15:162–171.

81. Pinto dos Santos J, et al. Impact of dialysis room and reuse strategies on the incidence of HCV infection in HD units. *Nephrol Dial Transplant* 1996;11:2017–2022.

82. Huraib S, et al. High prevalence of and risk factors for hepatitis C in haemodialysis patients in Saudi Arabia: a need for new dialysis strategies. *Nephrol Dial Transplant* 1995;10:470–474.

83. Geerlings W, et al. Report on the management of renal failure in Europe, XXIII. *Nephrol Dial Transplant* 1994;9:6–25.

84. Tokars JI, et al. National surveillance of dialysis associated diseases in the United States, 1997. *Semin Dial* 2000;13:75–85.

85. Dussol B, et al. Hepatitis C virus infection among chronic dialysis patients in the south of France: a collaborative study. *Am J Kidney Dis* 1995;25:399–404.

86. Medici G, et al. Anti-hepatitis C virus positivity and clinical correlations in hemodialyzed patients. *Nephron* 1992;61:363–364.

87. Hardy NM, et al. Antibody to hepatitis C virus increases with time on dialysis. *Clin Nephrol* 1992;38:44–48.

88. Oguchi H, et al. Hepatitis virus infection (HBV and HCV) in eleven Japanese hemodialysis units. *Clin Nephrol* 1992;38:36–43.

89. Sivapalasingam S, et al. High prevalence of hepatitis C infection among patients receiving hemodialysis at an urban dialysis center. *Infect Control Hosp Epidemiol* 2002;23:319–324.

90. Selgas R, et al. Prevalence of hepatitis C antibodies (HCV) in a dialysis population at one center. *Perit Dial Int* 1992;12:28–30.

91. Dussol B, et al. Hepatitis C virus infection among chronic dialysis patients in the south-east of France. *Nephrol Dial Transplant* 1995;10: 477–478.

92. McIntyre PG, et al. Hepatitis C virus infection in renal dialysis patients in Glasgow. *Nephrol Dial Transplant* 1994;9:291–295.

93. Huang CC, et al. The prevalence of hepatitis C virus antibodies in patients treated with continuous ambulatory peritoneal dialysis. *Perit Dial Int* 1992;12:31–33.

94. Chan TM, et al. Hepatitis C infection among dialysis patients: a comparison between patients on maintenance haemodialysis and continuous ambulatory peritoneal dialysis. *Nephrol Dial Transplant* 1991; 6:944–947.

95. Brugnano R, et al. Antibodies against hepatitis C virus in hemodialysis patients in the central Italian region of Umbria: evaluation of some risk factors. *Nephron* 1992;61:263–265.

96. Jonas MM, et al. Hepatitis C infection in pediatric dialysis population. *Pediatrics* 1992;89:707–709.

97. Cantu P, et al. Prevalence of antibodies against hepatitis C virus in a dialysis unit. *Nephron* 1992;61:337–338.

98. Barril G, et al. Prevalence of hepatitis C virus in dialysis patients in Spain. *Nephrol Dial Transplant* 1995;10[Suppl 6]:78–80.

99. Cendoroglo-Neto M, et al. Incidence of and risk factors for hepatitis B virus and hepatitis C virus infection among haemodialysis and CAPD patients: evidence for environmental transmission. *Nephrol Dial Transplant* 1995;10:240–246.

100. Yoshida CFT, et al. Hepatitis C virus in chronic hemodialysis patients with non-A, non-B hepatitis. *Nephron* 1992;60:150–153.

101. Weinstein T, et al. Hepatitis C infection in dialysis patients in Israel. *Isr Med Assoc J* 2001;3:174.

102. Gilli P, et al. Non-A, non-B hepatitis and anti-HCV antibodies in dialysis patients. *Int J Artif Organs* 1990;13:737–741.

103. Pascual J, et al. Nosocomial transmission of hepatitis C virus (HCV) infection in a hemodialysis (HD) unit during two years of prospective follow-up. *J Am Soc Nephrol* 1992;3:386(abst).

104. Bruguera M, et al. Incidence and features of liver disease in patients on chronic hemodialysis. *J Clin Gastroenterol* 1990;12:298–302.

105. Jadoul M, et al. Incidence and risk factors for hepatitis C seroconversion in hemodialysis: a prospective study. *Kidney Int* 1993;44: 1322–1326.

106. Corcoran GD, et al. Hepatitis C virus infection in hemodialysis patients: a clinical and virological study. *J Infect Dis* 1994;28: 279–285.

107. Jeffers LJ, et al. Hepatitis C infection in two urban hemodialysis units. *Kidney Int* 1990;38:320–322.

108. Stuyver L, et al. Hepatitis C virus in a hemodialysis unit: molecular evidence for nosocomial transmission. *Kidney Int* 1996;49:889–895.

109. Halfon P, et al. Use of phylogenetic analysis of hepatitis C virus (HCV) hypervariable region 1 sequences to trace an outbreak of HCV in an autodialysis unit. *J Clin Microbiol* 2002;40:1541–1545.

110. Grethe S, et al. Molecular epidemiology of an outbreak of HCV in a hemodialysis unit: direct sequencing of HCV-HVR1 as an appropriate tool for phylogenetic analysis. *J Med Virol* 2000;60:152–158.

111. Olmer M, et al. Transmission of the hepatitis C virus in a hemodialysis unit: evidence for nosocomial infection. *Clin Nephrol* 1997;47: 263–270.

112. Sullivan DG, et al. Investigating hepatitis C virus heterogeneity in a high prevalence setting using heteroduplex tracking analysis. *J Virol Methods* 2001;96:5–16.

113. Zeuzem S, et al. Phylogenetic analysis of hepatitis C virus isolates from hemodialysis patients. *Kidney Int* 1996;49:896–902.

114. Kiyosawa K, et al. Hepatitis C in hospital employees with needlestick injuries. *Ann Intern Med* 1991;115:367–369.

115. Mitsui T, et al. Hepatitis C virus infection in medical personnel after needlestick accident. *Hepatology* 1992;16:1109–1114.

116. Alter MJ, et al. National surveillance of dialysis-associated diseases in the United States, 1989. *ASAIO Trans* 1991;37:97–109.

117. Niu MT, et al. Outbreak of hemodialysis-associated non-A, non-B hepatitis and correlation with antibody for hepatitis C virus. *Am J Kidney Dis* 1992;19:345–352.

118. Garcia-Valdescasas J, et al. Strategies to reduce the transmission of HCV infection in hemodialysis (HD) units. *J Am Soc Nephrol* 1993; 4:347(abst).

119. Jadoul M, et al. Universal precautions prevent hepatitis C virus transmission: a 54-month follow-up of the Belgian multicenter study. *Kidney Int* 1998;53:1022–1025.

120. Alfurayh O, et al. Hand contamination with hepatitis C virus in staff looking after hepatitis C-positive hemodialysis patients. *Am J Nephrol* 2000;20:103–106.

121. Petrosillo N, et al. Prevalence of infected patients and understaffing

have a role in hepatitis C virus transmission in dialysis. *Am J Kidney Dis* 2001;37:1004–1010.

122. Da Porto A, et al. Hepatitis C virus in dialysis units: a multicenter study. *Nephron* 1992;61:309–310.

123. Mitwalli A, et al. Hepatitis C in chronic renal failure patients. *Am J Nephrol* 1992;12:288–291.

124. Rais-Jalali G, et al. Anti-HCV seropositivity among haemodialysis patients of Iranian origin. *Nephrol Dial Transplant* 1999;14:2055–2056.

125. Delarocque-Astagneau E, et al. Outbreak of hepatitis C virus infection in a hemodialysis unit: potential transmission by the hemodialysis machine? *Infect Control Hosp Epidemiol* 2002;23:328–334.

126. Taskapan H, et al. Patient to patient transmission of hepatitis C virus in hemodialysis units. *Clin Nephrol* 2001;55:477–481.

127. Lombardi M, et al. Results of a national epidemiological investigation on HCV infection among dialysis patients. (Survey by the Italian Branch of EDTNA/ERCA.) *J Nephrol* 1999;12:322–327.

128. Valtuille R, et al. Decline of high hepatitis C virus prevalence in a hemodialysis unit with no isolation measures during a 6-year follow-up. *Clin Nephrol* 2002;57:371–375.

129. Aucella F, et al. Systemic monitor disinfection is effective in limiting HCV spread in hemodialysis. *Blood Purif* 2000;18:110–114.

130. Barril G, et al. Autoclaving eliminates hepatitis C virus from a hemodialysis monitor contaminated artificially. *J Med Virol* 2000;60:139–143.

131. Yuasa T, et al. The particle size of hepatitis C virus estimated by filtration through microporous regenerated cellulose fibre. *J Gen Virol* 1991;72:2021–2024.

132. Hubmann R, et al. Hepatitis C virus—does it penetrate the haemodialysis membrane? PCR analysis of haemodialysis ultrafiltrate and whole blood. *Nephrol Dial Transplant* 1995;10:541–542.

133. Caramelo C, et al. Evidence against transmission of hepatitis C virus through hemodialysis ultrafiltrate and peritoneal fluid. *Nephron* 1994;66:470–473.

134. Noiri E, et al. Hepatitis C virus in blood and dialysate in hemodialysis. *Am J Kidney Dis* 2001;37:38–42.

135. Mizuno MHT, et al. Dialysis-membrane-dependent reduction and adsorption of circulating hepatitis C virus during hemodialysis. *Nephron* 2002;91:235–242.

136. Lombardi M, et al. Is the dialysis membrane a safe barrier against HCV infection? *Nephrol Dial Transplant* 1995;10:578–579.

137. Taal MW, et al. Hepatitis C virus infection in chronic haemodialysis patients—relationship to blood transfusions and dialyser re-use. *S Afr Med J* 2000;90:621–625.

138. Moyer LA, et al. Hepatitis C virus in the hemodialysis setting: a review with recommendations for control. *Semin Dial* 1994;7:124–127.

139. Tokars JI, et al. Infection control in hemodialysis units. *Infect Dis Clin North Am* 2001;15:797–812.

140. CDC. Recommendations for preventing transmission of infections among chronic hemodialysis patients. *MMWR* 2001;50:1–41.

141. Stehman-Breen C, et al. Risk of death among chronic dialysis patients infected with hepatitis C virus. *Am J Kidney Dis* 1998;32:629–634.

142. Nakayama E, et al. Prognosis of anti-hepatitis C virus antibody-positive patients on regular hemodialysis therapy. *J Am Soc Nephrol* 2000;11:1896–1902.

143. Pereira BJG, et al. Effect of hepatitis C infection and renal transplantation on survival in end-stage renal disease. *Kidney Int* 1998;53:1374–1381.

144. Lindsay KL. Therapy of hepatitis C: overview. *Hepatology* 1997;26[Suppl 1]:71S–77S.

145. Management of hepatitis C: NIH consensus statement online 1997, March 24–26;15:1–41.

146. Nieforth KA, et al. Use of an indirect pharmacodynamic stimulation model of MX protein induction to compare in vivo activity of interferon alfa-2a and a polyethylene glycol-modified derivative in healthy subjects. *Clin Pharmacol Ther* 1996;59:636–646.

147. Xu Z-X, et al. Single-dose safety/tolerability and pharmacokinetics (PK/PD) following administration of ascending doses of pegilated interferon (PEG-INF) and interferon a-2a (INF a-2a) to healthy subjects. *Hepatology* 1998;28:702A.

148. Zeuzem S, et al. Peginterferon alfa-2a in patients with chronic hepatitis C. *N Engl J Med* 2000;343:1666–1672.

149. Heathcote EJ, et al. Peginterferon alfa-2a in patients with chronic hepatitis C and cirrhosis. *N Engl J Med* 2000;343:1673–1680.

150. Lindsay KL, et al. A randomized, double-blind trial comparing pegylated interferon alfa-2b to interferon alfa-2b as initial treatment for chronic hepatitis C. *Hepatology* 2001;34:395–403.

151. Knodell RG, et al. Formulation and application of a numerical scoring system for assessing histological activity in asymptomatic chronic active hepatitis. *Hepatology* 1981;1:431.

152. Management of hepatitis C: 2002. NIH consensus statement online 2002, June 10–12;19:116.

153. Rao VK, et al. Clinical and histological outcome following interferon treatment of chronic viral hepatitis, in uremic patients, before and after renal transplantation (abst), 14th annual meeting of the American Society of Transplant Physicians, Chicago, 1995, May 15–17.

154. Pol S, et al. Efficacy and tolerance of alpha-2b interferon therapy on HCV infection of hemodialyzed patients. *Kidney Int* 1995;47:1412–1418.

155. Rostaing L, et al. Preliminary results of treatment of chronic hepatitis C with recombinant interferon alpha in renal transplant patients. *Nephrol Dial Transplant* 1995;10:93–96.

156. Casanovas TT, et al. Interferon may be useful in hemodialysis patients with hepatitis C virus chronic infection who are candidates for kidney transplant. *Transplant Proc* 1995;27:2229–2230.

157. Koenig P, et al. Interferon treatment for chronic hepatitis C virus infection in uremic patients. *Kidney Int* 1994;45:1507–1509.

158. Duarte R, et al. Interferon-alpha facilitates renal transplantation in hemodialysis patients with chronic viral hepatitis. *Am J Kidney Dis* 1995;25:40–45.

159. Harihara Y, et al. Interferon therapy in renal allograft recipients with chronic hepatitis C. *Transplant Proc* 1994;26:2075.

160. Raptopoulou-Gigi M, et al. Interferon-alpha2b treatment of chronic hepatitis C in haemodialysis patients. *Nephrol Dial Transplant* 1995;10:1834–1837.

161. Ozgur O, et al. Recombinant alpha-interferon in renal allograft recipients with chronic hepatitis C. *Nephrol Dial Transplant* 1995;10:2104–2106.

162. Rostaing L, et al. Pharmacokinetics of alfa-interferon-2b in chronic hepatitis C virus patients undergoing chronic hemodialysis or with normal renal function: clinical implications. *J Am Soc Nephrol* 1998;9:2344–2348.

163. Hanafusa T, et al. Retrospective study on the impact of hepatitis C virus infection on kidney transplant patients over 20 years. *Transplantation* 1998;66:471–476.

164. Rodrigues A, et al. Limited benefit of INF-alpha therapy in renal graft candidates with chronic viral hepatitis B or C. *Transplant Proc* 1997;29:777–780.

165. Yasumura T, et al. Long-term outcome of recombinant INF-a treatment of chronic hepatitis C in kidney transplant recipients. *Transplant Proc* 1997;29:784–786.

166. Chan TM, et al. Interferon treatment for hepatitis C virus infection in patients on haemodialysis. *Nephrol Dial Transplant* 1997;12:1414–1419.

167. Davis G, et al. Factors predictive of a beneficial response to therapy of hepatitis C. *Hepatology* 1997;26[Suppl 1]:122S–127S.

168. Tokumoto T, et al. Effect of interferon-alpha treatment in hemodialysis patients and renal transplant recipients with chronic hepatitis C. *Transplant Proc* 1999;31:2887–2889.

169. Brouwer JT, et al. Treatment of chronic hepatitis C: efficacy of interferon dose and analysis of factors predictive of response. Interim report of 350 patients treated in a Benelux multicenter study, 44th annual meeting of the American Association for the Study of Liver Diseases, Chicago, November 4–7, 1993.

170. Huraib S, et al. Interferon-alpha in chronic hepatitis C infection in dialysis patients. *Am J Kidney Dis* 1999;34:55–60.

171. Uchihara M, et al. Interferon therapy for chronic hepatitis C in

hemodialysis patients: increased serum levels of interferon. *Nephron* 1998;80:51–56.

172. Espinosa M, et al. Interferon therapy in hemodialysis patients with chronic hepatitis C virus infection induces a high rate of long-term sustained virological and biochemical response. *Clin Nephrol* 2001; 55:220–226.

173. Hanrotel C, et al. Virological and histological responses to one year alpha-interferon-2a in hemodialyzed patients with chronic hepatitis C. *Nephron* 2001;88:120–126.

174. Poynard T, et al. A comparison of three interferon alpha-2b regimens for the long-term treatment of chronic non-A, non-B hepatitis. *N Engl J Med* 1995;332:1457–1462.

175. Black M, et al. Alpha-interferon treatment of chronic hepatitis C: need for accurate diagnosis in selecting patients. *Ann Intern Med* 1992;116:86–88.

176. Chan TM, et al. Chronic hepatitis C after renal transplantation: treatment with alpha-interferon. *Transplantation* 1993;56: 1095–1098.

177. Campistol JM, et al. Efficacy and tolerance of interferon-alpha2b in the treatment of chronic hepatitis C virus infection in haemodialysis patients: pre- and post-renal transplantation assessment. *Nephrol Dial Transplant* 1999;14:2704.

178. Casanovas TT, et al. Efficacy of interferon for chronic hepatitis C virus-related hepatitis in kidney transplant candidates on hemodialysis: results after transplantation. *Am J Gastroenterol* 2001;96: 1170–1177.

179. Bruchfeld A, et al. Ribavirin treatment in dialysis patients with chronic hepatitis C virus infection—a pilot study. *J Viral Hepat* 2001; 8:287–292.

180. Manns MP, et al. Peginterferon alfa-2b plus ribavirin compared to interferon alfa-2b plus ribavirin for the treatment of chronic hepatitis C 24 weeks treatment analysis of a multicenter, multinational phase III randomized controlled trial. *Hepatology* 2000;32:297A(abst).

181. Fried MW, et al. Pegylated (40kDa) interferon alfa-2a (PEGASYS) in combination with ribavirin: efficacy and safety results from a phase III, randomized, actively-controlled multicenter study. *Gastroenterology* 2001;120:A55(abst).

182. Alter HJ. Transfusion transmitted hepatitis C and non-A, non-B, non-C. *Vox Sang* 1994;67:19–24.

183. Alter MJ, et al. Risk factors for acute non-A, non-B hepatitis in the United States and association with hepatitis C virus infection. *JAMA* 1990;264:2231–2235.

184. Koretz RL, et al. Non-A, non-B posttransfusion hepatitis: comparing C and non-C hepatitis. *Hepatology* 1993;17:361–365.

185. Muerhoff AS, et al. Genomic organization of GB viruses A & B: two new members of the Flavi-viridae associated with GB agent hepatitis. *J Virol* 1995;69:5621–5630.

186. Deinhardt F, et al. Studies on the transmission of disease of human viral hepatitis to marmoset monkeys. I: transmission of disease, serial passage and description of liver lesions. *J Exp Med* 1967;125: 673–688.

187. Simons JN, et al. Identification of two flavivirus-like genomes in the GB hepatitis agent. *Proc Natl Acad Sci* 1995;92:3401–3405.

188. Simons JN, et al. Isolation of novel virus-like sequences associated with human hepatitis. *Nature* 1995;1:564–569.

189. Leary TP, et al. Sequence and genomic organization of GBV-C: a novel member of the flaviviridae associated with human non-A-E hepatitis. *J Med Virol* 1996;48:60–67.

190. Linnen J, et al. Molecular cloning and disease association of hepatitis G virus: a transfusion-transmissible agent. *Science* 1996;271: 505–508.

191. Zuckerman AJ. Alphabet of hepatitis viruses. *Lancet* 1996;347: 558–559.

192. Tacke M, et al. Detection of antibodies to putative hepatitis G virus envelope protein. *Lancet* 1997;349:318–320.

193. Cheung RC, et al. Hepatitis G: is it a hepatitis virus? *West J Med* 1997;167:23–33.

194. Szabo A, et al. GBV-C/HGB infection in renal dialysis and transplant patients. *Nephrol Dial Transplant* 1997;12:2380–2384.

195. Casteling A, et al. GB virus C prevalence in blood donors and high risk groups for parenterally transmitted agents from Gauteng, South Africa. *J Med Virol* 1998;55:103–108.

196. Kallinowski B, et al. Clinical impact of GB-C virus in haemodialysis patients. *Nephrol Dial Transplant* 1998;13:93–98.

197. Sheng L, et al. High prevalence of hepatitis G virus infection compared with hepatitis C virus infection in patients undergoing chronic hemodialysis. *Am J Kidney Dis* 1998;31:218–223.

198. Love A, et al. Hepatitis G virus infection in Iceland. *J Virol Hepatol* 1999;6:255–260.

199. Hwang SJ, et al. Seroprevalence of GB virus C/hepatitis C virus-RNA and anti-envelope antibody in high-risk populations in Taiwan. *J Gastroenterol Hepatol* 2000;15:1171–1175.

200. Pilot-Matias TJ, et al. Expression of the GB virus C E2 glycoprotein using the Semliki Forest virus vector system and its utility as a serologic marker. *Virology* 1996;225:282–292.

201. Nubling CM, et al. Frequencies of GB virus C/hepatitis G virus genomes and of specific antibodies in German risk and non-risk populations. *J Med Virol* 1997;53:218–224.

202. Schulte-Frohlinde E, et al. Significance of antibodies to recombinant E2 protein of hepatitis G virus in hemodialysis patients. *J Viral Hepat* 1998;5:341–344.

203. Schlauder GG, et al. Molecular and serological analysis in the transmission of the GB hepatitis agents. *J Med Virol* 1995;46:81–90.

204. Jarvis LM, et al. Infection with hepatitis G virus among recipients of plasma products. *Lancet* 1996;348:1352–1355.

205. Tagariello G, et al. Hepatitis G viral RNA in Italian haemophiliacs with and without hepatitis C infection [letter]. *Lancet* 1996;348: 760–761.

206. Neilson J, et al. Hepatitis G virus in long-term survivors of haematological malignancy [letter; comment]. *Lancet* 1996;347:1632–1633.

207. Masuko K, et al. Infection with hepatitis GB virus C in patients on maintenance hemodialysis. *N Engl J Med* 1996;334:1485–1490.

208. Tsuda F, et al. Infection with GB virus C (GBV-C) in patients with chronic liver disease or on maintenance hemodialysis in Indonesia. *J Med Virol* 1996;49:248–252.

209. Sampietro M, et al. Hepatitis G virus in hemodialysis patients. *Kidney Int* 1997;51:348–352.

210. Murthy BVR, et al. Predictors of GBV-C infection among patients referred for renal transplantation. *Kidney Int* 1998;53:1769–1774.

211. Shibuya A, et al. Prevalence of hepatitis G virus RNA and anti-E2 in Japanese haemodialysis population. *Nephrol Dial Transplant* 1998;13: 2033–2036.

212. Desassis JF, et al. Prevalence of present and past hepatitis G virus infection in a French haemodialysis centre. *Nephrol Dial Transplant* 1999;14:2692–2697.

213. Okuda M, et al. GB virus C/hepatitis G viremia and antibody response to the E2 protein of hepatitis G virus in hemodialysis patients. *J Clin Gastroenterol* 2000;30:425–428.

214. Furusyo N, et al. Lower hepatitis G virus infection prevalence compared to hepatitis B and C virus infection prevalences. *Dig Dis Sci* 2000;45:188–195.

215. Fabrizi F, et al. GBV-C/HGV infection in end-stage renal disease: a serological and virological survey. *J Nephrol* 2000;13:68–74.

216. Stark K, et al. Hepatitis G virus RNA and hepatitis G virus antibodies in renal transplant recipients: prevalence and risk factors. *Transplantation* 1997;64:608–612.

217. Fabrizi F, et al. Hepatitis G virus infection in chronic dialysis patients and kidney transplant recipients. *Nephrol Dial Transplant* 1997;12: 1645–1651.

218. Raengsakulrach B, et al. High prevalence of hepatitis G viremia among kidney transplant patients in Thailand. *J Med Virol* 1997;53:162–166.

219. Berthoux P, et al. High prevalence of hepatitis G virus (HGV) infection in renal transplantation. *Nephrol Dial Transplant* 1998;13:2909–2913.

220. Dawson GJ, et al. Prevalence studies of GB virus-C infection using reverse transcriptase-polymerase chain reaction. *J Med Virol* 1996;50: 97–103.

221. Stark K, et al. Detection of the hepatitis G virus genome among injecting drug users, homosexual and bisexual men, and blood donors. *J Infect Dis* 1996;174:1320–1323.

222. Seme K, et al. Prevalence of hepatitis G virus infection in Slovenian

hemodialysis patients as determined by the detection of viral genome and E2 antibodies. *Nephron* 1998;79:426–429.

223. Tribl B, et al. GBV-C/HGV in haemodialysis patients: anti-E2 antibodies and GBV-C/HGV-RNA in serum and peripheral blood mononuclear cells. *Kidney Int* 1998;53:212–216.

224. Schroter M, et al. GB virus C/hepatitis G virus infection in hemodialysis patients: determination of seroprevalence by a four-antigen recombinant immunoblot assay. *J Med Virol* 1999;57:230–234.

225. Dussol B, et al. Prevalence of hepatitis G virus infection in kidney transplant recipients. *Transplantation* 1997;64:537–539.

226. Murthy BVR, et al. GB hepatitis agent among cadaver organ donors and their recipients. *Transplantation* 1997;63:346–351.

227. Murthy BVR, et al. Impact of pre-transplantation GB virus-C (GBV-C) infection on the outcome of renal transplantation. *J Am Soc Nephrol* 1997;8:1164–1173.

228. Feucht HH, et al. Vertical transmission of hepatitis G [letter] [see comments]. *Lancet* 1996;347:615–616.

229. Moaven LD, et al. Mother-to-baby transmission of hepatitis G virus. *Med J Aust* 1996;165:84–85.

230. Kao JH, et al. GB virus-C/hepatitis G virus infection in prostitutes: possible role of sexual transmission. *J Med Virol* 1997;52:381–384.

231. Tanaka T, et al. Acute hepatitis caused by sexual or household transmission of GBV-C. *J Hepatol* 1997;27:1110–1112.

232. Dai CY, et al. Epidemiology and clinical significance of chronic hepatitis-related viruses infection in hemodialysis patients from Taiwan. *Nephron* 2002;90:148–153.

233. Ashby M, et al. Prevalence of hepatitis G infection in chronic hemodialysis patients. *J Am Soc Nephrol* 1996;7:1471(abst).

234. Fernandez J, et al. Hepatitis G virus infection in hemodialysis patients and its relationship with hepatitis C virus infection. *Am J Nephrol* 2000;20:380–384.

235. Badalamenti S, et al. High prevalence of HGV, a novel hepatitis virus, among hemodialysis patients. *J Am Soc Nephrol* 1996;7:1472(abst).

236. Cabrerizo M, et al. Hepatitis G virus (HGV) infection in hemodialysis patients. *J Am Soc Nephrol* 1996;7:1478(abst).

237. Izopet J, et al. Impact of HGV infection in hemodialysis patients [abstr.]. *J Am Soc Nephrol* 1996;7:1483.

238. Charrel R, et al. Prevalence of hepatitis G virus (HGV) infection among 32 transplant recipients. *J Am Soc Nephrol* 1996;7:1904(abst).

239. Cabrerizo M, et al. GBV-C/HGV-RNA in serum and peripheral blood mononuclear cells in hemodialysis patients. *Kidney Int* 1999; 56:1120–1128.

240. Anastassopoulou CG, et al. Molecular epidemiology of GB virus C/hepatitis G virus in Athens, Greece. *J Med Virol* 2000;61:319–326.

241. Lopez-Alcorocho JM, et al. Prevalence of hepatitis B, hepatitis C, GB virus C/hepatitis G and TT viruses in predialysis and hemodialysis patients. *J Med Virol* 2001;63:103–107.

242. Hinrichsen H, et al. Prevalence of and risk factors for hepatitis G (HGV) infection in haemodialysis patients: a multicenter study. *Nephrol Dial Transplant* 2002;17:271–275.

243. Gartner BC, et al. High prevalence of hepatitis G virus (HGV) infections in dialysis staff. *Nephrol Dial Transplant* 1999;14:406–408.

244. Fiordalisi G, et al. High prevalence of GB virus C infection in a group of Italian patients with hepatitis of unknown etiology. *J Infect Dis* 1996;174:181–183.

245. Yoshiba M, et al. Detection of GBV-C hepatitis virus genome in serum from patients with fulminant hepatitis of unknown aetiology. *Lancet* 1995;346:1131–1132.

246. Tameda Y, et al. Infection with GB virus C (GBV-C) in patients with fulminant hepatitis. *Hepatology* 1996;25:842–847.

247. Heringlake S, et al. Association between fulminant hepatic failure and a strain of GBV virus C. *Lancet* 1996;348:1626–1629.

248. Alter MJ, et al. Acute non-A-E hepatitis in the United States and the role of hepatitis G virus infection. *N Engl J Med* 1997;336:741–746.

249. Alter HJ, et al. The incidence of transfusion-associated hepatitis G virus infection and its relation to liver disease. *N Engl J Med* 1997; 336:747–754.

250. Kanda T, et al. Detection of GBV-C RNA in patients with non-A-E fulminant hepatitis by reverse-transcription polymerase chain reaction. *Hepatology* 1997;25:1261–1265.

251. Fried MW, et al. Hepatitis G virus co-infection in liver transplantation recipients with chronic hepatitis C and nonviral chronic liver disease. *Hepatology* 1997;25:1271–1275.

252. Pessoa MG, et al. Hepatitis G virus in patients with cryptogenic liver disease undergoing liver transplantation. *Hepatology* 1997;25: 1266–1270.

253. Berg T, et al. GB virus C infection in patients with chronic hepatitis B and C before and after liver transplantation. *Transplantation* 1996; 62:711–714.

254. Tanaka E, et al. Effect of hepatitis G virus infection on chronic hepatitis C [see comments]. *Ann Intern Med* 1996;125:740–743.

255. Bouthot BA, et al. Predictors of GB virus-C (GBV-C) infection in patients referred for renal transplantation, American Society of Transplant Physicians, Chicago, May 10–14, 1997.

256. Murthy BVR, et al. Impact of GB virus-C (GBV-C) infection on clinical outcomes in renal transplantation candidates, American Society of Transplant Physicians, Chicago, May 10–14, 1997.

257. Zaidi Y, et al. Aplastic anaemia after HGV infection [letter]. *Lancet* 1996;348:471–472.

258. Byrnes JJ, et al. Hepatitis G-associated aplastic anaemia [letter]. *Lancet* 1996;348:472.

259. Mushahwar IK, et al. Clinical implications of GB virus C. *J Med Virol* 1998;56:1–3.

260. Mushahwar IK. Tissue tropism of GBV-C and protective immunity of anti-GBV-C E2, VIII International Symposium on Viral Hepatitis, Madrid, Spain, 1998.

261. Mushahwar IK, et al. Tissue tropism of GBV-C and HCV. Abstracts of the XIX U.S.–Japan Hepatitis Joint Panel Meeting, U.S.–Japan Cooperative Medical Science Program., Pacific Grove, CA, 1998.

262. Manolopoulos S, et al. Influence of GB virus C viraemia on the clinical, virological and histological features of early hepatitis C-related hepatic disease. *J Hepatol* 1998;28:173–178.

263. Tucker TJ, et al. The hepatitis G virus? GBV-C is associated with glomerulonephritis. *S Afr Med J* 1998;88:286–287.

264. Berthoux P, et al. Membranoproliferative glomerulonephritis with subendothelial deposits (type 1) associated with hepatitis G virus infection in a renal transplant recipient. *Am J Nephrol* 1999;19:513–518.

265. UNAIDS. The Report on the Global HIV/AIDS Epidemic. United Nations Program on HIV/AIDS & the XIV:1–44 International Conference on AIDS, Barcelona, July 7–12, 2002.

266. CDC. *HIV/AIDS Surveillance Rep* 2001;13(1):1–44.

267. Bourgoignie JJ, et al. The clinical spectrum of renal disease associated with human immunodeficiency virus. *Am J Kidney Dis* 1988;12: 131–137.

268. Bourgoignie JJ, et al. AIDS associated nephropathy. *Adv Nephrol* 1988;17:113–124.

269. Kimmel PL, et al. Continuous ambulatory peritoneal dialysis and survival of HIV infected patients with end-stage renal disease. *Kidney Int* 1993;44:373–378.

270. Rubin J. Prevalence of HIV virus among patients undergoing continuous ambulatory peritoneal dialysis. *ASAIO Trans* 1989;35:144–145.

271. U.S. Renal Data System. USRDS 1993 Annual data report. Bethesda, MD: The National Institutes of Health, National Institute of Diabetes and Digestive and Kidney Diseases, 1993.

272. U.S. Renal Data System. USRDS 1997 Annual data report. Bethesda, MD: National Institutes of Health, National Institute of Diabetes and Digestive and Kidney Diseases, 1997.

273. United States Renal Data System. USRDS Annual data report. Bethesda, MD: The National Institutes of Health, National Institutes of Diabetes and Digestive and Kidney Diseases, 2001.

274. Remuzzi G, et al. Hematologic consequences of renal failure. In: Brenner BM, ed. *The kidney,* vol II. Philadelphia: WB Saunders, 1996:2170–2186.

275. Reiser IW, et al. The incidence and epidemiology of human immunodeficiency virus infection in 320 patients treated in an inner-city hemodialysis center. *Am J Kidney Dis* 1990;16:26–31.

276. Rao TKS, et al. The types of renal disease in the acquired immunodeficiency syndrome. *N Engl J Med* 1987;316:1062–1068.

277. Carbone L, et al. Course and prognosis of human immunodeficiency virus-associated nephropathy. *Am J Med* 1989;87:389–395.

278. Ortiz C, et al. Outcome of patients with human immunodeficiency virus on maintenance hemodialysis. *Kidney Int* 1988;34:248–253.

279. Tebben JA, et al. Outcome of HIV infected patients on continuous ambulatory peritoneal dialysis. *Kidney Int* 1993;44:191–198.

280. Ifudu O, et al. Uremia therapy in patients with end-stage renal disease and human immunodeficiency virus infection: has the outcome changed in the 1990s? *Am J Kidney Dis* 1997;29:549–552.

281. Perinbasekar S, et al. Predictors of survival in HIV-infected patients on hemodialysis. *Am J Nephrol* 1996;16:280–286.

282. Ahuja TS, et al. Highly active antiretroviral therapy improves survival of HIV-infected hemodialysis patients. *Am J Kidney Dis* [Online] 2000;36:574–580.

283. Valeri A, et al. Acute and chronic renal disease in hospitalized AIDS patients [see comments]. *Clin Nephrol* 1991;35:110–118.

284. Abbott KC, et al. Human immunodeficiency virus/acquired immunodeficiency syndrome-associated nephropathy at end-stage renal disease in the United States: patient characteristics and survival in the pre highly active antiretroviral therapy era. *J Nephrol* 2001;14:377–383.

285. Schoenfeld P, et al. Survival of ESRD patient with HIV infection. *J Am Soc Nephrol* 1995;6:561(abst).

286. Winston J, et al. HIV-1 viral burden in HIVAN patients on highly-active anti-retroviral therapy (HAART). *J Am Soc Nephrol* 1998;9:103A(abst).

287. Schoenfeld P, et al. Patients with HIV infection and end-stage renal disease. *Adv Ren Replace Ther* 1996;3:287–292.

288. Curi MA, et al. Hemodialysis access: influence of the human immunodeficiency virus on patency and infection rates. *J Vasc Surg* 1999;29:608–616.

289. Fontana D, et al. Can choice of dialyser membrane have a beneficial effect on HIV load in the HIV-infected dialysis patient? *Nephrol Dial Transplant* 2002;17:529–530.

290. Tokars J, et al. National surveillance of dialysis associated diseases in the United States, 1993. *ASAIO J* 1996;42:219–229.

291. Marcus R, et al. Prevalence and incidence of human immunodeficiency virus among patients undergoing long-term hemodialysis: the Cooperative Dialysis Study Group. *Am J Med* 1991;90:614–619.

292. Cendoroglo M. HIV-1 and HIV-2 infection in end-stage renal disease patients treated by hemodialysis, CAPD and renal transplantation (post-graduate thesis). Division of Nephrology, Department of Medicine. Sao Paulo, Brazil: Federal University of Sao Paulo, 1992:115.

293. Fabrizi F, et al. Epidemiology of human immunodeficiency virus (HIV) infection in dialysis: recent insights. *Int J Artif Organs* 2001;24:425–433.

294. Anonymous. Recommendations for providing dialysis treatment to patient infected with human T-lymphotropic virus type III/lymphadenopathy virus. *MMWR* 1986;35:376–378, 383.

295. Dyer E. Argentinian doctors accused of spreading AIDS. *BMJ* 1993;307:584.

296. Velandia M, et al. Transmission of HIV in dialysis centre [see comments]. *Lancet* 1995;345:1417–1422.

297. El Sayed NM, et al. Epidemic transmission of human immunodeficiency virus in renal dialysis centers in Egypt. *J Infect Dis* 2000;181:91–97.

298. Ippolito G, et al. The risk of occupational exposure to blood and body fluids for health care workers in the dialysis setting: Italian Multicenter Study on Nosocomial and Occupational Risk of Infections in Dialysis. *Nephron* 1995;70:180–184.

299. CDC. Surveillance of healthcare workers with HIV/AIDS infection. Fact sheet. Atlanta: Centers for Disease Control and Prevention, 2002.

300. Gerberding JL. Management of occupational exposures to bloodborne viruses [review]. *N Engl J Med* 1995;332:444–451.

301. Bell DM. Occupational risk of human immunodeficiency virus infection in healthcare workers: an overview. *Am J Med* 1997;102:9–15.

302. Ippolito G, et al. The risk of occupational human immunodeficiency virus infection in health care workers: Italian Multicenter Study—the Italian Study Group on Occupational Risk of HIV infection. *Arch Intern Med* 1993;153:1451–1458.

303. Anonymous. Case-control study of HIV seroconversion in health-care workers after percutaneous exposure to HIV-infected blood—France, United Kingdom, and United States, January 1988–August 1994. *MMWR Morb Mortal Wkly Rep* 1995;44:929–933.

304. Cardo DM, et al. A case-control study of HIV seroconversion in health care workers after percutaneous exposure. Centers for Disease Control and Prevention Needlestick Surveillance Group. *N Engl J Med* 1997;337:1485–1490.

305. Mast ST, et al. Efficacy of gloves in reducing blood volumes transferred during simulated needlestick injury. *J Infect Dis* 1993;168:1589–1592.

306. D'Amico R, et al. Effect of zidovudine postexposure prophylaxis on the development of HIV-specific cytotoxic T-lymphocyte responses in HIV-exposed healthcare workers. *Infect Control Hosp Epidemiol* 1999;20:428–430.

307. U.S. Public Health Service. Updated U.S. Public Health Service Guidelines for the management of occupational exposures to HBV, HCV, and HIV and recommendations for postexposure prophylaxis. *MMWR Morb Mortal Wkly Rep* 2001;50:1–52.

308. Gerberding JL. Prophylaxis for occupational exposure to HIV. *Ann Intern Med* 1996;125:497–501.

309. Williams PF, et al. Continuous ambulatory peritoneal dialysis fluid: another fluid positive for HIV antibody [letter]. *BMJ Clin Res Ed* 1986;293:885.

310. Scheel PJ, et al. Survival of human immunodeficiency virus in peritoneal dialysis effluent. *Perit Dial Int* 1995;15[Suppl]:81(abst).

311. Scheel PJ, et al. Survival of human immunodeficiency virus on peritoneal dialysis exchange tubing. *Perit Dial Int* 1995;15[Suppl]:81.

312. Schoenfeld P, et al. Acquired immunodeficiency syndrome and renal disease: report of National Kidney Foundation–National Institutes of Health Task Force on AIDS and kidney disease. *Am J Kidney Dis* 1990;16:14–25.

313. Scheel PJJ, et al. Disposal of dialysate in HIV-positive patients: an update. *Adv Ren Replace Ther* 1996;3:298–301.

314. CDC. Nosocomial transmission of multidrug-resistant tuberculosis among HIV-infected persons—Florida and New York. *MMWR* 1991;40:585.

315. Tsai CC, et al. Prevention of SIV infection in macaques by (R)-9-(2-phosphonylmethoxypropyl)adenine. *Science* 1995;270:1197–1199.

316. Tsai CC, et al. Effectiveness of postinoculation (R)-9-(2-phosphonylmethoxypropyl) adenine treatment for prevention of persistent simian immunodeficiency virus SIVmne infection depends critically on timing of initiation and duration of treatment. *J Virol* 1998;72:4265–4273.

317. Bottiger D, et al. Prevention of simian immunodeficiency virus, SIVsm, or HIV-2 infection in cynomolgus monkeys by pre- and postexposure administration of BEA-005. *AIDS* 1997;11:157–162.

318. Otten RA, et al. Efficacy of postexposure prophylaxis after intravaginal exposure of pig-tailed macaques to a human-derived retrovirus (human immunodeficiency virus type 2). *J Virol* 2000;74:9771–9775.

319. Fahrner R, et al. Safety of zidovudine (ZDV) administered as postexposure prophylaxis to health careworkers (HCW) sustaining HIV-related occupational exposure (OE) (abst). Program and abstracts—interscience conference on antimicrobial agents and chemotherapy. Washington, DC: American Society of Microbiology, 1994:133.

320. Puro V, et al. Zidovudine prophylaxis after accidental exposure to HIV: the Italian experience. The Italian Study Group on Occupational Risk of HIV Infection. *AIDS* 1992;6:963–969.

321. Tokars JI, et al. Surveillance of HIV infection and zidovudine use among health care workers after occupational exposure to HIV-infected blood. The CDC Cooperative Needlestick Surveillance Group [see comments]. *Ann Intern Med* 1993;118:913–919.

322. Connor EM, et al. Reduction of maternal-infant transmission of human immunodeficiency virus type 1 with zidovudine treatment. Pediatric AIDS Clinical Trials Group Protocol 076 Study Group [see comments]. *N Engl J Med* 1994;331:1173–1180.

323. Sperling RS, et al. Maternal viral load, zidovudine treatment, and the risk of transmission of human immunodeficiency virus type 1 from mother to infant. Pediatric AIDS Clinical Trials Group Protocol 076 Study Group. *N Engl J Med* 1996;335:1621–1629.

324. Shaffer N, et al. Short-course zidovudine for perinatal HIV-1 transmission in Bangkok, Thailand: a randomised controlled trial. Bangkok Collaborative Perinatal HIV Transmission Study Group. *Lancet* 1999;353:773–780.

325. Wade NA, et al. Abbreviated regimens of zidovudine prophylaxis and perinatal transmission of the human immunodeficiency virus. *N Engl J Med* 1998;339:1409–1414.

326. Guay LA, et al. Intrapartum and neonatal single-dose nevirapine compared with zidovudine for prevention of mother-to-child transmission of HIV-1 in Kampala, Uganda: HIVNET 012 randomised trial. *Lancet* 1999;354:795–802.

327. Jochimsen EM. Failures of zidovudine postexposure prophylaxis. *Am J Med* 1997;102:52–55, discussion 56–57.

328. Ippolito G, et al. Simultaneous infection with HIV and hepatitis C virus following occupational conjunctival blood exposure. *JAMA* 1998;280:28.

329. Weiss SH. Risks and issues for the health care worker in the human immunodeficiency virus era. *Med Clin North Am* 1997;81:555–575.

330. Jochimsen EM, et al. Investigations of possible failures of postexposure prophylaxis following occupational exposures to human immunodeficiency virus. *Arch Intern Med* 1999;159:2361–2363.

331. Wang SA, et al. Experience of healthcare workers taking postexposure prophylaxis after occupational HIV exposures: findings of the HIV Postexposure Prophylaxis Registry. *Infect Control Hosp Epidemiol* 2000;21:780–785.

332. Anonymous. Update: Provisional Public Health Service recommendations for chemoprophylaxis after occupational exposure to HIV. *MMWR Morb Mortal Wkly Rep* 1996;45:468–480.

β₂-MICROGLOBULIN-ASSOCIATED AMYLOIDOSIS OF END-STAGE RENAL DISEASE

WILLIAM J. STONE

Amyloidosis refers to a group of disease processes in which organ damage results from the deposition of a beta-pleated sheet protein. Tissue sections from patients with an amyloidosis will both stain with Congo red and demonstrate characteristic fibrils on electron micrographs. Table 23.1 lists the common amyloidoses (1). Each amyloid is a polymer of a distinct protein subunit. The second letter of the abbreviation for each amyloidosis usually refers to the subunit (e.g., *L* for *light chain*-associated amyloid).

An unusual amyloidosis was discovered in the mid-1980s, approximately 10 years after the advent of the widespread use of chronic hemodialysis to treat end-stage renal disease (ESRD) in developed countries (2,3). At first this illness was mistaken for AA amyloidosis because the amyloid protein was permanganate-sensitive. Pretreatment of histologic sections containing this amyloid with potassium permanganate abolished Congo red staining (4,5). However, this new amyloidosis seemed to affect only the skeletal system, unlike AA (4,6). When immunoperoxidase-labeled anti-AA antibodies were employed on sections of bony amyloidosis from renal failure patients, there was no reaction (4,5). Furthermore, the electron-microscopic appearance of the fibrils differed from AA amyloidosis in that the renal failure fibrils were shorter and more curved (Table 23.2) (4,7). Finally,

complete sequencing of the subunit protein showed that it was identical to β₂-microglobulin (B2M) (8). Immunoperoxidase staining for B2M was positive in the amyloid lesions and negative in controls (4). Thus the amyloidosis of renal failure is now termed *AB2M*.

CLINICAL PRESENTATIONS OF AB2M

Usually, AB2M amyloidosis gains the attention of the attending nephrologist when the patient begins complaining of pain in the spine or extremities (Table 23.3). These complaints may be initially difficult to differentiate from those of other illnesses accompanying chronic renal failure. Many dialysis patients have skeletal problems related to aging, osteomalacia, prior steroid therapy, hyperparathyroidism, metastatic calcification, or a number of less common processes. Carpal tunnel syndrome is frequently seen in the nonuremic population, so the dialysis patient with median nerve compression may not have AB2M considered in the differential diagnosis.

This chapter discusses each category of clinical presentation. More than one category may be found in any individual patient

TABLE 23.1. CLASSIFICATION OF AMYLOIDOSIS

Type	Protein Subunit	Associated Diseases
AL	Immunoglobulin light chain	"Primary" amyloidosis
		Multiple myeloma
		Other paraproteinemias
AA	Protein AA (acute-phase reactant)	Osteomyelitis
		Subacute endocarditis
		Tuberculosis
		Rheumatoid arthritis
		Familial Mediterranean fever
ATTR	Mutant transthyretin	Familial polyneuropathic amyloidosis, types I and II
AE	Procalcitonin	Medullary thyroid carcinoma
AB	B-protein precursor (Pre A4)	Alzheimer's disease
		Down syndrome
		Hereditary cerebral amyloidosis
AS	Transthyretin	Senile amyloidosis
AB2M	β₂-microglobulin	Chronic renal failure

TABLE 23.2. HISTOLOGIC DIFFERENTIATION OF FOUR COMMON AMYLOIDOSES

Type of Amyloidosis	Permanganate-Sensitive Congo Red Staining	Fibrils on EM	Immunohistochemistry		
			Anti-AA	Anti-TTR	Anti-B2M
AL	No	Straight	–	–	–
AA	Yes	Straight	+	–	–
AF	No	Straight	–	+	–
AB2M	Yes	Curved	–	–	+

Anti-AA, antibody to AA protein; anti-B2M, antibody to β_2-microglobulin; anti-TTR, antibody to transthyretin.

with AB2M. Unfortunately, AB2M now represents the most crippling complication of ESRD. It severely limits lifestyle and rehabilitation of long-term dialysis patients.

CARPAL TUNNEL SYNDROME

Carpal tunnel syndrome (CTS) is a common condition in the nonuremic population (0.1%) and causes disabling pain and numbness in the hand. Certain occupations that involve repetitive hand motion have an incidence of as much as 15% of CTS (9). CTS is even more frequently seen in maintenance dialysis patients (up to 30%) regardless of modality of treatment (10–12). This increase is undoubtedly due to AB2M.

The median nerve passes through a tunnel in the wrist and proximal palm. The tunnel is composed of walls of bone and ligaments, but it also carries flexor tendons. Enlargement or destruction of any of these three structures could compress the nerve. Additionally, edema, inflammation, neoplastic growth or deposition of acellular material could impinge on this nerve and its blood supply.

Patients with CTS complain of an unpleasant feeling in the affected hand, including numbness, a tingling sensation, and frank pain. At first these symptoms may be reversed by shaking or warming the hand. However, the pain and dysesthesia grow steadily worse in duration and intensity. The whole hand may seem to be involved to the patient, or arm pain may predominate. Nocturnal exacerbations are common, as well as worsening during hemodialysis treatments.

Physical examination is not always reliable, but Tinel's and Phalen's signs should be elicited. Tinel's sign is a tingling sensation in a distal limb when a supplying nerve is percussed; Phalen's sign is positive if there is tingling in the distribution of the median nerve when the wrist is flexed or extended for 30 to 60 seconds. There is a broad differential diagnosis, including

neuropathy related to underlying disease such as diabetes mellitus and cervical spine disease. Studies of nerve conduction velocity are diagnostic.

The first reports of CTS in dialysis patients did not associate it with amyloidosis. Frequently, the dialysis arteriovenous fistula was blamed, even though the process was often bilateral. By the mid-1980s a relationship was noted between the duration of hemodialysis and the appearance of CTS (13–15). Some centers reported a 100% incidence of CTS in patients dialyzed over 20 years. Infiltration of the tendons and ligaments with amyloid was seen at surgical exploration (13–15). The deposits were pale and resembled granulation tissue.

Many centers have noted a much lower incidence of AB2M-related CTS in patients dialyzed chronically against noncellulosic membranes. After 15 years of maintenance hemodialysis, 40% of patients had CTS who had only cellulosic membrane exposure, as compared with a 20% incidence of CTS in patients only exposed to a biocompatible membrane (16). The lower incidence appears to be due to better B2M removal by convective transport and/or membrane adsorption. Polyacrylonitrile, polysulfone, and polymethylmethacrylate membranes have better B2M clearances than do cellulosic membranes (16–18). Additionally, bioincompatible reactions are reduced with these membranes, resulting in decreased B2M production because of less cellular injury during hemodialysis. Older age appears to be another risk factor for CTS in dialysis patients (16).

Although splinting and steroid injections into the carpal tunnel may have transient benefit in CTS patients, our experience and that of others has been that surgical release of the entrapped median nerve is the best therapy. This can be done as an outpatient procedure and should be accompanied by a biopsy of involved tissue for amyloid studies. Surgery must not be postponed too long, or permanent nerve damage may result. Immediate surgical decompression is necessary for any patient whose symptoms of CTS become continuous. Recurrence after successful surgery is all too frequent and may necessitate reexploration.

PERIPHERAL ARTHROPATHY

The mechanism of arthropathy appears to be infiltration of the bone and synovium with amyloid fibrils. Free fibrils may also be seen with Congo red stains of synovial fluid of affected patients (14). The joint fluid is serous, sterile, and noninflammatory.

TABLE 23.3. CLINICAL PRESENTATIONS OF AB2M

1. Carpal tunnel syndrome (hand and forearm pain, numbness)
2. Osseous involvement (bone pain, fractures)
3. Large-joint arthropathy (swelling, pain, decreased mobility)
4. Spondyloarthropathy (neck and lumbar pain, nerve compression)
5. Tendon rupture/contracture (trigger finger)
6. Subcutaneous masses (widely distributed)
7. Renal calculi (renal colic)

Protein concentration is low and glucose levels are normal (19). Erosions and cystic lesions are often present in nearby bones and reflect deposits of AB2M. This is particularly well shown on MRI: lesions that appear interosseous on plain radiographs can be shown to be contiguous with well-defined erosions of the articular surface by magnetic resonance studies (20).

Pain and stiffness in a number of large joints are commonly seen in chronic dialysis patients. Muñoz-Gomez and colleagues reported seven chronic hemodialysis patients with pain, swelling, and effusion in large joints for more than 3 months (21). Knees, shoulders, elbows, hips, wrists, and ankles were involved. Similar findings were reported by Kurer et al. (10). Shoulder involvement was most common, and many patients had concomitant CTS and bone cysts. Symmetric or asymmetric arthropathy could be seen in any of these joints. Bilateral disease was demonstrated in 65% of wrists, 30% of hips, and 20% of shoulders in one study (16).

Laurent et al. found shoulder pain in 49% of their maintenance hemodialysis patients that correlated strongly with the duration of dialysis and presence of CTS (14). Patients dialyzed less than 5 years rarely had either syndrome. There was a progressive increase in CTS and shoulder pain with increased duration of dialysis, until both were uniformly present in those dialyzing more than 18 years. Additionally, 95% of patients who had AB2M found at the time of CTS surgery had shoulder pain, but only 28% of amyloid-negative patients had painful shoulders (14). They noted a small group of patients who improved when switched from hemodialysis to continuous ambulatory peritoneal dialysis (CAPD).

An important autopsy study by Jadoul et al. evaluated the prevalence of AB2M in the biopsied large joints of maintenance hemodialysis (HD) patients (22). The prevalence of AB2M escalated from 21% after 0 to 2 years of HD to 100% by 13 years of HD. Independent risk factors for AB2M were age at HD onset and duration of HD. The sternoclavicular joint was judged to be the best site to biopsy because of high sensitivity and accessibility. The same group also studied peritoneal dialysis (PD) patients and found an AB2M prevalence of 31% after 27 months of PD (23). There was no difference between PD and HD when matched for age and duration of dialysis. Thus AB2M deposition begins early in the course of dialysis at a time when patients have few clinical manifestations.

Treatment of AB2M arthropathy has involved low-dose daily oral glucocorticoids and palliative surgical procedures. Oral nonsteroidals and intraarticular steroids have limited roles.

Konishiike et al. studied 24 patients with intense shoulder pain who had been receiving hemodialysis a mean of 14.0 years (24). Twenty-one shoulders in 18 patients were treated with open or endoscopic resection of the coracoacromial ligament. Severing the coracoacromial ligament does not usually produce adverse effects in the shoulder; however, if the shoulder is already unstable, the ligament cannot be severed or the instability will become worse. Sixteen patients had resection of both the coracoacromial and transverse humeral ligaments. Pain at night and during hemodialysis was relieved following these procedures. Amyloid deposits were found in 19 of 21 subacromial bursae and 15 of 16 biopsies of the tenosynovium of the biceps groove (24).

Okutsu and colleagues treated intractable shoulder pain in 29 long-term hemodialysis patients (48 shoulders) (25). Using an endoscope they found proliferation and amyloid infiltration of the subacromial bursae and surrounding ligaments. The subacromial space was significantly decreased. Resection of the coracoacromial ligament increased the subacromial space and relieved pain in all patients. AB2M was found in 87% of the resected ligaments and 86% of the bursae removed (25).

Two studies of the effect of successful renal transplantation on AB2M arthropathy have revealed similar results (26,27). Seventeen patients with biopsy-proven AB2M amyloidosis had improved shoulder stiffness within the first week after grafting, possibly due to steroids in the immunosuppressive regimen (26). In the seven patients who lost their grafts after a mean of 47 months, shoulder pain and stiffness as well as CTS rapidly returned as they resumed hemodialysis. Another 14 patients who had been on hemodialysis for a mean of 16 years were evaluated for the number of painful joints before and after renal transplantation (27). Although 72 painful joints were reduced to 15 after grafting, 14 new arthropathies developed. Three of 14 patients were actually worse than before transplantation. Articular AB2M deposits were identified in two of these patients at 2 and 10 years following successful renal allografting. The number and size of bone cysts and subchondral erosions were unchanged by renal transplantation in this study.

TENDONS

Kurer and colleagues reviewed 83 patients hemodialyzed more than 10 years (10). Five of them presented with "trigger fingers" after 8 to 14 years of dialysis. Tenosynovitis of the finger flexors was successfully treated by surgical release in all cases. All tendons and sheaths were infiltrated with amyloid. Four other patients were seen in a more advanced state of finger contracture and stiffness with a heavier burden of amyloid. Each had hemodialyzed more than 15 years. Full excision was not possible and only some hand function was regained after surgery. These authors described six other patients out of the 83 who ruptured seven tendons after slight trauma. Quadriceps, finger flexor, finger extensor, calcaneal, and supraspinatus tendons were involved with amyloid (10). Surgical repair was successful in five of five patients.

Trigger finger was commonly associated with CTS according to Laurent (14) and usually did not require surgery. Others have spoken of the "dialysis hand" caused by AB2M. This consists of trigger finger, carpal tunnel syndrome, wrist arthropathy, and subcutaneous masses of amyloid over the dorsum of the wrist.

SPONDYLOARTHROPATHY

Cervical pain heralds the clinical appearance of a destructive spondyloarthropathy (DSA) in long-term dialysis patients. Although more than one pathogenic process may be involved, deposition of AB2M plays a dominant role. As in large joints and the long bones, deposition of amyloid begins years earlier but does not reach symptomatic levels until after 5 to 10 years

TABLE 23.4. FEATURES OF AB2M-RELATED DESTRUCTIVE SPONDYLOARTHROPATHY

1. Neck or back pain
2. Disk space narrowing
3. Erosion of the vertebral margins
4. Vertebral body destruction
5. Spondylolisthesis
6. Paralysis is rare

of chronic dialysis. Ohashi and colleagues did careful studies of autopsy specimens from 41 ESRD patients in Japan (28). Thirty-six of the 41 had undergone dialysis for periods ranging from 1 month to 18 years mainly using cuprophane membranes. The intervertebral disks from the entire spine of each patient were examined for the presence of AB2M. AB2M was not found in the vertebral disks of the five nondialyzed patients or in any patient who had dialyzed for less than 1.5 years. Beginning at 1.6 years of maintenance dialysis there was a progressive accumulation of AB2M in the vertebral disks. The cervical disks were first affected, followed by lumbar and upper thoracic involvement. The middle and lower thoracic spine was the last area to be infiltrated by amyloid. Both the extent throughout the vertebral column and the severity of individual lesions increased as the amount of time on dialysis lengthened. The authors felt that the parts of the spine that received the most mechanical stress were the first to be infiltrated by AB2M.

Maruyama et al. surveyed 405 maintenance hemodialysis patients for the presence of DSA (29). Most patients had dialyzed using the cuprophane membrane. Standard radiographs were taken of the entire spine. These were searched for erosions of the vertebral rim, reactive sclerosis, and narrowing of the disk space. Thirty-seven patients (9.1%) were affected. MRI, CT scans, and radionuclide bone scans were also done in some

patients. DSA most involved the lower cervical spine. AB2M was confirmed in 15 of 29 patients in whom biopsy of a disk or other tissue was available. Risk factors for DSA were older age at onset of dialysis, duration of hemodialysis, cystic bone lesions, and CTS. The authors also carefully discussed the differential diagnosis of neck pain in dialysis patients.

Fiocchi and colleagues found that nine of 50 (18%) patients who had hemodialyzed more than 5 years had evidence of DSA (30). All had involvement of the lower cervical spine. Three patients had major alterations in the lower thoracic spine at T 9–10, and two patients had L 4–5 abnormalities. Radiologic findings included narrowing of the disk space, erosion of the vertebral margins, subchondral sclerosis, and spondylolisthesis. Osteophytes were not seen. Pain was prominent in eight of nine patients, and paraparesis was seen in one. Seven of nine had cystic lesions in the extravertebral skeleton. Three patients died and had histologic confirmation of AB2M vertebral involvement at autopsy.

This process may be so severe as to cause paralysis and death. Allard and co-workers reported two patients with fatal DSA after 15 to 17 years of chronic hemodialysis (31). One patient had neck pain and spastic paraplegia. The other developed neck pain and quadriparesis. Chassagne et al. described a similar patient of their own and found two other cases in the literature (32). These three were proven to be due to AB2M.

In summary, neck or lumbar pain in a long-term dialysis patient should alert the nephrologist to the possible presence of DSA due to AB2M (Table 23.4). The differential diagnosis mainly centers on infection and degenerative vertebral diseases of other etiologies. MRI and CT scans are the best diagnostic tests (Fig. 23.1), but plain radiographs are helpful when these newer imaging modalities are unavailable. The major therapy involves stabilizing neurosurgical procedures if there is severe pain or other evidence of nerve root compression. Results of

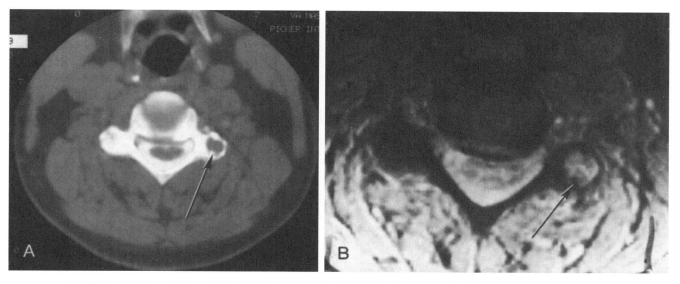

FIG. 23.1. A: CT scan at the axial level of the C 4–5 disk. A lytic lesion is seen in the left articular process *(arrow)*. **B:** MRI at the same level in the same long-term hemodialysis patient. The defect demonstrates internal increased soft-tissue signal *(arrow)*, presumably due to AB2M. This patient had biopsy-proven AB2M in his carpal tunnel.

renal transplantation have been disappointing. Four of five patients with pretransplant cervical DSA had progression of disease following renal allografting (27). One of these required cervical spine surgery for C6 root compression after transplantation.

INVOLVEMENT OF THE NONAXIAL SKELETON

AB2M first gained clinical recognition when enlarging cystic lesions of the long bones and pelvis resulted in pathologic fractures (6,33). Material from the autopsy of a patient, who had hemodialyzed for 9 years before suffering consecutive fractures of both femoral necks, provided the first proof that dialysis-associated amyloid was a polymer of intact β_2-microglobulin (B2M) (8). The areas favored for the development of the cystic lesions of AB2M include the acetabulum, femur, humerus, tibia, pelvis, and carpal bones (Figs. 23.2 and 23.3). Other skeletal regions may be less commonly affected.

Kurer et al. examined 83 patients, who had received maintenance hemodialysis for more than 10 years, for the presence of cystic bone lesions (10). Bone cysts were seen in 42 patients (51%), and most were free of symptoms. Areas most affected were the carpal bones and phalanges, but long bones were also involved. Eight of the 42 suffered pathologic fractures—five in the femoral neck (one bilateral), two in the scaphoid, and two in cervical vertebrae. Stabilization procedures by orthopedic surgeons were eventually successful in the femoral and vertebral fractures, but total hip replacements were needed after nonunion occurred in three patients.

Van Ypersele and coworkers studied 221 patients receiving hemodialysis for more than 5 years (16). They compared patients dialyzed against cellulosic membranes to those treated only with AN69 membranes. Radiographs of shoulders, hips,

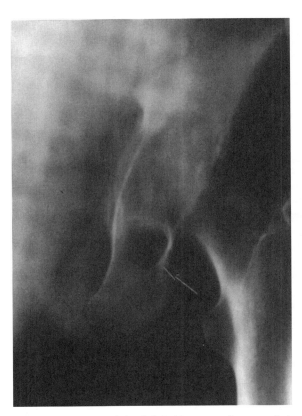

FIG. 23.3. A tomogram of the left ischium revealing a well-circumscribed lytic defect without internal calcification *(arrow)*. This occurred in a chronic hemodialysis patient maintained for more than 10 years on cuprophane dialysis.

hands, and wrists were examined for the presence of bone cysts of at least 5 mm in diameter at the wrist and 10 mm at the shoulder. Twenty patients had bony cysts after a range of 56 to 171 months of dialysis. Degrees of involvement were wrists, 100% (bilateral in 65%); hips, 53% (bilateral in 30%); and shoulders, 36% (bilateral in 20%). Bone amyloidosis developed in three of 115 (2.6%) patients dialyzing with AN69 membranes and 17 of 106 (16%) patients dialyzing against cellulosic membranes.

Onishi and colleagues reviewed bone biopsy specimens from 224 maintenance hemodialysis patients (1 to 22 years of dialysis) (34). Most of these were iliac crest biopsies analyzed previously in their earlier studies of renal osteodystrophy. Congo red stains and anti-B2M antibody immunohistochemical testing were performed. AB2M deposits were found in 8% of the 224 patients. Bone amyloid was absent in all patients hemodialyzed less than 6 years but was found in 3% of patients dialyzing 6 to 10 years and in 19% of patients who dialyzed more than 10 years. Seven femoral head specimens from patients with femoral neck fractures were also examined for the presence of AB2M. Six of seven (86%) were positive. It has also been our own experience that 80% of femoral fractures in dialysis patients are due to AB2M (33).

The effects of renal transplantation on bone cysts have been studied in two reports from France. The number and size of

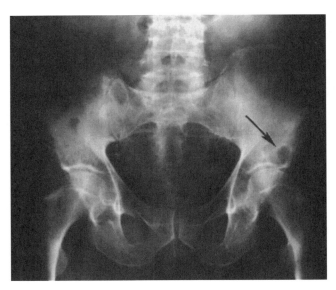

FIG. 23.2. A large circumscribed lytic area is seen in the left acetabulum *(arrow)*. The patient had received maintenance hemodialysis versus cuprophane membranes for more than 20 years.

cysts stayed remarkably constant after successful allografting of 17 patients, suggesting no progression but also no regression of these lesions (26). One patient with bone cysts developed a hip fracture 2 years after transplantation. Another 14 patients evaluated over a mean of 54 months following transplantation also demonstrated no change in bone cysts (27).

We recommend performing yearly skeletal surveys on maintenance dialysis patients. Views should include the wrists, pelvis, femurs, humeri, and cervical spine. Prophylactic orthopedic surgical procedures can be scheduled if cystic or infiltrative lesions threaten skeletal integrity.

RENAL CALCULI

"Matrix" stones have been seen occasionally in hemodialysis patients for many years. These were never carefully analyzed until Bommer et al. found a microfibrillar protein to be the main component of seven matrix stones from hemodialysis patients (35). They reported that this material was not Tamm-Horsfall protein but that it was similar to amyloid. They could not demonstrate a beta-pleated sheet structure by x-ray diffraction. These stones also contained small amounts of calcium oxalate. This same group was later able to show that this protein reacted with antibodies to B2M and had an analogous N-terminal amino acid sequence to B2M (36).

Digenis and coworkers summarized the situation in an editorial (37). They concluded that the passage of renal calculi was not uncommon in dialysis patients who still made urine (>100 mL daily). From 5% to 9% of dialysis patients form stones that consist of a protein matrix like AB2M along with some calcium oxalate. Renal CT scans may show further stones fixed in the renal parenchyma that may never pass. Matrix stones may also be associated with acquired renal cystic disease (38).

SUBCUTANEOUS MASSES

Tumorlike subcutaneous masses have been observed uncommonly in long-term hemodialysis patients and identified as containing AB2M. These masses are firm but not hard, relatively immobile, and nonfluctuant. There is no tenderness or inflam-

mation. They have been seen in the popliteal space, in the gluteal regions, near the wrists, in the vulva, and in the groin (39–41). Surgical excision was often needed for patient comfort.

SYSTEMIC DEPOSITS

Scanty, small deposits of AB2M are seen in small and large blood vessels in patients with AB2M heavily involving the skeletal system (42–44). Both arteries and veins can be infiltrated. Rarely, large visceral deposits are seen (44). Usually these lesions are not clinically significant.

DIAGNOSTIC TESTS IN AB2M
Imaging

Table 23.5 summarizes radiologic imaging of the skeleton. Conventional radiographs show radiolucent lesions, usually with thin sclerotic margins, in association with soft-tissue masses (20) (Figs. 23.1 to 23.3). Favored areas are the pelvis, carpal bones, shoulder, and femur. Lesions tend to increase in size and in number as time on dialysis lengthens. Most pathologic fractures occur in the femoral neck. Conventional radiography is best used in initial diagnosis or as a screening procedure.

MRI and CT scans are both useful in evaluating extensive lesions of the nonaxial skeleton and particularly in spondyloarthropathy (20,29,45). MRI is the single best test if available. Amyloid lesions can be differentiated from inflammatory masses and hyperparathyroidism by MRI (20).

Radionuclide bone scans often do not detect small lesions and underestimate the extent of AB2M, in our experience, but they may have a role in some patients (46,47). A new radionuclide imaging method employing ^{131}I-B2M has been used in Europe (48). Positive scans were found in 13 of 14 patients who had dialyzed more than 10 years. All scans were negative in those dialyzed less than 5 years.

Ultrasound may have a limited role, especially when MRI is unavailable. Ultrasound may be used to image the shoulder or to direct joint aspiration (49). Ultrasound is not helpful in determining the extent of bony lesions or in spondyloarthropathy.

TABLE 23.5. SKELETAL IMAGING IN AB2M

Skeletal Study	Advantages	Disadvantages	Role
Conventional radiographs	Inexpensive Readily available	Radiation exposure Underestimation of the extent of lesions	Screening
CT scan	Present in most hospitals	More expensive, not 100% available; cuts limit imaging and defining extent of lesions	Imaging of extensive lesions when MRI not available
Radionuclide Bone scan	Inexpensive Readily available	Many false negatives	None
MRI	Imaging in all planes; more sensitive than CT scan	Most expensive; not always available	Imaging of extensive lesions, particularly of the spine
Radioiodinated B2M scans	Promising early results; still experimental	Not available	Unknown
Ultrasound	Inexpensive; readily available	Limited applications	Imaging of large joints such as the shoulder

Biopsy

Although a clinical diagnosis of AB2M may be made based on radiologic changes and physical findings in a maintenance dialysis patient, definitive diagnosis rests on biopsy information. On light microscopy of tissue biopsies with Congo red staining, the typical appearance of apple-green birefringence under polarized light is seen (4,34). This is nonspecific and occurs in all amyloidoses. Pretreatment of sections from AB2M patients with potassium permanganate abolishes this reaction as in AA amyloidosis (4,6,43). Immunohistochemical studies with anti-B2M antibodies label involved tissues from AB2M patients but are negative in patients with other types of amyloidosis (4,42). Table 23.2 summarizes these changes. Antibodies to other types of amyloidosis do not stain tissues in patients with AB2M.

Electron-microscopic examination of biopsies from AB2M patients reveal a different type of fibril when compared with AA or AL amyloidosis. The AB2M fibrils are shorter, slightly thicker, and more curved than AA or AL amyloids. AB2M fibrils are often arranged in bundles (4,7) (Fig. 23.4).

Preferred biopsy sites would include accessible cystic bone lesions, soft-tissue masses, and synovium of involved joints. The sternoclavicular joint is high in yield if cartilage is present in the sample (50). All tissue resected by surgeons at carpal tunnel exploration, at fixation of fractures, or in procedures performed on the vertebral column should be submitted for AB2M studies. Particularly important is that nephrologists insist that patients undergoing CTS surgery or other surgical procedures have biopsy material removed for examination. Orthopedic surgeons who are not forewarned may only unroof the tunnel containing the median nerve without sampling involved tissue. Biopsies that have not been very useful include skin, abdominal fat, and deep organ (e.g., liver).

PATHOGENESIS OF AB2M

The major factor leading to disabling skeletal amyloidosis in maintenance dialysis patients appears to be the greatly increased circulating levels of B2M. These high B2M levels result from loss of proteases in renal tubular epithelium due to progressive nephron destruction (51). Concentrations of B2M in serum can be 30 to 50 times normal in ESRD patients (52). Intact B2M will also form amyloid fibrils in vitro (53). However, the degree of serum B2M elevation in an individual patient does not predict the presence of clinically significant AB2M (47), but the duration of a high B2M level does. Among the important unknowns are the mechanisms leading to the polymerization of B2M into amyloid fibrils and what causes the peculiar localization of the AB2M protein almost exclusively in bone and joints in contrast to other common amyloidoses. Studies of van Ypersele and colleagues have illustrated the sequence of events in joint deposits of AB2M (50). Early, cartilage-restricted AB2M consisted of small deposits after a mean dialysis duration of 39 months. Larger cartilaginous deposits were accompanied by synovial and/or capsular AB2M in the absence of macrophages. This occurred after 56 months of dialysis. The last stage was that of large cartilaginous deposits with macrophages around synovial and capsular deposits after a mean of 111 months of dialysis. Protein misfolding may be a key step in amyloidogenesis (54). Partially folded protein molecules tend to self-assemble into insoluble amyloid fibrils. This is protein-specific and concentration-dependent. The extremely high circulating B2M levels in ESRD patients would predict fibrillogenesis by this mechanism.

Older patient age and the number of years on dialysis increase the risk of developing AB2M (10,29,34), emphasizing the added risks of exposure to high circulating levels of B2M over long periods of time and aging bone. Other possible factors (Table 23.6) include high bone turnover renal osteodystrophy, chronic dialysis against cellulosic membranes (bioincompatibility), loss of residual renal function, B2M itself as a growth factor, glycated or fragmented B2M, and skeletal accumulation of iron or aluminum (19,47,55–57). Onishi et al. presented evidence from their study of uremic bone biopsies that high-turnover osteodystrophy correlated best with the presence of AB2M (34). There was a decreased incidence of low bone turnover states (aplastic, osteomalacic) in their AB2M-positive patients. Additionally, they found no correlation between either the localization of iron in bone marrow or aluminum in bone with the location of AB2M deposits. In agreement with us they felt that neither metal was important in the pathogenesis of

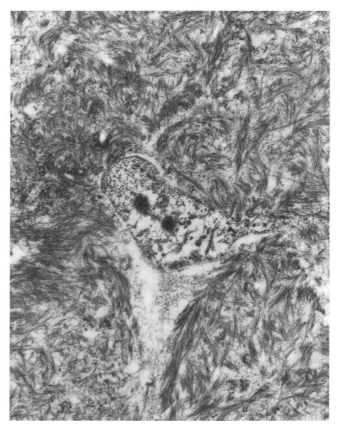

FIG. 23.4. Ultrastructural study of AB2M amyloid from the humerus of a 71-year-old man who was dialyzed thrice weekly for 9 years versus cellulosic membranes. The fibers are arranged in short bundles and have a curved appearance.

TABLE 23.6. FACTORS POSSIBLY INVOLVED IN THE PATHOGENESIS OF AB2M

1. Greatly increased circulating levels of B2M
   a. Innate tendency to polymerize
   b. B2M as bone-remodeling factor (IL-6)
2. Older patient age (other bone diseases more prevalent in aging)
3. Bioincompatibility with cellulosic membranes
   a. Cytokines (IL-1, TNF-alpha)
   b. Reactive oxygen species
   c. Formation of B2M polymers
   d. Anaphylotoxins derived from complement
   e. Eicosanoids
4. Loss of residual renal function
5. High-turnover renal osteodystrophy
6. Years of dialysis
7. Use of impure dialysate

B2M, β₂-microglobulin; IL-1, interleukin-1; IL-6, interleukin-6; TNF-alpha, tumor necrosis factor alpha.

AB2M. Although we have sequenced only one patient's AB2M subunit, it was found to be intact B2M (8). Campistol et al. have also found intact B2M in dialysis amyloid deposits (58). No lower-molecular-weight products of B2M were found by them in four AB2M-laden patient samples. Others have proposed that partially degraded or glycated B2M participated in the formation of AB2M polymer, but we have no direct evidence of our own favoring either theory (55,57). Bioincompatibility effector molecules may include reactive oxygen species, eicosanoids, anaphylotoxic components of complement and cytokines (59,60). IL-l and TNF-alpha have been called more powerful bone-resorbing factors than parathormone (61). These cytokines may be found in increased concentrations in ESRD patients. Enhanced bone resorption must play a role in the creation of the cystic lesions of bone in AB2M. IL-6 gene expression and release are increased by B2M and result in bone mineral dissolution (56).

THERAPY

Before discussing therapy, a brief consideration of the magnitude of the problem is in order. B2M is generated at a rate of 150 to 200 mg/d both in normal and uremic subjects (52,62). Loss of renal tubular catabolism because of greatly decreased or absent glomerular filtration of B2M leads to the immense increase in circulating B2M concentrations in renal failure. Levels of 30 to 50 times normal are usual. Standard peritoneal dialysis regimens remove less than 100 mg/d (63). Cellulosic membrane hemodialysis (HD) may slightly increase generation and does not decrease serum levels (60). Using more biocompatible membranes (polysulfone, polymethylmethacrylate [PMMA], or polyacrylonitrile) in HD, hemofiltration (HF), or hemodiafiltration (HDF) modes removes more B2M and decreases serum levels somewhat (by 30% to 50%) (17,18). HF and HDF remove the most B2M (64,65). However, the patient is still left with a B2M level of 10 to 20 times normal. To begin to normalize serum B2M concentrations, virtually continuous treatment would be needed with any of these modalities. This is nei-

ther acceptable to patients nor economically feasible. HF and HDF offer no clear benefit over current biocompatible HD regimens carried out at high blood-flow rates (300 to 400 mL/min). HD combined with a B2M adsorption column has shown promise in preliminary studies (66).

A further distressing feature concerns the amount of B2M built up in AB2M polymer, probably directly related to the duration of renal failure/dialysis. This accumulated amyloid polymer may not be affected by simple removal of circulating B2M monomer by extracorporeal methods. Restoration of normal B2M levels by renal transplantation does not lessen skeletal AB2M (26,27).

What is of proven therapeutic benefit? Certainly orthopedic surgery or neurosurgery consultants are extremely helpful in the presence of pathologic fractures, ruptured tendons, contractures, carpal tunnel syndrome, spinal cord compression, and dysfunctional shoulders. Occasionally, urologists may be needed to treat matrix stone disease and plastic surgeons may be called upon to resect subcutaneous masses. Although each is quite necessary in the particular setting, none of these consultants can address the primary problem.

Renal transplantation is an obvious treatment. A normally functioning renal allograft catabolizes B2M and quickly restores circulating B2M concentrations to normal range (17). However, there is an increasing shortage of donor kidneys. Long-term dialysis patients are often not on transplant lists because of personal choice, difficulties in matching, multiple failed prior allografts, or advanced age. This bevy of impediments makes transplantation therapy of AB2M even more improbable.

When successful renal transplantation has been realized, a stabilization of the complications of AB2M has occurred (26,27). It is not yet clear whether skeletal lesions will improve with long-term viability of renal allografts (67). If it is true that lesions of AB2M do not regress but merely stabilize following a successful renal transplant and restoration of renal catabolism of B2M, then the infusion of recombinant renal proteases into dialysis patients would appear unlikely to succeed as well. It would be very costly (68).

Another strategy dictated by the former observation would be to enhance organ procurement so that acceptable transplant candidates can be grafted early in dialysis and not allowed to accumulate AB2M. Finally, pharmaceutical companies are developing agents that will bind specifically to protein intermediates to prevent them from aggregating into fibrils (54).

Because there will never be a time when every ESRD patient can receive a successful renal transplant in the first few years of dialysis, a better method of extracorporeal B2M removal is mandatory to prevent this crippling and sometimes fatal complication. Until that method becomes available, it is necessary to employ HD, HF, or HDF strategies that will delay the development of AB2M. There is some evidence that the prevalence and severity of AB2M are decreasing (69). Each treatment should employ biocompatible membranes with good B2M clearances at high blood flows (high *Kt/V* values), along with ultrapure dialysate and parenteral replacement fluids (free of endotoxin) (60,70,71).

Each patient receiving dialysis, HF, or HDF therapy for more than 5 years should be surveyed annually for the development of

TABLE 23.7. SPECIFIC RECOMMENDATIONS REGARDING MANAGEMENT OF AB2M AMYLOIDOSIS

1. Renal transplantation if possible
2. Biocompatible membrane hemodialysis or hemodiafiltration at high blood flows (increased B2M clearances) using ultrapure dialysate
3. Annual bone survey
4. Prompt surgical intervention
   a. Fractures
   b. Ruptured tendons
   c. Contractures
   d. Carpal tunnel syndrome
   e. Spinal cord or nerve root compression
   f. Dysfunctional shoulders
5. Prophylactic joint replacement or internal fixation
   a. Large lytic lesions
   b. Loss of 50% or more of long bone cortex

skeletal lesions, spondyloarthropathy, peripheral arthropathy, and carpal tunnel syndrome. Prompt surgical intervention should be sought when it is indicated. The onset of bone pain may be an important clue to microfractures that may later progress to displaced fractures. When half or more of the long bone diameter is involved by endosteal lesions, considerable weakening occurs. Prophylactic internal fixation has been advised when there are lytic lesions of more than 3 cm in diameter and in which 50% or more of the surrounding cortex has been destroyed (33). Hip fractures are best treated with total joint replacement, since there is great difficulty in successfully nailing bone involved with amyloid (10,33).

CONCLUSION

In summary, AB2M amyloidosis must be added to the list of causes of renal osteodystrophy. It is a disabling condition for which there is imperfect treatment. Of current options, early renal transplantation offers the most hope. Table 23.7 summarizes our current recommendations.

ACKNOWLEDGMENTS

The author appreciates the efforts of Ms. Maurine Burton in the preparation of this manuscript. Dr. William Witt assisted in the preparation of the radiologic studies.

REFERENCES

1. Gertz MA, et al. Primary systemic amyloidosis—a diagnostic primer. *Mayo Clin Proc* l989;64:1505–1519.
2. Gorevic PD, et al. β_2- microglobulin is an amyloidogenic protein in man. *J Clin Invest* 1985;76:2425–2429.
3. Gejyo F, et al. B2-microglubulin: a new form of amyloid protein associated with chronic hemodialysis. *Kidney Int* 1986;30:385–390.
4. Casey TT, et al. Tumoral amyloidosis of bone of beta2-microglobulin origin in association with long-term hemodialysis. *Hum Pathol* 1986;17:73l–738.
5. Shirahama T, et al. Histochemical and immunohistochemical charac-

terization of amyloid associated with chronic hemodialysis as B_2-microglobulin. *Lab Invest* 1985;53:705–709.
6. Bardin T, et al. Hemodialysis-associated amyloidosis and β_2- microglobulin. *Am J Med* 1987;83:419–424.
7. Nishi S, et al. Electron-microscopic and immunohistochemical study of β_2—microglobulin-related amyloidosis. *Nephron* 1990;56:357–363.
8. Gorevic PD, et al. Polymerization of intact B2-microglobulin in tissue causes amyloidosis in patients on chronic hemodialysis. *Proc Natl Acad Sci* 1986;83:7908–7912.
9. Katz JN, et al. The carpal tunnel syndrome: diagnostic utility of the history and physical examination findings. *Ann Intern Med* 1990;112: 321–327.
10. Kurer MHJ, et al. Musculoskeletal manifestations of amyloidosis. *J Bone Joint Surg (Br)* 1991;73B:271–276.
11. Word-Sims WS, et al. Carpal tunnel syndrome in the dialysis patient. *Semin Dial* 1990;3:47–51.
12. Benz RL, et al. Carpal tunnel syndrome in dialysis patients: comparison between continuous ambulatory peritoneal dialysis and hemodialysis populations. *Am J Kidney Dis* 1988;11:473–476.
13. Spertini F, et al. Carpal tunnel syndrome: a frequent, invalidating, long-term complication of chronic hemodialysis. *Clin Nephrol* 1984; 21:98–101.
14. Laurent G, et al. Dialysis related amyloidosis. *Kidney Int* 1988;33 (Suppl 24):S32–S34.
15. Spencer JD. Amyloidosis as a cause of carpal tunnel syndrome in hemodialysis patients. *J Hand Surg* 1988;13B:402–405.
16. Van Ypersele de Strihou C, et al. Effect of dialysis membrane and patient's age on signs of dialysis-related amyloidosis. *Kidney Int* 1991;39:1012–1019.
17. Acchiardo S, et al. B2-microglobulin levels in patients with renal insufficiency. *Am J Kidney Dis* 1989;13:70–74.
18. Canaud B, et al. Failure of a daily haemofiltration programme using a highly permeable membrane to return B2-microglobulin concentrations to normal in haemodialysis patients. *Nephrol Dial Transplant* 1992;7:924–930.
19. Kleinman KS, et al. Amyloid syndromes associated with hemodialysis. *Kidney Int* 1989;35:567–575.
20. Cobby MJ, et al. Dialysis-related amyloid arthropathy: MR findings in four patients. *Am J Roentgenol* 1991;157:1023–1027.
21. Muñoz-Gomez J, et al. Amyloid arthropathy in patients undergoing periodical haemodialysis for chronic renal failure: a new complication. *Ann Rheum Dis* 1985;44:729–733.
22. Jadoul M, et al. Histological prevalence of B2-microglobulin amyloidosis in hemodialysis: a prospective post-mortem study. *Kidney Int* 1997;51:1928–1932.
23. Jadoul M, et al. Prevalence of histological B2-microglobulin amyloidosis in CAPD patients compared with hemodialysis patients. *Kidney Int* 1998;54:956–959.
24. Konishiike T, et al. Shoulder pain in long-term hemodialysis patients. *J Bone Joint Surg (Br)* 1996;78B:601–605.
25. Okutsu I, et al. Endoscopic management of shoulder pain in long-term haemodialysis patients. *Nephrol Dial Transplant* 1991;6:117–119.
26. Mourad G, et al. Renal transplantation relieves the symptoms but does not reverse B2-microglobulin amyloidosis. *J Am Soc Nephrol* 1996; 7:798–804.
27. Bardin T, et al. Dialysis arthropathy: outcome after renal transplantation. *Am J Med* 1995;99:243–248.
28. Ohashi K, et al. Cervical discs are most susceptible to beta2-microglobulin amyloid deposition in the vertebral column. *Kidney Int* 1992;41: 1646–1652.
29. Maruyama H, et al. Clinical studies of destructive spondyloarthropathy in long-term hemodialysis patients. *Nephron* 1992;61:37–44.
30. Fiocchi O, et al. Radiological features of dialysis amyloid spondyloarthropathy. *Int J Artif Organs* 1989;12:216–222.
31. Allard JC, et al. Fatal destructive cervical spondyloarthropathy in two patients on long-term dialysis. *Am J Kidney Dis* 1992;19:81–85.
32. Chassagne P, et al. Fatal destructive cervical spondyloarthropathy. *Am J Kidney Dis* 1992;20:199–200.
33. DiRaimondo CR, et al. Pathologic fractures associated with idiopathic

amyloidosis of bone in chronic hemodialysis patients. *Nephron* 1986; 43:22–27.

34. Onishi S, et al. Beta2-microglobulin deposition in bone in chronic renal failure. *Kidney Int* 1991;39:990–995.
35. Bommer J, et al. Urinary matrix calculi consisting of microfibrillar protein in patients on maintenance hemodialysis. *Kidney Int* 1979;16: 722–728.
36. Linke RP, et al. Amyloid kidney stones of uremic patients consist of beta2-microglobulin fragments. *Biochem Biophys Res Comm* 1986;136: 665–671.
37. Digenis GE, et al. Kidney stones in chronic dialysis patients. *Semin Dial* 1992;5:11–12.
38. Gehrig JJ, et al. Acquired cystic disease of the end-stage kidney. *Am J Med* 1985;79:609–620.
39. Reese W, et al. B₂-microglobulin and associated amyloidosis presenting as bilateral popliteal tumors. *Am J Kidney Dis* 1988;12:323–325.
40. Floege J, et al. Subcutaneous amyloid-tumor of beta2-microglobulin origin in a long-term hemodialysis patient. *Nephron* 1989;53:73–75.
41. Athanasou NA, et al. Subcutaneous deposition of beta₂-microglobulin amyloid in a long-term haemodialysis patient. *Nephrol Dial Transplant* 1990;5:878–881.
42. Athanasou NA, et al. Joint and systemic distribution of dialysis amyloid. *Q J Med* 1991;287:205–214.
43. Noel LH, et al. Tissue distribution of dialysis amyloidosis. *Clin Nephrol* 1987;27:175–178.
44. Gal R, et al. Systemic distribution of B₂-microglobulin-derived amyloidosis in patients who undergo long-term hemodialysis. *Arch Pathol Lab Med* 1994;188:718–721.
45. Rafto SE, et al. Spondyloarthropathy of the cervical spine in long-term hemodialysis. *Radiology* 1988;166:201–204.
46. Sethi D, et al. Technetium-99-labelled methylene diphosphonate uptake scans in patients with dialysis arthropathy. *Nephron* 1990;54: 202–207.
47. Stone WJ, et al. Beta2-microglobulin amyloidosis in long-term dialysis patients. *Am J Nephrol* 1989;9:177–183.
48. Floege J, et al. Imaging of dialysis-related amyloid (AB-amyloid) deposits with ¹³¹I-B₂-microglobulin. *Kidney Int* 1990;38:1169–1176.
49. McMahon LP, et al. Shoulder ultrasound in dialysis related amyloidosis. *Clin Nephrol* 1991;35:227–232.
50. Van Ypersele de Strihou C, et al. Morphogenesis of joint B₂-microglobulin amyloid deposits. *Nephrol Dial Transplant* 2001;16(Suppl 4):3–7.
51. Carone FA, et al. Renal tubular transport and catabolism of proteins and peptides. *Kidney Int* 1979;16:271–278.

52. Revillard JP, et al. Structure and metabolism of beta2-microglobulin. *Contr Nephrol* 1988;62:44–53.
53. Connors LH, et al. In vitro formation of amyloid fibrils from intact B₂-microglobulin. *Biochem Biophys Res Comm* 1985;131:1063–1068.
54. Taubes G. Misfolding the way to disease. *Science* 1996;271:1493–1495.
55. Floege J, et al. B₂-microglobulin-derived amyloidosis: an update. *Kidney Int* 2001;59(Suppl 78):S164–S171.
56. Balint E, et al. Role of interleukin-6 in B₂-microglobulin-induced bone mineral dissolution. *Kidney Int* 2000;57:1599–1607.
57. Floege J, et al. Dialysis related amyloidosis: a disease of chronic retention and inflammation? *Kidney Int* 1992;42(Suppl 38):S78–S85.
58. Campistol JM, et al. Polymerization of normal and intact B₂-microglobulin as the amyloidogenic protein in dialysis amyloidosis. *Kidney Int* 1996;50:1262–1267.
59. Zaoui PM, et al. Effects of dialysis membranes on beta2-microglobulin production and cellular expression. *Kidney Int* 1990;38:962–968.
60. Zingraff J, et al. Can the nephrologist prevent dialysis-related amyloidosis? *Am J Kidney Dis* 1991;18:1–11.
61. Mundy GR. Hypercalcemia of malignancy revisited. *J Clin Invest* 1988;82:1–6.
62. Odell RA, et al. Beta2-microglobulin kinetics in end-stage renal failure. *Kidney Int* 1991;39:909–919.
63. DiRaimondo CR, et al. Beta2-microglubulin in peritoneal dialysis patients: serum levels and peritoneal clearances. *Perit Dial Int* 1988;8: 43–47.
64. Van Ypersele de Strihou C, et al. Dialysis amyloidosis. *Adv Nephrol* 1988;17:401–422.
65. Lornoy W, et al. On-line hemodiafiltration: remarkable removal of B₂-microglobulin—long-term clinical observations. *Nephrol Dial Transplant* 2000;15(Suppl 1):49–54.
66. Nakai S, et al. Outcomes of hemodiafiltration based on Japanese dialysis patient registry. *Am J Kidney Dis* 2001;38(Suppl 1):S212–S216.
67. Sethi D, et al. Persistence of dialysis amyloid after renal transplantation. *Am J Nephrol* 1989;9:173–l74.
68. Figueroa ML, et al. A less costly regimen of alglucerase to treat Gaucher's disease. *N Engl J Med* 1992;327:1632–1636.
69. Schwalbe S, et al. B₂-microglobulin associated amyloidosis: a vanishing complication of long-term hemodialysis? *Kidney Int* 1997;52: 1077–1083.
70. Schiffl H, et al. Clinical manifestations of AB-amyloidosis: effects of biocompatibility and flux. *Nephrol Dial Transplant* 2000;15:840–845.
71. Kuchle C, et al. High-flux hemodialysis postpones clinical manifestations of dialysis-related amyloidosis. *Am J Nephrol* 1996;16:484–488.

24

ENDOCRINE DISORDERS IN DIALYSIS PATIENTS

R. TYLER MILLER

Patients with renal insufficiency or who are receiving dialysis may develop the same endocrine disorders that are found in the general population, including thyroid, adrenal, and pituitary diseases. In these situations, the symptoms of the endocrine disease may overlap and be confused with the symptoms of renal failure. Patients with renal failure are also subject to endocrine disorders that arise as a consequence of their renal disease. These disorders include infertility, impotence, growth hormone resistance, and disorders of mineral and bone metabolism. Additionally, uremia and metabolic acidosis, which frequently accompany renal failure uremia, cause a generalized hormone insensitivity syndrome, a situation that contributes to illness in dialysis patients and complicates the diagnosis of many endocrine disorders. In this chapter, adrenal, and pituitary diseases will be discussed because they occur in patients with renal failure, may not be suspected, and may be difficult to diagnose because many tests of endocrine function are altered, or are impossible to carry out in renal failure. Fertility and impotence will also be considered because these are important problems for many patients. In each section, the physiology of the endocrine system, the most common diseases that affect it, and the diagnosis and therapy if they differ from diagnosis and therapy in the normal patient population will be reviewed. Disorders of vitamin D, PTH, bone, and lipids are considered elsewhere.

THYROID DISORDERS

An appropriate supply of thyroid hormone is essential for normal metabolism, cardiovascular function, mental status, and muscle strength. Diagnosis of thyroid disease in patients on dialysis is complicated by the fact that renal failure can produce many of the same findings as thyroid disease and is often caused or accompanied by diseases such as diabetes, connective-tissue diseases, and liver disease. These conditions can confound physical findings or alter standard tests used to evaluate thyroid function. Thyroid physiology, the effects of renal failure, the most common thyroid disorders, and their evaluation and management will be described in this section.

Thyroid Physiology

Thyroid function is regulated at multiple levels to ensure that only minimal variation in thyroid hormone levels occurs. The complexity of regulation of thyroid hormone reflects its importance as a regulator of development as well as metabolism and essential systemic functions. The synthesis and secretion of thyroid hormone are primarily controlled by the hypothalamus and pituitary. Although T_4 is the predominant circulating form of thyroid hormone, T_3 is the biologically active form and is responsible for the negative feedback at the levels of the hypothalamus and pituitary that can reduce thyroid-releasing hormone (TRH) and thyroid-stimulating hormone (TSH) secretion. TRH is produced in the hypothalamus and stimulates TSH by the thyrotrophic cells in the anteromedial region of the pituitary. TRH production and secretion increase in response to reduced circulating levels of T_3. TSH is the primary trophic hormone for the thyroid gland and is responsible for its size, vascularity, and amount of thyroid hormone production as well as the release of thyroid hormone.

Iodine, an essential substrate of thyroid hormone synthesis that is concentrated in the thyroid by an active transport mechanism, contributes to control of thyroid hormone synthesis and release. Excess iodine inhibits iodine uptake and thyroid hormone synthesis by the thyroid. High levels or acute high doses (such as those given with Lugol's solution or with radio contrast) reduce hormone synthesis and secretion. The primary route of iodine excretion is the kidney, and as renal insufficiency progresses, one would expect iodine to be retained. Dialysis patients have increased serum inorganic iodine and thyroid iodine content as well as an increased incidence of enlarged thyroid glands, but the full physiologic implications of this situation are not understood (1).

Both T_4 and T_3 are produced in the thyroid, but T_4 is the predominant secreted form. T_3 levels in the systemic circulation primarily reflect peripheral conversion of T_4 to T_3 by a monodeiodinase, a metabolic step that is also subject to regulation. Several proteins in the blood bind and transport thyroid hormone, including thyroid-binding globulin (TBG), prealbumin, and albumin. Except in rare circumstances, the effects of the other proteins are negligible compared with those of TBG. Loss of thyroid hormone through hemo- or peritoneal dialysis is negligible under normal circumstances (1). Finally, the sensitivity of tissues to thyroid hormone can be altered through changes in thyroid hormone receptor expression (2).

Serum thyroid hormone levels vary with changes in the concentration of serum thyroid hormone-binding proteins. In states

TABLE 24.1. CHANGES IN THYROID FUNCTION TESTS IN EUTHYROID/SICK, HYPOTHYROID, AND THYROTOXIC STATES

	Normal	Euthyroid/Sick	Hypothyroid	Thyrotoxic
TSH	0.5–5 mU/mL	Normal to slightly increased	Increased	Decreased
T_3	1.1–2.9 nmol/L	Decreased	Decreased	Increased
T_4	64–154 nmol/L	Decreased	Decreased	Increased
FT_4I	0.85–1.10	Slightly decreased	Decreased	Increased
rT_3	0.15–0.61 nmol/L	Increased	Decreased to normal	Normal

Reference values for TSH (0.5–5 mU/mL or 0.5–5 μU/mL), T_3 (1.1–2.9 nmol/L or 75–220 ng/dL), T_4 (64–154 nmol/L or 4–11 μg/dL), FT_4I (0.86–1.10), and reverse T_3 (rT_3, 0.15–0.61 nmol/L or 10–40 ng/dL) are given as the normal values (2). The direction of the change in the serum value is shown under the heading for each condition. In many situations, not all values will be abnormal but may be at the upper or lower limits of the normal range.

such as liver disease (acute and chronic hepatitis, primary biliary cirrhosis), HIV infection, use of estrogen, tamoxifen, or pregnancy, TBG levels are increased, which will be reflected in increased total thyroid hormone. In the nephrotic syndrome, following administration of androgens, or high-dose glucocorticoids, and in major systemic illnesses or acromegaly, TBG levels are decreased, and total serum thyroid hormone levels are reduced. In the absence of other complicating factors, the free serum T_3 level, the biologically important parameter, is normal.

Peripheral conversion of T_4 to T_3 is controlled by at least three enzymes, types 1 (5′), 2 (5′), and 3 (5′) deiodinases. Type 1 is expressed in liver, kidney, thyroid, the central nervous system, and the pituitary, and is responsible for conversion of T_4 to T_3 in these tissues. This enzyme is primarily responsible for systemic T_3 levels but may also produce rT_3, a metabolically inactive form of T_3. The peripheral conversion of T_4 to T_3 (presumably through inhibition of this enzyme) is reduced in a number of conditions that are important in nephrology, including renal failure, malnutrition, liver disease, other systemic illnesses, and following trauma or surgery (euthyroid sick syndrome) (Table 24.1). Drugs that impair conversion of T_4 to T_3 include glucocorticoids, propranolol (>200 mg/d), amiodarone, and oral cholecystographic agents. The type 2 deiodinase is expressed in the central nervous system, pituitary, brown fat, and placenta. In states (see later) where peripheral conversion of T_4 to T_3 is reduced, this enzyme may maintain the central nervous system, pituitary, brown fat, and placenta in a relatively euthyroid state through in situ production of T_3. Type 3 deiodinase is expressed in the central nervous system, placenta, and skin, and is the primary source of reverse T_3 (rT_3). Reverse T_3 is an inactive metabolite of T_4 that increases in some conditions, including burns, trauma, and uremia. The fact that local concentrations of T_3 may differ because of differential regulation of the deiodinases can make it difficult to determine if a hypothyroid state exists.

Measurement of Thyroid Function

The suspicion of thyroid disease is raised by the patient's history and physical findings, and confirmed with laboratory measurement of thyroid hormone levels. Below are described the most commonly used assays with an emphasis on the laboratory characterization of the euthyroid sick syndrome because renal failure produces this pattern of laboratory values in up to 65% of dialysis patients (Fig. 24.1) (3). Sensitive assays are available for measuring T_4, T_3, rT_3, and TSH, and these measurements are

the clinical tests used most commonly to establish the diagnosis of thyroid hormone excess or deficiency. Total serum T_4, T_3, and rT_3 are measured by radioimmunoassay (RIA). The normal ranges are 64 to 142 nmol/L (5 to 11 μg/dL) for T_4 and 1.1 to 2.9 nmol/L (70 to 190 ng/dL) for T_3. Total T_3 levels are more useful than those of T_4 because an elevated total serum T_3, the active hormone, is found in thyrotoxicosis and this finding is required for that diagnosis. However, the normal range is broad enough so that some patients who have physiologic evidence of thyrotoxicosis may have serum T_3 levels that are within the normal range. The normal levels of rT_3 are lower than those of T_3, but variable. rT_3 is measured in special circumstances (see later). Its level increases with alterations in peripheral deiodinase activity in systemic illnesses. T_4 is tightly bound by serum proteins (primarily TBG), and the level of total T_4 changes substantially with changes in the level of TBG. TBG may change markedly with disease or nutritional state. A high or low total T_4 level may not be meaningful if the level of the thyroid hormone-binding protein is also high or low. Renal failure and dialysis do not directly affect TBG levels, although these levels may be reduced with persistent nephrotic range proteinuria, with high rates of peritoneal protein loss, or after androgen administration for anemia in patients who might not also be receiving erythropoietin.

The biologically active form of the hormone is that which is free in the serum and not protein bound. Unfortunately, true free thyroid hormone levels are difficult to measure clinically, so alternative assays have been developed. These assays, the free T_4 index (FT_4I) or free T_3 index (FT_3I) do not directly measure free hormone, but reflect it. The serum samples are incubated with a radioactive tracer (T_3 or T_4) and the binding of the tracer to a solid-phase thyroid hormone-binding matrix is measured. The value is corrected for variability among different assays by dividing it by the control value of serum from a normal person who has normal amounts of TBG. The free hormone levels can then be estimated by multiplying the fraction of free hormone by the total hormone concentration, which is the FT_4I or FT_3I. Generally, if a patient is euthyroid, increases or decreases in serum thyroid hormone-binding proteins are compensated for by hypothalamic and pituitary feedback mechanisms, and the biologically active free hormone (T_3) levels remain normal.

Interpretation of the FT_4I or FT_3I has caused confusion because of terminology and because it has limitations. The assay is called the FT_4I or FT_3I based on whether T_4 or T_3 is used as the tracer. Because T_4 and T_3 both bind to TBG and the solid-phase hormone-binding resin, this assay does not distinguish between T_4 and T_3, but it does allow correction for different lev-

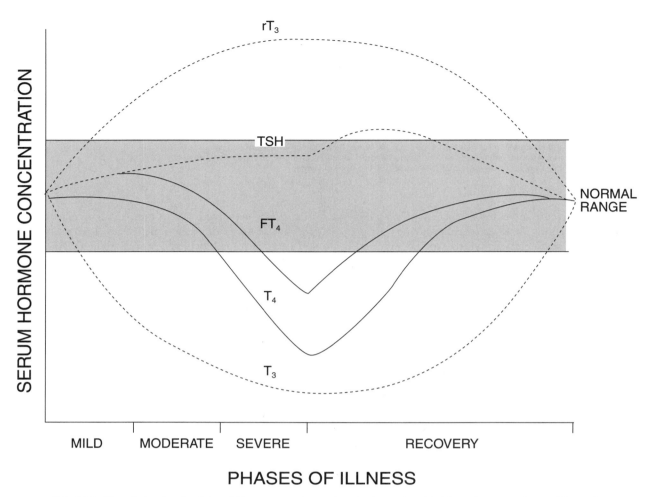

FIG. 24.1. The varying levels of thyroid hormones, TSH, and FT₄ in the euthyroid-sick syndrome. Patients with renal failure and receiving dialysis treatment may have thyroid function test values that correspond to any severity of illness shown on the graph when they do not have intrinsic thyroid, pituitary, or hypothalamic pathology. (From Brent GA, et al. Effect of nonthyroidal illness on thyroid function tests. In: Van Middlesworth L, ed. *The thyroid gland: a practical and clinical treatise.* Chicago: Year Book Medical, 1986:83–110, and Larsen PR, et al. The thyroid. In: Wilson JD, et al., eds. *Williams textbook of endocrinology.* Philadelphia: WB Saunders, 1992:357–487.)

els of thyroid-binding proteins in the serum. In states of pure thyroid disease, the lack of specificity for T_4 or T_3 is not a problem because the level of free T_3 is a function of the level of free T_4. However, in conditions such as renal failure, malnutrition or other systemic diseases (euthyroid sick syndrome), the activity of the peripheral deiodinases is altered, and conversion of T_4 to T_3 is not regulated normally. In these situations, additional indices of thyroid function are required but still may not fully characterize thyroid function.

Sensitive assays exist that allow direct measurement of TSH, the trophic hormone from the pituitary that participates in feedback regulation of thyroid function. TSH levels are a function of T_3 biologic activity in the hypothalamus, where TRH production and release respond to T_3 levels, and T_3 biologic activity in the pituitary, where TSH secretion and release are directly controlled by T_3. In primary thyroid disease, if T_3 levels are reduced, TSH levels rise. If T_3 levels are elevated, TSH levels are suppressed. However, hypothyroidism can occur as a result of a fail-

ure of the hypothalamopituitary axis, resulting in low TSH levels, and thyrotoxicosis can result from increased secretion of TSH such as from a pituitary tumor. The normal range for TSH is 0.5 to 5 mU/mL. Patients who are thyrotoxic have serum TSH levels below 0.5 mU/mL, and patients who are hypothyroid have serum levels above 5 mU/mL. If pituitary failure is suspected, a TRH stimulation test can be performed.

Dialysis patients have at least one systemic illness, chronic renal failure, and frequently others, such as malnutrition and diabetes. These chronic illnesses (and others) alter the activity of peripheral deiodinases and cause an abnormal pattern of thyroid function tests, termed the *euthyroid-sick syndrome* (3). The euthyroid sick syndrome is characterized by reduced total and free serum T_3 and increased serum rT_3 as a result of increased peripheral deiodination of T_4 to rT_3. The degree of reduction of the serum T_3 level corresponds to the severity of the systemic illness. In mild to moderately severe illnesses, T_3 is reduced, rT_3 is increased, but T_4, FT_4I (or FT_3I), and TSH levels are normal.

With severe illness, the T_4 and FT_4I (or FT_3I) levels may fall in the subnormal range. During recovery from a severe illness, the TSH level may rise to levels slightly above normal before normalizing. Consequently, thyroid hormone levels in dialysis patients must be interpreted using a euthyroid-sick pattern as normal.

Whether patients with the euthyroid-sick syndrome are in fact physiologically hypothyroid is unknown. T_4, T_3, rT_3, and FT_4I or FT_3I levels reflect systemic metabolism of T_4, whereas TSH levels reflect hypothalamic and pituitary levels of T_3. TSH levels do not suggest that T_3 levels are low, but the conversion of T_4 to T_3 in the tissue responsible for sensing T_3 activity (hypothalamus and pituitary) is mediated by a deiodinase whose activity does not appear to change with systemic illness. In contrast, systemic measurement of thyroid hormones reflects metabolism by different deiodinases whose activity does change with systemic illness. Consequently, the CNS and pituitary may be euthyroid while the remainder of the body is hypothyroid. Administration of L-T_4 to severely ill patients has been studied but has not altered their outcomes (4,5). Survivors could be identified by their high baseline T_3/T_4 ratios. Despite administration of L-T_4, there was no benefit to this patient population in survival. Preliminary studies in dialysis patients suggest that treatment of dialysis patients with low doses of T_3 results in a less favorable nitrogen balance and increased protein degradation (1).

Thyroid Diseases

Thyroid diseases can be separated into those that cause increased hormone levels (thyrotoxicosis), decreased hormone levels (hypothyroidism), nonfunctional nodules, and inflammatory diseases of the thyroid.

Thyrotoxicosis

Thyrotoxicosis is a physiologic condition that results from excess thyroid hormone. The precise manifestations of thyrotoxicosis depend on the magnitude of hormone excess, the age of the patient, and the presence of other illnesses, such as cardiovascular disease and diabetes. In general, the effects of thyroid hormone excess represent an exaggeration of its normal physiologic response and are usually most prominent on metabolism and on the cardiovascular and nervous systems.

Elevated thyroid hormone levels cause an increase in metabolic rate that is reflected in increased calorie utilization, oxygen consumption, heat generation, and increased basal body temperature. Protein synthesis and breakdown are increased, but degradation exceeds synthesis leading to decreased body mass and weight loss. Many such patients have an abnormal glucose tolerance that may simulate diabetes mellitus. Lipid metabolism is also altered with both increased synthesis and degradation of lipids, but degradation exceeds synthesis. Free fatty acid levels are increased, whereas triglyceride and cholesterol levels are decreased. The metabolic manifestations of thyrotoxicosis may be difficult to detect in patients with renal disease and those who are on dialysis because they overlap with those of renal failure or with chronic diseases such as diabetes mellitus that are com-

monly found in the dialysis population. Although renal failure patients rarely are hyperthermic, they commonly are catabolic and glucose intolerant.

Thyroid hormone has a direct cardiostimulatory activity that leads to increased cardiac output through resting tachycardia (greater than 90), and combined increased heart rate and stroke volume with decreased peripheral resistance. The increased cardiac output is a response to supply the increased oxygen demands and the requirement to dissipate heat. These patients also have increased blood pressure and a widened pulse pressure. Because of the high frequency of hypertension and alterations in total body volume in dialysis patients, these findings may not be valuable in identifying patients with thyrotoxicosis. However, arrhythmias, congestive heart failure, and a change in pattern of angina may provide excellent clues to the presence of thyrotoxicosis. Supraventricular arrhythmias, especially atrial fibrillation, are common and may be the presenting complaint in patients with thyrotoxicosis. In the absence of preexisting heart disease, congestive heart failure is uncommon with thyrotoxicosis but occurs commonly in patients who do have a compromised heart. Patients with thyrotoxicosis are commonly resistant to the effects of digitalis. The frequency, pattern, or severity of angina is frequently increased in thyrotoxic patients with coronary artery disease. Patients may complain of shortness of breath in the absence of congestive heart failure. This sensation may be due to reduced lung compliance and muscle weakness in some circumstances.

Thyrotoxicosis usually produces prominent effects in the nervous system. Patients complain of nervousness that is characterized by a short attention span, restlessness, and compulsion to move despite fatigue. These patients often have fast, jerky movements, and a fine rhythmic tremor of hands and tongue. They are emotionally labile and often complain of insomnia. Psychiatric disorders occur including manic-depressive, schizoid, and paranoid states. In patients with seizure disorders, the seizure threshold is lowered, resulting in increased frequency of seizures. The hyperkinetic state described is uncommon in dialysis patients, but fatigue, restlessness, inattention, psychiatric and emotional disturbances, and changes in seizure frequency occur often. Consequently, the existence of any one of these findings in a patient may not be helpful in suggesting thyrotoxicosis, but their appearance in a patient who was previously stable may be of diagnostic value.

Common gastrointestinal symptoms include increased gastrointestinal motility (faster gastric and intestinal emptying and transit times) with less-well-formed stools, and increased stool frequency. Overt diarrhea is rare. Patients usually note increased appetites, although appetite may be decreased in severe cases or in the elderly. Patients with renal failure usually have decreased bowel motility, so apparent normalization of bowel function may be due to thyrotoxicosis. Hepatic dysfunction with elevated transaminases has been reported in thyrotoxicosis, possibly due in part to increased O_2 extraction in the splanchnic bed (6).

Increased levels of thyroid hormone alter the structure and function of muscle and bone. Patients complain of proximal muscle weakness and fatigability. These symptoms are usually partly due to wasting and loss of muscle mass, but are also due to primary changes in the muscles. Myopathy is more common in men than in women. In patients with normal renal function, thyrotoxicosis leads to loss of bone mass with increased urinary excretion of Ca and PO_4, and increased hydroxyproline turnover with reduced levels of PTH and vitamin D. In dialysis patients, the effects of excess thyroid hormone on bone mass presumably are similar, but they have not been reported.

Causes of Thyrotoxicosis

Dialysis patients develop thyrotoxicosis for the same reasons as nondialysis patients. The causes include Graves' disease or toxic diffuse goiter, toxic multinodular goiter, and increased secretion of TSH due to a pituitary adenoma, increased secretion of TRH, or resistance of either the hypothalamus or pituitary to T_3. Graves' disease is the most common cause of thyrotoxicosis and is an autoimmune disease that results from circulating autoantibodies (long-acting thyroid-stimulating antibodies, or LATS) that appear to be directed against a component of the thyroid cell membrane. The disease is characterized not only by thyrotoxicosis, but also by an infiltrative ophthalmopathy-producing exophthalmos, and dermopathy. Toxic multinodular goiter usually arises in a multinodular thyroid gland. The thyrotoxicosis is usually less severe than in Graves' disease, but it occurs in an older population, so cardiovascular symptoms may be more prominent (2). Thyroid nodules may be more common in patients receiving chronic dialysis (7).

Diagnosis of Thyrotoxicosis

Thyrotoxicosis may not be suspected in dialysis patients because the symptoms of thyrotoxicosis may be ascribed to other underlying illnesses such as cardiovascular disease, hypertension, and volume overload. Many of the symptoms may be masked by medications such as beta blockers or other blood pressure medications. Weight loss may be masked by retained fluid or ascribed to gastroparesis. Nevertheless, new symptoms that are consistent with thyrotoxicosis, particularly cardiovascular symptoms, should suggest the possibility of thyrotoxicosis. The complaint or finding of increasing neck size or a lump in the anterior neck is particularly valuable in identifying patients who may be thyrotoxic. Thyrotoxicosis is caused by elevated T_3, and a diagnosis of thyrotoxicosis normally requires elevated levels of T_3, so T_3 should be measured. If thyrotoxicosis is caused by primary overproduction of thyroid hormone by the entire gland (Graves' disease) or by nodules (95% of cases), the TSH level should be suppressed. If thyrotoxicosis is caused by overproduction of TSH (pituitary tumor, hypothalamic lesion, or ectopic production, 5% of cases), the TSH level will be elevated.

Treatment of Thyrotoxicosis

The immediate treatment of thyrotoxicosis in patients with renal failure is the same as that for other patients and includes the use of beta blockers, dexamethasone, and agents that block thyroid hormone synthesis and release (propylthiouracil and methimazole). In patients with renal failure, propylthiouracil can cause granulocytopenia, agranulocytosis, rheumatic syndromes, and hepatitis. However, the doses of both propylthiouracil and methimazole are not changed in dialysis patients. [131]I may also be used, and it is cleared by both peritoneal and hemodialysis (8).

Hypothyroid States

Hypothyroidism occurs for three general reasons: (a) there is a loss of functional thyroid tissue; (b) there is a loss of trophic activity by TSH; and (c) there is defective hormone synthesis (as with iodine deficiency). Loss of trophic activity in pituitary or hypothalamic lesions represents approximately 5% of all cases of hypothyroidism. The symptoms of hypothyroidism are generally the opposite of those of thyrotoxicosis. They are even more difficult to identify in renal failure and dialysis because, like renal failure, hypothyroidism results in generalized constitutional symptoms and gradual loss of function.

In hypothyroidism the metabolic rate slows, resulting in decreased oxygen consumption; heat generation decreases; appetite decreases; and the rate of protein synthesis is reduced. The latter may be due to decreased effectiveness of growth hormone and insulin-like growth factor 1 (IGF-1, also known as somatomedin C). The oral glucose tolerance test is flat, and the peak insulin response is delayed. The rate of degradation of insulin is decreased, leading to an increased sensitivity to exogenous insulin. Patients also have increased capillary permeability, which leads to peripheral edema. Cholesterol and triglyceride circulating concentration levels are elevated as a consequence of their decreased clearance, and HDL levels are reduced. Superficially, none of these findings is specific for hypothyroidism but they are seen in dialysis patients.

Hypothyroidism reduces heart rate and myocardial contractility, diminishing pulse pressure and reducing cardiac output. The heart is enlarged and a pericardial effusion frequently develops. Pleural effusions are also common. EKG abnormalities include sinus bradycardia, prolonged PR interval, reduced amplitude of the P wave and QRS complex, and nonspecific ST-segment and T-wave changes. These changes may contribute to congestive heart failure. Other than the bradycardia, these findings are commonly seen to progress slowly over months and are commonly seen in patients on dialysis services.

In hypothyroidism gastrointestinal motility is decreased and constipation is a frequent complaint. The mucosa of the GI tract is atrophic, causing reduced absorption, but the decreased transit time partially compensates for the decreased absorption rate. Ascites consisting of mucopolysaccharide- and protein-rich fluid is common. Superficially, these findings are not pathognomonic for hypothyroidism and can occur for a variety of reasons in the dialysis population.

The most prominent symptoms in hypothyroidism are frequently found in the nervous system. They include reduced cognitive function, deterioration of memory, slow speech, syncope, and coma. Psychiatric symptoms may include paranoia or depression. Speech is thick and slurred as a consequence of infiltration of the larynx and tongue by mucopolysaccharides. Movements are slow and appear uncoordinated, and may be further compromised by compression of peripheral nerves by myxedematous deposits. Reflexes are slow due to altered nerve responses, including decreased relaxation. Myxedematous patients complain of stiff, sore muscles, but muscle strength usually remains intact.

Causes of Hypothyroidism

Loss of functional thyroid tissue occurs following ablation of hyperactive thyroid tissue (such as following ablative therapy for

Graves' disease with ^{131}I), idiopathic hypothyroidism, or the late stages of Hashimoto's thyroiditis (autoimmune thyroiditis). Excess iodine inhibits thyroid function by inhibiting thyroid uptake of iodine and thyroid hormone synthesis and release. Since the primary route of excretion of iodine is the urine, one might expect high levels of iodine to accumulate in patients with renal failure. Regulation of iodine metabolism in renal failure and dialysis patients has not been studied systematically, but iodine (^{131}I) is removed by hemo- and peritoneal dialysis (8). One report exists of three cases of hypothyroidism due to iodine accumulation in dialysis patients eating a high-iodine diet (9). Radiocontrast agents may also represent an iodine load for dialysis patients that could affect thyroid function. Another group possibly at risk for hypothyroidism is made up of patients with iron overload syndromes (10).

Diagnosis of Hypothyroidism

Many of the symptoms of hypothyroidism are nonspecific and overlap with those of chronic renal failure (11). Consequently, hypothyroidism may not be suspected and may go undiagnosed. Patients who are at particular risk for hypothyroidism are those who have a history of previous ablative treatment of thyroid disease, possibly those with other autoimmune endocrine diseases, or those whose general condition deteriorates for unexplained reasons. The physical signs of hypothyroidism, such as delayed reflexes in a diabetic patient or a slow pulse in patients taking beta blockers, may also be difficult to identify in dialysis patients. Nevertheless, delayed reflexes are valuable in making the diagnosis of hypothyroidism as long as other neurologic disorders are not present. If a patient is not taking medications that could slow the heart rate, then heart rate is also valuable in screening patients for hypothyroidism. Measurement of circulating thyroid hormone levels will usually reveal a sick-euthyroid pattern with a variable (low or normal) T_4, low RT_3U, low T_3, and normal or mildly elevated TSH. However, dialysis patients who are truly hypothyroid will have elevations of TSH with normal hypothalamopituitary function, so primary hypothyroidism can be diagnosed with a serum TSH in most situations. Whether mild elevations of TSH represent subclinical hypothyroidism or whether this state represents a euthyroid central nervous system and pituitary with a hypothyroid periphery is not clear (2). Normal patients with minimal elevations of their TSH levels (10 to 15 mU/mL) are usually not symptomatic. Isolated hypothyroidism is unusual in pituitary or hypothalamic lesions (see later), but if hypothyroidism is due to pituitary or hypothalamic failure (tumors, following radiation therapy, trauma), the TSH level will be extremely low (<0.5 mU/mL). In these situations, evaluation of the pituitary and hypothalamus structure with either CT or MRI scans and function with TSH and TRH stimulation tests is indicated. Corroborative evidence of hypothalamic or pituitary disease with reduced FSH, luteinizing hormone (LH), growth hormone (GH), and cortisol levels should also be sought.

Treatment of Hypothyroidism

Thyroid replacement therapy in hypothyroid patients on chronic dialysis is the same as that in other populations. In general, patients with renal disease are at risk for cardiovascular dis-

ease if they have not already been diagnosed with it. Consequently, their thyroid hormone should be replaced slowly to avoid precipitating angina or congestive heart failure, unless the patient is comatose or severely ill with another diagnosis. The usual replacement dose of thyroid extract is 120 mg/d, and for levothyroxine (T_4) it is 112 to 150 µg/d. Some physicians use T_3 (liothyronine or ctyomel, replacement dose 50 to 100 µg/d), but levothyroxine (T_4) has the advantage that the body can regulate its conversion to T3 and the serum half-life is longer (12). A role for T_3 in euthyroid-sick patients has not been established (2). The effectiveness and dosing of thyroid replacement therapy is usually followed by measuring serum TSH because no other physiologic or symptomatic parameter is sufficiently sensitive.

ANTERIOR PITUITARY DISORDERS

The anterior pituitary gland integrates information from the brain (hypothalamus) and feedback from peripheral hormones to control production of its trophic hormones (13,14). The hormones produced by the anterior pituitary, adrenocorticotropic hormone (ACTH), GH, prolactin, TSH, FSH, and LH, all have specific effects on different tissues in the body, and their excess production as well as loss of their production produces specific syndromes. In general, syndromes of pituitary hormone excess can be related to individual hormones because they are individually controlled, and produced in distinct cell types. In contrast, deficiency syndromes involve multiple or all of the hormones secreted because they are caused by processes that destroy the hypothalamus and/or pituitary. Prolactin is the exception because its synthesis and release are under tonic inhibitory control by the hypothalamus. Chronic renal failure alters the regulation and response to GH, prolactin, FSH, and LH. The biology of these hormones is complex and not fully understood in normal conditions, and remains only partially characterized in dialysis patients. TSH was discussed earlier in the section on thyroid disease.

Physiology

The anterior pituitary contains cells that produce several hormones, including ACTH, GH, prolactin, TSH, FSH, and LH. Each hormone is produced by an individual cell type. Functioning tumors of the pituitary are usually clonal and produce one hormone of the anterior pituitary. The venous system that drains the hypothalamus forms a plexus in the anterior pituitary so that peptide-releasing factors descending from the hypothalamus control the activity of the pituitary cells and the release of ACTH, growth hormone (GH), prolactin (PRL), TSH, FSH, and LH. The six peptide-releasing factors are the following:

- Corticotrophin-releasing factor (CRF), which stimulates ACTH release
- TRF, which stimulates TSH release
- Gonadotropin-releasing hormone (GnRH), which simulates FSH and LH release
- Growth hormone–releasing hormone (GHRH), which stimulates GH release

- Somatostatin, which inhibits secretion of all the pituitary hormones but is most potent in inhibiting GH release
- Prolactin inhibitory activity (PRIH), which tonically inhibits prolactin release

The latter may be several factors, including dopamine. These hormones are also subject to regulation at the level of the pituitary by direct feedback mechanisms.

Growth Hormone

Growth hormone has a variety of growth-promoting and metabolic effects (13,14). It is produced in the somatotrophs of the pituitary and is secreted under the dual control of GHRH (stimulatory) and somatostatin (inhibitory), which results in a pulsatile pattern of release. GHRH secretion is increased by dopamine, serotonin, alpha-adrenergic agonists, hypoglycemia, exercise, protein-rich food, and emotional stress, and is inhibited by beta-adrenergic agonists, free fatty acids, IGF-1, and GH. GH is carried in the serum primarily by a binding protein growth hormone–binding protein (GHBP) that is derived from the GH receptor. Although GH has direct differentiating effects on some cell types, most of its effects are through stimulation of production of somatomedins or insulin-like growth factors I and II (IGF-1 and IGF-2). IGF-1 appears to replicate many of the biologic effects of GH, but the function of IGF-2 is less well defined. IGF-1 is produced locally in small quantities in response to GH, but the liver appears to be the main site of production. IGF is carried in the serum by a six-member family of binding proteins (IGFBP 1–6), and is so tightly bound that only approximately 1% of the hormone is free.

The growth-promoting effects of GH are primarily to increase cell number and produce a positive nitrogen balance, with accumulation of Ca, Mg, K, Na, and PO_4. Before puberty and the closure of epiphyses, GH increases bone length and thickness, and produces a proportional increase in the size of other organs and tissues except the CNS. In adulthood (after the closure of epiphyses), bones cannot grow in length, and only become thicker, whereas other organs increase in size. Like insulin, GH is an anabolic hormone, but in contrast to insulin, it leads to carbohydrate intolerance, inhibits lipogenesis, increases mobilization of fat, and promotes ketosis. In nondiabetic patients with even low amounts of insulin present, these effects of GH are anabolic, but in diabetic patients, its effects are diabetogenic. In the absence of insulin, GH does not have anabolic activity. GH levels increase with exercise, hypoglycemia, and sleep.

Growth hormone excess causes gigantism if it occurs before puberty, and acromegaly if it occurs after epiphyseal closure. The most common cause of GH excess is a microadenoma of the pituitary. Growth hormone deficiency may occur as a consequence of hypothalamic disease or as a result of loss of GH receptors (Laron dwarfism). If it occurs in infancy or childhood, growth failure results. In adults who are fully grown at the time GH deficiency develops, the consequences appear to be minimal and may involve mild loss of muscle mass and impaired nutrient utilization, but the condition has not been studied well.

Chronic renal failure alters the GHRH–GH–IGF-1 system such that uremic patients appear to be insensitive to GH and IGF-1 (15–19). This resistance to GH and IGF-1 may explain why acromegaly is so rare in dialysis patients. This field is complicated because the nutritional and metabolic status of the patient and chronic illnesses alter the GH/IGF axis. Consequently, the relative importance of malnutrition, acidosis, uremic toxins, and decreased clearance of peptides by the kidney is difficult to determine. This is an area of intense investigation in both clinical and basic science. Most of the recent information is from the pediatric literature because of interest in the growth retardation found in pediatric renal failure and dialysis patients. In the adult population, insensitivity to GH and IGF-1 may contribute to the catabolism and wasting that commonly occur. Information on the mechanisms of resistance to GH and IGF-1 has not been completely established in humans. Some information is available from human studies, and more can be inferred from animal disease models.

In renal failure, GH levels are increased because of reduced clearance of GH by the kidney and an increased number of secretory bursts. In one study, the circulating concentrations in controls were 0.7 μg/mL versus 1.22 μg/mL in dialysis patients (15). In prepubertal patients, secretion is increased, but in pubertal patients and presumably adults, it is decreased (17,20). The level of GHBP (which reflects hepatic GH receptor expression levels) is reduced, providing a possible mechanism for GH insensitivity. Studies in humans and experimental animals suggest that metabolic acidosis is sufficient to confer resistance to GH (18,21,22). Dialysis patients are resistant to the short-term metabolic effects of IGF-1, IGF-1-stimulated reductions in plasma insulin, cortisol, C-peptide, and amino acid levels (23). Although the levels of IGF-1 are normal to slightly reduced, the levels of IGFBP (particularly IGFBP-2, -3, and -5) are increased (24). Because these IGFBPs bind IGF-1 tightly, the bioavailability of IGF-1 is reduced (17). The levels of the IGFBPs appear to be increased because of their reduced clearance by the kidney. In experimental systems, excess IGFBP is sufficient to inhibit the growth-promoting effects of IGF-1 (17). The half-life ($t1/2$) and volume of distribution of recombinant human IGF-1 are reduced in dialysis patients (25). Low-molecular-weight substances in uremic serum also appear to inhibit the action of IGF-1 (17,26).

The biologic effects of GH and IGF-1 are inhibited at many levels in uremia, and tissue resistance to these hormones may contribute to morbidity and mortality in this patient population. Long-term (4 to 8 years) administration of recombinant hGH (achieving supranormal levels and increasing IGF-1 levels) to children with chronic renal insufficiency and failure can restore linear growth so that they achieve normal height (27,28). This therapy does not have adverse effects on Ca, PO_4, or bone metabolism, and for patients with renal insufficiency, the rate of progression of renal disease was not accelerated (27,28). Factors that contribute to a favorable response to hGH are increased height at the initiation of therapy, young age at the start of therapy, and shorter duration of dialysis treatment (28).

The role for recombinant hGH in the treatment of adults on dialysis is less clear. Although patients without renal failure who are GH deficient respond favorably to its administration, it may not be beneficial for all dialysis patients. Erythropoietin may sensitize the pituitary to the effects of GHRH (29,30). Patients treated with hGH for 6 months show an increase in muscle mass, hand grip strength, albumin levels, and increased bone turnover with a decrease in bone density and total body mineral content (31–33). These studies are preliminary and of relatively short duration, so the potential complications of elevated levels of GH and IGF-1 that include insulin resistance and glucose intolerance, hypertension, cardiomyopathy, and an increased incidence of colonic polyps, were not evaluated. Optimal treatment of acidosis may also restore the sensitivity of patients to GH and IGF-1. The leptin system does not appear to play a major role in the catabolic state of dialysis patients (34,35).

Prolactin

Prolactin is produced by the lactotrophs in the pituitary, and it is secreted in a pulsatile fashion. In contrast to other pituitary hormones, prolactin is under tonic negative control by inhibitory factors from the hypothalamus. Its normal function in women is to promote lactation in cooperation with estrogen and progesterone, but its function in men is not established. Increased prolactin levels are caused by dopamine antagonists, oral contraceptives, diseases of the hypothalamus or pituitary that interfere with tonic suppression of prolactin secretion, and tumors. Up to 30% of pituitary tumors are prolactin-secreting. Prolactin is a stress response hormone, and its blood levels may rise with stress or pain. Normal prolactin levels are 2 to 15 μg/mL, levels in dialysis patients are often in the range of 15 to 50 μg/mL, and levels over 250 μg/mL are suggestive of first-trimester pregnancy or a prolactin-secreting tumor (14,15). In women excess production of prolactin results in galactorrhea, suppression of menstrual cycles, and infertility, and in men it results in infertility (36).

In dialysis patients, prolactin levels are elevated because of increased secretion and decreased clearance (15,36). Elevated prolactin levels may be responsible for some of the gonadal abnormalities found in renal failure. Recent reports indicate that erythropoietin reduces prolactin levels by mechanisms that may be independent of the improvement in anemia (37). Sexual function in dialysis patients has improved in response to bromocriptine, a dopamine agonist that suppresses prolactin production (38).

FSH, LH, and Gonadal Function

Follicle-stimulating hormone (FSH) and luteinizing hormone (LH) are secreted by the same pituitary cell, the gonadotrope. Their secretion is controlled by the integration of signals from luteinizing hormone-releasing hormone (LHRH) and feedback signals from estrogen, progesterone, and androgens, and gonadal peptides such as inhibin (14). Pulsatile, rather than continuously elevated, levels of LHRH are required for normal gonadal function. The frequency and amplitude of the pulses are controlled by the hypothalamus through hypothalamic function and feedback mechanisms from the periphery. LH controls production of estrogen and progesterone in the ovary and testosterone in the testis. FSH stimulates Sertoli cells to produce sperm and expression of LH receptors by Leydig cells. In women, FSH stimulates follicle development. These systems are

abnormal in both men and women with renal failure or on dialysis. Although psychologic factors may contribute to sexual dysfunction, abnormalities at the levels of the hypothalamus and gonads are probably the predominant cause.

Reproduction in Women

Female dialysis patients frequently exhibit amenorrhea, dysmenorrhea, dysfunctional uterine bleeding, and cystic ovarian disease. These disorders occur because of disruption of normal menstrual cycles at the level of the hypothalamus and ovary (36,39). LH levels are tonically elevated because of increased release, the estrogen-induced LH surge does not occur, and FSH levels are normal or slightly elevated (39). Suppression of pulsatile LHRH secretion by prolactin may contribute to this problem. Additionally, the ovaries have a subnormal steroidogenic response to LH. The frequency of menstruation has risen from 10% to 20% 20 years ago to approximately 40% at this time, but these cycles are generally thought to be anovulatory (40).

Conception occurs with a frequency of approximately 0.3% to 2.2% per year in Western countries, although these numbers represent estimates, because accurate records are not kept (40–44). The frequency of conception on dialysis appears to be increasing, which may reflect improved dialysis techniques and beneficial effects of erythropoietin. Of the patients who conceive and progress to the first trimester, approximately 50% deliver viable infants. In two studies of patients who were treated with dialysis when they were pregnant, those who conceived before starting dialysis delivered viable infants in 73.6% to 80% of the cases, and those who conceived on dialysis delivered viable infants in 40.2% to 50% of cases (41,44). Pregnancies are complicated by intrauterine death, hypertension, intrauterine growth retardation, premature labor, premature birth of babies with low birth weights for gestational age, and an increased frequency of congenital malformations, and neonatal care is an important factor in the survival of these infants (41–44). Deliveries of viable infants occur at approximately 32 weeks, and the outcome improves with longer gestation. The infants weigh on the order of 1,200 to 1,550 g at birth. An increased dose of dialysis appears to be beneficial, with reports of weekly *Kt/V* values of 6 to 8, on dialysis 5 to 6 days per week (41–43). Increased doses of erythropoietin are required to maintain hemoglobin levels in an acceptable range, and transfusions are sometimes required (41,44). In many cases, patients are hospitalized around week 20 of gestation for management of blood pressure, dialysis fluid balance, nutrition, and anemia.

Evaluation of women receiving dialysis for amenorrhea, dysmenorrhea, or dysfunctional uterine bleeding should be carried out in consultation with a gynecologist. The evaluation should include a thorough pelvic examination and Pap smear, and may include measurement of serum prolactin, LH and FSH levels, a pelvic ultrasound, and endometrial biopsy.

Reproduction in Men

In men, erectile dysfunction, impotence, decreased libido, and decreased sperm count are manifestations of uremia. LH is elevated due to increased secretion and decreased clearance. The increased LH production may be caused by low levels of testosterone synthesis by the testes. FSH levels are usually normal but may be high, with severe testicular dysfunction. Presumably, increased prolactin levels would interfere with normal regulation of LHRH secretion. Evaluation of men for impotence should include measurement of serum prolactin, testosterone, FSH, and LH levels. Correction of anemia with erythropoietin may improve the function of the hypothalamo–pituitary–testicular axis in dialysis patients (45). Patients should also be evaluated for autonomic neuropathy and peripheral vascular disease, since these two entities are relatively common in dialysis patients, especially those with hypertension and diabetes.

In contrast to women whose primary reproductive endocrinologic defect appears to be hypothalamic, hypogonadism is more prominent in men (46). These men, who have reduced testosterone levels, may respond to replacement testosterone. Erectile dysfunction is common in dialysis patients, affecting 70% to 80% of men (47). The incidence is higher in men with diabetes and who have been on dialysis for long periods, and these men tend to have reduced testosterone levels and reduced penile blood flow. Approximately 80% of men with erectile dysfunction respond to sildenafil (Viagra) (48). The level of penile blood flow is the most important parameter for predicting a response to sildenafil.

ACTH

ACTH stimulates steroidogenesis in the glomerulosa and fasciculata layers of the adrenal glands. ACTH is derived from proopiomelanocortin (POMC), a peptide that is produced by the corticotrope cells of the anterior pituitary and cleaved to ACTH and β-lipotropin (LPH). ACTH is further cleaved into α-melanocyte-stimulating hormone (α-MSH or ACTH 1–13) and ACTH-like peptide (ACTH 18–39). β-lipotropin is processed to lipotropin (LPH) and β-endorphin. Secretion of ACTH is stimulated by corticotropin-releasing hormone (CRH) and vasopressin. Negative feedback control is provided by suppression of CRH, vasopressin, and ACTH secretion by cortisol, and inhibition of CRH secretion by ACTH. ACTH is secreted in a pulsatile fashion in a diurnal pattern that is maximal in the early morning and minimal in the evening.

In dialysis patients, ACTH levels are normal or slightly increased compared to normal controls, and its metabolism does not appear to be altered. Normal and abnormal responses to dexamethasone and metyrapone suppression tests have been reported. The circadian rhythms and levels of cortisol are normal, and the response of the adrenals to ACTH stimulation is normal. Consequently, a number of the tests of pituitary–adrenal function used in normal patients are applicable to dialysis patients.

DISORDERS OF THE ADRENAL CORTEX

The adrenal cortex produces two physiologically important steroid hormones, cortisol and aldosterone. Aldosterone's primary physiologic effect is on the kidneys, where it acts on the distal nephron to promote Na reabsorption and K and H excre-

tion. Aldosterone also affects transport in the colon, but disorders of aldosterone metabolism in dialysis patients have not been reported. Consequently, this section will deal with glucocorticoid excess or insufficiency.

Glucocorticoids are essential for life and affect glucose and lipid metabolism, the immune system, and bone and mineral metabolism. No tissue or organ system—including the cardiovascular, gastrointestinal, or central nervous system—functions normally in the absence of glucocorticoids. Glucocorticoid activity is required for glycogen synthesis and maintenance of glycogen stores, gluconeogenesis, and has a permissive effect on lipolysis. The effects of glucocorticoids on the immune system under normal physiologic conditions are not fully understood, but pharmacologic concentrations decrease the number of peripheral lymphocytes, inhibit T-cell activation, result in macrophage proliferation, and inhibit the actions of a number of mediators of inflammation, including chemokines, prostaglandins, and histamine. Glucocorticoids affect bone formation by reducing osteoblast numbers, decreasing intestinal Ca reabsorption, and increasing serum PTH levels.

Adrenal Insufficiency

In the general population, primary adrenal insufficiency usually presents as an adrenal crisis following some form of stress, such as surgery or an acute illness. Patients usually complain of anorexia, nausea, vomiting, and weakness with a history of weight loss. The findings may include volume depletion, hypotension and shock, hypoglycemia, fever, and possibly hyperpigmentation. This constellation of findings is caused by loss of both cortisol and aldosterone. The loss of aldosterone is largely responsible for the symptoms and findings related to volume depletion. Patients who are receiving replacement therapy but who encounter a physiologic stress can also develop adrenal crisis (19,49).

Dialysis patients have minimal renal function and therefore do not develop the salt-losing nephropathy associated with adrenal insufficiency. Presumably, if dialysis patients develop adrenal insufficiency, they present more like patients with secondary adrenal insufficiency (pituitary lesions with loss of ACTH production) or tertiary adrenal insufficiency (hypothalamic lesions with loss of CRF production). In these patients, adrenal crisis is rare, and they present with an insidious onset of generalized symptoms of malaise and signs and symptoms of hypoglycemia.

Primary adrenal insufficiency is caused by tuberculosis, fungal diseases, metastases from tumors, and autoimmune disease (Table 24.2). Since dialysis patients are at increased risk for tuberculosis, they are also presumably at increased risk for adrenal insufficiency due to tuberculosis. Autoimmune adrenalitis is associated with polyglandular autoimmune syndromes I and II, which are associated with mucocutaneous candidiasis and hypoparathyroidism, and thyroid disorders and insulin-dependent diabetes, respectively. Primary autoimmune polyglandular syndrome type II is more common than the autosomal recessive type I syndrome. Patients with HIV infections and with cytomegalovirus, *Mycobacterium avium intracellulare*, cryptococcus, or Kaposi's sarcoma may manifest partial adrenal

TABLE 24.2. TESTS FOR PRIMARY OR SECONDARY ADRENAL INSUFFICIENCY

	Normal	Primary Adrenal Insufficiency	Pituitary/Hypothalamic Insufficiency
ACTH (8 A.M.)	4.5–20 pmol/L	Increased	Low or normal range
Cortisol (8 A.M.)	275–550 nmol/L	≤275 nmol/L	Low or normal range
Cortrisyn stim	≥550 nmol/L after 30–60 min	≤550 nmol/L after 30–60 min	Normal or low if adrenals are atrophic
Metyapone	8 A.M. ACTH ≥17 pmol/L, 11-deoxycortisol 210–660 nmol/L	8 A.M. ACTH ≥17 pmol/L, 11-deoxycortisol < 210 nmol/L	8 A.M. ACTH ≤17 pmol/L, 11-deoxycortisol ≤210 nmol/L

Reference values or normal responses are shown for a normal patient's ACTH (4.5–20 pmol/L or 20–80 pg/mL), Cortisol (8 A.M., 275–550 nmol/L or 10–20 µg/dL). The CRF stimulation may be used to distinguish hypothalamic from pituitary disease (49).
ACTH, adrenal corticotrophic hormone; CRF, corticotropin releasing factor.

insufficiency. Adrenal insufficiency can be precipitated by keto-conazole because it inhibits cortisol synthesis, or rifampin, because it increases cortisol metabolism (49). Secondary or tertiary adrenal insufficiency is associated with destructive lesions of the pituitary or hypothalamus, such as tumors, postradiation therapy, trauma, or use of anticoagulants. In these situations, other pituitary hormones are usually lost in addition to ACTH. Adrenal insufficiency is also caused by long-term use of glucocorticoids for immune suppression, as in patients with systemic lupus erythematosus, other glomerular diseases, or renal transplantation.

Renal failure and dialysis do not alter the diurnal variation of cortisol or the adrenal response to ACTH (19). Consequently, morning and evening cortisol levels, and the ACTH stimulation test can be used to demonstrate adrenal or hypothalamic–pituitary–adrenal function. The simplest test for primary adrenal insufficiency is the ACTH stimulation test. Plasma cortisol is measured before, 30 minutes after, and 60 minutes after intravenous injection of 250 µg of synthetic ACTH (ACTH 1–24). A cortisol value of more than 20 µg/dL or 550 nmol/L at any of the time points in the test indicates normal adrenal function. If partial adrenal insufficiency is suspected, prolonged ACTH stimulation tests may be of value because this test can assess adrenal reserve. The overnight, single-dose metyrapone suppression test with measurement of serum cortisol, 11-deoxycortisol, and ACTH is useful for making a diagnosis of complete or partial pituitary–adrenal insufficiency, and is the most sensitive test of pituitary–adrenal reserve (49). Patients may have a normal response of ACTH and cortisol to hypoglycemia but have an abnormal response to metyrapone suppression. Metyrapone blocks conversion of 11-deoxycortisol, a compound that has no glucocorticoid activity and that does not participate in feedback to cortisol. As cortisol production decreases, ACTH rises, and stimulates the production of cortisol precursors that can be measured as 11-deoxycortisol. Metyrapone (30 mg/kg body weight) is given orally at midnight, and 8 A.M. cortisol, 11-deoxycortisol, and ACTH levels are measured. A normal response is a rise in 11-deoxycortisol to 210 to 660 nmol, and a level of ACTH greater than 17 pmol/L. If the cortisol level is normal or greater than 210 nmol/L in the 8 A.M. sample, the dose of metryapone was inadequate to block cortisol synthesis. A normal response to the metyrapone suppression test excludes abnormalities of the hypothalamo–pituitary–adrenal axis. ACTH release can also be measured in response to CRF to document intact pituitary func-

tion (49). Patients who are Addisonian may become symptomatic with the metyrapone suppression test, so it should be supervised. If primary adrenal insufficiency is suspected, a CT scan of the abdomen to evaluate the size of the adrenal glands is warranted.

Adrenal Hyperfunction

The adrenal glands may overproduce aldosterone or cortisol. Overproduction of aldosterone is caused by adrenal adenomas of the glomerulosa layer (either single or multiple). In patients with renal failure who are on dialysis, it is not clear if aldosterone excess causes clinical abnormalities. Consequently, this section will deal with glucocorticoid excess or Cushing's syndrome. Cushing's syndrome may be caused by excess ACTH (usually due to a pituitary adenoma; see earlier), adrenal hyperplasia, or exogenous glucocorticoids for inflammatory diseases or antirejection therapy. Cushing's syndrome is comprised of centripetal obesity, glucose intolerance, weakness (due to proximal myopathy), hypertension, psychologic changes (depression or mania), bruisability, striae, osteopenia, menstrual irregularities or impotence, acne or oily skin, edema, and hirsutism. No one of these findings is diagnostic of cortisol excess, but the occurrence of several of them in the same patient is suggestive of Cushing's syndrome. In dialysis patients, hypertension and edema and menstrual irregularities or impotence may not be valuable, because they are so common in the dialysis population.

The diagnosis of Cushing's syndrome in dialysis patients can be based on most of the same criteria as the general population. Glucocorticoid use for inflammatory diseases of the kidney or as part of an antirejection regimen are probably the most common causes of Cushing's syndrome in the dialysis population. In the absence of such a history, glucocorticoid excess may be either primary or secondary. Renal failure and dialysis do not alter the diurnal variation of cortisol or the adrenal response to ACTH, so morning and evening cortisol levels can be used to demonstrate abnormal diurnal variation (loss of the evening fall) in cortisol. The distinction between primary and secondary or tertiary hypercortisolism can be made using the dexamethasone suppression test or the single-dose metyrapone test with measurement of serum 11-deoxycortisol and cortisol (49). Dexamethasone suppresses ACTH secretion through negative feedback at the levels of the pituitary and hypothalamus. The low-dose dexamethasone suppression test (1 mg P.O. between 11 P.M. and

TABLE 24.3. SERUM ASSAYS AND PROVOCATIVE TESTS FOR HYPERCORTISOLISM

	Normal	Primary Adrenal Overproduction	Pituitary or Hypothalamic
ACTH	4.5–20 pmol/L	Reduced	Increased
Cortisol	Normal diurnal variation (8 A.M. 220–660, 4 P.M. 50–410 nmol/L)	Loss of diurnal variation with elevated 4 P.M. values early, and generally elevated values late	Loss of diurnal variation with elevated 4 P.M. values early, and generally elevated values late
Low-dose dexamethasone suppression	8 A.M. cortisol ≤140 nmol/L, 8 A.M. ACTH ≤4.4 pmol/L	8 A.M. cortisol ≥220 nmol/L, low ACTH	8 A.M. cortisol ≥220 nmol/L, elevated ACTH
High-dose dexamethasone suppression	8 A.M. cortisol ≤140 nmol/L, 8 A.M. ACTH ≤4.4 pmol/L	8 A.M. cortisol ≥220 nmol/L, low ACTH	8 A.M. cortisol ≤140 nmol/L, 8 A.M. ACTH ≤4.4 pmol/L but may show only partial suppression
Metyrapone	8 A.M. ACTH ≥17 pmol/L, 11-deoxycortisol 210–660 nmol/L	8 A.M. ACTH no change to increased, 11-deoxycortisol no change to decreased	8 A.M. ACTH ≥17 pmol/L, 11-deoxycortisol 210–660 nmol/L

Reference values and normal responses are shown in the "normal" columns and are the same as those for Table 24.2 (49).

midnight with measurement of 8 A.M. cortisol and ACTH) is designed to distinguish patients with glucocorticoid excess for any reason from patients with normal hypothalamo–pituitary–adrenal function. If the patient is normal, the low dose of dexamethasone will suppress cortisol production, and the 8 A.M. plasma cortisol level should be less than 140 nmol/L (5 μg/dL) and the ACTH should be less than 4.4 pmol/L (20 pg/mL). Greater values for cortisol and ACTH will require the high-dose dexamethasone suppression test or the metyrapone suppression test. In patients with pituitary adenomas or increased hypothalamic activity, ACTH and cortisol secretion can be suppressed by high doses of dexamethasone (8 mg between 1 P.M. and midnight) so that 8 A.M. cortisol levels are less than 140 nmol/L (5 μg/dL), and ACTH levels may be undetectable. If the hypercortisolism is due to primary adrenal overproduction of steroids, it is not ACTH dependent and will not suppress with either the high or low dose of dexamethasone (Table 24.3).

The metyrapone suppression test can also be used to distinguish primary adrenal overproduction of cortisol from excess ACTH secretion due to pituitary or hypothalamic disease. Metyrapone blocks conversion of 11-deoxycortisol, a compound with no glucocorticoid activity and that does not participate in feedback, to cortisol. The reduced cortisol levels stimulate ACTH production, which in turn stimulates the cortisol synthetic pathway. A pituitary adenoma responds to reduced cortisol with increased ACTH production resulting in an increase in 11-deoxycortisol production. In contrast, in the presence of an adrenal adenoma, the hypothalamo–pituitary axis is atrophic, the increase in ACTH is minimal, and 11-deoxycortisol levels fall or do not change. Approximately half of adrenal adenomas and most adrenal carcinomas do not respond to ACTH. A normal adrenal gland may be atrophic and unable to respond to ACTH (49). If a pituitary or hypothalamic lesion is suspected, structural evaluation of the pituitary and hypothalamus with CT or MRI scans is indicated.

REFERENCES

1. Lim VS. Thyroid function in patients with chronic renal failure. *Am J Kidney Dis* 2001;38:S80–S84.
2. Larsen PR, et al. The thyroid gland. In: Wilson JD, et al., eds. *Williams textbook of endocrinology*, 9th ed. Philadelphia: WB Saunders, 1998:389–515.
3. Brent GA, et al. Effect of nonthyroidal illness on thyroid function tests. In: Van Middlesworth L, ed. *The thyroid gland: a practical clinical treatise*. Chicago: Year Book Medical, 1986:83–110.
4. Becker RA, et al. Hypermetabolic low triiodothyronine syndrome of burn injury. *Crit Care Med* 1982;10:870–875.
5. Brent GA, et al. Thyroxine therapy in patients with severe nonthyroidal illness and low serum thyroxine concentration. *J Clin Endocrinol Metab* 1986;63:1–8.
6. Myers JD, et al. A correlative study of the cardiac output and the hepatic circulation in hypothyroidism. *J Clin Invest* 1950;29:1069–1077.
7. Miki H, et al. Thyroid nodules in female uremic patients on maintenance hemodialysis. *J Surg Oncol* 1993;54:216–218.
8. Culpepper RM, et al. Clearance of ^{131}I by hemodialysis. *Clin Nephrol* 1992;38:110–114.
9. Takeda S, et al. Iodine-induced hypothyroidism in patients on regular dialysis treatment. *Nephron* 1993;65:51–55.
10. Shirota T, et al. Primary hypothyroidism and multiple endocrine failure in association with hemochromatosis in a long-term hemodialysis patient. *Clin Nephrol* 1992;38:105–109.
11. Lim VS, et al. Thyroid dysfunction in chronic renal failure. *J Clin Invest* 1977;60:522–534.
12. Haynes RC. Thyroid and antithyroid drugs. In: Gilman AG, et al., eds. *The pharmacological basis of therapeutics*, 8th ed. New York: Pergamon, 1990:1361–1383.
13. Kuret JA, et al. Adenohypophyseal hormones and related substances. In: Gilman AG, et al., eds. *The pharmacological basis of therapeutics*, 8th ed. New York: Pergamon, 1990:1334–1360.
14. Thorner MO, et al. The anterior pituitary. In: Wilson JD, et al., eds. *Williams textbook of endocrinology*, 9th ed. Philadelphia: WB Saunders, 1998:249–340.
15. Veldhuis JD, et al. Neuroendocrine alterations in the somatotropic and lactotropic axes in uremic men. *Eur J Endocrinol* 1994;131:489–498.
16. Haffner D, et al. Metabolic clearance of recombinant human growth hormone in health and chronic renal failure. *Clin Invest* 1994;93:1163–1171.
17. Tonshoff B, et al. Derangements of the somatotropic hormone axis in chronic renal failure. *Kidney Int* 1997;51:S106–S113.
18. Kuemmerle N, et al. Growth hormone and insulin-like growth factor in non-uremic acidosis and uremic acidosis. *Kidney Int* 1997;51:S102–S105.
19. Emmanouel DS, et al. Endocrine abnormalities in chronic renal failure: pathogenic principles and clinical implications. *Semin Nephrol* 1981;1:151–174.
20. Tonshoff B, et al. Deconvolution analysis of spontaneous nocturnal growth hormone secretion in prepubertal children with preterminal

chronic renal failure and with end-stage renal disease. *Pediatr Res* 1995;37:86–93.

21. Maniar S, et al. Growth hormone action is blunted by acidosis in experimental uremia or acid load. *Clin Nephrol* 1997;46:72–76.
22. Kleinknecht C, et al. Acidosis prevents growth hormone-induced growth in experimental uremia. *Pediatr Nephrol* 1996;10:256–260.
23. Fouque D, et al. Impaired metabolic response to recombinant insulin-like growth factor-1 in dialysis patients. *Kidney Int* 1995;47:876–883.
24. Ulinski T, et al. Serum insulin-like growth factor binding protein (IGFBP)-4 and serum IGFBP-5 in children with chronic renal failure: relationship to growth and glomerular filtration rate. *Pediatr Nephrol* 2000;14:589–597.
25. Fouque D, et al. Pharmacokinetics of recombinant human insulin-like growth factor-1 in dialysis patients. *Kidney Int* 1995;47:869–875.
26. Kreig Jr RJ, et al. Growth hormone, insulin-like growth factor and the kidney. *Kidney Int* 1995;48:321–326.
27. Haffner D, et al. Effect of growth hormone treatment on the adult height of children with chronic renal failure. *N Engl J Med* 2000;343:923–930.
28. Hokken-Koelega A, et al. Long-term effects of growth hormone treatment on growth and puberty in patients with chronic renal insufficiency. *Pediatr Nephrol* 2000;14:701–706.
29. Diez JJ, et al. Growth hormone responses to growth hormone releasing hormone and clonidine before and after erythropoietin therapy in CAPD patients. *Nephron* 1996;74:548–554.
30. Cremagnanai L, et al. Recombinant human erythropoietin (rhEPO) treatment potentiates growth hormone (GH) response to growth hormone releasing hormone (GHRH) stimulation in hemodialysis patients. *Clin Nephrol* 1993;39:282–286.
31. Gram J, et al. The effect of recombinant human growth hormone treatment on bone and mineral metabolism in hemodialysis patients. *Nephrol Dial Transplant* 1998;13:1529–1534.
32. Jensen PB, et al. Growth hormone, insulin-like growth factors and their binding proteins in adult hemodialysis patients treated with recombinant human growth hormone. *Clin Nephrol* 1999;52:103–109.
33. Johannsson G, et al. Double-blind, placebo-controlled study of growth hormone treatment in elderly patients undergoing chronic hemodialysis: anabolic effect and functional improvement. *Am J Kidney Dis* 1999;33:709–717.
34. Garibotto G, et al. Effects of growth hormone on leptin metabolism and energy expenditure in hemodialysis patients with protein-calorie malnutrition. *JASN* 2000;11:2113.
35. Rodrigues-Carmona A, et al. Hyperleptinemia is not correlated with markers of protein malnutrition in chronic renal failure: a cross-sectional study in predialysis, peritoneal dialysis, and hemodialysis patients. *Nephron* 2000;86:274–280.
36. Mujais SK, et al. Pathophysiology of the uremic syndrome. In: Brenner BM, et al., eds. *The kidney,* 3rd ed. Philadelphia: WB Saunders, 1986:1587–1630.
37. Yeskan M, et al. Effect of recombinant human erythropoietin (r-HuEPO) therapy on plasma FT_3, FT_4, TSH, FSH, LH, free testosterone and prolactin levels in hemodialysis patients. *Int J Artif Organs* 1992;15:585–589.
38. Bommer J, et al. Improved sexual function in male hemodialysis patients on bromocriptine. *Lancet* 1979;2:496–497.
39. Lim VS, et al. Ovarian function in chronic renal failure: evidence suggesting hypothalamic anovulation. *Ann Int Med* 1980;93:21–27.
40. Hou S. Pregnancy in chronic renal insufficiency and end-stage renal disease. *Am J Kidney Dis* 1999;33:235–252.
41. Bagon J, et al. Pregnancy and dialysis. *Am J Kidney Dis* 1998;31:756–765.
42. Chao A-S, et al. Pregnancy in women who undergo long-term dialysis. *Am J Obstet Gynecol* 2002;187:152–156.
43. Toma H, et al. Pregnancy in women receiving renal dialysis or transplantation in Japan: a nationwide survey. *Nephrol Dial Transplant* 1999;14:1511–1516.
44. Okundaye I, et al. Registry of pregnancy in dialysis patients. *Am J Kidney Dis* 1998;31:766–773.
45. Tokgoz B, et al. Effects of long-term erythropoietin therapy on the hypothalamo–pituitary–testicular axis in male CAPD patients. *Perit Dial Int* 2001;21:448–454.
46. Palmer BF. Sexual dysfunction in uremia. *JASN* 1999;10:1381–1388.
47. Turk S, et al. Erectile dysfunction and the effects of sildenafil treatment in patients on hemodialysis and continuous ambulatory peritoneal dialysis. *Nephrol Dial Transplant* 2001;16:1818–1822.
48. Chen J, et al. Clinical efficacy of sildenafil in patients on chronic dialysis. *J Urol* 2001;165:819–821.
49. Orth DN, et al. The adrenal cortex. In: Wilson JD, et al., eds. *Williams textbook of endocrinology,* 9th ed. Philadelphia: WB Saunders, 1998:517–664.

25

GASTROINTESTINAL COMPLICATIONS IN END-STAGE RENAL DISEASE

GEORGE T. FANTRY AND DONNA S. HANES

Gastrointestinal symptoms are very common in patients with end-stage renal disease (ESRD), occurring in 77% to 79% of patients undergoing hemodialysis (1,2). Before the widespread use of dialysis, gastrointestinal complications accounted for a large part of the uremic syndrome. Uremia causes pathologic and physiologic changes throughout the gastrointestinal tract, which results in gastrointestinal disturbances involving both the upper and lower gastrointestinal tract as well as the pancreas, leading to a broad spectrum of gastrointestinal complaints (Table 25.1) (1). There is an increased frequency of gastroesophageal reflux disease (GERD), gastritis, gastrointestinal bleeding, pancreatitis, ascites, and constipation. These gastrointestinal complications of ESRD have a negative impact on quality of life, increase morbidity, and may contribute to death. This chapter reviews the pathophysiology, diagnosis, and management of these common gastrointestinal disorders in dialysis patients.

ESOPHAGUS

Upper gastrointestinal symptoms, including nausea, vomiting, heartburn, and epigastric pain, are common in patients with chronic renal failure. In addition to dialysis-related nausea and vomiting, potential esophageal causes of these symptoms include GERD or reflux esophagitis and esophageal motility disorders.

A number of studies have addressed the potential relationship between renal failure and GERD or esophagitis. In an autopsy series of 78 patients with ESRD, a high prevalence of mild to severe esophagitis (36%) was found (3). However, in prospective studies of patients with chronic renal failure on hemodialysis, the prevalence of esophagitis was much lower. In one study of 60 patients, esophagitis was found in 13% (4). In another study of 249 patients, esophagitis was seen in 6.8% (5). The prevalence rate of endoscopic esophagitis in these studies is similar to or slightly greater than that in the general population.

A more recent case-controlled study was performed to address the association between GERD and ESRD. In this study, 42 patients with ESRD and symptoms suggestive of GERD were evaluated with endoscopy and 24-hour pH monitoring (6). The prevalence of GERD in these patients was very

high (81%) and similar to that in controls, suggesting that upper gastrointestinal symptoms in patients with chronic renal failure are important in predicting the presence of GERD. Multivariate analysis showed that chronic ambulatory peritoneal dialysis (CAPD) was a risk factor for the development of GERD. A similar link between CAPD and GERD has been reported by other investigators (7). This association is likely due to increased intraabdominal pressure when the abdominal cavity is filled with dialysate fluid and its effect on lower esophageal sphincter pressure.

A high prevalence of hiatal hernia has been reported in patients with ESRD (1,8). Hiatal hernias are known to play a role in the pathophysiology of GERD by altering the antireflux barrier and by acting as a reservoir for potential acid refluxate. Nonspecific esophageal motility disorders have been identified in chronic hemodialysis patients (9–11); however, the clinical significance of these findings is uncertain.

A presumptive diagnosis of GERD can be made when esophageal symptoms such as heartburn and regurgitation are present, and empiric therapy with acid-suppressive therapy with a proton-pump inhibitor should be instituted. Symptom response to therapy confirms the diagnosis. Endoscopy should be performed in patients with persistent symptoms. Early endoscopy is indicated for unexplained nausea and vomiting or when alarm symptoms such as dysphagia are present.

STOMACH/DUODENUM

Dyspeptic symptoms are very common in patients with chronic renal failure leading to investigation for possible gastroduodenal pathology, such as gastritis, duodenitis, and peptic ulcer disease. Many decades ago a high prevalence of diffuse hemorrhagic gastritis and duodenitis was described in patients with fatal acute uremia (12,13). A subsequent autopsy study of chronic hemodialysis patients revealed a similar frequency of gastritis, which was less extensive and severe (3). More recent radiologic and endoscopic studies have confirmed a high prevalence of gastritis and duodenitis in patients on maintenance hemodialysis with endoscopic or histologic evidence of chronic superficial gastritis found in up to 60% to 70% of the patients (4,14,15). There is a strong association between *Helicobacter pylori* infec-

TABLE 25.1. PREVALENCE OF GASTROINTESTINAL SYMPTOMS IN PATIENTS ON HEMODIALYSIS

Symptoms	Percent
Nausea	74
Vomiting	68
Anorexia	64
Constipation	59
Heartburn	52
Abdominal distention	51
Abdominal pain	49
Diarrhea	25
Dysphagia	16

tion and gastritis; however, poor correlation between endoscopic and histologic findings was seen (14).

Physiologic abnormalities in the presence of ESRD, such as decreases in pancreatic and duodenal bicarbonate secretion and elevated serum gastrin levels, led to speculation of an association between chronic renal failure and peptic ulcer disease. Early clinical studies of small numbers of patients utilizing diagnostic radiology techniques suggested that chronic renal failure was a risk factor for the development of peptic ulcers, but more recent endoscopic studies in patients on chronic hemodialysis have found a prevalence of peptic ulcers similar to that of the general population (5,16,17). There is a difference in the clinical presentation and endoscopic features of peptic ulcers in uremic patients compared with patients with normal renal function. Uremic patients are more likely to be pain-free and to present with hemorrhage (18). In addition, uremic patients are more likely to have giant and multiple ulcers as well as *H. pylori*-negative and postbulbar duodenal ulcers (18,19).

Given the frequency of dyspepsia in patients with chronic renal failure and the known role of *H. pylori* as a pathogen in the development of gastritis and peptic ulcer disease, a number of studies have addressed the prevalence of *H. pylori* in ESRD. Most studies have demonstrated that the prevalence of *H. pylori* infection in patients with ESRD is similar to or possibly less than that of the general population (20–25). Dyspepsia is not associated with *H. pylori* infection in chronic renal failure patients (26), a finding that is similar to the lack of a clear association between *H. pylori* infection and functional dyspepsia in the general population. These findings suggest that other factors likely contribute to the development of gastritis and dyspepsia. Treatment of *H. pylori* infection with proton pump inhibitor–based triple therapy (omeprazole, amoxicillin, clarithromycin) is as effective in chronic renal failure patients on hemodialysis or CAPD as in those individuals with normal renal function (27,28).

Another potential cause of frequent dyspeptic symptoms—such as nausea, vomiting, abdominal bloating, early satiety, and anorexia—in dialysis patients is abnormal or delayed gastric emptying (26,29). Gastroparesis is a common complication of diabetes mellitus, the most common cause of chronic renal failure requiring dialysis, particularly in the presence of other end-organ damage such as chronic renal failure. In addition to diabetic gastroparesis, gastric emptying can be significantly delayed in nondiabetic dialysis patients as well (30,31). Potential causes

of abnormal gastric emptying in these patients include neuropathy directly related to the uremia and alterations in gastrointestinal hormones that can affect gastric emptying. The prevalence of dysmotility-like dyspepsia has been shown to be higher in CAPD patients than in hemodialysis patients (26). In CAPD patients, studies showing delayed gastric emptying when the abdominal cavity is filled with dialysate and absent when the abdominal cavity is empty suggest that increased intraabdominal pressure may play an important role (32). Delayed gastric emptying in patients with chronic renal failure is not associated with *H. pylori* infection (26,33).

Upper gastrointestinal symptoms due to gastroparesis may have an adverse effect on nutritional status and may be one of the important factors that lead to malnutrition in dialysis patients. Delayed gastric emptying in chronic hemodialysis patients is associated with changes in biochemical indicators of nutritional status such as albumin and prealbumin (30). Furthermore, treatment of gastroparesis in nondiabetic dialysis patients with promotility agents such as erythromycin or metoclopramide can significantly improve gastric emptying and short-term nutritional status as measured by serum albumin (31).

There are a couple of therapeutic options for the management of patients with dyspepsia. An empiric trial of a proton-pump inhibitor can be considered. Alternatively, a serum *H. pylori* antibody can be obtained. If the *H. pylori* antibody is positive, appropriate treatment with a 2-week course of proton-pump inhibitor–based triple therapy should be instituted. In patients with persistent dyspepsia, endoscopy is warranted. Early endoscopy should be pursued in older patients and in those with associated vomiting, anorexia, and unexplained weight loss. When empiric therapy fails and a diagnostic EGD is unrevealing, it may be useful to obtain a gastric emptying study to assess for gastroparesis that can be treated with a promotility agent such as metoclopramide.

GASTROINTESTINAL BLEEDING

Gastrointestinal bleeding is a common complication of ESRD, accounting for up to 8% to 12% of cases of upper gastrointestinal bleeding (34,35). The frequency of bleeding in chronic renal failure patients with underlying gastrointestinal pathology may be partially explained by a high occurrence of clotting abnormalities in this patient population (35). Most studies have found that peptic ulcer disease (gastric or duodenal ulcers) is the most common cause of upper gastrointestinal bleeding in chronic renal failure patients, accounting for 30% to 60% of bleeding episodes (34–36).

The association of chronic renal failure with bleeding upper gastrointestinal angiodysplasias is controversial. A few studies have shown that angiodysplasias of the stomach and duodenum are a significantly more common source of upper gastrointestinal bleeding in patients with chronic renal failure (34,35,37,38), with angiodysplasias identified as the cause of bleeding in 13% to 23% of patients (34,35). However, this has not been a universal finding (36,39,40). In one study, the prevalence of angiodysplasias as a cause of upper gastrointestinal bleeding was related to the duration of renal failure and the need for dialysis (34). The lesions are often multiple and can also be found in the small bowel and colon (35,37,41,42). Recurrent bleeding is frequent and more common in patients with chronic renal failure (35,38). In addition to acute gastrointestinal hemorrhage, patients with bleeding angiodysplasias often present with chronic gastrointestinal blood loss manifested by chronic anemia and hemoccult-positive stool (39). Erosive esophagitis and erosive gastritis may also be more common causes of upper gastrointestinal bleeding in chronic renal failure patients (35,36).

The diagnosis of angiodysplasias in the appropriate clinical setting is usually made by endoscopy with upper endoscopy and/or colonoscopy. The diagnosis of angiodysplasia can sometimes be difficult to make, as the lesions may be very small and hidden between or behind folds. A high index of suspicion for the possibility of angiodysplasias should be maintained in patients with recurrent acute bleeding episodes, which are undiagnosed after conventional endoscopy with upper endoscopy and colonoscopy, and in patients with chronic iron-deficiency anemia and hemoccult-positive stool. In this subset of patients, small bowel angiodysplasia is the most common cause of bleeding, and further evaluation with enteroscopy is warranted. When identified endoscopically, the lesions can be successfully treated with thermal therapy using contact probes or argon plasma coagulation.

Endoscopic intervention for gastrointestinal angiodysplasias is ineffective when the vascular lesions are diffuse, are inaccessible, or escape identification. Additionally, rebleeding is an important clinical issue after endoscopic therapy. This has led to trials of medical therapy with estrogen and progesterone to prevent recurrent bleeding from angiodysplasias. Potential mechanisms for the beneficial effect of estrogen on bleeding gastrointestinal telangiectasias include improvement in coagulation status with decreased bleeding time and improvement in the integrity of the vascular endothelial lining. Studies of hormonal therapy have had mixed results (42–44). In an uncontrolled trial of estrogen–progesterone therapy in seven patients with chronic renal failure and bleeding gastrointestinal telangiectasias, bleeding ceased in all patients and monthly transfusion requirements decreased (42). In a subsequent double-blind, placebo-controlled cross-over trial in ten patients, hormonal therapy significantly decreased transfusion requirements (43). However, in a more recent multicenter, randomized, placebo-controlled, double-blind trial of 72 patients, including eight patients with chronic renal failure, no significant difference in bleeding episodes or transfusion requirements was found in those patients receiving estrogen–progesterone therapy (44).

PANCREAS

Abnormal glandular morphology and pancreatic exocrine function are very common in ESRD. Approximately 70% of patients have abnormal pancreatic exocrine function (45). Investigators have demonstrated reduced duodenal amylase, lipase, bicarbonate, and protein levels in response to secretory stimulation tests (46). In addition, fecal chymotrypsin levels are significantly reduced in chronic kidney disease (47). These changes in excre-

tory pancreatic function are infrequently associated with ultrasonographic changes within the pancreas. Autopsy studies reveal a correlation between pancreatic disease and elevated intact PTH levels (48). Whether these abnormalities are part of the clinical spectrum of chronic pancreatitis or represent a distinct uremic pancreatopathy is unclear. Other possible causes of pancreatic disease in dialysis patients include hypercalcemia, hypertriglyceridemia, vascular insufficiency, and drug toxicity (such as long-standing diuretic use, antibiotics, and NSAIDS) (Table 25.2).

Patients with chronic kidney disease frequently have elevated serum amylase and lipase levels in the absence of clinical pancreatitis, probably related to reduced renal clearance. The kidney is responsible for 20% of the clearance of these enzymes. Serum amylase, lipase, and trypsin values remain normal until the creatinine clearance is less than 50 mL/min (49). The levels then rise to approximately two to three times normal, which may correlate with the duration of chronic renal failure (50). Total serum amylase, pancreatic amylase, and salivary amylase isoenzymes are elevated, but isoenzymes are not routinely measured in clinical practice (47,51). Serum amylase in asymptomatic patients rarely exceeds 500 IU/L and is unaffected by dialysis (49,52). The predialysis serum lipase activity is also increased in ESRD patients and rises further after hemodialysis. This effect is related to the lipolytic effect of intradialytic heparin and is dose related. Patients on CAPD and with peritonitis also have mild elevations in serum and peritoneal amylase (up to 100 IU/L); however, marked elevations, as seen in patients with pancreatitis or cholecystitis, are not found (53).

Acute pancreatitis has been reported to be more common in ESRD than in the general population. Several series report an incidence of 2.3% to 6.4% in renal failure patients (54,55). Pancreatitis is significantly more common in those with alcohol abuse, systemic lupus erythematosus, and polycystic kidney disease. It is not significantly associated with biliary tract disease, hyperlipidemia, or hypercalcemia. The mortality is 20% to 50%. Acute pancreatitis is significantly more common in patients on CAPD than in those on hemodialysis (55–57). The dialysate may be clear, hemorrhagic, or cloudy. It has been suggested that metabolic abnormalities related to absorption of glucose and buffer from dialysate, hypertrigylceridemia, or absorp-

TABLE 25.2. POTENTIAL CAUSES OF PANCREATIC DISEASE IN DIALYSIS PATIENTS

Alcoholism
Gallstones
Hyperparathyroidism
Hypercalcemia
Hypertriglyceridemia
Vascular insufficiency
Drug toxicity
    Diuretics
    Antibiotics
    Nonsteroidal antiinflammatory agents
    Heparin (transient)
    Dialysate
Systemic lupus erythematosus
Polycystic kidney disease

tion of a toxic substance in the dialysate, bags, or tubing may increase the risk of pancreatitis in CAPD patients (58).

Chronic pancreatitis can interfere with absorption and may result in malnutrition, vitamin deficiencies, and chronic wasting in dialysis patients. Histologic evidence of pancreatitis can be seen in greater than 50% of ESRD patients, 85% of which is chronic (59). Pathologic changes include calcifications, fibrosis, abscess formation, and deposition of hemosiderin. However, despite the frequency of chronic morphologic findings and functional abnormalities of the pancreas associated with ESRD, clinically significant chronic pancreatitis is rare. Most patients are asymptomatic; rarely, symptoms suggestive of malabsorption such as steatorrhea develop.

Diagnosing pancreatitis in dialysis patients can be very difficult. Dialysis patients frequently experience abdominal discomfort, nausea, and vomiting as a result of uremia or dialysis treatments. Nonspecific elevations of serum amylase and lipase are common. Therefore interpretation of hyperamylasemia must be approached with caution. Clinicians should maintain a high level of suspicion if values exceed three times the normal limit. Abdominal CT can be useful to confirm pancreatic inflammation and peripancreatic abnormalities suspicious for pancreatitis. Early diagnosis and therapy may reduce the progression or severity of disease. Acute pancreatitis is more likely to be severe and is associated with a worse prognosis in dialysis patients than in the general population (60). Using Ranson's criteria, the mortality for patients with three or more (including renal insufficiency) criteria approaches 70%, in comparison with 11% for patients without kidney disease. Complications such as pancreatic abscesses, pseudocysts, and necrosis occur with the same frequency as in the general population. However, dialysis patients develop twice as many systemic complications, such as cardiovascular and pulmonary complications, and sepsis (61). Treatment should be similar to that for nondialysis patients, including bowel rest, volume resuscitation as needed with frequent dialysis to maintain euvolemia, and pain control. Pain management strategies should avoid the use of Demerol, which may lower the threshold for seizures in ESRD.

NEPHROGENIC ASCITES

Nephrogenic ascites (NA) or idiopathic dialysis ascites (IDA) is an uncommon but important cause of morbidity in dialysis patients. By definition, it is a disorder that manifests as massive, refractory ascites in chronic hemodialysis patients where all other causes of ascites have been excluded (62). The incidence appears to be decreasing with improved volumetrically controlled dialysis and nutrition, and is center dependent (62,63). Most patients present with sustained volume overload, arterial hypertension, large interdialytic weight gains, minimal extremity edema, cachexia, and a history of dialysis-associated hypotension (62–65). NA is frequently associated with hyperparathyroidism, hypoalbuminemia, and uremia; has a male predominance; and is unrelated to age or race (66,67). It is associated with a grave prognosis, with a 1-year mortality rate of more than 30% (64) (Table 25.3).

The pathophysiology of NA is complex, probably multifactorial, and incompletely understood. Many patients have a his-

TABLE 25.3. CAUSES AND CHARACTERISTICS OF NEPHROGENIC ASCITES

Possible causes
  Sustained volume overload
  Impaired lymphatic drainage
  Elevated hepatic venous hydrostatic pressure
  Increased peritoneal membrane permeability resulting from
    Dialysate solutions
    Uremic toxins
    Hyperparathyroidism
    Hypoalbuminemia
    Circulating immune complexes
    Hemosiderosis
    Activation of the renin–angiotensin system
Clinical characteristics
  Refractory ascites in the absence of hepatic, neoplastic, or infectious disease
  Arterial hypertension
  Large interdialytic weight gains
  Minimal extremity edema
  Cachexia
  History of intradialytic hypotension
  Exudative ascites

Adapted from Hammond TC, et al. Nephrogenic ascites: a poorly understood syndrome. *J Am Soc Nephrol* 1994;5:1173–1177.

tory of previous CAPD, suggesting persisting abnormalities of the peritoneal membrane. However, the syndrome also occurs in patients even before the initiation of dialysis (64). The accumulation of ascites may occur up to 18 months preceding dialysis, to as late as 5 years after initiation of dialysis. The characteristics of the ascitic fluid indicate that the underlying pathogenesis is an alteration of the balance between peritoneal membrane permeability and impaired resorption due to peritoneal lymphatic obstruction, without a significantly elevated hepatic vein hydrostatic pressure (65,68). The ascitic fluid is straw colored and exudative, with a total protein of more than 3 g/dL; ratio of serum albumin to ascites albumin of less than 0.9 g/dL; and ascites total protein/serum total protein of more than 0.72. Thus NA must be differentiated from pancreatitis, malignancy, and tuberculous peritonitis (69). Changes in membrane permeability as a result of dialysis membranes and fluid, circulating immune complexes, iron deposition, abnormal sodium transport, or activation of the renin angiotensin system have been proposed (62,65,70–72). Histologic examination of the peritoneum typically demonstrates chronic inflammation, fibrosis, and mesothelial cell proliferation (63).

The diagnosis of NA is one of exclusion. Examination of the ascitic fluid is critical to establish an exudative pattern. Diagnostic paracentesis is central to establish the protein content and rule out infectious or neoplastic causes. Ultrasound or CT may help to delineate hepatic structure, but peritoneoscopy with biopsy is generally more definitive.

The treatment of NA is multimodal and includes intensive fluid restriction, daily hemodialysis for several weeks, frequent paracentesis, and optimization of protein nutrition. Other strategies have been employed with varying and unsatisfactory success. Ascites may respond to ascitic fluid reinfusion, peritoneal-venous shunts, CAPD, bilateral nephrectomy, intraperitoneal corticosteroids, and possibly ACE inhibitor therapy (63,68,73–76). However, renal transplant remains the definitive treatment for nephrogenic ascites and offers the best hope for cure. Patients experience complete resolution of ascites within 6 weeks of graft functioning but may recur after graft failure (77,78). Such measures can reverse the progressive course of cachexia and malnutrition, improve the quality of life, and improve survival.

CONSTIPATION

Functional constipation consists of decreased bowel frequency with fewer than three stools per week or frequent straining, incomplete evacuation, hard or lumpy stools, and the need for manual maneuvers. In the general population, the prevalence of constipation rises with age, affecting greater than 25% of patients over the age of 65 (79,80). Approximately 63% of hemodialysis patients experience constipation, possibly as a result of associated comorbidities, poor nutritional status, or medications (Table 25.4). Among CAPD patients, the prevalence is 29% and is age related (81). The lower rate of constipation in CAPD has been attributed to better metabolic and potassium control, and increased dietary fiber intake. In most patients, constipation is bothersome and may interfere with the quality of life; however, in rare instances, severe obstipation can be associated with colonic perforation and death.

Uremic patients with chronic constipation, abdominal pain, and distension should be evaluated for colonic pseudoobstruc-

TABLE 25.4. FACTORS COMMONLY ASSOCIATED WITH CONSTIPATION IN DIALYSIS PATIENTS

Drugs
  Analgesics
  Anticholinergics
    Antidepressants
      Anticholinergics
      Serotonin antagonists
    Antipsychotics
  Antihypertensives
    Calcium channel antagonists
  Calcium-containing drugs
    Iron supplements
    Aluminum binders
    Calcium acetate binders
    Calcium carbonate
  Opiates
Neurogenic disorders
  Autonomic neuropathy
  Diabetic enteropathy
  Interstinal pseudo-obstruction
Metabolic problems
  Hypercalcemia
  Hypocalcemia
  Hypothyroidism
Nutritional factors
  Malnutrition
  Dehydration
  Low dietary fiber
  Hyperkalemia
Inactivity

tion. This is associated with colonic perforation in up to 50% of cases, particularly if the bowel wall diameter exceeds 12 cm (82). Early endoscopic or surgical decompression may result in complete recovery. Aluminum hydroxide binders have been associated with 78% of these cases, as well as drugs and autonomic neuropathy (83). Plain abdominal films can be helpful to confirm the diagnosis, and CT scan or colonoscopy can rule out potential causes of mechanical obstruction. Antacid impactions should be considered in ESRD patients, who ingest a large volume of antacids for dyspepsia and control of phosphorus absorption, as stercoral ulceration and perforation are not uncommon (84).

The initial evaluation of a patient with constipation should include a careful history and physical examination, with emphasis on recent changes in bowel movements, and medications. If no cause is identified, imaging studies to rule out mass lesions, megacolon, and strictures may be useful. If these studies are normal, studies to assess for prolonged fecal transit time and pelvic floor dysfunction should be considered, in conjunction with consultation with a gastroenterologist.

Early and aggressive measures to reduce constipation are important, as uremic patients have a greater risk of developing diverticuli and perforation than the general population (85). This is particularly true in patients with polycystic kidney disease, nearly 80% of which have diverticuli, compared with 49% of patients with other causes of chronic kidney disease (86). Medical management of constipation in dialysis patients can begin with increasing dietary fiber and activity, and avoiding volume depletion. Medications should be tailored to reduce the number of drugs associated with constipation (Table 25.4). Bulk laxatives containing psyllium increase fecal mass and may also be added. Stool softeners with docusate sodium may improve the ability of water to enter the stool but are not very effective. Hyperosmolar, magnesium-containing compounds cause hypermagnesemia in renal failure and are contraindicated. Chronic use of aluminum binders may worsen constipation, renal osteodystrophy, and encephalopathy. Chronic use of intestinal wall stimulants such as bisacodyl may induce hypokalemia and protein malnutrition; their use should be restricted to short-term management only. Lactulose, sorbitol, and polyethylene glycol are helpful in dialysis patients and can be used occasionally for refractory constipation. For severe incapacitating constipation, surgical measures may be necessary.

REFERENCES

1. Farsakh NA, et al. Brief report: evaluation of the upper gastrointestinal tract in uraemic patients undergoing hemodialysis. *Nephrol Dial Transplant* 1996;11:847–850.
2. Hammer J, et al. Chronic gastrointestinal symptoms in hemodialysis patients. *Wien Klin Wochenschr* 1998;110:287–291.
3. Vaziri ND, et al. Pathology of gastrointestinal tract in chronic hemodialysis patients: an autopsy study of 78 cases. *Am J Gastroenterol* 1985;80:608–611.
4. Andriulli A, et al. Patients with chronic renal failure are not at risk of developing chronic peptic ulcers. *Clin Nephrol* 1985;23:245–248.
5. Margolis DM, et al. Upper gastrointestinal disease in chronic renal failure: a prospective evaluation. *Arch Intern Med* 1978;138:1214–1217.
6. Cekin AH, et al. Gastroesophageal reflux disease in chronic renal fail-

ure patients with upper GI symptoms: multivariate analysis of pathogenic factors. *Am J Gastroenterol* 2002;97:1352–1356.

7. Kim MJ, et al. Gastroesophageal reflux disease in CAPD patients. *Adv Perit Dial* 1998;14:98–101.

8. Fernandez M, et al. High incidence of hiatal hernia in patients with end-stage renal disease. *Clin Nephrol* 1996;46:218.

9. Francos GC, et al. Disorders of oesophageal motility in chronic haemodialysis patients. *Lancet* 1984;1:219.

10. Siamopoulos KC, et al. Esophageal dysfunction in chronic hemodialysis patients. *Nephron* 1990;55:389–393.

11. Dogan I, et al. Esophageal motor dysfunction in chronic renal failure. *Nephron* 1996;72:346–347.

12. Jaffe RN, et al. Changes of the digestive tract in uremia: a pathologic anatomic study. *Arch Intern Med* 1934;53:851–864.

13. Mason EE. Gastrointestinal lesions occurring in uremia. *Ann Intern Med* 1952;37:95–105.

14. Moustafa FE, et al. *Helicobacter pylori* and uremic gastritis: a histopathologic study and correlation with endoscopic and bacteriologic findings. *Am J Nephrol* 1997;17:165–171.

15. Fabbian F, et al. Esophagogastroduodenoscopy in chronic hemodialysis patients: 2-year clinical experience in a renal unit. *Clin Nephrol* 2002;58:54–59.

16. Kang JY, et al. Prevalence of peptic ulcer in patients undergoing maintenance hemodialysis. *Dig Dis Sci* 1988;33:774–778.

17. Andriulli A, et al. Patients with chronic renal failure are not at risk of developing chronic peptic ulcers. *Clin Nephrol* 1985;23:245–248.

18. Troskot B, et al. Giant peptic ulcers in patients undergoing maintenance hemodialysis. *Acta Med Croatica* 1995;49:59–64.

19. Kang JY, et al. Peptic ulcer and gastritis in uraemia, with particular reference to the effect of *Helicobacter pylori* infection. *J Gastroenterol Hepatol* 1999;14:771–778.

20. Ozgur O, et al. *Helicobacter pylori* infection in haemodialysis patients and renal transplant recipients. *Nephrol Dial Transplant* 1997;12:289–291.

21. Gladziwa U, et al. Prevalence of *Helicobacter pylori* in patients with chronic renal failure. *Nephrol Dial Transplant* 1993;8:301–306.

22. Davenport A, et al. Prevalence of *Helicobacter pylori* in patients with end-stage renal failure and renal transplant recipients. *Nephron* 1991;59:597–601.

23. Jaspersen D, et al. Significantly lower prevalence of *Helicobacter pylori* in uremic patients than in patients with normal renal function. *J Gastrenterol* 1995;30:585–588.

24. Krawczyk W, et al. Frequency of *Helicobacter pylori* infection in uremic hemodialyzed patients with antral gastritis. *Nephron* 1996;74:621–622.

25. Ala-Kaila K, et al. Gastric *Helicobacter* and upper gastrointestinal symptoms in chronic renal failure. *Ann Med* 1991;23:403–406.

26. Schoonjans R, et al. Dyspepsia and gastroparesis in chronic renal failure: the role of *Helicobacter pylori*. *Clin Nephrol* 2002;57:201–207.

27. Mak SK, et al. Efficacy of a 1-week course of proton-pump inhibitor-based triple therapy for eradicating *Helicobacter pylori* in patients with and without chronic renal failure. *Am J Kidney Dis* 2002;40:576–581.

28. Suleymanlar I, et al. Response to triple treatment with omeprazole, amoxicillin, and clarithromycin for *Helicobacter pylori* infections in continuous ambulatory peritoneal dialysis patients. *Adv Perit Dial* 1999;15:79–81.

29. Van Vlem B, et al. Delayed gastric emptying in dyspeptic chronic hemodialysis patients. *Am J Kidney Dis* 2000;36:962–968.

30. De Schoenmakere G, et al. Relationship between gastric emptying and clinical and biochemical factors in chronic hemodialysis patients. *Nephrol Dial Transplant* 2001;16:1850–1855.

31. Ross EA, et al. Improved nutrition after the detection and treatment of occult gastroparesis in nondiabetic dialysis patients. *Am J Kidney Dis* 1998;31:62–66.

32. Schoonjans R, et al. Gastric emptying of solids in cirrhotic and peritoneal dialysis patients: influence of peritoneal volume load. *Eur J Gastroenterol Hepatol* 2002;14:395–398.

33. Kao CH, et al. Delayed gastric emptying and *Helicobacter pylori* infection in patients with chronic renal failure. *Eur J Nucl Med* 1995;22:1282–1285.

34. Chalasani N, et al. Upper gastrointestinal bleeding in patients with chronic renal failure: role of vascular ectasia. *Am J Gastroenterol* 1996;91:2329–2332.

35. Zuckerman GR, et al. Upper gastrointestinal bleeding in patients with chronic renal failure. *Ann Intern Med* 1985;102:588–592.

36. Tsai C, et al. Investigation of upper gastrointestinal hemorrhage in chronic renal failure. *J Clin Gastroenterol* 1996;22:2–5.

37. Clouse RE, et al. Angiodysplasia as a cause of upper gastrointestinal bleeding. *Arch Intern Med* 1985;145:458–461.

38. Navab F, et al. Angiodysplasia in patients with renal insufficiency. *Am J Gastroenterol* 1989;84:1297–1301.

39. Cappell MS, et al. Changing epidemiology of gastrointestinal angiodysplasia with increasing recognition of clinically milder cases: angiodysplasia tend to produce mild chronic gastrointestinal bleeding in a study of 47 consecutive patients admitted from 1980–1989. *Am J Gastroenterol* 1992;87:201–206.

40. Alvarez L, et al. Investigation of gastrointestinal bleeding in patients with end-stage renal disease. *Am J Gastroenterol* 1993;88:30–33.

41. Marcuard SP, et al. Gastrointestinal angiodysplasia in renal failure. *J Clin Gastroenterol* 1988;10:482–484.

42. Bronner MH, et al. Estrogen-progesterone therapy for bleeding gastrointestinal telangiectasias in chronic renal failure. *Ann Intern Med* 1986;105:371–374.

43. Van Cutsem E, et al. Treatment of bleeding gastrointestinal vascular malformations with oestrogen-progesterone. *Lancet* 1990;335:953–955.

44. Junquera F, et al. A multicenter, randomized, clinical trial of hormonal therapy in the prevention of rebleeding from gastrointestinal angiodysplasia. *Gastroenterology* 2001;121:1073–1079.

45. Bartos B, et al. The function of the exocrine pancreas in chronic renal disease. *Digestion* 1970;3:33–37.

46. Sachs EF, et al. Pancreatic exocrine hypofunction in the wasting syndrome of end-stage renal disease. *Am J Gastroenterol* 1983;78:170–176.

47. Ventrucci M, et al. Alterations of exocrine pancreas in end-stage renal disease: do they reflect a clinically relevant uremic pancreatopathy? *Dig Dis Sci* 1995;40:2576–2581.

48. Avram RM, et al. Pancreatic disease in uremia and parathyroid hormone excess. *Nephron* 1982;32:60–62.

49. Collen MJ, et al. Serum amylase in patients with renal insufficiency and renal failure. *Am J Gastroenterol* 1990;85:1377–1380.

50. Bardella MT, et al. Serum amylase and isoamylase in chronic renal failure. *Int J Artif Organs* 1987;10:259–262.

51. Tsianos EV, et al. The value of alpha-amylase and isoamylase determination in chronic renal failure patients. *Int J Pancreatol* 1994;15:105–111.

52. Vaziri ND, et al. Pancreatic enzymes in patients with end-stage renal disease maintained on hemodialysis. *Am J Gastroenerol* 1988;83:410–412.

53. Caruana RJ, et al. Serum and peritoneal fluid amylase levels in CAPD: normal values and clinical usefulness. *Am J Nephrol* 1987;7:169–172.

54. Padilla B, et al. Pancreatitis in patients with end-stage renal disease. *Medicine* 1994;73:8–20.

55. Rutsky EA, et al. Acute pancreatitis in patients with end-stage renal disease without transplantation. *Arch Intern Med* 1986;146:1741–1745.

56. Pannekeet MM, et al. Acute pancreatitis during CAPD in the Netherlands. *Nephrol Dial Transplant* 1993;8:1376–1381.

57. Bruno MJ, et al. Acute pancreatitis in peritoneal dialysis and hemodialysis: risk, clinical course, outcome and possible aetiology. *Gut* 2000;46:385–389.

58. Caruana RJ, et al. Pancreatitis: an important cause of abdominal symptoms in patients on peritoneal dialysis. *Am J Kidney Dis* 1986;7:135–140.

59. Araki T, et al. Histologic pancreatitis in end-stage renal disease. *Int J Pancreatol* 1992;12:263–269.

60. Joglar FM, et al. Outcome of pancreatitis in CAPD and HD patients. *Perit Dial Int* 1995;15:264–266.

61. Pitchumoni CS, et al. Acute pancreatitis in chronic renal failure. *Am J Gastroenterol* 1996;91:2477–2482.

62. Gluck Z, et al. Ascites associated with end-stage renal disease. *Am J Kidney Dis* 1987;10:9–18.

63. Singh S, et al. Ascites in patients on maintenance hemodialysis. *Nephron* 1974;12:114–120.

64. Mauk PM, et al. Diagnosis and course of nephrogenic ascites. *Arch Intern Med* 1988;148:1577–1579.

65. Hammond TC, et al. Nephrogenic ascites: a poorly understood syndrome. *J Am Soc Nephrol* 1994;5:1173–1177.

66. Gutch CF, et al. Refractory ascites in chronic dialysis patients. *Clin Nephrol* 1974;2:59–62.

67. Nasr EM, et al. Is nephrogenic ascites related to secondary hyperparathyroidism? *Am J Kidney Dis* 2001;37:E16.

68. Han SH, et al. Nephrogenic ascites: analysis of 16 cases and review of the literature. *Medicine* 1998;77:233–245.

69. Tannenberg AM. Ascites in dialysis patients. In: Nissenson AR, et al., eds. *Dialysis therapy.* Philadelphia: Hanley & Belfus, 1993:299–301.

70. Gotloib L, et al. Ascites in patients undergoing maintenance hemodialysis. *Am J Med* 1976;61:465–470

71. Twardowski ZJ, et al. Circulating immune complexes: possible toxins responsible for serositis (pericarditis, pleuritis, peritonitis) in renal failure. *Nephron* 1983;35:190–195.

72. Besbas N, et al. Peritoneal hemosiderosis in pediatric patients with nephrogenic ascites. *Nephron* 1992;62:292–295.

73. Rubin J, et al. Continuous ambulatory peritoneal dialysis: treatment of dialysis-related ascites. *Arch Intern Med* 1981;14:1093–1095.

74. Roy-Chaudhury P, et al. ACE inhibitors in the management of hemodialysis ascites. *Nephrol Dial Transplant* 1994;9:1695–1696.

75. Tse KC, et al. Peritoneal dialysis in patients with refractory ascites. *Perit Dial Int* 2001;21:626–627.

76. Buselmeier TJ, et al. Local steroid treatment of intractable ascites in dialysis patients. *Proc Clin Dial Transplant Forum* 1975;5:9–11.

77. Popli S, et al. Hemodialysis ascites in anephric patients. *Clin Nephrol* 1981;15:203–205.

78. Melero M, et al. Idiopathic dialysis ascites in the nineties: resolution after renal transplantation. *Am J Kidney Dis* 1995;26:668–670.

79. Thompson WG, et al. Functional bowel disorders and functional abdominal pain. *Gut* 1999;45(Suppl):II43.

80. Talley NJ, et al. Prevalence of gastrointestinal symptoms in the elderly: a population-based study. *Gastroenterology* 1992;102:895.

81. Yasuda G, et al. Prevalence of constipation in continuous ambulatory peritoneal dialysis patients and comparison with hemodialysis patients. *Am J Kidney Dis* 2002;39:1292–1299.

82. Nanni G, et al. Ogilvie's syndrome (acute colonic pseudo-obstruction). *Dis Colon Rectum* 1982;132:66–69.

83. Adams DL, et al. Lower gastrointestinal tract dysfunction in patients receiving long-term hemodialysis. *Arch Intern Med* 1982;142:303–306.

84. Welch JP, et al. Management of antacid impactions in hemodialysis and renal transplant patients. *Am J Surg* 1980;139:561–568.

85. Flynn CT, et al. Renal failure and angiodysplasia of the colon. *Ann Intern Med* 1985;103:154–157.

86. Scheff RJ, et al. Diverticular disease in patients with chronic renal failure due to polycystic kidney disease. *Ann Intern Med* 1980;28:202–206.

RENAL OSTEODYSTROPHY

DONALD J. SHERRARD

This chapter presents a practical approach to the problems of renal osteodystrophy by first presenting the background for the difficulties clinicians face today. We then examine the present pattern of bone disease, together with factors that contribute to the picture and current concepts of prevention and treatment. Finally, we use renal osteodystrophy as a starting point to discuss transplant-related bone disorders.

HISTORICAL BACKGROUND

Predialysis Era

Probably the first connection between renal disease and bone disease was made in nineteenth-century London when it was discovered that patients with Bright's disease developed rickets that responded to fish liver oil. It would be many years before vitamin D was discovered to be the active principal substance in fish liver oil, and considerably later that vitamin D deficiency was clarified and treated. Thus what was later termed *renal rickets* was the first form of rickets to be treated with vitamin D.

In the 1930s and 1940s, several workers described the marked parathyroid enlargement found at autopsy in patients dying of renal failure. At that time, this was of little clinical significance, as the fatal consequences of uremia placed such information in the category of "useless minutia."

Early Dialysis Period

Once dialysis provided prolonged survival for subjects with end-stage renal disease (ESRD), the "minutia" observed in previous times suddenly assumed importance. However, neither hyperparathyroidism nor vitamin D deficiency first attracted clinical attention to calcium metabolism. Scribner and his coworkers observed that the first dialysis patients were "turning to stone," as the patients accumulated huge metastatic calcifications (Fig. 26.1). In studying this problem, they described its association with an elevated calcium × phosphate product (1). During a conversation with a local gastroenterologist, Scribner learned that an occasional consequence of vigorous antacid therapy was hypophosphatemia. He then experimented with dietary phosphate restriction and the use of aluminum-containing antacids to further inhibit phosphate absorption. In the early 1960s, it was known that both magnesium and calcium salts could be absorbed with serious clinical consequences. At that time aluminum was said to be "nonabsorbable," so any toxicity from aluminum was considered unlikely. The use of phosphate-binding antacids and low-phosphate diets resulted in the disappearance of the tumorous calcium deposits (2).

In the mid-1960s dialysis patients began to develop features of hyperparathyroidism, particularly bone pain, cystic bone lesions, subperiosteal resorption on x-ray, and hypercalcemia. This form of hyperparathyroidism was called "tertiary" because the parathyroid glands apparently became autonomous after prolonged "secondary" hyperparathyroidism due to persistent hypocalcemia (3).

Attempts to prevent this development focused on the hypocalcemia and included supplemental oral calcium and high doses of vitamin D. Because it took so much vitamin D to correct the hypocalcemia, patients were thought to be vitamin D resistant. No one knew, of course, that the form of vitamin D in use was a precursor that required liver and kidney activation. The reason such high doses were required was that the precursor (and its liver metabolite) was weakly active (i.e., it could bind to and activate D receptors to a small extent). Unfortunately, when toxicity (hypercalcemia) occurred, it persisted for several months as a result of the prolonged half-life of vitamin D precursors.

Because of the hazards of vitamin D, clinicians sought better ways of correcting the hypocalcemia, ultimately settling on a high-dialysate calcium to provide the solution. For this reason the standard dialysate calcium of the period (and until very recently) was 3.25 to 3.50 mEq/L, a value guaranteed to result in substantial transfer of calcium into the patient. Very early studies of parathyroid hormone (PTH) metabolism documented that this high-dialysate calcium did suppress parathyroid hormone.

When such measures failed to control the hyperparathyroidism, parathyroidectomy was necessary. The initial reports often described total parathyroidectomy (4). Later subtotal parathyroidectomy was used, and then the variant of transplant of remnant tissue to the arm (5). Recently, total parathyroidectomy has been advocated again, particularly for patients not eligible for renal transplantation (6,7).

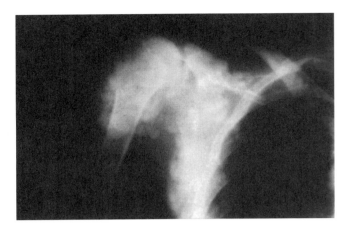

FIG. 26.1. X-ray showing large calcium deposit in the shoulder of a dialysis patient with chronic elevation of the calcium × phosphate product.

Later Dialysis Period

The renal patients' refractoriness to vitamin D, in part, stimulated investigators to assess vitamin D metabolism (8). It was soon learned that the liver and kidney both played a role and the final active metabolite, 1,25 (OH)₂ vitamin D (1,25D), was produced in the kidney. Later studies showed that PTH was the trophic hormone for 1,25D production and that hypophosphatemia and hypocalcemia also could stimulate its synthesis (9,10). Finally, it was shown that 1,25D participated with calcium in the feedback inhibition of PTH and was very effective in reversing hyperparathyroid bone disease (11,12).

Because vitamin D is important in the healing of osteomalacia in patients without renal failure, 1,25D was first used in dialysis patients with osteomalacia. This therapy was unsuccessful, and "vitamin D resistance" was again reported in uremic subjects. Only this time the investigators were referring to the failure of this peculiar form of osteomalacia to respond to what is now known to be the active form of the vitamin.

Epidemiologic studies soon showed an association between this fracturing osteomalacia and aluminum contamination of dialysate (13). Subsequent studies demonstrated that oral aluminum (the primary phosphate binder) was also involved. Indeed, it was soon recognized that oral aluminum in any form was absorbed (albeit in small amounts) and that a combination

of prolonged exposure and lack of renal excretion led to a large cumulative body burden. Because of several other toxic manifestations in addition to the bony effects, aluminum was largely abandoned in favor of calcium salts as a phosphate binder (2). Subsequently, the recognition that calcium accumulation contributed to vascular calcification has led to the development of newer binders, containing neither aluminum nor calcium, such as sevelamer (14,15).

CURRENT STATUS OF RENAL OSTEODYSTROPHY

Early Renal Failure

Bone disease begins quite early in renal failure (16) in response to the abnormalities of PTH and 1,25D that develop when kidney function is reduced as little as 30% (i.e., with a serum creatinine of 1.5 to 2.0 mg/dL). These early changes are rarely severe and do not lead to symptomatic disease unless the patient is a child, has a very prolonged course, or has some other metabolic problem affecting calcium metabolism. With any of those exceptions, which place additional stress on the skeleton, patients may develop the more severe lesions described in the following discussion early in the course of their renal disease and require specific treatment.

Bone Disease with Advanced Renal Failure

Five histologically specific bone lesions (Table 26.1) develop in dialysis patients (16–20). They fall into three general classes:

1. Normal-/high-bone-turnover disorders, including mild and severe hyperparathyroidism.
2. Low-turnover bone lesions, including osteomalacia and the aplastic lesion.
3. Mixed uremic osteodystrophy, which has features suggestive of both high and low turnover, and, depending on its cause, may be either low or high turnover or even change from one category to the other.

Because bone resorption and bone formation are in equilibrium in the nongrowing individual, bone turnover is defined by bone formation. Clinically, bone formation is determined by giving the patient two doses of tetracycline 2 weeks apart and then viewing a bone biopsy (21) section with fluorescent microscopy (Table 26.2). The administered tetracycline shows

TABLE 26.1. TYPES OF BONE DISEASE IN RENAL FAILURE AND CHARACTERISTIC HISTOLOGIC FEATURES

Disorder	Feature
Normal-/high-turnover disorders	
Mild bone disease	Increased osteoid surface
Osteitis fibrosa	Marrow fibrosis
Low-turnover disorders	
Aplastic (adynamic)	Low bone formation
Osteomalacia	Increased unmineralized osteoid
Mixed uremic osteodystrophy	Marrow fibrosis and increased unmineralized osteoid

TABLE 26.2. OBTAINING A BONE BIOPSY

Labeling schedule
    Tetracycline 1,000 mg (15 mg/kg) PO 3 weeks before biopsy
    Demeclocycline 600 mg (9 mg/kg) PO 1 week before biopsy
Characteristics of biopsy (iliac crest)
    Site: 2 cm posterior to anterior superior iliac spine
    Size: >3 × 8 mm
    Cancellous (trabecular) bone should predominate
Fixation[a]
    Place sample in 10% buffered formalin for 8–24 hours
    Transfer to 70% ethanol for shipping

[a]If osteoclast evaluation is important specimens should be kept cold (32–40°F), but not frozen.

up as two fluorescent bands (Fig. 26.2) on the bone surface. Measuring the length of the bands and the distance between them can quite accurately measure bone formation rate (much as foresters can measure tree growth by measuring between a tree's growth rings) and infer bone turnover.

The normal-/high-turnover lesions are first categorized as such by the bone formation measurement. Other features include an increase in osteoblasts (the bone-forming cells), bone surface covered with osteoid, osteoclasts (bone-resorbing cells), eroded (resorbing) surface, marrow fibroblasts, and marrow fibrosis. With the least severe, mild hyperparathyroidism, one may see only a modest increase in bone-forming surface (osteoid) and a high normal bone formation. In the most severe form, for which the term *osteitis fibrosa* is used, a very high bone formation is accompanied by marked increases in all the other histologic features. Marrow fibrosis may be so severe in some cases as to displace other marrow elements. Many of the histologic features occur in response to PTH, which stimulates all the cellular elements involved to proliferate and hyperfunction. The degree to which these features develop is generally proportional to the elevation of PTH and the length of time it has been elevated. Symptoms such as bone pain, muscle weakness, and occasionally fractures reflect both the severity of the PTH elevation and the resultant bone disease. In a large study (18), we noted that 45 patients had mild and 57 had severe hyperparathy-

roidism out of a total of 259 unselected patients. Those with more severe disease had a longer duration of renal failure (Fig. 26.3).

Similarly, the low-turnover lesions are initially identified by the bone formation assessment. Then they are categorized as *osteomalacic,* in which there is a marked excess of unmineralized osteoid, or *aplastic* (also referred to as adynamic), in which osteoid volume is not increased. Adynamic (aplastic) lesions were originally thought to be caused by aluminum toxicity (or rarely, iron toxicity). It is now clear that aluminum does cause the osteomalacic lesion, but it more frequently causes the adynamic disorder. In our study of 259 patients (18), we described osteomalacia in only 11; in ten of these patients the osteomalacia was due to aluminum (>25% bone surface). On the other hand, of 128 patients who had the aplastic disorder, in 88 patients it was not due to aluminum (<25% bone surface). The major etiologic factor was hypoparathyroidism (presumably resulting from excessive correction of hyperparathyroidism); diabetes and age may also have contributed. In contrast to high bone turnover, the aluminum-induced disorders (either the osteomalacia or the adynamic lesion) were often accompanied by bone pain, fracture, or muscle weakness.

A commonly occurring problem associated with the low-turnover disorders when they are not due to aluminum is an increased incidence of asymptomatic hypercalcemia. Contrary to previous thinking, which characterized aplastic disorder as benign, recent data show that it carries long-term consequences. In the study mentioned earlier, 34% of the patients had aplastic (adynamic) lesions without significant aluminum deposition (20). These patients were reevaluated 5 years after the initial evaluation. The results show that most of these patients developed bone pain and fracture and may also have had an increased mortality.

Finally, we identified mixed uremic osteodystrophy in 18 of our 259 patients. Mixed uremic osteodystrophy is characterized by an increase in unmineralized osteoid to the extent seen in osteomalacia and an increase in marrow fibrosis to the extent seen in the severe hyperparathyroid disorder (osteitis fibrosa). In our study, bone formation was high in this group, probably

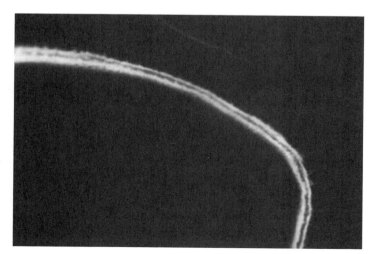

FIG. 26.2. Photomicrograph (×640) showing two tetracycline labels on the cancellous bone surface. (Reprinted with permission from Sherrard DJ, et al. Single-dose tetracycline labeling for bone histomorphometry. *Am J Clin Pathol* 1989;91:682–687.)

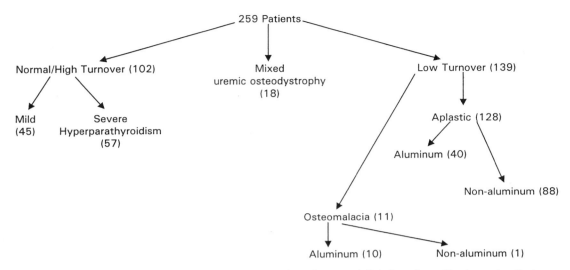

FIG. 26.3. Distribution of various bone lesions in an unselected group of dialysis patients. Numbers of patients are in parentheses. (Reprinted with permission from Sherrard DJ, et al. The spectrum of bone disease in end-stage renal failure—an evolving disorder. *Kidney Int* 1993;43:436–442.)

because the PTH level was very high. The high PTH was almost certainly due to inadequate calcium replacement. Appropriate calcium balance is essential for the maintenance of mineral homeostasis and the support of adequate bone mineralization. Therefore the lack of adequate calcium replacement results in a large amount of unmineralized osteoid as in our patients. So although calcium was being deposited at a very high rate, the overstimulated osteoblasts were forming osteoid at an even higher rate. Mixed uremic osteodystrophy has also been described with a normal or low bone formation. Such a picture may be seen when aluminum toxicity and hyperparathyroidism are combined to produce normal bone formation or even a low bone formation if aluminum toxicity dominates the picture.

Factors Relating to Type of Bone Disease

Diabetes, aluminum, age, and the parathyroid status may influence the pattern of bone disease. In addition, the type of dialysis appears to play an important role. In our study described earlier, roughly half the patients were treated with hemodialysis and half were treated with peritoneal dialysis (18). Of the peritoneal dialysis patients, 66% had low-turnover lesions, while 62% of the hemodialysis patients had high turnover lesions. This difference, which may have been related to the better calcium maintenance in the peritoneal dialysis patients, was highly significant.

Amyloid

Although the problem of amyloid is discussed extensively in Chapter 23, it needs to be remembered that it does involve the skeleton. β_2-Microglobulin amyloid deposits may be found at subperiosteal locations, infiltrating cortical or cancellous bone, within cartilage and osteoid, or even free in the marrow space (22). Large cystic deposits can be seen in the long bones, clavicles, phalanges, carpal or tarsal bones, and pelvis. Fractures

through these cysts or into infiltrates in the femoral head are particularly common and heal with difficulty.

Amyloid deposits may be seen as an additional problem superimposed on any of the bone lesions described earlier. Of particular note, these large, often cystic deposits are commonly misdiagnosed by radiologists as the "brown tumors" of osteitis fibrosa cystica (severe hyperparathyroid bone disease). In fact, cysts, particularly large cysts, are distinctly uncommon in uremic hyperparathyroidism. When hyperparathyroid cysts do occur, they are more likely to be found in the mandible or skull, and they are usually quite small (22,23). So when the radiologist finds cystic bone lesions, they are most likely amyloid.

Prevention

In early renal disease there are rarely any symptoms related to renal osteodystrophy. The primary goal is to prevent the development of hyperparathyroidism. The major risk of the therapy is that the progression of the renal disease might be accelerated.

Before Dialysis

Prevention of hyperparathyroidism involves correcting the reversible causes of PTH elevation (Table 26.3)—specifically, elevated phosphate, low calcium, and low calcitriol levels (16). As soon as the renal function begins to fall, phosphate restriction is important. This may increase production of calcitriol by residual kidney tissue (low phosphate stimulates and high phosphate suppresses renal 1,25D production); lowering the calcium × phosphate product may slow the progression of renal failure. In addition, phosphate has been shown to have a direct effect on parathyroid cell proliferation and hormone secretion in rats (24–27). Therefore early aggressive phosphate restriction will likely prevent or delay the onset of PTH hypersecretion and parathyroid cell proliferation. If phosphate remains elevated

TABLE 26.3. CAUSES OF PTH ELEVATION IN RENAL FAILURE

Reversible causes
    Hyperphosphatemia
    Hypocalcemia
    Low 1,25D levels
Irreversible causes
    Uremic resistance to PTH
    Decreased PTH metabolism
    Decreased number of 1,25D receptors*
    Decreased number of calcium receptors
Artifacts in PTH elevation: use of assay that measures PTH
    metabolites
    C-terminal assay
    Mid-region assay
Effect on calcium levels and through a direct effect on the
    parathyroids.

*The number of 1,25D receptors increases (but not to normal) with 1,25D treatment.

despite dietary restriction, phosphate binders are indicated. Calcium acetate and calcium carbonate are the preferred agents. Once they are needed (usually when the creatinine is >4.0 mg/dL), it is important to monitor both renal function and calcium × phosphate more closely because a high product (>50) is likely to accelerate the progression of renal disease (26).

When this therapy fails to maintain calcium levels, calcitriol should be added. Minimal doses should be used first and the dose should be increased slowly, probably no more often than every 2 months. Calcitriol will increase gut absorption of both calcium and phosphate, so their levels will need to be monitored closely and therapy adjusted promptly if elevations occur.

Although this therapy will help prevent the later development of hyperparathyroidism and is therefore important, it must be remembered that it does place the kidneys at risk. Hyperparathyroidism is a serious and difficult complication to manage, but its prevention should not be achieved at the cost of precipitating ESRD prematurely. It is far better to undertreat than overtreat, and the preservation of kidney function should be the primary goal at this stage, with the prevention of hyperparathyroidism a secondary goal. In pursuit of these sometimes conflicting goals, one should attempt to maintain normal phosphate (3.5 to 5.5 mg/dL) and total calcium levels (8.5 to 9.5 mg/dL) with the judicious use of calcium salts (for phosphate binding and calcium supplementation) and calcitriol. Both are usually needed to suppress PTH. It is unnecessary to follow the expensive ionized calcium because it correlates so highly with the total calcium. An increased calcium × phosphate product or increased calcium alone will aggravate renal failure and must be closely assessed (26). At the same time, monitoring the PTH will define whether therapy is working.

In this context, familiarity with the PTH measurement used is important to be sure that the assay has been characterized in renal failure. Such nonspecific tests as the C-terminal and mid-molecule assays largely measure inactive PTH metabolites that are retained in renal failure, and thus do not reflect the true state of parathyroid metabolism in uremic subjects (Table 26.3). In addition, there appears to be a state of parathyroid resistance in uremic subjects so that even if one uses the more precise "intact hormone" assays the goal should be to reduce PTH to no less

than about twice the upper normal limit (28,29). The data suggest that the normal range of intact PTH should be shifted to 100 to 300 pg/mL in dialysis patients to prevent the development of the aplastic lesion, on the one hand, and hyperparathyroidism, on the other.

For several years it has been known that the "intact" PTH measured a mixture of the 1–84 amino acid sequence (the actual PTH molecule) and a variety of other fragments, mostly the 6–84 amino acid sequence. It turns out that about 50% of the intact PTH measurement represents the actual PTH molecule, about 50% is the 6–84 fragment, and a tiny amount is other metabolites. Although measurements of the 1–84 sequence correlate very highly with the intact value reported by various laboratories (r values between 0.92 and 0.97), the situation is further complicated by the fact that the 6–84 fragment inhibits response to the active hormone (30).

In addition, there have been recent concerns about the adequacy of intact PTH as a surrogate marker of the bone lesions in ESRD patients. Although a decade ago the intact assay was a strong predictor, with values of less than 100 suggesting low-turnover bone disorders and those of more than 300 suggesting high turnover lesions (28,29), this no longer appears to be the case. It has been suggested that this might result from the recent change in therapy in regard to parenteral vitamin D, since these agents may have direct effects on bone, independent of their effects on PTH (33,34). An attempt to improve this situation was the recently proposed "ratio," in which combining the intact and whole (1–84 amino acid sequence) was said to resolve the issue (31). Unfortunately, this has not been supported by subsequent reports (32). Current investigations may clarify this problem. However, at this point we are stuck with the use of intact PTH as the best noninvasive indicator of renal osteodystrophy. It appears to continue being reliable at the low range to predict low-turnover bone disorders but is questionable at high ranges in predicting high turnover and may require other measures (e.g., bone biopsy, alkaline phosphatase) to be confident about the bone lesion (31,32).

It is extremely rare for pre-ESRD patients to develop symptoms of renal osteodystrophy (fractures, bone pain, arthropathy) or metastatic calcifications as a result of the disturbances of calcium metabolism associated with uremia. Should any of these occur at this stage, the patient should be evaluated as if renal disease were not present. In other words, such events as an atraumatic fracture or bone pain should be aggressively evaluated and not attributed to renal osteodystrophy. Hypercalcemia, of course, may well occur if patients are being treated with both calcium salts and calcitriol. If it persists for more than a week after these agents are stopped, the patient should be assessed for other causes than renal osteodystrophy.

Management of Dialysis Patients

Once ESRD occurs and the patient needs chronic dialysis treatment there is less need to worry about modest elevations of the calcium or calcium × phosphate product. Although the failing kidney appears particularly susceptible to such developments, other organs are less vulnerable. Therefore therapeutic goals are somewhat less strict (Table 26.4).

TABLE 26.4. PREVENTION OF HYPERPARATHYROIDISM IN DIALYSIS PATIENTS: THERAPEUTIC GOALS

Phosphate <5.5 mg/dL
Calcium 8.4–9.5 mg/dL
Intact PTH two to four times upper limit of normal

In general, the same approach as outlined earlier for predialysis patients should be continued. Dietary phosphate restriction is the foundation on which all other treatment is based. Compliant patients will be able to achieve phosphate levels below 7.0 mg/dL without phosphate binders and below 6.5 with binders at the time they start dialysis. Those patients who do not achieve phosphate goals are usually either confused by the dietary regimen or noncompliant. The best evidence of noncompliance is when the phosphate levels of such patients subside—often to surprisingly low levels—once the patient is confined in the hospital (personal observation). After many years of prolonged noncompliance and high phosphate levels, tissue phosphate levels become so elevated that the serum level remains too high, despite subsequent months of adherence to an appropriate regimen. Such patients often require parathyroidectomy to achieve reasonable levels.

Few patients will be able to achieve adequate phosphate levels through diet restriction alone without becoming protein malnourished. Although Medicare recommendations suggest maintaining phosphate below 6.0 mg/dL, the current data on vascular calcification and cardiovascular mortality in relation to calcium, phosphate, and calcium × phosphate product strongly support a much lower goal. Many patients will require substantial quantities of binders, often 1 g or more of calcium carbonate form with each meal (or equivalent amounts of acetate). To use this amount but avoid hypercalcemia, a dialysate calcium of 2.0 or 2.5 mEq/L is almost always necessary. Either in combination with a calcium binder or by itself, sevelamer is a useful (though costly) alternative. We have observed that many patients eating a traditional oriental diet do not seem to have a problem with phosphate control; in fact, they often suffer from hypophosphatemia.

An important aspect of phosphate binder therapy is to give the binder with the phosphate. If the patient eats little or no breakfast or perhaps only drinks a cup of coffee, the patient will not need any binders at that time. On the other hand, if most food (and most phosphate) is eaten at one meal, that is when the binders should be consumed. (One patient we saw in consultation was drinking a glass of milk with his noon meal because he had been told to take binders, and he felt that he should provide some phosphate "so the binders could work"!)

Aluminum compounds may sometimes be useful. In the initial management of a neglected or previously noncompliant patient, aluminum in conjunction with calcium compounds is often effective. Phosphate levels will fall more rapidly. If such therapy is used, patients must be specifically cautioned against using citrate in any form (particularly Shohl's solution, Alka Seltzer, or even large amounts of citric juices), because citrate markedly enhances aluminum absorption (35). After achieving phosphate control, aluminum compounds should be discontinued, if possible.

What the maximum dose of aluminum ought to be is unclear, but toxicity is commonly seen with a cumulative dose of aluminum of 2 kg over a period of 1 or more years. The maximum dose may depend on the individual dialysis patient—for example, whether the patient has diabetes or concomitantly uses aluminum-containing phosphate binders or antacids (36). Patients should be monitored for symptoms of aluminum toxicity such as dementia, bone pain, or fracture. A random plasma aluminum of more than 40 µg/L had been thought to be suggestive of aluminum toxicity. However, recent data show that a random level may not be an adequate screening tool, particularly in patients on hemodialysis. In our 259 patients who had bone biopsies (141 patients on continuous ambulatory peritoneal dialysis/continuous cyclic peritoneal dialysis [CAPD/CCPD] and 116 on hemodialysis), eight patients had aluminum bone toxicity with plasma levels of less than 20 µg/L. At this point, there does not appear to be any plasma aluminum level that adequately rules out aluminum toxicity, and one must still rely on the cumbersome deferoxamine challenge test (18).

If a calcium compound is used as the primary phosphate binder, few patients will need additional calcium supplements to maintain the calcium level. Most will need an active vitamin D metabolite to control PTH. This may be administered in three different regimens. In the conventional mode, calcitriol is given daily or twice daily at whatever dose is needed to maintain the serum calcium level between 8.5 and 9.5 mg/dL. Pulse dosing is generally reserved for patients who become hypercalcemic with conventional schedules. Studies suggest that pulse dosing, either intravenously or orally (1 to 3 µg, three times a week), may suppress PTH more easily with less risk of hypercalcemia (37). Recent studies suggest that parenteral paricalcitol is superior to calcitriol in that fewer episodes of hypercalcemia and elevated calcium × phosphate product are seen with its use (38). In the hypocalcemic patient, PTH suppression depends on correction of hypocalcemia through oral calcium supplementation, phosphate control, and adequate vitamin D levels. Hypocalcemia is best corrected with both oral calcium and oral calcitriol.

Whichever technique is used, the goal should be to suppress the intact PTH level between 150 and 300 pg/mL (two to five times the upper limit of the normal range for subjects without renal failure). Because of PTH resistance in uremia, greater suppression than this results in bone formation rates below the normal range, probably an undesirable result (26). PTH levels should be monitored at least quarterly to assess control.

For compliant patients treated this way, a few will develop either hyperparathyroidism, bone disease, or metastatic calcifications. Noncompliant or neglected patients may present with any of these problems, and the following section deals with how to proceed in these situations.

SPECIFIC CLINICAL PROBLEMS, WORKUP, AND MANAGEMENT

Hypercalcemia

Perhaps the most common clinical problem faced in most dialysis patients is hypercalcemia. In fact, if hypercalcemia does not occur at least occasionally, then the patients are probably not being managed appropriately (i.e., if the physician is "pushing" therapy, hypercalcemia will result from time to time). The most common cause of hypercalcemia in dialysis patients is the conventional therapy with calcium and calcitriol. If doses of these agents are not advanced too quickly (e.g., monthly changes should be adequate), problems are less likely. Most patients monitored monthly will not develop severe hypercalcemia (i.e., total calcium will be less than 12 mg/dL) and will not be symptomatic. If the patient is only on oral calcium or if the hypercalcemia does not remit when vitamin D is discontinued, other causes must be considered (Fig. 26.4).

A common but infrequently described problem that may cause acute hypercalcemia in the previously stable uremic patient is bed rest. When a normal person goes to bed, bone formation decreases rapidly and bone resorption slows down less quickly. The result is that calcium entry into bone is decreased while its efflux is maintained (39,40). In the normal individual, this excess calcium is excreted in the urine, and hypercalcemia is

extremely rare. In the dialysis patient this excretory route is not available, so the calcium accumulates in the extracellular fluid, often causing hypercalcemia. Activity corrects this situation. If that is not possible, then an inhibitor of bone resorption such as calcitonin, etidronate, or pamidronate might be helpful, though only the latter is approved for this problem in dialysis patients. Pamidronate has been shown to be safe in this setting (41).

Next to be considered is hyperparathyroidism or one of the low-turnover bone diseases. If the patient has hyperparathyroidism, the alkaline phosphatase will often be greater than 1.5 times the upper normal limit and the intact PTH level will be more than five times the upper normal limit. If hyperparathyroidism is identified, suppression may be attempted with intravenous or oral calcitriol pulse therapy (usually 1 to 3 μg after each dialysis) (37,38). Unlike conventional daily dosing, pulse therapy does not routinely worsen the hypercalcemia. Therapy may be continued as long as neither worsening hypercalcemia nor other complications develop. Perhaps 50% of patients respond to such therapy. In the other 50%, parathyroidectomy (33) will probably be necessary because of persistent hypercalcemia. (Details about this surgery and postoperative management are discussed later.)

On the other hand, if PTH is less than twice the upper limit of normal, hyperparathyroidism is not the problem. From the perspective of renal osteodystrophy, the most likely cause is a low-turnover bone lesion such as the aplastic lesion or osteomalacia. Hypercalcemia occurs because the bones are not taking up calcium and any administered calcium remains in the extracellular fluid. It does not require very much calcium supplementation to cause hypercalcemia if the calcium is distributed only in the relatively small extracellular compartment.

The low-turnover bone lesions (18) may result from oversuppression of PTH and continued calcium administration or occasionally from aluminum use. Aluminum is associated with toxicity not only to bone but also to brain and erythropoietic marrow. As discussed earlier, a random plasma aluminum level of 40 μg/L or even lower does not exclude aluminum bone disease (ABD). Although a random value of more than 100 μg/L strongly suggests ABD, in a patient with lower values whose clinical history suggests ABD, the deferoxamine (DFO) test will be helpful. In this test a baseline aluminum level is obtained before a midweek dialysis. During the last 2 hours of that dialysis deferoxamine is administered intravenously at a dose of 5 mg/kg (42–44). Before the next dialysis plasma aluminum is measured again. If the difference between the two values is greater than 150 μg/L, the diagnosis of aluminum toxicity is confirmed.

Treatment will depend on ancillary symptoms. If the patient has no symptoms, the treatment will be simply to eliminate all sources of aluminum. Similarly, if anemia or refractoriness to erythropoietin (EPO) is the only symptom, merely eliminating all aluminum intake is probably sufficient. On the other hand, if bone pain, fractures, or dementia to any degree are present, DFO therapy is indicated. Such therapy should be administered at a low dose (e.g., 5 mg/kg at the end of dialysis once a week) for a short time (2 to 3 months) and then repeated if symptoms recur. The high incidence of infections in dialysis patients treated with higher doses of DFO (particularly mucormycosis,

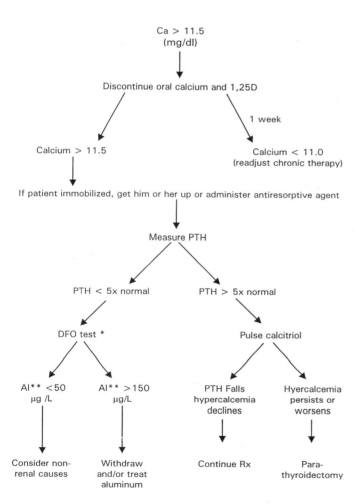

*DFO = deferoxamine
**Al = serum aluminum level

FIG. 26.4. Flow diagram for the evaluation and management of hypercalcemia in patients with renal failure.

which has been 95% fatal) mandates this cautious, conservative approach (45).

If aluminum excess is not present, the patient probably has the adynamic disorder without aluminum. Again, this condition is not as benign, as was once thought. These patients still appear to be at risk for future complications, including hypercalcemia, and bone pain or fracture. Treatment will include withdrawal of calcium and calcitriol. Lowering the calcium in the dialysate bath may stimulate PTH secretion, but further data are needed in this group of patients (46).

If these causes of hypercalcemia can be excluded, then one must think of disorders that cause hypercalcemia in the patient without kidney failure (47,48). Malignancy would be first on the list. Sarcoid and other granulomatous diseases (in which 1,25D is produced in excess from giant cells) might be strongly considered in black patients or in patients with an unknown cause of renal failure. A high 1,25D level would be strongly suggestive of sarcoid and unheard of in a chronic uremic patient not receiving supplemental 1,25D. Next, one would need to consider the many causes of hypercalcemia in the general population.

Bone Pain, Fracture, Poor Healing of Fracture

Patients experience bone pain at weight-bearing joints, particularly the hips, knees, ankles, and lower spine or ribs. This pain is usually seen with weight bearing and is relieved by rest. The disorders that cause bone pain are the same as those that cause pathologic fractures or poor healing of fractures, so this group of complaints will be considered together (Fig. 26.5).

Often these complaints are associated with hypercalcemia. When that is the case, one may follow the workup noted earlier for hypercalcemia. Management for bone pain or fracture in conjunction with hypercalcemia must be much more aggressive than for asymptomatic hypercalcemia, however. For instance, if hyperparathyroidism is present, it is unlikely that patients will respond to medical therapy; parathyroidectomy will almost always be required. Similarly, if aluminum intoxication is associated with fracture and hypercalcemia, deferoxamine chelation therapy will usually be necessary. Because of the serious concerns about infection with deferoxamine (45), therapy should be brief (perhaps 3 months in duration) and at a very low dose, such as 5 mg/kg given weekly at the end of a dialysis. A month after such a course is completed repeat assessment can determine if a second session might be worthwhile.

If hypercalcemia is not present (Fig. 26.4), the differential diagnosis still includes aluminum toxicity, hyperparathyroidism, mineral deficiency, β_2-microglobulin amyloidosis (uremia-related disorders), cancer, and other causes unrelated to renal failure (e.g., osteoporosis). The first two disorders may be pinpointed by the diagnostic criteria noted earlier. If aluminum intoxication is present, by those criteria, chelation therapy may be necessary for the fracture to heal. However, the serious complications of infection with deferoxamine treatment must be kept in mind. Hyperparathyroidism without hypercalcemia often responds to 1,25D and calcium. This therapy should be tried for at least 2 months to see if the fracture heals before parathyroidectomy is considered.

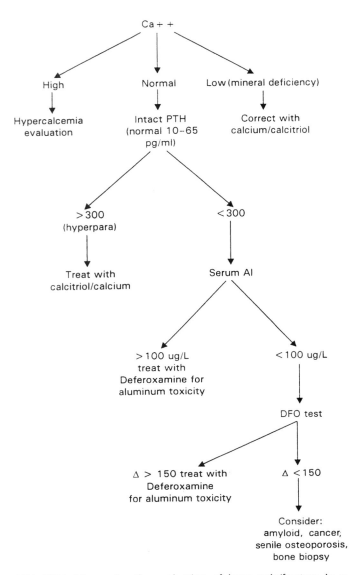

FIG. 26.5. Schema for the evaluation of bone pain/fracture in a chronic dialysis patient.

If the diagnosis still is unclear, amyloidosis must be considered in the presence of bone cysts or polyarthralgia. A history of carpal tunnel syndrome is usually obtained. Ultrasound studies often show thickening of the capsule at the shoulder joint. A bone biopsy may identify the characteristic amyloid fibrils or exhibit a positive Congo red stain. However, because of the patchy nature of the lesion, it may be missed (see Chapter 23).

If still lacking a clear-cut diagnosis at this point, one must consider either doing a bone biopsy (primarily to exclude aluminum toxicity or hyperparathyroidism) or pursuing a possible occult malignancy. A patient with either hypercalcemia or bone fracture from malignancy has little likelihood of prolonged survival (48), so such an evaluation is of marginal value. On the other hand, the bone biopsy may well reveal a treatable pathology.

If a clinician decides to perform a bone biopsy, the procedure should be discussed ahead of time with the laboratory that will assess the biopsy. Few hospital pathology laboratories are equipped or have the expertise to interpret bone histology, but several national laboratories and numerous excellent regional laboratories provide this service. It is particularly important that tetracycline labeling be performed. The sample should be obtained from the iliac crest, should contain a substantial amount of cancellous (trabecular) bone, and should be handled properly (Table 26.2). Random samples from fracture sites or obtained at surgery or autopsy are not useful for bone histology, though they may be helpful in the diagnosis of malignancy.

Metastatic Calcifications, Calciphylaxis

If the calcium × phosphate product is high enough, all patients will form calcium deposits. There is, however, a striking difference in patient sensitivity to different products. Few dialysis patients will have difficulties with products less than 70, and many patients tolerate products over 100 for years without obvious distress. The response, then, is highly variable.

With a high calcium × phosphate product, deposits in the skin may produce intolerable itching. Curiously, it takes several months of good phosphate control before such symptoms are relieved. The patient will often argue that control was tried (usually for a week or two) and did not work. Because patients may need 3 months of good control before itching is relieved (and chemistries are reasonable), this attitude must be countered and corrected.

Tumorlike calcifications also occur with high products (1). These generally form around joints and may interfere with joint function. Infection of one of these masses is a life-threatening complication. The infection will usually not be treatable without removal of the involved mass.

Deposits in vessels take the form of medial calcinosis. These deposits may aggravate preexisting atherosclerotic lesions and contribute to ischemia. Gangrenous digits have been reported to result. Both good phosphate control and parathyroidectomy have been reported to be beneficial (49–52). Recent concerns about vascular calcification related to calcium loading and hyperphosphatemia have led to searches for new binders and lower target values for these chemistries (14,15,51).

Calcium deposits have also been described in the lungs and heart. In the lungs, calcium is found in the alveolar capillary basement membrane. A progressive, restrictive lung disease occurs that has been fatal in all recognized cases. Occasionally, this lesion is seen on x-rays as a diffuse, fine, granular deposit, but a negative x-ray does not rule out the lesion. The lesion should be suspected in patients with a progressive, restrictive pulmonary lesion associated with a high calcium × phosphate product. Small deposits also occur in the heart and may impinge on the conduction system, causing arrhythmias.

None of these conditions is necessarily associated with calciphylaxis, a disorder characterized by evidence of soft-tissue calcification, vascular calcifications, and ischemic skin necrosis (49). The skin lesions are the hallmark of the disease. These lesions are usually seen in association with high phosphate levels; the lesions may occur in dialysis or transplant patients and rarely in patients without renal disease. The lesions sometimes respond to parathyroidectomy and are probably prevented by good phosphate control. Recent data suggest that protein C

deficiency is an important predisposing factor in patients who develop this rare syndrome, but this observation has not yet provided any useful therapeutic maneuvers (50).

In summary, there is a variable sensitivity to calcium phosphate product in dialysis patients. Some patients will develop tissue calcification at much lower levels than others. Phosphate control is preventive. Parathyroidectomy will result in mobilization of much of the deposited calcium, presumably with translocation to the bone. If patients resume their poor compliance, the lesions will inevitably recur and no treatment will work.

Parathyroidectomy

At present, numerous potential options are available for parathyroidectomy (4,7): total parathyroidectomy, total parathyroidectomy with transplant of a remnant into the arm, or subtotal parathyroidectomy leaving a remnant in the neck.

Our own preference is to do a total parathyroidectomy in patients who are not transplant candidates because of the frequency of recurrence in patients who have subtotal resections (7). In patients who are likely to be transplanted, our preference is to identify all glands and remove all but the smallest. Surgeons must remember that 5% of people have fewer than four glands and 10% have more than four. Therefore finding three glands and removing them all will be excessive 5% of the time and inadequate 10% of the time.

We do not favor the transplantation of tissue into the arm because of the difficulty in knowing what to do when there is

Recurrence—in which case one must prove that there is no residual tissue in the neck

Local invasion by the transplanted tissue, as is commonly seen

Occasional occurrence of malignancy in these transplanted remnants (5)

For similar reasons, we do not like leaving a remnant of a gland in the neck. There are numerous examples of wide seeding of parathyroid tissue in the neck (parathyromatosis) when glands are transected in situ.

We reported five patients with secondary hyperparathyroidism complicated by parathyromatosis. Two had subtotal parathyroidectomy and three had total parathyroidectomy with autotransplantation. All required repeated surgeries for recurrent hyperparathyroidism. Some had evidence of soft-tissue calcification or muscle weakness, whereas others had multiple fractures. Two out of the five patients eventually died of complications (6).

The hungry bone syndrome occurs in many parathyroidectomized uremic patients who have successful surgeries. In this syndrome, the sudden decrease in PTH levels results in an almost immediate, rapid decrease in bone resorption. Bone formation continues at a very high rate. Thus large amounts of calcium continue to enter the skeleton, but little comes out. When this occurs an excellent guide to the amount of calcium patients will require postoperatively is provided by the weight of the parathyroid tissue removed. For every gram of tissue resected, patients will require 1 g of calcium chloride over the following 24 hours. (The gluconate compound provides much less elemental calcium.) This rule has been useful in the management of more than 50 patients with removed tissue weighing from 1.5 to 17 g. The infusion should be started as soon as the patient reaches the recovery room. At this infusion rate, patients with successful surgery will maintain a total calcium between 8.5 and 10.5 mg/dL. Calcium must be measured every 6 hours for the first day or two. If calcium levels rise when on this therapy, it usually means that the surgery has been inadequate. This infusion rate will generally be necessary for the first day or two, then a gradual reduction can occur over the next 2 or 3 days until the patient can be maintained on oral calcium and calcitriol.

High doses of oral calcium (up to 10 g daily) and calcitriol (up to 4 μg daily) may be necessary for as long as 1 to 2 months after surgery. Gradual reductions to more conventional doses will then be dictated by the serum calcium level, which will need to be monitored frequently until the patient is taking reasonable doses of both compounds.

Recently, we have observed that patients who have received high-dose parenteral vitamin D before parathyroidectomy (in an attempt to suppress PTH) may not develop hungry bone syndrome (Sherrard, personal observation). This may be another example of vitamin D's effect on bone being independent of its effect on PTH (33,34).

RENAL TRANSPLANTATION AND BONE DISEASE

Strictly speaking, bone disease that follows renal transplantation is not renal osteodystrophy, but it is a major problem that many nephrologists must frequently face (53). Therefore a brief review of the condition, together with considerations for prevention and management, follows.

The bone diseases associated with transplantation are not unique to kidney transplants but occur with other kinds of transplants as well (54). Cyclosporine has been implicated, but its relationship to bone disease remains controversial (55,56). Steroids play a known major role in these conditions. Steroids increase bone resorption and decrease bone formation by numerous mechanisms, not surprisingly resulting in serious bony complications. Two kinds of bone disease occur in transplant patients: avascular necrosis (aseptic necrosis) and osteopenia (steroid-related osteoporosis) (54,57–61).

Avascular Necrosis

Avascular necrosis (AVN) affects all weight-bearing joints, particularly the hip. In this disorder, the weight-bearing surface of the concave component (such as the femoral head) fails. This bone dies and is not replaced. The death of this segment of bone results in additional stress being placed on adjacent bone, which may also collapse, resulting in a larger lesion. Often multiple lesions occur, such as bilateral hip disease or disease of the knee and ankle simultaneously. In one case of bilateral AVN of the hips, the shoulder joints also failed when the patient was forced to use crutches, which converted the shoulder to a weight-bearing joint.

AVN occurs in 5% to 30% of transplant patients, usually in the first year after transplant, though it may occur later (57–59). AVN occurs more frequently in patients who receive high doses of steroid. There are several theories about the etiology of the disease, but none are proven. The cause may vary from case to case or be multifactorial. The leading theory today is that steroids induce fat cells to proliferate in the marrow space with resultant marked increases in intraosseous pressure. This pressure allegedly interferes with perfusion at the site and the ischemic bone dies. A flaw with this theory is that the pressure measurements were all done after the disease had developed, so it is unclear whether the high pressure was the cause or the result of the injury.

The diagnosis of AVN is usually made after the patient begins to complain of pain in the hip. For obscure reasons, patients initially may experience pain in the knee (51). Routine x-rays are usually negative at this stage, but as time progresses radiographs will show a defect in the femoral head. Bone scans are more helpful than x-rays but may still be negative for several weeks after symptoms begin. Magnetic resonance imaging (MRI) is definitive and often reveals the lesion even before symptoms develop (Fig. 26.6). For this reason it has been sug-

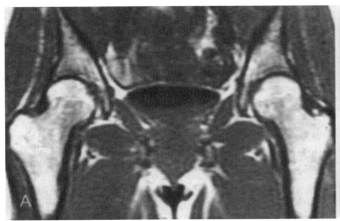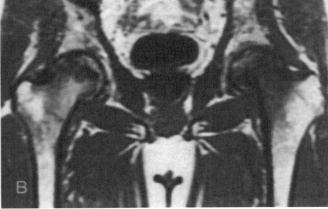

FIG. 26.6. Magnetic resonance images from a transplant patient. **A:** Normal femoral heads at the time of transplant. **B:** Avascular necrosis of the femoral heads 3 months after transplant.

gested that MRIs be monitored frequently so that the lesion can be detected earlier. Because there is no specific therapy for the condition, at this point MRIs do not appear necessary.

Prevention of AVN involves using the lowest possible dose of steroids. As cyclosporine has also been incriminated, replacing steroids with high doses of this agent is not a justifiable alternative (54). Newer agents that permit very low doses of steroids or even steroid-free regimens offer great hope, but no data have yet been reported to support this hope. Other sensible but unproven approaches include aggressive treatment of renal osteodystrophy before transplant and careful monitoring and maintenance of calcium and phosphate following transplant. Many transplant patients have renal wasting of calcium and phosphate with significant hypocalcemia and hypophosphatemia. The physician should correct such abnormalities with calcium, phosphate, and vitamin D supplements as necessary.

Once AVN occurs, hip replacement will usually be required. With a small, asymptomatic lesion, inactivity and limited weight bearing may permit healing and recovery. Lesions greater than about 5 mm, however, usually will not respond to this conservative approach. In these lesions some orthopedists recommend decompressing the femoral head by inserting a needle up the femoral neck into the diseased area of the femoral head, allowing the high intraosseous pressure to be dissipated (57–59). No controlled studies document the efficacy of this approach, though supportive anecdotal reports exist.

Steroid-Related Osteoporosis

Steroid-related osteoporosis is less dramatic than AVN but is equally difficult to manage. Data suggest that almost all transplant patients will eventually develop osteoporosis. This form of osteoporosis is usually recognized when the transplant patient begins to fracture. Initial fractures may be associated with mild trauma, but often are not. Any bones may be involved, but the metatarsal bones often fracture first. Subsequently, fractures occur in vertebrae, wrists, other long bones, and the femoral neck (56). When fractures begin to occur, routine x-rays usually show osteopenia, which generally means a reduction of total body calcium of greater than 30%. Specific measurements of bone density (e.g., dual energy x-ray analysis) will show bone density to be often as low as 50% of age-matched controls (56). Bone biopsy reveals a marked decrease in all bone cells and, in some cases, a relatively greater bone resorption than bone formation. With this histologic picture it is not surprising that fractures in these patients are often slow to heal.

The etiology of the bone loss with steroids is multifactorial (56,60). A variety of growth factors are suppressed, resulting in impaired osteoblast function. It is likely, though less well established, that osteoclast function is stimulated. In addition, renal calcium and phosphate wasting occur, and gut absorption of calcium is also decreased.

As with AVN, prevention involves treating renal osteodystrophy before transplant and counteracting and correcting the calcium abnormalities that occur after the transplant. Serum calcium and phosphate need to be maintained with appropriate dietary supplements. Vitamin D will often be needed to bring serum levels of calcium and phosphate up to normal. Thiazides,

which increase tubular reabsorption of calcium, may help if there is severe renal calcium wasting.

Preventive therapy appears increasingly important. Early studies by Cunningham have shown that pamidronate given at the time of transplant may eliminate the bone loss that so commonly occurs (61). Similar efficacy has been reported for heart transplantation, and others have found pamidronate very effective in preventing bone loss in patients treated with steroids for a variety of reasons (62). Its safety is well established in patients with renal disease (41). This inhibitor of bone resorption may prove a boon to transplant patients in the future if steroids continue to be a mainstay of immunosuppressive therapy.

Clearly, there is little to offer the transplant patient who is already having fractures. We must be aggressive about treating bone disease before transplantation and about correcting the known posttransplant abnormalities as well as possible. This is an area that demands additional research, both into better immunosuppressive protocols and into ways of counteracting steroid toxicity.

ACKNOWLEDGMENTS

This study was supported by funds from the General Medical Research Services of the Department of Veterans Affairs.

REFERENCES

1. Johnson C, et al. Roentgenographic manifestations of chronic renal disease treated by periodic hemodialysis. *Am J Roentgenol* 1967;101: 915–926.
2. Sherrard DJ. Aluminum—much ado about something. *N Engl J Med* 1991;324:558–559.
3. Kurokawa K. Calcium-regulating hormones and the kidney. *Kidney Int* 1987;32:760–771.
4. Ogg CS. Parathyroidectomy in the treatment of secondary renal hyperparathyroidism. *Kidney Int* 1973;4:168–173.
5. Hampl H, et al. Recurrent hyperparathyroidism after total parathyroidectomy and autotransplantation in patients with long-term hemodialysis. *Miner Electrolyte Metab* 1991;17:256–260.
6. Stehman-Breen G, et al. Secondary hyperparathyroidism complicated by parathyromatosis. *Am J Kidney Dis* 1996;28:502–507.
7. Kaye M, et al. Elective total parathyroidectomy without autotransplant in end-stage renal disease. *Kidney Int* 1989;35:1390–1399.
8. Audran M, et al. The physiology of the vitamin D endocrine system. *Semin Nephrol* 1986;6:4–20.
9. Fraser DR, et al. Unique biosynthesis by kidney of a biologically active vitamin D metabolite. *Nature* 1970;228:764–767.
10. Haussler MR, et al. Basic and clinical concepts related to vitamin D metabolism and action. *N Engl J Med* 1977;297:974–983, 1041–1050.
11. Russell J, et al. Suppression by $1,25(OH)_2 D_3$ of transcription of the pre-proparathyroid hormone gene. *Endocrinology* 1986;119: 2864–2867.
12. Madsen S, et al. Direct feedback regulation of PTH-secretion by 1,25 dihydroxyvitamin D_3 in renal failure: a controlled trial. *Proc EDTA* 1980;17:557–564.
13. Sherrard DJ, et al. Aluminum-related osteodystrophy. *Adv Intern Med* 1989;34:307–323.
14. Goodman WG, et al. Coronary artery calcification in young adults with end-stage renal disease who are undergoing dialysis. *N Engl J Med* 2000;342:1478–1483.
15. Chertow GM, et al. Sevelamer attenuates the progression of coronary

and aortic calcification in hemodialysis patients. *Kidney Int* 2002;62: 245–252.

16. Malluche H, et al. Renal bone disease 1990: an unmet challenge for the nephrologist. *Kidney Int* 1990;38:193–211.

17. Andress DL, et al. The osteodystrophy of chronic renal failure. In: Schrier RW, et al., eds. *Diseases of the kidney,* 5th ed. Boston: Little, Brown, 1993:2759–2788.

18. Sherrard DJ, et al. The spectrum of bone disease in end-stage renal failure—an evolving disorder. *Kidney Int* 1993;43:436–442.

19. Pei Y, et al. Risk factors for renal osteodystrophy: a multivariant analysis. *J Bone Miner Res* 1995;10:149–158.

20. Hercz G, et al. Aplastic osteodystrophy: follow-up after 5 years. *J Am Soc Neph* 1994;5:851A.

21. Sherrard DJ, et al. Single-dose tetracycline labeling for bone histomorphometry. *Am J Clin Pathol* 1989;91:682–687.

22. Onishi S, et al. β₂-microglobulin deposition in bone in chronic renal failure. *Kidney Int* 1991;39:990–995.

23. Kleinman KS, et al. Amyloid syndromes associated with hemodialysis. *Kidney Int* 1989;35:567–575.

24. Parfitt AM. The hyperparathyroidism of chronic renal failure: a disorder of growth. *Kidney Int* 1997;52:3–9.

25. Slatopolsky E, et al. Phosphorus restriction prevents parathyroid gland growth: high phosphorus directly stimulates PTH secretion in vitro. *J Clin Invest* 1996;97:2534–2540.

26. Ibels LS, et al. Preservation of function in experimental renal disease by dietary restriction of phosphate. *N Engl J Med* 1978;298:122–126.

27. Denda M, et al. Phosphorus accelerates the development of parathyroid hyperplasia and secondary hyperparathyroidism in rats with renal failure. *Am J Kidney Dis* 1996;28:596–602.

28. Quarles LD, et al. Intact parathyroid hormone overestimates the presence and severity of parathyroid-mediated osseous abnormalities in uremia. *J Clin Endocrinol Metab* 1992;75:145–150.

29. Wang W, et al. Relationship between intact I-84 parathyroid hormone and bone histomorphometric parameters in dialysis patients without aluminum toxicity. *Am J Kidney Dis* 1995;26:836–844.

30. Goodman WG, et al. Perspectives on parathyroid hormone (PTH), PTH-derived peptides, and new PTH assays in renal osteodystrophy. *Kidney Int* 2003;63:1–11.

31. Goodman WG, et al. Development of adynamic bone in patients with secondary hyperparathyroidism after intermittent calcitriol therapy. *Kidney Int* 1994;46:1160–1166.

32. Monier-Faugere MC, et al. Improved assessment of bone turnover by the PTH-(1-84)/large C-PTH fragments in ESRD patients. *Kidney Int* 2001;60:1460–1468.

33. Andress DL, et al. Intravenous calcitriol in the treatment of refractory osteitis fibrosa of chronic renal failure. *N Engl J Med* 1989;321:274–279.

34. Coen G, et al. PTH 1–84 and PTH "7-84" in the non-invasive diagnosis of renal bone disease. *Am J Kid Dis* 2002;40:348–354.

35. Coburn JW, et al. Calcium citrate markedly enhances aluminum absorption from aluminum hydroxide. *Am J Kidney Dis* 1991;17: 708–711.

36. Kausz A, et al. Screening plasma aluminum levels in relation to aluminum bone disease among asymptomatic dialysis patients. *Am J Kid Dis* 1999;34:688–693.

37. Martin KJ, et al. Pulse oral calcitriol for the treatment of hyperparathyroidism in patients on continuous ambulatory peritoneal dialysis: preliminary observations. *Am J Kidney Dis* 1992;19:540–545.

38. Sprague S, et al. Suppression of PTH secretion in hemodialysis patients: comparison of paricalcitol with calcitriol. *Am J Kid Dis* 2001; 38:S551–S556.

39. Arnaud SB, et al. Effects of 1 week head-down tilt bed rest on bone formation and the calcium endocrine system. *Aviat Space Environ Med* 1992;63:14–20.

40. Stewart AF, et al. Calcium homeostasis in immobilization: an example of resorptive hypercalciuria. *N Engl J Med* 1982;306:1136–1140.

41. Machado CE, et al. Safety of Pamidronate in patients with renal failure and hypercalcemia. *Clin Nephrol* 1996;45:175–179.

42. Pei Y, et al. Non-invasive prediction of aluminum bone disease in hemodialysis and peritoneal dialysis patients. *Kidney Int* 1992;41: 1374–1382.

43. Milliner DS, et al. Use of deferoxamine infusion test in the diagnosis of aluminum-related osteodystrophy. *Ann Intern Med* 1984;101: 775–780.

44. D'Haese PC, et al. Use of low deferoxamine test to diagnose and differentiate between patients with aluminum related bone disease, increased risk for aluminum toxicity or aluminum overload. *Nephrol Dial Transplant* 1995;10:1874–1884.

45. Windus DW, et al. Fatal *Rhizopus* infections in hemodialysis patients receiving deferoxamine. *Ann Intern Med* 1987;107:678–680.

46. Hercz G, et al. Aplastic osteodystrophy without aluminum: the role of "suppressed" parathyroid function. *Kidney Int* 1993;44:860–866.

47. Potts JT. Hypercalcemia. In: Braunwald E, et al., eds. *Principles of internal medicine.* New York: McGraw-Hill, 1987:1870–1882.

48. Ralston SH, et al. Cancer-associated hypercalcemia: morbidity and mortality. *Ann Intern Med* 1990;112:499–504.

49. Gipstein RM, et al. Calciphylaxis in man. *Arch Intern Med* 1976;136: 1273–1280.

50. Mehta RL, et al. Skin necrosis associated with acquired protein C deficiency in patients with renal failure and calciphylaxis. *Am J Med* 1990; 88:252–257.

51. Block GA, et al. Association of serum phosphorus and calcium × phosphate product with mortality risk in chronic hemodialysis patients: a national study. *Am J Kid Dis* 1998;31:601–617.

52. Cassidy MJD, et al. Renal osteodystrophy and metastatic calcification in long-term continuous ambulatory peritoneal dialysis. *Q J Med* 1985; 54/213:29–48.

53. Julian BA, et al. Musculoskeletal complications after renal transplantation: pathogenesis and treatment. *Am J Kidney Dis* 1992;19:99–120.

54. Rich GM, et al. Cyclosporin A and prednisone associated osteoporosis in heart transplant recipients. *J Heart Lung Transplant* 1992;11: 950–958.

55. Dumoulin G, et al. Lack of evidence that cyclosporine treatment impairs calcium-phosphorus homeostasis and bone remodeling in normocalcemic long-term renal transplant recipients. *Transplantation* 1995;59:1690–1694.

56. Lukert BP, et al. Glucocorticoid-induced osteoporosis: pathogenesis and management. *Ann Intern Med* 1990;112:352–364.

57. Nielsen HE, et al. Aseptic necrosis of bone following renal transplantation. *Acta Med Scand* 1977;202:27–35.

58. Felsen DT, et al. A cross-study evaluation of association between steroid dose and avascular necrosis of bone. *Lancet* 1987;1:902–906.

59. Ficat RP. Idiopathic bone necrosis of the femoral head: early diagnosis and treatment. *J Bone Joint Surg* 1985;67B:3–9.

60. Rickers H, et al. Corticosteroid-induced osteopenia. *Clin Endocrinol* 1982;16:409–415.

61. Fan S, et al. Pamidronate therapy for prevention of bone loss following renal transplantation. *Kidney Int* 2000;58:682–690.

62. Boutsen Y, et al. Primary prevention of glucocorticoid induced osteoporosis with intravenous pamidronate and calcium. *J Bone Min Res* 2001;16:104–112.

ACID–BASE CONSIDERATIONS IN END-STAGE RENAL DISEASE

F. JOHN GENNARI

Maintenance of normal body pH and P_{CO_2} depends on daily replenishment of body alkali stores that are either consumed, neutralizing strong acids produced by normal body metabolism, or lost in the stool (1–4). This task is normally accomplished by the kidneys through an incompletely defined system of sensors and effectors that regulate H^+ and NH_4^+ secretion in the renal tubules (4). The result is acid balance, achieved by reabsorption of all the filtered HCO_3^- and, in addition, excretion of just enough acid (primarily as NH_4^+) to generate the new HCO_3^- needed to replenish the HCO_3^- lost from the body (Fig. 27.1). This renal process is flexible, responding rapidly to changes in acid production, and precise, maintaining blood $[HCO_3^-]$ remarkably constant from day to day.

As kidney disease progresses, renal regulation of acid balance is lost and metabolic acidosis ensues, due to a failure both to match endogenous acid production with acid excretion and to recapture filtered HCO_3^-. Initiation of renal replacement therapy addresses this problem not by removing H^+ but by adding

HCO_3^- to the body on a regular basis. As discussed in this chapter, the net addition of HCO_3^- during dialysis therapy is regulated not by any physiologic feedback mechanism but by the physical principles of diffusion and convection (5–8). This switch has major implications for acid–base homeostasis, changing the way one thinks about both normal and disordered acid balance.

GENERAL PRINCIPLES

Regardless of the alkali source added to the dialysis bath or infused during renal replacement therapy, a new equilibrium is achieved that is driven primarily by variations in endogenous acid production, just as in individuals with normal renal function (5,7,8). The fundamental reason for this linkage is that the net gain of HCO_3^- is directly related to the transmembrane concentration gradient. Thus the lower the concentration of HCO_3^- in the body fluids at the onset of treatment, the greater will be the net entry of alkali. In patients receiving renal replacement therapy, the prevailing serum $[HCO_3^-]$ is determined jointly by the characteristics of the dialytic process and by endogenous acid production. Because the dialysis prescription is fixed, the variable component is endogenous acid production, which likely accounts for most of the variability in serum $[HCO_3^-]$ in end-stage renal disease (ESRD) patients (5,7,8). Although less flexible than functioning kidneys, this property of dialysis allows for variations in endogenous acid production to be matched by variable amounts of net HCO_3^- addition during treatment. The details of how this equilibrium is achieved are discussed later, first for peritoneal dialysis and then for various forms of hemodialysis.

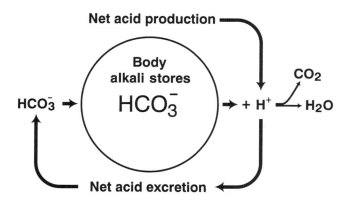

In steady state: Net acid excretion = Net acid production

FIG. 27.1. Normal acid–base balance. Net acid production, comprising endogenous acid production and the difference between the alkali added by the diet and the alkali lost in the stool, adds new H^+ to the body fluids. These ions react with HCO_3^-, yielding CO_2 and H_2O. In the steady state, through an as yet undefined signal, the kidney adjusts net acid excretion (NH_4^+ plus titratable acid excretion minus any HCO_3^- lost in the urine) to match net acid production, thereby adding back an equivalent amount of HCO_3^-.

ACID–BASE HOMEOSTASIS IN PERITONEAL DIALYSIS

Alkali Source

To replenish alkali stores with peritoneal dialysis, the bath solution contains the HCO_3^- precursor, lactate, in most instances. (A new delivery system using HCO_3^- as the alkali source is discussed at the end of this section.) Lactate ions in the bath dif-

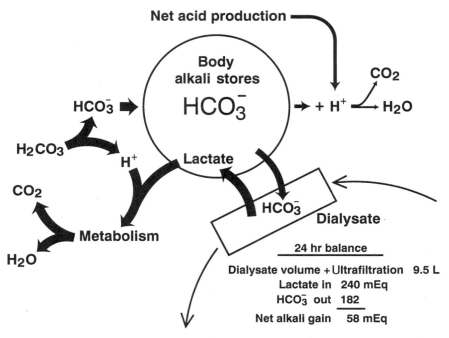

FIG. 27.2. Acid balance in peritoneal dialysis. Net acid production consumes body HCO_3^- stores, yielding CO_2 and H_2O. To replenish HCO_3^- stores, lactate is added from the dialysis fluid and metabolized to produce new HCO_3^- ions. A large portion of the new HCO_3^- is lost by diffusing back into the peritoneal dialysis fluid. Because the rate of HCO_3^- loss is dependent on the transmembrane concentration gradient, a new steady state is achieved. As shown in the example, the serum [HCO_3^-] is at a level at which the difference between lactate added and HCO_3^- lost each day is equal to daily net acid production.

fuse into the extracellular compartment and enter cells coupled to H^+, generating new HCO_3^- in the extracellular fluid (Fig. 27.2). To retain the newly gained HCO_3^-, the intracellular lactate (and H^+) must be metabolized to CO_2 and water or to a stable neutral compound such as glucose. In fact, under most conditions virtually all lactate is metabolized, primarily in the liver, to generate an equivalent amount of new HCO_3^- (9). Until recently, the lactate in peritoneal dialysis solutions was racemic (containing both D- and L-lactate). The L-lactate is metabolized readily, but D-lactate is more slowly metabolized (through conversion to L-lactate), leading to small but measurable levels of this form in the blood (10,11). This delay in metabolism is of no clinical significance; nonetheless, D-lactate has been removed from most peritoneal dialysis solutions (12). The concentration of lactate in peritoneal dialysis solutions was initially set empirically at 35 mM, but most bath solutions now have a concentration of 40 mM because it results in more nearly normal serum [HCO_3^-] (13,14).

Acid–Base Balance

The process by which acid–base balance is achieved in peritoneal dialysis is illustrated in Fig. 27.2. The rate of lactate entry from the bath to the patient is determined by its transmembrane concentration gradient, its permeability across the peritoneal membrane, and the total surface area available for exchange. The added lactate is rapidly metabolized, and serum levels do not increase notably during dialysis, allowing a large and favorable concentration gradient (~39 mEq/L) to be maintained. During a standard 6-hour dwell time, approximately 75% of the lactate in the bath is absorbed and metabolized, yielding an equivalent amount of new HCO_3^- (9). Because the bath contains no HCO_3^-, this anion diffuses from the patient to the bath down its concentration gradient (7,9). Its rate of diffusion is governed by the same principles that determine lactate entry, but because it is not metabolized in the bath its concentration rises. After 6 hours of dwell time, bath [HCO_3^-] is approximately 80% of serum [HCO_3^-] (9). The net alkali gained for any given time period is equal to the difference between the HCO_3^- lost during the treatment and the lactate added and metabolized (7,9).

In the quantitative example shown in Fig. 27.2, four 2-L exchanges are carried out each day, resulting in the ultrafiltration of 1.5 L (total dialysate volume plus ultrafiltration = 9.5 L/d). Assuming a serum [HCO_3^-] of 24 mEq/L, such a treatment regimen will result in the addition of 240 mEq of lactate and the loss of 182 mEq of HCO_3^- each day, based on the equilibrium values discussed earlier. The difference, 58 mEq, is the net alkali gained. If this amount is less than the daily consumption of HCO_3^- by net acid production, serum [HCO_3^-] will fall and the amount of HCO_3^- lost will fall as well, leading to greater net alkali addition. If the net alkali added exceeds the amount of HCO_3^- consumed, then serum [HCO_3^-] will rise, and the

TABLE 27.1. STEADY-STATE ACID–BASE VALUES IN PATIENTS RECEIVING PERITONEAL DIALYSIS

Type	Bath [Lactate] (mM)	N	Venous [total CO₂] (mEq/L)	Reference
CAPD[a]	35	31	23.9 ± 4.0	14
CAPD	40	25	27.4 ± 3.3	14
	40	8	26.0 ± 3.3	13
	40	20	26.3 ± 2.5	6
	40	8	28.8 ± 3.0	9
	40	17	24.0 ± 3.1	7
CCPD	40	13	27.9 ± 2.0	—[b]

Type	Bath [Lactate] (mM)	N	Arterial [HCO₃⁻] (mEq/L)	pH	PCO₂ (mmHg)	Reference
CAPD	40	69	22.1 ± 3.1 —	—	—	12
CAPD[c]	0	9	22.0 ± 2.6	7.37 ± .04	37.9 ± 3.3	17
CAPD[d]	0	9	25.9 ± 2.0	7.42 ± .04	39.0 ± 3.6	17

[a]CAPD, four exchanges/day; CCPD, overnight cycling peritoneal dialysis.
[b]Gennari, new observations.
[c]HCO₃⁻ bath, 34 mEq/L.
[d]HCO₃⁻ bath, 39 mEq/L.

amount of this anion lost will rise as well, reducing net alkali addition. Thus a new steady state is achieved whereby the prevailing serum [HCO₃⁻] is determined largely by net acid production (7,8).

An experimental assessment of these theoretical considerations has been carried out in patients receiving peritoneal dialysis (9). The patients studied had higher values for steady-state serum [HCO₃⁻] than in the example in Fig. 27.2, and as a result had an average net gain of alkali of only 31 mEq/d. This gain, however, coupled with the net alkali content of the diet, equaled estimated net acid production, and thus the patients were in acid balance. A surprising finding in this study is that the bulk (65% to 70%) of acid production was accounted for by organic acids produced and lost into the bath solution. In fact, nonlactate organic anion loss was essentially equal to net alkali gain in these patients. Sulfate production was lower than expected, based on dietary protein intake, and was entirely counterbalanced by dietary net alkali. The low sulfate production in these patients remains unexplained.

These measurements confirm that, in the steady state, acid balance is achieved as predicted by the theoretical considerations presented earlier. From this analysis, it is apparent that variations in serum [HCO₃⁻] among patients receiving peritoneal dialysis are primarily due to changes in net acid production reflective of differences in diet and tissue catabolism. On average, however, blood pH and [HCO₃⁻] values are usually within or very close to the normal range found in individuals with functioning kidneys (Table 27.1).

Overnight Cycling Peritoneal Dialysis

Peritoneal dialysis using four 6-hour exchanges a day has largely been supplanted with overnight cycling, using an automated exchange device. This new technique uses shorter dwell times and allows for a much larger volume of fluid to be exchanged, enhancing urea clearance. Because the rate of diffusion of HCO₃⁻ across the peritoneal membrane appears to be slightly higher than lactate (see earlier), one might predict that shorter

dwell times would decrease net alkali gain, resulting in a lower steady-state serum [HCO₃⁻]. Although no formal studies have been carried out comparing the two forms of peritoneal dialysis, overnight cycling appears to have no impact on serum [HCO₃⁻]. In our program, all patients are on overnight cycling, and mean serum [total CO₂] is 28 mEq/L, a value virtually identical to that reported with manual four-exchange peritoneal dialysis (Table 27.1).

Peritoneal Dialysis with HCO₃⁻ Bath

Bicarbonate is the ideal alkali replacement for all dialysis bath solutions but has not been used in peritoneal dialysis because of the problem of precipitation with calcium at alkaline pH values. This technical problem has been overcome by using a two-compartment dialysis bath bag (15,16). One compartment contains the HCO₃⁻ solution and the other, the calcium solution. The two compartments are mixed just as the solution is infused into the peritoneal space, where the prevailing CO₂ tension keeps the pH in a range that prevents calcium precipitation. When this system is used, serum [HCO₃⁻] is, not surprisingly, directly related to bath [HCO₃⁻], with more optimal acid–base status achieved when bath [HCO₃⁻] is increased from 34 to 39 mEq/L (Table 27.1) (17). The increase in serum [HCO₃⁻] after the switch to the bath solution with the higher [HCO₃⁻] is also inversely correlated with endogenous acid production (estimated from protein catabolic rate) (17), again demonstrating the dependence of steady-state serum [HCO₃⁻] on endogenous acid production.

Although average serum [total CO₂] in patients using lactate-based peritoneal dialysis solutions is essentially normal (Table 27.1), it has been argued that [total CO₂] is below the normal range in many patients and that the normal average value is due to a small subset of patients with metabolic alkalosis (12). In fact, average arterial [HCO₃⁻] in patients receiving standard peritoneal dialysis with a lactate-containing bath may be lower than normal (Table 27.1). As discussed later, increasing serum [HCO₃⁻] in patients receiving peritoneal dialysis has been demonstrated to improve muscle metabolism and well-being (18,19). Despite these arguments, the additional expense and inconvenience of the HCO_3^-–based solution has not gained wide acceptance. Perhaps the most practical argument for its use is in patients with infusion pain. In such patients, the use of a HCO_3^-–containing bath, either as the sole alkali or combined with lactate, markedly reduces this troublesome symptom (20).

ACID–BASE HOMEOSTASIS IN HEMODIALYSIS

Conventional hemodialysis is an intermittent treatment, in contrast to the continuous nature of peritoneal dialysis. As a result, there is no day-to-day steady state with regard to alkali stores and serum $[HCO_3^-]$. As diagrammed in Fig. 27.3, alkali is added as rapidly as possible during a 3- to 4-hour treatment three times a week. This added alkali is then gradually dissipated during the period between treatments, as HCO_3^- is consumed by endogenous acid production. Thus, from an acid–base perspective, hemodialysis patients undergo a continuous back-and-forth fluctuation from postdialysis metabolic alkalosis to predialysis metabolic acidosis. Given this fluctuation in serum $[HCO_3^-]$ (by as much as 7 to 8 mEq/L from the end of one dialysis to the beginning of the next), it is important to note when acid–base status is assessed. By convention, one usually reports the predialysis value and, ideally, the nadir predialysis value obtained after the longest interval between treatments (Table 27.2).

Alkali Source

The alkali source used for hemodialysis has come full circle, from HCO_3^- in the 1950s to mid-1960s, to acetate from the mid-1960s through the 1980s, and back to HCO_3^- in the 1990s. When hemodialysis was first developed, the bath solution contained HCO_3^- in a concentration of 27 mEq/L (21), but the concentration was empirically increased to 35 mEq/L over the next decade to improve alkali transfer (22). To prevent

precipitation of $CaCO_3$, bath pH was adjusted to 7.4 by aeration with a carbon dioxide/oxygen gas mixture. Acetate was first introduced as an alkali precursor in 1964 (23). This organic anion was chosen because it was metabolized readily by most tissues in the body (24), allowing for rapid HCO_3^- production during treatment. Because its use obviated the need for aerating the bath with CO_2, acetate simplified bath preparation and quickly replaced HCO_3^- as an alkali source.

This change created a bidirectional dynamic similar to that for peritoneal dialysis with lactate, but more rapid and impressive in magnitude. Almost as quickly as acetate is converted to HCO_3^- during hemodialysis, the new HCO_3^- is lost back into the bath (5). As a result, the only way to add alkali is to overcome its rate of metabolic removal and raise the acetate concentration in the blood. After the dialysis session is over, this unmetabolized acetate is converted to HCO_3^- and retained by the patient. By trial and error, a bath acetate concentration of 37 mEq/L was settled on to achieve this goal. This concentration represented a compromise between providing sufficient substrate for HCO_3^- generation during each treatment and limiting the rate of acetate delivery to an amount that could be metabolized without producing toxic levels (25–27).

Despite the ease of bath preparation, alkali repletion using acetate is a remarkably inefficient process. During a 4-hour hemodialysis treatment, for example, more than 700 mEq of HCO_3^- is lost into the bath (5,26). This large HCO_3^- loss limits alkali replenishment, so that patients receiving this form of dialysis have predialysis serum $[HCO_3^-]$ values of less than 18 mEq/L, on average (5,6,26,28). As blood-flow rates and dialyzer membrane permeability increased, the amount of acetate delivered also increased, and serum acetate concentration reached toxic levels, causing hypotension and other symptoms (25,27,29–32). An additional problem was CO_2 loss from the patient to the bath, an effect that decreased ventilatory drive and contributed to dialysis-induced hypoxemia (32,33).

Because of these problems, HCO_3^- was again introduced as the source for alkali replenishment in the early 1980s (34,35).

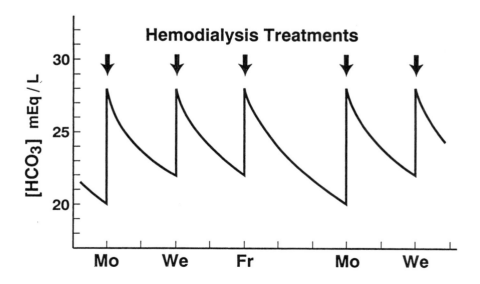

FIG. 27.3. Schematic representation of the pattern of serum [HCO₃⁻] in a patient receiving hemodialysis treatments three times weekly (Monday, Wednesday, Friday). Serum [HCO₃⁻] is only intermittently lower than normal, and only falls to its nadir once a week at the end of the long interval between treatments.

TABLE 27.2. STEADY-STATE PREDIALYSIS ACID–BASE VALUES IN PATIENTS RECEIVING CONVENTIONAL HEMODIALYSIS[a]

Year	N	[Total CO2] (mEq/L)	Reference
1990[b]	22	21.4 ± 2.4	6
1993	38	19.0 ± 3.1	45
1996[b]	44	20.4 ± 2.0	7
1999	995	21.6 ± 3.4	41
2000[c]	7123	22.8 ± 3.5	40
2002[b]	80	22.9 ± 3.3	—[d]

Year	N	[HCO3−] (mEq/L)	pH	Pco2 (mmHg)	Reference
1982	10	18.9 ± 2.5	7.37 ± .09	33 ± 2.5	34
1983	10	20.2[e]	7.40 ± .04	33 ± 1.2	47
1985	16	19.8 ± 1.2	7.37 ± .02	36 ± 1.9	31

[a]Three times weekly with a bicarbonate bath (final concentration 32–36 mEq/L).
[b]Values obtained after longest interval between treatments.
[c]Midweek predialysis value.
[d]Gennari, new observations.
[e]Calculated from mean pH and Pco2.

Reintroduction of HCO_3^- into the bath solution was made possible by a new technology, the use of a proportioning system that allows continuous production of dialysate from concentrated salt solutions during treatment. In such a system, $NaHCO_3$ is added to the rest of the bath solution just prior to delivery to the dialysis membrane. At the moment of HCO_3^- addition, the pH of the bath is reduced by the presence of a small amount of acetic acid. The acetic acid reacts rapidly with the added HCO_3^-, yielding a mixture of HCO_3^- (most commonly at a final concentration of 35 mEq/L), acetate (4 mEq/L), and CO_2 (4 mmol/L, equivalent to a Pco2 of 133 mm Hg). The high Pco2 in the bath falls rapidly as it diffuses across the dialysis membrane, raising the post-filter blood Pco2 to approximately 50 mm Hg (36). The inward diffusion of CO_2 reverses the loss from the patient that occurred with acetate dialysis (see earlier) but has no impact on systemic Pco2 or ventilation (26,36). The acetate produced by this reaction also diffuses across the dialysis membrane into the blood, providing a small additional source of new HCO_3^- as it is metabolized.

Reintroduction of HCO_3^- into the hemodialysis bath solution increased predialysis serum [HCO3−] by 3 to 4 mEq/L (31,32,34,35,37,38), and decreased patient symptoms (31,32,34,39). By 1990, this technology essentially completely replaced acetate hemodialysis. The subsequent discussion of acid–base homeostasis in patients receiving hemodialysis will only cover baths containing HCO_3^-. For further information about the dynamics of acid–base equilibrium when acetate is the sole buffer substance in the bath, the reader is referred to earlier reviews (5,6,26,27).

Virtually all bath solutions currently used for conventional hemodialysis combine 39 mEq/L of HCO_3^- with 4 mmol/L of acetic acid, yielding a final bath [HCO3−] of 35 mEq/L and [acetate] of 4 mEq/L when mixed. Assuming the acetate enters the blood and is completely metabolized, this combination is equivalent to a total alkali concentration of 39 mEq/L. As will

be discussed further later, newer dialysis machines provide the ability to vary bath [HCO3−] from 25 mEq/L to 40 mEq/L.

Acid–Base Balance

Although the transient events are more complex than in peritoneal dialysis, a similar equilibrium is almost certainly established between net acid production and alkali addition in patients receiving chronic intermittent hemodialysis. The amount of HCO_3^- added from the bath to the patient during a hemodialysis session is primarily dependent on the dialysance of this anion (a function of dialysis membrane surface area and permeability) and the transmembrane concentration gradient (Fig. 27.4). Because the bath [HCO3−] is fixed, as are the surface area and permeability of the membrane, the variable factor in this relationship is serum [HCO3−]. The serum [HCO3−] at the beginning of each treatment is determined primarily by the rate of acid production in the interdialytic period (see later). The lower the initial value, the greater the initial rate of HCO_3^- addition, and vice versa.

The total amount of HCO_3^- added during each hemodialysis treatment is determined not only by the initial transmembrane concentration gradient, but also by the rate of change in the gradient. To the extent that newly added HCO_3^- is retained in the extracellular compartment, its concentration in the blood will rise, diminishing the gradient across the dialysis membrane as the treatment progresses. The minute-to-minute change in this gradient is determined by the extent to which the added HCO_3^- is consumed by the rapid production of H^+ from body buffers (Fig. 27.4). The immediate buffer response to rapid alkalinization of the body fluids includes not only the release of H^+ from nonbicarbonate buffers, but also the stimulation of organic acid production (4,5,7,37,38).

Increases in organic acid production can produce almost unlimited amounts of new H^+ to titrate and remove added HCO_3^- from the extracellular compartment. If the organic anions produced by this titration are retained, they eventually will be metabolized and will regenerate the HCO_3^- titrated by their formation. Organic anions, however, readily cross the dialysis membrane and are lost into the dialysate soon after their formation (Fig. 27.4) (37,38). At blood-flow rates much lower than are now customarily used, losses of 30 to 50 mEq of organic anions have been measured during a standard hemodialysis treatment (37,38). Because many more organic acids are produced than were measured in these studies, and because blood flow and therefore clearance rates have increased, it seems likely that organic anion losses are now even higher (7). The magnitude of this response to added HCO_3^- remains undefined, but it is clear that organic acid production and loss of the organic anions formed can have a major influence on net alkali addition during hemodialysis (7).

The transmembrane HCO_3^- concentration gradient could also be influenced if the blood returning to the dialyzer contained an admixture of slowly mixing pools with differing [HCO3−], but whether this occurs to any measurable degree is unknown. Finally, it is conceivable that there are ionic constraints on HCO_3^- diffusion, despite the presence of a favorable concentration gradient, as it competes with Cl^- and negatively

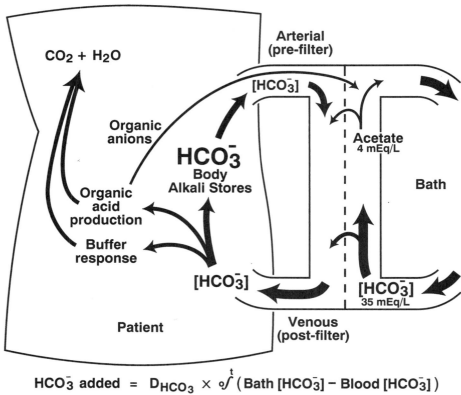

$$HCO_3^- \text{ added} = D_{HCO_3} \times \int^t (\text{Bath } [HCO_3^-] - \text{Blood } [HCO_3^-])$$

In steady state: Alkali gained = Net acid production

FIG. 27.4. Alkali addition and disposition during hemodialysis. During each hemodialysis treatment, body HCO_3^- stores are replenished by the addition of HCO_3^- and acetate from the bath. The added HCO_3^- is partially consumed by titration with body buffers and by organic acid production. The remaining HCO_3^- is added to the pool and raises $[HCO_3^-]$ in the blood returning to the hemodialysis membrane, reducing the transmembrane concentration gradient and thereby limiting further HCO_3^- addition. The total amount of HCO_3^- added is determined by its dialysance (D_{HCO_3}) and by the integral over the time of treatment of the transmembrane concentration gradient. Because the variable component of the transmembrane gradient is serum $[HCO_3^-]$, a new steady state is achieved at a serum $[HCO_3^-]$ at which the alkali added with each treatment is equivalent to net acid production.

charged proteins for charge balance with the cations in the blood, particularly during the latter half of the treatment. These factors probably influence net alkali addition to much less than do the buffer and organic acid responses, but their contribution remains undefined.

Assuming the factors controlling alkali addition during hemodialysis are constant from treatment to treatment, the amount of HCO_3^- added with each treatment is determined primarily by the steady-state predialysis serum $[HCO_3^-]$. This value, in turn, is determined by the rate of endogenous acid production in the period between treatments, and by the amount of fluid retained (see later).

In the steady state, a new equilibrium is achieved, in which the interplay between intradialytic and interdialytic events serves to maintain predialysis serum $[HCO_3^-]$ relatively constant. One should, of course, put the term *steady state* in parentheses, as the predialysis value for serum $[HCO_3^-]$ is the nadir in a descending trend, with the peak value occurring immediately after dialysis and falling gradually until the next session (Fig. 27.3). Because of the complex nature of the response to alkali addition

during hemodialysis and its variability from patient to patient, as well as differences in net acid production and fluid retention between treatments, predialysis serum $[HCO_3^-]$ varies more widely in patients receiving hemodialysis than in individuals with normal renal function (6,7,40,41).

Determinants of Postdialysis Serum $[HCO_3^-]$

Figure 27.5 shows the pattern and magnitude of the increase in serum $[HCO_3^-]$ during a single hemodialysis treatment. This figure shows the increase in serum $[HCO_3^-]$ induced by 4 hours of hemodialysis in seven stable patients, treated using a high-flux membrane with a blood-flow rate of 400 mL/min and a dialysate flow rate of 500 mL/min (7). The striking feature shown in this figure is that serum $[HCO_3^-]$ changes little, if at all, during the last 2 hours of dialysis, despite an 8 to 10 mEq/L gradient for HCO_3^- entry across the dialysis membrane. This pattern has been confirmed by other investigators (36,42). While the observations shown in Fig. 27.4 are characteristic, serum $[HCO_3^-]$ actually falls during dialysis in a small subset of

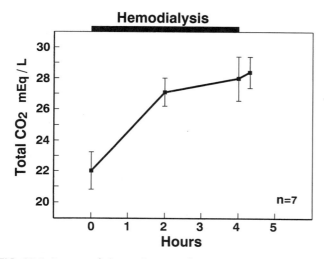

FIG. 27.5. Pattern of change in serum [total CO_2] during 4 hours of hemodialysis treatment, based on measurements in seven stable, non-diabetic patients. In these patients, [total CO_2] was measured before dialysis, after 2 hours, at the end of dialysis, and 15 minutes after completion of dialysis. The brackets around the data points are equal to ±1 standard error. Note that virtually the entire increase in [total CO_2] occurs during the first 2 hours of treatment.

TABLE 27.3. ESTIMATED EFFECT OF ENDOGENOUS ACID PRODUCTION AND FLUID RETENTION ON PREDIALYSIS SERUM [HCO_3^-] IN PATIENTS RECEIVING CONVENTIONAL HEMODIALYSIS

Acid Production (mEq/day)	Fluid Retention[a] (L/Interval)	Predialysis [HCO_3^-][b] (mEq/L)
40	2	23.4
80	2	20.4
120	2	17.3
60	0	23.1
60	3	21.3
60	6	19.8

Assumptions: weight = 70 kg; postdialysis serum [HCO_3^-] = 28 mEq/L; HCO_3^- buffer space = 0.5 × body weight (kg).
[a]Liters retained during longest interval between treatments.
[b]After longest interval between treatments (68 hr).

patients (7). The fall in these patients most likely is due to a surge in organic acid production, resulting from tissue hypoxia and hypotension, but this remains unproven.

Although the factors responsible for determining end-dialysis serum [HCO_3^-] remain to be completely elucidated, this value is of critical importance because it sets the platform from which [HCO_3^-] slowly falls in the period between treatments. Assuming no intervening events, the postdialysis serum [HCO_3^-] is normally determined primarily by the specific dialysis prescription for any given patient.

Determinants of Predialysis Serum [HCO_3^-]

In the interval between hemodialysis sessions, the two major determinants of the rate of fall in serum [HCO_3^-] are the rate of endogenous acid production and the rate of fluid retention. Endogenous acid production between treatments is determined primarily by diet; patients ingesting a diet low in sulfur-containing proteins will have low rates of endogenous acid production and vice versa (1,2). Although there is no information on the effect of specific diets on predialysis serum [HCO_3^-], a clear inverse correlation between normalized protein catabolic rate (an indirect measure of dietary protein intake in the steady state) and predialysis serum [HCO_3^-] is evident in patients receiving hemodialysis (40,41,43).

Based on these observations and a few assumptions, one can estimate the magnitude of the effect of variations in endogenous acid production on predialysis serum [HCO_3^-]. If one assumes that all the acid produced is retained and that the buffer space for the retained H^+ is 50% of body weight [an assumption supported by measurements in dialysis patients (43)], such an analysis predicts that variations in acid production will alter predialysis serum [HCO_3^-] by as much as 6 mEq/L (Table 27.3).

Given these assumptions, variations in daily acid production can mean the difference between a normal and frankly acidotic predialysis serum [HCO_3^-] level in patients receiving exactly the same dialysis prescription. Although the major determinant of endogenous acid production is dietary protein intake, the catabolic state of the patient will also influence acid production.

For the analysis shown in the first half of Table 27.3, we have assumed that 2 L of fluid is retained between each treatment, highlighting the importance of the second factor, fluid retention between runs. For any given rate of endogenous acid production, fluid retained without proportionate alkali between treatments will also decrease predialysis serum [HCO_3^-]. This is a "dilution acidosis," caused by an increase in the fluid compartment in which the existing HCO_3^- stores are distributed. Using a fixed value for endogenous acid production of 60 mEq/d, keeping the same assumptions for buffering, and assuming that changes in ECF fluid volume do not have any special effects on the buffer response, one can also predict the effect of variations in fluid retention on predialysis serum [HCO_3^-]. As shown in the lower portion of Table 27.3, this effect is almost as profound as changes in acid production. This theoretical analysis also has experimental support; a difference of only 1 L in fluid retention between dialysis treatments has been shown to affect predialysis serum [HCO_3^-] by more than 1 mEq/L (44). The implications of these effects for the management of acid–base equilibrium in patients receiving hemodialysis are obvious and discussed further later.

Normal Values for Pre-Dialysis Serum [HCO_3^-]

The average predialysis serum [HCO_3^-] (or [total CO_2]) for stable patients receiving three hemodialysis treatments a week ranges from 19 to 23 mEq/L (Table 27.2) (6,7,40,41,45). These values are lower than those in individuals with normal renal function and in patients receiving peritoneal dialysis therapy, and they show a much wider range of values. The respiratory response to hypobicarbonatemia is normal in ESRD (5,27,28, 31,37,46), and therefore P_{CO_2} is appropriately reduced when serum [HCO_3^-] is low. As a result, average blood pH is only either within the normal range or only slightly reduced (Table

27.2) (31,34,38,47). Little attention has been paid to the very mild acidemia found in most patients receiving conventional hemodialysis because it is only present intermittently and had been assumed to have no adverse effects (5). However, as discussed later, it appears that even a mild and intermittent acidosis can have deleterious effects on bone and muscle metabolism, and may be a risk factor for mortality.

EFFECTS OF METABOLIC ACIDOSIS ON BONE AND MUSCLE METABOLISM, AND ON MORTALITY

In two randomized prospective studies, a steady-state predialysis serum [HCO$_3^-$] of less than 19 mEq/L was associated with impaired parathyroid hormone responsiveness to changes in serum calcium concentration and with more severe bone disease (48,49). In one of these studies, predialysis serum [HCO$_3^-$] was increased from 15.6 to 24 mEq/L by increasing bath [HCO$_3^-$] (Table 27.4), and this change arrested the progression of both high- and low-turnover bone disease, despite otherwise equivalent management (49). In the second study, predialysis serum [HCO$_3^-$] was increased from 18.6 to 25.3 mEq/L using the same approach (Table 27.4), and this maneuver improved the sensitivity of parathyroid hormone to changes in serum calcium concentration (48).

In addition to worsening bone disease and blunting the responsiveness of the parathyroid gland to changes in calcium, a low predialysis serum [HCO$_3^-$] also appears to have adverse effects on protein metabolism. In one study, a low predialysis serum [HCO$_3^-$] (18.5 mEq/L) was associated with high muscle protein turnover, a measure of muscle catabolism, and raising this value to 24.8 mEq/L by increasing bath [HCO$_3^-$] (Table 27.4) reduced protein turnover (50). The same group of investigators demonstrated a similar reduction in protein turnover in patients receiving peritoneal dialysis in whom steady-state serum [HCO$_3^-$] was increased from 19 to 26 mEq/L by giving oral NaHCO$_3^-$ supplements (18). These results have been supported by several other studies showing a beneficial effect on increasing predialysis serum [HCO$_3^-$] on muscle metabolism (51–53).

In addition to effects on bone and muscle metabolism, the relative risk of death in hemodialysis patients increases in patients with low values for predialysis serum [HCO$_3^-$] (as compared with a reference group with values between 20 and 22.5 mEq/L) (54). In a large group of patients (almost 20,000) the risk increased by 10% for values between 17.5 and 20 mEq/L, and rose even more dramatically for lower values. In the same study, the relative risk for mortality also increased in patients with predialysis values of more than 22.5 mEq/L. Although this seems an argument against increasing predialysis [HCO$_3^-$], it is not. All the patients in this study were dialyzed against a bath with the same [HCO$_3^-$] three times a week. Thus the patients with higher predialysis serum [HCO$_3^-$] were probably malnourished due to poor protein intake or had superimposed metabolic alkalosis (see later).

Management of Patients with Low Serum [HCO$_3^-$]

Given the evidence cited earlier, some have advocated increasing predialysis serum [HCO$_3^-$] to 24 mEq/L or higher in all dialysis patients (55). Although this recommendation remains controversial, it seems clear that one should assess the cause of the low predialysis serum [HCO$_3^-$] in patients with persistent values of less than 19 mEq/L. This assessment should include an analysis of both the events between treatments and during dialysis. The rate of serum fall [HCO$_3^-$] between treatments can be assessed by comparing the end-dialysis value with the next predialysis value. As discussed earlier, the key factors influencing the rate of decline are nutrition (specifically, protein intake) and fluid retention. If dietary adjustments are called for, one must be careful to ensure that overall nutrition remains adequate, as protein malnutrition will certainly not be beneficial for the patient (54). If fluid retention is excessive, a reduction in intake between treatments should be encouraged, recognizing that this is a difficult undertaking. For completeness, one should also determine whether patients are losing large amounts of HCO$_3^-$ in their urine (if they still have significant urine output) or in their stool (diarrhea states, see later). To assess intradialysis events, measurement of serum [HCO$_3^-$] pre- and postdialysis can easily answer the question of whether the added alkali has been retained or consumed by excessive organic acid production.

Regardless of the cause, predialysis serum [HCO$_3^-$] can now easily be increased by increasing bath [HCO$_3^-$] (42,45, 48–52,55). Table 27.4 summarizes the results of studies in which bath [HCO$_3^-$] was increased to improve predialysis

TABLE 27.4. IMPROVING PREDIALYSIS SERUM [HCO$_3^-$] IN CONVENTIONAL HEMODIALYSIS: TECHNIQUES AND RESULTS

N	Duration (months)	[HCO$_3^-$] (mEq/L)		Technique	Reference
		Baseline	Treatment		
11	18	15.6	24.0	↑ Bath [HCO$_3^-$] to 40–48 mEq/L	49
38	3	19.0	24.8	↑ Bath [HCO$_3^-$] to 39 mEq/L	45
8	1	18.6	25.3	↑ Bath [HCO$_3^-$] to 40 mEq/L	48
6	1	18.5	24.8	↑ Bath [HCO$_3^-$] to 40 + oral NaHCO$_3$	50
9	1	20.0	25.0	↑ Bath [HCO$_3^-$] to 40 + oral NaHCO$_3$	42
12	6	18.8	23.1	↑ Bath [HCO$_3^-$] to 36 + oral NaHCO$_3$	51
21	6	20.4	23.3	↑ Bath [HCO$_3^-$] to 40 mEq/L	52
25	6	22.5	26.7	↑ Bath [HCO$_3^-$] to 40 mEq/L	52

serum [HCO_3^-]. These studies demonstrate that postdialysis [HCO_3^-] is directly related to bath [HCO_3^-], and this value in turn exerts a parallel effect on the nadir serum [HCO_3^-] before the next treatment. In these studies, postdialysis serum [HCO_3^-] increased to 30 to 34 mEq/L, but this relative alkalemia was not associated with any adverse events.

An alternative (or supplemental) approach is to administer oral sodium bicarbonate on a daily basis. This supplement will effectively increase predialysis serum [HCO_3^-] (42,50,51,56), or steady-state serum [HCO_3^-] in peritoneal dialysis patients (18). The potential problems with bicarbonate supplementation include patient compliance and stimulation of thirst with a resultant increase in weight gain between treatments (56).

Given the wide range in predialysis serum [HCO_3^-] in hemodialysis patients (40,41), some have recommended individualizing bath alkali concentration to achieve normal acid–base values before dialysis in every patient (57). This task is relatively simple to achieve now that machines are available to allow one to vary bath [HCO_3^-] for each individual treatment. An alternative approach is simply to increase bath [HCO_3^-] in all concentrates (55).

DAILY HEMODIALYSIS

The use of daily hemodialysis treatments, either in critically ill inpatients or in stable outpatients, readily normalizes serum [HCO_3^-] and pH (58–60). In stable outpatients receiving daily slow nocturnal hemodialysis treatments, the difference between pre- and postdialysis serum [HCO_3^-] is reduced to less than 1 mEq/L and bath [HCO_3^-] has been reduced to 28 to 32 mEq/L to avoid metabolic alkalosis (Pierratos, personal communication) (see Chapter 11). These results are not surprising, given the dynamic changes in serum [HCO_3^-] described earlier for intermittent hemodialysis. No long-term data have been published evaluating the effect of this change in serum [HCO_3^-] on morbidity and mortality.

CONTINUOUS RENAL REPLACEMENT THERAPIES

Continuous hemofiltration, hemofiltration plus dialysis, and slow low-efficiency hemodialysis are all currently used for the treatment of renal failure in critically ill patients (61–63). With these techniques, the same principles hold with regard to acid–base homeostasis as discussed earlier for conventional hemodialysis. With continuous hemofiltration HCO_3^- loss is related to the serum concentration and the ultrafiltration rate, as well as to the ongoing rate of endogenous acid production. Replacement is achieved with a continuous infusion of either a HCO_3^- or lactate-containing solution (63,64), and serum [HCO_3^-] is readily maintained within the range of normal (60). With continuous slow, low-efficiency dialysis, serum [HCO_3^-] becomes essentially equal to the concentration in the dialysis bath solution and the latter must be reduced to 24 to 28 mEq/L to prevent the development of metabolic alkalosis (65).

Hemofiltration and Hemodiafiltration

Hemofiltration uses the principle of convection rather than diffusion for toxin removal, and can be used as an intermittent therapy. To achieve adequate toxin removal, high-volume ultrafiltration occurs during the procedure, necessitating the rapid infusion of replacement fluids (at approximately 100 mL/min) (66). Although acetate-containing solutions were originally used for this procedure, replacement solutions containing HCO_3^- are necessary for adequate acid–base homeostasis (66). The high-volume ultrafiltration and rapid infusion of replacement solutions make the technique more complex and subject to risk than conventional hemodialysis, and it is rarely used now.

Hemodiafiltration combines the high convective characteristics of intermittent hemofiltration with a bath solution containing either acetate or HCO_3^- (67,68). For this treatment, replacement solutions containing HCO_3^- are necessary to achieve positive net alkali addition, and the procedure has the same complexity as hemofiltration and little advantage over conventional hemodialysis from an acid–base perspective.

Acetate-free biofiltration is a hemodiafiltration technique in which the dialysate contains no HCO_3^- or acetate but does contain other key solutes (69). High-volume ultrafiltration is carried out, and isotonic $NaHCO_3$ is continually infused into the postfilter blood. One proposed advantage for this procedure is the removal of all acetate from the bath, but there is no evidence that the small amount of acetate currently used in bath solutions has any clinically important toxicity. As opposed to regular hemodiafiltration where the replacement solution contains all electrolytes, only $NaHCO_3$ is reinfused with this procedure, allowing for high concentrations of HCO_3^- to be used. Using this technique, one can predictably increase serum [HCO_3^-] to the level desired in each patient (69). As discussed earlier, the same goal can be achieved with conventional hemodialysis by adjusting the bath [HCO_3^-] in a simpler way, and acetate-free biofiltration is only rarely used for the treatment of ESRD.

ACID–BASE DISORDERS IN PATIENTS WITH END-STAGE RENAL DISEASE

Thus far, we have considered the factors determining the "normal" values for serum [HCO_3^-] in patients receiving renal replacement therapy. This section is directed at identifying and managing acute or chronic superimposed deviations in acid–base balance, or acid–base disorders, in this population of patients. Such disorders are heralded by deviations from the expected normal values for serum [HCO_3^-] and P_{CO_2} (Tables 27.1 and 27.2). In general, a change in serum [HCO_3^-] of 3 mEq/L or greater from the usual value should signal the presence of a new acid–base disorder.

Given the wide variation in predialysis serum [HCO_3^-] in this unique group of patients, identification of superimposed disorders seems a formidable task. Fortunately, however, an ongoing log of monthly values for serum [total CO_2] is available in most cases to use for comparison with a suspected abnormal value. Identifying an abnormality in P_{CO_2} is a more difficult undertaking because no laboratory trail exists for this parameter.

The ventilatory response to variations in serum [HCO$_3^-$] is normal in patients with renal failure (5,27,28,31,37,38), so one can use the following formulas to estimate the expected P$_{CO_2}$ for any given serum [HCO$_3^-$] if one has a clinical suspicion that a ventilatory problem is present:

For serum [HCO$_3^-$] values 24 mEq/L or less:

$$P_{CO_2} \text{ (mm Hg)} = 40 - 1.3 \times (24 - [HCO_3^-]) \quad (1)$$

For serum [HCO$_3^-$] values greater than 24 mEq/L:

$$P_{CO_2} \text{ (mm Hg)} = 40 + 0.7 \times ([HCO_3^-] - 24) \quad (2)$$

Although these equations should be considered only as approximations, they can be used as benchmarks for determining whether a measured P$_{CO_2}$ deviates significantly from the expected value. Given the variability in the ventilatory response to a given serum [HCO$_3^-$], one should consider the measured P$_{CO_2}$ to be abnormal only if it is 5 mm Hg or more from the expected value.

Once an abnormal P$_{CO_2}$ or serum [HCO$_3^-$] has been identified, the approach to characterizing the abnormality is the same as that in patients with normal renal function:

1. Identify the primary disorder (e.g., metabolic acidosis or alkalosis, respiratory acidosis or alkalosis).
2. Determine whether the adaptive response is appropriate.
3. Determine the cause of the disorder.

Although the general approach is the same, the diagnostic process is actually simpler than that in patients with normal renal function (Fig. 27.6). In ESRD patients, for example, there is no renal adaptive response to respiratory acid–base disorders. In addition, one need not consider renal forms of either metabolic acidosis or alkalosis in the differential diagnosis. The approach to each of the four cardinal acid–base disorders is discussed in following sections.

Metabolic Acidosis

A new metabolic acidosis is diagnosed in an ESRD patient when serum [HCO$_3^-$] falls by 3 mEq/L or more from the usual value in that patient (6). Unlike patients with normal renal function, one does not have to consider the possibility that chronic respiratory alkalosis is responsible, because the reduction in [HCO$_3^-$] induced by hypocapnia requires a functioning kidney. Although a primary respiratory alkalosis cannot be the cause of the low serum [HCO$_3^-$] in ESRD patients, blood pH and P$_{CO_2}$ should be measured to determine whether the ventilatory response to metabolic acidosis is appropriate. In patients with functioning fistulas this information can be gained without a separate arterial puncture (5,70). The normal adaptive response to metabolic acidosis results in a decrease in P$_{CO_2}$ of 1.3 mm Hg for each 1 mEq/L fall in serum [HCO$_3^-$] (equation 1 above) (46). If the measured P$_{CO_2}$ deviates from the expected value by more than 5 mm Hg, then the patient has a mixed disorder (see later). If the fall in P$_{CO_2}$ is within the expected range, then the patient has an uncomplicated metabolic acidosis (Fig. 27.6), and attention should be directed at diagnosing its cause.

Causes

Metabolic acidosis can be produced either by the sudden addition of a new acid to the body fluids or by the loss of HCO$_3^-$ (Table 27.5). As shown in the table, the major consideration is acid generation as a result of abnormalities in body metabolism, or through toxin-induced stimulation of acid production. The only site for HCO$_3^-$ losses in these individuals without renal function is from the gastrointestinal tract.

Separation of the causes of metabolic acidosis by assessment of whether the anion gap is increased or not is less useful in

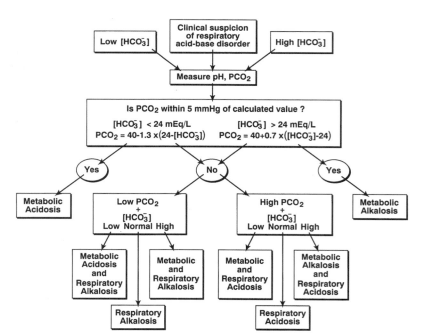

FIG. 27.6. Approach to the evaluation of acid–base disorders in patients with ESRD. The terms "low [HCO$_3^-$]" and "high [HCO$_3^-$]" in the diagram refer to values that are 3 mEq/L or more either lower or higher than the average values found in patients receiving renal replacement therapy (Tables 27.1, 27.2).

TABLE 27.5. CAUSES OF METABOLIC ACIDOSIS IN END-STAGE RENAL DISEASE

Increased Anion Gap	No Increase in Anion Gap
Diabetic ketoacidosis	Gastrointestinal alkal loss
Lactic acidosis	Diarrhea
Alcoholic ketoacidosis	Pancreatic drainage
Toxin ingestions	Hemofiltration
Methyl alcohol	NaCl replacement
Ethylene glycol	Ammonium chloride ingestion
Salicylates	
Paraldehyde	
Other causes	
Catabolic state	
High protein intake	
High intradialytic fluid intake	

ESRD patients than in patients with functioning kidneys. The anion gap is often already increased in these patients (6), and metabolic acidosis is virtually always associated with a further increase. The most useful tool is a baseline anion gap to allow assessment of any change, but with serum $[Na^+]$ not routinely measured in many dialysis centers, this value may not be available. In the absence of baseline data, an anion gap of more than 20 mEq/L should be considered abnormally high.

Organic Acidoses

The most common cause of a new metabolic acidosis in ESRD patients is a pathologic process that leads to overproduction of one or more organic acids. Diabetic ketoacidosis is the most common culprit, but one also should consider other causes such as alcoholic ketoacidosis, lactic acidosis, and toxin ingestions (Table 27.5). The organic acids produced by these disorders titrate and replace HCO_3^- in the body fluids, causing the anion gap to increase as the anions of these acids accumulate in the serum. In contrast to patients with functioning kidneys, ESRD patients cannot excrete these newly formed anions and they remain available to be metabolized, regenerating the HCO_3^-

that was consumed, once the pathologic process leading to their generation is reversed. This sequence of events is illustrated in Fig. 27.7 in an ESRD patient with diabetes mellitus who developed diabetic ketoacidosis (6). In this patient, the ketoacidosis rapidly lowered serum $[HCO_3^-]$ and increased the anion gap. Insulin therapy alone decreased the anion gap and increased serum $[HCO_3^-]$ from 14 to 25 mEq/L over 10 hours. Note that this recovery occurred without an intervening dialysis and it required only minimal fluid replacement and no exogenous alkali; these patients lose neither fluid nor organic anions when they develop ketoacidosis.

Although diabetic ketoacidosis is rapidly reversed by insulin therapy, production of other organic acids cannot be so easily halted. Thus dialysis is often required both to remove the organic anions and to rapidly replace them with HCO_3^-. Hemodialysis therapy is particularly useful when toxin ingestions lead to metabolic acidosis in anephric individuals, as this mode of therapy is the most effective in removing the offending toxins. In some types of lactic acidosis, production of lactic acid cannot be halted (71,72), and hemodialysis in this setting offers a means to replace HCO_3^- rapidly without causing fluid overload. Unfortunately, the rapid alkalinization accomplished by hemodialysis may simply serve to accelerate lactic acid production (72). As with all organic acidoses, reversal of the cause of the increase in acid production is key to sustained correction of the metabolic acidosis.

Other Causes

As discussed earlier, an increase in dietary protein intake or an increase in body protein catabolism will reduce predialysis serum $[HCO_3^-]$ (Table 27.3). Because the increase in endogenous acid production engendered is associated with anions other than chloride, this type of acidosis also increases the anion gap. An increase in fluid retention between hemodialysis treatments will also lower predialysis serum $[HCO_3^-]$ by diluting body alkali stores (Table 27.3). Neither an increase in ECF fluid volume nor an increase in protein catabolism is likely to produce a severe metabolic acidosis. If serum $[HCO_3^-]$ falls by more than

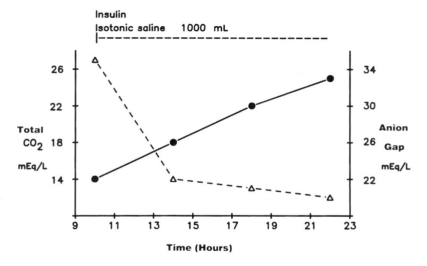

FIG. 27.7. Correction of diabetic ketoacidosis in a patient with ESRD without HCO_3^- administration or dialysis treatment. Serum [total CO_2] and serum anion gap were restored to preacidosis levels by the administration of insulin and 1 L of isotonic saline. (Reprinted with permission from Gennari FJ. Acid–base disorders in end-stage renal disease: part I. *Semin Dial* 1990;3:81–85.)

6 to 8 mEq/L acutely, one can be virtually certain that an organic acidosis is responsible.

Induction of metabolic acidosis from gastrointestinal HCO_3^- losses requires the development of severe diarrhea, or could occur from surgical drainage of fluid rich in pancreatic secretion. This form of metabolic acidosis does not increase the anion gap above the usual level, as the acidosis is associated with the disproportionate loss of HCO_3^- and therefore an increase in serum $[Cl^-]$. Inadvertent replacement of alkali in the bath with a chloride-containing solution is a technique error that will induce a severe metabolic acidosis without increasing the anion gap (73). An extremely rare cause of metabolic acidosis without a further increase in the anion gap is the deliberate or accidental ingestion of ammonium chloride. In patients with no renal function, renal tubular acidosis need not be considered as a cause of metabolic acidosis.

In patients treated with continuous hemofiltration, metabolic acidosis can be induced if an inappropriate replacement solution is used. If Ringer's lactate is used in a patient who is unable to metabolize this organic anion, the resulting metabolic acidosis will be associated with an increase in the anion gap, even though the acidosis is induced by HCO_3^- loss through hemofiltration. If sodium chloride is used as the replacement solution, then the acidosis will be associated with hyperchloremia and no increase in anion gap.

Metabolic Alkalosis

Metabolic alkalosis is diagnosed by the finding of an increase in serum $[HCO_3^-]$. In ESRD patients chronic respiratory acidosis is not a consideration, because the increase in serum $[HCO_3^-]$ engendered by sustained respiratory acidosis requires renal function. Metabolic alkalosis is generated by the selective loss of HCl from the body fluids (e.g., from vomiting or nasogastric drainage) or by the addition of new alkali. Unlike patients with functioning kidneys, the disorder is sustained once initiated, regardless of dietary intake (74). In addition, because the hypokalemia associated with metabolic alkalosis is primarily caused by renal K^+ losses, serum $[K^+]$ is unchanged from its usual value when metabolic alkalosis occurs in ESRD patients (75). Renal causes of metabolic alkalosis (e.g., Bartter's syndrome, primary hyperaldosteronism) need not be considered, nor is it necessary to partition the causes into chloride-sensitive and chloride-resistant groups.

An increase in serum $[HCO_3^-]$ of 3 mEq/L or more from the usual value in an ESRD patient is the working rule for diagnosing a new metabolic alkalosis, but because serum $[HCO_3^-]$ is lower than that of individuals with normal renal function, the diagnosis is often not recognized unless a much larger increase is present (some 8 to 10 mEq/L). One should not overlook smaller increases in serum $[HCO_3^-]$, however, because mortality rises in patients dialyzed with a standard bath solution who have predialysis serum $[HCO_3^-]$ values only 2 to 3 mEq/L higher than average (54). Although one does not have to consider chronic respiratory acidosis as a cause of the increase in serum $[HCO_3^-]$, one should measure blood pH and P_{CO_2} to ensure that the respiratory response to the metabolic alkalosis is in the expected range. The normal response to an increase in serum $[HCO_3^-]$ is

hypoventilation: for each 1 mEq/L increase in $[HCO_3^-]$, P_{CO_2} increases by 0.7 mm Hg (see equation 2 earlier). If the measured P_{CO_2} is within 5 mm Hg of the expected value, the patient has an uncomplicated metabolic alkalosis (Fig. 27.6). If the value deviates from this range, the patient has a mixed disorder (see later).

Causes

Table 27.6 presents the causes of metabolic alkalosis in ESRD patients. Note that there is no partition of the causes into chloride-responsive and chloride-resistant groups. There are only two categories to consider: loss of acid or the addition of new alkali. The former occurs only with vomiting or nasogastric drainage, and the diagnosis is almost always immediately apparent. However, bulimic patients may deny vomiting (75). The potential sources of alkali range from $NaHCO_3$ to certain anionic amino acids (Table 27.6). Administration of $NaHCO_3$ in a dose of 2 mEq/kg body weight will increase serum $[HCO_3^-]$ by 4 to 5 mEq/L (4,56). Calcium salts containing carbonate, acetate, or citrate only add alkali to the body to the extent that calcium is ionized and absorbed. Thus they rarely cause significant metabolic alkalosis.

A rare cause of metabolic alkalosis in ESRD patients is the combined use of sodium polystyrene sulfonate (kayexelate) and aluminum hydroxide (76). Aluminum hydroxide is usually converted to aluminum phosphate or chloride by gastric acid, and a portion of these salts dissociate in the duodenum, allowing aluminum ions to bind to HCO_3^- secreted by the pancreas. When kayexelate is present, however, aluminum ions bind to it instead, forming a compound that does not dissociate. As a result, no HCO_3^- is neutralized or bound, and this alkali is reabsorbed by the small intestine and retained in the body fluids.

Management

Management of metabolic alkalosis in ESRD patients should be directed at removing the cause. Treatment of the cause of vomiting and removal of any sources of exogenous alkali in most instances will lead to eventual correction of the disorder. If these interventions fail to correct the disorder and if the high serum $[HCO_3^-]$ is causing symptoms or interfering with management

---

TABLE 27.6. CAUSES OF METABOLIC ALKALOSIS IN END-STAGE RENAL DISEASE

Vomiting
Nasogastric drainage
Exogenous alkali/alkali precursor
   $NaHCO_3$
   $KHCO_3$
   $CaCO_3$
   Lactate
   Acetate
   Citrate
   Glutamate
   Proprionate
Aluminum hydroxide + kayexelate

(e.g., ventilator dependence), serum $[HCO_3^-]$ can be reduced by decreasing bath $[HCO_3^-]$, an option easily managed with the newer dialysis machines now available. Metabolic alkalosis in the anephric patient in the intensive care unit can also be corrected by using continuous hemofiltration and replacing losses with only sodium chloride (74) or by using slow, low-efficiency hemodialysis with a bath $[HCO_3^-]$ of 25 mEq/L.

Respiratory Acidosis

Respiratory acidosis is caused by alveolar hypoventilation and is manifest by an increase in arterial PCO_2. The normal adaptive response to this disorder has two separable components (77). The first is an acute buffer response that leads to only a very slight increase in serum $[HCO_3^-]$; the second and major component involves an adjustment in renal HCO_3^- generation. In ESRD patients no adaptation occurs in response to an increase in PCO_2; therefore none of the laboratory data normally collected in these patients will signal its presence. One must have a clinical suspicion for the disorder and then measure blood pH and PCO_2 to confirm it (Fig. 27.6). A PCO_2 value of 5 mm Hg or higher than the expected value for the prevailing serum $[HCO_3^-]$ establishes the diagnosis (see equations 1 and 2). One need not evaluate whether the serum $[HCO_3^-]$ is appropriate; serum $[HCO_3^-]$ is determined by the dialysis treatment rather than by PCO_2.

Because no renal adaptation occurs, hypercapnia leads to a sustained and severe acidemia in patients with ESRD. For example, a patient with a sustained PCO_2 level of 55 mm Hg and normal renal function will have only a minor reduction in blood pH, because this increment in PCO_2 will induce an increase in serum $[HCO_3^-]$ to 30 to 33 mEq/L through renal mechanisms. By contrast, an ESRD patient with the same PCO_2 level may have a predialysis serum $[HCO_3^-]$ of 20 mEq/L, with a resultant blood pH of 7.18.

Management

The management of respiratory acidosis should be directed at reversing the hypercapnia if at all possible. If the PCO_2 cannot be reduced to a safe level, one should use a dialysis modality that maximizes serum $[HCO_3^-]$, such as daily or continuous hemodialysis or peritoneal dialysis. Bicarbonate supplementation is also an option, but this therapy may lead to fluid overload, further embarrassing pulmonary gas exchange.

Respiratory Alkalosis

Respiratory alkalosis is caused by alveolar hyperventilation and is manifest by a decrease in arterial blood PCO_2. The normal adaptive response to this disorder has two separable components, acute and chronic (77). As in the case of respiratory acidosis, this distinction does not apply in patients with ESRD. The chronic response requires renal function and the acute response is overwhelmed by the effect of dialysis on serum $[HCO_3^-]$. Thus severe alkalemia can occur as a result of hyperventilation. Because the usual laboratory measurements obtained in ESRD patients do not change notably, one must

have a clinical suspicion that the disorder is present and measure blood pH and PCO_2 to establish the diagnosis. The presence of a PCO_2 level that is 5 mm Hg or more lower than expected for the prevailing serum $[HCO_3^-]$ indicates the presence of respiratory alkalosis (see equations 1 and 2, and Fig. 27.6).

Causes and Management

Many pathologic events can cause respiratory alkalosis (Table 27.7). In contrast to patients with normal renal function who can tolerate hypocapnia without serious complications, patients with renal failure can develop severe and sustained life-threatening alkalemia. Blood pH levels greater than 7.70 have been reported in patients with sustained respiratory alkalosis receiving peritoneal dialysis therapy (78,79). In one patient with sustained respiratory alkalosis receiving conventional hemodialysis, we observed an arterial pH greater than 7.80. If hypocapnia cannot be corrected, one can attempt to reduce serum $[HCO_3^-]$ by continuous hemofiltration without alkali replacement (using only saline) in an intensive care unit setting, but mortality is high if the problem persists.

Mixed Acid–Base Disorders

Mixed acid–base disorders occur when two or more primary acid–base abnormalities are present at the same time. In patients with ESRD, the spectrum of possible mixed disorders is narrower than in patients with renal function, because of the absence of any compensation for hypo- and hypercapnia (Table 27.8). The most common mixed disorders are a combination of metabolic and respiratory disturbances. These are diagnosed by measuring PCO_2 and using equations 1 and 2 to determine if the value is appropriate for the concomitantly measured serum $[HCO_3^-]$. If the serum $[HCO_3^-]$ is low (metabolic acidosis), the ventilatory response can be inadequate (superimposed respiratory acidosis) or greater than expected (respiratory alkalosis). The former is more common and can be associated with severe

TABLE 27.7. CAUSES OF RESPIRATORY ALKALOSIS

Hypoxemia
Central nervous system disorders
 Anxiety–hyperventilation syndrome
 Stroke
 Infection
 Trauma
 Tumor
Pulmonary disease
 Pneumonia
 Pulmonary edema
 Pulmonary embolus
 Interstitial fibrosis
Other causes
 Gram-negative sepsis
 Hepatic failure
 Pregnancy
Drugs
 Salicylates
 Nicotine

TABLE 27.8. MIXED ACID–BASE DISORDERS IN END-STAGE RENAL DISEASE

Mixed metabolic and respiratory disorders
$\downarrow$ [HCO_3^-]
P_{CO_2} > expected – metabolic + respiratory acidosis[a]
P_{CO_2} < expected – metabolic acidosis + respiratory alkalosis
$\uparrow$ [HCO_3^-]
P_{CO_2} > expected – metabolic alkalosis + respiratory acidosis
P_{CO_2} < expected – metabolic + respiratory alkalosis
Metabolic acidosis + alkalosis
Anion gap $\uparrow$ without equivalent $\downarrow$ in [HCO_3^-]
(Δanion gap – Δ[HCO_3^-] > 5 mEq/L)
Triple disorders
Metabolic acidosis + alkalosis +:
P_{CO_2} > expected – respiratory acidosis
P_{CO_2} < expected – respiratory alkalosis

[a]Using formulas 1 and 2 (see text and Fig. 27.6).

acidemia. Urgent intubation and assisted ventilation is needed for such patients in addition to management of the metabolic acidosis. If the serum [HCO_3^-] is high (metabolic alkalosis), this disorder can also be associated with an inadequate or greater than normal ventilatory response. When primary hyperventilation (respiratory alkalosis) complicates metabolic alkalosis, life-threatening increases in pH can occur. Attention should be directed at increasing P_{CO_2} if possible, or urgently reducing serum [HCO_3^-].

More rarely, a mixed metabolic alkalosis and acidosis can occur. The sequence that might cause such a disorder in a dialysis patient would be the administration of exogenous alkali, increasing serum [HCO_3^-], followed by the development of a lactic acidosis or diabetic ketoacidosis. Such a sequence might fortuitously result in a serum [HCO_3^-] at or near normal levels, but the disorder is uncovered by finding an increase in the anion gap. If the respiratory response to the final serum [HCO_3^-] in such a patient is abnormal, then a triple disorder is diagnosed.

SUMMARY

From an acid–base perspective, two issues should be addressed in the management of ESRD patients. First, one must understand the forces determining the steady-state serum [HCO_3^-] and modify these forces as necessary to prevent the complications of metabolic acidosis. The available evidence indicates that intervention should be undertaken in those individuals with predialysis or steady-state serum [HCO_3^-] levels of less than 19 mEq/L.

Second, one must recognize and treat superimposed acid–base disorders in these patients. The approach to diagnosing these disorders is actually simpler in patients with no renal function. One need not consider metabolic acid–base disorders caused by changes in renal alkali or acid excretion, nor need one consider renal adaptive responses to respiratory acidosis or alkalosis. The laboratory data normally accumulated in these patients facilitate the quick identification of changes in serum [total CO_2] caused by either metabolic acidosis or alkalosis, but respiratory acid–base disorders must be suspected on clinical grounds. Diagnosis and

management of uncomplicated acid–base disorders is straightforward. Although relatively uncommon, mixed disturbances can occur in patients with renal failure, and their recognition and management can be life-saving.

REFERENCES

1. Kurtz I, et al. Effect of diet on plasma acid–base composition in normal humans. *Kidney Int* 1983;24:670–680.
2. Lennon EJ, et al. The effects of diet and stool composition on the net external acid balance of normal subjects. *J Clin Invest* 1966;45:1601–1607.
3. Relman AS, et al. Endogenous production of fixed acid and the measurement of the net balance of acid in normal subjects. *J Clin Invest* 1961;40:1621–1630.
4. Gennari FJ, et al. Renal regulation of acid–base homeostasis: integrated response. In: Seldin DW, et al., eds. *The kidney: physiology and pathophysiology,* 3rd ed. Philadelphia: Lippincott Williams & Wilkins, 2000:2015–2053.
5. Gennari FJ. Acid–base balance in dialysis patients. *Kidney Int* 1985;28:678–688.
6. Gennari FJ. Acid–base disorders in end-stage renal disease: part I. *Semin Dial* 1990;3:81–85.
7. Gennari FJ. Acid–base homeostasis in end-stage renal disease. *Semin Dial* 1996;9:404–411.
8. Gennari FJ. Acid–base balance in dialysis patients. *Semin Dial* 2000;13:235–239.
9. Uribarri J, et al. Acid–base balance in chronic peritoneal dialysis patients. *Kidney Int* 1995;47:269–273.
10. Graham KA, et al. Acid–base regulation in peritoneal dialysis. *Kidney Int* 1994;48(Suppl):S47–S50.
11. Yasuda T, et al. D-Lactate metabolism in patients with chronic renal failure undergoing CAPD. *Nephron* 1993;63:416–422.
12. Feriani M. Use of different buffers in peritoneal dialysis. *Semin Dial* 2000;13:256–260.
13. Mandelbaum JM, et al. Six months' experience with PD-2 solution. *Dial Transplant* 1983;12:259–260.
14. Nolph KD, et al. Multicenter evaluation of a new peritoneal dialysis solution with a high lactate and a low magnesium concentration. *Perit Dial Bull* 1983;3:63–65.
15. Feriani M, et al. Continuous ambulatory peritoneal dialysis with bicarbonate buffer—a pilot study. *Perit Dial Int* 1993;13:S88–S91.
16. Feriani M, et al. Short-term clinical study with bicarbonate-containing peritoneal dialysis solution. *Perit Dial Int* 1993;13:296–301.
17. Feriani M, et al. Clinical experience with a 39 mmol/L bicarbonate-buffered peritoneal dialysis solution. *Perit Dial Int* 1997;17:17–21.
18. Graham KA, et al. Correction of acidosis in CAPD decreases whole body protein degradation. *Kidney Int* 1996;49:1396–1400.
19. Stein A, et al. Role of an improvement in acid–base status and nutrition in CAPD patients. *Kidney Int* 1997;52:1089–1095.
20. Mactier RA, et al. Bicarbonate and bicarbonate/lactate peritoneal dialysis solutions for the treatment of infusion pain. *Kidney Int* 1998;53:1061–1067.
21. Murphy WP, et al. Use of an artificial kidney III: current procedures in clinical hemodialysis. *J Lab Clin Med* 1952;40:436–444.
22. Brandon JM, et al. Prolongation of survival by periodic prolonged hemodialysis in patients with chronic renal failure. *Am J Med* 1962;33:538–544.
23. Mion CM, et al. Substitution of sodium acetate for sodium bicarbonate in the bath fluid for hemodialysis. *Trans Am Soc Artif Intern Organs* 1964;10:110–113.
24. Mudge GH, et al. Sodium acetate as a source of fixed base. *Proc Soc Exp Biol Med* 1949;71:136–139.
25. Kveim MH, et al. Utilization of exogenous acetate during hemodialysis. *Trans Am Soc Artif Intern Organs* 1975;21:138–143.
26. Tolchin N, et al. Metabolic consequences of high mass-transfer hemodialysis. *Kidney Int* 1977;11:366–378.

27. Vreman HJ, et al. Acetate metabolism and acid–base homeostasis during hemodialysis: influence of dialyzer efficiency and rate of acetate metabolism. *Kidney Int* 1980;(Suppl 10):S62–S74.
28. Cohen E, et al. Patterns of metabolic acidosis in patients with chronic renal failure: impact of hemodialysis. *Int J Artif Organs* 1988;11:440–448.
29. Vinay P, et al. Acetate metabolism and bicarbonate generation during hemodialysis: 10 years of observation. *Kidney Int* 1987;31:1194–1204.
30. Kveim MH, et al. Acetate metabolizing capacity in man. *J Oslo City Hosp* 1980;30:101–104.
31. Hakim RM, et al. Effects of acetate and bicarbonate dialysate in stable chronic dialysis patients. *Kidney Int* 1985;28:535–540.
32. Graefe U, et al. Less dialysis-induced morbidity and vascular instability with bicarbonate in dialysate. *Ann Intern Med* 1978;88:332–336.
33. Hunt JM, et al. Gas exchange during dialysis: contrasting mechanisms contributing to comparable alterations with acetate and bicarbonate buffers. *Am J Med* 1984;77:255–260.
34. Man NK, et al. Effect of bicarbonate-containing dialysate on chronic hemodialysis patients: a comparative study. *Artif Organs* 1982;6:421–428.
35. Ward RA, et al. Effects of long-term bicarbonate hemodialysis on acid–base status. *Trans Am Soc Artif Intern Organs* 1982;28:295–298.
36. Symreng T, et al. Ventilatory and metabolic changes during high efficiency hemodialysis. *Kidney Int* 1992;41:1064–1069.
37. Gotch FA, et al. Hydrogen ion balance in dialysis therapy. *Artif Organs* 1982;6:388–395.
38. Ward RA, et al. Hemodialysate composition and intradialytic metabolic, acid–base and potassium changes. *Kidney Int* 1987;32:129–135.
39. Diamond SM, et al. Acetate dialysate versus bicarbonate dialysate: a continuing controversy. *Am J Kidney Dis* 1987;9:3–11.
40. Chauveau P, et al. Acidosis and nutritional status in hemodialyzed patients: French Study Group for Nutrition in Dialysis. *Semin Dial* 2000;13:241–246.
41. Uribarri J, et al. Association of acidosis and nutritional parameters in hemodialysis patients. *Am J Kidney Dis* 1999;34:493–499.
42. Harris DC, et al. Correcting acidosis in hemodialysis: effect on phosphate clearance and calcification risk. *J Am Soc Nephrol* 1995;6:1607–1612.
43. Uribarri J, et al. Acid production in chronic hemodialysis patients. *J Am Soc Nephrol* 1998;9:114–120.
44. Fabris A, et al. The importance of ultrafiltration on acid–base status in a dialysis population. *ASAIO Trans* 1988;34:200–201.
45. Oettinger CW, et al. Normalization of uremic acidosis in hemodialysis patients with a high bicarbonate dialysate. *J Am Soc Nephrol* 1993;3:1804–1807.
46. Bushinsky DA, et al. Arterial PCO_2 in chronic metabolic acidosis. *Kidney Int* 1982;22:311–314.
47. Henrich WL, et al. High sodium bicarbonate and acetate hemodialysis: double-blind crossover comparison of hemodynamic and ventilatory effects. *Kidney Int* 1983;24:240–245.
48. Graham KA, et al. Correction of acidosis in hemodialysis patients increases the sensitivity of the parathyroid glands to calcium. *J Am Soc Nephrol* 1997;8:627–631.
49. Lefebvre A, et al. Optimal correction of acidosis changes progression of dialysis osteodystrophy. *Kidney Int* 1989;36:1112–1118.
50. Graham KA, et al. Correction of acidosis in hemodialysis decreases whole-body protein degradation. *J Am Soc Nephrol* 1997;8:632–637.
51. Kooman JP, et al. The influence of bicarbonate supplementation on plasma levels of branched-chain amino acids in haemodialysis patients with metabolic acidosis. *Nephrol Dial Transplant* 1997;12:2397–2401.
52. Williams AJ, et al. High bicarbonate dialysate in haemodialysis patients: effects on acidosis and nutritional status. *Nephrol Dial Transplant* 1997;12:2633–2637.
53. Bergstrom J, et al. Plasma and muscle free amino acids in maintenance hemodialysis patients without protein malnutrition. *Kidney Int* 1990;38:108–114.
54. Lowrie EG, et al. Death risk in hemodialysis patients: the predictive value of commonly measured variables and an evaluation of death rate differences between facilities. *Am J Kidney Dis* 1990;15:458–482.
55. Kraut JA. Disturbances of acid–base balance and bone disease in end-stage renal disease. *Semin Dial* 2000;13:261–266.
56. Van Stone JC. Oral base replacement in patients on hemodialysis. *Ann Intern Med* 1984;101:199–201.
57. Thews O. Model-based decision support system for individual prescription of the dialysate bicarbonate concentration in hemodialysis. *Int J Artif Organs* 1992;15:447–455.
58. Buoncristiani U, et al. Daily dialysis: long-term clinical metabolic results. *Kidney Int* 1988;24(Suppl):S137–S140.
59. Buoncristiani U. Fifteen years of clinical experience with daily haemodialysis. *Nephrol Dial Transplant* 1998;13(Suppl 6):148–151.
60. Zimmerman D, et al. Continuous veno-venous haemodialysis with a novel bicarbonate dialysis solution: prospective cross-over comparison with a lactate buffered solution. *Nephrol Dial Transplant* 1999;14:2387–2391.
61. Forni LG, et al. Continuous hemofiltration in the treatment of acute renal failure. *N Engl J Med* 1997;336:1303–1309.
62. Marshall MR, et al. Sustained low-efficiency dialysis for critically ill patients requiring renal replacement therapy. *Kidney Int* 2001;60:777–785.
63. Manns M, et al. Continuous renal replacement therapies: an update. *Am J Kidney Dis* 1998;32:185–207.
64. McLean AG, et al. Effects of lactate-buffered and lactate-free dialysate in CAVHD patients with and without liver dysfunction. *Kidney Int* 2000;58:1765–1772.
65. Melanson TM, et al. Slow low-efficiency dialysis normalizes metabolic profiles in ICU patients. *J Am Soc Nephrol* 2001;12:271A.
66. Santoro A, et al. Regulation of base balance in bicarbonate hemofiltration. *Int J Artif Organs* 1994;17:27–36.
67. Biasioli S, et al. Different buffers for hemodiafiltration: a controlled study. *Int J Artif Organs* 1989;12:25–30.
68. Feriani M, et al. Effect of dialysate and substitution fluid buffer on buffer flux in hemodiafiltration. *Kidney Int* 1990;39:711–717.
69. Santoro A, et al. Analysis of the factors influencing bicarbonate balance during acetate-free biofiltration. *Kidney Int* 1993;41(Suppl):S184–S187.
70. Santiago-Delpin EA, et al. Blood gases and pH in patients with artificial arteriovenous fistulas. *Kidney Int* 1972;1:131–133.
71. Fields AL, et al. Chronic lactic acidosis in a patient with cancer: therapy and metabolic consequences. *Cancer* 1981;47:2026–2029.
72. Fraley DS, et al. Stimulation of lactate production by administration of bicarbonate in a patient with a solid neoplasm and lactic acidosis. *N Engl J Med* 1980;303:1100–1102.
73. Brueggemeyer CD, et al. Dialysate concentrate: a potential source for lethal complications. *Nephron* 1987;46:397–398.
74. Rimmer JM, et al. Metabolic alkalosis. *J Intensive Care Med* 1987;2:137–150.
75. Gennari FJ. A normal serum bicarbonate in a woman receiving chronic hemodialysis. *Semin Dial* 1991;4:59–61.
76. Madias NE, et al. Metabolic alkalosis due to absorption of "nonabsorbable" antacids. *Am J Med* 1983;74:155–158.
77. Madias NE, et al. Respiratory alkalosis and acidosis. In: Giebisch G, et al., eds. *The kidney: physiology and pathophysiology.* Philadelphia: Lippincott Williams & Wilkins, 2000:2131–2166.
78. Gennari FJ. Acid–base disorders in end-stage renal disease: part II. *Semin Dial* 1990;3:161–165.
79. Kenamond TG, et al. Severe recurrent alkalemia in a patient undergoing continuous cyclic peritoneal dialysis. *Am J Med* 1986;81:548–550.

DYSLIPIDEMIA IN DIALYSIS PATIENTS

ROBERT D. TOTO

Cardiovascular (CV) disease is the leading cause of death in the U.S. dialysis population, accounting for nearly 70% of all deaths (1). The incidence rate of myocardial infarction is several-fold higher in end-stage renal disease (ESRD) as compared with an age-matched non-ESRD population (2). Atherosclerosis is accelerated in maintenance dialysis patients, but the causes are incompletely understood and are not explained by an increased prevalence of traditional risk factors such as hypertension. Instead, both a constellation of CV risk factors prevalent in chronic kidney disease before dialysis initiation as well as factors associated with maintenance dialysis therapy likely contribute (2–5). The latter include hemodialysis-induced platelet activation and adherence and production of proinflammatory cytokines. A key risk factor observed in all dialysis patients is dyslipidemia. The contribution of dyslipidemia to atherosclerosis in dialysis patients is not entirely clear. Nevertheless it is a ubiquitous finding in dialysis patients and is thought to play an important role in this process. Observational data from hemodialysis populations suggest that the use of statins can be associated with lower cardiovascular death rate (6). However, it is unknown whether this effect is due to lipid lowering per se. To date there are no controlled clinical trials examining the effect of lipid-lowering therapy on cardiovascular outcomes in maintenance dialysis patients. Therefore it is still unknown whether lipid-lowering therapy can reduce cardiovascular mortality in this high-risk group. The purpose of this chapter is to discuss current understanding of the causes and treatment of dyslipidemia in dialysis patients.

RISK FACTORS FOR CARDIOVASCULAR DISEASE IN DIALYSIS PATIENTS

Dialysis patients are at very high risk for coronary heart disease (see Chapter 18 for a separate discussion). Table 28.1 illustrates both traditional and nontraditional risk factors, including the metabolic syndrome. The latter is a common metabolic disturbance in dialysis patients associated with dyslipidemia and increased cardiovascular death risk. Most patients on dialysis are older and have dyslipidemia, hypertension, insulin resistance, hyperhomocysteinemia, increased plasma calcium–phosphate product and elevated C-reactive protein level and oxidative stress (7) (Fig. 28.1). Nearly 80% of dialysis patients have demonstrable left ventricular hypertrophy, a known independent risk factor for sudden cardiac death (8,9). Hypertension in dialysis patients increases both morbidity and mortality (10–13). Insulin resistance is independently associated with increased risk of cardiovascular death in nonuremic patients (14–16). Elevated calcium × phosphate product is associated with increased mortality risk and may exacerbate vascular calcification, thereby contributing to coronary ischemia (17–20). Elevated plasma homocysteine level is an independent risk factor for myocardial infarction and cardiovascular morbidity in dialysis patients (21–25). These factors appear early on in chronic kidney disease and worsen progressively in those who progress to ESRD and together conspire to promote atherosclerosis leading to excessive cardiac and cerebrovascular death. The relative risk for cardiovascular death ranges from 10- to 1,000-fold higher

TABLE 28.1. RISK FACTORS FOR CORONARY HEART DISEASE IN ESRD PATIENTS

Traditional	Nontraditional	Metabolic Syndrome
Age	Lipoprotein (a)	Atherogenic dyslipidemia
	Small dense LDL-cholesterol	Elevated triglycerides (>150 mg/dL)
Hypertension	Apolipoproteins (CIII, B, A)	Small LDL-cholesterol
LDL-cholesterol	hsC-reactive protein	Elevated non-LDL-cholesterol (>130 mg/
HDL-cholesterol	PAI-1, fibrinogen,	Low HDL-cholesterol (<40 mg/dL in
	homocysteine	men women)
Insulin resistance	TNF-alpha	
Family history	F-isoprostanes	High-normal blood pressure
Cigarette smoking		Insulin resistance ± impaired fasting glucose
		Proinflammatory or prothrombotic state

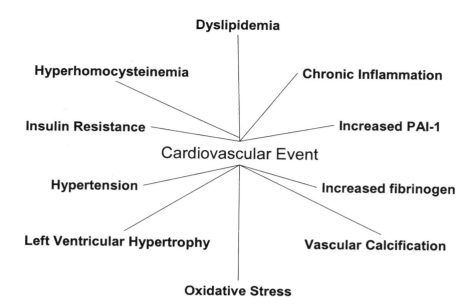

FIG. 28.1. Risk factors for cardiovascular morbidity and mortality in dialysis patients.

than that for normal individuals (2,26). Early intervention that reduces these risk factors in patients with chronic kidney disease may in turn reduce overall cardiovascular disease burden. Among these factors, dyslipidemia is a major modifiable risk factor that when treated is known to reduce cardiovascular morbidity and mortality in nondialysis populations.

NORMAL STRUCTURE AND FUNCTION OF LIPOPROTEINS

Lipoproteins are composed of lipid components, including cholesterol, triglycerides and phospholipids, and protein components, or apoproteins. They function as transporters of lipids to and from peripheral tissues and the liver. Apoproteins transport lipids in the plasma; activated enzymes that metabolize lipids and in some cases serve as ligands for cellular uptake of lipoproteins then determine the final metabolic disposition of the lipoproteins. Normal intravascular metabolism of lipoproteins via the endogenous (fasting and postprandial) pathway is illustrated in Fig. 28.2A. Both pathways are altered in dyslipidemic dialysis patients.

Very-Low-Density Lipoprotein (VLDL) and VLDL Remnants

VLDL and VLDL remnants are triglyceride-rich particles synthesized and secreted by the liver. They transport cholesterol, triglyceride, and other lipoproteins, and are precursors for LDL. In the circulation nascent VLDL particles exchange both lipid and apoproteins with high-density lipoprotein (HDL) particles and acquire apolipoprotein CII (Apo CII) from HDL. Acquisition of Apo CII is a critical step in the activation of lipoprotein lipase, which in turn mediates lipolysis of VLDL triglycerides (Fig. 28.2A). This process liberates fatty acids and glycerol from

VLDL and results in formation of VLDL remnants. VLDL remnants (IDL) undergo further lipolysis by endothelial lipoprotein lipase and subsequently by hepatic triglyceride lipase (HTGL) to form low-density lipoprotein (LDL). Because VLDL particles contain apoliprotein B, the ligand for the LDL receptor, VLDL, and VLDL remnants may be removed from plasma by hepatic LDL receptors.

Low-Density Lipoprotein Metabolism

LDL particles are synthesized from VLDL remnants and exist in two major populations in plasmas: (a) larger LDL particles and (b) small, dense LDL particles. Small, dense LDL particles are thought to be more atherogenic than larger particles. Hepatic uptake of LDL by LDL receptors accounts for about 70% of LDL clearance. The remainder is taken up by nonhepatic tissues, including scavenger receptors on monocytes and macrophages in the vascular wall, which contributes to atherosclerotic plaque formation (27).

High-Density Lipoprotein and Reverse Cholesterol Transport

HDL particles facilitate movement of cholesterol from peripheral tissues to liver by transfer of cholesterol and cholesterol esters to LDL and VLDL (Fig. 28.2). Movement of cholesterol from tissues to the liver is known as reverse cholesterol transport. HDL may be taken up by peripheral tissues and liver by specific HDL receptors (28–31). HDL particles activate delipidation of VLDL, LDL, and chylomicrons by transfer of apoproteins AI and CII. HDL can be divided into two major particle forms, namely, HDL_2 and HDL_3. Nascent HDL forms HDL_3 and subsequently HDL_2 by esterification of cholesterol via lecithin–cholesterol acyltransferase (LCAT) in the circulation. Cholesterol esters primarily in HDL_2 are exchanged for triglycerides carried

Overview of Lipoprotein Metabolism

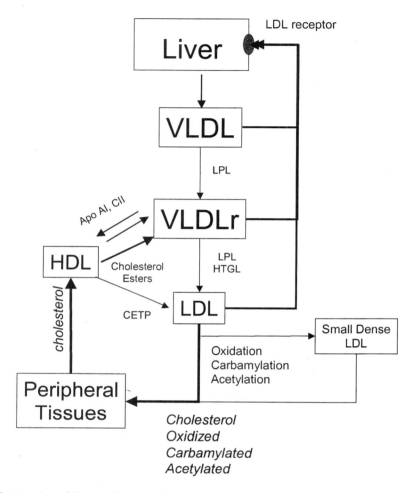

FIG. 28.2. Left: Overview of lipoprotein metabolism. Endogenous lipoprotein metabolism pathways are shown. The liver synthesizes and secretes very-low-density lipoprotein (VLDL) into the circulation, where it is delipidated by endothelial lipoprotein lipase (LPL) to form VLDL remnants (VLDLr), which are in turn metabolized by LPL and hepatic triglyceride lipase (HTGL) to form low-density lipoprotein (LDL). High-density lipoprotein (HDL) serves to move cholesterol from tissues to the liver by transferring tissue cholesterol to LDL and VLDLr particles. These particles are in turn removed from plasma by hepatic LDL receptors. Cholesterol ester transfer protein (CETP) facilitates this transfer process known as reverse cholesterol transport. Apolipoproteins A1 and CII are bidirectionally transferred from HDL to VLDLr particles as indicated. ApoA1 is important for normal HDL function and Apo CII is a potent activator of LPL. When Apo CII is deficient LPL activity is impaired. As indicated at the bottom of the figure, LDL molecules may be further modified by addition of oxygen, carbamyl, or acetyl groups to form oxidized, carbamylated, and acetylated LDL particles. These particles are believed to be more atherogenic than unmodified LDL particles.

on VLDL, VLDL remnants, and chylomicrons by cholesterol ester transfer protein (CETP). CETP functions to transfer cholesterol esters between VLDL and HDL particles in plasma to maintain normal composition and function of these lipoproteins.

A low concentration of HDL impairs transfer of Apo AI and CII, resulting in defective metabolism of VLDL and increased plasma triglyceride level (31). Low plasma HDL level is an independent risk factor for coronary artery disease mortality, presumably because of defective cholesterol transport via the reverse cholesterol transport pathway (31,32). Conversely, increased plasma levels of HDL cholesterol are associated with decreased risk of atherosclerotic cardiovascular disease (30).

Abnormal Lipoprotein Metabolism in Uremia

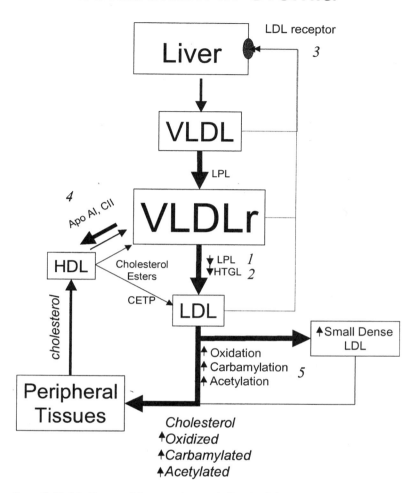

FIG. 28.2. *(Continued)* **Right:** Abnormal lipoprotein metabolism in dialysis patients. Impaired VLDL metabolism is a major cause of increased lipoprotein remnant formation in hemodialysis patients. In uremia, lipoprotein lipase activity is decreased (1) resulting in increased VLDLr. Defective HTGL activity is also in part responsible for increased VLDLr (2) and for increased synthesis of small, dense LDL. Impaired hepatic LDL receptor activity can increase VLDLr and LDL by reducing uptake from the plasma (3). In addition, defective transfer of Apo CII from HDL to VLDL partially explains the defect in lipolysis, since Apo CII is a necessary co-factor for normal LPL activity (4). Compositional abnormalities in the HDL subfraction levels are low in uremia as a consequence of decreased synthesis. This reduction in synthesis may be related to decrease in transfer of Apo AI or Apo AII from VLDL owing to impaired LPL activity. The abnormal increase in oxidation, carbamylation, and acetylation of LDL increases uptake by peripheral tissues (5). These abnormalities together contribute to accelerated atherosclerosis in dialysis patients.

Lipoprotein (a)

Lipoprotein (a) [Lp(a)] is a cholesterol ester-rich lipoprotein composed of a single molecule of LDL covalently linked by a disulfide bond to apolipoprotein a [apo(a)] (33,34). Apo(a) is composed of a heavily glycated protein with many repeating ("kringle") domains and contains a protease moiety in the C-terminal region of the molecule highly homologous with plasminogen. Lp(a) is synthesized exclusively in the liver and the synthetic rate is the major determinant of plasma Lp(a) level in normal individuals (35).

The function of Lp(a) is unknown; however, increased plasma Lp(a) concentration is associated with increased risk of coronary artery disease (36). It has very low affinity for the LDL receptor, and plasma concentration is independent clearance rate. Unlike LDL, the concentrations of Lp(a) are remarkably stable and are not influenced by age, sex, diet, body weight, and most drugs (34,37).

DYSLIPIDEMIAS IN DIALYSIS PATIENTS

Dyslipidemias represent a heterogeneous group of lipid disorders encompassing abnormal levels of lipids and lipoproteins and abnormal lipoprotein composition, metabolism, and function (7,32,34,38–42). ESRD is associated with major abnormalities in lipoprotein metabolism and composition that engender an atherogenic lipid profile (Table 28.2). Both increases in apolipoprotein B–containing lipoproteins [very-low-density lipoprotein (VLDL), low-density lipoprotein (LDL), and lipoprotein(a) (Lp(a)] as well as decreases in apolipoprotein (a) containing lipoproteins [high-density lipoprotein (HDL)] together increase atherosclerotic cardiovascular disease risk. In addition, increased levels of small, dense LDL are present in peritoneal and hemodialysis patients. Both the incidence and the severity of hyperlipidemia in hemodialyzed patients with myocardial infarction are higher than those without infarction, suggesting that dyslipidemia is a key factor in accelerating atherosclerosis in uremia (10,20,41,43–46).

The Adult Treatment Panel III (ATPIII) guidelines for prevention of coronary artery disease recognize the metabolic syndrome as an important risk factor complex necessitating treatment (47). Metabolic syndrome is defined as the presence of any three of the following: (a) atherogenic dyslipidemia consisting of low HDL cholesterol, elevated plasma triglyceride level, increased small LDL cholesterol particles, and elevated non-HDL cholesterol level; (b) high normal blood pressure; (c) insulin resistance + impaired fasting glucose; (d) obesity (waist circumference >40 inches in men and >36 inches in women); (e) proinflammatory or prothrombotic state (Table 28.3). The metabolic syndrome is present in a high proportion of dialysis patients with or without diabetes. In summary, multiple cardiovascular risk factors are prevalent in progressive renal disease and often persist after renal replacement therapy. The following sections describe normal lipid metabolism and abnormal metabolism caused by uremia in ESRD.

Increased VLDL Remnants and Hypertriglyceridemia

The most common dyslipidemia in dialysis patients is increased VLDL-remnant particles (VLDL-r) (48–52). VLDL-r are present in all patients on dialysis even in the absence of overt eleva-

TABLE 28.2. DYSLIPIDEMIAS IN DIALYSIS PATIENTS

Abnormal plasma concentration
  Hypertriglyceridemia
  Increased VLDL and IDL (VLDL remnants)
  Cholesterol enrichment of VLDL and apolipoprotein B
  Decreased HDL-cholesterol and apolipoprotein AI
  Increased Apo CIII
  Decreased Apo CII
  Increased small density LDL-cholesterol
Abnormal lipoprotein composition
  Increased TG content in VLDL, LDL, HDL
  Increased cholesterol content of VLDL
  Presence of ApoC and ApoE in LDL particles
  Presence of ApoB 48 in VLDL

TABLE 28.3. ATP III RECOMMENDED GOALS FOR OPTIMAL LIPID MANAGEMENT

Lipid/lipoprotein	Concentration (mg/dL)
LDL cholesterol	
Optimal	<100
Near optimal	100–129
Borderline high	130–159
High	160–189
Very high	≥190
HDL cholesterol	
Low	<40
High	>80
Triglycerides	
Normal	<150
Borderline high	150–199
High	200–499
Very high	>500
Atherogenic dyslipidemia	
Raised triglycerides	≥150
Small LDL	In excess
Reduced HDL-cholesterol level	<40 (men)
	<50 (women)

tion in triglyceride level (42). Mild to moderate hypertriglyceridemia (250 to 500 mg/dL) is typical in hemodialysis patients and occurs in about 30% of patients on hemodialysis and 40% to 50% of patients on peritoneal dialysis (42,53–59). On average, triglyceride levels are somewhat higher in CAPD patients because systemic glucose loading stimulates hyperinsulinemia and consequent increase in hepatic triglyceride synthesis (60,61). Both increased synthesis (62,63) and decreased catabolism of VLDL contribute to increased VLDL-remnant levels in dialysis patients, but decreased catabolism of VLDL is the predominant mechanism (42). Decreased plasma lipoprotein lipase, hepatic triglyceride lipase, and adipose tissue lipase activities are all impaired in dialysis patients (64–70). Down-regulation of tissue lipoprotein lipase also contributes to the defective VLDL lipolysis. Apolipoprotein CIII, an inhibitor of lipoprotein lipase, is increased, and apolipoprotein CII, an activator of lipoprotein lipase, is decreased in dialysis patients (71,72). The latter mechanism is due to decreased transfer of Apo CII, from HDL₂ to VLDL. Defective clearance of VLDL remnants via LDL receptor activity ascribed to carbamylation of apoB and advanced glycation of the receptor also contribute to this dyslipidemia (73–76).

Atherogenicity of VLDL Remnants in Dialysis Patients

VLDL remnants are atherogenic lipoprotein particles (32,77–81) associated with increased risk of coronary artery disease (80,82–87). VLDL remnants in dialysis patients are both triglyceride- and cholesterol-enriched particles that penetrate the vascular endothelium. They may be taken up by nonreceptor-mediated mechanisms and can engender formation of small, dense LDL particles (see later). Also, abnormal intravascular metabolism responsible for increased VLDL-remnant levels in dialysis patients is associated with low HDL cholesterol. In diabetic patients with ESRD, VLDL cholesterol is increased and cholesterol/triglyceride ratio content in VLDL is highest in those with overt macrovascular disease.

Low-HDL Cholesterol

Reduction in plasma HDL cholesterol is a major and common dyslipidemia in dialysis patients, and part of the metabolic syndrome complex. This reduction results from decreased HDL_2 subfraction in uremic patients (51,88). Black patients treated with hemodialysis and peritoneal dialysis tend to exhibit higher total HDL and HDL_2 levels than age-matched whites (89,90). This difference may be due to differences in plasma HDL_2 cholesterol levels. Compositional abnormalities in the HDL subfractions include reductions free cholesterol ester, apolipoproteins I and II content. Decreased plasma HDL levels in ESRD are probably caused by decreased synthesis that impairs the ability of HDL to esterify and transport free cholesterol from tissues and Apo B-100 containing lipoproteins (i.e., VLDL and LDL) (91).

Increased LDL Cholesterol and Small, Dense LDL Particles

Hypercholesterolemia is less common than hypertriglyceridemia in dialysis patients. It is present in about 20% of patients on maintenance dialysis. Hypercholesterolemia seems to occur more commonly in diabetics than in nondiabetics on dialysis. Increased LDL cholesterol in dialysis patients probably results from increased VLDL-r and impaired LDL receptor function (92).

The distribution of LDL particles from larger to smaller, denser particles occurs in uremia. Total LDL cholesterol is generally less than 130 mg/dL in dialysis patients, but more than one-third of patients have a larger fraction of total LDL distributed in small, dense LDL particles (84,93). Small, dense LDL is more atherogenic than lighter, less dense LDL particles.

Compositional abnormalities in LDL also occur in dialysis patients. Thus LDL particles may be triglyceride-enriched as a result of coexisting abnormalities in HDL metabolism, cholesterol ester transfer protein (CETP) activity, or a combination of these two abnormalities (34,94–96). Also, increased amounts of oxidized LDL (97) and carbamylated LDL particles are present (32,38,75,76,93,98). These alterations facilitate LDL particle uptake by macrophages, which in turn form foam cells, even in the absence of markedly elevated plasma levels of LDL. Increased scavenger receptor activity on monocytes and macrophages in dialysis patients also accelerates this process (99–101).

Lipoprotein (a)

Plasma Lp(a) concentration is elevated in dialysis patients (34,37,102–104) and decreases after renal transplantation (105). Since increased levels of Lp(a) constitute an independent risk factor for coronary artery disease in nonuremic populations, this lipoprotein may be atherogenic in ESRD. The mechanism of increased Lp(a) in uremia is unknown, but increased synthesis is the most likely explanation. However, decreased clearance

of Lp(a) via LDL-receptor- or nonreceptor-mediated mechanisms is responsible for increased levels has not been studied in uremia. In contrast to nondialysis patients, increased synthesis of small Lp(a) isoforms is not responsible for increased plasma concentrations in dialysis patients (34,106,107). Serum albumin concentration may also regulate Lp(a) in dialysis patients, as increasing albumin in peritoneal dialysis patients tends to lower plasma Lp(a) levels (105). Dialysis does not lower plasma Lp(a) levels.

Chylomicronemia

Hemodialysis patients have postprandial chylomicronemia caused by a severe defect in chylomicron-remnant clearance (108). Impaired lipoprotein lipase activity is thought to be responsible for this defect. Whether chylomicrons play an important role in atherogenesis in dialysis patients is unknown.

MANAGEMENT OF DYSLIPIDEMIA

Measurement and Monitoring of Plasma Lipid Levels

Fasting plasma lipid total cholesterol, LDL cholesterol, HDL cholesterol, and triglyceride levels should be measured in dialysis patients routinely to screen for and monitor dyslipidemia. Most nephrologists obtain routine plasma lipid levels with the monthly laboratory studies in a dialysis center, and in many cases these are nonfasting values. Obtaining a fasting level can be inconvenient for many patients. However, because hypertriglyceridemia is prevalent in dialysis patients and postprandial triglyceride level is an inaccurate estimate, a fasting sample is preferred. For patients with borderline abnormal levels the fasting lipid profile should be repeated to confirm abnormalities before initiating interventions. If LDL cholesterol is not a part of the routine laboratory panel, the Friedwald equation [LDL = (total cholesterol − HDL − triglyceride levels)/5] can be used to calculate LDL cholesterol level. This formula has been validated in dialysis patients with triglyceride levels of less than 500 mg/dL (109).

It is important to monitor blood levels of LDL cholesterol, HDL cholesterol, and triglycerides, preferably after a 12-hour fast. These levels can be monitored every 2 to 3 months to determine efficacy of the regimen. In addition, because pharmacologic lowering may be associated with potentially serious side effects, patients should be monitored carefully (see later). Routine measurement of Lp(a) is not recommended, as there is no current target level for dialysis patients.

ATP III Guidelines for Prevention of Coronary Heart Disease

The Adult Treatment Panel III guidelines for primary and secondary prevention of coronary heart disease utilize a stepwise approach to assessing risk and selecting appropriate intervention (Table 28.3) (47). The first step is to calculate the 10-year coronary heart disease risk using the Framingham formula (110,111). However, the Framingham risk score probably underestimates the 10-year risk in hemodialysis patients, and chronic kidney disease with diabetes (and perhaps in nondiabetics) is a coronary heart disease risk equivalent. In a patient without a documented coronary event, a condition that increases the 10-year risk for a new coronary artery disease event is considered to be a coronary heart disease risk equivalent. ESRD may be such a condition; however, ESRD is not included as a coronary risk equivalent in the current ATP III guidelines (47). Still, if a dialysis patient is deemed to be in this category of risk, then it seems reasonable to include a more aggressive approach to lipid lowering in such a patient. Diabetes mellitus type 2 is considered a coronary heart disease, and because more than one-third of dialysis patients are diabetics, this group of dialysis patients should be treated to a more aggressive LDL goal of less than 100 mg/dL (see later).

General Approach to Management of Dialysis Patients

Precise treatment guidelines for dyslipidemia in ESRD have yet to be established because of the lack of information concerning the relative risk of common dyslipidemias. At this time, no study directly assesses whether aggressive lipid-lowering therapy reduces coronary artery disease in dialysis patients. Also, no study has shown that lowering VLDL triglyceride or correcting low HDL levels reduces cardiovascular risk in dialysis patients. However, the high rate of cardiovascular complications in this population provides a compelling reason to consider treatment for patients with (a) persistent severe hypertriglyceridemia (>500 mg/dL), (b) LDL cholesterol level above 130 mg/dL for lower risk and >100 mg/dL for high risk, and (c) HDL cholesterol levels <40 mg/dL. Still, in patients with severe hypertriglyceridemia, with increased LDL cholesterol levels, and with low HDL it is desirable to modify dialysis and dietary treatment to manage lipid abnormalities. Given the lack of clinical trial data in dialysis patients, one must exercise clinical judgment, tailoring therapy for an individual patient.

The goal of therapy is to normalize plasma levels of triglyceride, LDL, and HDL cholesterol levels. Dietary counseling is an important first step for such patients; however, it should not be expected that diet alone will normalize cholesterol or triglyceride levels in most patients.

Diet and Exercise

Reduction in dietary carbohydrate to approximately one-third of total calories alone or in combination with high polyunsaturated-to-saturated fat ratio of 2:1 lowers triglyceride levels in dialysis patients (63,112). In contrast, dietary modification to lowering protein intake has no benefit on plasma triglyceride levels and is not advisable in dialysis patients (113). For patients with mild hypertriglyceridemia (200 to 500 mg/dL) a renal dietician should obtain dietary history and adjust dietary carbohydrate to about one-third of the diet whenever feasible. This may limit the effect, especially in peritoneal dialysis patients who receive obligate glucose load during dialysis. Reducing saturated fat intake to 10% of total daily caloric intake is desirable to lower LDL cholesterol level and should be encouraged. Sub-

stitution of monounsaturated fats for saturated fat is possible and helps to allow a decrease in dietary carbohydrate content while maintaining an energy intake of 35 kcal/kg/d. Still, normalizing triglyceride and cholesterol levels with diet is often not achievable in dialysis patients.

Exercise in dialysis patients is possible in many and desirable in most. There are no clinical trials demonstrating benefit of exercise alone on lipids in ESRD patients. However, routine aerobic exercise can raise HDL cholesterol and lower triglyceride level.

High-Flux Membranes

Initiation of maintenance hemodialysis is associated with a reduction in VLDL triglyceride levels in many patients (54), but abnormal VLDL-remnant metabolism persists (114). High-flux hemodialysis using polysulfone membranes improves fasting plasma lipid profiles compared with cellulosic membranes (114–116). Careful longitudinal studies designed to determine whether long-term hemodialysis normalizes VLDL triglycerides or HDL$_2$ levels have not been performed. Dialysis with polyamide membranes has also been shown to reduce triglyceride and raise HDL levels as compared with cellulosic membranes (115). In the Hemodialysis study, use of a high-flux membrane was associated with lower cardiovascular mortality (117). Whether or not this observation is explained by changes in plasma lipid profiles has not yet been determined. Still, it seems reasonable to avoid using cellulosic membranes in preference to high-flux membranes in dialysis patients with hypertriglyceridemia.

Low-Molecular-Weight Heparin

Several studies have shown that systemic heparin use during dialysis is associated with depletion of lipoprotein lipase activity and therefore may contribute to excess VLDL remnants. Theoretically, replacement of heparin with the low-molecular-weight mixtures could improve dyslipidemia by not interfering with lipolysis of VLDL. Studies examining the potential benefit of low-molecular-weight heparins on plasma lipids in dialysis patients yield conflicting results (118–120). Small numbers of subjects, limited duration, and lack of outcome data limit the application of these results. Thus low-molecular-weight heparin is not recommended as a replacement for heparin to improve lipid profiles in dialysis patients.

PHARMACOLOGIC TREATMENT OF SPECIFIC HYPERLIPIDEMIAS

Hypertriglyceridemia

Fibric acid derivatives effectively lower VLDL triglycerides by decreasing hepatic VLDL synthesis and enhancing lipoprotein lipase (Table 28.4) Metabolites of these drugs are excreted by the kidney, requiring dose adjustment in dialysis patients. Gemfibrozil is effective for lowering triglyceride level and can be given daily at a starting dose of 300 mg orally twice daily. Dose titration up to a total of 1,200 mg per can be undertaken over a period of 1 to 2 months with repeated measurement of fasting

TABLE 28.4. TREATMENT OPTIONS FOR DYSLIPIDEMIA IN DIALYSIS PATIENTS

Dyslipidemia Pattern	Treatment/Drug of Choice	Alternative
Hypertriglyceridemia (<500 mg/dL)	Dietary counseling, high-flux dialyzer	Weight loss if obese
Hypertriglyceridemia (>500 mg/dL)	Gemfibrozil 300–600 mg TIW	Clofibrate 200–400 mg TIW
Hypercholesterolemia (130 mg/dL)	Statin 10–40 mg/d	Nicotinic acid 1–2 g/d
Combined hyperlipemia[a]	Statin 10–40 mg/d	Nicotinic acid 1–2 g/d
Low HDL (<35 mg/dL) and N1 TG	Exercise, moderate ETOH[b]	Clofibrate, Fenofibrate
Low HDL and high TG	Gemfibrozil 300–600 mg/d, weight loss	Clofibrate, Fenofibrate
Metabolic syndrome	Statin 10–40 mg/d	Weight loss if obese

[a]Both hypercholesterolemia and hypertriglyceridemia.
[b]For example, two 4-oz. glasses of wine daily.

triglyceride. Clofibrate is effective and generally well tolerated by dialysis patients (67,69,121). However, awareness of muscle injury symptoms and surveillance for creatine phosphokinase (CPK) levels should be initially monitored weekly and at regular intervals thereafter. Clofibrate should be given in doses of 200 mg three times per week. The reason for the less frequent dosing is the tendency for this drug to accumulate in ESRD. High doses of clofibrate (1,500 mg/d) should be avoided because of increased incidence of adverse effects, including myositis, gait disturbances, abdominal discomfort, diarrhea, and malaise. Adverse events are usually reversible and can be managed by discontinuation or dose adjustment. Fenofibrate reduces plasma cholesterol and triglycerides in nonrenal conditions and in those with moderate renal failure (122,123). However, it has not been tested in dialysis patients. Fibric acids must be used with caution in dialysis patients because of their propensity to cause muscle injury. Therefore educating patients concerning these side effects and monitoring plasma creatine phosphokinase levels on a monthly basis are important management considerations (124,125).

Nicotinic Acid

Nicotinic acid in doses of 1 to 2 g/d may be used to lower VLDL triglyceride (and cholesterol) levels in dialysis patients. Nicotinic acid reduces plasma triglyceride level by decreasing hepatic VLDL synthesis/secretion. The dose must be titrated slowly, beginning with doses of 250 mg three times daily and titrating up to the 1 to 2 g/d over a period of 1 to 2 months. Upward-dose titration may be performed on a weekly basis until the maximum dose is achieved. It should be noted that these doses usually cause palmar itching, and in some patients orthostatic hypotension, hyperglycemia, hyperuricemia, and occasionally hepatic toxicity. For these reasons blood glucose, uric acid, and liver enzyme tests should be monitored with monthly laboratory measurements.

Hypercholesterolemia

HMG-CoA Reductase Inhibitors (Statins)

Statins are the most effective and well-tolerated agents for lowering plasma LDL cholesterol level and are the drug class of choice for hypercholesterolemia. This class of agents has been shown to reduce coronary artery disease mortality in both pri-

mary and secondary prevention trials in nondialysis populations (122,126–128). In a large observational study of maintenance hemodialysis patients, Seliger et al. demonstrated that incident hemodialysis patients whose medical regimen included a statin had a lower cardiovascular mortality after 2 years of follow-up (6). Whether this was associated with cholesterol lowering or not is unclear. Die Deutsche Diabetes Dialyse study is an ongoing randomized double-blind placebo controlled trial designed to determine whether statin therapy improves survival in type 2 diabetics on dialysis (129). The results of this study will provide important new information for management of dyslipidemia in diabetic dialysis patients.

Routine once-daily statin therapy in doses of 10 to 40 mg usually results in a 20% to 30% decrease in plasma LDL cholesterol level in both hemodialysis and peritoneal dialysis patients (130–132). Statins also lower triglyceride and in some cases increase HDL cholesterol levels. The blood LDL cholesterol goal in all diabetics should be less than 100 mg/dL. Although an LDL cholesterol level of 100 to 130 mg/dL may be acceptable in low-risk patients, as mentioned earlier, the Framingham risk scores probably underestimate overall coronary heart disease risk in dialysis patients. Therefore it is reasonable to aggressively treat LDL cholesterol to less than 100 mg/dL in most patients on dialysis.

Statins are generally safe in dialysis patients. The most serious side effect of these agents is myopathy, so symptoms and signs of myopathy should be monitored monthly. The agent should be discontinued immediately if there is clinical (muscle cramps, pain, tenderness, weakness) or biochemical (increased plasma creatine phosphokinase level) evidence of myopathy. As with fibrates, routine monthly CPK and liver enzyme tests should be monitored while on statin therapy.

Nicotinic Acid

As noted earlier, nicotinic acid also reduces LDL cholesterol and can be used in patients with a contraindication to an HMG-CoA reductase inhibitor. Nicotinic acid may be used for management of hypercholesterolemia using doses identical to those described earlier. This agent should be avoided in diabetic patients because of the tendency to increase blood glucose.

Bile Acid-Binding Resins

Bile acid-binding resins are powerful agents and are effective for lowering plasma cholesterol. However, they should not be used in patients with uremic dyslipidemia because of their potential to increase the synthesis and secretion of VLDL from the liver. This would serve to exacerbate the metabolism of VLDL and its remnants, which could worsen atherosclerosis. Moreover, patients poorly tolerate these agents, and their use should be limited to statin- and niacin-intolerant dialysis patients.

Low-HDL Cholesterol

As mentioned already, low plasma HDL cholesterol level is commonly associated with increased VLDL remnants and hypertriglyceridemia in dialysis patients. Thus maneuvers that tend to lower triglyceride levels also tend to increase HDL cholesterol level. Therapy with gemfibrozil aimed at increasing HDL cholesterol levels has been shown to reduce cardiovascular morbidity and mortality in nondialysis populations (133). In addition, treatment of hypertriglyceridemic hemodialysis patients with clofibrate may increase plasma HDL levels (67,69). Weight loss in obese patients, moderate alcohol consumption, and aerobic exercise increase HDL cholesterol in nondialysis patients. Weight loss and exercise are recommended. Prescribing moderate alcohol consumption—for example, one or two glasses of wine on a daily basis—may be reasonable in some patients. These maneuvers may also improve HDL cholesterol level.

Combined Hyperlipidemia

Combined hypercholesterolemia and hypertriglyceridemia may be effectively treated with an HMG-CoA reductase inhibitor because the increase in LDL receptor removes VLDL, VLDL remnants, and LDL from the circulation. Both simvastatin and atorvastatin lower LDL cholesterol and triglycerides in nondialysis patients. The adverse side effect profile of these agents is superior to fibric acids and nicotinic acid. Therefore this class should be tried first in patients with combined hyperlipidemia. If there is insufficient response to therapy, treatment with fibric acid derivative may be used instead of a statin. Combination therapy with a statin and a fibric acid derivative should be done with extreme caution because of increased risk of myopathy.

Metabolic Syndrome

In dialysis patients with the metabolic syndrome more aggressive treatment of dyslipidemia is probably warranted. Treatment of the metabolic syndrome is relevant and applicable to the dialysis population. In patients with atherogenic dyslipidemia in the setting of the metabolic syndrome, LDL is still the target. However, elevated VLDL cholesterol may contribute to coronary heart disease, particularly when triglycerides are elevated. Therefore the non-HDL cholesterol (= total cholesterol − HDL cholesterol) is a secondary target. The goal is to reduce the non-HDL cholesterol to less than 30 mg/dL above the LDL target. For example, if the LDL cholesterol goal were 100 mg/dL, then the non-HDL cholesterol goal would be 130 mg/dL. When possible, treatment should be aimed at underlying causes, including obesity and diabetes mellitus and hypertension. Statin therapy to reduce non-HDL cholesterol may be employed in this situation unless there is a contraindication. Treatment regimes should

therefore include intensifying weight reduction in men with a waist circumference of more than 102 cm (>40 inches) and women with a waist circumference of more than 88 cm (>35 inches) by diet and regular exercise (minimum of 30 minutes of aerobic exercise three times per week). It should be noted that physical activity programs are extremely important and can be applied to many dialysis patients.

Adjunctive Therapies

In addition to specific lipid-lowering therapy, drugs designed to reduce atherogenicity may be considered. Vitamin E is known to reduce LDL oxidation and to inhibit macrophage adhesion to endothelium. The Secondary Prevention of Cardiovascular Events (SPACE) trial was a double-blind randomized placebo-controlled trial involving nearly 200 maintenance hemodialysis patients with a prior history of a cardiovascular event (44). The study demonstrated an improvement in survival among those randomized to 800 IU of vitamin E. Others have not yet confirmed this benefit. Given the low toxicity of vitamin E, it may be advisable to treat dialysis patients with vitamin E at this dose level. However, the results of this small study have not yet been confirmed. High doses of B vitamins—including folic, B-6, and B-12—have been shown to significantly lower homocysteine levels in dialysis patients. However, this has not translated into improved outcomes (134). These adjunctive therapies may lower CV mortality and are generally safe.

REFERENCES

1. USRDS. U.S. Renal Data System, USRDS 2002 Annual Data Report: Atlas of End-Stage Renal Disease in the United States, National Institutes of Health, National Institute of Diabetes and Digestive and Kidney Diseases, Bethesda, MD, 2002.
2. Sarnak MJ, et al. Cardiovascular disease and chronic renal disease: a new paradigm. *Am J Kidney Dis* 2000;35(Suppl 1):S117–S131.
3. Lindner A, et al. Accelerated atherosclerosis in prolonged maintenance hemodialysis. *N Engl J Med* 1974;290:697–701.
4. Mailloux LU, et al. Hypertension in patients with chronic renal disease. *Am J Kidney Dis* 1998;32:S120–S141.
5. Longenecker JC, et al. Validation of comorbid conditions on the end-stage renal disease medical evidence report: the CHOICE study—choices for healthy outcomes in caring for ESRD. *J Am Soc Nephrol* 2000;11(3):520–529.
6. Seliger L, et al. HMG-CoA reductase inhibitors are associated with reduced mortality in ESRD patients. *Kidney Int* 2002;61:297–304.
7. Mathur S, et al. Accelerated atherosclerosis, dyslipidemia, and oxidative stress in end-stage renal disease. *Curr Opin Nephrol Hypertens* 2002;11:141–147.
8. Culleton BF, et al. Cardiovascular disease and mortality in a community-based cohort with mild renal insufficiency. *Kidney Int* 1999;56:2214–2219.
9. Levey AS, et al. Controlling the epidemic of cardiovascular disease in chronic renal disease: what do we know? What do we need to learn? Where do we go from here? National Kidney Foundation Task Force on Cardiovascular Disease. *Am J Kidney Dis* 1998;32:853–906.
10. Mailloux LU, et al. The impact of co-morbid risk factors at the start of dialysis upon the survival of ESRD patients. *ASAIO J* 1996;42:164–169.
11. Mailloux LU, et al. Hypertension in the ESRD patient: pathophysiology, therapy, outcomes, and future directions. *Am J Kidney Dis* 1998;32:705–719.

12. Vincenti F, et al. The role of hypertension in hemodialysis-associated atherosclerosis. *Am J Med* 1980;68:363–369.
13. Charra B, et al. Control of hypertension and prolonged survival on maintenance hemodialysis. *Nephron* 1983;33:96–99.
14. Cheng SC, et al. Association of hypertriglyceridemia and insulin resistance in uremic patients undergoing CAPD. *Perit Dial Int* 2001; 21:282–289.
15. Dzurik R, et al. The prevalence of insulin resistance in kidney disease patients before the development of renal failure. *Nephron* 1995;69: 281–285.
16. Haffner SM, et al. Insulin sensitivity in subjects with type 2 diabetes: relationship to cardiovascular risk factors—the Insulin Resistance Atherosclerosis Study. *Diabetes Care* 1999;22:562–568.
17. Goodman WG, et al. Coronary-artery calcification in young adults with end-stage renal disease who are undergoing dialysis. *N Engl J Med* 2000;342:1478–1483.
18. Cozzolino M, et al. Role of calcium-phosphorus product and bone-associated proteins in vascular calcification in renal failure. *J Am Soc Nephrol* 2001;12:2511–2516.
19. Chertow GM, et al. Sevelamer attenuates the progression of coronary and aortic calcification in hemodialysis patients. *Kidney Int* 2002;62: 245–252.
20. Raggi P, et al. Cardiac calcification in adult hemodialysis patients: a link between end-stage renal disease and cardiovascular disease? *J Am Coll Cardiol* 2002;39:695–701.
21. Okamura T, et al. Plasma level of homocysteine is correlated to extracranial carotid-artery atherosclerosis in non-hypertensive Japanese. *J Cardiovasc Risk* 1999;6:371–377.
22. Friedman AN, et al. Plasma total homocysteine levels among patients undergoing nocturnal versus standard hemodialysis. *J Am Soc Nephrol* 2002;13:265–268.
23. Liaugaudas G, et al. Renal insufficiency, vitamin B_{12} status, and population attributable risk for mild hyperhomocysteinemia among coronary artery disease patients in the era of folic acid–fortified cereal grain flour. *Arterioscler Throm Vasc Biol* 2001;21:849–851.
24. Bostom AG. Homocysteine: "expensive creatinine" or important modifiable risk factor for arteriosclerotic outcomes in renal transplant recipients? *J Am Soc Nephrol* 2000;11:149–151.
25. Bostom AG, et al. Hyperhomocysteinemia and traditional cardiovascular disease risk factors in end-stage renal disease patients on dialysis: a case-control study. *Atherosclerosis* 1995;114:93–103.
26. Sarnak MJ, et al. Epidemiology, diagnosis, and management of cardiac disease in chronic renal disease. *J Thromb Thrombolysis* 2000;10: 169–180.
27. Goldstein J, et al. Familial hypercholesterolemia. In: Scriver CR, ed. *The metabolic basis of inherited disease.* New York: McGraw-Hill, 1989:1215–1250.
28. Acton S, et al. Identification of scavenger receptor SR-BI as a high density lipoprotein receptor. *Science* 1996;271:518–520.
29. Gu X, et al. Scavenger receptor class B, type I–mediated [3H]cholesterol efflux to high and low density lipoproteins is dependent on lipoprotein binding to the receptor. *J Biol Chem* 2000;275: 29993–30001.
30. Krieger M, et al. Influence of the HDL receptor SR-BI on atherosclerosis. *Curr Opin Lipidol* 1999;10:491–497.
31. Breckenridge WC, et al. Hypertriglyceridemia associated with deficiency of apolipoprotein C-II. *N Engl J Med* 1978;298:1265.
32. Shoji T, et al. Atherogenic lipoproteins in end-stage renal disease. *Am J Kidney Dis* 2001;38:S30–S33.
33. Scanu AM, et al. Lipoprotein(a): heterogeneity and biological relevance. *J Clin Invest* 1990;85:1709–1715.
34. Kronenberg F, et al. Lipoprotein metabolism in renal replacement therapy: a review. *Isr J Med Sci* 1996;32:371–389.
35. Dieplinger H, et al. Genetics and metabolism of lipoprotein(a) and their clinical implications (Part 1). *Wien Klin Wochenschr* 1999;111:5–20.
36. Kostner GM, et al. Lipoprotein Lp(a) and the risk for myocardial infarction. *Atherosclerosis* 1981;38:51–61.
37. Dieplinger H, et al. Elevated plasma concentrations of lipoprotein(a) in patients with end-stage renal disease are not related to the size polymorphism of apolipoprotein(a). *J Clin Invest* 1993;91:397–401.
38. Quaschning T, et al. Abnormalities in uremic lipoprotein metabolism and its impact on cardiovascular disease. *Am J Kidney Dis* 2001;38: S14–S19.
39. Shah B, et al. Dyslipidemia in patients with chronic renal failure and in renal transplant patients. *J Postgrad Med* 1994;40:57–60.
40. Mittman N, et al. Dyslipidemia in renal disease. *Semin Nephrol* 1996;16:202–213.
41. Wanner C, et al. Inflammation, dyslipidemia and vascular risk factors in hemodialysis patients. *Kidney Int* 1997;62(Suppl):S53–S55.
42. Joven J, et al. Lipoprotein heterogeneity in end-stage renal disease. *Kidney Int* 1993;43:410–418.
43. Ansari A, et al. Cardiac pathology in patients with end-stage renal disease maintained on hemodialysis. *Int J Artif Organs* 1993;16:31–36.
44. Boaz M, et al. Secondary prevention with antioxidants of cardiovascular disease in endstage renal disease (SPACE): randomised placebo-controlled trial. *Lancet* 2000;356:1213–1218.
45. Karnik JA, et al. Cardiac arrest and sudden death in dialysis units. *Kidney Int* 2001;60:350–357.
46. Chertow GM, et al. Cost-effectiveness of cancer screening in end-stage renal disease. *Arch Intern Med* 1996;156:1345–1350.
47. Grundy SM. United States Cholesterol Guidelines 2001: expanded scope of intensive low-density lipoprotein-lowering therapy. *Am J Cardiol* 2001;88:23J–27J.
48. Savdie E, et al. Impaired plasma triglyceride clearance as a feature of both uremic and posttransplant triglyceridemia. *Kidney Int* 1980;18: 774–782.
49. Senti M, et al. Lipoprotein abnormalities in hyperlipidemic and normolipidemic men on hemodialysis with chronic renal failure. *Kidney Int* 1992;41:1394–1399.
50. Attman PO, et al. Lipoprotein abnormalities as a risk factor for progressive nondiabetic renal disease. *Kidney Int* 1999;71(Suppl): S14–S17.
51. Attman P, et al. Serum apolipoprotein profile of patients with chronic renal failure. *Kidney Int* 1987;32:368–375.
52. Chan MK, et al. Lipid abnormalities in uremia, dialysis, and transplantation. *Kidney Int* 1981;19:625–637.
53. Bagdade J, et al. Effects of chronic uremia, hemodialysis, and renal transplantation on plasma lipids and lipoproteins in man. *J Lab Clin Med* 1976;87:37–48.
54. Chan PCK, et al. Apolipoprotein B turnover in dialysis patients: its relationship to pathogenesis of hyperlipidemia. *Clin Nephrol* 1989;31: 88–95.
55. Cramp DG. Plasma lipid alterations in patients with chronic renal disease. *Crit Rev Clin Lab Sci* 1982;17:77–101.
56. Norbeck H, et al. Serum lipid and lipoprotein concentrations in chronic uremia. *Acta Med Scand* 1976;200:487–492.
57. Cianciaruso B, et al. Lipid abnormalities in patients with different degrees of chronic renal failure. *Contrib Nephrol* 1984;41:438–440.
58. Strapans I, et al. Apoprotein composition in plasma lipoproteins in uremic patients on hemodialysis. *Clinica Chimica Acta* 1979;93: 135–143.
59. Grundy SM. Management of hyperlipidemia in renal disease. *Kidney Int* 1990;37:847–853.
60. Cattran DC, et al. Defective triglyceride renal in lipemia associated with peritoneal dialysis and haemodialysis. *Ann Intern Med* 1976;85: 29–33.
61. Dieplinger H, et al. Plasma cholesterol metabolism in end-stage renal disease. *J Clin Invest* 1986;77:1071–1083.
62. Murase T, et al. Inhibition of lipoprotein lipase by uremic plasma, a possible cause of hypertriglyceridemia. *Metabolism* 1975;24: 1279–1286.
63. Sanfellipo M, et al. Transport of very low density lipoprotein triglyceride (VLDL-TG): comparison of hemodialysis and hemofiltration. *Kidney Int* 1979;16:878–886.
64. Applebaum-Bowden D, et al. Postheparin plasma triglyceride lipases in chronic hemodialysis: evidence for a role for hepatic lipase in lipoprotein metabolism. *Metabolism* 1979;28:917–924.
65. Chan MK, et al. Pathogenic roles of post-heparin lipases in lipid abnormalities in hemodialysis patients. *Kidney Int* 1984;25:812–818.
66. Goldberg A, et al. Adipose tissue lipoprotein lipase in chronic hemo-

dialysis: role in plasma triglyceride metabolism. *J Clin Endocrinol Metab* 1978;47:1173–1182.

67. Goldberg A, et al. Increase in lipoprotein lipase during clofibrate treatment of hypertriglyceridemia in patients on hemodialysis. *N Engl J Med* 1979;301:1073–1076.

68. Mordasini R, et al. Selective deficiency of hepatic triglyceride lipase in uremic patients. *N Engl J Med* 1977;297:1362–1366.

69. Pasternack A, et al. Normalization of lipoprotein lipase and hepatic lipase by gemfibrozil results in correction of lipoprotein abnormalities in chronic renal failure. *Clin Nephrol* 1987;27:163–168.

70. Vaziri ND, et al. Downregulation of tissue lipoprotein lipase expression in experimental chronic renal failure. *Kidney Int* 1996;50:1928–1935.

71. Wakabayashi Y, et al. Decreased VLDL apoprotein CII/apoprotein CIII ratio may be seen in both normotriglyceridemic and hypertriglyceridemic patients on chronic hemodialysis treatment. *Metabolism* 1987;36:815.

72. Moberly JB, et al. Apolipoprotein C-III, hypertriglyceridemia and triglyceride-rich lipoproteins in uremia. *Miner Electrolyte Metab* 1999;25:258–262.

73. Bucala R, et al. Modification of low density lipoprotein by advanced glycation end products contributes to the dyslipidemia of diabetes and renal insufficiency. *Proc Natl Acad Sci USA* 1994;91:9441–9445.

74. Makita Z, et al. Reactive glycosylation endproducts in diabetic uraemia and treatment of renal failure. *Lancet* 1994;343:1519–1522.

75. Horrko S, et al. Carbamylation-induced alterations in low-density lipoprotein metabolism. *Kidney Int* 1992;41:1175–1181.

76. Maggi E, et al. Enhanced LDL oxidation in uremic patients: an additional mechanism for accelerated atherosclerosis? *Kidney Int* 1994;45:876–883.

77. Vega GL, et al. Management of primary mixed hyperlipidemia with lovastatin. *Arch Intern Med* 1990;150:1313–1319.

78. Vega GL, et al. Increased catabolism of VLDL-apolipoprotein B and synthesis of bile acids in a case of hypobetalipoproteinemia. *Metabolism* 1987;36:262–269.

79. Kameda K, et al. Increased frequency of lipoprotein disorders similar to type III hyperlipoproteinemia in survivors of myocardial infarction in Japan. *Atherosclerosis* 1984;51:241–249.

80. Tatami R, et al. Intermediate-density lipoprotein and cholesterol-rich very low density lipoprotein in angiographically determined coronary artery disease. *Circulation* 1981;64:1174–1184.

81. Grundy SM, et al. Hypertriglyceridemia: causes and relation to coronary heart disease. *Semin Thromb Hemost* 1988;14:149–164.

82. Brown G, et al. Regression of coronary artery disease as a result of intensive lipid-lowering therapy in men with high levels of apolipoprotein B. *N Engl J Med* 1990;323:1298.

83. Burke SW, et al. Cardiac complications of end-stage renal disease. *Adv Ren Replace Ther* 2000;7:210–219.

84. Coresh J, et al. Association of plasma triglyceride concentration and LDL particle diameter, density, and chemical composition with premature coronary artery disease in men and women. *J Lipid Res* 1993;34:1687–1697.

85. Koch M, et al. Apolipoprotein B, fibrinogen, HDL cholesterol, and apolipoprotein(a) phenotypes predict coronary artery disease in hemodialysis patients. *J Am Soc Nephrol* 1997;8:1889–1898.

86. Patsch W, et al. Associations of allelic differences at the A-I/C-III/A-IV gene cluster with carotid artery intima-media thickness and plasma lipid transport in hypercholesterolemic-hypertriglyceridemic humans. *Arterioscler Thromb* 1994;14:874–883.

87. Varghese K, et al. Coronary artery disease among diabetic and non-diabetic patients with end-stage renal disease. *Ren Fail* 2001;23:669–677.

88. Hsia SL, et al. Defect in cholesterol transport in patients receiving maintenance hemodialysis. *J Lab Clin Med* 1985;106:53–61.

89. Joven J, et al. Apoprotein A-1 and high density lipoprotein subfractions in patients with chronic renal failure receiving hemodialysis. *Nephron* 1985;40:451–454.

90. Haffner SM, et al. Increased lipoprotein(a) concentrations in chronic renal failure. *J Am Soc Nephrol* 1992;3:1156–1162.

91. Fuh MMT, et al. Effect of chronic renal failure on high-density lipoprotein kinetics. *Kidney Int* 1990;37:1295–1300.

92. Vaziri ND, et al. Down-regulation of hepatic LDL receptor expression in experimental nephrosis. *Kidney Int* 1996;50:887–893.

93. Quaschning T, et al. Non-insulin-dependent diabetes mellitus and hypertriglyceridemia impair lipoprotein metabolism in chronic hemodialysis patients. *J Am Soc Nephrol* 1999;10:332–341.

94. Ambrosch A, et al. Compositional and functional changes of low-density lipoprotein during hemodialysis in patients with ESRD. *Kidney Int* 1998;54:608–617.

95. Ambrosch A, et al. Small-sized low-density lipoproteins of subclass B from patients with end-stage renal disease effectively augment tumor necrosis factor-alpha-induced adhesive properties in human endothelial cells. *Am J Kidney Dis* 2002;39:972–984.

96. O'Neal D, et al. Low-density lipoprotein particle size distribution in end-stage renal disease treated with hemodialysis or peritoneal dialysis. *Am J Kidney Dis* 1996;27:84–91.

97. Sevanian A, et al. Contribution of an in vivo oxidized LDL to LDL oxidation and its association with dense LDL subpopulations. *Arterioscler Thromb Vasc Biol* 1996;16:784–793.

98. Makita Z, et al. The role of advanced glycosylation end-products in the pathogenesis of atherosclerosis. *Nephrol Dial Transplant* 1996;(Suppl 5):31–33.

99. Kusuhara M, et al. Oxidized LDL stimulates mitogen-activated protein kinases in smooth muscle cells and macrophages. *Arterioscler Thromb Vasc Biol* 1997;17:141–148.

100. Ding G, et al. Oxidized LDL stimulates the expression of TGF-beta and fibronectin in human glomerular epithelial cells. *Kidney Int* 1997;51:147.

101. O'Byrne D, et al. Low-density lipoprotein (LDL)-induced monocyte-endothelial cell adhesion, soluble cell adhesion molecules, and autoantibodies to oxidized-LDL in chronic renal failure patients on dialysis therapy. *Metabolism* 2001;50:207–215.

102. Cressman MD, et al. Elevated Lp(a) levels and abnormal Apo(a) density distribution accompany the increased risk of cardiovascular disease in hemodialysis patients. *Circulation* 1992;86:2172.

103. Cressman MD, et al. Lipoprotein(a) is an independent risk factor for cardiovascular disease in hemodialysis patients. *Circulation* 1992;86:475–482.

104. Kandoussi AM, et al. Apo(a) phenotypes and lp(a) concentrations in renal transplant patients. *Nephron* 1998;80:183–187.

105. Yang WS, et al. Effect of increasing serum albumin on serum lipoprotein(a) concentration in patients receiving CPAD. *Am J Kid Dis* 1997;30:507–513.

106. Kronenberg F, et al. The low molecular weight apo(a) phenotype is an independent predictor for coronary artery disease in hemodialysis patients: a prospective follow-up. *J Am Soc Nephrol* 1999;10:1027–1036.

107. Kronenberg F, et al. Multicenter study of lipoprotein(a) and apolipoprotein(a) phenotypes in patients with end-stage renal disease treated by hemodialysis or continuous ambulatory peritoneal dialysis. *J Am Soc Nephrol* 1995;6:110–120.

108. Weintraub M, et al. Severe defect in clearing postprandial chylomicron remnants in dialysis patients. *Kidney Int* 1992;42:1247–1252.

109. Nauck M, et al. Is the determination of LDL cholesterol according to Friedewald accurate in CAPD and HD patients? *Clin Nephrol* 1996;46:319–325.

110. Framingham. Risk score, www.intmed.mcw.edu/clincalc/heartrisk.html. Web site. 2002.

111. Wilson P, et al. Prediction of coronary heart disease using risk factor categories. *Circulation* 1998;97:1837–1847.

112. Cattran DC, et al. Dialysis hyperlipemia: response to dietary manipulations. *Clin Nephrol* 1980;13:177–182.

113. Attman P-O, et al. Effect of protein-reduced diet on plasma lipids, apolipoproteins and lipolytic activities in patients with chronic renal failure. *Am J Nephrol* 1984;4:92–98.

114. Seres DS, et al. Improvement of plasma lipoprotein profiles during high-flux dialysis. *J Am Soc Nephrol* 1993;3:1409–1415.

115. De Precigout V, et al. Improvement in lipid profiles and triglyceride removal in patients on polyamide membrane hemodialysis. *Blood Purif* 1996;14:170–176.

116. Blankestijn PJ. Hemodialysis using high flux membranes improves lipid profiles. *Clin Nephrol* 1994;42(Suppl 1):S48–S51.

117. Eknoyan, et al. Effect of dialysis dose and membrane flux in maintenance hemodialysis. *N Engl J Med* 2002;347:2010–2019.

118. Stefoni S, et al. Standard heparin versus low-molecular-weight heparin: a medium-term comparison in hemodialysis. *Nephron* 2002;92:589–600.

119. Yang C, et al. Low molecular weight heparin reduces triglyceride, VLDL and cholesterol/HDL levels in hyperlipidemic diabetic patients on hemodialysis. *Am J Nephrol* 1998;18:384–390.

120. Lai KN, et al. Effect of low molecular weight heparin on bone metabolism and hyperlipidemia in patients on maintenance hemodialysis. *Int Soc Artif Organs* 2002;24:447–455.

121. Grutzmacher P, et al. Lipid lowering treatment with bezafibrate in patients on chronic haemodialysis: pharmacokinetics and effects. *Klin Wochenschr* 1986;64:910–916.

122. Levin A, et al. A randomized placebo-controlled double-blind trial of lipid-lowering strategies in patients with renal insufficiency: diet modification with or without fenofibrate. *Clin Nephrol* 2000;53:140–146.

123. Guay D. Update on fenofibrate. *Card Drug Rev* 2002;20:281–302.

124. Pierides AM, et al. Clofibrate-induced muscle damage in patients with chronic renal failure. *Lancet* 1975;2:1279–1282.

125. Kijima Y, et al. Untoward effects of clofibrate in hemodialyzed patients. *Correspondence* 1977;296:515.

126. Sacks F, et al. The effect of pravastatin on coronary events after myocardial infarction in patients with average cholesterol levels. *N Engl J Med* 1996;335:1001–1009.

127. Scandinavian Simvistatin Survival Study Group. Scandinavian randomized trial of cholesterol lowering in 4,444 patients with coronary heart disease. *Lancet* 1994;344:1383–1389.

128. Shepherd J, et al. Prevention of coronary heart disease with pravastatin in men. *N Engl J Med* 1996;334:1333–1335.

129. Wanner C, et al. Rationale and design of a trial improving outcome of type 2 diabetics on hemodialysis. Die Deutsche Diabetes Dialyse Studie Investigators. *Kidney Int* 1999;71(Suppl):S222–S226.

130. Saxenhofer H, et al. Effects of simvastatin in plasma lipid profile in patients undergoing continuous peritoneal dialysis (CP). *Kidney Int* 1991;39:1330.

131. DiPaolo B, et al. Therapeutic effects of simvastatin on hyperlipidemia in CAPD patients: one-year, alternate day dosage, corticosteroid Rx reduces rate of further relapses in adult minimal change nephrosis. *ASAIO Trans* 1990;36:M578–M580.

132. Wanner C, et al. Effects of HGM-CoA reductase inhibitors in hypercholesterolemic patients on hemodialysis. *Kidney Int* 1991;39:754–760.

133. Robins SJ, et al. VA-HIT Study Group. Veterans Affairs High-Density Lipoprotein Intervention Trial. Relation of gemfibrozil treatment and lipid levels with major coronary events: VA-HIT—a randomized controlled trial. *JAMA* 2001;285:1585–1593.

134. Bostom AG, et al. High dose-B-vitamin treatment of hyperhomocysteinemia in dialysis patients. *Kidney Int* 1996;49:147–152.

DIALYSIS CONSIDERATIONS IN THE PATIENT WITH ACUTE RENAL FAILURE: ICU DIALYSIS

ANDREW E. BRIGLIA

Major changes have occurred in the medical management of intensive care unit (ICU) patients over the past two decades. Extracorporeal blood purification (ECBP) has undergone significant changes in its role for replacing renal function and its application in nonrenal indications has grown (1) (Table 29.1). Reviews on acute renal failure (ARF) and ECBP in the ICU have been recently published (2–4), and complications of extracorporeal therapy have been thoroughly described (5,6). The purpose of this chapter is to characterize existing ECBP methodologies, including hybrid circuits, and to describe ECBP in specific disease states commonly encountered in ICU patients.

HOW IS THE APPLICATION OF ECBP DIFFERENT IN THE ICU?

Acute renal failure (ARF) in the ICU has a reported incidence of 1% to 25% (7,8), and a higher incidence (31%) has been reported in trauma patients admitted to the ICU (9). The mortality rate from ARF, which has generally been accepted as greater than 50% (10,11), may be improving based on studies conducted recently (12,13). In a 3-year multicenter cohort study [Project to Improve Care in Acute Renal Disease (PICARD)], the mean BUN and creatinine concentrations were 52 and 2.8 mg/dL, respectively, on admission; 63 and 3.3 mg/dL at time of the nephrology consultation; and 85 and 4.6 mg/dL at time of hemodialysis (HD) initiation (intermittent hemodialysis (IHD) 26%, continuous renal replacement therapy (CRRT) 22%, both 17%). Mortality was 32% for the entire cohort (44% in dialyzed versus 23% in nondialyzed patients, p <0.001). ARF was defined as an increase in serum creatinine concentration of at least 0.5 mg/dL with baseline less than 1.4 and ARF superimposed on chronic renal failure (A/CRF) as an increase in serum creatinine of at least 1.0 with baseline of more than 1.5 to 4.9. Higher mortality was observed in men (44% versus 34%) and with increase in age more than 65 (39% versus 34%) (14). However, hospitalized patients with ARF are more likely to have a worse outcome than those without renal dysfunction (8) or end-stage renal disease (ESRD). Clermont and coworkers conducted a prospective evaluation of 1,530 patients

(254 patients with ARF, 57 with ESRD, and 1,219 with no renal dysfunction) admitted to eight ICUs and found that of the ARF patients considered severe enough to require dialysis, 57% died. The overall mortality was 23% for patients with ARF, 11% for those with ESRD, and 5% for patients with no renal dysfunction (15). The lasting effects of ARF extend beyond the hospital setting, as 2.7% to 33% of patients with ARF who survive hospitalization will be considered dialysis dependent (10,13).

Because there are a variety of definitions for ARF, depending upon the study (16), some authors (7) have proposed a tiered consensus approach that separates early and late acute renal injury (ARI) from chronic renal failure. Such a model takes into consideration factors such as the degree of injury and renal dysfunction as well as the time component of injury. While this approach may be less than ideal, it may help categorize patients in studying outcomes of ARF and determine the timing of application of renal replacement therapy (RRT) modalities. In addition, the ideal markers of renal injury are undefined, since traditional markers—namely, urea and serum creatinine concentrations—vary with somatic mass, gender, volume status, gastrointestinal blood loss, parenteral nutrition, and hypercatabolism. Moreover, other parameters such as concurrent organ dysfunction, anemia, and nutrition also affect mortality (7,17).

The ideal quantification of ECBP dose in ARF is also debated. ARF severity scoring, such as the Cleveland Clinic Foundation (CCF) model, may facilitate ECBP prescription (18), since dialysis dose delivery can affect outcome in certain patients (19) (Fig. 29.1). The traditional single-pool urea kinetic model assumes that urea is uniformly distributed in one pool and that urea generation is kept constant. The Kt/V_{urea} is a three-point approach that takes into consideration dialyzer clearance (K), duration of treatment (t), and urea distribution volume (V_{urea}), which is assumed to be 50% to 60% of body weight. As an alternative to single-pool urea kinetics, some investigators have utilized equivalent renal clearance (EKR) as an integral approach to patients with hypercatabolic ARF. EKR is the quotient of urea generation rate (G) divided by normalized PCR (nPCR) and is expressed in milliliters per minute. This kinetic model has been applied to hemofiltration. For specific values of

TABLE 29.1. POTENTIAL INDICATIONS FOR RENAL REPLACEMENT THERAPY (RRT) IN THE ICU

Nonobstructive oliguria
Severe acidemia (pH <7.1) due to metabolic acidosis
Azotemia (blood urea >30 mmol/L or >100 mg/dL)
Hyperkalemia (plasma potassium >6.5 mmol/L) or rapidly rising
   potassium
Suspected uremic organ involvement (pericarditis, encephalopathy,
   neuropathy, or myelopathy)
Progressive severe dysnatremia (sodium >160 or <115 mmol/L)
Hyperthermia (core temperature >39.5°C)
Clinically significant organ edema (especially lung)
Overdose with dialyzable drug
Coagulopathy requiring large amounts of blood products in patients
   with or at risk of pulmonary edema/adult respiratory distress
   syndrome
Hepatic failure
Congestive heart failure

Adapted with permission from Burchardi H. Renal replacement therapy (RRT) in the ICU: criteria for initiating RRT. In: Ronco C, et al., eds. *Blood purification in intensive care.* Contributions to Nephrology. Basel: Karger, 2001:171–180.

initial BUN and nPCR, increasing the ultrafiltration rate from 1.5 to 3.5 L/h results in an 85% to 95% increase in EKR for patients on continuous venovenous hemofiltration (CVVH) (20). In addition, CVVH provides 8% greater urea clearance than sustained low-efficiency dialysis (SLED) and 60% greater urea clearance than intermittent hemodialysis (IHD). The EKR for middle molecules such as inulin and β_2-microglobulin (β_2-m) in CVVH is approximately twofold greater than IHD and fourfold greater than SLED (21).

The Hemodialysis (HEMO) study recently showed no influence of dialysis dose or flux on survival in patients with ESRD (overall cohort, 1,846 patients). Among women, however, increased dialysis dose was associated with increased survival, and the use of high-flux dialyzer filters (β_2-M clearance >20 mL/min) was associated with a 20% reduction in cardiac death (22). Because prior evidence suggests that an inverse relationship exists between delivered dialysis dose and outcome in patients with

ESRD in the United States (23–29), it has been suggested that the prescription and delivery of dialysis for ARF should be targeted to ESRD goals (30). Thus quantification techniques that are employed in ESRD have been extrapolated to patients with ARF (23). These quantification techniques assume that, like ESRD, ARF is a steady-state process. In fact, urea distribution volume (V_{urea}) is often higher (65% of total body weight versus 50% to 60% in steady-state ESRD patients), as is normalized protein catabolic rate (nPCR) (1.5 g/kg/d in ARF versus 1.25 g/kg/d in ESRD), as a consequence of volume overload, hypercatabolism, and increased urea generation in patients with ARF (23). A model designed by Clark et al., which plots time-averaged blood urea nitrogen (BUN_a) for intermittent hemodialysis (IHD) and steady-state BUN (BUN_s) for continuous renal replacement therapy (CRRT) against nPCR (normalized for daily therapy dose Kt/V_{urea}) (23) indicates that by increasing frequency of IHD treatments, one can approach the efficiency of CRRT in providing steady-state urea clearance. Table 29.2 lists factors to be considered in ARF renal replacement therapy (RRT) determination (23). Prescription and delivery of hemodialysis are known to be affected by several factors, including hemodynamic status, degree of catabolism, variable extracellular fluid volume, and coagulation status. One study found that the following factors affect single-pool Kt/V (spKt/V):

1. Blood flow Q_b (0.2 unit higher spKt/V per 100 mL/min increase)
2. Gender (0.15 units higher spKt/V in female patients)
3. Vascular access (0.1 unit lower spKt/V with femoral catheter use)
4. Body weight (0.07 unit lower spKt/V per 10-kg increase)
5. Dialyzer surface area (0.03 units higher spKt/V per 0.1 m² dialyzer surface area increase) (31)

Indeed, more frequent hemodialysis has been advocated. Schiffl and colleagues randomized 160 patients to receive hemodialysis on either a daily (N = 80) or alternate-day (N = 80) basis. All patients had ARF secondary to acute tubular necrosis, and patients who required CRRT or who had cardiogenic shock and hepatorenal syndrome were excluded. Patients in each arm

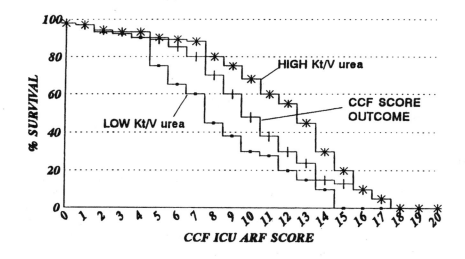

FIG. 29.1. Dialysis dose and outcome in ARF. The Cleveland Clinic Foundation (CCF) ARF Severity Scoring model was found to be highly predictive of survival (78% in those with scores less than 4 and 0% in those with scores more than 15) in 512 critically ill patients, regardless of dialysis dose. Higher delivered dialysis dose (urea reduction ratio more than 58% in IHD and time-averaged concentration of urea less than 45 mg/dL in CRRT) appeared to have the greatest survival impact in those with intermediate scores. (With permission from Paganini EP, et al. Establishing a dialysis therapy/patient outcome link in the intensive care unit for patients with acute renal failure. *Am J Kidney Dis* 1996;28(Suppl 3): S81–S89.)

TABLE 29.2. RENAL REPLACEMENT THERAPY (RRT) PRESCRIPTION FACTORS IN ARF

Substrate Removal	Renal Replacement Therapy (RRT) Prescription Factors in ARF
Plasma concentration	Extent of protein hypercatabolism
Dialyzer membrane porosity	Body size / total body water (including effect of volume overload)
Dialysate and ultrafiltration rate	Access recirculation
Blood flow	Desired level of metabolic control
Modality (CRRT vs. IHD)	Ability of chosen RRT to achieve treatment goal
	Achieving delivery of prescribed RRT

Adapted with permission from Clark WR, et al. The role of renal replacement therapy (RRT) quantification in acute renal failure. *Am J Kid Dis* 1997;30(Suppl 4):S10–S14.
CRRT, continuous renal replacement therapy; IHD, intermittent hemodialysis.

were equally distributed with regard to age, gender, etiology of renal failure, and APACHE (Acute Physiology and Chronic Health Evaluation) III scores. Similarly, hemodialysis sessions were prescribed to provide similar duration, blood-flow rate, and delivered Kt/V_{urea} per session. Patients who received daily hemodialysis had lower mortality (22%) than those in the alternate-day group (37%) ($p = .01$), and resolution of ARF occurred sooner in those who received daily therapy (daily HD 9 ± 2 versus alternate-day HD 16 ± 6, $p = .001$) (32). Although this study supports prescription of more frequent dialysis, it has been criticized for excluding patients whose severity of illness led them to require CVVHD and delivery of lower dialysis dose to the alternate-day HD group (weekly delivered Kt/V_{urea} 3.0 ± 0.6 alternate-day versus 5.8 ± 0.4 daily) (33). In addition, the ideal timing of initiation of ECBP is uncertain. Retrospective data by Gettings et al. suggest that earlier CRRT (BUN <60 mg/dL) was associated with greater survival (39% versus 20%) than later initiation (BUN >60 mg/dL) in posttraumatic ARF ($p = 0.041$) (34). Choice of dialyzer membrane also influences ECBP prescription. Although evidence suggests that greater survival, increased recovery of renal function, and need for fewer dialysis sessions are associated with synthetic versus cellulosic membranes (35,36), some controversy still exists over ideal membrane composition (37). However, a recent metaanalysis favors use of synthetic membranes in patients with ARF (38). Selection between CRRT and intermittent hemodialysis (IHD) is also debated. A metaanalysis by Kellum et al. evaluated 13 studies, of which three were randomized. These authors found no difference in mortality between intermittent and continuous modalities. However, adjustment for severity of illness yielded a lower mortality rate in patients treated with CRRT [cumulative relative risk (RR) 0.72 (0.60 to 0.87), $p < 0.01$] (39). Similarly, Mehta and coworkers conducted a prospective multicenter trial that randomized 136 patients with ARF (BUN ≥40 mg/dL, serum creatinine ≥2.0 mg/dL, or a sustained rise in serum creatinine ≥1 mg/dL) to receive either IHD or CRRT [continuous venovenous hemodialysis (CVVHD)]. Although IHD was associated with lower mortality (41.5% IHD versus 59.5% CVVHD, $p < 0.02$), CRRT was associated with shorter median ICU length of stay (CRRT 17.1 versus IHD 26.3 days, $p < 0.01$). Moreover, following adjustment for certain factors, CRRT was associated with greater recovery of renal function (CRRT 92.3% versus IHD 59.4%, $p < 0.01$) (40). The reader is

directed to Chapter 13 for a more in-depth description of CRRT modalities and prescription. The Acute Dialysis Quality Initiative has been recently created to develop a consensus and evidence-based approach for the management of ARF (41). From this consortium, a list of guidelines pertaining to CRRT patient selection, prescription, operational characteristics, and solute control has emerged (42).

ECBP: CURRENT TECHNOLOGY, HYBRID CIRCUITS, AND EMERGING MODALITIES

Because CRRT has been promoted as a way to achieve more gradual, physiologic solute and volume control and because conventional hemodialysis is often associated with intradialytic hypotension, several researchers have modified conventional hemodialysis to create a more favorable hemodynamic profile. Their efforts have led to the development of sustained low-efficiency dialysis (SLED) and extended daily dialysis (EDD). These techniques combine CRRT with conventional IHD to provide prolonged dialysis treatments with low rates of solute and fluid clearance (43). These modalities can be performed with conventional dialysis machines such as the Fresenius 2008H (Fresenius Medical Care, Lexington, MA) or the Althin Drake-Willock System 1000 or Althin Tina (Althin Medical, Inc., Miami, FL). Treatments are typically run from 6 to 12 hours with lower blood flows and dialysate flows than those prescribed for conventional hemodialysis (43–47). EDD was initiated at the University of California–Davis in 1997. SLED was introduced at the University of Arkansas in 1998 and has recently been utilized at the University of Maryland. A sample prescription is outlined (43–47) (Table 29.3). Either technique has the advantage of providing slower therapy to patients with hemodynamic compromise for whom CRRT is indicated but nurse staffing limitations prevent institution of CRRT. In addition, the use of SLED or EDD is potentially cost-saving, as on-line production of dialysate occurs and standard blood tubing is utilized. Moreover, EDD and SLED may save nurse staffing, since one dialysis nurse can manage more than one treatment at a time. EDD and SLED are hemodynamically well tolerated, are easier to manage than CRRT, and are capable of delivering adequate dialysis without inducing urea disequilibrium (45,46). Slow, continuous dialysis with the Fresenius 2008H machine has also been described (47).

TABLE 29.3 SLED/EDD: PRESCRIPTION

Dialysate flow (Qd): 300 mL/min
Blood flow (Qb): 100–200 mL/min
Vascular access: 11.5°F, 20 cm dual-lumen catheter
Dialyzer: Fresenius F4 (Fresenius Medical Care)
Anticoagulation: heparin 25,000 units in 250 mL NS @ 200–750 U/hr
  (or hourly boluses)
Ultrafiltration: 100–500 mL/hr
Dialysate temperature: 35.5°C
Dialysate composition: profiled sodium, potassium, bicarbonate
Days/hours operation: 7 a.m. to 7 p.m., Monday through Saturday

Adapted with permission from Marshall MR, et al. Hybrid renal replacement modalities for the critically ill. *Contrib Nephrol* 2001;132:252–257.
SLED, sustained low-efficiency dialysis; EDD, extended daily dialysis.

Hemofiltration/Hemodiafiltration

Hemofiltration and hemodiafiltration are achieving increasing interest in their application to several disease states, particularly sepsis and hepatic failure (see later). Hemofiltration is primarily a convective technique in which the ultrafiltrate is either partially or completely replaced with sterile solution [infused either prefilter (predilution) or postfilter (postdilution)]. Hemodiafiltration is a hybrid between hemofiltration and hemodialysis, and as such, incorporates a countercurrent dialysate solution within the hemofiltration circuit. Convective techniques such as hemofiltration and hemodiafiltration lead to accumulation of solutes along the surface of the filtering membrane. As a consequence, higher ultrafiltration rates lead to solute concentration polarization (48–50). This phenomenon describes the formation of a protein layer along the blood–membrane interface that occurs linearly along the hollow fiber with increasing transmembrane pressure (TMP). As a consequence, there is greater concentration of solutes along the membrane than in bulk plasma flow. This tends to favor removal of large-molecular-weight substances (30,000 to 70,000 daltons) but also allows for backdiffusion of solutes from the ultrafiltrate side into the blood compartment. Factors that tend to increase concentration polarization include increasing ultrafiltration rate, low blood flow, and postdilution replacement fluids. Evidence suggests that the use of predilution substitution fluids may preserve sieving coefficients of both small-molecular-weight (urea, creatinine) and middle-molecular-weight (vancomycin, inulin, and β_2-M) molecules despite increasing ultrafiltration rates from 20 to 60 mL/min (or 17 to 51 mL/h/kg in a 70-kg patient) (51). Use of predilution substitution fluids in hemofiltration may reduce the anticoagulation requirement but may require as much as a twofold increase in substitution fluid rate (Q_S) to maintain small solute clearance (52). Studies comparing these modalities as they apply to specific disease states will be discussed in more detail later. Unfortunately, few data exist that compare use of hemodialysis with hemofiltration in ICU-related ARF.

Peritoneal Dialysis

Peritoneal dialysis (PD) is a safe and inexpensive renal replacement modality in ARF and has been referred to as an "internal CAVHD (continuous arteriovenous hemodialysis) system" (53). This therapy has been demonstrated to have the same mortality as conventional hemodialysis, or possibly better, and may contribute to recovery of renal function by virtue of its stable hemodynamic profile (54–58). Obviously, PD is not practical in ARF patients with abdominal trauma, surgical intervention to the abdomen, and ileus (53,59). Swartz and coworkers found that the main complications encountered with PD in the ARF setting were hyperglycemia (57%), mechanical difficulties such as poor catheter drainage (52%) and mild bleeding (26%), and asymptomatic positive peritoneal cultures (26%). Cardiac deaths were identified more often in PD than in HD patients. However, this likely reflects a bias toward greater application of PD in this population (53,56). Although typical volumes of peritoneal dialysate (e.g., 2 to 3 L every 6 hours) provide less clearance of small-molecular-weight molecules (e.g., urea and creatinine) than hemodialysis, clearance may be increased by augmenting exchange volumes to ≥1.5 to 2.0 L/h. In addition, PD has the capability of removing middle molecules such as proteins (5 to 20 g/d) to which toxins may be bound (60), as well as chemical mediators such as platelet activator inhibitor-1 (PAI-1) (53,61). Use of a dual-cuff chronic PD catheter is advocated in ARF (53). Several hybrid circuits have been developed to increase solute removal efficiency with PD, including external dialysis of the peritoneal effluent (62,63) and continuous flow peritoneal dialysis (CFPD) (64). The reader is referred to Chapters 14 and 15 for more detailed discussion of PD.

Therapeutic Plasma Exchange

Therapeutic plasma exchange (TPE) and plasmapheresis have received growing attention in the ICU. These techniques differ in that TPE is a single-step process where plasma is filtered by means of a highly porous filter (e.g., Plasma-Flo filter produced by Asahi: Apheresis Technologies, Palm Harbor, FL) or by centrifugation to allow removal of large-molecular-weight or protein-bound substances. In turn, the effluent is replaced by albumin, fresh-frozen plasma, cryoprecipitate, or starch (e.g., 6% Hetastarch, Baxter Anesthesia & Critical Care, New Providence, RI). Plasmapheresis, on the other hand, is a dual-step procedure whereby separated plasma is further exposed to an adsorptive column, after which the processed plasma is returned to the patient, rather than being discarded (65). TPE and plasmapheresis are advocated for removal of substances that are ≥15,000 daltons and that are not easily removed by conventional hemodialysis or hemofiltration alone. Examples of these substances are immune complexes (molecular weight >300,000 daltons), immunoglobulins (e.g., IgG 160,000 daltons), myeloma light chains (Bence-Jones protein 10,000 to 25,000 daltons), cryoglobulins, endotoxin (100 to $2,400 \times 10^3$ daltons), and lipoproteins (1.3×10^6 daltons) (66). Therapy is generally prescribed on the basis of estimated plasma volume [EPV = (0.065 × wt in kg) × (1 − hematocrit)] (67). In addition, TPE can be provided with a modification of conventional dialysis machines, a process that is referred to as membrane plasma separation (MPS) (68–71). Plasma exchange therapy has been utilized with hematologic disorders such as thrombotic microangiopathy (thrombotic thrombocytopenic purpura and hemolytic–uremic syndrome) (72–76), cryoglobulinemia, and hyperviscosity syndrome (77). In addition, this modality has been employed in neurologic disorders such as Guillain-Barré syndrome, myasthenia gravis, and chronic inflammatory demyelinating polyneuropathy (78). Plasma exchange has become standard therapy for patients with anti-GBM antibody-mediated glomerulonephritis (Goodpasture's syndrome) (79–83), and there is some literature supporting efficacy in other renal diseases such as myeloma cast nephropathy (84,85), other forms of rapidly progressive glomerulonephritis (not associated with anti-GBM-antibody), and postrenal transplantation (recurrent focal segmental glomerulosclerosis and renal allograft rejection) (86). TPE has also been applied to cases of sepsis and hepatic failure (see later).

Bioartificial Renal Tubule Assist Device

The bioartificial renal tubule assist device (RAD) applies cell engineering to create a hollow fiber tubule that duplicates proximal convoluted tubule (PCT) function (87–89). The initial device was inoculated with porcine renal PCT cells. Since then, models utilizing canine PCT cells and human cadaveric kidney PCT cells have also been developed. Confluent growth of the cells is noted within 7 to 10 days, and monolayer integrity and performance are maintained for 6 months. Electron microscopy demonstrates epithelial differentiation, including formation of microvilli, intercellular infoldings, and endocytotic vesicles (87). Figure 29.2 illustrates the device (87). A number of tubular functions have been documented (87), including vectorial fluid transport and several metabolic (ammoniagenesis, gluconeogenesis, IL-10 production, and transport of sodium, glucose, and paraaminohippurate (PAH)) and endocrinologic (1-OH vitamin D_3 activity) properties. The device has been applied to a canine model of sepsis, where increments in IL-10 (an antiinflammatory cytokine) and mean arterial pressure have been documented (90,91). More reliable models of animal sepsis are being utilized, and the precise dose of cell therapy remains to be defined (90). Ultrafiltration membranes composed of silicone are also being developed to facilitate tissue engineering of nephronal units (92). In time, these filters may become implantable, thereby making the RAD a portable device. The bioartificial kidney (BK) synthetic hemofiltration cartridge has been combined in series with a renal tubule-assist device containing 10^9 human renal tubule cells in a conventional CVVH circuit. It has been used in phase I/II clinical trials and has demonstrated alterations in inflammatory cytokines in patients with ARF and multiorgan dysfunction (93).

Sorbent-Based Therapy

Sorbents have achieved new interest in the treatment of acute renal failure in the setting of sepsis and hepatic encephalopathy, because many of the putative toxins associated with these disease states (e.g., bile acids, bilirubin, aromatic amino acids, fatty acids) are "middle-molecular-weight" substances (molecular weight 600 to 30,000 daltons) that are highly bound by albumin. Sorbents are characterized as either specific or nonspecific. The former rely on tailored ligands or antibodies that have high target specificity. Nonspecific adsorption, on the other hand, usually refers to charcoals and resins that rely on hydrophobic interaction, ionic (electrostatic) attraction, hydrogen bonding, and van der Waals interactions to bind toxins. These agents have high adsorptive capacity (>500 m²/g) and are inexpensive to produce compared with specific adsorptive agents. However, they are associated with thrombocytopenia and neutropenia (94). Hemoperfusion has been employed most for cases of toxic ingestion and is reviewed in greater detail in Chapter 38. Activated carbons, or charcoals, are either uncoated or coated with substances, such as cellulose nitrate, cellulose acetate, methacrylic hydrogel, or petroleum/polyhema. Ion exchange columns, another type of specific adsorptive material, are designed to exchange one ion for another. Nonionic porous resins, in turn, have been developed with varieties such as cross-linked polystyrene amberlite (XAD-2, XAD-4) and a new item, Betasorb, which is composed of polystyrene divinylbenzene resin. The Betasorb column is capable of removing molecules of 4 to 30 kDa molecular weight (such as β_2-microglobulin, angiogenin, leptin, TNF-α, and IL-1β), and it can be placed in series with a hemodialysis filter (95). Lastly, a hemoperfusion cartridge composed of polymyxin B-immobilized fibers has been described for use in sepsis because of its affinity for endotoxin (96,97).

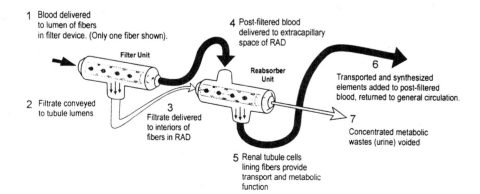

1 Blood delivered to lumen of fibers in filter device. (Only one fiber shown).

Filter Unit

2 Filtrate conveyed to tubule lumens

3 Filtrate delivered to interiors of fibers in RAD

Reabsorber Unit

4 Post-filtered blood delivered to extracapillary space of RAD

5 Renal tubule cells lining fibers provide transport and metabolic function

6 Transported and synthesized elements added to post-filtered blood, returned to general circulation.

7 Concentrated metabolic wastes (urine) voided

FIG. 29.2. Bioartificial renal tubule assist device (RAD). The RAD (labeled as reabsorber unit in this figure) is placed in series with a filter unit. (With permission from Humes HD, et al. The bioartificial renal tubule assist device to enhance CRRT in acute renal failure. *Am J Kidney Dis* 1997;30:S28–S31.)

SPECIAL CIRCUMSTANCES

Sepsis

Sepsis is a condition in which an imbalance of inflammatory and antiinflammatory mediators develops, and patients may fluctuate between these two phases (Fig. 29.3) (98). Data compiled from the Cleveland Clinic Foundation indicate that patients with ARF requiring HD demonstrate a frequency of infections and sepsis at 62.9% and 26.1%, respectively, compared with 23.7% and 13.2% of those patients with ARF who do not require dialysis (99) [N = 22,589 (1993–2000)]. Prospective data collected in a cohort of 398 patients with ARF at five U.S. centers showed that 75.2% of patients who died had sepsis at the time of death. The authors concluded that ARF may play a role in perpetuating sepsis (100). Some have equated the inability of these patients to respond normally to an endotoxin challenge to a state of "immunoparalysis." At the afferent limb of the sepsis cascade, lipopolysaccharide (LPS) is capable of activating both circulating soluble factors and monocytes. In the latter case, LPS binds to "toll-like" receptors, which in turn bind to other receptors and adhesion molecules to ultimately activate nuclear factor kappa B (NF-κB), a substance that can be inhibited by agents such as cyclosporine, glucocorticoids, and angiotensin-converting enzyme inhibitors. Once it is transported to the nucleus, NF-κB increases the formation of inflammatory cytokines such as tumor necrosis factor alpha (TNF-α); interleukins (IL)-1, 6, and 8; and platelet activating factor (PAF) (101) (Fig. 29.4). Many of these cytokines are water-soluble, which makes them amenable for removal from the circulation by ECBP techniques. In addition, since many of these cytokines are categorized as middle-molecular-weight compounds (Table 29.4) (102), continued interest in convective methods of removal (hemofiltration and hemodiafiltration) has surfaced. Moreover, continuous hemofiltration has been advocated as a means of reducing peak plasma levels of cytokines as they appear sequentially over time ("peak concentration hypothesis") (103).

Much of the cytokine clearance associated with convective techniques may be attributable to adsorption. De Vriese and colleagues found that the greatest decrement in serum cytokine concentration occurred after 1 hour of start of CVVH and after change of the membrane. Convective elimination of these mediators was also found to be augmented by increasing blood flow from 100 to 200 mL/min with an AN69 membrane (104). The impact of hemofiltration on survival was observed by Ronco and coworkers in patients with multiorgan dysfunction syndrome (MODS) and renal dysfunction (105). These investigators demonstrated that when convective rates were increased from 20 mL/kg/h to 35 mL/kg/h (or from ~1,500 mL/h to 2,500 mL/h in a 70-kg adult), mortality was reduced from 59% to 42% (p = .0013). On the other hand, there was no significant decrease in mortality by increasing convective rates further to 45 mL/kg/h (~3,000 mL/h in a 70-kg adult). This has led some researchers to question whether it is time to move from a "renal" dose of hemofiltration (or CVVH) to a "septic" dose. Bellomo and his coworkers studied the effects of high-volume hemofiltration (HVHF) (>50 to 100 L of fluid replacement daily) in eight patients with sepsis. They demonstrated significantly greater reductions in serum concentrations of C3a (an anaphylatoxin) and vasopressor requirements than occurred with patients on CVVH at conventional rates of ultrafiltration (103,106,107). Other authors have found favorable effects in patients treated with HVHF, and still others have described cytokine removal with super-high-flux filters (108). Honore and coworkers have described short-term high-volume hemofiltration (STHVH) consisting of isovolemic hemofiltration with 35 L of replacement solution administered over 4 hours followed by CVVH with a fluid exchange rate of 24 L/d (109,110). Journois et al. evaluated pediatric patients following cardiac surgery and found that those treated with ultrafiltration rates of 4.9 L/m²/h demonstrated significantly less postsurgical blood loss, were extubated sooner, and had overall improved alveolar–arterial oxygen gradients than controls (111). Oudemans-Van Straaten

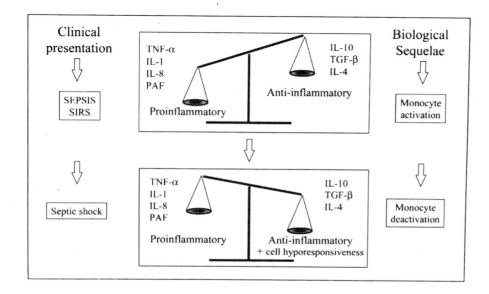

FIG. 29.3. Biologic phases of sepsis. This figure depicts the proinflammatory and antiinflammatory phases of sepsis. The systemic inflammatory response syndrome (SIRS) is met with a compensatory antiinflammatory response (CARS), which leads to a state of "immunoparalysis," in which cells are incapable of mounting a response to lipopolysaccharide (LPS). (With permission from Ronco C, et al. Use of sorbents in acute renal failure and sepsis. *Contrib Nephrol* 2001;133:180–193.)

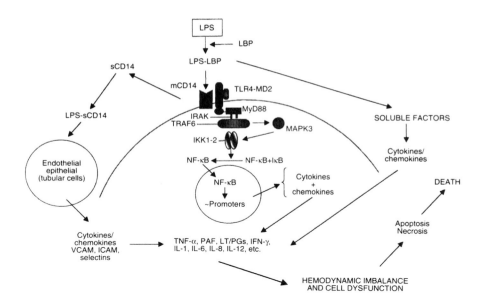

FIG. 29.4. ARF and the sepsis syndrome: mediators of cellular origin. LPS, lipopolysaccharides; LBP, LPS-binding protein; mCD14, membrane CD14 receptor; sCD14, soluble CD14; MyD88, adaptor protein; IRAK, interleukin-1 receptor-associated kinase; TRAF6, tumor necrosis factor-associated factor-6; MAPK3, mitogen-activated protein kinase-3; IKK1-2, IκB kinase-1 and -2; NF-κB, nuclear factor-κB; IκB, inhibitor of NF-κB; TNFα, tumor necrosis factor-α; PAF, platelet activating factor; LT/PGs, leukotrienes/prostaglandins; IFNγ, interferon γ; IL, interleukin; VCAM, vascular cell adhesion molecule; ICAM, intracellular adhesion molecule. (With permission from Schor N. Acute renal failure and the sepsis syndrome. *Kidney Int* 2001;61:764–776.)

and coworkers found improved hemodynamic parameters, such as increased cardiac index, stroke volume, and mean arterial pressure in patients with multiorgan dysfunction (two-thirds of these patients were classified as having shock) in whom hemofiltration was initiated (112). These patients also experienced reduced requirements in vasopressor (dopamine) dose. Similarly, Lonnemann demonstrated attenuation of immunoparalysis in mononuclear cells (defined as restored ability to produce TNF-α in response to endotoxin) when hemofiltration was prescribed. However, this effect was attenuated after 24 hours, presumably due to saturated membrane adsorption. It is important to note that the effects on whole blood mononuclear cells were more sustained in patients given high flux hemodialysis with polysulfone filters (113).

Although these studies and animal data (114,115) support use of ECBP, particularly hemofiltration, in patients with sepsis,

other human studies evaluating survival are not as favorable. Cole and coworkers evaluated 24 patients (12 hemofiltration: 12 control, ten with septic shock in each group). Survival was identical (eight of 12 patients) in each group, and mean APACHE II scores (21.8 ± 4.0 HF: 22.2 ± 6.4, *p* = .91) were not different. Serum concentrations of C3, C5a, IL-6, IL-8, IL-10, and TNF-α were measured at baseline and at 2, 24, 26, 48, and 72 hours. However, CVVH was not associated with overall reduction in these mediators or with improvement in pressor requirements, oxygenation, or Multiple Organ Dysfunction Score (MODS). The authors concluded that CVVH utilizing a fluid exchange rate of 2 L/h was insufficient to modulate soluble mediators of sepsis and that CVVH cannot be advocated for this purpose unless severe ARF is also present (116). In addition, Bouman and colleagues found no effect of high ultrafiltrate volumes (72 to 96 L/d) or early initiation (within 7 hours of study

TABLE 29.4. CONVECTIVE REMOVAL OF MEDIATORS

Mediator	Molecular Weight (Daltons)	Sieving Coefficient
AA mediators	600	0.5–0.91
Bradykinin	1,100	
Endothelin	2,500	0.19
C3a/C5a	11,000	0.11–0.77
Factor D	24,000	
MDS	600–30,000	
LPS	67,000	
LPS fragments	<1,000–20,000	
TNF-alpha (trimer)	17,000 (54,000)	0.0–0.2
STNFr	30,000–50,000	<0.1
IL-1	17,500	0.07–0.42
IL-1ra	24,000	0.28–0.45
IL-6	22,000	
IL-8	8,000	0.0–0.48
IL-10	18,000	0.0
INF-gamma	20,000	

With permission from Schetz M. Non-renal indications for continuous renal replacement therapy. *Kidney Int* 1999;56:S88–S94.

inclusion) of hemofiltration on survival at 28 days in a cohort of 106 oliguric ICU patients (117). Data collected from other groups have further suggested that hemofiltration does not decrease plasma concentrations of cytokines in systemic inflammatory response syndrome (SIRS) (118) or in trauma patients with multiple organ dysfunction and absence of ARF (119). Moreover, markers of endothelial injury (soluble tissue factor, thrombomodulin, E-selectin, and endothelin-1) do not appear to be affected by CVVH (120). Finally, limited prospective (121,122) and retrospective studies comparing continuous hemofiltration with intermittent hemodialysis have not demonstrated a clear advantage of one modality over the other. Therefore the application of convective techniques in sepsis as immunomodulating therapy is not clearly established, and more trials are required to define the role of these modalities in cases of sepsis where renal failure is absent.

Circuits combining plasma filtration, adsorptive columns, and hemofilters have been designed (Fig. 29.5). Coupled plasma filtration-adsorption (CPFA), in particular, has been employed in sepsis (98,123). This technique processes blood through a plasma filter, which is positioned in sequence with a hemofilter. In addi-

tion, a sorbent cartridge is placed in parallel with the plasma filter, which processes the filtered effluent and then returns it to the hemofilter. Several authors have reported adsorption of cytokines, amelioration of the immunoparalysis state accompanying sepsis, and improvement in cardiovascular parameters with this technique; however, no improvement in overall outcome has been demonstrated with CPFA (124,125). Therefore, it remains experimental. Hemolipodialysis is yet another sorbent-based technology that uses a dialysis solution that is saturated with liposomes, which consist of a spherical arrangement of a phospholipid bilayer that is embedded with molecules of vitamin E. The solution bathing the liposomes contains vitamin C as well as other electrolytes (126). This technique is undergoing research for application in the removal of lipid-soluble, hydrophobic, and protein-bound toxins that are found in sepsis. The addition of antioxidants, such as vitamins C and E, is believed to possess potential as a free radical "sink" (126).

Rhabdomyolysis

Rhabdomyolysis is a complication of myocyte necrosis secondary to either traumatic or nontraumatic causes, including ethanol, strenuous exercise, crush injury, or inherited defects in cellular metabolism (127–130). The diagnosis of rhabdomyolysis-associated ARF is generally made on the finding of myoglobinuria [which is characterized by discoloration of the urine and the finding of positive blood on urinary benzidine dipstick, which does not distinguish between myoglobin, hemoglobin, and red blood cells (RBCs)], and absence of RBCs on urine sediment. It is important to note that hemoglobin (64,000 daltons) is structurally related to myoglobin and can induce ARF (129). Once it occurs, rhabdomyolysis can cause ARF by the following mechanisms:

1. Tubular obstruction by myoglobin casts;
2. Tubular cell damage by lipid oxidant injury mediated by the heme group of myoglobin;
3. Vasoconstriction (131).

ARF caused by rhabdomyolysis was originally described during World War II (128) and is found in more than 50% of patients admitted with CK levels of more then 5,000 IU/L (131). Renal dysfunction has been estimated to occur in 16.5% to 33% of cases, and the incidence of dialysis has been estimated at 31% to 61% (132). The definitive approach to renal replacement therapy in rhabdomyolysis has not been established. Both plasma exchange and charcoal hemoperfusion have been utilized. The former was associated with only 10% clearance of serum myoglobin in a porcine model (133). Although myoglobin may be more amenable to removal by convection rather than diffusion due to its molecular weight (17,000 daltons), the timing and application of either hemofiltration or hemodialysis in this situation remains investigational. Renal replacement therapy may be indicated for hyperkalemia, a common electrolyte complication of tissue necrosis. However, comparison between conservative management with volume expansion and alkalinization and renal replacement therapy is limited, if at all available. Recovery of renal function is expected within 3 months of the initial insult, if the patient survives (134).

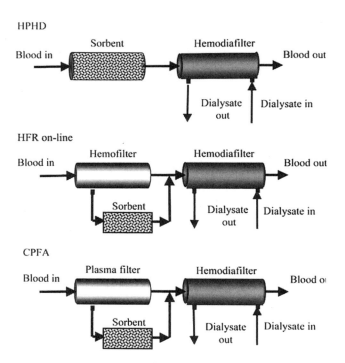

FIG. 29.5. Sorbent applications. **Top:** The sorbent unit is placed in series before the hemodiafilter. The system is defined as hemoperfusion-hemodialysis (HPHD). **Middle:** The sorbent unit is placed parallel to the hemofilter and processes ultrafiltrate produced by the hemofilter. The hemofilter is then placed in series with the hemodiafilter. The system is used for on-line hemodiafiltration and is defined as hemodiafiltration with endogenous ultrafiltrate regeneration (HFR on-line). **Bottom:** The sorbent unit is placed parallel to a plasma filter and processes the filtrate produced by the plasma filter. The plasma filter, in turn, is placed in series with the hemodiafilter. The system is used for critically ill patients with septic shock and is defined as coupled plasma filtration adsorption (CPFA). (With permission from Ronco C, et al. Use of sorbents in acute renal failure and sepsis. *Contrib Nephrol* 2001;133:180–193.)

Amyot et al. (135) report the case of a patient with hyperosmolar state, rhabdomyolysis (peak creatine kinase level 313,500 IU/L), and ARF (creatinine 8.2 mg/dL). CVVH was initiated, and serum myoglobin levels decreased from 92,000 µg/L to 28,600 µg/L after 16 hours of therapy. The mean clearance of myoglobin was 22 mL/min, with a mean ultrafiltration rate of 2,153 ± 148 mL/h and later decreased to 14 mL/min. The sieving coefficient (the percentage of the concentration of a plasma solute that appears in the ultrafiltrate) for myoglobin was reduced from 0.6 during the first 9 hours of therapy with a 0.9 m^2 surface area AN69 membrane to 0.4 during the subsequent 7 hours. Sieving coefficients for urea, creatinine, and phosphorus, on the other hand, remained stable at 1.0 during the first 16 hours of CVVH treatment. Bastani and coworkers (136) have reported removal of serum myoglobin in CVVH using a high-flux F80 polysulfone membrane and ultrafiltration rate of 1 L/h, and others have employed continuous hemodiafiltration as well (137,138). It is important to note that still other authors detected rapid decreases in serum myoglobin levels independent of changes in renal function or method of ECBP (102,139,140). Because myoglobin has minimal nephrotoxic capability in the absence of aggravating factors such as volume depletion, acidosis, and aciduria (130,132,141), prophylactic renal replacement therapy based on the presence of an elevated CPK alone cannot be recommended. Moreover, not all rhabdomyolysis leads to ARF, and the prognosis of rhabdomyolysis-induced ARF is benign (142).

The mainstay of therapy has focused on attenuating precipitation factors with intravenous fluid resuscitation (0.45% normal saline with 75 mEq/L sodium bicarbonate, 6 to 10 L/d, ± mannitol 15% at 10 mL/h, ± allopurinol) (129). The addition of mannitol may increase renal blood flow and glomerular filtration rate (GFR), reduce intratubular cast obstruction, and along with allopurinol, scavenge free radicals (129). These conservative measures are recommended to mitigate or prevent progression of aciduria, myoglobin-induced iron release (iron causes free radical production), and uric acid–myoglobin tubular cast formation.

Refractory Congestive Heart Failure and Cardiopulmonary Bypass

Refractory congestive heart failure generally represents an extreme in the spectrum of decompensated cardiac function, in which impaired cardiorenal dynamics lead inevitably to neurohormonal upregulation of the renin–angiotensin–aldosterone axis and progressive sodium and water retention. Consequently, patients develop overt edema and pulmonary volume overload, which may ultimately become resistant to conventional measures such as inotropic and diuretic agents. Often patients require renal replacement therapy to control ensuing azotemia, electrolyte abnormalities, and extravascular volume overload. There is growing evidence that convective therapies can be provided to patients with congestive heart failure that has become refractory to diuretic treatment. A recent study by Marenzi and coworkers evaluated 24 patients with New York Heart Association functional class IV heart failure (17 subjects with ischemic heart disease and seven with idiopathic dilated cardiomyopa-

thy) in the cardiac intensive care unit who were receiving different doses of inotropic, diuretic, and afterload-reducing agents (143). Hemodynamic data were obtained via pulmonary artery catheterization after each liter of ultrafiltrate was obtained and 24 hours after completion of the procedure. The mean treatment time was 9 ± 3 hours, and the range of ultrafiltration was 4,300 to 7,000 mL. Relief of pulmonary edema, ascites, and peripheral edema was documented, and patients were found to have improved response to subsequent diuretic therapy (mean dose of furosemide reduced from 380 ± 157 mg/d to 112 ± 70 mg/d after ultrafiltration). Moreover, mean right atrial pressure and pulmonary artery wedge pressure were reduced in a 1:1 ratio, and pulmonary artery pressure was also decreased. Other parameters, such as heart rate, systemic arterial pressure, cardiac output, and systemic vascular resistance did not change. Down-regulation of the neurohormonal axis (144–146) and, possibly, removal of myocardial depressant factors (147) have been postulated as mechanisms responsible for improvement. In more severe cases of decompensated heart failure, cardiogenic shock ensues, resulting in compromised renal blood flow and renal insufficiency with or without multiorgan failure (148). Because of compromised hemodynamic status in many of these patients, CVVH has become a favored RRT modality to remove excess sodium and water, relieve left ventricular preload, and down-regulate neurohormonal activation, so that renal perfusion is restored. Several authors have described their experience with both intermittent and continuous hemofiltration (149–155). Figure 29.6 illustrates the hemodynamic parameters of a patient with CHF due to dilated cardiomyopathy and coexistent renal failure (148). In addition, isolated ultrafiltration (145,156–158) and peritoneal dialysis (159) have been applied in this setting. As such, convective modalities may hold future promise in serving as a bridge to cardiac transplantation or insertion of ventricular assist devices in patients with severely decompensated congestive heart failure. Marenzi et al. (160) also demonstrated decreases in plasma renin (39%), aldosterone (50%), and norepinephrine (47%), and an increase in urine output by 500% in patients given hemofiltration targeted to remove 500 mL/h until right atrial pressure had declined to 50% baseline. Hemofiltration has also been used to attenuate fluid overload incurred as a consequence of cardiopulmonary bypass (CPB) intra- and postoperatively (161,162), and there is evidence in the pediatric literature that modulation of the inflammatory response associated with CPB occurs with hemofiltration. The negatively inotropic effects of TNF-α and IL-1-β make them targets for removal in this setting, since these substances may exert their effects by decreasing intramyocardial nitric oxide and cGMP (163,164). Still, others have reported significantly less postoperative anemia, hypoalbuminemia, and thrombocytopenia, with hemofiltration provided during CPB (164). Moreover, large pleural effusions were also reported to be less common, and less than 1% of exogenously administered vasoactive drugs were removed in cases of hemofiltration (165). The provision of ultrafiltration alone in moderate (New York Heart Association functional class II–III) congestive heart failure results in removal of extravascular lung water, reduction of pulmonary blood volume, and improvement in ventricular dynamics. Isolated ultrafiltration removes

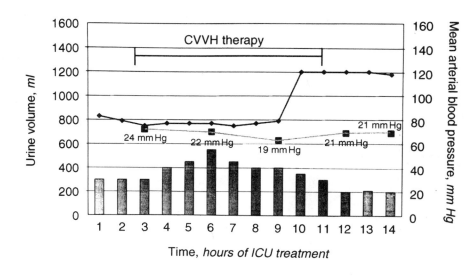

FIG. 29.6. Time course of continuous venovenous hemofiltration (CVVH) treatment in a patient with severe congestive heart failure and massive volume overload. Hemofiltration with a lactate-buffered replacement solution was provided at 1,000 mL/h (substitution fluid rate: 750 mL/h; net ultrafiltration rate: 250 mL/hour). Columns represent urine output, (♦) represent mean arterial pressure, and (■) represent central venous pressure. Although urine output improves in response to hemofiltration, mean arterial pressure remains the same or increases during therapy, and central venous pressures remain nearly the same. (With permission from Braüse M, et al. Congestive heart failure as an indication for continuous renal replacement therapy. *Kidney Int* 1999;56(Suppl 72):S95–S98.)

fluid, which is nearly isosmotic and isonatric with plasma, creating more efficient solute and volume removal than with diuretics (urine sodium ~100 mEq/L with furosemide administration) (166–168). The induction of transient hypovolemia by ultrafiltration is also believed to temporarily up-regulate the renin–angiotensin–aldosterone system, making angiotensin-converting enzyme inhibitors (ACE-I) more effective in sustaining body weight reduction than in individuals who are provided ultrafiltration but are not concurrently treated with ACE-I. Generally, high-flux membranes (K_{UF} >20 mL/h × mm Hg × m²) made of polysulfone, polyamide, polymethylmethacrylate, or polyacrylonitrile are used (168). Continuous convection (CVVH and SCUF) is often favored over intermittent ultrafiltration (IUF) because of its more gradual reduction of plasma volume and more physiologic equilibration of fluid between the interstitial spaces (Fig. 29.7) (168). Convection may soon be accomplished via a long-term indwelling catheter that is capable of direct plasma extraction (168). The intracorporeal

plasma separation system (IPSS) has been engineered to be a hollow fiber system that provides increased surface area per unit length fiber. The filtration topography of the microfibers allows for higher shear flow rate and lower viscosity from blood in the vena cava (3 to 6 L/min) as opposed to lower shear flow and higher viscosity within each individual hollow fiber of a conventional extracorporeal circuit. This ultimately translates to reduced transmembrane pressure (20 mm Hg, versus 50 to 100 mm Hg in conventional hemofiltration) and increased plasma water removal (60% versus 15% to 20% with whole blood in a conventional extracorporeal circuit). The catheter itself consists of approximately 130 hollow fibers 1.5 cm long. Graded differences in the fiber itself not only allow for decreased path tortuosity for filtered fluid but also exclude cellular components from blood (Fig. 29.8) (169). This modality allows for slow plasma water removal (~2 L/d) and has potential application in patients with congestive heart failure or other chronic volume overload states (169).

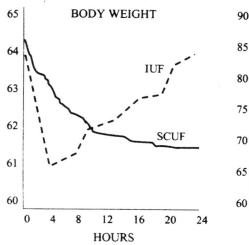

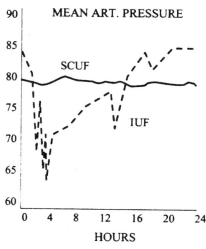

FIG. 29.7. Typical example of the hemodynamic response to fluid withdrawal in continuous and intermittent ultrafiltration. SCUF, slow continuous ultrafiltration; IUF, isolated ultrafiltration. (With permission from Ronco C, et al. Extracorporeal ultrafiltration for the treatment of overhydration and congestive heart failure. *Cardiology* 2001;96:155–168.)

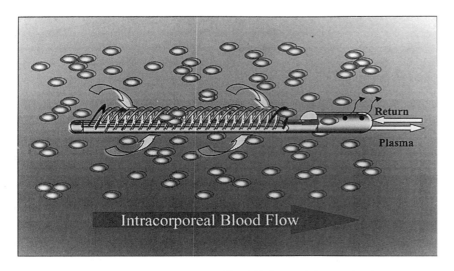

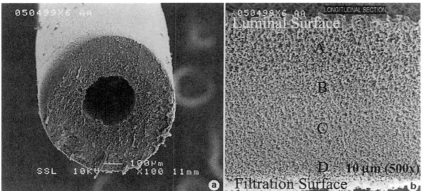

FIG. 29.8. A: Intracorporeal plasma separation system (IPSS). In contrast to standard HD hollow-fiber filters, blood flows outside the IPSS hollow fibers, and plasma is drawn into the fibers by applied transmembrane pressure. (With permission from Handley H, et al. Intravenous catheter for intracorporeal plasma filtration. *Blood Purif* 2002;20:61–69.) **B:** Scanning electron micrograph (SEM) of intracorporeal hollow fibers used for plasma separation in vivo. **(a)** Cross section (×100) of the fiber; **(b)** view (× 500) of the wall of the fiber, illustrating an asymmetric pore size distribution with four quadrants of pore sizes (A–D). (With permission from Handley H, et al. Intravenous catheter for intracorporeal plasma filtration. *Blood Purif* 2002; 20:61–69.)

Hepatic Failure

The etiologies of combined hepatic and renal failure are manifold and have been described by several authors (170–172). The choice of the ECBP modality that is to be used is governed by the nature of the toxin to be removed (Table 29.5) (173). However, no single ECBP technique can remove all toxins associated with hepatic failure (173,174) because of their large differences in molecular weight. In addition, currently utilized ECBP methodologies do not replace the synthetic and metabolic functions of the liver and may, in fact, remove regenerative substances as well (173,174). Indeed, some forms of hepatic failure, such as hepatorenal syndrome, are only cured by orthotopic liver transplantation (OLT). In such a case, dialysis has been traditionally considered as ineffective and to be used solely as a bridge to OLT for a limited time period (172,175–177). Several modalities have been utilized for patients with hepatic failure. For example, both isolated ultrafiltration and hemofiltration have been prescribed to remove sodium and water from patients who have refractory edema and nephrotic syndrome (178). Continuous venovenous hemofiltration (CVVH) has been used in combined hepatic failure and acute renal failure to remove middle-molecular-weight molecules, which are believed to be responsible for hepatic encephalopathy. High-pressure liquid chromatography (HPLC) performed on the serum of one such patient demonstrated reduction in molecules in the 45-to 60-kDa range, which was correlated with improvement in coma scale (Fig. 29.9) (179).

The Molecular Adsorbent Recirculating System (MARS) is currently used in Europe for the removal of albumin-bound toxins from patients with hepatic failure (Fig. 29.10). The patient's blood is dialyzed against an albumin-based dialysate. This dialysate is, in turn, regenerated by dialysis against a bicarbonate-buffered bath and further through adsorption in charcoal and ion exchange columns. Albumin-bound toxins are subsequently exchanged across a high-flux membrane (180). Several trials have demonstrated favorable endpoints, such as improved hepatic encephalopathy grade, increased synthetic ability with increased serum clotting factor concentrations, improved urine volume, and decreased plasma renin levels (181–189). At the time of this writing, the device is pending approval by the Food and Drug Administration for use in the United States (Steffen R. Mitzner, personal communication).

Hemodiabsorption, also known as liver dialysis, has been developed as a hybrid circuit of dialysis and sorbent-based therapy. The device (Biologic-DT Hemocleanse, Inc., West Lafayette, IN) provides hemodialysis with a suspension of pulverized sorbents replacing the usual dialysate solution. The main advan-

TABLE 29.5. TOXINS ASSOCIATED WITH HEPATIC FAILURE: RELATION TO BLOOD PURIFICATION

Small-molecular-weight toxins removable by hemodialysis
1. Ammonia
2. False neurotransmitters
3. Gamma-aminobutyric acid (GABA)
4. Octopamine (false neurotransmitter)

Middle-molecular-weight substances removable by hemofiltration
1. Cytokines (IL-6, IL-1, TNF)
2. Middle molecules[a]

Albumin-bound or large-molecular-weight toxins removable by plasma exchange
1. Aromatic amino acids[b]
2. Bile acids
3. Bilirubin
4. Endotoxin
5. Endotoxin-induced substances such as nitrous oxide, cytokines (IL-6, IL-1, TNF-α)
6. Indols[a]
7. Merctans[a,b]
8. Phenols[a,b]
9. Short-chain fatty acids[b]

Substances removable by hemoperfusion
1. Bile acids[a]
2. Bilirubin (conjugated and unconjugated)[a]
3. Cytokines (IL-6, IL-1, TNF)
4. Mercaptans[a,b]
5. Phenols[a,b]

With permission from Kaplan AA, et al. Extracorporeal blood purification in the management of patients with hepatic failure. *Semin Nephrol* 1997;17:576–582.
[a]Phenolic acids, fatty acids, and mercaptans have all been shown to inhibit sodium/potassium ATPase activity and may contribute to the cerebral edema associated with severe hepatic encephalopathy.
[b]Albumin bound.

tage of this technique is that it provides a large surface area for adsorption (300,000 m²) using a cellulose-based membrane with molecular-weight cutoff of 5,000 daltons. The sorbent dialysate suspension consists of 140 g of powdered charcoal in addition to 80 g of polystyrene sulfonate and physiologic amounts of sodium, chloride, bicarbonate, and calcium. Future sorbent suspensions may contain isoleucine (a branched-chain amino acid that is deficient in hepatic encephalopathy) and more selective cation exchangers, such as zirconium silicates (190). Several trials have evaluated patients with fulminant hepatic failure and acute on chronic hepatic failure (A-on-C) (188,191–197). Liver dialysis treatments were conducted for 6 hours daily for 1 to 5 days at blood-flow rates of 180 to 225 mL/min. The procedure was found to significantly improve outcome for A-on-C patients (defined as return to previous level of chronic hepatic insufficiency or improvement in physical condition to allow transplantation) (71.5% versus control 35.7%, *p* = .036). However, there was no significant improvement in outcomes for fulminant hepatic failure (FHF) (defined as a trend toward normal hepatic function). The reasons for this are not entirely clear but may be related to a higher frequency of sepsis and SIRS in the FHF cohort (190). One complication that is associated with hemodiabsorption is platelet loss during treatment, and liver dialysis may accentuate coagulopathy and risk of bleeding in patients with disseminated intravascular coagulation (DIC). Because of the limited ability of a charcoal-based sorbent to remove albumin-bound toxins, a new hemodiabsorption system has been developed to incorporate a plasma filter module (PF-Liver Dialysis) (190). Once blood is exposed to the sorbent dialysate in the cellulose filter, it is subjected to a plasma filter where alterations in transmembrane pressure allow for plasma protein–bound toxins to mix with a sorbent suspension. The plasma is then returned to the blood with the albumin-bound toxins removed (push–pull pheresis) (190).

Hemoperfusion involves exposure of blood to a column that is filled with sorbents such as activated charcoal [removes water-soluble substances such as γ-amino butyric acid (GABA), mercaptans, and inhibitors of Na⁺/K⁺-ATPase] and ion exchange resins [remove protein-bound (bile acids and aromatic amino acids) and lipid-soluble substances]. The largest study of hemoperfusion in hepatic failure evaluated patients with FHF and found no survival advantage regardless of treatment time (grade II encephalopathy: 5 hours = 51%, 10 hours = 50%; grade IV encephalopathy: no HP = 39.3%, 10 hours = 34.5%) (174,198). Hemoperfusion columns are limited in that they are saturated rapidly, making column changes at 3- to 5-hour intervals necessary (190). Moreover, hemoperfusion has been associated with loss of platelets, fibrinogen, and other clotting factors (190,191).

Therapeutic plasma exchange (TPE) has been applied to hepatic failure because of its ability to remove albumin-bound macromolecular substances such as endotoxin, aromatic amino acids, and certain bile constituents. It has been shown to be successful in a small cohort of patients with cholestatic liver disease (199), but when used alone as an ECBP modality in FHF, it has little impact on survival (200,201). However, TPE has been successfully combined with hemodiafiltration to improve hepatic encephalopathy and neurologic status in patients with FHF and A-on-C who are awaiting OLT (202–204).

Tumor Lysis Syndrome

Tumor lysis syndrome (TLS) occurs as a consequence of cytoreductive therapy in rapidly growing, radiochemotherapy-sensitive neoplasms (205). Uric acid, xanthine, and phosphate are believed to be crucial mediators of ARF, as these substances are capable of precipitating within the renal tubule and causing intraluminal obstruction (205). Approximately 25% of patients with B-cell acute lymphoblastic leukemia (ALL) and Burkitt's lymphoma require hemodialysis after chemotherapy (206). In addition, ARF may occur more frequently in patients with a lactate dehydrogenase index (LDH value at diagnosis divided by the upper limit of normal) of more than 3.3 (207). Early initiation of hemodialysis has been advocated to remove purine byproducts and phosphate. Renal replacement therapy can also modify some of the accompanying electrolyte abnormalities of TLS, which include hyperphosphatemia, hyperkalemia, and hypocalcemia (208). Because of their low molecular weight, uric acid and phosphate are amenable to removal by diffusive therapy (102). However, CVVH has been used to prevent phosphate rebound after conventional hemodialysis in a child with T-cell ALL (209). CVVH has also been used to prevent ARF in three

BLOOD PURIFICATION FOR HEPATIC FAILURE

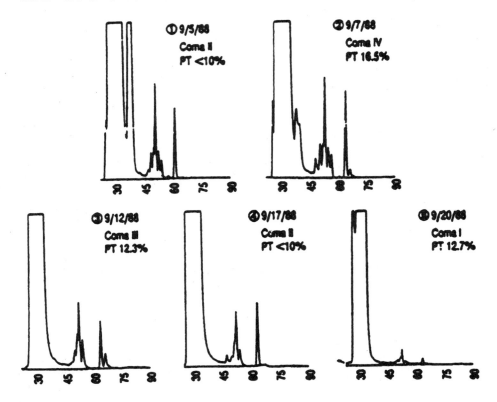

FIG. 29.9. CVVH in hepatic failure. Daily change in the HPLC profile of sera, coma grade, and prothrombin time (PT) during continuous hemofiltration in a patient with fulminant hepatic failure. (With permission from Matsubara S, et al. Continuous removal of middle molecules by hemofiltration in patients with acute liver failure. *Crit Care Med* 1990;18:1331–1338.)

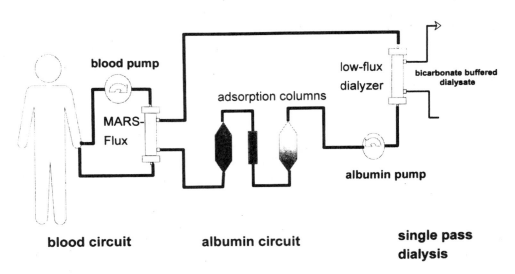

FIG. 29.10. Schematic of MARS. (With permission from Mitzner SR, et al. Extracorporeal detoxification using the molecular adsorbent recirculating system for critically ill patients with liver failure. *JASN* 2001;12:S75–S82.)

children with abdominal Burkitt's lymphoma and two children with T-cell ALL (208). In this study CVVH was initiated at a mean time of 10.5 hours before the start of chemotherapy and was continued for a mean of 85 hours (range, 70 to 91 hours). Only one child developed transient ARF in this cohort.

Adult Respiratory Distress Syndrome

Adult respiratory distress syndrome (ARDS) has been clinically defined in the past as low arterial oxygen (PaO_2 <75 mm Hg) in the setting of high inspired oxygen requirement (FiO_2 >0.5), diffuse pulmonary infiltrates, and pulmonary capillary wedge pressure (PCWP) <18 mm Hg (210). The application of ECBP, namely, hemofiltration and ultrafiltration, has been controversial in this area. Retrospective studies have shown improvement in patients treated with continuous therapies (211,212). Laggner and coworkers prospectively applied hemofiltration to nine patients with ARDS and found a nonsignificant reduction in PCWP (14 ± 2 before to 12 ± 2 mmHg after) and a nonsignificant elevation in PaO_2/FiO_2 ratio (95 ± 27 to 132 ± 79). Furthermore, hemofiltration was accompanied by a significant decrease in cardiac output (50 ± 10 to 34 ± 14 L/min, p <0.05), which was reflected in a trend toward decreased oxygen delivery (DO_2 492 ± 143 to 376 ± 163 mL/min/m^2) (213). Cosentino et al. utilized CAVH with bicarbonate-based replacement solution, a polyamide filter, and mean ultrafiltration rate of 12.0 ± 0.8 L/d in 15 patients (six control, nine CAVH). Although there was no improvement in hemodynamic and gas exchange parameters in the treatment group, these researchers found a nonsignificant trend of increased survival in patients who received CAVH (56% versus 17% in control group, p = .29) (214). Application of convection-based extracorporeal therapy has been believed to reduce accumulation of extravascular lung water by decreasing hydrostatic pressure within the pulmonary circulation (102). Consistent with this postulate, Humphrey et al. demonstrated improved survival in a retrospective evaluation of 40 ARDS patients whose PCWP was reduced by at least 25% with diuretics, dialysis, and ultrafiltration (75% treatment versus 29% control) (215). It is also possible that accumulation of extravascular lung water occurs as a consequence of ischemia–reperfusion injury in other organ systems, resulting in down-regulation of epithelial sodium channels and aquaporin-5 (216) as well as release of macrophage-derived inflammatory mediators (e.g., cytokines, complement components, and arachidonic acid derivatives) (217). Similarly, biomechanical alterations induced by increased alveolar capillary pressure (which can lead to fracturing of small capillaries and fluid extravasation) and high levels of positive end-expiratory pressure (PEEP) (which can produce antinatriuresis) may contribute to the pathogenesis of extravascular lung water accumulation in ARDS. Induction of hypothermia (30.5°C) in a patient with posttraumatic ARF has been reported with CAVH (218). The cooling effect was associated with decreased minute ventilation and reduced oxygen consumption by 70% independent of changes in fluid balance, which remained positive throughout the treatment period. Induction of permissive hypercapnia with administration of bicarbonate-containing replacement solution may have also contributed to the improvement in lung function (218).

Contrast-Mediated Nephropathy

Radiocontrast medium–induced nephropathy (RCIN) is an ongoing concern in the ICU. The syndrome occurs as a consequence of several features, including a brief episode of vasodilation followed by intrarenal vasoconstriction, tubular cell epithelial toxicity and luminal obstruction, and renal medullary ischemia (219–221). Although mild decreases in glomerular filtration rate (GFR) have been observed in most patients who are exposed to radiocontrast media, more substantial decrements in renal function have been associated with several preexisting factors as well as the volume of contrast injected (<100 mL associated with no acute renal failure requiring dialysis) (222). The use of low-osmolality and isoosmolality media as alternatives to high-osmolality media is controversial. Although low-osmolality and isoosmolality media are one-third to one-half of the osmolality of the high-osmolality agents, they are still capable of inducing renal medullary ischemia (221,223). Moreover, there is evidence that low-osmolality agents may only confer benefit in patients with existing abnormal renal function (serum creatinine >1.6 mg/dL) (221,224). A recent trial demonstrated that of 439 patients with baseline serum creatinine of more than 1.8 mg/dL, 161 (37%) developed ≥25% increase in serum creatinine concentration, and 31 patients required hemodialysis after coronary intervention (in-hospital mortality 22.6%). The 1-year mortality rate was 45.2% for those requiring dialysis, 35.4% for those who did not require dialysis, and 19.4% for those with no increase in serum creatinine concentration (p = .001) (219). Several interventions have been employed to prevent or ameliorate renal dysfunction incurred by intravenous radiocontrast media, including saline with or without furosemide and mannitol, calcium channel antagonists, dopamine, fenoldopam, atrial natriuretic peptide, and acetylcysteine (219,225,226). Both hemodialysis and peritoneal dialysis have been found to remove contrast media (227–230). Of the extracorporeal blood purification modalities, hemodiafiltration appears to have the greatest extraction ratio (0.81 ± 0.1) compared with high-flux dialysis (0.74 ± 0.1), low-flux hemodialysis (0.64 ± 0.1), and hemofiltration (0.62 ± 0.1) (p <0.05 for all). Several studies clearly demonstrate removal of iodinated radiocontrast material (228,231–234), but they are uncontrolled case series with varying intervals between contrast exposure and ECBP (30 minutes to 25 hours) and differences in dialyzer membrane composition (with some preference for polysulfone over cuprophane filters) (233). Vogt and coworkers randomized 113 patients with abnormal renal function to receive either intravenous saline [1 mL/kg/h 12 hours before and after intravenous contrast administration (N = 58) or saline before and hemodialysis after contrast administration (N = 55)] (235). All patients had moderately to severely impaired renal function (serum creatinine concentration >2.3 mg/dL), and all received nonionic, low-osmolality contrast media (20 to 740 mL, mean 176 ± 133 mL). Angiotensin-converting enzyme inhibitors and diuretics were postponed on the day of contrast agents and were withheld until after the procedure, and no patients received acetylcysteine, dopamine, mannitol, or furosemide during the study. Hemodialysis with a high-flux polysulfone membrane (F60 or F70, Fresenius Medical Care, Lexington, MA) was started between 30 and 280 minutes (median, 120 minutes) after the first bolus of radiocontrast was given to those in the hemodialysis group. Most (48/55) received isovolemic dialysis (mean duration, 3.1 ± 0.7 hours). Primary endpoints were need for hemodialysis 1 to 6 days after contrast administration, cardiovascular events (myocardial infarction, cerebrovascular accident, or pulmonary edema) or dialysis-related complications, or death. For patients in the hemodialysis group, the baseline serum creatinine was 3.6 ± 1.3 mg/dL, which decreased to 3.1 ± 1.1 mg/dL after 24 hours and peaked to 3.6 ± 1.4 mg/dL at 96 hours (p = .04). In the patients of the nonhemodialysis group, the serum creatinine level increased from 3.5 ± 1.2 mg/dL at baseline to a peak of 3.6 ± 1.4 mg/dL at 96 hours (p = .98). While there was a significant difference in the quantity of contrast given between nonhemodialysis and prophylactic hemodialysis groups (143 ± 115 mL non-HD versus 210 ± 143 mL, p = .007), no beneficial effect of hemodialysis was found for patients who received more than 150 mL of contrast media. Moreover, there was no significant influence of contrast volume more than 150 mL on the development of RCIN. Twenty-two patients (nine in the non-HD group and 13 in the HD group, p = .35) developed RCIN (defined as an increase in serum creatinine concentration of 0.5 mg/dL or more than 25% above baseline at any time), and 11 (three non-HD and eight HD, p = .12) required subsequent dialysis treatments. Of this group, three required permanent hemodialysis (one in non-HD and two in HD group, p = .44). The reasons for the lack of benefit of prophylactic hemodialysis in this cohort are unknown. Delay of institution of therapy (>20 minutes) and reduced renal perfusion due to osmotic shifts (decrease in plasma osmolality from removal of contrast media leads to a shift of water from the intravascular to the interstitial and intracellular compartments), along with twofold greater incidence in coronary angiography in the hemodialysis group were suggested as possible causes by the authors. Furthermore, the two groups showed no differences in the prevalence of cardiovascular endpoints (235).

Acute Brain Injury

Patients who develop brain injury either in the setting of multiple trauma or as part of a systemic illness can develop acute renal failure as a consequence of sepsis and nephrotoxin exposure. Similarly, conditions such as infection, vasculitis, hemolytic uremic syndrome (HUS), and malignant hypertension (as with scleroderma renal crisis) may cause acute renal failure (236). As a consequence, brain edema occurs. This further complicates matters in a patient requiring ECBP, since conventional hemodialysis has the potential to increase brain water content (237,238). The mechanism for this has been eloquently described (236,239–241) and is related to relatively slower removal of urea from the cerebrospinal fluid than from the plasma. This creates an osmotic gradient, and water moves from plasma to brain tissue (236). At the same time, urea removal from cerebral tissue leads to formation of intracellular idiogenic osmoles (236,240,241). It is important to note that infusion of bicarbonate from dialysate leads to increased plasma pH. Since bicarbonate is a charged molecule, it must be converted to carbon dioxide to cross the blood-brain barrier. Thus, paradoxical intracellular acidosis ensues, and further formation of idiogenic

osmoles occurs (236,242,243). Moreover, intracerebral hypoxia leads to production of lactic acid and vasodilatory substances that increase intracerebral pressure (ICP) (236,244,245). To maintain cerebral perfusion pressure and cerebral blood flow without increasing ICP, Davenport and colleagues recommend initiating conventional hemodialysis with a blood flow rate of 50 mL/min, which can be incremented to a maximum rate of 200 mL/min if the patient remains hemodynamically stable. In addition, dialysate containing high sodium (e.g., 140 to 150 mEq/L) and low bicarbonate (e.g., 30 mEq/L) concentrations should be used to limit osmotic gradients and increases in plasma pH, respectively. The dialysate solution should be cooled to 35.5°C to improve cardiovascular stability (236,246). Davenport further recommends an initial treatment time of 2 hours, with 100 mL 20% mannitol infused during the second hour of treatment. This time may be cautiously increased; however, patients usually require daily therapy. HD is performed with a synthetic low-flux filter that has been primed with human albumin to both coat the dialyzer membrane and maintain effective circulating plasma volume. Anticoagulation of the circuit poses the obvious risk of intracerebral hemorrhage. Therefore, systemic anticoagulation should be avoided, and regional anticoagulation with agents such as trisodium citrate or prostacyclin may be considered (236,247–249). It is important to note that prostacyclin may reduce cerebral perfusion pressure and increase ICP due to its vasodilatory properties (236,250,251). CRRT may be particularly useful in acute brain injury since continuous venovenous hemo(dia)filtration [CVV(HD)F] may impart greater intracranial stability than intermittent hemodialysis or hemofiltration due to less profound changes in serum osmolality, urea, and bicarbonate concentrations. CRRT also has the advantage of allowing improved cardiovascular stability based on thermal losses of the CRRT circuit (251).

Lactic Acidosis

Lactic acidosis receives considerable attention in the ICU because of its association with poor outcome (236,252–255). Approximately 25% to 30% of exogenous lactate is removed by the kidneys, and the liver assumes 53% of the clearance. The kidneys perform this task through lactate metabolism in the renal cortex. However, urinary excretion can lead to elimination of as much as 10% to 12% of renal lactate under conditions of hyperlactatemia (236,252,253). It is believed that the kidneys' ability to metabolize lactate is increased during acidosis, whereas hepatic lactate metabolism in this case is blocked via stimulation of phosphoenolpyruvate carboxykinase, an enzyme in the gluconeogenesis cascade. Levraut and colleagues (236,256) compared endogenous lactate clearance with lactate clearance during CRRT [continuous venovenous hemodiafiltration (CVVHDF)] in ten patients. Although the median endogenous lactate clearance was 1,379 mL/min, the median lactate clearance with bicarbonate-buffered CRRT was only 24.2 mL/min, thus contributing less than 3% to the overall lactate clearance. This occurred despite a hemofilter sieving coefficient of approximately 1.0 (levels of lactate in ultrafiltrate nearly the same as the plasma concentration) (236,252,253,256). Therefore CRRT with bicarbonate-buffered solutions should not be considered as a method of treating lactic acidosis or as a modality that disguises hyperlactatemia and tissue hypoxia. Although some researchers (102,236,257–259) have reported benefit of extracorporeal lactate clearance by hemofiltration or hemodiafiltration, others (256) support the notion that increased lactate clearance is a reflection of improved endogenous acid–base and metabolic status achieved during extracorporeal therapy.

ROLE OF NEPHROLOGISTS IN THE ICU

The breadth of knowledge and technologies available for ICU patients has increased dramatically and has resulted in growing opportunities. Subspecialists, in and of themselves, have finite knowledge bases, and therefore complement one another with the unique clinical expertise that each brings to the bedside. Nephrologists, because of their ongoing, daily contact with renal pathophysiology, are uniquely positioned to diagnose renal dysfunction and conservatively manage what are often inevitable consequences of renal failure, including extracellular fluid overload, acid–base complications, and electrolyte disorders. If conservative measures fail, it is the nephrologist who is most experienced to determine which patients require dialysis, when to initiate therapy, and perhaps most important, which patients are unsuitable candidates for renal replacement therapy. Moreover, the nephrologist is trained in urea kinetic modeling and offers expertise in dialysis prescription (260,261). However, competition may arise between specialists over particular aspects of therapeutic intervention, raising questions regarding who is best suited to provide care (260). This conflict has occasionally developed as intensivists seek to manage all aspects of management of ICU patients. Moreover, the age of managed care has made it more fiscally appealing for intensivists to conduct all of their own procedures. Subsequently, some intensivists have developed a "closed" ICU approach (261), where management is directed by a critical care specialist who chooses to consult other specialists.

This approach has been embraced in Australia, where intensivists perform CRRT without nephrology consultation (262). Cole and coworkers (262) conducted a prospective 3-year multicenter observational study involving 24 Australian ICUs. CRRT was initiated in 110 of 116 patients with severe ARF, defined as any degree of renal dysfunction deemed worthy of commencement of CRRT by the treating physician (62% had persistent oliguria or anuria). In addition, seven dialysis-dependent patients were enrolled, six of whom received CRRT while in the ICU. Patients were not randomized for severity scoring; however, SAPS and APACHE II were not different between survivors and nonsurvivors. The actual mortality rate was 49.2%, and 11 survivors were dialysis dependent at the time of hospital discharge. The results of this trial raise several concerns regarding the inherent inception bias incurred by initiating CRRT instead of IHD. One wonders whether the same or better results could not have been achieved with IHD. In addition, no mention is made of dialysis dose prescription or dose delivery, factors that may affect the outcome of renal replacement therapy in ARF. Prospective trials comparing both outcome and costs for patients receiving renal replacement therapy in the presence ("traditional" ICU) or absence ("closed" ICU) of nephrologic

consultation are lacking in the United States. The concept of "closed" ICUs is particularly alarming when one considers that only 2.7% of all intensivists have received sustained nephrology training (263). This raises concern both from a risk management standpoint and, potentially, from a cost management perspective. The provision of daily CRRT, particularly for patients with nonrenal indications in whom renal replacement therapy may yield little therapeutic benefit, will likely increase costs of supplies compared with intermittent hemodialysis (IHD) (264). However, further investigation of the potential for increased recovery of renal function with CRRT must be considered. In addition, costs of IHD and CRRT may, when extrapolated over a long period of time, be nearly equal (265).

CONCLUSION

ECBP in the ICU has changed dramatically over the past several decades as both new modalities and hybrid circuits have emerged. With time, considerable research will be invested in targeting extracorporeal renal replacement therapy to fulfill the unique needs posed by specific disease states and clinical entities, opening the way for further applications of these therapies in both renal, and potentially nonrenal, indications. More prospective, controlled trials are required to determine at what time ECBP should be initiated, what dose should be delivered, and which modality (convection or diffusion, continuous or intermittent) best serves the ICU patient with ARF.

ACKNOWLEDGMENTS

The author expresses his gratitude to Ms. Geetha Stachowiak for her expertise in the preparation of this manuscript.

REFERENCES

1. Buchardi H. Renal replacement therapy (RRT) in the ICU: criteria for initiating RRT. In: Ronco C, et al., eds. *Blood purification in intensive care: contributions in nephrology.* Basel: Karger, 2001:171–180.
2. Briglia A, et al. Acute renal failure in the intensive care unit: therapy overview, patient risk stratification, complications of renal replacement, and special circumstances. *Clin Chest Med* 1999;20:347–366.
3. Al Khafaji A, et al. Acute renal failure and dialysis in the chronically critically ill patient. *Clin Chest Med* 2001;22:165–174.
4. Manns M, et al. Continuous renal replacement therapies: an update. *Am J Kidney Dis* 1998;32:185–207.
5. Ronco C. FAPM. Complications of RRT in the ICU. In: Lamiere NMR, ed. *Complications of dialysis.* New York: Marcel Dekker, 2000: 625–641.
6. Leunissen KML, et al. Acute dialysis complications. In: Lamiere NMR, ed. *Complications of dialysis.* New York: Marcel Dekker, 2000:69–88.
7. Bellomo R, et al. Acute renal failure: time for consensus. *Intensive Care Med* 2001;27:1685–1688.
8. Vincent JL. Incidence of acute renal failure in the intensive care unit. *Contrib Nephrol* 2001;132:1–6.
9. Vivino G, et al. Risk factors for acute renal failure in trauma patients. *Intensive Care Med* 1998;24:808–814.
10. Chertow GM, et al. Prognostic stratification in critically ill patients with acute renal failure requiring dialysis. *Arch Intern Med* 1995;155: 1505–1511.

11. Brivet FG, et al. Acute renal failure in intensive care units: causes, outcome, and prognostic factors of hospital mortality—a prospective, multicenter study. French Study Group on Acute Renal Failure. *Crit Care Med* 1996;24:192–198.

12. McCarthy JT. Prognosis of patients with acute renal failure in the intensive care unit: a tale of two eras. *Mayo Clin Proc* 1996;71:117–126.

13. Nash K, et al. Hospital-acquired renal insufficiency. *Am J Kidney Dis* 2002;39:930–936.

14. Mehta RL, et al. Refining predictive models in critically ill patients with acute renal failure. *J Am Soc Nephrol* 2002;13:1350–1357.

15. Clermont G, et al. Renal failure in the ICU: comparison of the impact of acute renal failure and end-stage renal disease on ICU outcomes. *Kidney Int* 2002;62:986–996.

16. Novis BK, et al. Association of preoperative risk factors with postoperative acute renal failure. *Anesth Analg* 1994;78:143–149.

17. Paganini EP. Dialysis is not dialysis is not dialysis! Acute dialysis is different and needs help! *Am J Kidney Dis* 1998;32:832–833.

18. Paganini EP, et al. Severity scores and outcomes with acute renal failure in the ICU setting. *Contrib Nephrol* 2001;(132):181–195.

19. Paganini EP, et al. Establishing a dialysis therapy/patient outcome link in the intensive care unit for patients with acute renal failure. *Am J Kidney Dis* 1996;28(Suppl 3):S81–S89.

20. Liao Z. Determinants of effective treatment dose in CVVH. *J Am Soc Nephrol* 2002;13:236A.

21. Liao Z, et al. Dose capabilities of renal replacement therapies in acute renal failure (ARF). *J Am Soc Nephrol* 2002;13:237A.

22. Eknoyan G. Effect of dialysis dose and membrane flux in maintenance hemodialysis. *N Engl J Med* 2002;347:2010–2019.

23. Clark WR, et al. The role of renal replacement therapy quantification in acute renal failure. *Am J Kidney Dis* 1997;30:S10–S14.

24. Collins AJ, et al. Urea index and other predictors of hemodialysis patient survival. *Am J Kidney Dis* 1994;23:272–282.

25. Hakim RM, et al. Effects of dose of dialysis on morbidity and mortality. *Am J Kidney Dis* 1994;23:661–669.

26. Parker TF III, et al. Survival of hemodialysis patients in the United States is improved with a greater quantity of dialysis. *Am J Kidney Dis* 1994;23:670–680.

27. Clark WR, et al. A comparison of metabolic control by continuous and intermittent therapies in acute renal failure. *J Am Soc Nephrol* 1994;4:1413–1420.

28. Clark WR. Solute control by extracorporeal therapies in acute renal failure. *Am J Kidney Dis* 1996;28(Suppl 3):S21–S27.

29. Clark WR. Extracorporeal therapy requirements for patients with acute renal failure. *J Am Soc Nephrol* 1997;8:804–812.

30. Evanson JA, et al. Prescribed versus delivered dialysis in acute renal failure patients. *Am J Kidney Dis* 1998;32:731–738.

31. Rao M. Patient- and dialysis-related variables predict dialysis delivery in acute renal failure. *J Am Soc Nephrol* 2002;13:643A.

32. Schiffl H, et al. Daily hemodialysis and the outcome of acute renal failure. *N Engl J Med* 2002;346:305–310.

33. Bonventre JV. Daily hemodialysis—will treatment each day improve the outcome in patients with acute renal failure? *N Engl J Med* 2002;346:362–364.

34. Gettings LG, et al. Outcome in post-traumatic acute renal failure when continuous renal replacement therapy is applied early vs. late. *Intensive Care Med* 1999;25:805–813.

35. Schiffl H, et al. Biocompatible membranes in acute renal failure: prospective case-controlled study. *Lancet* 1994;344:570–572.

36. Hakim RM, et al. Effect of the dialysis membrane in the treatment of patients with acute renal failure. *N Engl J Med* 1994;331:1338–1342.

37. Jorres A, et al. Haemodialysis-membrane biocompatibility and mortality of patients with dialysis-dependent acute renal failure: a prospective randomised multicentre trial. International Multicentre Study Group. *Lancet* 1999;354:1337–1341.

38. Subramanian S, et al. Influence of dialysis membranes on outcomes in acute renal failure: a meta-analysis. *Kidney Int* 2002;62:1819–1823.

39. Kellum JA, et al. Continuous versus intermittent renal replacement therapy: a meta-analysis. *Intensive Care Med* 2002;28:29–37.

40. Mehta RL, et al. A randomized clinical trial of continuous versus intermittent dialysis for acute renal failure. *Kidney Int* 2001;60:1154–1163.

41. Kellum JA, et al. Acute dialysis quality initiative (ADQI). *Contrib Nephrol* 2001;(132):258–265.

42. Ronco C, et al. The Acute Dialysis Quality Initiative: the New York conference. *Adv Ren Replace Ther* 2002;9:248–251.

43. Marshall MR, et al. Hybrid renal replacement modalities for the critically ill. *Contrib Nephrol* 2001;132:252–257.

44. Marshall MR, et al. Sustained low-efficiency dialysis for critically ill patients requiring renal replacement therapy. *Kidney Int* 2001;60:777–785.

45. Marshall MR, et al. Urea kinetics during sustained low-efficiency dialysis in critically ill patients requiring renal replacement therapy. *Am J Kidney Dis* 2002;39:556–570.

46. Kumar VA, et al. Extended daily dialysis: a new approach to renal replacement for acute renal failure in the intensive care unit. *Am J Kidney Dis* 2000;36:294–300.

47. Schlaeper C, et al. High clearance continuous renal replacement therapy with a modified dialysis machine. *Kidney Int* 1999;72(Suppl):S20–S23.

48. Clark WR, et al. Factors influencing therapy delivery in acute dialysis. *Contrib Nephrol* 2001;(132):304–312.

49. Henderson LW. Biophysics of UF and HF. In: Jacobs C, ed. *Replacement of renal function by dialysis*. Boston: Kluwer Academic, 1995:114–118.

50. David S, et al. Hemofiltration: predilution versus postdilution. *Contrib Nephrol* 1992;96:77–85.

51. Huang Z. Effect of ultrafiltration rate on hemofilter performance in predilution hemofiltration. *J Am Soc Nephrol* 2002;13:237A.

52. Huang Z. Determinants of solute clearance in hemodiafiltration (HDF). *J Am Soc Nephrol* 2002;13:237A.

53. Ash SR. Peritoneal dialysis in acute renal failure of adults: the safe, effective, and low-cost modality. *Contrib Nephrol* 2001;(132):210–221.

54. Ash SR, et al. Peritoneal dialysis for acute and chronic renal failure: an update. *Hosp Pract (Off Ed)* 1983;18:179, 183, 187.

55. Orofino L, et al. Survival of acute renal failure (ARF) on dialysis: review of 82 patients. *Rev Clin Esp* 1976;141:155–160.

56. Swartz RD, et al. Complications of the HDF and PD in ARF. *ASAIO J* 1980;3:98.

57. Firmat J, et al. Peritoneal dialysis in acute renal failure. *Contrib Nephrol* 1979;17:33–38.

58. Struijk DG, et al. Experiences with acute peritoneal dialysis in adults. *Ned Tijdschr Geneeskd* 1984;128:751–755.

59. Rottembourg J. Residual renal function and recovery of renal function in patients treated by CAPD. *Kidney Int* 1993;40(Suppl):S106–S110.

60. Ash SR. The sorbent suspension in reciprocating dialyzer for use in peritoneal dialysis. In: Maher JF, et al., eds. *Frontiers in peritoneal dialysis*. New York: Field, Rich & Associates, 1986:148–156.

61. Bergstein JM, et al. Role of plasminogen-activator inhibitor type 1 in the pathogenesis and outcome of the hemolytic uremic syndrome. *N Engl J Med* 1992;327:755–759.

62. Shinaberger JH, et al. Acute renal failure, Viet Nam, 1965: transglobal treatment. *Mil Med* 1965;130:1078–1081.

63. Stephen RL, et al. Recirculating peritoneal dialysis with subcutaneous catheter. *Trans Am Soc Artif Intern Organs* 1976;22:575–585.

64. Diaz-Buxo JA. Continuous flow peritoneal dialysis: clinical applications. *Blood Purif* 2002;20:36–39.

65. Berlot G, et al. Plasmapheresis in sepsis. *Contrib Nephrol* 2001;(132):391–399.

66. Kaplan AA. *A practical guide to therapeutic plasma exchange*. Cambridge, MA: Blackwell Science, 1999:3–9.

67. Kaplan AA. A simple and accurate method for prescribing plasma exchange. *ASAIO Trans* 1990;36:M597–M599.

68. Kaplan AA. *A practical guide to therapeutic plasma exchange*. Cambridge, MA: Blackwell Science, 1999:23–26.

69. Gurland HJ, et al. A comparison of centrifugal and membrane-based apheresis formats. *Int J Artif Organs* 1984;7:35–38.

70. Gurland HJ, et al. Comparative evaluation of filters used in membrane plasmapheresis. *Nephron* 1984;36:173–182.
71. Gerhardt RE, et al. Acute plasma separation with hemodialysis equipment. *J Am Soc Nephrol* 1992;2:1455–1458.
72. Moake JL. Thrombotic microangiopathies. *N Engl J Med* 2002;347:589–600.
73. Bell WR, et al. Improved survival in thrombotic thrombocytopenic purpura-hemolytic uremic syndrome: clinical experience in 108 patients. *N Engl J Med* 1991;325:398–403.
74. Rock GA, et al. Comparison of plasma exchange with plasma infusion in the treatment of thrombotic thrombocytopenic purpura: Canadian Apheresis Study Group. *N Engl J Med* 1991;325:393–397.
75. Byrnes JJ, et al. Thrombotic thrombocytopenic purpura and the haemolytic–uraemic syndrome: evolving concepts of pathogenesis and therapy. *Clin Haematol* 1986;15:413–442.
76. Ruggenenti P, et al. Renin-angiotensin system, proteinuria, and tubulointerstitial damage. *Contrib Nephrol* 2001;(135):187–199.
77. Kaplan AA. Hematologic disorders. *A practical guide to therapeutic plasma exchange.* Malden, MA: Blackwell Press, 1999:110–138.
78. Kaplan AA. Neurologic disorders. *A practical guide to therapeutic plasma exchange.* Malden, MA: Blackwell Press, 1999:89–109.
79. Balow JE. Plasmapheresis: development and application in treatment of renal disorders. *Artif Organs* 1986;10:324–330.
80. Baumgartner I, et al. Recovery from life threatening pulmonary hemorrhage in Goodpasture's syndrome after plasmapheresis and subsequent pulse dose cyclophosphamide. *Clin Nephrol* 1995;43:68–70.
81. Lockwood CM, et al. Recovery from Goodpasture's syndrome after immunosuppressive treatment and plasmapheresis. *Br Med J* 1975;2:252–254.
82. Johnson JP, et al. Plasmapheresis and immunosuppressive agents in antibasement membrane antibody-induced Goodpasture's syndrome. *Am J Med* 1978;64:354–359.
83. Rosenblatt SG, et al. Treatment of Goodpasture's syndrome with plasmapheresis: a case report and review of the literature. *Am J Med* 1979;66:689–696.
84. Zucchelli P, et al. Controlled plasma exchange trial in acute renal failure due to multiple myeloma. *Kidney Int* 1988;33:1175–1180.
85. Johnson WJ, et al. Treatment of renal failure associated with multiple myeloma: plasmapheresis, hemodialysis, and chemotherapy. *Arch Intern Med* 1990;150:863–869.
86. Kaplan AA. Renal disease. *A practical guide to therapeutic plasma exchange.* Malden, MA: Blackwell Science, 1999:178–196.
87. Humes HD, et al. The bioartificial renal tubule assist device to enhance CRRT in acute renal failure. *Am J Kidney Dis* 1997;30:S28–S31.
88. Humes HD. Bioartificial kidney for full renal replacement therapy. *Semin Nephrol* 2000;20:71–82.
89. Humes HD, et al. Tissue engineering of a bioartificial renal tubule assist device: in vitro transport and metabolic characteristics. *Kidney Int* 1999;55:2502–2514.
90. Fissell WH, et al. Bioartificial kidney alters cytokine response and hemodynamics in endotoxin-challenged uremic animals. *Blood Purif* 2002;20:55–60.
91. Fissell WH. Bioartificial kidney (BK) protects against septic shock in uremic animals. *J Am Soc Nephrol* 2002;13:326A.
92. Fissell WH. Initial characterization of a nanoengineered ultrafiltration membrane. *J Am Soc Nephrol* 2002;13:602A.
93. Weitzel. Early results with the bioartificial kidney in ICU patients with acute renal failure. *J Am Soc Nephrol* 2002;13:642A.
94. Winchester JF. Sorbent hemoperfusion in end-stage renal disease: an in-depth review. *Adv Ren Replace Ther* 2002;9:19–25.
95. Winchester JF, et al. The next step from high-flux dialysis: application of sorbent technology. *Blood Purif* 2002;20:81–86.
96. Nakamura T, et al. Effect of polymyxin B–immobilized fiber hemoperfusion on sepsis-induced rhabdomyolysis with acute renal failure. *Nephron* 2000;86:210.
97. Kunitomo T, et al. Endotoxin removal by toraymyxin. *Contrib Nephrol* 2001;(132):415–420.
98. Ronco C, et al. Use of sorbents in acute renal failure and sepsis. *Contrib Nephrol* 2001;(133):180–193.
99. Thakar. Renal dysfunction and frequency of sepsis and serious infections after cardiac surgery. *J Am Soc Nephrol* 2002;13:243A.
100. Mehta RL. Sepsis influences outcomes from acute renal failure. *J Am Soc Nephrol* 2002;13:246A.
101. Schor N. Acute renal failure and the sepsis syndrome. *Kidney Int* 2001;61:764–776.
102. Schetz M. Non-renal indications for continuous renal replacement therapy. *Kidney Int* 1999;56:S88–S94.
103. Reiter K, et al. High-volume hemofiltration in sepsis: theoretical basis and practical application. *Nephron* 2002;92:251–258.
104. De Vriese AS, et al. Cytokine removal during continuous hemofiltration in septic patients. *J Am Soc Nephrol* 1999;10:846–853.
105. Ronco C, et al. Effects of different doses in continuous veno-venous haemofiltration on outcomes of acute renal failure: a prospective randomised trial. *Lancet* 2000;356:26–30.
106. Bellomo R. Preliminary experience with high volume HF in human septic shock. *Kidney Int* 1998;53(Suppl 66):S182–S185.
107. Bellomo R, et al. High-volume hemofiltration. *Contrib Nephrol* 2001;(132):375–382.
108. Uchino S, et al. Super high flux hemofiltration: a new technique for cytokine removal. *Intensive Care Med* 2002;28:651–655.
109. Honore PM, et al. Prospective evaluation of short-term, high-volume isovolemic hemofiltration on the hemodynamic course and outcome in patients with intractable circulatory failure resulting from septic shock. *Crit Care Med* 2000;28:3581–3587.
110. Honore PM, et al. Short-term high-volume hemofiltration in sepsis: perhaps the right way is to start with. *Crit Care Med* 2002;30:1673–1674.
111. Journois D, et al. High-volume, zero-balanced hemofiltration to reduce delayed inflammatory response to cardiopulmonary bypass in children. *Anesthesiology* 1996;85:965–976.
112. Oudemans-van Straaten. Outcome of critically ill patients treated with intermittent high volume hemofiltration: a prospective cohort analysis. *Intensive Care Med* 1999;25:814–821.
113. Lonnemann G, et al. Tumor necrosis factor-alpha during continuous high-flux hemodialysis in sepsis with acute renal failure. *Kidney Int* 1999;72(Suppl):S84–S87.
114. Yekebas EF, et al. Attenuation of sepsis-related immunoparalysis by continuous veno-venous hemofiltration in experimental porcine pancreatitis. *Crit Care Med* 2001;29:1423–1430.
115. Yekebas EF, et al. Impact of different modalities of continuous venovenous hemofiltration on sepsis-induced alterations in experimental pancreatitis. *Kidney Int* 2002;62:1806–1818.
116. Cole L, et al. A phase II randomized, controlled trial of continuous hemofiltration in sepsis. *Crit Care Med* 2002;30:100–106.
117. Bouman CS, et al. Effects of early high-volume continuous venovenous hemofiltration on survival and recovery of renal function in intensive care patients with acute renal failure: a prospective, randomized trial. *Crit Care Med* 2002;30:2205–2211.
118. Sander A, et al. Hemofiltration increases IL-6 clearance in early systemic inflammatory response syndrome but does not alter IL-6 and TNF alpha plasma concentrations. *Intensive Care Med* 1997;23:878–884.
119. Sanchez-Izquierdo JA, et al. Cytokines clearance during venovenous hemofiltration in the trauma patient. *Am J Kidney Dis* 1997;30:483–488.
120. Cardigan R, et al. Endothelial dysfunction in critically ill patients: the effect of haemofiltration. *Intensive Care Med* 1998;24:1264–1271.
121. Misset B, et al. A randomized cross-over comparison of the hemodynamic response to intermittent hemodialysis and continuous hemofiltration in ICU patients with acute renal failure. *Intensive Care Med* 1996;22:742–746.
122. Swartz RD, et al. Comparing continuous hemofiltration with hemodialysis in patients with severe acute renal failure. *Am J Kidney Dis* 1999;34:424–432.
123. Ronco C, et al. A pilot study of coupled plasma filtration with adsorption in septic shock. *Crit Care Med* 2002;30:1250–1255.
124. Berlot G, et al. Plasmapheresis in the critically ill patient. *Kidney Int* 1998;66(Suppl):S178–S181.
125. Reeves JH, et al. Continuous plasmafiltration in sepsis syndrome. *Crit Care Med* 1999;27:2096–2104.

126. Wratten ML, et al. Should we target signal pathways instead of single mediators in the treatment of sepsis? *Contrib Nephrol* 2001;(132):400–414.

127. Better OS, et al. Early management of shock and prophylaxis of acute renal failure in traumatic rhabdomyolysis. *N Engl J Med* 1990;322:825–829.

128. Bywaters. Crush injuries with impairment of renal function. *BMJ* 1941;1:427–432.

129. Vanholder R, et al. Rhabdomyolysis. *J Am Soc Nephrol* 2000;11:1553–1561.

130. Zager. Rhabdomyolysis and myohemoglobinuric acute renal failure. *Kidney Int* 2002;46:314–376.

131. Holt SG, et al. Pathogenesis and treatment of renal dysfunction in rhabdomyolysis. *Intensive Care Med* 2001;27:803–811.

132. Rice EK, et al. Heroin overdose and myoglobinuric acute renal failure. *Clin Nephrol* 2000;54:449–454.

133. Szpirt WM. Plasmapheresis is not justified in treatment of rhabdomyolysis and acute renal failure. *J Cardiovasc Surg (Torino)* 1997;38:557.

134. Oda Y, et al. Crush syndrome sustained in the 1995 Kobe, Japan, earthquake: treatment and outcome. *Ann Emerg Med* 1997;30:507–512.

135. Amyot SL, et al. Myoglobin clearance and removal during continuous venovenous hemofiltration. *Intensive Care Med* 1999;25:1169–1172.

136. Bastani B, et al. Significant myoglobin removal during continuous veno-venous haemofiltration using F80 membrane. *Nephrol Dial Transplant* 1997;12:2035–2036.

137. Berns JS, et al. Removal of myoglobin by CAVH-D in traumatic rhabdomyolysis. *Am J Nephrol* 1991;11:73.

138. Bellomo R, et al. Myoglobin clearance during acute continuous hemodiafiltration. *Intensive Care Med* 1991;17:509.

139. Wakabayashi Y, et al. Rapid fall in blood myoglobin in massive rhabdomyolysis and acute renal failure. *Intensive Care Med* 1994;20:109–112.

140. Shigemoto T, et al. Blood purification for crush syndrome. *Ren Fail* 1997;19:711–719.

141. Bywaters EG, et al. The production of renal failure following injection of solution containing myoglobin. *Q J Exp Physiol* 1994;33:53–70.

142. Woodrow G, et al. The clinical and biochemical features of acute renal failure due to rhabdomyolysis. *Renal Failure* 1995;17:467–474.

143. Marenzi G, et al. Circulatory response to fluid overload removal by extracorporeal ultrafiltration in refractory congestive heart failure. *J Am Coll Cardiol* 2001;38:963–968.

144. Kishore KK. Renal replacement therapy in congestive heart failure. *Semin Dial* 1997;10:259–266.

145. Agostino P, et al. Sustained improvement in functional capacity after removal of body fluid with isolated ultrafiltration in chronic cardiac insufficiency. *Am J Med* 1994;96:191–199.

146. Blake P, et al. Refractory congestive heart failure: overview and application of extracorporeal ultrafiltration. *Adv Ren Replace Ther* 1996;3:166–173.

147. Blake P, et al. Isolation of "myocardial depressant factor(s)" from the ultrafiltrate of heart failure patients with acute renal failure. *ASAIO J* 1996;42:M911–M915.

148. Brause M, et al. Congestive heart failure as an indication for continuous renal replacement therapy. *Kidney Int* 1999;72(Suppl):S95–S98.

149. Rimondini A, et al. Hemofiltration as short-term treatment for refractory congestive heart failure. *Am J Med* 1987;83:43–48.

150. Iorio L, et al. Daily hemofiltration in severe heart failure. *Kidney Int* 1997;51:62–65.

151. Biasioli S, et al. Intermittent venovenous hemofiltration as a chronic treatment for refractory and intractable heart failure. *Am Soc Artif Intern Organs J* 1992;38:M658–M663.

152. Coraim FI, et al. Continuous hemofiltration for the failing heart. *New Horizons* 1995;3:725–731.

153. Inoue T, et al. Hemofiltration as a treatment for patients with refractory heart failure. *Clin Cardiol* 1992;15:514–518.

154. Chapman A, et al. Continuous arteriovenous hemofiltration in patients with severe congestive heart failure. *Am J Med* 1987;83:1167–1168.

155. Kramer P, et al. A new and simple method for treatment of overhydrated patients resistant to diuretics. *Klin Wochenschr* 1977;55:1121–1122.

156. Simpson IA, et al. Ultrafiltration in the management of refractory congestive heart failure. *Br Heart J* 1985;55:344–347.

157. Agostino P, et al. Isolated ultrafiltration in moderate congestive heart failure. *J Am Coll Cardiol* 1993;21:424–431.

158. Forslund T, et al. Hormonal changes in patients with severe chronic congestive heart failure treated by ultrafiltration. *Nephrol Dial Transplant* 1992;7:306–310.

159. Tormey V, et al. Long-term successful management of refractory congestive cardiac failure by intermittent ambulatory peritoneal ultrafiltration. *Q J Med* 1996;89:683.

160. Marenzi G, et al. Interrelation of humoral factors, hemodynamics, and fluid and salt metabolism in congestive heart failure: effects of extracorporeal ultrafiltration. *Am J Med* 1993;94:49–56.

161. Baudouin SV, et al. Continuous veno-venous hemofiltration following cardio-pulmonary bypass. *Intensive Care Med* 1993;19:290–293.

162. Bent P, et al. Early and intensive continuous hemofiltration for severe renal failure after cardiac surgery. *Ann Thorac Surg* 2001;71:832–837.

163. Kumar A, et al. Role of nitric oxide and cGMP in human septic serum-induced depression of cardiac myocyte contractility. *Am J Physiol* 1999;276:R265–R276.

164. Bellomo R, et al. Intensive care unit management of the critically ill patient with fluid overload after open heart surgery. *Cardiology* 2001;96:169–176.

165. Bellomo R, et al. Effect of continuous venovenous hemofiltration with dialysis on hormone and catecholamine clearance in critically ill patients with acute renal failure. *Crit Care Med* 1994;22:833–837.

166. Agostini P. Sustained benefit from ultrafiltration in moderate congestive heart failure. *Cardiology* 2001;96:183–189.

167. Canaud. Slow isolated ultrafiltration for the treatment of congestive heart failure. *Am J Kidney Dis* 1996;28(Suppl 3):S67–S73.

168. Ronco C, et al. Extracorporeal ultrafiltration for the treatment of overhydration and congestive heart failure. *Cardiology* 2001;96:155–168.

169. Handley H, et al. Intravenous catheter for intracorporeal plasma filtration. *Blood Purif* 2002;20:61–69.

170. Eckardt KU. Renal failure in liver disease. *Intensive Care Med* 1999;25:5–14.

171. Epstein M. Hepatorenal syndrome in the kidney in liver disease. In: Epstein M, ed. *The kidney in liver disease.* Philadelphia: Hanley & Belfus, 1996:75–108.

172. Green J, et al. Circulatory disturbance and renal dysfunction in liver disease and in obstructive jaundice. *Isr J Med Sci* 1994;30:48–65.

173. Kaplan AA, et al. Extracorporeal blood purification in the management of patients with hepatic failure. *Semin Nephrol* 1997;17:576–582.

174. Briglia AE, et al. Hepatorenal syndrome: definition, pathophysiology, and intervention. *Crit Care Clin* 2002;18:345–373.

175. Ellis D, et al. Renal failure and dialysis therapy in children with hepatic failure in the perioperative period of orthotopic liver transplantation. *Clin Nephrol* 1986;25:295–303.

176. Sandy D, et al. Acute dialytic support in patients with end-stage liver disease awaiting liver transplantation. *J Am Soc Nephrol* 1996;7:1462A.

177. Perez GO. Dialysis, hemofiltration, and other extracorporeal techniques in the treatment of the renal complications disease. *The kidney in liver disease.* Philadelphia: Hanley & Belfus, 1996:517–528.

178. Davenport A. Ultrafiltration in diuretic-resistant volume overload in nephrotic syndrome and patients with ascites due to chronic liver disease. *Cardiology* 2001;96:190–195.

179. Matsubara S, et al. Continuous removal of middle molecules by hemofiltration in patients with acute liver failure. *Crit Care Med* 1990;18:1331–1338.

180. Mitzner SR, et al. Extracorporeal detoxification using the molecular adsorbent recirculating system for critically ill patients with liver failure. *J Am Soc Nephrol* 2001;12(Suppl 17):S75–S82.

181. Awad SS, et al. Preliminary results of a phase I trial evaluating a non–cell based extracorporeal hepatic support device. *ASAIO J* 2000;46:220.

182. Novelli G, et al. Use of MARS in the treatment of acute liver failure: preliminary monocentric experience. *ASAIO J* 2000;46:234.

183. Stange J, et al. Molecular adsorbent recycling system (MARS): clinical results of a new membrane-based blood purification system for bioartificial liver support. *Artif Organs* 1999;23:319–330.

184. Mitzner SR, et al. Improvement of hepatorenal syndrome with extracorporeal albumin dialysis MARS: results of a prospective, randomized, controlled clinical trial. *Liver Transplant* 2000;6:277–286.

185. Stange J, et al. Liver support by extracorporeal blood purification: a clinical observation. *Liver Transplant* 2000;6:603–613.

186. Schmidt LE, et al. Improvement of systemic vascular resistance and arterial pressure in patients with acute or chronic liver failure during treatment with the molecular adsorbent recycling system (MARS). *Hepatology* 2000;32:401A.

187. Kreymann B, et al. Albumin dialysis: effective removal of copper in a patient with fulminant Wilson disease and successful bridging to liver transplantation: a new possibility for the elimination of protein-bound toxins. *J Hepatol* 1999;31:1080–1085.

188. Ash SR. Extracorporeal blood detoxification by sorbents in treatment of hepatic encephalopathy. *Adv Ren Replace Ther* 2002;9:3–18.

189. Jost U. Einsatz eines zellfreien Leberunterstutzungssystems zur Elimination albumin-gebundener toxischer Substanzen beim akuten Leberversagen. *Germ Interdisciplin J Intensive Care Med* 2000;37:435.

190. Ash SR. Extracorporeal blood detoxification by sorbents in treatment of hepatic encephalopathy. *Adv Ren Replace Ther* 2002;9:3–18.

191. Ash SR, et al. Clinical effects of a sorbent suspension dialysis system in treatment of hepatic coma (the BioLogic-DT). *Int J Artif Organs* 1992;15:151–161.

192. Ash SR. Hemodiabsorption in treatment of acute hepatic failure and chronic cirrhosis with ascites. *Artif Organs* 1994;18:355–362.

193. Wilkinson AH, et al. Hemodiabsorption in treatment of hepatic failure. *J Transpl Coord* 1998;8:43–50.

194. Hughes RD, et al. Evaluation of the BioLogic-DT sorbent-suspension dialyser in patients with fulminant hepatic failure. *Int J Artif Organs* 1994;17:657–662.

195. Ellis AJ, et al. Temporary extracorporeal liver support for severe acute alcoholic hepatitis using the BioLogic-DT. *Int J Artif Organs* 1999;22:27–34.

196. Mazariegos GV, et al. Preliminary results: randomized clinical trial of the BioLogic-DT in treatment of acute hepatic failure (AHF) with coma. *Artif Organs* 1997;21:529.

197. Kramer L, et al. Biocompatibility of a cuprophane charcoal-based detoxification device in cirrhotic patients with hepatic encephalopathy. *Am J Kidney Dis* 2000;36:1193–1200.

198. O'Grady JG, et al. Controlled trials of charcoal hemoperfusion and prognostic factors in fulminant hepatic failure. *Gastroenterology* 1988;94:1186–1192.

199. Omokawa S, et al. Therapeutic plasmapheresis for cholestatic liver diseases: study of 9 cases. *Prog Clin Biol Res* 1990;337:233–236.

200. Lepore MJ, et al. Plasmapheresis with plasma exchange in hepatic coma. II. Fulminant viral hepatitis as a systemic disease. *Arch Intern Med* 1972;129:900–907.

201. Lepore MJ, et al. Plasmapheresis with plasma exchange in hepatic coma: methods and results in five patients with acute fulminant hepatic necrosis. *Ann Intern Med* 1970;72:165–174.

202. Yoshiba M, et al. Favorable effect of new artificial liver support on survival of patients with fulminant liver failure. *Artif Organs* 1996;20:1169–1172.

203. Sadamori H, et al. High-flow-rate haemodiafiltration as a brain-support therapy proceeding to liver transplantation for hyperacute fulminant hepatic failure. *Eur J Gastroenterol Hepatol* 2002;14:435–439.

204. Sadahiro T, et al. Usefulness of plasma exchange plus continuous hemodiafiltration to reduce adverse effects associated with plasma exchange in patients with acute liver failure. *Crit Care Med* 2001;29:1386–1392.

205. Zager RA. Acute renal failure in the setting of bone marrow transplantation. *Kidney Int* 1994;46:1443–1458.

206. Bowman WP, et al. Improved survival for children with B cell (sIg+) acute lymphoblastic leukemia (B-ALL) and stage IV small non-cleaved cell lymphoma. *Proc ASCO* 1992;11:277.

207. Griffin TC, et al. Treatment of advanced stage diffuse, small non-cleaved cell lymphoma in childhood: further experience with total therapy B. *Med Pediatr Oncol* 1994;23:393–399.

208. Saccente SL, et al. Prevention of tumor lysis syndrome using continuous veno-venous hemofiltration. *Pediatr Nephrol* 1995;9:569–573.

209. Sakarcan A. Hyperphosphatemia in tumor lysis syndrome: role of hemodialysis and continuous veno-venous HF. *Pediatr Nephrol* 1994;8:351–353.

210. Pepe PE, et al. Clinical predictors of the adult respiratory distress syndrome. *Am J Surg* 1982;144:124–130.

211. Barzilay E, et al. Use of extracorporeal supportive techniques as additional treatment for septic-induced multiple organ failure patients. *Crit Care Med* 1989;17:634–637.

212. Coraim FJ, et al. Acute respiratory failure after cardiac surgery: clinical experience with the application of continuous arteriovenous hemofiltration. *Crit Care Med* 1986;14:714–718.

213. Laggner AN, et al. Influence of ultrafiltration/hemofiltration on extravascular lung water. *Contrib Nephrol* 1991;93:65–70.

214. Cosentino F, et al. Continuous arteriovenous hemofiltration in the adult respiratory distress syndrome: a randomized trial. *Contrib Nephrol* 1991;93:94–97.

215. Humphrey H, et al. Improved survival in ARDS patients associated with a reduction in pulmonary capillary wedge pressure. *Chest* 1990;97:1176–1180.

216. Rabb H, et al. Downregulation of the water channel aquaporin 5 in the lung following renal ischemic reperfusion injury occurs independent of reperfusion products. *J Am Soc Nephrol* 1999;10:639A.

217. Rabb H, et al. Molecular mechanisms underlying combined kidney-lung dysfunction during acute renal failure. *Contrib Nephrol* 2001;(132):41–52.

218. Moonka R, et al. Hypothermia induced by continuous arteriovenous hemofiltration as a treatment for adult respiratory distress syndrome: a case report. *J Trauma* 1996;40:1026–1028.

219. Gruberg. The prognostic implications of further renal function deterioration within 48 hours of interventional coronary procedures in patients with pre-existing chronic renal insufficiency. *J Am Soc Nephrol* 2002;36:1542–1548.

220. Albert SG, et al. Analysis of radiocontrast-induced nephropathy by dual-labeled radionuclide clearance. *Invest Radiol* 1994;29:618–623.

221. Murphy SW, et al. Contrast nephropathy. *J Am Soc Nephrol* 2000;11:177–182.

222. McCullough PA, et al. Acute renal failure after coronary intervention: incidence, risk factors, and relationship to mortality. *Am J Med* 1997;103:368–375.

223. Liss P, et al. Injection of low and iso-osmolar contrast medium decreases oxygen tension in the renal medulla. *Kidney Int* 1998;53:698–702.

224. Rudnick MR, et al. Nephrotoxicity of ionic and nonionic contrast media in 1196 patients: a randomized trial. The Iohexol Cooperative Study. *Kidney Int* 1995;47:254–261.

225. Solomon R, et al. Effects of saline, mannitol, and furosemide to prevent acute decreases in renal function induced by radiocontrast agents. *N Engl J Med* 1994;331:1416–1420.

226. Tepel M, et al. Prevention of radiographic-contrast-agent-induced reductions in renal function by acetylcysteine. *N Engl J Med* 2000;343:180–184.

227. Lehnert T, et al. Effect of hemodialysis after contrast medium administration in patients with renal insufficiency. *Nephrol Dial Transplant* 1998;13:358–362.

228. Moon. HD for elimination of the nonionic contrast medium iohexol after angiography in patients with impaired renal function. *Nephron* 1995;70:430–437.

229. Solomon R. Contrast-medium-induced acute renal failure. *Kidney Int* 1998;53:230–242.

230. Brooks. Removal of iodinated contrast material by peritoneal dialysis. *Nephron* 1973;12:10–14.

231. Ueda J, et al. Elimination of ioversol by hemodialysis. *Acta Radiologica* 1996;37:826–829.

232. Waaler A, et al. Elimination of iohexol, a low osmolar nonionic contrast medium, by hemodialysis in patients with chronic renal failure. *Nephron* 1990;56:81–85.

233. Matzkies FK, et al. Influence of dialysis procedure, membrane surface

and membrane material on iopromide elimination in patients with reduced kidney function. *Am J Nephrol* 2000;20:300–304.

234. Furukawa T, et al. Elimination of low osmolality contrast media by hemodialysis. *Acta Radiologica* 1996;37:966–971.

235. Vogt B, et al. Prophylactic hemodialysis after radiocontrast media in patients with renal insufficiency is potentially harmful. *Am J Med* 2001;111:692–698.

236. Davenport A. Renal replacement therapy in the patient with acute brain injury. *Am J Kidney Dis* 2001;37:457–466.

237. Winney RJ, et al. Changes in brain water with haemodialysis. *Lancet* 1986;2:1107–1108.

238. Ronco C, et al. Brain density changes during renal replacement in critically ill patients with acute renal failure: continuous hemofiltration versus intermittent hemodialysis. *J Nephrol* 1999;12:173–178.

239. Kennedy AC, et al. The pathogenesis and prevention of cerebral dysfunction during dialysis. *Lancet* 1964;1:790–793.

240. Arieff AI, et al. Central nervous system pH in uremia and the effects of hemodialysis. *J Clin Invest* 1976;58:306–311.

241. Arieff AI. Dialysis disequilibrium syndrome: current concepts on pathogenesis and prevention. *Kidney Int* 1994;45:629–635.

242. Rosen F, et al. Studies on the nature and specificity of the induction of several adaptive enzymes responsive to cortisol. *Adv Enzyme Regul* 1964;2:115–135.

243. Goldsmith DJA, et al. Bicarbonate therapy and intracellular acidosis. *Clin Sci* 1997;93:593–598.

244. Davenport A, et al. Early changes in intracranial pressure during haemofiltration treatment in patients with grade 4 hepatic encephalopathy and acute oliguric renal failure. *Nephrol Dial Transplant* 1990; 5:192–198.

245. Davenport A. The management of renal failure in patients at risk of cerebral edema/hypoxia. *New Horiz* 1995;3:717–724.

246. Jost CM, et al. Effects of cooler temperature dialysate on hemodynamic stability in "problem" dialysis patients. *Kidney Int* 1993;44: 606–612.

247. Davenport A. Renal replacement therapy in the patient with acute brain injury. *Am J Kidney Dis* 1996;30:S20–S27.

248. Ward DM. The approach to anticoagulation in patients treated with extracorporeal therapy in the intensive care unit. *Adv Ren Replace Ther* 1997;4:160–173.

249. Ohtake Y, et al. Nafamostat mesylate as anticoagulant in continuous hemofiltration and continuous hemodiafiltration. *Contrib Nephrol* 1991;93:215–217.

250. Davenport A, et al. The effect of prostacyclin on intracranial pressure in patients with acute hepatic and renal failure. *Clin Nephrol* 1991;35:151–157.

251. Yagi N, et al. Cooling effect of continuous renal replacement therapy in critically ill patients. *Am J Kidney Dis* 1998;32:1023–1030.

252. Benjamin E. Continuous venovenous hemofiltration with dialysis and lactate clearance in critically ill patients. *Crit Care Med* 1997;25:4–5.

253. Bellomo R. Bench-to-bedside review: lactate and the kidney. *Critical Care* 2002;6:322–326.

254. Mizock BA, et al. Lactic acidosis in critical illness. *Crit Care Med* 1992;20:80–93.

255. Madias NE. Lactic acidosis. *Kidney Int* 1986;29:752–774.

256. Levraut J, et al. Effect of continuous venovenous hemofiltration with dialysis on lactate clearance in critically ill patients. *Crit Care Med* 1997;25:58–62.

257. Barton IK, et al. Successful treatment of severe lactic acidosis by haemofiltration using a bicarbonate-based replacement fluid. *Nephrol Dial Transplant* 1991;6:368–370.

258. Kirschbaum B, et al. Lactic acidosis treated with continuous hemodiafiltration and regional citrate anticoagulation. *Crit Care Med* 1990; 20:349–353.

259. Forni G, et al. Lactate intolerance with continuous venovenous hemofiltration: the role of bicarbonate-buffered hemofiltration. *Clinical Intensive Care* 1998;9:40–42.

260. Charytan C, et al. Role of the nephrologist in the intensive care unit. *Am J Kidney Dis* 2001;38:426–429.

261. Paganini EP. Continuous renal replacement therapy: a nephrological technique, managed by the nephrologist. *Semin Dial* 1996;9:200–203.

262. Cole. A prospective multicenter study of the epidemiology, management, and outcome of severe acute renal failure in a "closed" ICU system. *Am J Respir Crit Care Med* 2000;162:191–196.

263. Corhick R. Data management and services at the American Board of Medical Specialties. Data management and services at the American Board of Medical Specialties, 1995–1997. 1995.

264. Hoyt DB. CRRT in the area of cost containment: is it justified? *Am J Kidney Dis* 1997;30:S102–S104.

265. Moreno L. Continuous renal replacement therapy: cost considerations and reimbursement. *Semin Dial* 1996;9:209–214.

MALNUTRITION AND INTRADIALYTIC PARENTERAL NUTRITION IN END-STAGE RENAL DISEASE PATIENTS

MARSHA WOLFSON

Numerous studies have documented a significant incidence of protein-energy malnutrition in hemodialysis and peritoneal dialysis patients (1–8). Markers of poor nutritional status, particularly low serum albumin levels, are predictors of increased morbidity and mortality in this population (9–15). Thus it is imperative that assessment of nutritional status and early nutritional intervention become a routine part of the management of dialysis patients (Fig. 30.1). The impact of inflammation on these markers of nutritional status may further influence the development of malnutrition, so it is also important for health care providers to understand the relationship between inflammation and nutritional status (16,17).

This chapter outlines common causes of malnutrition in the patient with end-stage renal disease (ESRD) and discusses methods of nutritional assessment. The baseline nutritional requirements for hemodialysis and peritoneal dialysis patients are presented as a necessary prelude to managing the malnourished dialysis patient. A diagnostic and therapeutic approach is outlined that entails early and periodic nutritional assessment and aggressive nutritional counseling and support. Finally, methods of nutritional intervention such as oral supplements, intradialytic parenteral nutrition, and use of amino acid dialysate are discussed.

The National Kidney Foundation's K/DOQI initiative has also addressed the concerns of malnutrition. The recommendations from that initiative will be summarized where appropriate (18).

SCOPE OF THE PROBLEM

A number of studies have documented malnutrition as a common occurrence in a large subset of the dialysis population (1–8,15). Cross-sectional and longitudinal nutritional measurements reveal that more than one-third of adult hemodialysis patients display signs of moderate to severe protein calorie malnutrition (1–5,8). Available data suggest a similar frequency of malnutrition in the peritoneal dialysis population (5–8,15). A cross-sectional study compared the nutritional status of hemodialysis and peritoneal dialysis patients in eight centers in Italy (8). The subjective global nutritional assessment indicated a greater proportion of malnourished CAPD patients than hemodialysis patients (42.3% versus 30.8%). This difference diminished with age and the authors could not exclude selection bias as a contributing factor. Nevertheless, the study confirmed once again the high prevalence of malnutrition in the ESRD patient.

It should be emphasized that the assessment of nutritional status in dialysis patients is confounded by the lack of uniform criteria for malnutrition in this population and the difficulties in separating abnormal nutritional parameters due to malnutrition from those caused by inflammation or uremia per se. Nevertheless, the problem of malnutrition is undoubtedly widespread in the dialysis population. Moreover, the incidence of malnutrition can be expected to rise as the age and medical complexity of these patients increases.

Many studies have demonstrated a strong association between malnutrition and increased morbidity and mortality (9–15). A low serum albumin is one of the most consistent and powerful predictors of mortality in the dialysis population. Lowrie et al. analyzed a large amount of data on 12,000 hemodialysis patients in centers throughout the United States (10). Of all the laboratory values examined, the serum albumin correlated most strongly with the probability of death. Interestingly, a low serum creatinine and cholesterol were also associated with an increased risk of death, and both the serum albumin and creatinine were directly correlated with treatment time. Thus inadequate dialysis leading to malnutrition and increased mortality might be suggested by these results. The Canada–USA (CANUSA) study, a 2-year prospective observational study of nutrition and adequacy of dialysis in patients commencing therapy on peritoneal dialysis (15), also found a significant relationship between the serum albumin and mortality and morbidity. In addition, it demonstrated that nutrition status, as evaluated by a modified version of the Subjective Global Assessment, was directly related to morbidity and mortality.

The correlation of markers of malnutrition with poor outcome does not necessarily establish a cause–effect relationship. For example, comorbid illnesses may cause malnutrition and increase mortality independently. In addition, it is as yet unclear through what mechanisms malnutrition may lead to increased

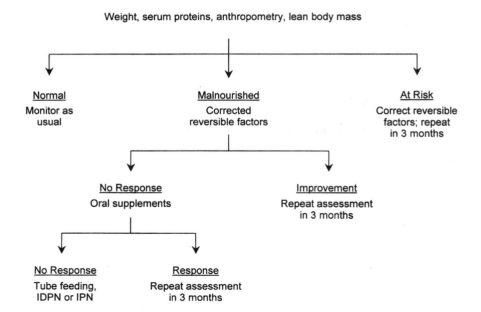

FIG. 30.1. Nutritional assessment.

mortality, as malnutrition per se is rarely indicated as the direct cause of death in ESRD patients. Controlled prospective studies examining the influence of nutritional intervention on outcome are needed to further clarify the relationship of malnutrition to mortality. Nevertheless, until proven otherwise it would seem reasonable to assume that malnutrition likely contributes significantly to the high morbidity and mortality of this population.

CAUSES OF MALNUTRITION IN THE ESRD PATIENT

Table 30.1 summarizes the various factors that may contribute to malnutrition in the ESRD patient. Careful dietary histories on dialysis patients reveal that their caloric intake is often significantly less than the recommended 35 kcal/kg body wt/d

TABLE 30.1. CAUSES OF MALNUTRITION IN THE DIALYSIS PATIENT

Decreased intake
  Inadequate dialysis
  Delayed gastric emptying
  Dietary restrictions
  Depression
Intercurrent illness
Metabolic/endocrine disturbances
  Insulin resistance
  Catabolic effects of parathyroid hormone
  Resistance to insulin growth factor 1
  Metabolic acidosis
  Altered amino acid metabolism
Effects of dialysis
  Amino acid losses into dialysate
  Protein losses (peritoneal dialysis)
  Catabolic effects of blood-membrane interactions

(1,2). Hospitalized dialysis patients have been documented to have inadequate protein and energy intake, resulting in significant deterioration in nutritional parameters (19). Nausea, vomiting, and decreased appetite may be present in some patients because of delayed gastric emptying or other gastrointestinal problems. In addition, food may not be palatable because of dietary restrictions. Finally, depression, a frequent problem in the dialysis patient, is often accompanied by decreased food intake.

Inadequate dialysis may be an important contributory factor in causing malnutrition. A number of studies have demonstrated a positive correlation between protein nitrogen appearance (PNA, formally known as the protein catabolic rate, or PCR) and clearance as measured by Kt/V in hemodialysis and peritoneal dialysis patients (20–24). However, others have criticized this as simply a mathematical artifact due to common factors used in calculating Kt/V and the PNA (25,26).

A correlation between Kt/V and other nutritional parameters such as the serum albumin has been less consistent. Undoubtedly this is because inadequate dialysis is only one of many factors that impact nutritional status. In addition, the method of calculating V in the malnourished patient may be important. If the actual body weight is used, the underweight malnourished patient will have a relatively low V and thus may have an adequate Kt/V. Yet if the patient's ideal body weight is used, the Kt/V may be inadequate (27). The exact mechanism for inadequate dialysis leading to malnutrition is unclear, but substances within the middle-molecule weight range in uremic plasma have been shown to induce a dose-dependent suppression of appetite in rats (28). Further support for an association between dialysis dose and nutrition comes from a recent publication demonstrating improvement in dietary intake and nutritional status in a small group of patients treated with daily hemodialysis (29).

A variety of metabolic and endocrine disturbances associated with renal failure may also have an impact on nutritional status

(30,31). It is well recognized that there is resistance to the actions of insulin, a potent anabolic hormone, in renal failure (32). Although serum levels of growth hormone and its mediator, insulin growth factor 1 (IGF-1), are increased, there is evidence that an inhibitor of the biologic activity of IGF-1 is present in uremia (33). Thus the anabolic effects of growth hormone and its mediators are probably diminished.

Parathyroid hormone (PTH) is commonly increased in dialysis patients and has well-described effects on bone and calcium and phosphorus metabolism. Less well appreciated is the fact that elevated PTH levels may also increase protein wasting and promote negative nitrogen balance. The precise mechanism for this is unclear; however, one study showed a direct effect of PTH on amino acid and protein metabolism in skeletal muscle preparations from the rat (34).

Metabolic acidosis is also a stimulus for protein breakdown. May et al. demonstrated that even relatively minor degrees of acidemia resulted in increased muscle protein breakdown in the rat with chronic renal failure (34). This process was dependent on an increase in glucocorticoid production, as adrenalectomy prevented the increase in proteolysis. Correction of metabolic acidosis in patients with chronic renal failure or patients on hemodialysis or peritoneal dialysis results in a decrease in protein degradation (36–38). Mitch et al. have shown that metabolic acidosis stimulates protein degradation in the rat via the ATP-dependent pathway involving ubiquitin and proteosomes (39). There is also some evidence that metabolic acidosis decreases the level of IGF-1, an anabolic hormone (40,41). More recently, increasing the serum bicarbonate level in patients treated with peritoneal dialysis by increasing the lactate concentration of the dialysis solution demonstrated improved nutritional status and decreased hospitalization (42,43). This suggests that correction of even mild metabolic acidosis may have a beneficial effect on both nutritional status and outcome.

Dialysate losses are another important contributing factor in the development of malnutrition. Protein losses in peritoneal dialysis patients average between 5 and 15 g/d and increase further during episodes of peritonitis (44). For hemodialysis patients, negative nitrogen balance occurs on dialysis days and is most likely due to a combination of amino acid losses into the dialysate and increased catabolism (45,46). Free amino acid losses average about 8 g per hemodialysis session (47–49). The type of membrane is important, as losses are greater with high-flux membranes and increase further as the membrane is reused. In addition, substantial albumin losses of up to 20 g have been reported with bleach-processed polysulfone dialyzers (50). Protein losses were reduced when bleach was removed from the reuse procedure.

Several studies have shown that the hemodialysis procedure per se enhances protein catabolism (48,51–53). Gutierrez et al. studied the metabolic effect of blood contact with the dialysis membrane by measuring the release of free amino acids from leg tissue in a group of normal volunteers undergoing sham hemodialysis (51). Amino acid efflux from the leg increased following exposure of blood to the regenerated cellulose membrane, representing increased protein catabolism. Of interest, exposure of blood to the synthetic polyacrylonitrile membrane did not result in increased release of amino acids, and pretreat-

ment with indomethacin prevented the rise in amino acid release with the regenerated cellulose-based membrane. The authors postulated that release of cytokines such as interleukin-1 during blood–membrane contact enhances protein breakdown. Prostaglandins were thought possibly to be mediators in this process, as reflected by the protective effect of indomethacin. Finally, the composition of the membrane and degree of complement activation were postulated to play a role in affecting protein catabolism.

Löfberg et al. also examined the metabolic effect of hemodialysis by measuring muscle ribosome and amino acid content during a single hemodialysis session in a small group of chronic hemodialysis patients (52). Muscle alanine concentration and ribosome content decreased, indicating a fall in capacity for protein synthesis. The authors again postulated a role for cytokine release. In summary, amino acid losses in conjunction with the protein catabolic effect of the hemodialysis procedure itself probably account for the negative nitrogen balance observed in patients on hemodialysis days.

Leptin, a polypeptide encoded by the *ob* gene, is increased in patients with ESRD (54). In addition, several cross-sectional studies have demonstrated an association between elevated leptin levels and decreased dietary intake in maintenance dialysis patients, suggesting that hyperleptinemia may be one cause of anorexia and decreased dietary intake in these patients (54).

A number of recent publications have postulated an association between malnutrition, inflammation, and cardiovascular disease (55). While this entire area is beyond the scope of this chapter, it is important to appreciate the impact of inflammation on nutritional status. Bistrian has reviewed the association between nutritional status and inflammation in ESRD (16). The data suggest that hypoalbuminemia is more likely to occur as a response to inflammation than as a response to inadequate dietary protein intake. This is discussed in greater detail later.

NUTRITIONAL ASSESSMENT

Accurate nutritional assessment at regular intervals is critical for identifying malnourished patients and monitoring the results of therapy. Table 30.2 summarizes recommendations for assessing

TABLE 30.2. NUTRITIONAL ASSESSMENT

Patient interview
 Recent weight changes, changes in appetite, gastrointestinal symptoms, medical illnesses, eating patterns, food preferences
 Medications with nutritional implications (steroids, insulin, etc.)
 Assessment of food intake
 Patient recall, food diary
Physical examination
 Assessment of dry weight, evaluation of skin, hair, mucous membranes
Anthropometry
 Height, weight, arm circumference, triceps skinfold
Laboratory tests
 Glucose, sodium, potassium, BUN, creatinine, albumin, transferrin, hematocrit, whole blood count, total lymphocyte count
 Calculate protein nitrogen appearance with kinetic modeling

nutritional status in the dialysis population. A variety of methods are available for the assessment of nutritional status in the dialysis patient. Selection and interpretation of these tests must be made in light of the effects of uremia per se and other clinical conditions on these parameters. In general, most of the usual methods of assessing nutritional status can be applied to patients with ESRD with minor adaptations (56,57). In particular, the potential effects of renal insufficiency per se on various nutritional parameters should be kept in mind when interpreting the results. The K/DOQI guidelines are helpful in outlining the usefulness of various nutritional parameters and their interpretation (18).

History and Physical Examination

The history and physical examination can often provide important clues about the nutritional status of the patient. Symptoms such as nausea, vomiting, or anorexia should be carefully evaluated. In addition, recent weight gain or loss should be identified. The history should address concomitant clinical problems such as alcoholism, diabetes, and gastrointestinal disease, which may impact the patient's nutritional status. Psychosocial issues such as access and the affordability of food, ability to prepare meals, and role of family members in food preparation should be explored. Signs or symptoms of depression should be identified, as clinical depression often results in a disinterest and decrease in caloric intake. The physical examination should include an assessment of the patient's volume status, as it is the patient's "dry weight" that should be compared with the recommended body weight.

An accurate assessment of the patient's food intake is a very important component of the nutritional assessment. Patient recall should cover a relatively short period of time, such as 3 days, and should include dialysis and nondialysis days. A food diary is very useful, especially if the patient weighs the portions of food. The intake of protein, fat, and carbohydrate can then be calculated from standard food tables. Dietary protein intake can also be estimated by calculating the protein nitrogen appearance using kinetic modeling as discussed in Chapter 7. It should be emphasized, however, that the PNA will reflect protein intake only if the patient is in neutral nitrogen balance.

Panels of Nutritional Measures

The K/DOQI Clinical Practice Guidelines for Nutrition in Chronic Renal Failure recommend that a panel of nutritional measures be used to assess nutritional status in maintenance dialysis patients. This is because no single measure provides a comprehensive indication of nutritional status and because different measures, such as measures of visceral protein pools, dietary intake, and measures of body composition, identify different aspects of nutritional status. Use of panels of nutritional status may identify the presence of malnutrition with greater sensitivity and specificity than any single measure alone. These measures should be carried out monthly for serum albumin and body weight, every 4 months for the standard NHANES body weight, and every 6 months for the subjective global assessment. Dietary history should be obtained every month in hemodialysis patients and every 3 to 4 months for peritoneal dialysis patients (18).

The guidelines further recommend the predialysis serum albumin, the percentage of postdialysis (in hemodialysis patients) or postdrain (in peritoneal dialysis patients) body weight, the percentage of standard (NHANES II) body weight, the subjective global assessment and dietary intake as assessed by dietary interview or diaries, and the normalized protein equivalent of nitrogen appearance (nPNA) in all dialysis patients (18).

Measures that can be used to confirm or extend the data obtained in the first category include the predialysis serum prealbumin, and a variety of anthropometric measurements, including skinfold thickness and mid-arm muscle area, and dual-energy x-ray absorptiometry (18). A further description of these measures follows.

Anthropometric Measurements and Assessment of Lean Body Mass

Anthropometric measurements provide a rapid, noninvasive, and reproducible method for evaluating body fat and protein stores. The dietitian can easily carry out these measurements. Body fat is estimated by measuring skinfold thickness at the triceps or subscapular area; midarm circumference can provide an estimate of the muscle mass. The results of these measurements are compared with the reference standards obtained from healthy adults during the National Health and Nutrition Examination Surveys (NHANES II) from 1976 to 1980.

A multicenter cooperative study was undertaken to establish anthropometric norms for the dialysis population (58). Stringent selection criteria were used to ensure that only stable maintenance dialysis patients were included in the study. The data from this study provide important information on anthropometric measurements in the "healthy" maintenance dialysis population and give a good frame of reference. As a general rule, patients whose measurements are greater than 95% of normal are considered to be adequately nourished, whereas values between 70% and 90% indicate the patient is at risk for malnutrition, and values of less than 70% represent significant malnutrition.

Although anthropometry is relatively simple and quick to carry out, it has several limitations. For one thing, there is interoperator error, making it necessary for the same person to carry out these measurements if they are to be used longitudinally. It also lacks precision.

More sophisticated measures of body composition include bioelectric impedance analysis (BIA) and dual-energy x-ray absorptiometry (DEXA) (59,60). These methods are more expensive in that they require special equipment and skilled operators, and one must differentiate between body fat and body water when using them. The best time for carrying out these measurements is immediately after the patient's midweek hemodialysis procedure. In CAPD patients, the best time is after a midday exchange, following the drain and before the instillation of the next exchange of dialysate.

Serum Proteins

Serum proteins are generally depressed as the body's protein stores are depleted. Serum albumin, prealbumin, and transferrin levels are most frequently used as markers of nutritional status. Many investigators have shown that serum albumin levels are depressed in maintenance dialysis patients who manifest other signs of malnutrition (1–8). In addition, serum albumin levels usually improve as nutritional repletion is accomplished (61). However, the serum albumin concentration may also be depressed in patients who have acute inflammation, because hepatic albumin synthesis may be reduced as the liver increases production of acute phase reactants (62,63). Bistrian recently reviewed the interaction between nutrition and inflammation in patients with ESRD and pointed out that dialysis patients, unlike those with acute trauma or major burns, may have mild but prolonged inflammation due to a variety of causes. This may lead to the development of protein-energy malnutrition. Serum albumin concentrations fall due to reduced hepatic albumin synthesis, as well as an increase in the albumin catabolic rate and extracellular fluid extravasation lowering the normal intravascular to extravascular ratio (16,18). It is unlikely, according to Bistrian, that reduced protein intake and albumin losses into dialysate could account for the reduction in serum albumin concentration in the absence of an inflammatory response causing these metabolic changes in albumin metabolism (16).

Serum transferrin levels are often difficult to interpret, as abnormalities in iron stores may affect levels independent of nutritional status. Serum prealbumin and retinol-binding protein (RBP) are also used as indices of nutritional status. However, RBP and prealbumin levels are usually increased in patients with renal failure, and because of this, serum prealbumin is often normal regardless of nutritional status. To use serum prealbumin levels to assess protein nutritional status, it is best to obtain a baseline level and then follow it serially. Generally, serum prealbumin levels below 30 mg/dL should be evaluated for protein energy malnutrition (17). Like serum albumin, prealbumin can be affected by the concomitant presence of inflammation.

Plasma Amino Acids

Plasma amino acids have also been used to assess nutritional status. Unfortunately, even well-nourished dialysis patients display abnormalities in the plasma amino acid pattern (64). Alterations in the intermediary metabolism and changes in renal excretion of amino acids compound the effects of protein malnutrition on amino acid levels. For these reasons, we do not routinely recommend using this test for assessing nutritional status.

NUTRITIONAL RECOMMENDATIONS

An understanding of the baseline nutritional needs of the dialysis patient is necessary before discussing various nutritional interventions.

Nutrition for Hemodialysis Patients

Table 30.3 summarizes the nutritional recommendations for hemodialysis patients. As mentioned earlier, protein requirements increase following initiation of maintenance hemodialysis

TABLE 30.3. NUTRITIONAL RECOMMENDATIONS FOR HEMODIALYSIS PATIENTS

Energy	35 kcal/kg body wt/d
Protein	1.2 g/kg body wt/d
Carbohydrate	Approximately 35% of nonprotein calories
Fat	Polyunsaturated to saturated ratio of 2:1
Calcium	1.0–1.5 g of elemental calcium
Phosphorus	800–1,200 mg
Sodium, potassium, and water	Individualize, depending on fluid balance and serum potassium

because of dialysate losses and catabolism associated with the dialysis procedure. As a result, protein intake should be liberalized to approximately 1.2 g/kg body wt/d of high biological protein (18,65). A caloric intake of 35 kcal/kg body wt/d is required to prevent protein breakdown and maintain neutral nitrogen balance in patients under 60 years of age and between 30 and 35 kcal/kg for patients who are older than 60 (18,66).

Approximately 35% of the nonprotein calories should be made up of carbohydrate and the remainder of fat. A polyunsaturated-to-saturated ratio of about 2:1 is recommended to minimize the lipid abnormalities associated with uremia.

Most patients will require some restriction of sodium, potassium, phosphorus, and fluid intake. Water-soluble vitamins are lost in the dialysate and should be routinely supplemented as outlined in Table 30.4 (67).

Nutrition for Peritoneal Dialysis Patients

Protein losses and glucose absorption from the dialysate may have important nutritional consequences in the peritoneal dialysis patient. Protein losses into the dialysate average between 5 g and 15 g daily and consist primarily of albumin (44,68–70). Most patients can maintain normal total albumin mass by increasing albumin synthesis and decreasing albumin degradation (68). Although there is large individual variation, daily losses usually do not vary in any given patient. Permeability characteristics of the membrane influence protein losses, as rapid transporters tend to have lower serum albumin levels (71). During episodes of peritonitis, protein losses may increase by as much as 50% to 100% and often remain elevated for several weeks following successful treatment of the episode.

TABLE 30.4. RECOMMENDATIONS FOR DAILY VITAMIN SUPPLEMENTATION FOR DIALYSIS PATIENTS

Vitamin B$_6$	10 mg/d
Vitamin C	100 mg/d
Folic acid	1 mg/d
Vitamin A	None
Thiamine	Usual recommended daily allowance
Riboflavin	Usual recommended daily allowance
Vitamin B$_{12}$	Usual recommended daily allowance
Pantothenic acid	Usual recommended daily allowance

TABLE 30.5. NUTRITIONAL RECOMMENDATIONS FOR PERITONEAL DIALYSIS PATIENTS

Energy (oral plus dialysate)	35–45 kcal/kg body wt/d
Protein	1.2–1.3 g/kg body wt/d
Carbohydrate (oral)	35% of ingested nonprotein calories
Fat	Polyunsaturated to saturated ratio of 2:1
Calcium	1.0–1.5 g of elemental calcium
Phosphorus	800–1,200 mg
Sodium, potassium, and water	Individualize, depending on fluid balance and serum potassium

Energy derived from glucose absorption may account for as much as 700 kcal/d or up to 30% of the patient's caloric intake (72,73). The quantity of glucose absorbed is directly proportional to the amount infused and is relatively constant from day to day in a given patient. On average, about 70% of the infused glucose is absorbed. An estimate of calories derived from the absorbed glucose can be calculated using the following formula:

$$y = 11.3x - 10.9$$

where

y equals the amount of glucose absorbed per liter of dialysate.
x equals the average daily concentration of glucose in the dialysate in g/dL.

For example, a CAPD patient undergoing four exchanges per day with two 2-L exchanges of 1.5% (1.3 g/dL) and two 2-L exchanges of 4.25% (3.76 g/dL) will have an average dialysate concentration of 2.53 g/dL. The daily amount of glucose absorbed can be calculated as follows:

Glucose absorbed per liter = 11.3(2.53) − 10.9 = 17.7 g

or

$$17.7 \text{ g/L} \times 8 \text{ L/d} = 142 \text{ g/d}$$

Of interest, von Baeyer et al. found that patients decreased their oral carbohydrate intake to compensate for the glucose load from the dialysate (72). The potential nutritional consequences of the continuous carbohydrate load include an increase in serum triglyceride levels and weight gain (74–76). Reducing the use of 4.25% glucose bags and encouraging regular exercise and a low-fat diet may help minimize these complications.

Table 30.5 outlines the specific dietary recommendations for the peritoneal dialysis patient. The protein intake should be at least 1.2 to 1.3 g/kg/d and the total nonprotein caloric requirement (including the calories from the dialysate glucose) is similar to that of maintenance hemodialysis patients (18,77–79). In general, peritoneal dialysis patients need fewer restrictions on sodium, potassium, and fluid intake than hemodialysis patients.

APPROACH TO THE MALNOURISHED PATIENT

Identifying the reversible causes of malnutrition is the critical first step in evaluation. Medical illnesses that may adversely affect nutritional status, such as poorly controlled diabetes, gastroparesis, or occult infection, should be identified and treated.

Significant acidemia (pH less than 7.35, or HCO_3 less than 20) should be corrected. The possibility of mental depression should be explored and appropriate referral and treatment initiated if indicated. Social issues that affect access and preparation of food such as transportation, cost, and help in meal preparation should be addressed. Often caloric intake can be increased with careful meal planning and attention to ethnic and personal food preferences.

Ensuring adequacy of dialysis is also extremely important. The quantity of delivered dialysis should be regularly assessed and increased if necessary as a very important component of the treatment of malnutrition.

Once reversible causes of malnutrition have been identified and corrected, nutritional intervention should be considered. Various options are available, including oral supplements, enteral feedings, parenteral nutrition, and intraperitoneal nutrition. A stepwise approach from least invasive to more invasive is recommended, depending upon the severity of malnutrition and the ability of the patient to increase intake via the oral route. Drugs to enhance appetite have been used with varying degrees of success. Recent studies with recombinant growth hormone show that it is effective in enhancing protein anabolism and promoting positive nitrogen balance (80).

Thus far, the studies that have examined the effectiveness of supplemental interventions on improving nutritional status and morbidity and mortality are conflicting. Differing patient populations, varying degrees of patient malnutrition, and different methodologies are some of the problems that make it difficult to compare study results. Longer-term prospective studies with larger, well-defined patient populations are required to identify which patients will benefit from nutritional intervention.

Oral Nutritional Supplements and Enteral Feeding

The gastrointestinal tract should be used whenever feasible for nutritional support, as it is the most physiologic way of providing nutrients and is the most cost-effective route. Unfortunately, there are limited data on the value of oral nutritional supplements in improving nutritional status (81). Several studies have examined the effectiveness of protein or amino acid supplements in hemodialysis patients (61,82–84).

Tepper et al. provided two hemodialysis patients with increasing amounts of essential amino acids to ingest orally during each hemodialysis treatment (83). Dialysate losses were proportional to the quantity of amino acids ingested and overall counterbalanced the loss of free amino acids during the dialysis run. More recently, Tietze et al. supplemented 19 hemodialysis patients with a fish protein rich in essential amino acids in a randomized double-blind crossover study (84). During the 3 months of fish supplementation, the serum amino acid profile improved toward normal, with an overall increase in the essential amino acids. In addition, dry weight and mean arm muscle circumference increased significantly. Fedje et al. carried out a trial in almost 100 maintenance dialysis patients with oral supplementation for up to 3 months. They found improvements in serum albumin in those patients with decreased albumin concentrations at the start of the study. Body weight and several

TABLE 30.6. ORAL NUTRITIONAL SUPPLEMENTS

Name	Cost[a] per 8 oz	kcal	Protein (g)	Carbohydrates (g)	Potassium (mg)	Phosphorus (mg)	Sodium (mg)
Ensure	$1.22	255	9.2	36	390	133	212
Nepro	$3.52	475	16.6	52.8	250	165	200
Magnacal	$1.68	470	17.7	47	300	189	190
Renal Sustacal	$1.19	240	14.5	33	490	220	220

[a]Cost may vary in different areas.

anthropometric variables were also improved (80). Further studies are needed to better define those patients who might benefit from oral protein or amino acid supplementation and to refine the optimal composition.

A variety of enteral products are available that may be prescribed as oral supplements or enteral feedings. These products contain varying amounts of carbohydrate, protein, and fat, in addition to differing quantities of electrolytes (Table 30.6). We generally recommend one to two cans per day if the supplement is given orally. Careful attention to the amounts of sodium, potassium, and phosphorus are required when prescribing these supplements.

Total Parenteral Nutrition

Total parenteral nutrition (TPN) should be considered for the malnourished patient who is unable to tolerate enteral feeding. The majority of patients who fall in this category are hospitalized with an intercurrent illness. However, TPN may occasionally be required for the chronically malnourished outpatient who is unable to tolerate oral or enteral supplements. In this latter group of patients, the alternative of intradialytic parenteral nutrition is discussed later. Table 30.7 outlines specific guidelines for prescribing TPN in the ESRD patient (85,86).

For patients hospitalized with an intercurrent illness, energy requirements may be as high as 50% to 100% over normal resting expenditure. To minimize protein breakdown, a total nonprotein caloric intake of 35 to 40 kcal/kg should be provided. A 10% to 20% lipid infusion providing up to one-third of the caloric intake will prevent essential fatty acid deficiency and provide a concentrated source of calories. Glucose should provide the remainder of the nonprotein calories. Protein intake should be between 1.2 and 1.5 g/kg body wt/d, and in most cases may be provided with a standard mix of essential and nonessential amino acids. More frequent dialysis may be required if the blood urea nitrogen increases with the protein load. However, this is preferable to protein restriction and the risk of providing inadequate nutrition.

Impairment of fluid and electrolyte excretion often requires modification of the TPN formulation. Fluid administration can be minimized by using concentrated solutions of amino acids (10% to 15%), glucose (D70), and lipid infusions (20%). Potassium, phosphorus, and magnesium should be added to the TPN with caution, and blood levels should be monitored closely. The amount of acetate in the TPN often must be increased to compensate for the metabolic acidosis associated with renal failure. Water-soluble vitamins should be routinely supplemented, as losses occur during dialysis (67). Supplementation of fat-soluble vitamins is not required because of decreased excretion and the potential risk of vitamin A toxicity (87). Trace minerals should be supplemented if prolonged parenteral nutrition is anticipated.

Use of Intradialytic Parenteral Nutrition

Providing parenteral nutrition to selected hemodialysis patients during the dialytic procedure to compensate for amino acid losses into the dialysate and provide additional nutritional supplementation has become a fairly common practice. Intradialytic parenteral nutrition, or IDPN, has been evaluated in several studies to determine the long-term value of this procedure. Careful review of these studies reveals mixed results (4,9,57,88–90). Only a few studies have been able to demonstrate improvement in more than one nutritional parameter with long-term administration, and the improvement is usually minimal (4,88,89). There were small increments in body weight in one study (57) and an improvement in the plasma amino acid profile in another (88).

Although most of the studies do not demonstrate any particular benefit to the procedure in terms of altering morbidity or mortality in this patient population, there have been two retrospective analyses of the use of IDPN in uncontrolled patients that indicate that mortality is reduced (91,92). Because neither study was prospective or controlled, they are difficult to interpret. However, they do provide limited evidence that IDPN may benefit some hemodialysis patients.

TABLE 30.7. SUGGESTED GUIDELINES FOR TOTAL PARENTERAL NUTRITION IN DIALYSIS PATIENTS

Protein	1.2–1.5 g/kg body wt/d of 8.5% to 15% amino acid solution (essential and nonessential)
Calories	35–40 kcal/d
Electrolytes	
Sodium	Approximately 70 mEq/L
Potassium, phosphorus, and magnesium	Add only if blood levels fall
Acetate or bicarbonate	Adjust as needed for acidemia
Vitamins and trace minerals	Supplement water-soluble vitamins and trace minerals. No need to supplement fat-soluble vitamins

IDPN treatment provides minimal supplementation, in that approximately 70% of the infused amino acids are retained (48) and it is administered only three times per week. However, there may be benefit in preventing further nutritional losses from the hemodialysis procedure. Severely malnourished patients may not tolerate oral nutritional supplementation well. In addition, severely depressed serum albumin levels may be associated with decreased gastrointestinal absorption of nutrients. In patients with such very low serum albumin levels, IDPN would not provide sufficient nutrients; TPN is indicated in these patients. However, in patients with moderate malnutrition who are intolerant of further oral supplementation secondary to anorexia, a short course of IDPN may improve nutritional status enough to permit more physiologic oral supplementation.

A recent study demonstrated that a solution comprised of amino acids and 20% lipids resulted in improvement in anthropometry, serum albumin, prealbumin, anthropometry, and skin test reactivity (90). In addition, the authors noted significant improvement in food intake while the patient was administered IDPN. It is possible that the improvement in nutritional status in this study was primarily due to the increase in appetite that was associated with the provision of supplemental nutrition. It is unclear from this study whether oral supplementation would not have been as beneficial, as all the patients were able to consume food.

IDPN is carried out by infusing a solution of 500 mL of a 10% general amino acid solution combined with 500 mL of 50% dextrose. The solution is infused into the venous drip chamber evenly during the entire 4-hour hemodialysis procedure. For patients who are dialyzed for shorter periods of time with high-flux equipment, there may need to be some alteration of the dialysis schedule to permit adequate infusion of nutrients without provoking complications such as painful cramps in the arm containing the fistula due to the high osmolality of the infusate. Although this phenomenon is not well understood, it is a frequent complaint in patients receiving IDPN. It is possible that the high osmolality of the solution as it is rapidly infused results in rapid fluid shifts from muscle cell to interstitium, causing the cramps. Rapid infusion of glucose may also be associated with hypoglycemia when the infusion is suddenly terminated. This may be prevented by giving the patient a small meal at the termination of the dialysis procedure. However, this is not always practical in patients who are often nauseated or have anorexia at the termination of dialysis. A more long-term complication of IDPN with glucose is the possible development of abnormal liver function tests. This is the result of excessive glucose or fat calories causing fatty deposition in the liver (93).

The complications associated with glucose infusion may be eliminated by the use of lipids as the calorie source. Lipids instead of glucose may eliminate the problems associated with rapid or excessive glucose infusion, but lipid infusions should also be closely monitored. In patients with acute renal failure, there was intolerance to the rapid infusion of lipids over 4 hours, resulting in some degree of hypertriglyceridemia in each of 12 patients studied (94). This also may be a problem in patients with ESRD who have an equally great propensity for difficulty in metabolizing fat infusions. In the study by Cano et al. that used lipids, the authors do not report the post- or intradialytic

triglyceride levels (89). However, there did not seem to be any long-term consequences of lipid infusion in this study.

Because rapid lipid infusions may also result in abnormal liver function tests and compromised reticuloendothelial system function (94), there is also a concern that the already immunosuppressed patient with ESRD and malnutrition may have further compromise of the immune system with IDPN over a long period of time. There have been no studies to evaluate this potential problem in the patient with ESRD.

It is recommended that IDPN be reserved for the moderately to severely malnourished patient who cannot increase oral intake. The physician should be aware that IDPN is quite expensive, and, generally, stringent criteria are applied to obtain reimbursement. The charges are quite variable and can range as high as $350 per therapy session. Medicare reimbursement is not uniform, which often limits reimbursement to those patients with private insurance. In the study by Chertow et al. (91), which included a large U.S. database, approximately 7% of patients were treated with IDPN. This is substantially lower than the percentage of patients treated with maintenance hemodialysis with malnutrition, suggesting that only patients with severe malnutrition receive this form of therapy.

IDPN should be closely monitored in terms of glucose control, hepatic function, and if lipids are used, triglyceride levels. As soon as patients can tolerate an increase in oral intake, supplementation with a variety of commercially available oral preparations designed for patients with ESRD should be undertaken.

Growth Hormone

Growth hormone (GH) is a single-chain polypeptide secreted by the anterior pituitary gland. It is an anabolic hormone that stimulates protein synthesis, increases nitrogen balance, and plays a critical role in postnatal growth. GH antagonizes the glucose-lowering action of insulin and enhances lipolysis and the release of free fatty acids. Many of these effects are mediated through the synthesis and release of insulin-like growth factor I (IGF-1).

The recent development of recombinant human growth hormone (rhGH) provides the potential for using the hormone in clinical practice. Several clinical studies have examined the nutritional impact of rhGH (95–98). Manson et al. studied four normal volunteers in eight paired studies, during which the subjects received parenteral nutrition with energy intakes varying between 30% and 100% of required amounts (95). Growth hormone was administered during one period of 7 days and saline during the control period. Growth hormone resulted in positive nitrogen balance and increased protein synthesis. The authors concluded that growth hormone administration resulted in a hormonal environment that promoted nitrogen retention and protein synthesis.

Ziegler et al. administered rhGH for 1 week to 11 malnourished patients who received hypocaloric parenteral nutrition (60% of caloric requirements) (96). As compared with the control phase, growth hormone induced significant nitrogen retention and increased IGF-1 levels by three to four times. Jiang et al. subsequently used rhGH in postoperative patients in a randomized, placebo-controlled double-blind trial (97). Uptake of amino acids, as measured by flux studies across the forearm, was increased in those patients receiving rhGH. In addition, there was less nitrogen loss, and lean body mass and hand grip force was better preserved.

The preceding studies in patients with normal renal function demonstrate the potential for rhGH as a component of the nutritional support regimen. Studies examining the use of rhGH in renal failure are more limited. Mehls et al. found that rhGH promoted growth and increased food utilization efficiency in uremic rats (79). In children with chronic renal failure or ESRD, rhGH has also been shown to increase growth velocity (98,99). Ziegler et al. studied the effects of rhGH in five adult hemodialysis patients and found that rhGH caused a significant decrease in urea generation and protein catabolic rate (100). Similar results were seen in ten stable peritoneal dialysis patients treated with growth hormone for 7 days in a prospective cross-over design (101). Urea generation and PCR decreased, in addition to small decreases in serum phosphorus and potassium levels and a rise in serum glucose levels (102). Finally, recombinant IGF-1 was administered to six malnourished peritoneal dialysis patients for 20 days and was found to result in a sustained increase in nitrogen balance during the treatment period (103).

Although these results are encouraging, the studies are small and of short term. In view of the expense of this drug, longer-term studies using greater numbers of ESRD patients are required to identify the subset of patients who would benefit from such an intervention. Additional studies may also help clarify whether the use of rhGH in selected patients would affect various nutritional parameters and quality of life or result in an improvement in morbidity and mortality. It is important to point out that currently, rhGH is not indicated for the treatment of malnutrition.

Amino Acid Dialysate for the Malnourished CAPD Patient

The use of amino acid dialysate provides a unique method of nutritional supplementation for the peritoneal dialysis patient. Replacement of one or more exchanges per day with amino acid dialysate is attractive for several reasons. First of all, as a nutritional supplement it could offset the protein and amino acid losses that occur into the dialysate. Second, the potential complications of the dialysate glucose load, such as hyperlipidemia, weight gain, and glucose intolerance, could be ameliorated.

A number of studies have examined the use of amino acid dialysate in peritoneal dialysis patients (104–114). Approximately 75% to 90% of the infused amino acids are absorbed, with peak serum levels occurring 30 to 60 minutes after infusion (104,105). Ultrafiltration has generally been shown to be within the range of that achieved with glucose-containing solutions. Most studies have used solutions containing a mixture of essential and nonessential amino acids with an electrolyte composition similar to that of the standard glucose-containing solutions. In most cases, one exchange per day is replaced with the amino acid solution.

The impact of amino acid dialysate on nutritional status, glucose metabolism, and hyperlipidemia has been variable. In the nondiabetic fasting patient, glucose levels remain stable during the dwell period with the amino acid dialysate as compared with a rise in blood glucose with the glucose-containing dialysate. Interestingly, insulin levels increase to similar levels with both types of dialysate, presumably due to the stimulation of insulin release by the absorbed amino acids (113). Effects on nutritional status and the lipid profile have been conflicting. Most studies suffer from relatively small patient numbers and short durations of observation. Although one study showed an improvement in low-density lipid (LDL) cholesterol levels over a 12-week period (109), most have failed to show significant changes, and one study even found an unfavorable fall in high-density lipid (HDL) cholesterol levels (108).

The effects on nutritional status have also been variable. In one recent study, nitrogen balance studies were conducted in the hospital in 19 malnourished peritoneal dialysis patients (114). After a baseline period of 15 days, the patients began on one or two dialysate exchanges per day containing amino acids for a 20-day period. Nitrogen balance became significantly positive as compared with baseline during treatment with the amino acid dialysate. In addition, the fasting amino acid profile became more normal and total protein and transferrin levels increased. Overall, the patients tolerated the amino acid dialysate well, although some patients developed a mild metabolic acidosis (mean pH, 7.35). This study confirmed earlier studies documenting an improvement in the amino acid profile of the blood toward normal with a rise in essential amino acids during treatment with amino acid dialysate.

Some, but not all, studies have shown improvement in other nutritional parameters, such as anthropometric measurements, serum albumin levels, and nitrogen balance. Side effects have occurred primarily with the higher concentrations of amino acids and include a rise in BUN, anorexia, nausea, and vomiting. In addition, it is not uncommon for a slight fall in serum bicarbonate and pH to occur.

In summary, the use of amino acid dialysate appears to be a promising nutritional intervention for malnourished peritoneal dialysis patients. At this time it is still quite expensive and is not consistently reimbursed. The cost is approximately $150 per bag of dialysis solution when amino acids are added to currently available peritoneal dialysis solutions. This therapy is often reserved for malnourished patients who fail a trial of oral supplements. Further study is needed to identify the patient subset that will benefit from this intervention and to further refine the amino acid composition.

Other Nutritional Interventions

The use of appetite stimulants may be appropriate for patients with anorexia. Appetite stimulants have been shown to improve serum albumin in a small study in patients treated with either hemodialysis or CAPD; however, the experience was limited (114).

Anabolic steroids may also be used to enhance some aspects of nutritional status. Nandrolone decanoate, 100 mg IM, weekly for 6 months versus placebo was reported to improve lean body mass and to increase both serum creatinine and exercise capacity in one study of maintenance dialysis patients.

However, other measures of nutritional status were not improved (115).

Because delayed gastric emptying may be one of the causes of malnutrition, use of agents to increase gastric emptying has been studied. In those patients with persistent hypoalbuminemia despite a prescribed increase in dietary intake and who also demonstrated delay in gastric emptying, serum albumin improved (116).

It is important to point out that all drugs have side effects and not all the drugs mentioned are approved for use in the applications reported. However, because of the serious consequences of malnutrition, it is appropriate to consider the risks and benefits of newer interventions in individual patients who suffer from malnutrition.

REFERENCES

1. Thunberg BJ, et al. Cross-sectional and longitudinal nutritional measurements in maintenance hemodialysis patients. *Am J Clin Nutr* 1981;34:2005–2012.
2. Wolfson M, et al. Nutritional status and lymphocyte function in maintenance hemodialysis patients. *Am J Clin Nutr* 1984;39:547–555.
3. Schoenfeld PY, et al. Assessment of nutritional status of the National Cooperative Dialysis Study population. *Kidney Int* 1983;23(Suppl 13):80–88.
4. Bilbrey GL, et al. Identification and treatment of protein calorie malnutrition in chronic hemodialysis patients. *Dial Transplant* 1989;18:669–700.
5. Marckmann P. Nutritional status of patients on hemodialysis and peritoneal dialysis. *Clin Nephrol* 1988;29:75–78.
6. Buchwald R, et al. Evaluation of nutritional status in patients on continuous ambulatory peritoneal dialysis (CAPD). *Perit Dial Int* 1989;9:295–301.
7. Young GA, et al. Nutritional assessment of continuous ambulatory peritoneal dialysis patients: an international study. *Am J Kidney Dis* 1991;17:462–471.
8. Cianciaruso B, et al. Cross-sectional comparison of malnutrition in continuous ambulatory peritoneal dialysis and hemodialysis patients. *Am J Kidney Dis* 1995;26:475–486.
9. Acchiardo SR, et al. Malnutrition as the main factor in morbidity and mortality of hemodialysis patients. *Kidney Int* 1983;24(Suppl 16):199–203.
10. Lowrie EG, et al. Death risk in hemodialysis patients: the predictive value of commonly measured variables and an evaluation of death rate differences between facilities. *Am J Kidney Dis* 1990;15:458–482.
11. Kopple JD. Effect of nutrition on morbidity and mortality in maintenance dialysis patients. *Am J Kidney Dis* 1994;24:1002–1009.
12. Avram MM, et al. Predictors of survival in continuous ambulatory peritoneal dialysis patients: the importance of prealbumin and other nutritional and metabolic markers. *Am J Kidney Dis* 1994;23:91–98.
13. Spiegel DM, et al. Serum albumin: a predictor of long-term outcome in peritoneal dialysis patients. *Am J Kidney Dis* 1994;23:283–285.
14. Iseki K, et al. Impact of the initial levels of laboratory variables on survival in chronic dialysis patients. *Am J Kidney Dis* 1996;28:541–548.
15. Churchill DN, et al. Adequacy of dialysis and nutrition in continuous peritoneal dialysis: association with clinical outcomes. *J Am Soc Nephrol* 1996;7:198–207.
16. Bistrian BR. Interaction between nutrition and inflammation in end-stage renal disease. *Blood Purif* 2000;18:333–336.
17. Kaysen GA. Inflammation nutritional state and outcome in end-stage renal disease. *Miner Electrolyte Metab* 1999;25:242–250.
18. Ikizler TA, et al. Nitrogen balance in hospitalized chronic hemodialysis patients. *Kidney Int* 1996;50(Suppl 57):S53–S56.
19. Lindsay RM, et al. A hypothesis: the protein catabolic rate is dependent upon the type and amount of treatment in dialyzed uremic patients. *Am J Kidney Dis* 1989;13:382–389.
20. Lindsay RM, et al. Which comes first, *KtV* or PCR—chicken or egg? *Kidney Int* 1992;42(Suppl 38):S32–S36.
21. Lynn RI, et al. The effect of *KtV*urea on nitrogen appearance and appetite in peritoneal dialysis. *Perit Dial Int* 1995;15(Suppl):S50–S52.
22. McCusker FX, et al. How much peritoneal dialysis is required for the maintenance of a good nutritional state? *Kidney Int* 1996;50(Suppl 56):S56–S61.
23. Harty J, et al. The influence of small solute clearance on dietary protein intake in continuous ambulatory peritoneal dialysis patients: a methodologic analysis based on cross-sectional and prospective studies. *Am J Kidney Dis* 1996;28:553–560.
24. Stein S, et al. The correlation between *KtV* and protein catabolic rate—a self-fulfilling prophecy. *Nephrol Dial Transplant* 1994;9:743–745.
25. Harty J, et al. Dialysis adequacy and nutritional status in continuous ambulatory peritoneal dialysis: is there a link? *Semin Dial* 1995;8:62–67.
26. Jones MR. Etiology of severe malnutrition: results of an international cross-sectional study in continuous ambulatory peritoneal dialysis patients. *Am J Kidney Dis* 1994;23:412–420.
27. Anderstam B, et al. Middle-sized molecule fractions isolated from uremic ultrafiltrate and normal urine inhibit ingestive behavior in the rat. *J Am Soc Nephrol* 1996;7:2453–2460.
28. Galland R, et al. Short daily hemodialysis rapidly improves nutritional status in hemodialysis patients. *Kidney Int* 2001;60:1555–1560.
29. Kopple JD, et al. Amino acid and protein metabolism in renal failure. *Am J Clin Nutr* 1978;31:1532–1540.
30. Feinstein EI, et al. Severe wasting and malnutrition in a patient undergoing maintenance dialysis. *Am J Nephrol* 1985;5:398–405.
31. DeFronzo RA, et al. Glucose intolerance in uremia: site and mechanism. *Am J Clin Nutr* 1980;33:1438–1445.
32. Phillips LS, et al. Somatomedin inhibitor in uremia. *J Clin Endocrinol Metab* 1984;59:764–772.
33. Garber AJ. Effects of parathyroid hormone in skeletal muscle protein and amino acid metabolism in the rat. *J Clin Invest* 1983;71:1806–1821.
34. May RC, et al. Mechanisms for defects in muscle protein metabolism in rats with chronic uremia. *J Clin Invest* 1987;79:1099–1103.
35. Papdoyannakis NJ, et al. The effect of the correction of metabolic acidosis on nitrogen and potassium balance of patients with chronic renal failure. *Am J Clin Nutr* 1984;40:623–627.
36. Graham KA, et al. Correction of acidosis in hemodialysis decreases whole body protein degradation. *J Am Soc Nephrol* 1997;8:632–637.
37. Graham KA, et al. Correction of acidosis in CAPD decreases whole body protein degradation. *Kidney Int* 1996;49:1396–1400.
38. Mitch WE. Metabolic acidosis stimulates protein metabolism in uremia. *Miner Electrolyte Metab* 1996;22:62–65.
39. Challa A, et al. Effect of metabolic acidosis on the expression of insulin-like growth factor and growth hormone receptor. *Kidney Int* 1993;44:1224–1227.
40. Brüngger M, et al. Effect of chronic metabolic acidosis on the growth hormone/IGF-1 endocrine axis: new cause of growth hormone insensitivity in humans. *Kidney Int* 1997;51:216–221.
41. Stein A, et al. Role of an improvement in acid–base status and nutrition in CAPD patients. *Kidney Int* 1997;52:1089–1095.
42. Williams AJ, et al. High bicarbonate dialysate in hemodialysis patients: effects on acidosis and nutritional status. *Nephrol Dial Transplant* 1997;12:2633–2637.
43. Blumenkrantz MJ, et al. Protein losses during peritoneal dialysis. *Kidney Int* 1981;19:593–602.
44. Borah MF, et al. Nitrogen balance during intermittent dialysis therapy of uremia. *Kidney Int* 1978;14:491–500.
45. Lim VS, et al. The effect of interdialytic interval on protein metabolism: evidence suggesting dialysis-induced catabolism. *Am J Kidney Dis* 1989;14:96–100.
46. Kopple JD, et al. The free and bound amino acids removed by hemodialysis. *Trans Am Soc Artif Organs* 1973;19:309–313.

47. Wolfson M, et al. Amino acid losses during hemodialysis with infusion of amino acids and glucose. *Kidney Int* 1982;21:500–506.
48. Ikizler TA, et al. Amino acid and albumin losses during hemodialysis. *Kidney Int* 1994;46:830–837.
49. Kaplan AA, et al. Dialysate protein losses with bleach processed polysulphone dialyzers. *Kidney Int* 1995;47:573–578.
50. Gutierrez A, et al. Effect of in vivo contact between blood and dialysis membranes on protein catabolism in humans. *Kidney Int* 1990;38:487–494.
51. Gutierrez A, et al. Hemodialysis-associated protein catabolism with and without glucose in the dialysis fluid. *Kidney Int* 1994;46:814–822.
52. Löfberg E, et al. Ribosome and free amino acid content in muscle during hemodialysis. *Kidney Int* 1991;39:984–989.
53. Wolf G, et al. Leptin and renal disease. *Am J Kidney Dis* 2002;39:1–11.
54. Stenvinkel P, et al. Elevated serum levels of soluble adhesion molecules predict death in pre-dialysis patients: association with malnutrition, inflammation, and cardiovascular disease. *Nephrol Dial Transplant* 2000;15:1624–1630.
55. Blumenkrantz MJ, et al. Methods for assessing nutritional status of patients with renal failure. *Am J Clin Nutr* 1980;33:1567–1585.
56. Guarnieri G, et al. Simple methods for nutritional assessment in hemodialyzed patients. *Am J Clin Nutr* 1980;33:1598–1607.
57. Nelson EE, et al. Anthropometric norms for the dialysis population. *Am J Kidney Dis* 1990;16:32–37.
58. Segal KR. Estimation of extracellular and total body water by multiple-frequency bioelectrical-impedance measurement. *Am J Clin Nutr* 1991;54:26–29.
59. Stall SH. Comparison of five body composition methods in peritoneal dialysis patients. *Am J Clin Nutr* 1996;64:125–130.
60. Young GA, et al. The effects of calorie and essential amino acid supplementation on plasma proteins in patients with chronic renal failure. *Am J Clin Nutr* 1978;31:1802–1807.
61. Kaysen GA, et al. Mechanisms of hypoalbuminemia in hemodialysis patients. *Kidney Int* 1995;48:510–516.
62. Kaysen GA, et al. Determinants of albumin concentration in hemodialysis patients. *Am J Kidney Dis* 1997;29:658–668.
63. Bergström J, et al. Plasma and muscle free amino acids in maintenance hemodialysis patients without protein malnutrition. *Kidney Int* 1990;38:108–114.
64. Kluthe R, et al. Protein requirement in maintenance hemodialysis. *Am J Clin Nutr* 1978;31:1812–1820.
65. Slomowitz LA, et al. Effect of energy intake on nutritional status in maintenance hemodialysis patients. *Kidney Int* 1989;35:704–711.
66. Wolfson M. Use of water-soluble vitamins in patients with chronic renal failure. *Semin Dial* 1988;1:28–32.
67. Kaysen GA, et al. Albumin homeostasis in patients undergoing continuous ambulatory peritoneal dialysis. *Kidney Int* 1984;25:107–114.
68. Dulaney JT, et al. Peritoneal dialysis and loss of proteins: a review. *Kidney Int* 1984;26:253–262.
69. Lindholm B, et al. Protein and amino acid metabolism in patients undergoing continuous ambulatory peritoneal dialysis (CAPD). *Clin Nephrol* 1988;30(Suppl 1):59–63.
70. Burkart J. Effect of peritoneal dialysis prescription and peritoneal membrane transport characteristics on nutritional status. *Perit Dial Int* 1995;15(Suppl):S20–S35.
71. Grodstein GP, et al. Glucose absorption during continuous ambulatory peritoneal dialysis. *Kidney Int* 1981;19:564–567.
72. Baeyer H, et al. Adaptation of CAPD patients to the continuous peritoneal energy uptake. *Kidney Int* 1983;23:29–34.
73. Bouma SF, et al. Glucose absorption and weight change in 18 months of continuous ambulatory peritoneal dialysis. *J Am Diet Assoc* 1984;84:194–197.
74. Lindholm B, et al. Serum lipids and lipoproteins during continuous ambulatory peritoneal dialysis. *Acta Med Scand* 1986;220:143–151.
75. Lameire N, et al. Effects of long-term CAPD on carbohydrate and lipid metabolism. *Clin Nephrol* 1988;30(Suppl 1):53–58.
76. Blumenkrantz MJ, et al. Metabolic balance studies and dietary protein requirements in patients undergoing continuous ambulatory peritoneal dialysis. *Kidney Int* 1982;21:849–861.
77. Kopple JD, et al. Nutritional requirements for patients undergoing continuous ambulatory peritoneal dialysis. *Kidney Int* 1983;24(Suppl 16):295–302.
78. McCann LM, et al. Nutritional recommendations for patients undergoing continuous peritoneal dialysis. *Semin Dial* 1992;5:136–141.
79. Mehls O, et al. Improvement of growth and food utilization by human recombinant growth hormone in uremia. *Kidney Int* 1988;33:45–52.
80. Fedje L, et al. A role for oral nutrition supplements in the malnutrition of renal disease. *J Renal Nutr* 1996;6:198–202.
81. Hecking E, et al. Treatment with essential amino acids in patients on chronic hemodialysis: a double blind cross-over study. *Am J Clin Nutr* 1978;31:1821–1826.
82. Tepper T, et al. Loss of amino acids during hemodialysis: effect of oral essential amino acid supplementation. *Nephron* 1981;29:25–29.
83. Tietze IN, et al. Effect of fish protein supplementation on amino acid profile and nutritional status in haemodialysis patients. *Nephrol Dial Transplant* 1991;6:948–954.
84. Mirtallo JM, et al. Nutritional support of patients with renal disease. *Clin Pharm* 1984;3:253–263.
85. Feinstein EI. Parenteral nutrition in acute renal failure. *Am J Nephrol* 1985;5:145–149.
86. Muth I. Implications of hypervitaminosis A in chronic renal failure. *J Ren Nutr* 1991;1:2–8.
87. Heidlund A, et al. Long-term effects of essential amino acids supplementation in patients on regular hemodialysis treatment. *Clin Nephrol* 1975;3:235–239.
88. Piraino AJ, et al. Prolonged hyperalimentation in catabolic chronic dialysis therapy patients. *J Parenter Enteral Nutr* 1981;5:466–477.
89. Cano N, et al. Peridialytic parenteral nutrition with lipids and amino acids in malnourished hemodialysis patients. *Am J Clin Nutr* 1990;52:726–730.
90. Cappelli JP, et al. Effect of intradialytic parenteral nutrition on mortality rates in end-stage renal disease care. *Am J Kidney Dis* 1994;23:808–816.
91. Chertow GM, et al. The association of intradialytic parenteral nutrition administration with survival in hemodialysis patients. *Am J Kidney Dis* 1994;24:912–920.
92. Leaseburge LA, et al. Liver test alterations with total parenteral nutrition and nutritional status. *J Parenter Enteral Nutr* 1992;16:348–352.
93. Druml W, et al. Lipid metabolism in acute renal failure. *Kidney Int* 1983;(Suppl 16):139–142.
94. Jensen GL, et al. Parenteral infusion of large and medium chain triglycerides and reticuloendothelial system function in man. *J Parenter Enteral Nutr* 1990;14:467–471.
95. Manson JM, et al. Growth hormone stimulates protein synthesis during hypocaloric parenteral nutrition. *Ann Surg* 1988;208:136–142.
96. Ziegler TR, et al. Metabolic effects of recombinant human growth hormone in patients receiving parenteral nutrition. *Ann Surg* 1988;208:6–16.
97. Jiang ZM, et al. Low-dose growth hormone and hypocaloric nutrition attenuate the protein-catabolic response after major operation. *Ann Surg* 1989;210:513–525.
98. Koch VH, et al. Accelerated growth after recombinant human growth hormone treatment of children with chronic renal failure. *J Pediatr* 1989;115:365–371.
99. Tönshoff B, et al. Improvement of uremic growth failure by recombinant human growth hormone. *Kidney Int* 1989;36(Suppl 27):201–204.
100. Ziegler TR, et al. Growth hormone administration decreases urea generation in patients undergoing chronic hemodialysis. *Clin Res* 1990;38:355A.
101. Ikizler TA, et al. Short-term effects of recombinant human growth hormone in CAPD patients. *Kidney Int* 1994;46:1178–1183.
102. Shamir E, et al. Effect of insulin-like growth factor-1 (IGF-1) on nitrogen balance in malnourished CAPD patients. *J Am Soc Nephrol* 1995;6:587(abstr).
103. Gjessing J. Addition of amino acids to peritoneal-dialysis fluid. *Lancet* 1968;2:812.
104. Williams PF, et al. Amino acid absorption following intraperitoneal administration in CAPD patients. *Perit Dial Bull* 1982;2:124–130.

105. Oren A, et al. Effective use of amino acid dialysate over four weeks in CAPD patients. *Perit Dial Bull* 1983;3:66–72.

106. Pedersen FB, et al. Alternate use of amino acid and glucose solutions in CAPD. *Perit Dial Bull* 1985;5:215–218.

107. Bruno M, et al. CAPD with an amino acid dialysis solution: a long-term, cross-over study. *Kidney Int* 1989;35:1189–1194.

108. Dibble JB, et al. Amino-acid-based continuous ambulatory peritoneal dialysis (CAPD) fluid over twelve weeks: effects on carbohydrate and lipid metabolism. *Perit Dial Int* 1990;10:71–77.

109. Arfeen S, et al. The nutritional/metabolic and hormonal effects of eight weeks of continuous ambulatory peritoneal dialysis with a 1% amino acid solution. *Clin Nephrol* 1990;4:192–199.

110. Honda M, et al. Effect of short-term essential amino acid-containing dialysate in young children on CAPD. *Perit Dial Int* 1991;11:76–80.

111. Dombros NV, et al. Six-month overnight intraperitoneal amino-acid infusion in continuous ambulatory peritoneal dialysis (CAPD) patients—no effect on nutritional status. *Perit Dial Int* 1990;10:79–84.

112. Hanning RM, et al. Effectiveness and nutritional consequences of amino acid-based vs. glucose-based dialysis solutions in infants and children receiving CAPD. *Am J Clin Nutr* 1987;46:22–30.

113. Kopple JD, et al. Treatment of malnourished CAPD patients with an amino acid based dialysate. *Kidney Int* 1995;47:1148–1157.

114. Lien YH. Low dose megestrol increases serum albumin in malnourished dialysis patients. *Int J Artif Organs* 1996;19:147–150.

115. Johansen KL, et al. Anabolic effects of nandrolone decanoate in patients receiving dialysis. *JAMA* 1999;281:1275–1281.

116. Silang R, et al. Prokinetic agents increase plasma albumin in hypoalbuminemic chronic dialysis patients with delayed gastric emptying. *Am J Kidney Dis* 2001;37:287–293.

31

DISORDERS OF HEMOSTASIS IN DIALYSIS PATIENTS

GIUSEPPE REMUZZI, MIRIAM GALBUSERA, AND PAOLA BOCCARDO

Bleeding in uremia is more easily controlled since the introduction of dialysis (1,2). Hemorrhagic complications varying from ecchymoses, epistaxis, and bleeding from gums and venipuncture sites have been observed in about one-third of uremic patients. However, low-grade gastrointestinal bleeding may be even more common. Subdural hematoma occurs only occasionally in 5% to 15% of hemodialysis patients, whereas hemopericardium and subcapsular hematoma of the liver are less frequent. The advent of modern dialysis techniques and the use of erythropoietin to correct anemia definitively reduced the incidence of severe hemorrhages, but bleeding diathesis still represents a problem for uremic patients, particularly during surgery or invasive procedures such as biopsies.

CAUSES OF UREMIC BLEEDING

The causes of uremic bleeding have been the subject of a major debate since the 1970s. The pathogenesis is multifactorial (Table 31.1) and the major defects involve primary hemostasis (Fig. 31.1), that is, platelet–vessel wall and platelet–platelet interactions. The skin bleeding time is the best predictor of clinical bleeding (3). It depends on the platelet number, vascular integrity, activity of von Willebrand factor (vWF), and hematocrit, and thus gives an excellent overall assessment of primary hemostasis.

Platelet Abnormalities

Moderate thrombocytopenia is found in a majority of uremic patients, suggesting inadequate production or platelet overconsumption (4,5). Thrombocytopenia severe enough to cause bleeding is very rare (6,7). Numerous biochemical changes in platelets have been reported. Dense granule content is decreased in uremic platelet (8,9), and a storage pool defect, with reduction in platelet ADP and serotonin, is present. Decreased subnormal platelet ATP release in response to stimulation with thrombin (8) indicates a defect in granule secretion, confirmed by studies showing an impairment in the release of the α-granule proteins and β-thromboglobulin in platelets from dialysis patients (10). Intraplatelet cyclic AMP is enhanced in uremic patients (11), and the regulation of adenylate cyclase may also be

abnormal (12), possibly contributing to defective platelet aggregation and adhesion to injured vessels.

Calcium content is increased in uremic platelets (13), which also mobilize calcium abnormally in response to stimulation (14). Elevation in platelet cAMP and abnormal calcium mobilization suggested a possible role of parathyroid hormone (PTH) in uremic platelet dysfunction, since PTH inhibits platelet aggregation in vitro (15,16). However, the bleeding time does not correlate with serum concentrations of intact PTH or PTH fragments (17), suggesting that elevated PTH in renal failure patients is not likely to play a major role in the uremic platelet defect.

Several abnormalities of the platelet–platelet interaction have also been reported. Defective platelet aggregation in vitro in response to various stimuli such as ADP, epinephrine, collagen, and thrombin is documented in a great number of studies, although the degree of impairment of platelet aggregation in uremia varies considerably. In several reports platelet aggregation was found to be normal or increased (reviewed in 18). In addition, defective platelet thromboxane A_2 (TxA_2) production, in response to endogenous and exogenous stimuli (19,20), is not correctable by thrombin (20). In a subpopulation of uremics, irreversible platelet aggregation does not occur in response to platelet-activating factor (PAF) (21,22). This abnormality is independent of plasma factor(s) but is probably due to the platelets' reduced capacity to form TxA_2 in response to PAF.

Data are available that suggest the bleeding tendency in uremia is associated with excessive formation of nitric oxide (NO) (23), an endogenous vasoactive molecule that also inhibits platelet function (24,25). This is supported by the observation that in rats made uremic by extensive surgical ablation of renal mass, bleeding time is increased, which is associated with plasmatic levels higher than normal of stable NO metabolites, nitrites, and nitrates (26). The ex vivo platelet adhesion increased and prolonged bleeding time returns completely to normal when uremic rats are given N-monomethyl-L-arginine, a competitive inhibitor of NO synthesis. As documented by the increased NO synthase activity and high expression of both inducible NO synthase (iNOS) and endothelial NO synthase (eNOS) in the aorta of uremic animals, excessive formation of NO at systemic levels derives from vessels (26). In patients with chronic renal failure defective platelet aggregation was associated

TABLE 31.1. CAUSES OF UREMIC BLEEDING

Platelet abnormalities
  Subnormal dense granule content
  Reduction in intracellular ADP and serotonin
  Impaired release of the platelet alpha-granule protein and
    beta-thromboglobulin
  Enhanced intracellular cAMP
  Abnormal mobilization of platelet Ca2+
  Abnormal platelet arachidonic acid metabolism
  Abnormal ex vivo platelet aggregation in response to different
    stimuli
  Defective cyclooxigenase activity
  Abnormality of the activation-dependent binding activity of
    GP IIb–IIIa
  Uremic toxins, especially parathyroid hormone
Abnormal platelet–vessel wall interactions
  Abnormal platelet adhesion
  Increased formation of vascular PGI$_2$
  Altered von Willebrand factor
Anemia
  Altered blood rheology
  Erythropoietin deficiency
Abnormal production of nitric oxide
Drug treatment
  Beta-lactam antibiotics
  Third-generation cephalosporins
  Nonsteroidal antiinflammatory drugs

with increased platelet NO synthesis (27). The same study also found significantly higher plasma levels of L-arginine, the substrate for NO synthesis, in uremic patients compared with healthy volunteers. Uremic plasma potently induced in vitro NO synthesis in cultured human umbilical vein endothelial cells

as well as in human microvascular endothelial cells, suggesting that substances are accumulating in uremic plasma that up-regulate the NO synthetic pathway. The stimulatory activity found in uremic plasma is attributed to cytokines such as tumor necrosis factor α (TNFα) and IL-1β that are potent inducers of iNOS and circulate in increased amounts in the blood of patients with chronic renal failure either undialyzed or on maintenance hemodialysis (28).

Two adhesive proteins, fibrinogen and vWF, and two adhesion receptors, glycoprotein (Gp) Ib and the Gp IIb–IIIa complex, play a vital role in the formation of platelet thrombi at sites of vascular injury (Fig. 31.2) (29). At high shear rates, such as those found in the capillary circulation, contact is dependent on the binding of vWF to the platelet GP Ib (30,31). In patients with chronic renal failure a decrease in the total content of platelet GP Ib has been documented (32,33) accompanied by an increase in glycocalicin, a soluble proteolytic fragment of GP Ib, and is probably due to proteolytic damage to membrane GP Ib. The normal surface expression of this receptor and the total decrease in content account for a redistribution from the intraplatelet pool to the surface pool (32,34). The activation-dependent receptor function of the Gp IIb–IIIa complex is defective in uremia, as shown by decreased binding of both vWF and fibrinogen to stimulated platelets (34). The number of Gp IIb–IIIa receptors expressed on the platelet membrane is normal, but their activation is impaired. Removal of substances present in uremic plasma markedly improved the Gp IIb–IIIa defect. Thus a reversible abnormality of the activation-dependent binding to Gp IIb–IIIa caused by dialyzable toxic substance(s) is probably a major component of the altered platelet function in uremia.

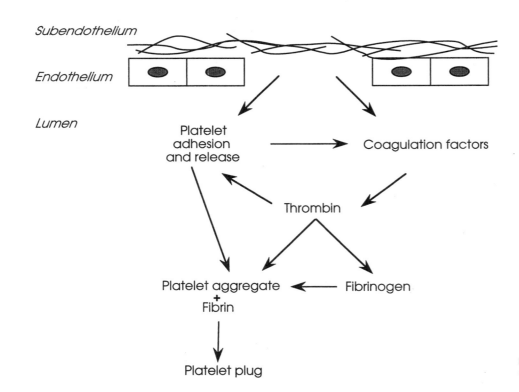

FIG. 31.1. Schematic representation of primary hemostasis.

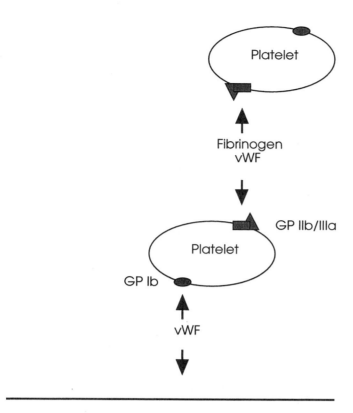

FIG. 31.2. Interaction of platelets with von Willebrand factor and fibrinogen.

The impaired Gp IIb–IIIa activation in uremia may explain the aggregation defect (35–37).

The evidence that several dialyzable "toxins"—including urea, creatinine, phenol, phenolic acids, or guanidinosuccinic acid (GSA)—may be involved in the genesis of the uremic platelet dysfunction (38–40) is not compelling. For example, an infusion of urea into healthy volunteers caused headache but did not influence bleeding time. Only a very high concentration was able to impair platelet aggregation and then only to a very limited extent. GSA, which accumulates in uremic plasma, inhibits the second wave of platelet aggregation to ADP when added to normal platelet-rich plasma (39). As recently demonstrated, GSA is involved in the generation of NO. GSA's effect of stimulating NO release provides a biological explanation for the data generated in the early 1970s showing that among uremic toxins, GSA was the only one that consistently inhibited platelet function to such a degree that it was defined as the "x" factor in the uremic bleeding (41,42). Phenolic acid, at the concentrations found in uremic plasma, also impairs kaolin-activated platelet factor 3 release and primary aggregation to ADP (38). All these observations suggest that reducing blood levels of these compounds may partially correct the abnormal hemostasis of patients with renal failure. However, no correlation has been found between bleeding time or platelet adhesion and the serum level of the dialyzable metabolites that mainly accumulate in uremia (40).

Abnormal Platelet–Vessel Wall Interaction

Platelet adherence to foreign surfaces is significantly impaired in nonthrombocytopenic patients with uremia (6,40,43), but this does not fully explain the prolonged bleeding time (40,44). Other studies of platelet adhesion using a perfusion chamber system have demonstrated a defect in the deposition of uremic platelet on the subendothelium (35,37). Formation of vascular prostacyclin (PGI_2), a potent vasodilator and inhibitor of platelet function, is increased in both uremic patients (45,46) and rats with experimental uremia (47,48). Plasma of uremic patients contains higher than normal amounts of a factor that stimulates vascular production of PGI_2 (49). This could be PTH, in view of findings that PTH increases urinary excretion of the PGI_2 metabolite, 6-keto PGF_1 (50).

Plasma levels of vWF are normal or elevated in renal failure (51), and qualitative abnormalities of vWF have not been uniformly observed (33,36,52,53). That a functional defect in the vWF–platelet interaction may play a role in the abnormal hemostasis of uremic patients rests on the findings that cryoprecipitate, a plasma derivative rich in factor VIII and vWF, and desmopressin, a synthetic derivative of antidiuretic hormone that releases autologous vWF from storage sites, both shortened the bleeding time of these patients.

Role of Anemia in Uremic Bleeding Tendency

Platelet adhesion and aggregation in flowing systems (54,55) are markedly potentiated by red blood cells. Erythrocytes enhance platelet function by releasing ADP (56), by inactivating PGI_2 (57), and by increasing platelet–vessel wall contact by displacing platelets away from the axial flow and toward the vessel wall (54).

The independent role of anemia in the bleeding tendency of uremia has been extensively investigated. A significant negative correlation was found between bleeding time and packed cell volume (PCV) (58). Despite a shorter bleeding time, a significant negative correlation between hematocrit and bleeding time was still demonstrable in 15 nonuremic anemic patients. These results were subsequently confirmed by other studies (59,60) that found that anemia was the main determinant of the prolonged bleeding time in uremic patients. Uremic bleeding time has been shortened and symptomatic hemostatic improvement achieved by treatment with recombinant human erythropoietin (rhEPO) (61,62). In one randomized study (63), the bleeding time became normal in all patients receiving erythropoietin as hematocrits increased to 27% to 32%. The role of erythropoietin deficiency as the primary underlying defect in anemia in renal failure was supported by data showing that partial correction of anemia by rhEPO was sufficient to correct defective primary hemostasis in uremia. There is good evidence that substances present in uremic serum, including polyamines, parathyroid hormone, and various cytokines, can inhibit erythropoiesis (64).

Role of Drugs in Uremic Bleeding

Uremic patients may be at an increased risk of bleeding complications caused by drug treatment. The risk of bleeding associated with the accumulation of β-lactam antibiotics in uremia has been highlighted (65). β-Lactam antibiotics apparently act by perturbing platelet membrane function and by interfering with ADP receptors (66,67). The prolonged bleeding time and the abnormal platelet aggregation are related to the dose and duration of treatment, and are promptly reversible after discontinuation. Third-generation cephalosporins may also inhibit platelet function and may lead to marked disturbance of blood coagulation (68,69).

Another risk of bleeding in uremic patients is associated with aspirin given to prevent vascular access thrombosis (70) or platelet activation on dialysis membranes (71). The beneficial effect of aspirin on vascular access thrombosis can be achieved with a moderate dose of aspirin (160 mg/d) that inhibits platelet thromboxane A_2 generation without affecting vascular PGI_2 formation (70). However, a moderate dose of ASA may prolong the bleeding time to a greater extent in uremic patients than in control subjects (72,73). This difference appears not to be related to the increased susceptibility of cyclooxygenase in uremic platelets. Furthermore, a temporal dissociation has been found in uremic patients between the prolongation of bleeding time and inhibition of serum thromboxane B_2 generation after aspirin. Indeed, aspirin seems to have two distinct inhibitory effects on platelet function in uremia: a transient effect that interferes with one of the determinants of bleeding time, and a lasting effect due to the irreversible blocking of platelet cyclooxygenase (73). However, the prolongation of bleeding time caused by aspirin may explain the frequency of gastrointestinal bleeding in uremic patients (74,75). Thus the use of aspirin for uremic patients treated with rhEPO to prevent thrombotic complications associated with an increasing hematocrit is highly questionable.

Nonsteroidal antiinflammatory drugs such as indomethacin, ibuprofen, naproxen, phenylbutazone, and sulfinpyrazone also inhibit platelet cyclooxygenase and disturb platelet function. However, in contrast to aspirin, the inhibitory effect of these compounds on platelet cyclooxygenase is readily reversible as the blood concentration of the drugs falls upon cessation of administration (76).

CONSEQUENCES OF THE BLEEDING TENDENCY IN UREMIA

The most common bleeding complications in uremia are petechial hemorrhages, blood blisters, and ecchymoses at the site of fistula access puncture or temporary venous access insertion. More serious bleeding problems are discussed later.

Gastrointestinal Bleeding

Before the advent of hemodialysis, gastrointestinal involvement was a common complication of uremia. Despite the universal application of hemodialysis, gastrointestinal bleeding is a common clinical problem requiring more than 300,000 hospitalizations annually in the United States, and upper gastrointestinal hemorrhage is the second leading cause of death in acute renal failure. Heparinization may play a role in this regard because mucosal lesions are more likely to bleed with the interruption of the normal clotting cascade. The most common causes of gastrointestinal bleeding are peptic ulcers (gastric or duodenal), hemorrhagic esophagitis, gastritis, duodenitis, and gastric telangiectasias (77–79). Angiodysplasia with gastrointestinal bleeding has been observed in the stomach, duodenum, jejunum, and colon (74,80). This abnormality, affecting the microcirculation of the gastrointestinal mucosa and submucosa, occurs more often in hemodialysis patients (81). Finally, dialysis patients suffering from HIV nephropathy may have specific lesions, such as Kaposi's sarcoma, cytomegalovirus colitis, and non-Hodgkin's lymphoma, that contribute to gastrointestinal bleeding (82).

Hemorrhagic Pericarditis

Pericarditis may develop in association with uremia (83,84) and may become hemorrhagic in the setting of defective hemostasis, creating the potential for cardiac tamponade. Pericarditis was frequent in the early days of hemodialysis but is now rare. The clinical features of this condition include normal cardiac shadow and increased jugular venous distention, with hypotension, shortness of breath, and a pericardial friction rub. Deaths caused by hemorrhagic pericarditis have been reported to be as high as 3% to 5% among dialysis patients (85,86).

Intracranial Hemorrhage

Subdural hematoma has been reported to occur in 5% to 15% of hemodialysis patients (87). It usually overlies the frontal or parietal lobe and is bilateral in approximately 15% of cases. Headache, vomiting, seizures, hypertension, drowsiness, confusion, and coma are usual symptoms. Head trauma, hypertension, and systemic anticoagulation are risk factors (87).

Prognosis is at least partly related to the stage of diagnosis, and the mortality rate may be as high as 90% in patients requiring emergency surgery.

Hemorrhagic Pleural Effusion and Retroperitoneal Bleeding

The development of pleural effusions in uremic patients is a relatively common occurrence. Anticoagulation treatment during dialysis may be a major risk factor in causing bleeding in patients with fibrinous pleuritis (88,89).

Spontaneous retroperitoneal bleeding is a rare complication in patients having chronic hemodialysis (90,91). Trauma, anticoagulation, and the presence of polycystic kidneys are predisposing factors. The symptoms and signs include sudden onset of pain in the abdomen, flank, back, or hip, with an associated drop in blood pressure. The hematocrit drops in the absence of any obvious blood loss. Computed tomography is useful in the diagnosis of retroperitoneal bleeding.

Subcapsular Liver Hematoma and Ocular Hemorrhage

Spontaneous subcapsular hematoma of the liver is a recognized complication in uremia (92). Typically, patients have right upper quadrant pain, fever, and sometimes elevated bilirubin and alkaline phosphatase accompanied by a falling hematocrit.

Intraocular hemorrhage can also occur in uremia, and spontaneous hyphema has been reported during dialysis (93). There is no visual loss and the hemorrhage generally resolves without any therapy. Intraocular bleeding with only temporary visual loss has been reported in a large percentage of transplant and dialysis patients after cataract surgery.

THERAPEUTIC STRATEGIES

The approach to uremic bleeding must be considered in two contexts: the prevention of bleeding in patients at high risk because of invasive procedures or surgery, and the treatment of patients with active bleeding. The strategy depends on the urgency of the situation, the severity of uremia, and the previous therapy employed.

Dialysis

Dialysis improves platelet functional abnormalities and reduces, but does not eliminate, the risk of hemorrhage (94). In addition, hemodialysis per se can contribute to platelet dysfunction and bleeding tendency through the platelet adhesion and activation induced by blood and artificial surface interactions and the systemic anticoagulation arising from heparin use. The risk of bleeding may be minimized by using peritoneal dialysis or alternative means to routine heparinization to prevent clotting in the extracorporeal circulation during hemodialysis.

Alternative strategies, developed specifically to anticoagulate patients at high risk of bleeding, include regional anticoagulation with heparin and protamine, low-dose heparin, hemodialysis without anticoagulation, regional anticoagulation with citrate, and the use of low-molecular-weight heparin (LMWH).

The earliest approach was regional heparinization (95–97). Heparin is given by constant infusion into the inlet line of the dialyzer. Simultaneously, protamine sulfate is infused into the outlet port before the blood returns to the patient. However, a rebound systemic anticoagulation has been reported several hours after the completion of dialysis, possibly because of dissociation of the heparin–protamine complex (98). This technique has been abandoned because of the above-mentioned complication together with technical complexity, and now low-dose heparin or heparin-free dialysis is used as an alternative. The rationale of low-dose heparinization is to obtain a balance between clotting in the dialyzer circuit and bleeding in patients with high risk of bleeding.

Patients at high risk of bleeding can also use a membrane such as an ethylene-vinyl alcohol copolymer hollow-fiber dialysis membrane, which does not require systemic anticoagulation with heparin, provided that blood flow is maintained at greater than 200 mL/min (99). Double access must be available, with separate needles for arterial and venous return, and blood products must be administered into a different intravenous line.

Multiple strategies have been described for citrate anticoagulation. In the first methods reported, anticoagulation was achieved by infusion of trisodium citrate into the blood line before, and infusion of calcium into the blood line after the dialysis, in combination with a calcium-free dialysate. These methods were relatively complex, and simpler approaches have been described. Comparative trials showed that this procedure may be safe and more effective than others in hemodialysis patients with an active or recently active bleeding focus (100–102). Serious and documented complications of citrate anticoagulation involved citrate intoxication, hyperaluminemia, hyperammonemia, hypernatremia, and profound metabolic alkalosis (103,104).

LMWH binds with antithrombin to enhance inhibition of factor Xa but does not contain the second binding sequence necessary for inhibiting thrombin activity. There are few long-term studies comparing the use of LMWH over unfractionated heparin in routine hemodialysis (105,106). Because only minor differences were detected, it remains unclear whether LMWH offers any advantage over anticoagulation with unfractionated heparin.

Different heparin-free hemodialysis protocols have been developed for patients at high risk of bleeding complications (107–109). Usually, these strategies employ flushes of 100 to 200 mL of saline every 15 to 60 min through the dialyzer (107,108,110). At the start of treatment some protocols use dialyzer primed with heparinized saline. This procedure, independent of the use of saline flushes or not, may be more successful when blood flow rate is maintained above 250 mL/min. The success of heparin-free dialysis, like that of low-dose heparin regimens, is compromised by poor dialysis technique. In addition, this procedure is associated with biochemical activation of the clotting system (107,110–112).

Dermatan sulfate has also been proposed as an anticoagulant agent during hemodialysis, because it causes less bleeding than heparin in animal models (113,114). The lower hemorrhagic property may be due to its reduced effect on platelets (115) and may also be attributed to a moderate prolongation of activated partial thromboplastin time (APTT) (116–118). Short-term clinical studies have been conducted in hemodialysis for chronic renal failure that tested fixed intravenous doses of dermatan sulfate against individualized heparin regimens (114,116). Dermatan sulfate suppressed both visible clot formation in the dialysis circuit and the generation of plasma markers of coagulation and platelet activation during the procedure (116–118). These effects were related to dermatan sulfate doses and plasma concentrations, which followed linear pharmacokinetics (114, 116–118). A comparative short-term clinical study was performed with 10 hemodialysis patients showing that dermatan sulfate dose can be individually titrated to suppress clot formation during hemodialysis as efficiently as does individualized heparin (119), but long-term comparative trials are warranted.

In the search for real alternatives to heparin, antiplatelet drugs such as sulfinpyrazone, adenosine, and PGE_1 have been used for regional infusion during extracorporeal circulation

(120,121), but they appear to have no advantage over heparin. Aspirin and dipyridamole analogs reduce fibrin and cellular deposition on the filter membrane but increase the risk of gastrointestinal bleeding (71,122).

PGI$_2$ showed some promise as a heparin alternative (123–125). However, such adverse reactions as headache, flushing, tachycardia, and chest and abdominal pain require careful hemodynamic monitoring and a physician's supervision (126–128). Thus the use of PGI$_2$ should be limited to patients at high risk of hemorrhage.

Correction of Anemia

Uremic patients are often severely anemic, and the severity of anemia appears to be related to the extent of the prolongation of bleeding time (59–61). Chronic renal failure patients with prolonged bleeding time consistently benefited from red cell transfusions. The beneficial effect was independent of changes in platelet function tests or in the level of vWF-related properties (59,60).

The cloning of the human erythropoietin gene (128,129) has provided recombinant human erythropoietin for clinical use. This treatment reverses the anemia of uremics, eliminating their dependency on transfusions (61,130–132). The progressive increase in hematocrit is accompanied by a significant decrease in the bleeding time (62,63,132). Although improvement in platelet adhesion to subendothelium was observed in some studies, no consistent changes in platelet number, platelet aggregability, markers of platelet activation in plasma, platelet TxA$_2$ formation, platelet adenine nucleotide content, global coagulation test results, antithrombin III, or cross-linked fibrin derivatives were reported (62,132,133).

Renal anemia is rapidly corrected by rhEPO therapy, but the dose required can vary greatly (see Chapter 32 for a full discussion). Current recommendations are to start with 50 to 100 IU/kg three times per week. With an intravenous dosage of 50 IU/kg three times per week, the rate of hemoglobin rise is approximately 1 g/dL every 4 weeks, and with 100 IU/kg three times per week it is 1.5 to 2 g/dL. Higher starting doses are used when there is the need to rapidly increase the level of hemoglobin. However, a rate of hemoglobin rise of more then 3 g/dL in any 4-week period should be avoided because of the possible exacerbation of hypertension. During the correction phase, the dosage of rhEPO must be adjusted monthly until the target is attained; the response to any change of dosage requires 4 weeks to be completely assessed.

A randomized study established that in uremic patients on rhEPO a threshold hematocrit between 27% and 32% effectively normalized bleeding time (Fig. 31.3) (63). rhEPO use, with hematocrit values of 36% to 39%, significantly improves quality of life, cardiac function, physical work capacity, cognitive function, and sexual function (134). However, the benefits and the risk of complete correction of anemia (hematocrit, 38% to 42%) and the optimal target concentration have not yet been established. The safety of the long-term maintenance of a normal hematocrit has been questioned as a consequence, in part, of the early termination of the Normal Hematocrit Cardiac Trial, in which the patients randomly assigned to the normal hematocrit group presented with a higher mortality and a higher incidence of nonfatal myocardial infarction (135,136).

Cryoprecipitate and Desmopressin

Cryoprecipitate is a plasma derivative rich in vWF, fibrinogen, and fibronectin that has traditionally been used in the treatment of hemophilia A, von Willebrand's disease, hypofibrinogenemia, and dysfibrinogenemia. The use of cryoprecipitate in uremic patients with a bleeding time greater than 15 minutes (137) was based on the observation that cryoprecipitate shortened the bleeding time of patients with platelet storage-pool disease. However, because this therapy carries the risk of transmitting blood-borne diseases, it was largely replaced by other approaches.

Desmopressin (1-deamino-8-D-arginine vasopressin) (DDAVP)—a synthetic derivative of the antidiuretic hormone—induces the release of autologous vWF from storage sites (138). In two randomized, double-blind, cross-over trials, DDAVP was effective at a dose of 0.3 µg/kg body weight given intravenously (138)—in 50 mL of physiologic saline over a period of 30 minutes (139)—or subcutaneously (Fig. 31.4) (140). Desmopressin can also be given by the intranasal route (141,142), which is well tolerated and quite safe. At 10 to 20 times the intravenous dose, intranasal desmopressin (3 µg/kg) shortens the prolonged bleeding time (141,142) and decreases clinical bleeding. Desmopressin loses its efficacy when repeatedly administered (143), probably due to a progressive depletion of vWF stores in endothelial cells.

Although remarkably free of serious side effects, DDAVP is reported to cause a mild to moderate decrease in platelet count, facial flushing, mild transient headache, nausea, abdominal cramps, and mild tachycardia, water retention, and hyponatremia. Rarely, thrombotic events followed DDAVP administration, particularly in patients with underlying advanced cardiovascular disease. Nonetheless, desmopressin is useful in the treatment of bleeding, and prophylactically in the prevention of bleeding during surgery or invasive procedures (144).

Conjugated Estrogens

The anecdotal observation of diminished gastrointestinal bleeding in uremic patients treated with conjugated estrogens and the improved hemostasis in von Willebrand's disease during pregnancy led to investigations of the effect of estrogens on bleeding tendency in uremia (53,145,146). One oral dose of 25 mg of conjugated estrogen preparation normalizes bleeding time for 3 to 10 days with no apparent ill effects (146). A controlled study showed that conjugated estrogens, given intravenously at the cumulative dose of 3 mg/kg divided over 5 consecutive days, produced a long-lasting reduction in the bleeding time in uremics. The estrogens were safe and well tolerated. The therapeutic activity could not apparently be ascribed to an effect on vWF multimeric structure, platelet aggregation in response to different stimuli (ADP, arachidonic acid, calcium ionophore A23187), or platelet TxB$_2$ generation.

At least 0.6 mg/kg estrogen was needed to reduce bleeding time (146), and four or five infusions spaced 24 hours apart were

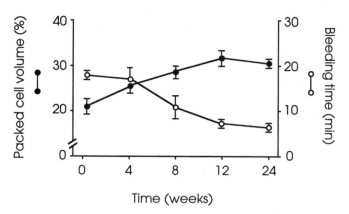

FIG. 31.3. Effect of recombinant human erythropoietin therapy on packed cell volume and bleeding time in uremic patients.

needed to reduce the bleeding time by at least 50%. The effect of estrogens on bleeding time in an experimental model of chronic uremia was completely reversed by NO precursor L-arginine (147), suggesting that the effect of estrogens on primary hemostasis in uremia might be mediated by changes in the NO synthesis pathway. Low-dose transdermal estrogen (estradiol 50 to 100 mg/24 h) applied as a patch twice weekly was found to reduce recurrent gastrointestinal bleeding with parallel improvement of bleeding time and no side effects (148). Thus estrogens may be a reasonable alternative to cryoprecipitate or desmopressin in the treatment of uremic bleeding, especially when a long-lasting effect is required.

THROMBOTIC COMPLICATIONS

Despite an underlying bleeding tendency, uremic patients are exposed to thrombotic complications of vascular access as a consequence of the hemodialysis procedure. Percutaneous cannulation, arteriovenous shunt, and native vein or prosthetic arteriovenous fistula, and fistulas made of artificial polymers used for chronic hemodialysis are particularly prone to thrombotic occlusion, which accounts for a substantial percentage of hospital admission of dialysis patients (149). Cardiovascular events related to thrombosis are a predominant cause of death and account for an important morbidity in uremic patients both on conservative treatments and on replacement of renal function by dialysis or transplantation. Hemostatic abnormalities consistent with a hypercoagulable state have been widely described in patients with end-stage renal failure (ESRD) on hemodialysis. Risk factors include enhanced platelet aggregability, increased plasma fibrinogen, factor VIII:C and vWF, decreased protein C anticoagulant activity and protein S, impaired fibrinolytic system activity, raised plasma lipoprotein(a), increased plasmatic concentration of homocysteine, and presence of lupus anticoagulant (reviewed in ref. 18).

Because platelet aggregation plays a major role in thrombus formation, antiplatelet agents have been used, with encouraging results. Aspirin, dipyridamole, ticlopidine, and sulfinpyrazone have proved useful in several studies. Fibrinolytic agents, such as streptokinase or urokinase, as well as recombinant tissue plasminogen activator have produced contrasting results.

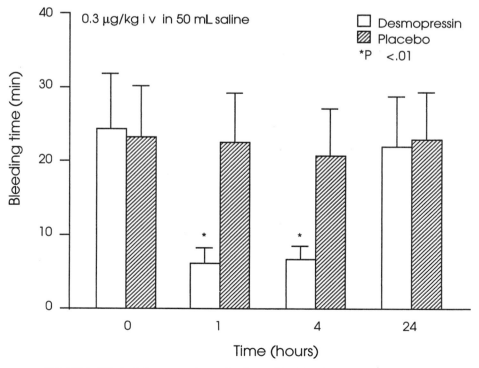

FIG. 31.4. Effect of desmopressin or placebo on bleeding time in uremic patients.

TABLE 31.2. GUIDELINES FOR THE MANAGEMENT OF HEMORRHAGIC COMPLICATIONS OF UREMIA

For all patients with hemorrhagic complications or undergoing major surgery, the adequacy of dialysis should be appropriately checked.

■ It is also advisable to change the dialysis schedule for 1 or 2 months in patients who have experienced severe hemorrhages (such as major gastrointestinal bleeding, hemorrhagic pericarditis, subdural hematomas) or who have undergone recent cardiovascular surgery so that heparin can be avoided. Acute bleeding episodes may be treated with desmopressin at a dose of 0.3 μg/kg, intravenously (added to 50 mL of saline over 30 min) or subcutaneously. Intranasal administration of this drug at a dose of 3 μg/kg is also effective and well tolerated.

■ Because the favorable effect of cryoprecipitate on bleeding time has not been uniformly observed, we do not recommend its use.

■ The effect of desmopressin lasts only a few hours, a major limitation to its use in treating severe hemorrhage. Desmopressin appears to lose efficacy when repeatedly administered. The ideal treatment of persistent chronic bleeding should have a long-lasting effect.

■ Conjugated estrogen treatment given by intravenous infusion in a cumulative dose of 3 mg/kg as daily divided doses (i.e., 0.6 mg/kg for 5 consecutive days) is the most appropriate way to achieve long-lasting hemostatic competence. Severely anemic patients should receive blood or red blood cell transfusions to improve hematocrit values.

■ Red blood cell transfusion is hemostatically effective only when the hematocrit rises above 30%.

■ As an alternative, bleeding in patients with renal failure and hematocrit less than 30% can be treated successfully with erythropoietin.

CONCLUSION

The pathogenesis of uremic bleeding has still not been fully elucidated. It has been attributed to abnormalities of primary hemostasis, particularly platelet dysfunction and impaired platelet–vessel wall interaction.

The current management includes an adequate dialysis schedule, and red cell transfusions or recombinant human erythropoietin for patients with severe anemia. Acute bleeding episodes may be treated with desmopressin, which is rapidly effective at least on bleeding time. Patients with gastrointestinal or intracranial bleeding or those undergoing major surgery may benefit from conjugated estrogen infusions, which are ideal for the treatment of dramatic bleeding because of their long-lasting effect (Table 31.2).

REFERENCES

1. Morgagni GB. *Opera Omnia. Ex Typographia Remondiniana.* Venezia, 1764.
2. Bright R. Reports of Medical Cases. London, 1827.
3. Mattix H, et al. Is the bleeding time predictive of bleeding prior to a percutaneous renal biopsy. *Curr Opin Nephrol Hypertens* 1999;8: 715–718.
4. Lindsay RM, et al. Platelet function in dialyzed and non-dialyzed patients with chronic renal failure. *Clin Nephrol* 1975;4:52–57.
5. Eknoyan G, et al. Platelet function in renal failure. *N Engl J Med* 1969;280:677–681.
6. Larsson SO. On coagulation and fibrinolysis in renal failure. *Scand J Haematol* 1971;15(Suppl):1–59.
7. Gafter U, et al. Platelet count and thrombopoietic activity in patients with chronic renal failure. *Nephron* 1987;45:207–210.
8. Di Minno G, et al. Platelet dysfunction in uremia: multifaceted defect partially corrected by dialysis. *Am J Med* 1985;79:552–559.
9. Eknoyan G, et al. Biochemical abnormalities of platelets in renal failure: evidence for decreased platelet serotonin, adenosine diphosphate and Mg-dependent adenosine triphosphatase. *Am J Nephrol* 1981;1: 17–23.
10. Kyrie PA, et al. Evidence for an increased generation of prostacyclin in the microvasculature and an impairment of the platelet alpha-granule release in chronic renal failure. *Thromb Haemostas* 1988;60: 205–208.
11. Vlachoyannis J, et al. Adenylate cyclase activity and cAMP content of human platelets in uremia. *Eur J Clin Invest* 1982;12:379–381.
12. Jacobsson B, et al. Abnormality of adenylate cyclase regulation in human platelet membranes in renal insufficiency. *Eur J Clin Invest* 1985;15:75–81.
13. Gura V, et al. Elevated thrombocyte calcium content in uremia and its correction by 1α(OH) vitamin D treatment. *Nephron* 1982;30: 237–239.
14. Ware JA, et al. Abnormalities of cytoplasmic Ca2+ in platelets from patients with uremia. *Blood* 1989;73:172–176.
15. Remuzzi G, et al. Parathyroid hormone inhibits human platelet function. *Lancet* 1981;2:1321–1323.
16. Benigni A, et al. Inhibition of human platelet aggregation by parathyroid hormone: is cyclic AMP implicated? *Am J Nephrol* 1985;5: 243–247.
17. Viganó G, et al. Hyperparathyroidism does not influence the abnormal primary haemostasis in patients with chronic renal failure. *Nephrol Dial Transplant* 1989;4:971–974.
18. Joist JH, et al. Abnormal bleeding and thrombosis in renal disease. In: Colman RW, et al., eds. *Hemostasis and thrombosis: basic principles and clinical practice.* Philadelphia: JB Lippincott, 1994:921–935.
19. Smith MC, et al. Impaired platelet thromboxane production in renal failure. *Nephron* 1981;29:133–137.
20. Remuzzi G, et al. Reduced platelet thromboxane formation in uremia: evidence for a functional cyclooxygenase defect. *J Clin Invest* 1983;71:762–768.
21. Macconi D, et al. Defective platelet aggregation in response to platelet-activating factor in uremia associated with low platelet thromboxane A2 generation. *Am J Kidney Dis* 1992;19:318–325.
22. Livio E, et al. Coagulation abnormalities in uremia. *Semin Nephrol* 1985;5:82–90.
23. Remuzzi G, et al. Role of endothelium-derived nitric oxide in the bleeding tendency of uremia. *J Clin Invest* 1990;86:1768–1771.
24. Ignarro LJ. Endothelium-derived nitric oxide: actions and properties. *Fed Am Soc Exp Biol J* 1988;3:31–36.
25. Radomski MW, et al. The role of nitric oxide and cGMP in platelet adhesion to vascular endothelium. *Biochem Biophys Res Comm* 1987; 148:1482–1489.
26. Aiello S, et al. Renal and systemic nitric oxide synthesis in rats with renal mass reduction. *Kidney Int* 1997;52:171–181.
27. Noris M, et al. Enhanced nitric oxide synthesis in uremia: implications for platelet dysfunction and dialysis hypotension. *Kidney Int* 1993;44:445–450.
28. Horl WH. Hemodialysis membrane: interleukins, biocompatibility, and middle molecules. *J Am Soc Nephrol* 2002;13:S62–S71.
29. Schmitt GW, et al. Alterations in hemostatic parameters during hemodialysis with dialyzers of different membrane composition and flow design. *Am J Med* 1983;83:411–418.
30. Weiss HJ, et al. Effect of shear rate in platelet interaction with subendothelium in citrated native blood. I. Shear-rate dependent decrease in adherence in von Willebrand's disease and the Bernard-Soulier syndrome. *J Lab Clin Med* 1978;92:750–764.
31. Sakariassen KS, et al. Platelet adherence to subendothelium of human arteries in pulsatile and steady flow. *Thromb Res* 1980;19:547–559.
32. Mezzano B, et al. Hemostatic disorder of uremia: the platelet defect, main determinant of the prolonged bleeding time, is correlated with indices of activation of coagulation and fibrinolysis. *Thromb Haemost* 1996;76:312–321.

33. Sloand EM, et al. Reduction of platelet glycoprotein Ib in uraemia. *Br J Haematol* 1991;77:375–381.

34. Benigni A, et al. Reversible activation defect of the platelet glycoprotein IIb–IIIa complex in patients with uremia. *Am J Kidney Dis* 1993; 22:668–676.

35. Castillo R, et al. Defective platelet adhesion on vessel subendothelium in uremic patients. *Blood* 1986;65:337–342.

36. Zwaginga JJ, et al. High von Willebrand factor concentration compensates a relative adhesion defect in uremic blood. *Blood* 1990;75: 1498–1508.

37. Escolar G, et al. Uremic platelets have a functional defect affecting the interaction of von Willebrand factor with glycoprotein IIb–IIIa. *Blood* 1990;76:1336–1340.

38. Rabiner SF, et al. The role of phenol and phenolic acid on the thrombocytopathy and defective platelet aggregation of patients with renal failure. *Am J Med* 1970;49:346–351.

39. Horowithz HI, et al. Further studies on the platelet inhibiting effect of guanidinosuccinic acid and its role in uremic bleeding. *Am J Med* 1970;49:336–340.

40. Remuzzi G, et al. Bleeding in renal failure: altered platelet function in chronic uraemia only partially corrected by haemodialysis. *Nephron* 1978;22:347–353.

41. Stein IM, et al. Guanidino succinic acid: the "X" factor in uremic bleeding? *Clin Res* 1968;16:397(abstr).

42. Horowitz HI. Uremic toxins and platelet function. *Arch Intern Med* 1970;126;823–826.

43. Rabiner SF. Bleeding in uremia. *Med Clin North Am* 1972;56: 221–223.

44. Eknoyan G, et al. Platelet function in renal failure. *N Engl J Med* 1969;280:677–681.

45. Remuzzi G, et al. Prostacyclin-like activity and bleeding in renal failure. *Lancet* 1977;2:1195–1197.

46. Remuzzi G, et al. Prostaglandins, plasma factors and haemostasis in uraemia. In: Remuzzi G, et al., eds. *Hemostasis, prostaglandins, and renal disease.* New York: Raven Press, 1980:273–281.

47. Leithner CH, et al. Enhanced prostacyclin availability of blood vessels in uraemic humans and rats. In: Robinson RHB, et al., eds. *Dialysis transplantation nephrology.* Proceedings of the 15th Congress of European Dialysis and Transplant Association. Tunbridge Wells, UK: Pitman Medical, 1978:418–422.

48. Zoja C, et al. Prolonged bleeding time and increased vascular prostacyclin in rats with chronic renal failure: effects of conjugated estrogens. *J Lab Clin Med* 1988;112:380–386.

49. Defreyn G, et al. A plasma factor in uraemia which stimulates prostacyclin release from cultured endothelial cells. *Thromb Res* 1980;19: 695–699.

50. Saglikes Y, et al. Effect of PTH on blood pressure and response to vasoconstrictor agonists. *Am J Physiol* 1985;248:F674–F681.

51. Deykin D. Uremic bleeding. *Kidney Int* 1983;24:698–705.

52. Turney JH, et al. Factor VIII complex in uremia and effects of hemodialysis. *Br Med J* 1981;282:1653–1656.

53. Livio M, et al. Conjugated estrogens for the management of bleeding associated with renal failure. *N Engl J Med* 1986;315:731–735.

54. Turnitto WT, et al. Red blood cells: their dual role in thrombus formation. *Science* 1980;207:541–543.

55. Sakariassen KS, et al. Platelet adherence to sub-endothelium of human arteries in pulsatile and steady flow. *Thromb Res* 1980;19:547–559.

56. Gaarder A, et al. Adenosine diphosphate in red cells as a factor in the adhesiveness of human blood platelets. *Nature* 1961;192:531–532.

57. Willems C, et al. Binding and inactivation of prostacyclin (PGI2) by human erythrocytes. *Br J Haematol* 1983;54:43–52.

58. Livio M, et al. Uraemic bleeding: role of anemia and beneficial effect of red cell transfusions. *Lancet* 1982;2:1013–1015.

59. Fernandez F, et al. Low hematocrit and prolonged bleeding time in uraemic patients: effect of red cell transfusions. *Br J Haematol* 1985; 59:139–148.

60. Aznar-Salatti J, et al. Serum obtained from uraemic patients modifies the reactivity towards platelets of extracellular matrices produced by endothelial cells. VIth International Symposium on the Biology of Vascular Cells, 1990;1:57(abstr).

61. Gordge MP, et al. Recombinant human erythropoietin corrects uraemic bleeding without causing intravascular haemostatic activation. *Thromb Res* 1990;57:171–182.

62. Moia M, et al. Improvement in the haemostatic defect of uraemia after treatment with recombinant human erythropoietin. *Lancet* 1987;2:1227–1229.

63. Viganò G, et al. Recombinant human erythropoietin to correct uremic bleeding. *Am J Kidney Dis* 1991;1:44–49.

64. Macdougall IC. Role of uremic toxins in exacerbating anemia in renal failure. *Kidney Int* 2001;59:S67–S72.

65. Andrassy K, et al. Uremia as a cause of bleeding. *Am J Nephrol* 1985; 5:313–319.

66. Fass RJ, et al. Platelet-mediated bleeding caused by broad-spectrum penicillins. *J Infect Dis* 1987;155:1242.

67. Shattil S, et al. Carbenicillin and penicillin G inhibit platelet function in vitro by impairing the interaction of agonists with the platelets surface. *J Clin Invest* 1980;65:329–337.

68. Bang N, et al. Effects of moxolactan on blood coagulation and platelet function. *Rev Infect Dis* 1982;4:S546–S554.

69. Bechtold H, et al. Evidence for impaired hepatic vitamin K metabolism in patients treated with N-methyl-thiotetrazole cephalosporin. *Thromb Haemost* 1984;51:358–361.

70. Harter HR, et al. Prevention of thrombosis in patients on hemodialysis by low dose of aspirin. *N Engl J Med* 1979;301:577–579.

71. Lindsay RM, et al. Reduction of thrombus formation on dialyzer membranes by aspirin and RA233. *Lancet* 1972;2:1287–1290.

72. Livio M, et al. Moderate doses of aspirin and risk of bleeding in renal failure. *Lancet* 1986;1:414–416.

73. Gaspari F, et al. Aspirin prolongs bleeding time in uremia by a mechanism distinct from platelet cyclooxygenase inhibition. *J Clin Invest* 1987;79:1788–1797.

74. Zuckerman GR, et al. Upper gastrointestinal bleeding in patients with chronic renal failure. *Ann Intern Med* 1985;102:588–592.

75. Boyle JM, et al. Acute upper gastrointestinal hemorrhage in patients with chronic renal disease. *Am J Med* 1983;75:409–412.

76. Harker LA, et al. Pharmacology of platelet inhibitors. *J Am Coll Cardiol* 1986;8:21B–32B.

77. Shepherd AM, et al. Peptic ulceration in chronic renal failure. *Lancet* 1973;1:1357–1359.

78. Margolis DM, et al. Upper gastrointestinal disease in chronic renal failure: a prospective evaluation. *Arch Intern Med* 1978;138: 1214–1217.

79. Dave PB, et al. Gastrointestinal telangiectasias: a source of bleeding in patients receiving hemodialysis. *Arch Intern Med* 1984;144: 1781–1783.

80. Boley SJ, et al. On the nature and aetiology of vascular ectasias of the colon: degenerative lesions of aging. *Gastroenterology* 1977;72:652–660.

81. Zuckerman GR, et al. Upper gastrointestinal bleeding in patients with chronic renal failure. *Ann Intern Med* 1978;138:1214–1217.

82. Dorothy CC. Gastrointestinal bleeding in dialysis patients. *Nephron* 1993;63:132–139.

83. Kumar S, et al. Pericarditis in renal disease. *Prog Cardiovasc Dis* 1980; 22:357–369.

84. Rutsky EA, et al. Treatment of uraemic pericarditis and pericardial effusion. *Am J Kidney Dis* 1987;10:2–8.

85. Comty CM, et al. Cardiac complications of regular dialysis therapy. In: Mather J, ed. *Replacement of renal function by dialysis.* Dordrecht, the Netherlands: Kluwer Academic, 1983.

86. Drueke T, et al. Uraemic cardiomyopathy and pericarditis. *Adv Nephrol Necker Hosp* 1980;9:33–70.

87. Bechar M, et al. Subdural hematoma during long term hemodialysis. *Arch Neurol* 1972;26:513–516.

88. Berger HW, et al. Uraemic pleural effusion: a study in 14 patients on chronic dialysis. *Ann Intern Med* 1975;82:362–364.

89. Galen MA, et al. Hemorrhagic pleural effusion in patients undergoing chronic dialysis. *Ann Intern Med* 1975;82:359–361.

90. Bhasin HK, et al. Spontaneous retroperitoneal hemorrhage in chronically hemodialyzed patients. *Nephron* 1978;22:322–327.

91. Milutinovich J, et al. Spontaneous retroperitoneal bleeding in patients on chronic hemodialysis. *Ann Intern Med* 1977;86:189–192.

92. Borra S, et al. Subscapular liver hematoma in a patient on chronic hemodialysis. *Ann Intern Med* 1980;93:574–575.

93. Slusher MM, et al. Letter: spontaneous hyphema during hemodialysis. *N Engl J Med* 1975;293:561.

94. Remuzzi G, et al. Altered platelet and vascular prostaglandin-generation in patients with renal failure and prolonged bleeding times. *Thromb Res* 1978;13:1007–1015.

95. Gordon LA, et al. Studies in regional heparinization. *N Engl J Med* 1956;255:1063–1066.

96. Maher JF, et al. Regional heparinization for hemodialysis. *N Engl J Med* 1963;268:451–456.

97. Lindholm DD, et al. A simplified method of regional heparinization during hemodialysis according to a predetermined dosage formula. *Trans Am Soc Artif Int Organs* 1964;10:92–97.

98. Blaufox MD, et al. Rebound anticoagulation occurring after regional heparinization for hemodialysis. *Trans Am Soc Artif Intern Organs* 1966;12:207–209.

99. Tolkoff-Rubin NE, et al. Successful hemodialysis of patients at high risk of hemorrhage using the ExVal dialyzer. *Dial Transplant* 1986;15:125–126.

100. Lowr JW, et al. Safety of regional citrate hemodialysis in acute renal failure. *Am J Kidney Dis* 1989;2:104–107.

101. Flanigan MJ, et al. Reducing the hemorrhagic complications of hemodialysis: a controlled comparison of low-dose heparin and citrate anticoagulation. *Am J Kidney Dis* 1987;9:147–153.

102. Janssen JFM, et al. Citrate compared to low molecular weight heparin anticoagulation in chronic hemodialysis patients. *Kidney Int* 1996;49:806–813.

103. Silverstein FJ, et al. Metabolic alkalosis induced by regional citrate hemodialysis. *ASAIO Trans* 1989;35:22–25.

104. Kelleher SP, et al. Severe metabolic alkalosis complicating regional citrate hemodialysis. *Am J Kidney Dis* 1987;9:235–236.

105. Schrader J, et al. Comparison of low molecular weight heparin to standard heparin in hemodialysis/hemofiltration. *Kidney Int* 1988;33:890–896.

106. Saltissi D, et al. Comparison of low-molecular-weight heparin (enoxaparin sodium) and standard unfractionated heparin for haemodialysis anticoagulation. *Nephrol Dial Transplant* 1999;14:2698–2703.

107. Ivanovich P, et al. Studies of coagulation and platelet functions in heparin-free hemodialysis. *Nephron* 1983;33:116–120.

108. Sanders PW, et al. Hemodialysis without anticoagulation. *Am I Kidney Dis* 1985;5:32–35.

109. Caruana RJ, et al. Heparin free dialysis: comparative data results in high-risk patients. *Kidney Int* 1987;31:1351–1355.

110. Casati S, et al. Hemodialysis without anticoagulants: efficiency and hemostatic aspects. *Clin Nephrol* 1984;21:102–105.

111. Romao JE, et al. Hemodialysis without anticoagulant: hemostasis parameters, fibrinogen kinetic, and dialysis efficiency. *Nephrol Dial Transplant* 1997;12:106–110.

112. Ambuhl PM, et al. Plasma hypercoagulability in hemodialysis patients: impact of dialysis and anticoagulation. *Nephrol Dial Transplant* 1997;12:2355–2364.

113. Nurmohamed MT, et al. A randomized cross-over study comparing the efficacy and safety of two dosages dermatan sulfate and standard heparin in six chronic hemodialysis patients. *Br J Haematol* 1990;76(Suppl):23.

114. Ryan KE, et al. Antithrombotic properties of dermatan sulphate (MF 701) in hemodialysis for chronic renal failure. *Thromb Haemost* 1992;68:563–569.

115. Fernandez F, et al. The hemorrhagic and antithrombotic effects of dermatan sulphate. *Br J Haematol* 1986;64:309–317.

116. Nurmohamed MT, et al. Clinical experience with a new anticoagulant (dermatan sulphate) in chronic hemodialysis patients. *Clin Nephrol* 1993;39:166–171.

117. Gianese F, et al. The pharmacodynamics of dermatan sulphate MF 701 during haemodialysis for chronic renal failure. *Br J Clin Pharmacol* 1993;35:335–339.

118. Nurmohamed MT, et al. No clinically relevant accumulation of der-

matan sulfate (DS) during chronic use in hemodialysis. *Thromb Haemost* 1993;69:1118(abstr).

119. Boccardo P, et al. Individualized anticoagulation with dermatan sulphate for haemodialysis in chronic renal failure. *Nephrol Dialysis Transplant* 1997;12:2349–2354.

120. Dawson A, et al. Sulfinpyrazone as a method of keeping dialysis membranes clean. In: Frost TH, ed. *Technical aspects of renal disease*. Bath, England: Pitman Press, 1978.

121. Shaarshmidt BF, et al. The use of calcium chelating agents and prostaglandin E1 to eliminate platelet and white blood cell losses resulting from hemoperfusion through charcoal albumin, agarose gel and neural and neutral and cation exchange resus. *J Lab Clin Nephrol* 1985;24:15–20.

122. Morring K, et al. Comparative evaluation of iatrogenic sources of blood loss during maintenance dialysis. In: *Proceedings of the 13th Congress of European Dialysis and Transplant Association*. Tunbridge Wells, UK: Pitman Medical, 1976:223.

123. Turney JH, et al. Platelet protection and heparin sparing with prostacyclin during regular therapy. *Lancet* 1980;2:219–222.

124. Arze RS, et al. Prostacyclin safer than heparin in haemodialysis. *Lancet* 1981;2:50.

125. Zusman RM, et al. Hemodialysis using prostacyclin instead of heparin as the sole antithrombotic agent. *N Engl J Med* 1981;304:934–939.

126. Swartz RD, et al. Epoprostenol (PGI, prostacyclin) during high-risk hemodialysis: preventing further bleeding complications. *J Clin Pharmacol* 1988;28:818–825.

127. Dubrow A, et al. Safety and efficacy of epoprostenol (PGI2) versus heparin in hemodialysis. *Trans Am Soc Artif Intern Organs* 1984;30:52–54.

128. Jacons J, et al. Isolation and characterization of genomic and cDNA clones of human erythropoietin-rich plasma in vivo. *J Clin Invest* 1984;74:434–441.

129. Lin FK, et al. Cloning and expression of the human erythropoietin gene. *Proc Nat Acad Sci USA* 1985;82:7580–7584.

130. Winearls CG, et al. Effect of human erythropoietin derived from recombinant DNA on the anaemia of patients maintained by chronic hemodialysis. *Lancet* 1986;2:1175–1178.

131. Eschbach JW, et al. Correction of the anemia and end-stage renal disease with recombinant human erythropoietin: results of a phase I and II clinical trial. *N Engl J Med* 1987;316:73–78.

132. Zwaginga JJ, et al. Treatment of uraemic anemia with recombinant erythropoietin also reduces the defects in platelet adhesion and aggregation caused by uraemic plasma. *Thromb Haemost* 1991;66:638–647.

133. Van Geet C, et al. Haemostatic effects of recombinant human erythropoietin in chronic haemodialysis patients. *Thromb Hamostas* 1989;61:117–121.

134. NKF-DOQI. Clinical practice guidelines: treatment of anemia of chronic renal failure. *Am J Kidney Dis* 1997;30:S192–S237.

135. Besarab A, et al. The effects of normal as compared with low hematocrit values in patients with cardiac disease who are receiving hemodialysis and epoetin. *N Engl J Med* 1998;339:584–590.

136. Minetti L. Erythropoietin treatment in renal anemia: how high should the target hematocrit be? *J Nephrol* 1997;10:117–119.

137. Janson PA, et al. Treatment of the bleeding tendency in uremia with cryoprecipitate. *N Engl J Med* 1980;303:1318–1322.

138. Mannucci PM, et al. 1-Deamino-8-D-arginine vasopressin: a new pharmacological approach to the management of haemophilia and von Willebrand's disease. *Lancet* 1977;1:869–872.

139. Mannucci PM, et al. Deamino-8-D—arginine vasopressin shortens the bleeding time in uremia. *N Engl J Med* 1983;308:8–12.

140. Viganó G, et al. Subcutaneous injection of desmopressin (DDAVP) shortens the bleeding time in uremia. *Am J Hematol* 1989;31:32–35.

141. Shapiro MD, et al. Intranasal deamino-8-D—argine vasopressin shortens the bleeding time in uremia. *Am J Nephrol* 1984;4:260–261.

142. Rydzewski A, et al. Shortening of the bleeding time after intranasal administration of 1-deamino-8-D—argine vasopressin to patients with chronic anemia. *Folia Haematol Int Mag Klin Morphol Blut Forsch* 1986;113:823–830.

143. Canavese C, et al. Reduced response of uraemic bleeding time to repeated doses of desmopressin. *Lancet* 1985;1:867–868.
144. Mannucci PM. Desmopressin (DDAVP) in the treatment of the bleeding disorders: the first 20 years. *Blood* 1997;90:2516–2521.
145. Liu YK, et al. Treatment of uraemic bleeding with conjugated oestrogen. *Lancet* 1984;2:887–890.
146. Viganó G, et al. Dose-effect and pharmacokinetics of estrogens given to correct bleeding time in uremia. *Kidney Int* 1988;34:853–858.
147. Zoja C, et al. L-Arginine, the precursor of nitric oxide, abolishes the effect of estrogens on bleeding time in experimental uremia. *Lab Invest* 1991;65:479–483.
148. Sloand JA, et al. Beneficial effect of low-dose transdermal estrogen on bleeding time and clinical bleeding in uremia. *Am J Kidney Dis* 1995;26:22–26.
149. Lazarus JM, et al. Medical aspects of hemodialysis. In: Brenner BM, et al., eds. *The kidney.* Philadelphia: WB Saunders, 1991:2223–2298.

TREATMENT OF ANEMIA IN DIALYSIS PATIENTS

ANATOLE BESARAB

HISTORICAL PERSPECTIVES

Since the initial observation of the progressive fading of the "healthy colors of the countenance" by Richard Bright in 1836 (1), anemia has been a hallmark of renal insufficiency. Bone marrow erythropoiesis in response to hypoxia was proposed in 1823 by Miescher (2). The concept of a "hemopoietin"—a humoral factor stimulating erythropoiesis—was postulated in 1906 by Carnot and Deflandre (3). Brown and Roth (4), in 1922, determined that the anemia of chronic nephritis resulted from reduced bone marrow red cell production. Bonsdorff and Jalavisto (5) coined the term "erythropoietin" in 1948 to describe an erythropoietic factor in the plasma of patients with congestive heart failure. The seminal work of Erslev (6,7) during the next 5 years confirmed and described the presence of an erythropoietic factor in the blood of anemic animals. In 1957, Jacobson et al. (8) showed that this factor was lacking in bilaterally nephrectomized animals. Erslev (9) then conclusively demonstrated the kidney to be a source of erythropoietin (EPO) in 1974 by demonstrating that isolated kidneys perfused with a serum-free medium respond to hypoxia by synthesizing EPO.

We now know erythropoiesis to be intricately and inextricably linked to the renal production of the hormone and recognize its deficiency as the prime but not sole cause of the anemia of renal disease. The fact that intense dialysis, androgens, and the administration of various growth factors can independently increase hemoglobin (Hb) levels merely reflects the effects of the metabolic environment on erythropoiesis.

The discovery, characterization, and commercial production of recombinant human erythropoietin (rhEPO or epoetin) have revolutionized treatment of anemia in patients with advanced renal disease. Recombinant EPO does not merely alleviate but even eliminates the anemia associated with kidney disease. The primary indication for rhEPO is the anemia associated with renal disease (10) although in recent years it has increasingly been used to treat the anemia of cancer (11).

A number of factors arising from chronic renal failure as well as its treatment may modify the need for and the response to EPO. The major issues regarding the clinical use of rhEPO in patients with renal disease are cost effectiveness, dosage, route of administration, and resistance to therapy (12). An important consideration is the degree of anemia and stage of renal disease at which EPO therapy should be initiated (13). Dosage deter-

mines the erythropoietic response and the magnitude of the increase in hematocrit (Hct). The dose that is used is determined by variability in dose needs among subjects and economic factors. This chapter reviews several aspects of therapy: (a) erythropoiesis in normal and in untreated end-stage renal disease (ESRD) patients, (b) the biochemistry and pharmacology of epoetin, (c) the benefits and hazards of epoetin therapy, (d) cost-effective use of epoetin based on pharmacodynamic principles, and (e) response resistance and iron management.

NORMAL ERYTHROPOIESIS

EPO is now known to be a multifunctional trophic factor with affects on general homeostasis. It has effects on the endothelial cell (EC) and on the central nervous system where it has some neurotrophic and neuroprotective function (14). Neurons in the ischemic retina are protected by expression of EPO receptors and by exogenous administration of rhEPO (15). However, its best characterized effects are in the bone marrow.

The pluripotent hematopoietic stem cell is capable of forming erythrocytes, leukocytes, and megakaryocytes (16,17). Under appropriate stimuli, these primitive cells have the capacity for both self-renewal and differentiation into committed progenitor cells. Renewal appears to occur by chance "stochastically" (18) and is initiated primarily by lineage, nonspecific cytokines such as interleukin 3 (IL-3), stem cell factor, insulin growth factor, and granulocyte-macrophage colony-stimulating factor (GM-CSF).

The transformation of a multipotential stem cell into a mature red blood cell (RBC) occurs in two morphologically distinct stages (Fig. 32.1). Only the first stage is responsive to EPO. This first stage begins with small mononuclear cells displaying a specific glycophosphoprotein CD34 on their surface (19), and then sequentially includes the committed erythroid progenitor, the primitive and mature burst-forming unit-erythroid (BFU-E), and the colony-forming unit-erythroid (CFU-E). In the second, the precursor stage, the cells appear as morphologically recognizable erythroblasts that mature into pronormoblasts and daughter erythrocytes.

Most multipotent committed progenitor cells exist in the resting G_0 stage of the cell cycle (20) and are stimulated into the G_1 stage by interleukins 1 and 6, and granulocyte colony-stim-

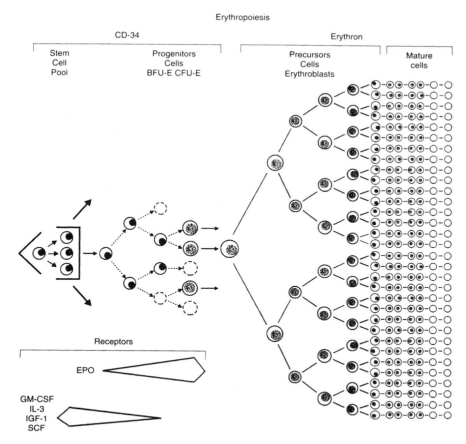

Erythropoiesis

FIG. 32.1. Model of red cell production. Erythropoiesis is partitioned into two stages. Erythropoietin (EPO) is needed in the first stage (from multipotential to progenitor cells in the burst-forming unit-erythroid) but not the second precursor cell stage. Site of action of EPO and other growth factors is shown. The stippling indicates potential apoptosis of progenitor cells. (From Erslev AJ, et al. Erythropoietin in the pathogenesis and treatment of the anemia of chronic renal failure. Editorial review. *Kidney Int* 1997;51:623–630, with permission.)

ulating factor (G-CSF). Under the influence of IL-3 and GM-CSF, they differentiate into primitive BFU-E. Peripheral demands for cellular production can only be met after this transformation of a multipotential stem cell to a unipotential progenitor cell. At this stage, the cells have lost most of their capacity for self-renewal but have gained receptors for EPO, which now becomes essential for the multiplication and differentiation of the BFU-E and CFU-E. There is an increasing dependence on, as well as sensitivity to, the effects of EPO with the progressive maturation from primitive BFU-E into CFU-E (21–23), to the point that the CFU-E will only survive and differentiate into a pronormoblast in the presence of EPO. Insulin or insulin-like growth factor 1 (IGF-1) is also required for CFU-E growth (24). In summary, EPO does not affect division or differentiation of the uncommitted pluripotent stem cell, but its constant presence is critical to the sustenance, multiplication, and differentiation of the committed erythroid progenitors. This concept is key with regard to clinical dosing practices.

Several other factors such as androgens, thyroid hormone, somatomedin, and catecholamines appear to augment the growth of CFU-E but are not essential (25). Other cytokines including interleukins 1α and 1β, interleukin 2, tumor necrosis factor alpha (TNF-α), and transforming growth factor beta (TGF-β) have a negative effect on erythropoiesis (26,27). These cytokines are significant mediators in the anemia of chronic diseases, may be activated by certain types of dialysis, and are invariably present during acute infection or inflammation. Their inhibitory effects produce resistance to exogenous EPO in renal failure patients.

EPO exerts its signal through the EPO receptor, a 55-kd transmembrane protein (28). Agents are being developed which are not epoetin like but can activate the receptor by molecular mimicry (29). Once activated, the receptor dimerizes, and tyrosine kinase activity via constitutively expressed JAK2 leads to phosphorylation of intracellular proteins (30), followed by activation of several signaling pathways that include STAT5, RAS, and phosphoinositol 3-kinase (31). EPO has also been shown to modulate calcium influx in erythroid cells through a transient receptor potential channel (32). Although the exact signals or pathways are still poorly understood, it is unlikely that the ultimate signals are transcription factors for genes involved in the synthesis of globin or other mature erythroid proteins; it is more likely that these signals maintain the viability of progenitor cells (33). In the absence of EPO, such cells undergo apoptosis and die before they reach the precursor cell stage. In the presence of EPO, they proliferate and eventually transform into precursor cells.

Erythroid progenitor cells exposed to optimal concentration of growth factors and EPO proliferate luxuriously and produce a "burst" of colonies (34). The kinetics of progenitor cell proliferation in vivo appears very similar but somewhat more restrained than those in vitro. A BFU-E even in the presence of large amounts of EPO will not produce a burst of thousands of CFU-E but merely 50 to 100 CFU-E (35). In the presence of a normal concentration of EPO (8 to 18 mU/mL), each BFU-E probably makes no more than 4 to 6 CFU-E.

At a certain level of maturation the CFU-E becomes activated and the cells are transformed into Hb-synthesizing morphologically recognizable erythroblasts (34). Further proliferation and maturation of these cells appear to be unaffected by EPO, proceeding at a fixed rate in the presence of adequate supplies of iron, folate, vitamin B_{12}, pyridoxine, ascorbic acid, and trace elements.

Until recently EPO was believed to have no affect on cells once they were released from the bone marrow. However, another EPO-dependent mechanism affecting circulating cells has been described. Hemolysis of recently formed RBCs occurs when EPO levels fall rapidly as with descent from altitude, thus permitting rapid adaptation when red cell mass is excessive for the new environment (36).

Erythropoietin: Regulation and Control of Production

Sheep plasma EPO was purified in 1971 (37). Six years later Miyake et al. purified human EPO (38). The years 1985 and 1986 saw the elucidation of its structure (39), sequencing of its mRNA (40), identification of the organs containing the mRNA (41,42), and the cloning and transfection of the human gene into Chinese hamster cells by Lin et al. (43), which allowed mass production of rhEPO for clinical use.

The kidneys produce more than 90% of EPO; the rest is produced largely by hepatocytes (25), with an insignificant contribution by macrophages. Bilateral nephrectomy virtually abolishes EPO production (8,44–46). In situ hybridization techniques have localized the messenger ribonucleic acid (mRNA) to interstitial cells (also known as the type I interstitial cell) (47,48) located near the base of proximal tubular cells, predominantly in the renal cortex (47). Under normal oxygen conditions interstitial cells positive for EPO mRNA are limited to the deep cortex and outer medulla. With increasing anemia, the number of positive cells increases in number and spreads into the superficial cortex (48). However, there are some studies suggesting a major role for the proximal tubule cells in epoetin production (49).

The kidney functions as a "critmeter" because it senses both oxygen tension and extracellular volume (50). Through EPO it regulates RBC mass and through salt and water excretion it regulates plasma volume. The kidney, thus, regulates the numerator and denominator of the "crit." It is able to dissociate changes in blood flow from those in oxygenation. The normal Hct of 40% to 50% is not random, but rather one that maximizes delivery of oxygen to the tissues.

The renal oxygen sensor that leads to increased production of EPO has for the past decade been believed to be a heme oxidase (51). This has been found to be too simplistic. The human EPO gene, on the long arm of chromosome 7, consists of five exons and four introns (52) but it is not directly regulated by molecular oxygen. Rather transcription is regulated by a hypoxia-inducible factor (HIF) acting on a hypoxia responsive element that is upstream of the gene (53,54). Studies have shown that hypoxia induces the production of HIF-1 (55–59) that binds to the oxygen-sensitive enhancer to induce gene transcription of mRNA. HIF factors have now been cloned. HIF-1 regulates the expression of many more genes apart from EPO [nitric oxide (NO) synthase, endothelin-1, adrenomedullin, vascular endo-

thelial growth factor (VEGF), platelet-derived growth factor (PDGF)]. These gene products provide adaptation to reduced oxygen supply. The HIF molecules exist as heterodimers composed of α- and β-subunits with the oxygen-regulated component on the α-subunit. Hydroxylation of a proline residue within the HIFα domain by specific oxidases is a crucial step in the oxygen-sensing mechanism and eventual gene transcription of epoetin and other proteins (60). Abundance of HIF is determined primarily by degradation rather than production. Degradation requires the presence of a normal von-Hippel-Lindau gene protein (pVHL) that binds to HIFα permitting rapid proteasomic degradation in the presence of oxygen. Cells lacking pVHL are unable to degrade the factor in the presence of oxygen (hypoxia is mimicked) (61).

Human EPO is a glycosylated protein with 165 amino acids and a molecular weight of 34 kd (62). Although the nonglycosylated form is biologically active in vitro, glycosylation is necessary for cellular secretion (63) and for biologic action in vivo to prevent rapid liver clearance (64). Because the primary function of EPO is to regulate the amount of oxygen available to the body by modulating the production of erythrocytes, it is natural that factors affecting its production do so by directly or indirectly affecting oxygen availability. EPO production is increased by conditions of reduced oxygen delivery and reduced by states of increased oxygen delivery.

In normal individuals, levels of EPO are remarkably constant under steady-state conditions, with average values of 10 to 18 mU/mL (range 8 to 25) in both adults and children (45,46,65).

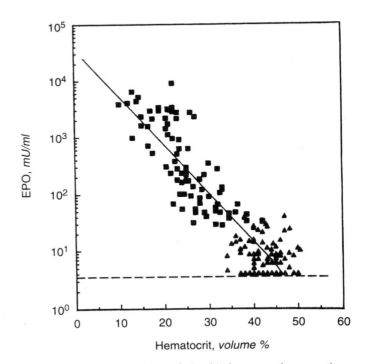

FIG. 32.2. Inverse logarithmic relationship between plasma erythropoietin levels and hematocrit. *j,* nonrenal anemias of various types, including those related to hemolysis, iron deficiency, and chronic inflammatory diseases; *m,* normal subjects without anemia. (From Erslev AJ. Erythropoietin. *N Engl J Med* 1991;324:1339–1344, with permission.)

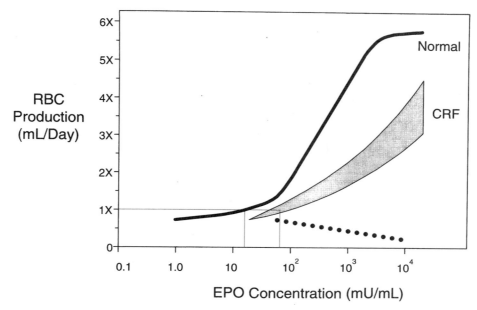

FIG. 32.3. Relationship of red cell production to erythropoietin (EPO) levels in normal and in renal failure patients. Red blood cell production is given as multiples of normal. In nonrenal anemias, the bone marrow response increases red cell production up to sixfold as EPO increases 100-fold or more. In renal failure, the dose response curve is shifted down and to the right. Basal production *(dotted line)* occurs at an EPO level of 15 mU/mL and 80 mU/mL in normal and end-stage renal disease subjects, respectively. The lower *dashed line* represents aplastic anemia.

EPO-producing cells are recruited in an on-off fashion (66); increased production of EPO results from the exponential recruitment of additional EPO synthesizing cells (66–68) as the hypoxic stimulus increases. This exponential recruitment of EPO-producing cells produces the inverse relationship between circulating EPO levels and Hct (Fig. 32.2). Levels can increase 100- to 1,000-fold in response to severe anemia. The maximum response of the bone marrow is limited to only a four- to sixfold increase of erythrocyte production (Fig. 32.3) (69). A negative feedback system resulting from the subsequent increase in oxygen-carrying capacity (increased Hct) turns off EPO production (70–72). Additional control elements exist that prevent an overshoot in erythrocyte production resulting from the long lifespan of red cells.

ANEMIA OF RENAL DISEASE: PATHOGENESIS

In progressive kidney disease, the degree of anemia is in general proportional to the severity of azotemia (73). Among patients, the correlation of Hct with glomerular filtration rate (GFR), blood urea nitrogen (BUN), or serum creatinine (Fig. 32.4) is imprecise (74). However, as renal function approaches that requiring replacement therapy, the Hct tends to plateau in the absence of complications or institution of rhEPO therapy. Most early dialysis patients had Hct values between 15% to 25%. The end-stage kidney continues to produce some EPO despite effective cessation of excretory function. The bilaterally nephrectomized patient invariably develops much lower levels of Hct (74).

Uncomplicated anemia of renal disease is normocytic and normochromic (75). Echinocytes, or burr cells, are the most frequently observed morphologic change in RBCs (76). Presence

of normal cellularity and maturation sequence in the bone marrow of dialysis patients is misleading inasmuch as erythropoiesis should be increased. Following acute blood loss or prolonged hypoxia, erythropoiesis in the marrow does increase to higher levels but not to the extent seen in nonuremic individuals.

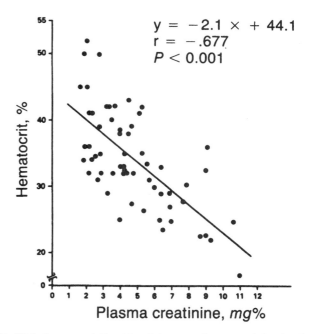

$$y = -2.1 \times + 44.1$$
$$r = -.677$$
$$P < 0.001$$

FIG. 32.4. Inverse relationship of hematocrit to creatinine level in patients with varying degrees of renal failure. (From McGonigle RSR, et al. Erythropoietin deficiency and erythropoiesis in renal insufficiency. *Kidney Int* 1984;25:437–444, with permission.)

Inadequate Erythropoietin Production

In nephric anemic dialysis patients, baseline EPO values are marginally higher than those of normal individuals, but these values are still much lower than those observed in nonuremic patients for similar degrees of anemia. The persistent observation of inappropriately low EPO levels in virtually all cases of chronic renal failure (45,65,77) indicates that the primary factor in the anemia of advanced renal failure is inadequate production of endogenous EPO by the diseased kidneys. Although acute blood loss or hemolysis can transiently increase plasma EPO levels two- to fivefold in dialysis patients, the levels are still lower than those achieved by normal individuals without renal disease sustaining similar degrees of blood loss. Diseased kidneys appear incapable of augmenting EPO production chronically in response to an appropriate anemic hypoxic stimulus (64,74,78, 79). Patients with autosomal dominant polycystic kidney disease are the exception and typically have higher EPO levels with less severe anemia (80,81). High EPO concentrations have been found in the fluid of cysts originating from proximal tubules with EPO mRNA identified in their interstitial cells (82).

The negative biofeedback loop between EPO and tissue oxygen delivery is present but impaired in renal failure. In stable dialysis patients, the Hct correlates directly rather than inversely with basal EPO levels (Fig. 32.5).

Shortened Erythrocyte Survival

Both mechanical and metabolic factors shorten the red cell lifespan in dialysis patients from a normal value of 120 days to 70

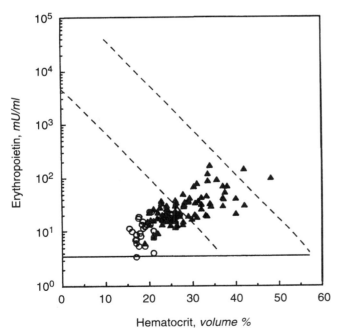

FIG. 32.5. Direct relationship of hematocrit to erythropoietin in endstage renal disease. (From Besarab A, et al. Dynamics of erythropoiesis following renal transplantation. *Kidney Int* 1987;32:526–536, with permission.)

to 80 days (83–86). A variety of metabolic abnormalities have been described (87–89) that support the Na$^+$-K$^+$ membrane pumps (89). Resulting changes in red cell shape and rigidity favor hemolysis. This hemolysis has been attributed to either uremic impairment of enzymatic activity (89) or decreased synthesis of Na$^+$-K$^+$ pump units by uremic reticulocytes (90,91). Because uremic red cells survive normally when transfused into healthy recipients (92) and normal red cells have a reduced lifespan in uremic individuals (83,93) and because erythrocyte lifespan can be normalized with intensive dialysis (94), retention of one or more uremic solutes in the plasma is believed to be responsible for the hemolysis. C-reactive protein levels, a marker for inflammation, are elevated in predialysis and more so in dialysis patients (95) Now that uremia has been recognized as an inflammatory state, the shortened red cell lifespan may also result from the hemolysis related to inflammation. Unrecognized blood loss will also decrease the "apparent" red cell survival. In well-dialyzed patients in whom blood losses are minimized, red cell survival can approach (but not achieve) normal (96).

Many processes can produce iatrogenic hemolysis. Drugs having strong oxidizing potential (primaquine, quinidine, sulfones, and nitrofurantoin) can induce hemolysis because of decreased activity of the hexose monophosphate shunt (97). Hemolysis can result from contamination of dialysate by chloramine from city tap-water sources (98,99); by copper (100), zinc (101), aluminum (102), and nitrates (103); and by formaldehyde from reprocessed dialyzer equipment (104). Fortunately these causes are mostly of historical significance. The dialysis process can produce hemolysis, through use of hypotonic dialysate (105), overheated dialysate (106), roller pump malocclusion (107), and mechanical disruption from dialysis needles (108). Severe hypophosphatemia can increase the susceptibility to hemolysis (109).

Rarely, long-term hemodialysis patients develop splenomegaly with markedly impaired red cell survival (110) and augmented erythrocyte destruction, as documented by radioisotope studies (111). Splenectomy should be reserved for those with either coexistent neutropenia or thrombocytopenia (112,113) or anemia resistant to rhEPO.

Blood Loss

In hemodialysis patients the true red cell lifespan can appear significantly shorter as a result of external blood losses. Measurement of red cell lifespan is affected both by the removal of senescent cells by the reticuloendothelial system and by extracorporeal losses resulting from vascular access puncture, residual blood in dialyzers, clotted dialyzers, phlebotomy for laboratory testing, and occasional blood leaks. Typical measurable losses approximate 60 mL of whole blood per week (114,115). Erythrocyte lifespan can approach normal in well-dialyzed patients when particular attention is paid to minimizing laboratory blood sampling (96). Such "routine" blood losses associated with hemodialysis contribute significantly to the iron deficiency of these patients, resulting in effective iron losses of between 1 to 3 g of iron per year. Such losses are obviously diminished in peritoneal dialysis.

Bleeding associated with renal insufficiency (116,117) has been known for decades. Common manifestations include telangiectasia and gastrointestinal angiodysplastic lesions (118). Functional abnormalities of platelets characterized by prolonged bleeding times, abnormal platelet aggregation and adhesiveness, and reduced platelet factor 3 release are well recognized (119). A reversible abnormality in the activation-dependent binding activity of glycoprotein IIb-IIIa occurs in uremia (119,120). Other defects include abnormalities in the multimeric structure of von Willebrand factor (vWF) (121) and acquired platelet storage pool deficiencies of adenosine diphosphate and serotonin (122). All these notwithstanding, anemia appears to be a major factor in sustaining the bleeding tendency, because prolonged bleeding times are corrected by red cell transfusions (123,124) and by the rise in Hct that occurs with therapeutic use of rhEPO (125,126).

Inhibition of Erythropoiesis

In the absence of significant overt blood loss, decreases in red cell survival alone do not fully account for the degree of anemia in progressive renal failure. If one examines the relationship of EPO levels to Hb and Hct levels in the earliest stages of kidney disease, EPO levels are appropriately increased for the degree of anemia until renal function drops below 40% of normal. Thereafter, EPO levels cannot be sustained and decrease progressively (73). Numerous in vitro studies have implicated an inhibitory effect of uremic serum on growth of erythroid precursors or on heme synthesis (127–131). Intensive dialysis can increase iron utilization and Hct without altering the level of circulating EPO (84,132).

Older studies tried to identify polar lipids, arsenic, vitamin A, spermine, spermidine, and parathyroid hormone (PTH) (128,131,133–138) as specific uremic inhibitors. More recent studies indicate that their role in the genesis of the anemia of renal failure is of very minor importance (139–144). In humans, acute ferrokinetic responses to rhEPO do not differ among hemodialysis patients, normal subjects, or patients with chronic renal failure restored to normal by transplantation (141). The improvement of anemia demonstrated following parathyroidectomy is due to the resolution of marrow fibrosis rather than the removal of erythropoietic inhibition (143).

Despite the clinical experience showing that exogenous EPO easily overcomes the effects of any such putative inhibitors, studies on uremic inhibitors continue because control of such factors could reduce the amount of rhEPO needed. Recent studies have focused on effects of albumin-bound furancarboxylic acid (145), activated monocytes, and polymorphonuclear leukocyte products (146) on erythropoiesis. T cells from uremic subjects may be unable to release general growth cytokines needed for optimal erythropoiesis (147). N-acetyl-seryl-lysyl-proline (AcsSDKP) is a physiologic inhibitor of hematopoiesis that is maintained at stable levels in patients without kidney disease. AcsSDKP levels increase almost twofold in patients not on dialysis and more than fivefold in patients on hemodialysis. Use of angiotensin-converting enzyme inhibitors increases AcsSDKP levels fourfold. At higher levels, AcsSDKP acts as a uremic toxin producing partial resistance to EPO. (148).

Nutritional Factors Contributing to Anemia

The patient with chronic renal failure or on maintenance dialysis is prone to anorexia, intercurrent illnesses, and dietary restrictions. Dialysis can also produce dialysate nutrient losses. All patients should be observed for malnutrition and vitamin deficiency syndromes. Folate deficiency in dialysis patients is uncommon (149) because routine use of supplements replaces dialysate losses. Prophylactic folate replacement is routine in most dialysis programs because the risk of vitamin B_{12} deficiency is uncommon in dialysis patients. Because of the water solubility of thiamin, pyridoxine, and B_{12}, deficiencies in one or more of these vitamins could develop from dialytic removal but no cases have been reported in dialysis patients. Currently, only pyridoxine supplementation is recommended—5 mg/day for those with progressive renal failure and 10 mg/day for dialysis patients (150).

THERAPY OF RENAL ANEMIA

Overview of Clinical Trials and the Cost of Therapy

Until the advent of epoetin therapy, anemia was considered a relatively minor problem for patients suffering from the many metabolic consequences of failing kidneys and was managed with transfusions or androgens. Treatment of anemia has assumed more importance given the increasing age of the ESRD population; these patients have more frequent and greater degrees of ischemic heart and peripheral vascular disease and are increasingly diabetics with both microvascular and macrovascular disease.

Clinical trials of rhEPO were initiated in 1985 to 1986, and replacement therapy with rhEPO quickly became the most rational therapy for anemia of chronic renal failure (151–154). These initial clinical trials convincingly demonstrated that the Hct could be increased by up to 10 points or more and could be maintained at a level above 30% in more than 90% of patients. Dialysis-treated patients increased their Hct in a dose-dependent manner (Fig. 32.6) (151). Maintenance intravenous (IV) doses needed three times a week to maintain steady-state Hct greater than 31% varied significantly among study patients (153): Fifteen percent require more than 150 U/kg, 20% less than 40 U/kg.

In clinical practice, significant improvement has been made in the management of the anemia (ESRD CPM Project Report 2002). More than 92% of hemodialysis patients and about 60% of Medicare-eligible patients on continuous ambulatory peritoneal dialysis (CAPD) were receiving rhEPO at the end of 1994 (155). Since then both epoetin dose and mean Hb have progressively increased, now reaching the target range of 33% to 38% achieved in clinical trials. As of the last quarter of 2001, mean Hb had reached 11.6 g/dL and epoetin dose exceeded 7,000 U/dose.

The expense of treating almost 90% of ESRD patients in the United States is a federal obligation (156). It has been estimated that total cost for ESRD care to Centers for Medicare & Medicaid Services (CMS) exceeded $8.3 to $8.6 billion in 1994, 8%

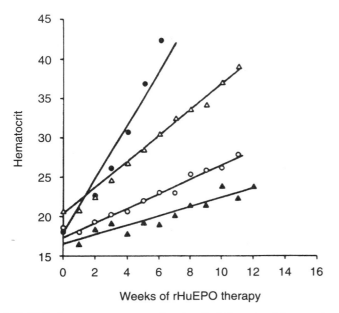

FIG. 32.6. Dose response curve showing that the rate of increase in hematocrit is a function of the administered epoetin dose. (From Eschbach JW, et al. Correction of the anemia of end-stage renal disease with recombinant human erythropoietin: results of combined phase I & II clinical trials. *N Engl J Med* 1987;316:73–78, with permission.)

of which was expended for epoetin (157). There have been many changes in the evolution of payment for epoetin in the United States (12,158–162). Within a few months of epoetin's general introduction, dosing levels for EPO were much lower than expected from the clinical trials (12,158,160). The initial reimbursement options contained financial incentives to constrain expenditures; providers skimped on its use to the detriment of patients' quality of care (162). Following a change in the payment method in 1991, dosing increased but without a corresponding proportional increase in Hct. Payment rewarding additional epoetin use has merely produced higher expenditures not improved anemia management. This lack of Hct response has led CMS through the networks to target anemia control as a health care quality improvement project (161). As a result of this program, iron deficiency in epoetin-treated patients has been largely eliminated. Different aspects of optimizing anemia relative to the current guidelines and targets are discussed in the section on management. A major need is to optimize the anemia management before patients reach the stage of kidney failure requiring dialysis (163).

Benefits, Hazards, and Outcomes of rhEPO Therapy: Transfusion Avoidance

Before epoetin therapy, up to 25% of hemodialysis patients were transfusion dependent (164), receiving up to 0.7 units of packed cells monthly (151–154). Such patients were at risk for iron overload and organ dysfunction. Patients who were iron-overloaded were treated with higher dose epoetin to accelerate iron removal through periodic phlebotomies (165–167). Both magnetic resonance imaging (MRI) (168) and computed tomography (CT) (169) were used to monitor therapy.

Most patients with transfusional iron overload have hemosiderosis, a state with minimal organ dysfunction (170,171), and not hemochromatosis. Even livers that contain more than 1,000 μg iron/100 mg dry tissue (normal is less than 200 μg/100 g dry tissue) show little fibrosis or damage (172). However, an additional reason for avoiding iron overload may be the increased susceptibility of dialysis patients to infection when iron overloaded (173,174). Use of the chelator desferrioxamine may also contribute to this infection risk (175,176).

Following epoetin therapy for the anemia of renal failure, the need for repeated transfusions has been virtually eliminated, and the risk of developing hemochromatosis from transfusions has vanished. In fact, the major problem for ESRD patients on maintenance epoetin therapy is the development of iron deficiency.

Given the infection risks of transfusion [human immunodeficiency virus (HIV), hepatitis C, and perhaps hepatis G] and the sensitization of potential transplant recipients, transfusions should be used prudently. Transfusions should not be withheld from uremic patients with symptomatic or refractory anemia, particularly those with underlying ischemic heart disease, because it takes weeks for epoetin to increase Hct. In situations of gastrointestinal bleeding, postoperative blood loss, or hemolysis, transfusions remain the mainstay of therapy.

Several studies have demonstrated that elimination of transfusions produces a marked reduction in the percentage panel reactive antibody (%PRA) as well as in anti-human leukocyte antigen (anti-HLA) specific antibody titers (177,178). Although blood transfusions are no longer a primary reason for allosensitization, they can increase the %PRA of patients previously sensitized by failed grafts or multiple pregnancies (179). If blood transfusions cannot be avoided, irradiated packed red blood (PRB) cells should be administered.

Hemodynamic and Cardiovascular Effects

The effect on the cardiovascular system and on physical activity is the major benefit correcting the anemia of renal failure. Uncorrected anemia produces a hyperdynamic state that contributes to the development of left ventricular hypertrophy (LVH) in renal failure (180) (see Chapter 17). Correction removes this anemic component but leaves unaffected any components arising from hypertension, hyperparathyroidism, or other structural abnormalities (181,182). Anemia also limits the myocardial oxygen supply, provoking angina pectoris or other ischemic events in those with coronary or peripheral vascular occlusive disease. Anemia and hypertension are, therefore, the major contributors to left ventricular dysfunction and congestive heart failure (182). Unfortunately, correction of anemia is frequently associated with de novo or worsening of hypertension in epoetin-treated patients.

Cardiovascular disease from hypertension and with LVH is a major risk factor for death (181) (see Chapter 17). The prevalence of LVH in ESRD patients starting dialysis may be as high as 73% (183). Anemia contributes to the development of LVH (184), and left ventricular mass and end-diastolic volume increase as compensatory mechanisms (185). The increase in cardiac output during anemia correlates well with the degree of anemia and is reversed when the Hct is increased to higher than 30% (186).

During partial correction of anemia in hemodialysis patients on sustained epoetin therapy, incomplete regression of LVH and volume occur (Fig. 32.7) (184,185,187–189). Mean decrease in left ventricular mass among 15 studies averaged 18% after a mean treatment time of 45 weeks as Hct was increased from an average of 20% to a range of 29% to 35% (189). In general, following rhEPO therapy, cardiac output and index decrease whereas peripheral systemic resistance increases (190). However, the effects on cardiac output are affected by changes in blood volume. If blood volume increases, cardiac output increases (191). In fact, such hypervolemia following correction of anemia can produce negative trends on left ventricular ejection fraction and function (192). To improve cardiac performance, blood volume expansion must be diligently prevented by appropriate changes in estimated dry weight (edema-free weight without hypotension) and by blood pressure control.

Before treatment, anemia produces a hyperdynamic state characterized by increased cardiac output and decreased peripheral vascular resistance (193). The low vascular resistance results from both hypoxic vasodilatation and lower blood viscosity. Reversal of anemia reverses these effects in normal (193) and dialysis individuals (186). Worldwide, new or worsening arterial hypertension develops in a subset of 20% to 40% of treated patients, with the greatest increases affecting daytime systolic and nighttime diastolic pressures (194,195). Increases in periph-

eral resistance range from 15% to 100%. Concomitant decreases in cardiac output vary from 10% to 35% (196–200). Individuals who become hypertensive or have worsening hypertension are unable to adapt to the increase in peripheral resistance by reducing cardiac output. A number of risk factors for this epoetin-induced hypertension have been proposed, including preexisting hypertension, severe anemia at initiation, rapid increase in Hct, high rhEPO doses given intravenously, and the presence of native kidneys.

Epoetin-induced Hypertension

Hypertension following epoetin therapy is likely to be multifactorial in origin (Table 32.1). The increase in peripheral resistance does not correlate with plasma renin activity nor with concentrations of angiotensin I or II (201). This does not exclude the participation of the renin-angiotensin system, because upregulation at the tissue level through increases in mRNA for renin and its substrate is possible (202). Catecholamines also do not correlate with mean blood pressure (203).

Chronic epoetin therapy was initially reported to raise plasma endothelin (ET-1) levels (204,205) and to leave prostaglandins unaltered while decreasing plasma atrial natriuretic peptide by 25% (205). High concentrations of EPO achieved during IV injection, greater than 1,000 mU/mL, increase ET-1 release from ECs in vitro (206). In EC culture systems, EPO directly stimulates EC proliferation as a competence factor and also accelerates ET-1 production in association with stimulation of DNA and protein syntheses (207).

The greater propensity for hemodialysis patients to develop hypertension was attributed to the route of administration. Higher peak EPO levels and, therefore, higher ET-1 levels are achieved in dialysis patients treated with IV compared with subcutaneous (SC) epoetin (204). However, other studies have shown that baseline ET-1 levels before epoetin therapy are elevated, do not increase during therapy, do not differ between the beginning and end of dialysis, and do not correlate with blood pressure

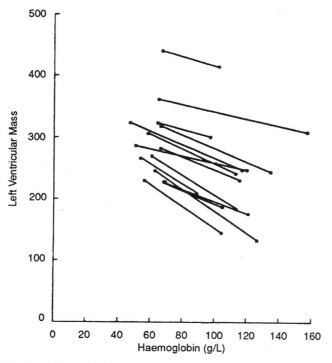

FIG. 32.7. Changes in hemoglobin compared with changes in left ventricular mass, determined by echocardiogram, in 14 patients with baseline left ventricular hypertrophy before starting recombinant human erythropoietin. (From Silberberg J, et al. Regression of left ventricular hypertrophy in dialysis patients following correction of anemia with recombinant human erythropoietin. *Can J Cardiol* 1990;6:1–4, with permission.)

TABLE 32.1. POSSIBLE ETIOLOGIES FOR HYPERTENSION AFTER CORRECTION OF ANEMIA IN ESRD

Lack of hypoxic vasodilation
Failure to downregulate cardiac output
Activation of pressor hormones/adrenergic system
    Renin-angiotensin (tissue level)
    Catecholamines
Increase in endothelin
Increase in vascular smooth muscle contraction
    Through increased cytosolic calcium
    Direct vasoconstrictor effect of rhEPO (?)
Changes in blood viscosity
    Increased whole blood viscosity
    Decreased red blood cell fluidity
Decrease in endothelial-derived relaxing factor (NO) action
    Diversion through binding to hemoglobin (less available)
    Impaired response to NO present
Expanded blood volume and extracellular fluid volume
Modulating effect of uremia
Genetic predisposition

NO, nitric oxide; rhEPO, recombinant human erythropoietin.

(203,208,209). Others have been unable to confirm the original findings of elevated levels following epoetin therapy, finding no changes or decreases in ET-1 levels during chronic EPO therapy (210,211). Thus, the exact role of vasoactive substances in the hypertension of post-EPO therapy remains undefined.

EPO also produces vascular smooth muscle contraction in renal and mesenteric artery preparations, suggesting a direct pressor effect (212,213). However, it does not alter arterial responses to K^+-induced depolarization, angiotensin II, $\alpha1$-agonists, or methoxamine (214). In a double-blind study, no change in arterial blood pressure, heart rate, or plasma ET-1 concentration within 60 minutes relative to the baseline values was observed after either EPO or placebo administration in nine hemodialysis patients (215). These results exclude a rapid effect on blood pressure, heart rate, and ET-1 concentration at therapeutic EPO doses that, when chronically administered, can clearly raise arterial blood pressure in ESRD patients. During SC epoetin therapy, blood levels of EPO are much lower than during IV epoetin therapy, but in our experience the incidence of blood pressure changes does not differ from that during IV therapy.

Loss of hypoxic vasodilatation (216) and changes in blood viscosity (201,217) following correction of anemia have also been postulated to be mechanisms increasing arterial pressure. Whole blood viscosity increases appropriately as Hct increases from 29% to 39%, whereas plasma viscosity remains normal and unchanged (218). Erythrocyte deformability (fluidity) also changes over a 30-week rhEPO treatment period (219). Corresponding to the period of rapid correction of anemia, erythrocyte fluidity decreases but then returns to basal levels during the maintenance phase. The epoetin-induced increase in Hb concentration could theoretically augment vascular resistance by diverting the endogenous vascular relaxation factor, NO (214,220).

Epoetin-induced hypertension usually develops within several weeks to months of starting epoetin therapy as the Hct is rising (200,201); it appears to be a time-dependent consequence of long-term epoetin administration. However, increases in blood pressure do not correlate with the increase in Hct, either in humans clinically (196) or in animals (214), and EPO-induced hypertension can be dissociated from the rise in erythrocyte mass (214,221). In animals, EPO therapy does impair hypotensive response to NO donors, suggesting an impaired vasodilatory response to NO (214). Other studies show that the endogenous NO activity is increased in rhEPO-treated rats, perhaps as a counterregulatory mechanism that limits the pressor effect (222). These observations have relevance to observations that some patients will exhibit severe hypertension with epoetin administration but not with red cell transfusions that produce identical Hct (223). Also, blood pressure remains unchanged in iron-deficient hemodialysis patients whose Hcts are increased from 25% to 32% with simple iron repletion (221).

A number of studies emphasize the important role of adequate control of body fluid and fluid gains in maintaining blood pressure control during epoetin therapy. Maintenance of normal blood volume requires equivalent decreases in plasma volume as red cell mass is increased to avoid changes in preload to the heart. In well-managed patients, measurements of ^{51}Cr-tagged erythrocytes and ^{125}I human serum albumin to measure erythrocyte mass and plasma volume shows that their sum (total blood volume) remains constant during rhEPO therapy (224,225). The importance of blood volume control on blood pressure is emphasized by the following study: in the absence of adjustments in antihypertensive medication, blood pressure remained unchanged in peritoneal dialysis patients but increased by 8 mm Hg in predialysis patients as anemia was corrected (226). Despite equal expansion of the red cell mass, plasma volume decreased in peritoneal dialysis but not in predialysis patients.

Interestingly, it has been observed that a hypertensive response to rhEPO does not occur when epoetin is used to treat other anemias or in nonrenal patients (patients with cancer) treated with epoetin for short or long periods (227–229). Experimental models indicate that rhEPO produces hypertension in a remnant model of renal failure but not in sham control animals (230). Thus, renal insufficiency appears to be a prerequisite for the development of hypertension during rhEPO therapy.

Effects on Survival and Hospitalization

Children are particularly likely to benefit from correction of anemia with epoetin (231,232). In adults undergoing hemodialysis, because anemia limits oxygen supply to the myocardium, it is not surprising that each decrease in Hb of 1 g/dL below 10 g/dL increases mortality by 18% (233). Epoetin therapy with partial correction of anemia has now been documented to improve exercise-induced ST-segment depression (234,235). Others have confirmed the decrease in cardiovascular disease and mortality if Hb is maintained above 10 g/dL with EPO therapy (233). Yang et al. (236) found that each decrease in Hct of 1% was associated with a 14% increase in mortality over a Hct range of 21% to 31%. Similarly, Lowrie et al. (237) found a stepwise increase in mortality as Hct fell below 30%. Individual analysis of a controlled European multicenter trial of the adverse events including death revealed a protective effect of rhEPO in high-risk cardiovascular dialysis patients (238). Some studies indicate that changes in cardiac morphometry and function require up to 1 year of therapy to achieve a maximum result (239).

In addition to beneficial effects on survival of adult dialysis patients, some studies now show a reduction in overall hospitalization in EPO-treated patients (240–242). The mean duration of hospitalization was 8.0 days for the EPO-treated group and 9.6 for the control group (240). For cardiac-related hospitalizations, the difference was 1.6 fewer days per patient-year at risk in EPO-treated patients (240). Fewer hospital days per patient-year at risk were also seen for infectious disease (1.8 days), gastrointestinal disease (1.2 days), and all other causes (4.0 days) (240). Only for hospitalizations related to vascular access complications did the difference favor the control group by 0.9 days (240). The EPO-treated group had 58 hospitalizations compared with 97 in the control group (240). Total costs of care for ESRD patients may, thus, be reduced in the long term through the use of epoetin (243).

Effects on Exercise Tolerance and Rehabilitation

Patients with renal failure typically demonstrate decreased exercise capacity compared with their age-matched healthy compatriots

(244), a decrease that affects many subjective aspects relating to quality of life (QOL). Metabolically, ESRD patients show low muscle mass and energy stores as well as histologic abnormality (245). Resting and exercise blood lactate levels are elevated, whereas oxygen consumption is decreased (246). The ratio of phosphocreatine to inorganic phosphate is lower in ESRD patients, a finding consistent with decreased oxidative metabolism (247). These findings could result from a variety of processes, including enhanced activity of the ubiquitin-proteasome pathway triggered by uremia, from acidosis, from cytokines generated during hemodialysis, or from infections (248).

Aerobic work capacity can be improved through correction of anemia (245–247,249–253). Although some of the benefit accrues from an increase in oxygen carrying capacity (252,253), some of it results from improvement in voluntary muscle function (245) as a result of a possible treatment-induced improvement in muscle oxidative phosphorylation (247). Improvement in exercise capacity during epoetin therapy also results from increased erythrocyte 2,3 DPG levels (254) that permit improved oxygen delivery to tissues (255–257). A variety of muscle functions improve, including voluntary contractions, force generation, and duration of force contraction, as well as histologic improvements in architecture and fiber diameter (244). Resting and maximal exercise-induced blood lactate levels improve (245) associated with improved aerobic metabolism (246).

However, increases in maximal uptake of oxygen are only half of those seen in normal subjects (258), and, in general, improvements in exercise or cardiopulmonary performance that are initially attained when anemia is corrected are not augmented at 1-year repeat testing (235). The increase in oxygen carrying capacity produced by rhEPO is accompanied by a significant reduction in peak blood flow to exercising muscle. This limits the gain in oxygen transport. Even after restoration of Hb, O_2 conductance from the muscle capillary to the mitochondria remains considerably below normal (259). Also, subnormal oxidative metabolism in hemodialysis patients apparently results from limited exchange of metabolites between blood and muscle rather than from any intrinsic oxidative defects in muscle (260).

Only one study has evaluated work capacity with full correction. Correction of anemia was defined as attainment of a Hct of 40% in men and 35% in women, with pretreatment Hct averaging about 30% (261). Sixty percent of patients with corrected anemia rated themselves as having increased energy compared with 42% of subjects with uncorrected anemia. Similarly, work capacity scores increased by one or more units in 61% of those subjects whose anemia was fully corrected compared with only 38% of the rhEPO-treated patients whose anemia was not fully corrected. Changes in work capacity were proportional to rhEPO dose.

It is likely that correction of anemia alone will not maximize exercise capacity and foster rehabilitation. Certainly higher Hcts may improve work capacity (261), but such levels may not be risk free. Even at Hb approaching normal, exercise capacity, although higher, remains subnormal compared with healthy subjects (262). Changes in well-being and physical performance have not generally translated into greater employment (263–265).

The role of anemia correction with regard to "rehabilitation" remains to be adequately addressed (266). The number of ESRD dialysis patients who are rehabilitated is far below the expectations set in 1973 when the ESRD program was started. Optimizing the Hct may only be one component of effective rehabilitation, in conjunction with maintenance or improvement in exercise capacity (267), maintenance of adequate dialysis, and appropriate changes in socioeconomic and health policies (268). Other factors such as deconditioning, neuropathy, and cardiovascular disease probably contribute as well, and programs emphasizing exercise training are needed (266). Poor rehabilitation outcomes in ESRD patients may simply result from initiating therapy for anemia too late in the clinical course of renal failure.

Effects on Quality of Life and Cognitive Functions

The earliest reports indicated that many of the symptoms attributed to uremia were really the result of anemia. Fatigue, cold intolerance, impotence, and mental sluggishness responded to correction of anemia. In patients with ESRD, correction of anemia with rhEPO therapy improves QOL indices, including those assessing global well-being and depression in hemodialysis patients (264) and CAPD patients (269). Renal patients who do not yet require dialysis also show improvement in QOL indices following rhEPO therapy (234,261,270).

QOL involves many aspects (including self-concept, interpersonal relations, and work), and these can be easily overwhelmed by medical problems. It is, therefore, noteworthy that substantial improvements in subjective symptoms were noted in a large double-blind phase II study (271). Clinically, important improvements were noted in fatigue, perceived strength, and global score of the Sickness Impact Profile; smaller degrees of improvement were noted in relationships and depression; and no change was noted in frustration or sleeping abnormalities. Disappointingly, no improvement in activities of daily living (ADLs) occurred with increase in Hct. A phase IV trial of over 1,000 patients receiving epoetin in clinical practice (272) confirmed many of these QOL effects even when a modest mean Hct of only 30.1% was achieved. Four of six domains of the Short Form-36 QOL questionnaire showed improvement.

Whether QOL indicators could be improved further by raising Hct above a level of 36% is currently debated. The data of Moreno et al. (273) indicate that both the Karnofsky functional scale and the Sickness Impact Profile correlate positively with the Hct between 29% and 35%. The Canadian Erythropoietin Study Group (250) could not demonstrate an increase in QOL when Hb was increased from 10.2 to 11.7 g/dL, suggesting that there was a plateau effect. However, Eschbach et al. (274) could show a further increase in QOL by normalizing Hct to 42%.

Improvement in cognition is highly sensitive to the Hct level and improves when anemic Hcts are increased into the 32% to 36% range (275–277). Quantitative electroencephalogram (EEG) and visual-event-related potential improve but do not become normal after partial correction of anemia with epoetin (278). Increasing the Hct to 42% with epoetin further improves brain and cognitive function (279), perhaps because maximum delivery of oxygen to the brain occurs within a Hct range of 40% to 45% (280). The recent report that neuronal cells carry the EPO receptor (281) and that EPO can be produced within the brain in a paracrine fashion is intriguing (282). Perhaps

EPO is needed to protect against hypoxia-induced neuronal damage. Certainly the epoetin doses needed for full correction of anemia are two- to threefold higher and the increased levels may permit EPO to cross into the central nervous system.

Endocrine Changes

Uremic men manifest a variety of biochemical hormonal abnormalities and sexual dysfunction. In general, sexual function improves with correction of anemia (283), but the mechanism producing this improvement is not clear. Initial reports suggested that high prolactin was decreased by correction of anemia (283,284). Correction of anemia also improves responsiveness to thyroid-releasing hormone (TRH) and gonadotrophin-releasing hormone (GnRH) of the thyroidal and gonadal axes, and it is this correction that may be important rather than any EPO levels achieved by therapy (285).

In elderly men, despite a significant erythropoietic response, no significant changes were seen in prolactin, testosterone, luteinizing hormone (LH), follicle-stimulating hormone (FSH), thyroid-stimulating hormone (TSH), free thyroxine, triiodothyronine, and IGF-1 levels (286). Only a small decrease in serum growth hormone concentrations occurred. Advanced age and chronic illness in these patients may have played a role in limiting the hormonal response. In addition, the total immunoreactive levels of gonadotrophins may be misleading, because anemia correction is associated with an increased ratio of bioactive to immunoreactive LH (287).

Metabolic Changes

Several studies have reported a positive nitrogen balance during epoetin therapy (288–290), but this alone does not improve growth in children or alter the abnormalities in amino acid metabolism (290). Decreased total cholesterol associated with a fall in apoprotein B and serum triglycerides followed correction of anemia in one study (291). This is an important observation in view of the risk of atherosclerotic complications in ESRD patients. Diabetic retinopathy improves with correction of anemia (292,293). Raising or maintaining red cell mass in the 33% to 36% Hct range may be effective adjunctive therapy for correcting hypoxia at the level of the retina.

Immune/Granulocyte Function

The incidence of life-threatening infection in ESRD patients over the past two decades has remained unchanged (294–296). Random and chemoattractant-induced granulocyte mobility, adherence, receptor expression, and phagocytosis are reduced in uremic patients (173,297–299). Chronic hemodialysis with complement-activating membranes further attenuates the ability of neutrophils to respond to phagocytic stimuli (300) or to express ¥-selectins (301). Chronic exposure of monocytes to membranes produces refractiveness to further stimuli (302), in part as a result of decreased Fc receptor function (303) and decreased monocyte-dependent IL-2 production by activated T cells (304). The end result is greater infection rates (305,306) with the use of cellulosic membranes.

Correction of anemia with epoetin improves many abnormalities in immune function. Positive changes in the number of natural killer cells and in helper to suppressor T-cell ratios (307), on immunoglobulin production by peripheral mononuclear cells (308), and on phagocytic function (309) occur following correction of anemia with epoetin. Correction of iron overload by epoetin may also be responsible for the observed improvement in phagocytic function (310) but not entirely (309,311).

In addition to granulocyte function, cell-mediated immunity and humoral function improve. Antibody titers to hepatitis B vaccine are eightfold higher in epoetin-treated patients, although the rate of seroconversion is unaffected (312). Cytokine secretion is decreased by anemia and corrected by increasing Hct whether by transfusion or epoetin treatment (313). However, the effect of epoetin on the overall incidence of infection has not been determined.

Miscellaneous Effects

Because of the improvement in QOL and brain function, changes in plasma levels of neuropeptides involved in central nervous system function have been examined. Corticotropin-releasing hormone, delta-sleep-inducing peptide, beta endorphin, methionine-enkephalin, and alpha-melanocyte-stimulating hormone were measured during epoetin-induced correction of anemia (314). Improvements in well-being, mood, and physical fitness occurred as expected, but the levels of the neuropeptides in plasma did not change.

Improvements in the skin circulation have been noted (315) in patients on long-term epoetin therapy, perhaps producing less sensation of being cold. De Marchi et al. (316) reported improvement in pruritus. We and others (317) are unimpressed by changes in pruritus following epoetin therapy.

Correction of anemia with transfusions improves hemodynamic tolerance to fluid removal during dialysis (318). EPO improves anemia, increases blood pressure, and ameliorates orthostatic hypotension in patients with primary autonomic failure (319). It should, therefore, stabilize blood pressure in hemodialysis patients, but there has been no prospective study of this effect.

Effects on Coagulation

Renal insufficiency is associated with a bleeding tendency (116,117) attributed to platelet function abnormalities, characterized by prolonged bleeding time, abnormal platelet aggregation and adhesiveness, and decreased platelet factor 3 release (117,320–322). Platelet adhesion to vessel subendothelium is decreased in dialysis patients (323). It is attributed to a platelet abnormality and a plasma factor that interfere with this process (324). It has been shown that a reversible abnormality in the activation-dependent binding activity of GP IIb-IIIa occurs in uremia and may be the major cause for the altered platelet function (Table 32.2) (119).

Additional coagulative abnormalities contribute to prolonged bleeding. These include abnormalities in the multimeric structure of vWF that affects the initial interaction with GP Ib and the subsequent activation of GP IIb-IIIa (120), a reaction

TABLE 32.2. EFFECTS OF ERYTHROPOIETIN ON COAGULATION

Decreased bleeding time
   Increased red cell number
   Transient increases in platelet number
Platelet reactivity and adhesion
   Increased plasma vWF activity
   Increased fibrinogen
   Decreased intracellular platelet calcium
Procoagulants
   Increased Factor VII and fibrinogen
   Inconsistent changes in protein S and C and antithrombin III

crucial for initiation of platelet thrombi. Uremic plasma also induces NO synthesis by cultured ECs that inhibits platelet function (325).

Following correction of anemia with epoetin, many of the hemostatic abnormalities improve. Both platelet adhesion and bleeding time, which correlates best with occurrence of clinical bleeding (320), are dependent on platelet number whose number are usually sufficient in uremic subjects. Both platelet adhesion and bleeding time are Hct-dependent and are dependent on the degree of anemia. Even before the advent of rhEPO, transfusion of washed filtered RBCs devoid of plasma or other cellular components partially corrected bleeding time and platelet adhesiveness (124). The therapeutic use of rhEPO confirmed that anemia per se was an important cause of the bleeding abnormalities in renal failure patients. The prolonged bleeding time corrects to normal as Hct increases above 30% (123–125,326). Transient increases in platelet count of 25,000 to 40,000 (327,328) occur commonly and seldom exceed normal limits. Changes in platelet reactivity and adhesiveness during epoetin therapy are variable (329–331). Epoetin therapy significantly increases plasma vWF activity, vWF antigen, and fibrinogen, but this effect appears to be indirect (120). Improvement in platelet function is probably more than a simple correction of the anemia (126,332). Uremic platelets do have a defect in intracellular calcium (333) that improves in response to epoetin therapy (332).

Changes in various procoagulant and anticoagulant factors following anemia correction have been inconsistent. Anemic hemodialysis patients have higher total but lower free protein S antigen levels than normal individuals (334). Both the antigen and functional activity of antithrombin III (ATIII) of uremic individuals are significantly lower than those of normal. No laboratory evidence of increased thrombogenesis resulting from reduction of natural coagulation inhibitors has been found in CAPD patients (335) or hemodialysis patients (336) receiving epoetin. Hemodialysis seems to activate synthesis of endogenous anticoagulation factors, because levels of protein C increase significantly and progressively (334,336). An increase in functional protein C reduces thrombosis risk. Partial correction of anemia with EPO does not further affect the levels of this clotting inhibitor during dialysis. During SC epoetin administered at 20 U/kg twice a week for over a year, bleeding time progressively decreased, vWF antigen or ristocetin cofactor did not change, and fibrinogen and factor VIII clotting activity increased (337).

The latter could increase clotting risk. However, another study showed no change in fibrinogen levels, ATIII activity, protein C activity, or protein S concentration by EPO treatment (338).

Whether there is an increased coagulative state following correction of anemia has clinical ramifications. Before epoetin therapy and consistent correction of anemia to a Hct greater than 30%, bleeding manifestations were a major concern. The feared complications included gastrointestinal bleeding (particularly from telangiectasias), pericarditis, hemorrhagic pleural effusions, spontaneous subcapsular hematomas, and spontaneous retroperitoneal bleeding (339). Now the concern is whether excessive thrombosis, particularly of vascular accesses, is or is not a major clinical and economic side effect of EPO therapy.

Thrombosis

Improvement in the bleeding time without change in the routine coagulation tests results primarily from the improvement in RBC mass. Early clinical studies reported that up to 11% of patients experienced clotting of dialyzers or lines following rhEPO therapy (152,250,340,341). As a consequence, hemodialysis heparin requirements increased by up to 50% at final target Hcts of 30% to 38% (153,249,340).

In U.S. studies, there was no apparent trend toward increased access thrombosis at Hcts up to 38% (151,153). Subsequently, small center studies (238,342) followed by larger studies (340,343) suggested an increased access thrombosis risk (see Chapter 4). In the Canadian multicenter trial (344) and one other clinical trial (154), an increased risk for thrombosis was noted. The risk appears to be greater in patients with synthetic bridge grafts (342,343,344) and in patients with previously known access dysfunction (340,345). Native fistulas did not appear to be at risk. However, this whole issue is controversial (346,347).

Thrombosis rate can be kept as low as 0.2 events per patient-year during epoetin therapy by using a vascular accesses surveillance program even while increasing mean Hct from 23% to 33% (348). Intraaccess flow is increasingly recognized as being crucial for the maintenance of access patency (349–353). Intraaccess fistula flow does not appear to change during epoetin therapy, despite the observed increase in whole blood viscosity and of Hcts into the range of 30% to 36% (354–356). Even at Hcts up to 42%, we have been unable to discern a change in access hemodynamics (356). A recent prospective analysis has not shown a risk for excessive thrombosis in epoetin-treated patients when Hcts are maintained in the low 30s (357). It is imperative that access monitoring be conducted on a regular basis to detect problems (358).

Aspirin can reverse the increase in in vitro platelet aggregation that occurs after epoetin therapy (359). The only study evaluating a potential effect of aspirin used a dose of 30 mg/day. No effect on access thrombosis was observed, but bleeding time did not change either (360).

Dialysis Efficiency

After correction of anemia, serum potassium, phosphate, and creatinine increase (361–365), but the magnitude of such changes is small. Aside from a change in the patient's appetite, the major reason for the observed (but inconsistent) effects in chemistries is a decrease in solute clearance. In vivo studies have found changes in dialyzer urea clearances because of a decrease in water flow as red cell mass increases. Clinical effects on the urea kinetic modeling parameter Kt/V are easily adjusted for by changing the dialysis prescription (362,364).

Dialyzer reuse efficiency decreases, despite 15% to 50% increases in heparin dosing (353,365). A recent study of high-flux hemodialysis noted an increase in treatment time from a mean of 140 to 169 minutes as Hct increased from 24% to 36% (366). With peritoneal dialysis, clearances of sodium, potassium, and urea and changes in protein loss or glucose absorption do not change after rhEPO therapy (367).

Other Side Effects

Flulike reactions have been reported in a minority of patients (151,152,154,340). The onset is within hours of administration and usually subsides within 12 hours. Slowing the rate of administration (340) can decrease the symptoms. Therapy is discontinued in less than 1% of treated patients because of this side effect.

SC injection is an effective route of administration. With the use of epoetin alfa, pain resulted from the hypertonic citrate in the formulation (368). Epoetin beta was tolerated better (369,370). Addition of benzyl alcohol to the alfa formulation has increased the tolerance to epoetin alfa in our experience. Using the highest concentration solution to minimize the volume that has to be subcutaneously injected also minimizes pain.

Correction of anemia to Hcts greater than 30% is associated with painless conjunctival injection (151,250). This so-called red eye is of cosmetic concern only.

Frequency of headache varies from 3% to 33%, averaging about 15% of treated patients (151–154,249,250,271,361), and the incidence does not differ from that of untreated or placebo-treated patients (250).

In the initial trials, development of encephalopathy or seizures was not uncommon (151,152,340) and may have resulted from less than optimal control of blood pressure. This is now much less often observed because of better appreciation of the need to control blood pressure during the ramp-up period. In most cases it is not related to the correction of anemia.

Pure Red Cell Aplasia

Development of pure red cell aplasia associated with the presence of neutralizing anti-EPO antibodies was reported in 13 patients from France treated with recombinant EPO (371). This complication, requiring transfusion, followed an initial response to epoetin and occurred after a successful duration or rhEPO use of 3 to 67 months, median 7 months. Of nine evaluable patients, six recovered some erythropoietic function following discontinuation of recombinant EPO, use of immunosuppressive therapy (immune globulin, plasmapheresis, corticosteroids), and/or renal transplantation. Cross reactivity to other epoetins (epoetin beta and darbepoetin) was noted.

Altered antigenicity of the European product (Eprex) because of a difference in manufacturing has been suggested. More than

80 patients with this complication have been noted in Europe, whereas it is rare in the United States (372,373). An intriguing possibility is that the route of administration may be important because this complication has been seen almost exclusively with SC injection. In one patient, wheals developed at the site of SC injection. Skin responses were evoked at the same site following IV epoetin injection indicating persistence of sensitized cells. The aplasia gradually improved following prednisone treatment (374). Recombinant epoetins are known to differ in their carbohydrate content (375), and these may account for the immunogenicity. Even human epoetin is not homogenous in its carbohydrate content by two-dimensional electrophoresis. Studies of recombinant human epoetins show up to 40 protein spots in the appropriate isoelectric and molecular weight ranges. Such techniques may need to be used to provide more homogeneous epoetin preparations (376).

Dosing, Pharmacokinetics, and Route of Administration

Target Hematocrit/Hemoglobin

A consideration of dosing first requires a consideration of the target Hb or Hct. Currently, the recommended target in the United States is a Hb between 11 to 12 g/dL (NKF–K/DOQI guidelines: anemia of chronic kidney disease: II. Target hematocrit/hemoglobin: guideline 4). With rhEPO it is possible to correct to any Hct without good data as to which Hct is optimal. The optimal Hct/Hb during EPO therapy in ESRD patients should be one that maximizes cardiovascular function and ADLs while minimizing risk. An optimal value is difficult to establish because the risk differs among individuals depending on their baseline cardiovascular function and on the presence or absence of cardiac or peripheral vascular disease. Similarly, the definition of what constitutes adequate ADL function may differ significantly in older sedentary patients as compared with younger, more active working or pediatric patients.

The reasons for focusing on the cardiovascular effects of rhEPO therapy are obvious. Cardiac disorders account for about 40% of deaths in ESRD patients (377). Cardiomyopathy, manifested by LVH and dilatation, and ischemic heart disease produce myocardial dysfunction. Optimal correction of anemia should remove any anemic component of this cardiomyopathy, leaving the contributions of structural abnormality (378) unaffected. As discussed previously, partial correction of anemia to a Hct of 30% to 36% produces incomplete reductions in LVH (185,187,188) and in left ventricular volume (185,188) and incomplete improvement in exercise-induced ST-segment depression (234). Complete normalization has been rarely attained except in children, perhaps the residual effect of access fistula shunt flow and myocardial fibrosis. Studies do show that the initial partial regression of LVH reverts after cessation of EPO therapy (379). and that regression to normal limits can be achieved only if anemia is corrected at earlier stages of anemia. The Canadian normalization study failed to prevent ventricular dilatation in patients who already had this complication suggesting that therapy may need to be started at milder stages of anemia.

QOL is closely related to the ability to perform physical ADLs. Reported increases in exercise and work capacity are proportional to the Hct increases but show wide interindividual variation. Few studies have attempted to examine whether additional increments occur as Hct is increased further from the 30s to the normal range (380). Treatment with rhEPO decreases overall hospitalization (240–242). Total costs of care for ESRD patients are also reduced in the long term through the use of rhEPO, in part because of a reduction in cardiovascular-related admissions (243).

The effects achieved by rhEPO therapy have until recently targeted Hcts of 27% to 38%. Different organs respond differently to correction of anemia, an effect that confounds the search for an optimal Hct. A few investigators have investigated outcomes and effects on various organ systems by increasing Hct further to 39% to 45%. Lim (261) reported that energy and work capacity improved more in those who were fully corrected (Hct 35% to 40%) than in those only partially corrected. Barany et al. (262) found that exercise capacity did increase further with normalization of Hb but that the increase remained subnormal compared with rhEPO-treated healthy subjects. Eschbach et al. (274) increased the Hct from a mean of 32.6% to 42.0% and noted significant improvements in cardiac function and exercise capacity. Nissenson et al. (279) found better brain function at Hcts of 42% than at the lower clinical targets of 30% to 36%. On the other hand, a major trial of the effect of normalizing Hct in ESRD patients with coronary artery disease or congestive heart failure was halted without evidence of benefit (381). Higher Hcts alone may not have been responsible for the lack of benefit because a lower mortality was observed with increasing Hcts within each randomized group. This study was severely biased toward the elderly diabetic population. Currently, several trials are underway in Europe to determine whether higher Hb in a more general population of dialysis patients or earlier treatment of the anemia (predialysis) will be beneficial. Studies by Khan et al. (382) indicate that in an outpatient setting, hospitalization risk was associated with lower Hcts.

However, in the absence of clinical studies that define a dose response between Hcts of 30% to 45% on hard end points such as left ventricular mass, cardiac morbidity and mortality, and exercise capacity, the target Hct should be individualized. The real challenge is to determine the optimal Hct in a specific patient. Clearly, the morbidity and mortality data indicate that no patient should have a Hct less than 30% (241,242). Hcts greater than 36% may be beneficial in some. Until such studies are conducted in ESRD patients without cardiac disease, the upper limit for the target Hct should probably not be maintained above those typically achieved in clinical trials, 35% to 38%.

Economic Aspects

Cost and methods of reimbursement are important issues in determining the optimal target Hct. The history of payment for epoetin in the United States illustrates a dynamic evolution. Shortly after its introduction in 1989, conflict developed between marketplace economics and the delivery of socialized medicine for the ESRD population (12). The therapeutic target was initially set at a relatively low Hct of 30% to 33%, and reimbursement policy was based on a fixed payment per dose, without coverage for acquisition or administration costs. Less

than 50% of ESRD patients attained a Hct of 30% or more (158) because the mean dose used in practice, 120 U/kg/week, was only half of that used in clinical trials.

Analysis of fiscal data clearly showed that for-profit, freestanding providers prescribed EPO more often and at smaller doses than nonprofit or government facilities, a pattern consistent with minimizing losses (or maximizing profit) (383). Following implementation of a fee schedule varying with the dose administered, doses increased and Hct progressively increased (160), with the mean approaching 32% in well-managed units. The upper target limit was simultaneously extended to a Hct of 36%. Progressive increments in Hb have occurred since publication of the NKF-DOQI anemia guidelines, interrupted by periodic attempts by governmental agencies and third-party payers to micromanage anemia management.

Now, the major thrust is to meet the anemia management guidelines set forth by CMS in the United States (see the section on integration of anemia management). This is not an easy task because the variance in Hct of six points, 30% to 36%, is one half of that found in a population of normal individuals. In 1996, at a cost of $0.01 per unit and an average of 4,800 U/dose to achieve a mean Hct of 32%, the annual cost in the United States was almost $7,500 per patient-year. Estimated CMS costs for ESRD patients were in excess of $750 million (384). Both have increased with the increases in dosage to achieve higher targets and the rapid growth in the ESRD population.

The target Hct range remains lower, from 28% to 33%, in many parts of the world. In some countries, the net health costs of using epoetin have not been positive. In Canada, the net effect of epoetin use has been an increase in costs estimated to be Can$3425 per patient year of therapy (385). In England, even with the use of a low-dose SC approach, cost analysis similarly yielded a net cost of £1,200/year (386).

Only in the United States has there been evidence of a possible cost saving (243), but all such analyses are sensitive to the assumptions made.

Pharmacodynamics of Response

The initial clinical studies demonstrated that almost all epoetin-treated dialysis patients increase their Hct in a dose-dependent manner (Fig. 32.6). The appropriate dose in a given patient is one that permits attainment of the target Hct over the lifespan of the erythrocyte, because it satisfies both the initiation and maintenance requirements. Fig. 32.8 depicts a desired response. There are two phases, the corrective phase and the maintenance phase during which the same dose of EPO is used. During correction, the Hct increases from 24% to 34% over a period of 100 days. During maintenance, the Hct remains constant as new RBCs are formed at a rate equal to their removal rate. Note that there is significant variation in the Hct from week to week, and dosing changes should not be driven by two- to three-point changes during any 1- or 2-week interval. It is the trend over 4 to 6 weeks that is important.

The response to a given dose of epoetin among patients is variable. In part this variability reflects the observation that, even in normal individuals, a 10-fold variability in endogenous EPO levels among subjects evidently maintains the same normal

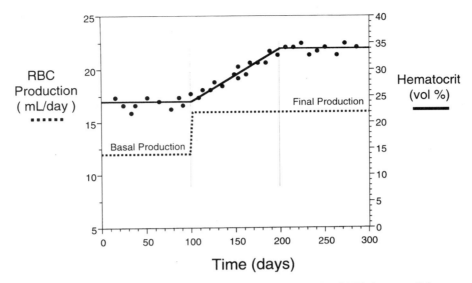

FIG. 32.8. Desired response to epoetin. Starting from a baseline hematocrit of 24%, hematocrit increases progressively and smoothly stabilizes at the desired target of 34% after a period equal to the average red cell survival of 100 days. The dose needed to initiate therapy is the dose needed to maintain hematocrit at target. Note that week-to-week hematocrit variations of three points are common, and 4 to 6 weeks are needed to establish trend. Baseline parameters are a blood volume of 5.0 L and red blood cell survival of 100 days.

red cell mass (387). This variation in EPO levels must indicate significant differences in bone marrow sensitivity among individuals to EPO. In ESRD patients, we (388) and others (153,154) have noted that the IV doses needed to attain a mean Hct of 34% to 35% show this same 10-fold variation, from 25 to 300 U/kg. Obviously, the dose needed for lower target Hb is lower (160), as commonly used by countries with limited resources.

The wide variability in the dose response of the bone marrow to EPO has resulted in the use of different dosing strategies. At one extreme is a dosing strategy that begins with very low doses, 20 U/kg subcutaneously, which are gradually increased to obtain the desired response (389). An intermediate approach uses a mean dose of 60 to 100 U/kg administered intravenously thrice weekly (390).

The clinical dilemma is that the sensitivity of a given patient is unknown at the beginning of therapy. In very sensitive patients, a rapid response will result in the Hct exceeding the target Hct (jeopardizing insurance reimbursement) and could increase the blood pressure and blood volume. By contrast, the less sensitive patients may experience a lag period, during which numerous dose adjustments must be made to initiate a response; this is often clinically frustrating and uneconomical. Presently, it is difficult to predict a dose of EPO required by an individual patient to initiate and maintain effective erythropoiesis. The route of administration may also affect the dose requirement at steady state.

Attempts have been made to use the tools of kinetic modeling to individualize dosing (388,389,391). One such attempt by Uehlenger, Gotch, and Steiner (392) involves the use of nomograms to determine a daily marrow RBC production for a given target Hct and then calculate an EPO dose based on predicted rates of RBC production and marrow sensitivity. The model

assumes mean population values for red cell survival, estimated blood volume, and, most importantly, bone marrow sensitivity to EPO. This procedure does not solve the dilemma of dosage adjustment nor the clinical problems resulting from extensive fluctuations around the desired response. However, the model developed does provide considerable insight into the determinants controlling the response to epoetin.

Epoetin induces an increase in the proliferation and differentiation of precursor cells. In a *steady state,* production and elimination of RBCs is equal. Production and elimination can be expressed as

$$\text{Production } P_{RBC} = S \times EPO$$
$$\text{Elimination } E_{RBC} = RBCm/T$$

where S is the marrow sensitivity (milliliters of RBCs produced per day per milliunits of EPO per milliliter of plasma), EPO is the serum concentration (mU/mL), RBCm is the RBC mass (milliliters of RBCs), and T is the RBC survival in days.

Combining the equations and rearranging yields

$$S = RBCm/T \times EPO$$

Given that the production of RBC at steady state is proportional to sensitivity of the bone marrow and EPO levels, then a response to a given dose should be a function of the variables of RBCm, T, and EPO. Because RBCm = (Hct) × (Blood volume) and if total blood volume and T remain unchanged during therapy, then S becomes proportional to Hct/EPO. Some individuals have termed this ratio the epoetin sensitivity index. How can this model be used?

As illustrated in Fig. 32.8, before epoetin therapy, the daily production of 12 mL of packed RBC maintains a Hct of 24% in an average 70-kg man. Before epoetin, elimination balances production. Elimination/destruction of RBC is a zero-order process in which a constant number of cells are removed daily, independent of the number of cells present. After epoetin administration, production of RBC is increased to 16 mL/day and exceeds the rate of destruction. As a result, RBCs accumulate and increase the percentage of blood volume consisting of red cells. This accumulation increases the Hct until the average RBC lifespan of the individual's cells is reached. The 16 mL of RBC formed T days previously begin to be removed at the same rate as they are being produced. As a result, the Hct abruptly plateaus and a new steady state is reached. In actuality, there is commonly a more gradual leveling off, because not all cells formed previously survive for precisely the same period. The goal of therapy is to attain the desired target Hct between 33% and 36% (Hb between 11 and 12 g/dL) with the least amount of titration of dosage.

The pharmacodynamic model permits analysis of the effect various factors have in response to a given dose of epoetin. An obvious variable is the red cell survival. The shorter the red cell survival, the lower will be the response to a given dose of epoetin if the other variables are constant. This is illustrated in Fig. 32.9. Three patients, each with a starting Hct of 24% and with the same sensitivity to EPO, are treated with the same dose of epoetin. A range of red cell survival varying from 40 days to a normal value of 120 days is depicted. Although red cell survival is generally believed to be short in renal failure, averaging about 60 to 80 days (392–394), it can also be within the normal range (395) in well-dialyzed nonbleeding patients. The patient with a short RBC lifespan of 40 days, whether resulting from hemolysis or external blood losses, never achieves a target Hct of at least 30%. This patient needs an increase in dose and aggressive iron management. The patient with a red cell survival averaging 80 days attains a Hct of 32%. However, the individual with a normal red cell survival may exceed the target Hct of 36%. Note that the plateau occurs in each and every case at the mean survival of the RBCs for each individual.

The relationship between survival of red cells and the response to epoetin is examined in more detail in Fig. 32.10. Although the baseline Hct is 24% in each and every case (bottom edge of the stippled area), the basal production (bottom edge of the black-shaded area) varies inversely with T, being 30 mL of packed cells per day at a T of 40 days, and 10 mL packed cells per day at a T of 120 days. The epoetin-induced increase in RBC production is the same (height of the black-shaded area), 6 mL packed cells per day. The effect on Hct engendered is depicted by the stippled area, with the final Hcts attained indicated by the upper edge. If the Hct in a treated patient plateaus prematurely (<60 days) without reaching the desired target range, it is imperative to determine whether hemolysis or external blood loss is responsible. If the plateau develops after a period of 60 to 80 days, inadequate dose is a more likely explanation for not reaching the target because of a lower sensitivity.

The previous considerations help explain the wide variation in the amount of epoetin needed to maintain Hct in the 32% to 38% range (153,154,388), as illustrated in Fig. 32.11. The epoetin dose needed to maintain Hcts within the six-point spread of 32% to 38% ranges from 12.5 U/kg to more than 500 U/kg given 3 times a week. The modal dose is 75 U/kg/dose. These findings lead to the evidence-based recommendation to initiate therapy with a fixed dose of 50 to 100 U/kg intravenously (390). When administered subcutaneously, the dose needed is frequently lower (see later) and a reasonable starting dose is 80 to 120 U/kg/wk in two to three divided doses.

The effect of variations in bone marrow sensitivity, S, on the pharmacodynamic response to epoetin is shown in Fig. 32.12. The red cell survival is assumed to be equal in three different patients receiving the same dose that increases the RBC production rate by differing amounts. Over the period of T equal to 100 days, one patient exceeds, one patient enters, and the last never attains the target Hct range.

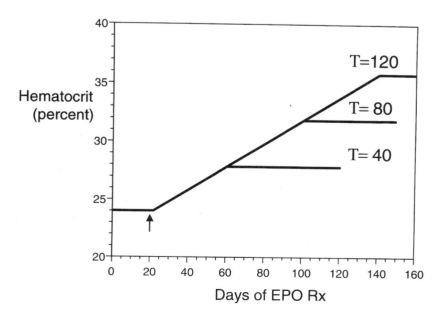

FIG. 32.9. Effect of red cell survival on the pharmacodynamic response to epoetin. A starting hematocrit of 24% is present before therapy and the effect of red cell survivals of 40, 80, and 120 days are compared. Bone marrow sensitivity and epoetin dose are equal for the three cases. In all cases production of red cells is increased by 5 mL packed cells per day from baseline values. Basal production and elimination/destruction rates, however, vary with the survival time (see Fig. 32.13). Note that steady-state hematocrit levels of 27% to 37% are achieved.

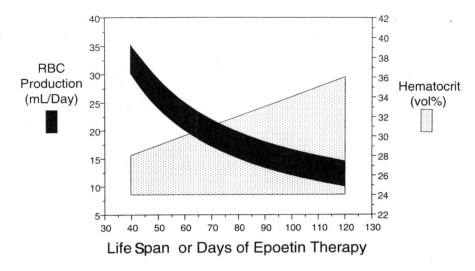

FIG. 32.10. Relationship of baseline survival of red blood cells to production rates and to the response to epoetin. The shorter the red cell lifespan, the greater is the baseline production rate needed to maintain a basal hematocrit of 24% (bottom edge of the *black-shaded* area), and the smaller is the epoetin-induced increase in hematocrit (top edge of *stippled area*).

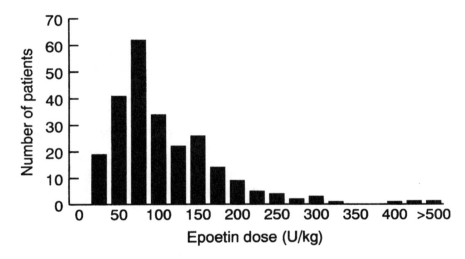

FIG. 32.11. Distribution of epoetin maintenance doses, administered intravenously three times a week to maintain a hematocrit between 32% and 38%. The dose refers to the upper value within each 25 U/kg dose range. (Adapted from Eschbach JW, et al. Recombinant human erythropoietin in anemic patients with end-stage renal disease: results of a phase III multicenter clinical trial. *Ann Intern Med* 1989:111:992–1000.)

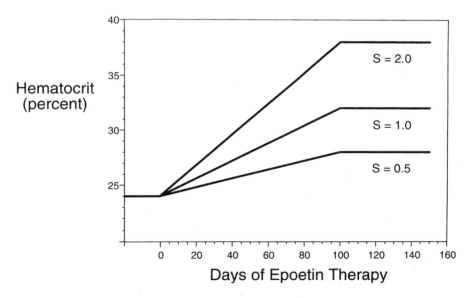

FIG. 32.12. Effect of intrinsic bone marrow sensitivity to epoetin (S) on the pharmacodynamic response to epoetin. For a constant red cell survival of 100 days, a fourfold difference in sensitivity produces final hematocrits varying from 27% to 38%.

Currently there are no readily available methods to predict either the response of any patient or the fraction of patients who will respond adequately to a given dose of epoetin before therapy. Pharmacodynamic modeling allows calculation of an individualized sensitivity by examining the change in Hct over a 6-week period. Over a longer time span of 8 to 14 weeks, red cell lifespan can also be estimated and appropriate adjustments in dose be made to achieve the desired Hct for any patient. Fig. 32.13 shows our results, in which the epoetin-induced increase in red cell production was estimated from pharmacodynamic measurements of red cell survival and blood volume. At any dose varying from 15 to 225 U/kg, three times a week, there is more than a fivefold variation in red cell production. A patient's Hct/Hb must be frequently monitored when initiating therapy, the rate of increase in Hct/Hb over a period of 4 to 6 weeks must be observed, and dosing changes should not be made more frequently than every 4 to 6 weeks unless the Hct increases by more than 1.5 points per week.

We have tried to determine whether the determinants of Hct-baseline/EPO and T could predict response to EPO (396). Red cell lifespan remained constant at 107 to 108 days before and during epoetin therapy (range 60 to 140 days) and was independent of *Kt/V*. The major source of variation in erythropoiesis parameters at baseline resulted from variations in the baseline pretherapy EPO levels. The dose requirements could be predicted from the ratio of Hct to EPO at baseline (*r* = 0.88). Three measurements of baseline EPO are needed to ensure accuracy. These data are promising, but it is premature to apply this method, because differences among EPO assays have not yet been explored.

The response to EPO is independent of the cause of renal failure (340). Some have suggested that those with diabetes respond slower and need higher doses than nondiabetics (397), but this has not been our experience. When the bone marrow is examined, 3 months of epoetin therapy decreases the myeloid to erythroid ratio from a baseline of 4.0 to a value of 2.4. Overall,

marrow cellularity increases (398). Importantly, marrow iron seen at baseline decreases markedly. Low pretreatment fibrinogen (no inflammation) and low baseline transferrin receptor (no ineffective red cell production) associated with 20% increases in receptor during epoetin therapy were the best predictors of response to treatment and achievement of a Hct greater than 30% (399). These measurements unfortunately are not routinely available. Steady-state levels of transferrin receptor, a quantitative measure of erythropoiesis (erythroblast pool of cells, Fig. 32.1), increase progressively and double after 6 to 8 weeks of therapy. When epoetin is discontinued, erythropoietic activity decreases (400).

Pharmacokinetic Considerations

More than 30 years ago, studies using crude preparations of EPO showed that there was a greater effect on red cell production when the EPO was administered in small portions rather than all at once (401,402). It appeared that the response was not dependent on the peak concentration of EPO but rather on the duration of time that EPO levels were maintained above a critical concentration. Our current knowledge of erythropoiesis explains this observation, because cells differentiating under the influence of EPO will undergo apoptosis if the levels decrease below a critical level needed to maintain them.

Many investigators have examined pharmacokinetic aspects of epoetin (388,403–406). Our results are shown in Table 32.3. Following IV administration, 15-minute and 1-hour plasma EPO levels correlate linearly with dose. At 15 minutes, each U/kg increases plasma levels by 19 mU/mL. We found an average apparent IV half-life of almost 7 hours (range 4 to 11 hours) (388). Total clearance averaged 8.0 mL/kg/hour (388), a value that does not differ from that of patients with normal renal function (403,407). The volume of distribution averaged 70 mL/kg, a value twice that of plasma.

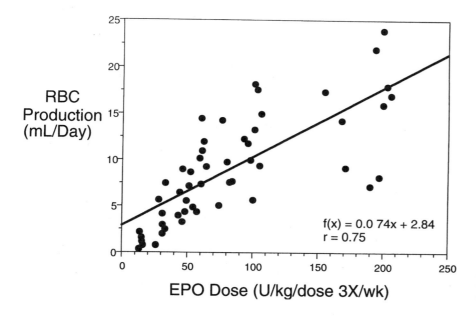

$$f(x) = 0.074x + 2.84$$
$$r = 0.75$$

FIG. 32.13. Relationship of epoetin-induced increase in red blood cell production to epoetin dose given three times a week. The variation in epoetin-induced increase in red cell production at any dose varies more than fivefold.

TABLE 32.3. PHARMACOKINETIC ASPECTS OF EPOETIN

Pharmacokinetic Parameter	Mean ± SEM	Range
Intravenous		
$T_{1/2}$ (h)	6.8 ± 0.3%	4.3–11.3
Clearance (mL/h/kg)	8.0 ± 0.4%	2.9–11.3
V_{dss} (mL/kg)	70.0 ± 5.2%	53–103
C_{max}/Dose	19.1 ± 1.3%	11.2–25.2
Subcutaneous		
Bioavailability (F)	48.8 ± 5.2%	14.5–96.5
T_{max} (h)	22.6 ± 3.4%	8–52
C_{max}/Dose	1.9 ± 0.3%	0.31–4.42

$T_{1/2}$, half-life measured from terminal elimination phase (4–44 h); V_{dss}, volume of distribution at steady state; C_{max}/Unit dose, maximum concentration adjusted for dose; Bioavailability (F), area under the curve for subcutaneous dose as a percentage of intravenous dose.

A variety of studies using radioactive tracers in animals indicate distribution to the bone marrow and spleen (408). The branched structures of the sugar chains are important, because desialiation produces rapid hepatic clearance (64) whereas replacement of the tetrantennary with biantennary sugar chains produces rapid renal clearance (409). Rapid clearance prevents maintenance of plasma levels and delivery of EPO to the target tissue. The only physiologic modulator of the half-life of EPO is the degree of bone marrow erythroid proliferation (410,411).

The temporal profile of subcutaneously administered epoetin differs from that of intravenously administered epoetin (Table 32.3; Fig. 32.14). We found that the bioavailability following SC administration was 48% of the IV dose (range 14.5 to 96.5), and the time to maximum concentration was delayed to 22.6 hours. C_{max}/dose following SC administration was only 10% of that seen after IV dosing. Our pharmacokinetic parameters were obtained following chronic administration of EPO and are similar to those found by others (405,407,412). Other studies indicate that the pharmacokinetic profiles do not change after a year or more of treatment (404).

Initial clinical trials focused on the thrice-weekly IV administration of epoetin in ESRD patients on dialysis. Its use has expanded to predialysis patients with progressive renal failure (413). The pharmacokinetic and pharmacodynamic findings suggest that the cost benefit may be improved by maintenance of EPO levels within a critical range, rather than by very high

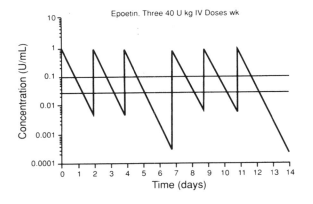

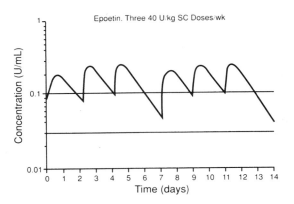

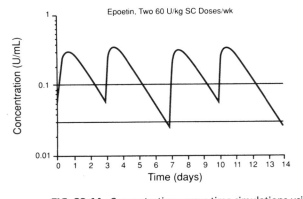

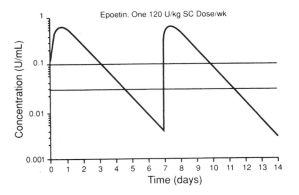

FIG. 32.14. Concentration versus time simulations using different routes and frequencies of epoetin administration. The concentrations represent the increments in EPO levels achieved by a dose of 40 U/kg. The target level is an increase in EPO of 30 to 100 mU/mL. Note that with thrice-weekly intravenous dosing the erythropoietin levels drop below the minimal needed to sustain erythropoiesis. This is not the case with thrice- or twice-weekly subcutaneous administration, although peak levels are much lower. With once a week subcutaneous dosing there are also significant periods of time with subtherapeutic erythropoietin levels. (From Besarab A, et al. Clinical pharmacology and economics of recombinant human erythropoietin in end-stage renal disease: the case for subcutaneous administration. *J Am Soc Nephrol* 1992;2:1405–1416, with permission.)

transient but less sustained levels. We, therefore, compared the pharmacokinetic characteristics of IV versus SC administration (concentration-time profiles) and different dosing strategies.

Typical pharmacokinetic simulations are shown in Fig. 32.14. A dose of 40 U/kg was chosen, representing the lower end of usual maintenance doses. From the pharmacodynamic models, an increase in EPO levels of only 30 to 100 mU/mL (Fig. 32.3) is needed to increase erythropoiesis twofold from baseline. The very high levels achieved immediately after IV administration following usual thrice-weekly IV doses are unnecessary to induce or sustain erythropoiesis in ESRD patients (414). Thrice-weekly IV dosing produces periods within each cycle, particularly in the 3-day interdialytic period, during which EPO levels fall below the critical incremental levels (top left panel of Fig. 32.14). During this period of relative EPO deficiency, some committed but still EPO-dependent cells undergo apoptosis and perish in the bone marrow. The only way to increase trough levels intravenously is to dose more frequently (impractical) or to increase the dose (cost ineffective).

For normal and renal failure patients, our simulations (388) and the studies of others (378, 407, 415–417) indicate that SC administration of epoetin produces a more favorable pharmacodynamic profile than does IV administration, despite incomplete absorption of epoetin. As shown in the upper right panel of Fig. 32.14, with SC dosing, levels are sustained in the interdialytic period. EPO-dependent cells do not perish in this period and this produces more sustained erythropoiesis. When the total dose per week is kept constant, less frequent dosing does produce intervals during which EPO levels fall below target.

The effect of variations in dosing frequency is shown in Fig. 32.15. In our studies, dosing once or twice a week, subcutaneously or intravenously, requires higher total weekly amounts than dosing three times a week (388). The longer half-life of the SC dose probably accounts for the ability to maintain more effective EPO levels at equal frequencies. Although we believe

that, in hemodialysis patients, the dosing period should not be extended beyond 7 days, this is controversial. Administering even smaller doses once a day subcutaneously is even better pharmacodynamically (418,419). Infusion of epoetin subcutaneously to chronic kidney disease (CKD) patients increased Hb by almost 3 g over weeks, whereas the same dose given once weekly produced a much smaller effect.

A wide range in overall absorption (15%–97%) accounts for the relative and variable differences between the two routes of administration in a given patient (388). Some studies have found a mean bioavailability of almost 50% for subcutaneously administered epoetin (388,420,421); others have found lower values in the 16% to 30% range (391,414,422,423). The only head to head comparison found minor and clinically unimportant differences in pharmacokinetics of epoetin alfa and epoetin beta (421). Pharmacokinetics do not change with time (424). Bioavailability may be greater when administered into the thigh, rather than the abdomen or arm (425,426).

It is of some interest for the model of erythropoiesis that patients receiving IV therapy only once a week continue to respond to therapy. Postdose levels exceed 8,000 to 1,000 mU/mL/hour following exceedingly high single doses of 425 U/kg. Enough progenitor cells appear to be stimulated while levels exceed the critical level result and terminally differentiate into a sufficient number of progeny. However, on average the total weekly dose needed to maintain the Hct is nearly double and is not cost effective.

The patient who is a poor absorber may not benefit from SC administration, and this patient's dose may be higher than with IV administration. Also, there are individuals whose endogenous EPO levels for adequate erythropoiesis are relatively high; these patients are more effectively treated intravenously. Most studies indicate that dosage requirements using the SC route are lower by 25% to 50% than those using the IV route (388,397,417,427–433), thus providing greater cost efficiency.

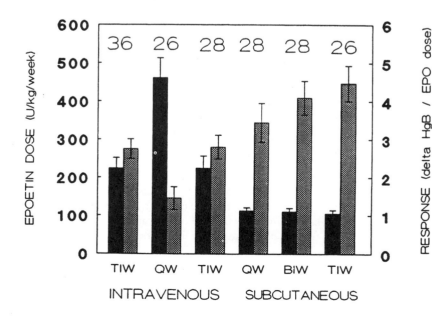

FIG. 32.15. Weekly epoetin dosage requirements *(black bars)* and normalized hemoglobin response *(crosshatched bars)* during sequential three times per week intravenous (TIW); once a week (QW) intravenous; return to three times a week intravenous; then once, twice (BIW), and thrice weekly subcutaneous administration. Hemoglobin is maintained between 10 to 12.5 g/dL and each dosing phase exceeds 90 days. Note that subcutaneous administration at equal frequency produces a 40% reduction in total dose without compromising the hemoglobin. Less frequent dosing, intravenous or subcutaneous, produces progressive increase in epoetin requirements. (From Besarab A, et al. Clinical pharmacology and economics of recombinant human erythropoietin in end-stage renal disease: the case for subcutaneous administration. *J Am Soc Nephrol* 1992;2:1405–1416, with permission.)

Kaufman et al. (434) convincingly proved in a randomized trial the superiority of the SC route. Besarab et al. (435) conducted a metaanalysis of SC versus IV epoetin in hemodialysis patients and concluded that both parallel and crossover studies showed a reduced dosage using the SC route. This could save $996 per patient annually. Although dosing at less than three times a week is frequent, particularly in predialysis or CAPD patients, we are concerned about compromise of cost efficacy.

In predialysis patients and those on some form of peritoneal dialysis, the preferred route of epoetin administration is SC. The IV route is inconvenient and costly in these patients. There is absolutely no need to switch routes when patients initiate on or switch to hemodialysis. Because of the easy availability of the IV route in hemodialysis patients, were it not for economic constraints epoetin would always be administered intravenously. However, the Dialysis Outcome Quality Initiatives committee recommends the SC route in all patients to satisfy the considerable pressure in the United States to reduce the dosage of this increasingly expensive drug.

Now that dead-space syringes and multidose 20,000 U vials are available, it is no longer necessary to adjust the dose to the nearest unit dose vial; thus, the volume injected subcutaneously can be kept low, reducing the degree of patient discomfort. If the IV route is used, it should be given during dialysis via the venous port downstream of the venous drip chamber (436). Administering the drug via the drip chamber traps up to 30% of the drug. Inappropriate handling to maximize the yield from each vial has been associated with an outbreak of *Serratia liquefaciens* bacteremia (437). Such pooling of epoetin alfa vials is inappropriate

Intraperitoneal administration is not recommended. Bioavailability is low (2%–12%), producing much lower serum levels than either IV or SC administration (412,420,422). Absorption of epoetin from the peritoneum seems to be the limiting factor when administered within the dialysate (412). About 80% of the administered dose is recovered in the peritoneal effluent at the end of a standard 4-hour dwell (68). Absorption is enhanced after intraperitoneal administration into a "dry" abdomen, but this interrupts dialysis (438).

Management of Anemia with Epoetin

Integration of Pharmacodynamic and Pharmacokinetic Principles

The variation among patient weekly epoetin needs is up to 10-fold when epoetin is administered thrice weekly. This variation is determined by differences in the patient's own intrinsic characteristics. Although some of the variation may arise from non-bone-marrow-dependent factors that influence red cell survival (e.g., red cell lifespan), the major portion reflects differences in bone-marrow responsiveness to the hormone. Different levels are needed to produce the necessary number of cells in otherwise comparable individuals. In addition, the models of erythropoiesis stress the importance of maintenance of sustained, moderately increased EPO levels during therapy. Thus, from a physiologic standpoint, the most effective route for epoetin therapy is frequent SC administration.

The dose needed to correct anemia is generally unknown in a given individual. Whether given intravenously or subcutaneously, the dose is affected by dosing frequency. The initial dose required is one that will attain the target Hct within a 2- to 4-month period (the lifespan of the RBC) by inducing a steady sustained increase in erythropoiesis. Fig. 32.16 presents data from Fig. 32.6 redrawn in a way that allows refinement of the dose. For example, if the desired increase in Hct is known to be 12 points and a mean RBC lifespan of 80 days is presumed, then the rate of rise needed is 0.15 points per day or 1.05 per week (Table 32.4). Usually the desired increase is smaller or slower and starting doses of 50 to 60 U/kg given three times a week are commonly used. The average dose from Fig. 32.16 is 75 U/kg intravenously three times a week. IV doses are typically up to a third higher than those used subcutaneously, and the dose is typically 80 to 100 U/kg/week divided among two or three doses. We discourage dosing at less frequent intervals in hemodialysis patients. Similarly, although less than three-times-a-week dosing has been found to be effective in both hemodialysis (430) and CAPD (439–441) patients, we believe that available data indicate compromise of cost effectiveness in a population of patients (although a few individual patients may benefit).

Because it is not possible to predict an individual's response, it is necessary to monitor each patient to optimize the dose (Table 32.4). In the presence of adequate iron stores, the goal is to obtain a 0.5- to 1.0-point increase in Hct per week. Therefore, during the induction phase Hct or Hb should be monitored weekly. More frequent monitoring is unnecessary. Adjustment should be made every 4 to 6 weeks.

Erythropoietic data suggest that changes in the erythroid compartments vary considerably in intensity and speed of response to epoetin therapy (400). The erythroblast pool is quantitatively the most important but also the slowest to respond. Drug dosage, therefore, should not be drastically lowered during the induction period or after reaching the target Hct because this produces a yo-yo or Ping-Pong effect. Dose modification should be performed gradually and in stages, because the full effect will not be seen for several months. A complete RBC lifespan must pass before the effect of a change in dosage can be fully assessed.

We advocate changes in epoetin of 25% to 30% of previous weekly dose or 10 U/kg/dose when titrating down for a Hct rise in excess of 1.5 points/week. The dose should be held only in the very rapid responder whose Hct rises more than two points per week or in those who develop difficult to control hypertension. In most patients, blood pressure can be managed effectively by reducing the dry weight followed by adding or increasing an antihypertensive agent if necessary. Only if these approaches fail to control hypertension should one consider holding or markedly reducing the dose of EPO.

Once a patient reaches the target Hct/Hb, the frequency of Hct or Hb monitoring can decrease. We favor monitoring every 2 weeks over monthly because of the variation in Hct that can occur unrelated to changes in Hb or RBC count and because of variations in interdialytic weight gain. In our experience the average patient has a standard deviation of 1.0 g/dL in the Hb level when measured over the course of a year. Changes in plasma volume change the Hct without changes in red cell mass.

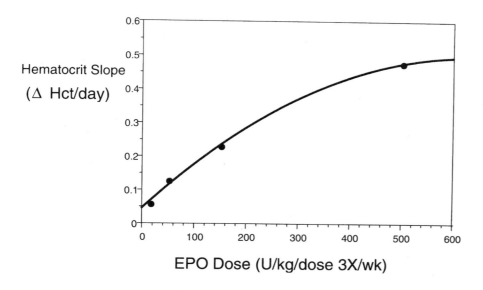

FIG. 32.16. Dose response curve showing the change in hematocrit per day at doses used in a major clinical trial. This figure can be used to estimate the intravenous dose needed to achieve a desired increase in hematocrit over a specified interval. Subcutaneous doses are one-third lower when given three times a week.

TABLE 32.4. PROTOCOL FOR CORRECTING ANEMIA

Step 1. Determine target hematocrit, and measure starting hematocrit
- Target hematocrit is 35%
- Starting hematocrit is 23%

Step 2. Determine rate of rise in hematocrit/day, assuming the red cell survival is 60–100 days
- 12 points over 12 weeks = 1.0 hematocrit point per week = 0.15 points per day

Step 3. Use Fig. 32.16 to determine the intravenous dose of epoetin needed given three times a week
- IV dose = 75 U/kg. In 70-kg patient, dose is rounded off to 5,000 U[a]
- Subcutaneous dose is 2/3 of IV dose and rounded off to 3,000 U three times a week

Step 4. Assure adequate iron availability for increased erythropoiesis (see Table 32.5)

Step 5. Measure hematocrit weekly to determine the dose
- Do not alter the dose for the first 6 weeks
- Use hematocrits from weeks 2–6 to determine increase in hematocrit per week

Step 6. If the hematocrit response is <1 point per week, increase the dose by 25%
- In this case, increase dose to 6,500 U IV or 4,000 U SC
- If the hematocrit response is greater than 1.5 points per week, decrease dose by 25%
- In this case, decrease dose to 3,500 U IV or 2,000 U SC

Step 7. Wait 4 more weeks and determine the hematocrit response. Project the hematocrit out to 12 weeks from the time of previous adjustment. Will hematocrit reach 33% to 36% at 12 weeks at this current dose?
Yes: Leave the dose unchanged
No: Will not reach Hct of 30%; increase the current dose by 25% (8,000 U IV, 5,000 U SC)
No: Will exceed Hct of 36%; decrease current dose by 25% (2,500 U IV, 1,500 U SC)

Step 8. Measure hematocrit weekly

Repeat steps 7 and 8 until hematocrit does not vary over a span of 4 weeks (steady state)

Monitor patient for iron deficiency, intercurrent resistance, or any other cause of epoetin resistance

[a]All doses should be rounded to the nearest 500 U if possible.

Samples should be collected just before the dialysis session. End dialysis samples will show a significant increase in Hct of up to six points because plasma volume is decreased at the end of hemodialysis, causing an increase in Hct (442). Hb and Hct increases by a g/dL and by three points, respectively, following dialysis (443). These increases from predialysis values correlated with percent change in body weight (ultrafiltration). At 24 hours following dialysis, Hct and Hb levels persisted at higher levels indicating slow reequilibration. The importance of this observation is that patients with Hct greater than 38% or Hb levels above 13 g/dL may be at risk from hemoconcentration effects particularly if they have large interdialytic weight gains. Samples can be collected at any time in peritoneal dialysis patients because the plasma volume is relatively constant during any given day; however, care should be taken to ensure the same posture.

Predictors of Response

Clinically, the earliest response to epoetin is an increase in reticulocyte count that can be seen within a week of initiating therapy (444). The corrected reticulocyte count correlates well with the change in the erythron transferrin uptake, but the increase in reticulocyte count poorly predicts the subsequent changes in Hct (445). Changes in reticulocyte count are transient, peaking at about 2 weeks then declining to levels approximately 1.5 to 2.0 times baseline. In general, a lag period of approximately 1 to 2 weeks is observed before Hb or Hct begins to increase following initiation of or a change in epoetin dosage. It is common to note dramatic decreases in the serum iron indices following onset of epoetin-induced erythropoiesis (446) and a tendency toward microcytosis (447) over the first month. Iron-deficient patients should be repleted before epoetin therapy. In general, studies of reticulocyte counts or transferrin receptors are not clinically useful, and the response can be more than adequately followed by examining sequential changes in Hct.

Optimizing the Response

Traditionally, the treatment of anemia of ESRD patients focused on blood loss and iron deficiency. These remain basic focuses, along with provision of adequate dialysis, avoidance of aluminum overload, and control of hyperparathyroidism. After more than a decade, reimbursement for epoetin in the United States is based on Hct levels and Hb levels. Hb levels are more reproducible. Hct can be factitiously increased by storage of blood samples at room temperature for more than 4 to 6 hours (448). The Core Indicator Project mandated by CMS in 1997 established a very tight range of Hcts (Fig. 32.17). On the one hand, the fraction of patients who have a Hct of less than 30% after 90 days of therapy with epoetin was mandated to be less than 15%. On the other hand, payment for epoetin administered in the third month of therapy would be denied if the rolling average for the previous 3 months exceeds 36.5%. This mandate resulted from the increasingly larger fraction of patients exceeding a Hb of 12 g/dL or Hct of 36%. Most dialysis centers responded by holding epoetin doses, thus inducing neocytolysis of recently formed cells. This contributed to the yo-yo effect. Subsequently, dialysis units adapted by decreasing the epoetin doses by 20% on a monthly basis and allowing for gradual return of over-target Hb levels. Although not enforced by all carriers, this Hct maintenance audit is still in effect.

The current concern is whether this policy will produce a reversal in the gains made over the past decade. Whether a tight enough distribution can be achieved that does not decrease the mean Hct/Hb remains to be determined. Achieving a tight distribution will require close attention to three facets of care: iron management, adequate dialysis, and close surveillance for inflammatory conditions. Of these, iron is the most important.

Newer Epoetins

The current standard of care is to administer epoetin two to three times per week. In practice in patients with CKD, this schedule of administration is achieved mainly in patients receiving hemodialysis, because of the three times weekly dialysis schedule. In patients receiving peritoneal dialysis and in patients in the predialysis stage, it is generally given once weekly, because of the less frequent contact between patient and caregiver and the inconvenience of frequent SC administration. The recommended dosage in all these patient groups is still three times weekly, however.

Current evidence indicates that erythropoiesis can only be maintained when levels of EPO are above a critical level, below which erythroid cells undergo apoptosis (33). Frequent dosing, however, places a considerable burden on health care staff and patients. Studies of EPO carbohydrate isoforms in animals demonstrated a positive relationship between the sialylated carbohydrate content of EPO and its half-life (that the higher the carbohydrate content, the longer the half-life) and in vivo biologic activity (449). Darbepoetin alfa (Aranesp, Amgen Inc., Thousand Oaks, California), a novel erythropoiesis stimulating protein (NESP), was developed as a longer acting erythropoietic agent using site-directed mutagenesis. It has two additional carbohydrate chains. It has been shown to have a threefold longer terminal elimination half-life compared with epoetin (25 vs. 8.5 hours) when administered IV and approximately twice as long (49 hours) when administered subcutaneously (450). The molecule was approximately 3.6-fold more biologically active than epoetin when each molecule was administered three times per week and 13 to 14 times as active when injected once a week (449). Darbepoetin does not accumulate over time when given repeatedly.

Clinical studies indicate that dosage interval can be increased using darbepoetin (451) when equal amounts of drug are used. Dialysis patients who were successfully maintained on epoetin were effectively and safely switched to darbepoetin alfa therapy when administered at a reduced dosing frequency compared with epoetin (452). All darbepoetin alfa patients receiving once-weekly dosing and 95% of patients assigned to once every other

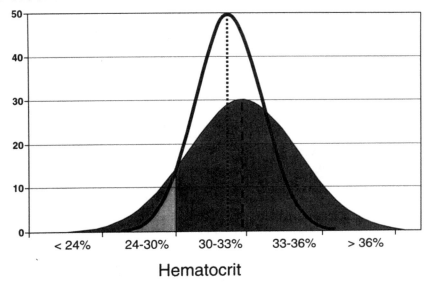

FIG. 32.17. Theoretical distribution curves of the fraction of patients attaining specified hematocrits during epoetin therapy. In clinical practice, 10% of patients have hematocrits greater than 36%, and 15% to 20% have hematocrits less than 30% (*shaded area* under wide distribution curve). Mean hematocrit approaches 33% (*bold dashed vertical line*). Avoidance of hematocrits greater than 36% (distribution curve shown as *solid line*) may cause a decrease in the mean hematocrit of the population (*dashed vertical line*).

week dosing were successfully maintained at their target Hb at these reduced dose frequencies (453). Twenty-eight of 34 patients were maintained with every 3-week dosing (454). Darbepoetin alfa is, thus, effective for correcting and maintaining Hb levels at once weekly, once every other week, and once every 3 weeks dose intervals. The need for fewer injections reduces the discomfort and burden on patients and reduces the number of times patients have to visit the clinic for injections. This is particularly important in rural areas, where the distances that patients have to travel can be substantial. The consistently predictable pharmacokinetic and efficacy profiles may also allow for less frequent testing of Hb levels. Darbepoetin alfa is well tolerated and has a safety profile comparable to that of epoetin.

An increase in the biologic half-life of epoetin can also be created by pegylating the molecule. Such pegylation increases the terminal half-life of the molecule to more than 50 hours administered IV and to almost 100 hours when administered SC.

Iron Management

The typical adult diet contains about 15 mg elemental iron per day, of which only 10% is absorbed. Obligate gastrointestinal losses of 1 to 2 mg per day occur. Additional losses of 6 to 7 mg of iron occur from trapped blood in the dialyzer and bloodlines. Usual annual iron losses in hemodialysis patients without other blood losses are about 2 g (in excess of normal total body stores of iron of approximately 1.2 g).

Dialysis patients have an increased frequency of clinical and subclinical gastrointestinal bleeding (455). Up to 7% of stable dialysis patients have a guaiac-positive stool when three consecutive stool specimens are analyzed (456). In the setting of other sources of blood loss such as gastrointestinal bleeding, menstruation, or surgical losses, yearly iron deficits of up to 6 to 8 g have been documented (145). Blood loss is further accentuated by hospitalization, where an average of 15.7 and 65 mL blood per day are taken from general medicine and intensive care unit patients, respectively (457). Therefore, the physician must review the necessity of blood tests and determine the minimal volume of blood needed for all tests, implement a plan assuring collection of the minimal amount of blood, and maximize the return of blood to the patient at the end of dialysis.

Suboptimal response to rhEPO commonly results from failure of an adequate delivery of iron to the erythron. Enhanced iron utilization resulting from EPO-induced RBC formation can quickly deplete iron stores. Although oral iron preparations remain the most common means to maintain iron stores (458,459), they frequently fail in hemodialysis patients. The USRDS Dialysis Morbidity and Mortality Study showed that 50% of patients receiving epoetin were iron deficient (460). Because erythropoiesis has to be stimulated to a greater than normal degree to compensate for blood losses and or shortened red cell survival, functional iron deficiency frequently develops.

Although a nomogram constructed by Van Wyck (461) can be used to estimate iron needs when correcting anemia, we prefer to calculate the amount on the basis of 1 mg of iron needed for each 1 mL of packed RBC; estimated weekly blood losses are summarized in Table 32.5. The increase in packed cells is estimated from the starting and target Hcts and the estimated blood

TABLE 32.5. PROTOCOLS FOR CALCULATING IRON NEEDS DURING CORRECTION OF ANEMIA AND AFTER ATTAINING TARGET HEMATOCRIT

Basic principles
- One mg of iron needed for each 1 mL of packed red blood cells (PRBCs) formed.
- Ongoing weekly losses of iron are at least 40 mg/week (range 25–100).
- Utilization of parenteral iron is approximately 80%–90% (iron dextran).

Correction phase

Step 1. Calculate the amount of packed red blood cells in mL (588) to be formed during anemia correction = mg iron needed for increased red cell mass.

(Desired Hct – Starting Hct) × Weight in kg × 70 mL/kg/100

Example: 70-kg person starting at Hct of 23% with desired target of 35% (35 – 23) × 72 × 70/100 = 588 mL PRBCs = 588 mg iron

Correction = 588/0.85 = 691, 700 mg

Step 2. Estimate the amount of iron lost over the period of anemia correction.

Interval = Red cell lifespan = 12 weeks

Iron lost = 14 × 40 = 560 mg

Correction = 588/0.85 = 660, 700 mg

Step 3. Determine serum ferritin level.

If ferritin >800 ng/mL, give only the amount needed to correct anemia.

100 mg once per week × 7 weeks = 700 mg

If ferritin <800 ng/mL, give the total amount of iron needed to correct anemia and replace ongoing stores.

100 mg per treatment × 2 weeks changing to 100 mg/wk for 8 weeks = 1,400 mg

Step 4. Check the iron indices monthly during the correction phase. Adjust iron as necessary.

Maintenance phase

Step 1. Give 25–100 mg of parenteral iron per week.

Step 2. Check iron indices monthly to quarterly.

Step 3. Adjust dosage to maintain a TSAT of 25%–50% and ferritin of 200–800 ng/mL.

Notes
- All iron dextran doses are given shortly after initiating dialysis and all iron studies are drawn prior to dialysis.
- CAPD patients have lower ongoing blood losses and usually no convenient IV access. As needed, they receive a single infusion of 500 to 1,000 mg iron dextran over 3 to 6 hours.
- Test dose of iron is used only with the very first dose of iron given.

CAPD, continuous ambulatory peritoneal dialysis; TSAT, transferrin saturation.

volume of the patient (70 to 80 mL/kg body weight). Ongoing blood losses during the period of correction are estimated at 600 to 700 mg of additional iron. The amount of iron dextran needed is corrected by 0.85 to compensate for less than 100% use of parenterally administered iron into red cells. The exact dosing then depends on whether the patient is iron replete (unusual in most patients starting dialysis) and unlikely to develop relative iron deficiency, using ferritin greater than 800 ng/mL as cutoff value for the iron-replete state.

During induction therapy in patients with ferritin less than 800 ng/mL, the total amount of iron is administered intravenously as 100 to 125 mg at each dialysis treatment for the first 2 weeks, changing to weekly doses thereafter. This prevents relative iron deficiency in the early stage yet avoids redistribution of the administered iron into tissue stores. Iron-replete patients receive only the amount of iron needed to correct the red cell mass as 62.5 to 125 mg weekly doses until the desired amount is given. Regular monitoring of iron status by measurement of serum ferritin and transferrin saturation (TSAT) is mandatory in the cost-effective management of anemia with epoetin and should be performed monthly.

In our experience, it is difficult for most dialysis patients to take more than 130 mg of elemental iron orally per day and avoid gastrointestinal intolerance. Our typical in-center hemodialysis patient invariably requires parenteral iron. As a result, once the maintenance period is reached, we have preferred to use a maintenance protocol of 25 to 125 mg of iron intravenously weekly, the dose adjusted in response to sequential iron indices. CAPD patients require less iron because of smaller ongoing blood losses. In most cases, administration of 500 or 1,000 mg slowly over 4 to 6 hours is sufficient, and adequate response can be maintained for 6 months to 1 year.

In traditional intermittent dosing regimens, IV iron dextran is given when TSAT or ferritin fall below 20% and 100 ng/mL, respectively. A number of studies have indicated that iron-replete patients receiving regular parenteral iron maintain better serum ferritin levels and require less recombinant human epoetin than patients receiving no parenteral iron supplementation or regular oral iron alone (462–468). Seven studies have shown an average increase in Hct of 14% with a concomitant decrease in epoetin doses of 38% by administering a prorated weekly dose of iron. In general, patients in these studies were considered to be iron replete because their TSAT exceeded 24% and ferritin ranged from 200 to 600 ng/mL.

In our own studies we have evaluated a maintenance regimen in which an initial iron dextran dose of 300 to 500 mg was followed by 25 to 100 mg every 1 to 2 weeks (to maintain a transferrin saturation between 30% and 50%) compared with a traditional intermittent dosing regimen (to maintain a transferrin saturation >20% or a ferritin level >200 ng/mL). The amount of recombinant EPO required in the maintenance group was more than 50% lower than that used in the intermittent group to achieve the same target Hb of 10 to 11 g/dL (469). In addition, adequate monitoring of iron indices could be performed weekly in those administered a maintenance regimen of less than 100 mg per week. With such a dosing regimen, it is not necessary to wait at least 2 weeks after the last iron dose to assess iron indices. An even more aggressive iron regimen was found to reduce epoetin also. Forty-two chronic dialysis patients were administered parenteral iron for 4 months to achieve a TSAT between 20% to 30% and a Hb concentration of 9.5 to 12.0 g/dL. They were then randomized to either 6 months of IV iron at a dose of 25 to 150 mg/week (control group) or to four to six doses of iron (100 mg) given over 2 weeks (to increase the TSAT to 30%), followed by 25 to 150 mg of iron weekly for 6 months to maintain a transferrin saturation between 30% and 50% (470). Although both regimens maintained adequate Hb levels, 40% less EPO was required in the high TSAT group. However, this regimen produced progressive elevations in serum ferritin level to an average of 730 ng/mL at month six with an average monthly iron administration of 400 mg/month, twice that in the control group. We have an arbitrary ceiling for ferritin of 1,000 ng/mL, above which parenteral iron is not used.

Currently iron dextran is used extensively in the United States, although other forms of iron are now available (463,466,467). Sodium ferric gluconate complex administered over eight consecutive dialysis days in equally divided doses for a total amount of 1.0 g significantly increased Hb levels (an increase of 1.3 g/dL at 30 days), serum ferritin, and iron saturation in 83 iron-deficient dialysis patients (471). Sodium ferric gluconate complex in sucrose may have fewer fatal adverse reactions than iron dextran and it's relatively as good or better than iron dextran (472). Cost-effectiveness may be the only factor preventing it from being preferred over iron dextran for most patients because it is one-third more expensive.

Iron sucrose (iron saccharate, Venofer), is also available (473). Administration of 200 mg/month of this formulation significantly increased Hct levels in 73 dialysis patients (of whom 64 were chronic hemodialysis patients (474). It also has been used as pulse therapy to correct iron deficiency (475). In these studies, iron sucrose was well tolerated, without any reported immediate or delayed reactions. Both sodium ferric gluconate complex (472) and iron sucrose (476) have been administered to iron-dextran allergic patients.

Some studies have indicated that more frequent administration of iron in smaller doses may also improve erythropoiesis. Administration of 6.25 to 21.3 mg of sodium ferric gluconate complex at every treatment compared with 62.5 mg every 1 to 4 weeks increased Hb levels and prevented an increase in ferritin levels (477). Administration of iron during each dialysis was also studied using a novel delivery system. Dialysis with a solution containing soluble ferric pyrophosphate, a chelated iron that readily diffuses into the blood compartment, was found to be safe and effective in a preliminary 6-month study of stable hemodialysis patients (478).

Controversy exists about the best method of assessing adequate iron stores and iron delivery to the bone marrow. The time-honored tests have been TSAT and serum ferritin. Although significant variation in the serum TSAT has been reported to arise from diurnal changes in the serum iron, this has not been a major problem in dosing patients receiving dialysis in the morning compared with those in the evening. Of more concern is the inability of either a TSAT greater than 20% or a serum ferritin greater than 100 ng/mL to reliably indicate absolute or functional iron deficiency (462,463,467,479–481). The latter occurs during epoetin therapy when the erythroid marrow responds and iron is removed from transferrin faster than the reticuloendothelial cell can release it to transferrin. As a result, the response lags or the epoetin dose needed to obtain the desired Hct is higher than it should be. In addition both ferritin and plasma transferrin are acute phase reactants. Thus, the degree of variation in TSAT and ferritin over time may be large without reflecting iron delivery or stores.

Other techniques have been sought to evaluate functional iron deficiency. These include protoporphyrins (482,483) and the percentage of hypochromic cells (484,485). In our opinion, these are probably of no greater use in clinical practice than the combined measurement of both TSAT and ferritin (486). A new method that measures the Hb content of reticulocytes holds greater promise (487), because the reticulocyte reflects bone marrow events affecting Hb synthesis within the previous several days. This test is in its third generation and was recently found to be useful and more sensitive in diagnosing iron deficiency (488).

Many physicians are concerned about the risks of using parenteral IV iron dextran. The incidence of severe life-threatening reactions to one or more doses in any patient is low, at less than 1% (489,490). The rate per number of injections is even lower at 0.1%. Decreasing the infusion rate to less than 10 mg/minute minimizes reactions.

Occasionally, patients are clearly iron overloaded but respond poorly to and require large doses of epoetin. Several options exist. Ascorbic acid, 500 mg given intravenously after hemodialysis one to three times a week, can mobilize tissue stores (491). Although serum ferritin remained unchanged, TSAT increased from 27% to 54 % and Hct increased from 27% to 32%. A control group with normal iron status and without resistance to EPO showed no changes in TSAT or Hct when challenged in the same manner with ascorbate. An alternative method uses desferrioxamine in patients with iron but without aluminum overload. Epoetin doses decreased dramatically from 400 to 25 U/kg while increasing Hb levels to and then maintaining them at 11 g/dL (492).

Iron overload has become uncommon with the decrease in transfusions. The persistent blood losses in hemodialysis patients can, over several years of epoetin treatment, produce iron deficiency even in those with initial serum ferritin greater than 5,000 ng/mL. It is now rare for any patient to be treated with phlebotomy after overdriving the bone marrow with epoetin (166,493,494).

Adequate Dialysis

It has been a clinical observation for more than three decades that many patients experience an increase in Hct values within 3 to 6 months of initiating dialysis (132,495–497). This can occur despite a decrease in EPO levels (497). In some patients, this effect is so profound that epoetin doses started before dialysis are markedly reduced or discontinued. Results of the National Cooperative Dialysis Study (498) found a lower Hct and a greater need for transfusions in patients whose dialysis was adjusted to keep their BUN high (low *Kt/V*). The beneficial effect of dialysis may operate through effects other than removal of inhibitors, such as improved nutrition, a decrease in inflammatory/infectious processes in well-dialyzed patients, less blood loss (by correction of uremic platelet dysfunction), or by improvement in RBC lifespan.

A recent study has demonstrated that increasing the dose of dialysis improves the response to epoetin (499) and that dialysis adequacy explains some of the variation in Hct among dialysis centers (500). Thus, the presence of still unidentified uremic toxins may reduce the erythropoietic effectiveness of rhEPO. Although the effect of these toxins can be easily overcome by increasing the amount of rhEPO administered, again it is more cost effective to provide adequate dialysis and to use the lowest epoetin dose necessary to achieve the target Hct. Recently studies have indicated improved iron utilization and less resistance to epoetin after patients on regular hemodialysis were transferred using on-line hemodiafiltration (501,502). The mechanism is

unclear but it may be related to the differential movement of non-protein-bound and protein-bound uremic solutes using the two differing dialysis techniques. Daily dialysis, reported to improve anemia management in dialysis patients, not only reduced non-protein-bound solutes but some protein-bound solutes as well (503).

The recent observation that IGF-1 can increase EPO-independent erythroid colony formation in an animal model of chronic renal failure (504) suggests important roles for other growth factors in the genesis of the anemia of renal failure, as well as the promise for therapeutic synergy effects of growth factors.

Resistance to Epoetin

Resistance to epoetin is defined as the requirement of a large dose during initiation (>150 U/kg three times a week) or the development of refractiveness to a previous efficacious dose with dosage escalation to maintain a target Hct. Biologic heterogeneity—variation in intrinsic sensitivity and in red cell survival—accounts for many instances of patients who require more than 450 U/kg/week to reach and then maintain a Hct greater than 30%. This was clearly proven in six patients who required large doses of epoetin to maintain their target Hct, but in whom studies of erythroid refractoriness, red cell survival, epoetin pharmacokinetics, PTH, and aluminum failed to disclose a reason for their large dose needs (505). Our experience is similar; about 10% of our patients need more than 450 U/kg/week of epoetin in the absence of any known state producing resistance.

At least nine separate conditions can produce epoetin resistance (506–508):

- *Absolute and relative iron deficiency* is the most common condition and has already been discussed. Blood loss should always be suspected in those requiring increasing doses or large maintenance doses of IV iron.
- *Infection and inflammation* is the second most common condition, and responsiveness can usually be restored on recovery. Inflammatory mediators may arise from the underlying process (27,509–511) or from hemodialysis (512). Key agents are TNF and IL-1 (506,513–515). Patients with failed transplants returning to dialysis frequently are resistant to epoetin (516) until the transplant is removed. Peritonitis in CAPD patients usually produces temporary impairment, but on occasion prolonged refractiveness may be seen (517,518). Chronic infection may be difficult to diagnose such as those associated with failed arteriovenous vascular access grafts (519).
- *Hyperparathyroidism* (143) is a less common cause, in which the relationship is between the degree of fibrosis and the amount of epoetin needed to maintain a target Hct. Serum levels of PTH do not correlate with epoetin dose.
- *Aluminum overload* has become a much less common cause of epoetin refractiveness (520–523) as non-aluminum-containing phosphate binders have increasingly replaced aluminum-containing agents.
- *Hemoglobinopathies* produce relative resistance. Experience in sickle cell disease has been disappointing (524,525). Therapy

of thalassemia requires prolonged high-dose epoetin therapy (526–528).

- Patients with *multiple myeloma* on dialysis also require higher dose epoetin (529).
- *Cofactor deficiency* can develop in patients who were initially responsive to epoetin. Evaluation of folate and vitamin B_{12} is needed in select cases (530–532). Macrocytosis is an inadequate differentiating feature.
- Hemolysis can be induced by residual *formaldehyde* in dialyzers, producing epoetin refractiveness (533). Patients with severe hemolysis across heart valves can require transfusions, despite use of large doses of epoetin (534). Emergence of EPO antibodies has been documented (370–374,535).
- *Malnutrition* is associated with low serum albumin levels that in turn are associated with low Hcts among dialysis patients. Malnutrition can be quickly worsened by inflammation (536). Acute phase reactants correlate with resistance to epoetin (537).

Response of Hemodialysis Compared with CAPD Patients

Many patients on CAPD can maintain higher Hcts than hemodialysis patients, whether they are just starting dialysis or transferring from hemodialysis (132,538–540). An increase to normal only occurs in those with the highest EPO levels (132). Partial amelioration occurs through a combination of increased red cell mass and decreased plasma volume (539). The National CAPD Registry found the average Hct in epoetin-untreated CAPD patients to be 29.4% with a median of 29% (540), values higher than those found in hemodialysis patients before the advent of epoetin (498).

CAPD patients have been shown to have a good response to epoetin (541–544). Indeed, they seem to require less epoetin to achieve a comparable Hct or have a higher Hct at comparable epoetin doses when compared with hemodialysis patients (543,545). Two reasons are probably responsible. First, CAPD patients are less deviated from their dry weight than are the hemodialysis patients when bloods are drawn; dilution of RBC mass is smaller. Second, the blood losses from the hemodialysis procedure effectively decrease red cell survival, and thus a higher production rate is needed to maintain the same Hct.

Modifiers of Erythropoiesis

Androgens

With the advent of rhEPO therapy, the use of anabolic steroids alone has been largely abolished. Two recent papers have explored the use of androgens along with rhEPO. One found synergy between epoetin and nandrolone decanoate with few side effects (546); the other found no synergy and many side effects (547). A third study found that the use of androgens in men younger than 50 years was as effective as epoetin and less costly (548).

In view of the known side effects of androgen therapy, particularly in women, its use alone or in combination with epoetin is not encouraged.

Carnitine

Some reports indicate that carnitine can improve epoetin response (549,550). More data are needed, because the study sample sizes have been extremely small. However, response to epoetin did correlate with serum carnitine levels (551).

Transfusions

Transfusions have been relegated to the treatment of acute episodes of symptomatic hypoxia. They should not be given if symptoms or signs are unlikely to be reversed by RBC transfusion (552).

Miscellaneous Considerations

Angiotensin-converting Enzyme Inhibitors

Angiotensin-converting enzyme (ACE) inhibitors have been used to control erythrocytosis, particularly that occurring after renal transplantation (553–555). Although some reports suggest that ACE inhibitors can decrease response to epoetin (556–560), others do not (561,562). In view of the importance of ACE inhibitors for cardiac remodeling and antihypertension treatment in hemodialysis patients, ACE inhibitor therapy for blood pressure control or heart failure should not be withheld to minimize epoetin dosage. The receptor antagonist losartan does not appear to change any indicator of erythropoiesis in normals and should be studied in ESRD patients receiving epoetin on dialysis (563).

Malignancy

Malignancy is frequently accompanied by increasing anemia. Larger doses of epoetin should be used, because patients without renal insufficiency frequently require larger doses than those received by patients with progressive renal insufficiency (564).

Intolerance to Subcutaneous Epoetin

Using small injection volumes with benzyl alcohol preservative in the stock epoetin vials (20,000 U/mL) minimizes intolerance to SC epoetin.

Intraperitoneal Epoetin

Intraperitoneal epoetin can be effectively used in small children by infusion of epoetin in 50 mL of fluid into a dry abdomen (565,566).

Intercurrent Illness or Surgery

Erythropoietic response is reduced during intercurrent illness or surgery. Our policy is to continue the epoetin therapy throughout the intercurrent illness. We generally stop the therapy after renal transplantation. Because EPO production may be delayed, particularly in the presence of delayed graft function, epoetin can reduce the need for postoperative transfusion; however, the amount of epoetin needed to maintain Hct levels is twofold greater than the amount needed before transplant (567).

REFERENCES

1. Bright R. Cases and observations, illustrative of renal disease accompanied with the secretion of albuminous urine. *Guys Hosp Rep* 1836; 1:338–379.
2. Remuzzi G, et al. Hematologic consequences of renal failure. In: Brenner BM, et al., eds. *The kidney.* Philadelphia: WB Saunders, 1995:2170–2176.
3. Carnot P, et al. Sur l'activite hematopoietizue de serum au cours de la regeneration du sang. *CR Seances Acad Sci (Paris)* 1906;143:384–386.
4. Brown GE, et al. The anemia of chronic nephritis. *Arch Intern Med* 1922;30:817–820.
5. Bonsdorff E, et al. A humoral mechanism in anoxic erythrocytosis. *Acta Physiol Scand* 1948;16:150–170.
6. Erslev AJ. Humoral regulation of red cell production. *Blood* 1953;8:349–357.
7. Erslev AJ. Blood and mountains. In: Wintrobe MM, ed. *Blood, pure and eloquent.* New York: McGraw-Hill, 1980:257–318.
8. Jacobson LO, et al. Role of the kidney in erythropoiesis. *Nature* 1957; 179:633–634.
9. Erslev AJ. In vitro production of erythropoietin by kidneys perfused with a serum-free solution. *Blood* 1974;44:77–85.
10. Fried W. Erythropoietin. *Ann Rev Nutr* 1995;15:353–77.
11. Gordon MS. Managing anemia in the cancer patient: old problems, future solutions. *Oncologist* 2002;7:331–341.
12. Besarab A, et al. Evolution of recombinant human erythropoietin usage in clinical practice in the United States. *ASAIO J* 1993;39:11–18.
13. Besarab A, et al. Defining a renal anemia management period. *Am J Kidney Dis* 2000;36[Suppl 3]:S13–S23.
14. Buemi M, et al. Erythropoietin and the brain: from neurodevelopment to neuroprotection. *Clin Sci* 2002;103:272–282
15. Junk AK, et al. Erythropoietin administrations protects retinal neurons from acute ischemia-reperfusion injury. *Proc Natl Acad Sci U S A* 2002;99:10659–10664.
16. Quesenberg P, et al. Hematopoietic stem cells. *New Engl J Med* 1979;301:755–760.
17. Ogawa M, et al. Renewal and commitments to differentiation of hematopoietic stem cells: an interpretive review. *Blood* 1983;61: 823–829.
18. Ogawa M. Differentiation and proliferation of hematopoietic stem cells. *Blood* 1993;81:2844–2853.
19. Krause DS, et al. CD34: structure, biology, and clinical utility. *Blood* 1996;87:1–13.
20. Spivak JL, et al. Cell cycle-specific behavior of erythropoietin. *Exp Hematol* 1996;24:141–150.
21. Gregory CG, et al. Three stages of erythropoietic progenitor cell differentiation distinguished by a number of physical and biological properties. *Blood* 1978;51:527–537.
22. Kannourakis S, et al. Fractionation of subsets of BFU-E from normal human bone marrow: responsiveness to erythropoietin, human placental-conditioned medium, or granulocyte-macrophage colony-stimulating factor. *Blood* 1988;71:758–765.
23. Gregory CJ. Erythropoietin sensitivity as a differentiation marker in the hemapoietic system: studies of three erythropoietic colony responses in cell culture. *J Cell Physiol* 1976;9:289–301.
24. Sawada K, et al. Human colony-forming units-erythroid do not require accessory cells but do require direct interaction with insulin-like growth factors 1 and/or insulin for erythroid development. *J Clin Invest* 1989;83:1701–1709.
25. Krantz SB. Erythropoietin. *Blood* 1991;77:419–433.
26. Faquin WC, et al. Effect of inflammatory cytokines on hypoxia-induced erythropoietin production. *Blood* 1992;79:1987–1994.
27. Means RT, et al. Inhibition of human erythroid colony-forming units by tumor necrosis factor requires beta interferon. *J Clin Invest* 1992; 91:416–419.
28. D'Andrea AD, et al. Expression cloning of the murine erythropoietin receptor. *Cell* 1989;57:277–285.
29. Wrighton NC, et al. Small peptides as potent mimetics of the protein hormone erythropoietin. *Science* 1996;273:458.
30. Klingmüller U, et al. Specific recruitment of SH-PTP1 to the erythropoietin receptor causes inactivation of JAK2 and termination of proliferative signals. *Cell* 1995;80:729–738.
31. Leyland-Jones B. Evidence for erythropoietin as a molecular targeting agent. *Semin Oncol* 2002;29[Suppl 11]:145–154.
32. Chu X, et al. Erythropoietin modulates calcium influx through TRCP2. *J Biol Chem* 2002;(Jul 11).
33. Koury MJ, et al. Erythropoietin retards DNA breakdown and prevents programmed death in erythroid progenitor cells. *Science* 1990; 248:378–381.
34. Stephenson JR, et al. Induction of hemoglobin-synthesizing cells by erythropoietin in vitro. *Proc Natl Acad Sci U S A* 1971;65: 1542–1546.
35. Adamson JW, et al. Analysis of erythropoiesis by erythroid colony formation in culture. *Blood Cells* 1978;4:89–103.
36. Rice L, et al. Neocytolysis on descent from altitude: a newly recognized mechanism for the control of red cell mass. *Ann Intern Med* 2002;134:710–712.
37. Goldwasser E, et al. Purification of erythropoietin. *Proc Natl Acad Sci* 1971;68:697–698.
38. Miyake T, et al. Purification of human erythropoietin. *J Biol Chem* 1977;252:5558–5564.
39. Lai P-H, et al. Structural characterization of human erythropoietin. *J Biol Chem* 1986;261:312–316.
40. Jacobs K, et al. Isolation and characterization of genomic and cDNA clones of human erythropoietin. *Nature* 1985;313:806–810.
41. Bondurat M, et al. Anemia induces accumulation of erythropoietin mRNA in the kidney and liver. *Mol Cell Biol* 1986;6:2731–2733.
42. Beru N, et al. Expression of the erythropoietin gene. *Mol Cell Biol* 1986;6:2571–2575.
43. Lin FK, et al. Cloning and expression of the human erythropoietin gene. *Proc Natl Acad Sci U S A* 1985;82:7580–7584.
44. Naets JP. Erythropoiesis in nephrectomized dogs. *Nature* 1958;181: 1134–1135.
45. Caro J, et al. Erythropoietin levels in uremic nephric and anephric patients. *J Lab Clin Med* 1979;93:449–458.
46. Radtke HW, et al. Serum erythropoietin concentrations in anephric patients. *Nephron* 1978;22:331–365.
47. Bachmann S, et al. Co-localization of erythropoietin mRNA and ecto-5'-nucleotidase immunoreactivity in peritubular cells of rat renal cortex indicates that fibroblasts produce erythropoietin. *J Histochem Cytochem* 1993;41:335–345.
48. Maxwell PH, et al. Identification of the renal erythropoietin-producing cells using transgenic mice. *Kidney Int* 1993;44:1149–1162.
49. Loya F, et al. Transgenic mice carrying the erythropoietin gene promoter linked to lacZ express the reporter in proximal convoluted tubule cells after hypoxia. *Blood* 1994;84:1831.
50. Donnelly S. Why is erythropoietin made in the kidney? The kidney functions as a critmeter. *Am J Kidney Dis* 2001;38:415–425.
51. Ratcliffe PJ, et al. Regulation of the erythropoietin gene. *Nephrol Dial Transplant* 1995;10[Suppl 2]:18.
52. Egrie JC, et al. The molecular biology of erythropoietin. In: Erslev AJ, et al., eds. *Erythropoietin—molecular, cellular, and clinical biology.* Baltimore: The Johns Hopkins University Press, 1991:21–40.
53. Beck I, et al. Enhancer element at the 3' flanking region controls transcriptional response to hypoxia in the human erythropoietin gene. *J Biol Chem* 1991;266:15563–15566.
54. Semenza GL, et al. Hypoxia-inducible nuclear factors bind to an enhancer element located 3' to the human erythropoietin gene. *Proc Natl Acad Sci U S A* 1991;88:5680–5684.
55. Madan A, et al. A 24-base-pair sequence 3' to the human erythropoietin gene contains a hypoxia-responsive transcriptional enhancer. *Proc Natl Acad Sci* 1993;90:3928–3932.
56. Madan A, et al. Regulated basal, inducible, and tissue specific human erythropoietin gene expression in transgenic mice requires multiple cis DNA sequences. *Blood* 1995;85:2735–2741.
57. Semenza GL, et al. A nuclear factor induced by hypoxia via de novo protein synthesis binds to the human erythropoietin gene enhancer at a site required for transcriptional activation. *Mol Cell Biol* 1992;12: 5447–5454.

58. Beck I, et al. Characterization of the hypoxia-responsive enhancer in the human erythropoietin gene shows presence of a hypoxia-inducible 120 KD nuclear DNA-binding protein in erythropoietin-producing and non-producing cells. *Blood* 1993;82:704–711.

59. Wang GL, et al. General involvement of hypoxia-inducible factor 1 in transcriptional response to hypoxia. *Proc Natl Acad Sci* 1993;90:4304–4308.

60. Wenger RH. Cellular adaptation to hypoxia: O2-sensing protein hydroxylases, hypoxia-inducible transcription factors, and O2-regulated gene expression. *FASEB J* 2002;16:1151–1162.

61. Wiesner MS, et al. Erythropoietin tumours and the von-Hippel-Lindau gene: towards identification and mechanism os and dysfunction of oxygen sensing. *Nephrol Dial Transplant* 2002;17:356–359.

62. Recny MA, et al. Structural characterization of natural human urinary and recombinant DNA-derived erythropoietin. *J Biol Chem* 1987;262:17156–17163.

63. Wang FF, et al. Some chemical properties of human erythropoietin. *Endocrinology* 1985;116:2286–2292.

64. Dube S, et al. Glycosylation at specific sites of erythropoietin is essential for biosynthesis, secretion, and biological function. *J Bio Chem* 1988;263:17516–17521.

65. Zaroulis CHG, et al. Serum concentration of erythropoietin measured by radioimmunoassay in hematologic disorders and chronic renal failure. *Am J Hematol* 1981;11:85–92.

66. Koury ST, et al. Quantitation of erythropoietin producing cells in kidneys of mice by in situ hybridization: correlation with hematocrit, renal erythropoietin mRNA, and serum erythropoietin concentration. *Blood* 1989;74:645–651.

67. Jelkmann W. Erythropoietin: structure, control of production, and function. *Physiol Rev* 1992;72:449–489.

68. Eckard K, et al. Distribution of erythropoietin producing cells in rat kidneys during hypoxic hypoxia. *Kidney Int* 1993;43:815–823.

69. Erslev AJ. Erythropoietin. *N Engl J Med* 1991;324:1339–1344.

70. Ratcliff PJ. Molecular biology of erythropoietin. *Kidney Int* 1993;44:887–904.

71. Fried W, et al. Observations on the regulation of erythropoietin production and of erythropoiesis during prolonged exposure to hypoxia. *Blood* 1970;36:607–616.

72. Fried W, et al. Regulation of the plasma erythropoietin level in hypoxic rats. *Exp Hematol* 1984;12:706–711.

73. Radtke HW, et al. Serum erythropoietin concentration in chronic renal failure: relationship to degree of anemia and excretory renal function. *Blood* 1979;54:877–884.

74. Kominami N, et al. The effect of total nephrectomy on hematopoiesis in patients undergoing chronic hemodialysis. *J Lab Clin Med* 1971;78:524–532.

75. Loge JP, et al. Characterization of the anemia associated with chronic renal insufficiency. *Am J Med* 1958;24:4–18.

76. Aherne WA. The "burr" red cell and azotemia. *J Clin Pathol* 1957;10:252–257.

77. Gurney CW, et al. The physiologic and clinical significance of erythropoietin. *Ann Intern Med* 1958;49:363–370.

78. Walle AJ, et al. Erythropoietin-circuit hematocrit feedback circuit in the anemia of end-stage renal disease. *Kidney Int* 1987;31:1205–1209.

79. Ross R, et al. Erythropoietin response to blood loss in hemodialysis patients is blunted but preserved. *ASAIO J* 1994;40:M880–M885.

80. Chandra M, et al. Serum immunoreactive erythropoietin levels in patients with polycystic kidney disease as compared with other hemodialysis patients. *Nephron* 1985;39:26–29.

81. Besarab A, et al. Dynamics of erythropoiesis following renal transplantation. *Kidney Int* 1987;32:526–536.

82. Eckard K-U, et al. Erythropoietin in polycystic kidneys. *J Clin Invest* 1989;84:1160–1166.

83. Chaplin H, et al. Red cell life-span in nephritis and in hepatic nephrosis. *Clin Sci* 1953;12:351–360.

84. Eschbach JW, et al. Erythropoiesis in patients with renal failure undergoing chronic dialysis. *N Engl J Med* 1967;276:653–658.

85. Hocken AG. Haemolysis in chronic renal failure. *Nephron* 1982;32:28–35.

86. Shaw AB. Haemolysis in chronic renal failure. *BMJ* 1967;2:213–216.

87. Lonergan ET, et al. Erythrocyte transketolase activity in dialyzed patients: a reversible metabolic lesion of uremia. *N Engl J Med* 1971;284:1399–1403.

88. Cole CH. Decreased ouabain-sensitive adenine triphosphatase activity in the erythrocyte membrane of patients with chronic renal disease. *Clin Sci* 1973;45:775–784.

89. Izumo H, et al. Erythrocyte Na, K pump in uremia: acute correction of a transport defect by haemodialysis. *J Clin Invest* 1984;74:581–588.

90. Welt LG, et al. An ion transport defect in erythrocytes from uremic patients. *Trans Assoc Am Physicians* 1964;77:169–171.

91. Cheng JT, et al. Mechanism of alteration of sodium potassium pump of erythrocytes from patients with chronic renal failure. *J Clin Invest* 1984;74:1811–1820.

92. Joske RA, et al. Isotope investigations of red cell production and destruction in chronic renal disease. *Clin Sci* 1956;15:511–522.

93. Ragen PA, et al. Radioisotope study of anemia in chronic renal disease. *Arch Intern Med* 1960;105:518–523.

94. Berry ER, et al. Effect of peritoneal dialysis on erythrokinetics and ferrokinetics of azotemic anemia. *Trans Am Soc Artif Intern Organs* 1965;10:415–419.

95. Ortega O, et al. Significance of high C-reactive proteins levels in predialysis patients. *Nephrol Dial Transplant* 2002;17:1105–1109.

96. Erslev AJ, et al. The rate and control of baseline red cell production in hematologically stable uremic patients. *J Lab Clin Med* 1995;126:283–286.

97. Rosenwund A, et al. Oxidative injury to erythrocytes, cell rigidity, and splenic hemolysis in hemodialyzed uremic patients. *Ann Intern Med* 1975;82:460–465.

98. Eaton JW, et al. Chlorinated urban water: a cause of dialysis-induced hemolytic anemia. *Science* 1973;181:463–464.

99. Tipple MA, et al. Illness in hemodialysis patients after exposure to chloramine contaminated dialysate. *ASAIO Trans* 1991;37:588–591.

100. Manzler AD, et al. Copper-induced acute hemolytic anemia: a new complication of home dialysis. *Ann Intern Med* 1970;73:409–412.

101. Petrie JJB, et al. Dialysis anaemia caused by sub acute zinc toxicity. *Lancet* 1977;1:1178–1180.

102. Short AIK, et al. Reversible microcytic hypochromic anemia in dialysis patients due to aluminum intoxication. *Proc Dur Dial Transplant Assoc* 1980;17:233–236.

103. Carlson DJ, et al. Methemoglobinemia from well water nitrates: a complication of home dialysis. *Ann Intern Med* 1970;73:757–759.

104. Orringer EP, et al. Formaldehyde-induced hemolysis during chronic hemodialysis. *N Engl J Med* 1976;294:1416–1420.

105. Said R, et al. Acute hemolysis due to profound hypo-osmolality: a complication of hemodialysis. *J Dial* 1977;1:447–452.

106. Schuett H, et al. Hemolysis in hemodialysis patients. *Dial Transplant* 1980;9:345–347.

107. Keshaviah P, et al. *Investigation of the risks and hazards associated with hemodialysis systems.* Silver Springs, MD: U.S. Department of Health and Human Services: Public Health Service/Food and Drug Administration/Bureau of Medical Devices, 1980.

108. Francos GC, et al. An unsuspected cause of acute hemolysis during hemodialysis. *Trans Am Soc Artif Intern Organs* 1983;24:140–145.

109. Iacob HS, et al. Acute hemolytic anemia with rigid red cells in hypophosphatemia. *N Engl J Med* 1971;285:1146–1150.

110. Neiman RS, et al. Hypersplenism in the uremic hemodialyzed patient. *Am J Clin Pathol* 1973;60:502–511.

111. Bischel MD, et al. Hypersplenism in the uremic hemodialyzed patient. *Nephron* 1972;9:146–161.

112. Bommer J, et al. Silicone induced splenomegaly: treatment of pancytopenia by splenectomy in a patient on hemodialysis. *N Engl J Med* 1981;305:1077–1079.

113. Hartley RA, et al. Splenectomy for anemia in patients on regular dialysis. *Lancet* 1971;2:1343–1345.

114. Longnecker RE, et al. Blood loss during maintenance hemodialysis. *Trans Am Soc Artif Intern Organs* 1974;20:135–138.

115. Lindsay RM, et al. Dialyzer blood loss. *Clin Nephrol* 1973;1:29–34.

116. Hassanein AA, et al. Relationship between platelet function tests in normal and uraemic subjects. *J Clin Invest* 1970;23:402–406.

117. Rabiner SF. Uremic bleeding. *Prog Hemost Thromb* 1972;1:233–250.

118. Clouse RE, et al. Angiodysplasia as a cause of upper gastrointestinal bleeding in uremia. *Arch Intern Med* 1985;145:458–461.

119. Benigni A, et al. Reversible activation defect of the platelet glycoprotein IIb-IIIa complex in patients with uremia. *Am J Kidney Dis* 1993; 22:668–676.

120. Gralnick HR, et al. Plasma and platelet von Willebrand factor defects in uremia. *Am J Med* 1988;85:806–810.

121. Savage B, et al. Modulation of platelet function through adhesion receptors. A dual role glycoprotein IIb-IIIa (integrin aIIbb3) mediated by fibrinogen and glycoprotein Ib-von Willebrand factor. *J Biol Chem* 1992;267:11300–11306.

122. Di Minno G, et al. Platelet dysfunction in uremia: multifaceted defect partially corrected by dialysis. *Am J Med* 1985;79:552–559.

123. Livio M, et al. Uraemic bleeding: role of anaemia and beneficial effect of red cell transfusions. *Lancet* l982;2:1013–1015.

124. Fernandez F, et al. Low hematocrit and prolonged bleeding time in uraemic patients: effect of red cell transfusion. *Br J Haematol* 1985;59:139–148.

125. Moia M, et al. Improvement in the haemostatic defect of uraemia after treatment with recombinant human erythropoietin. *Lancet* 1987;2:1227–1229.

126. Cases A, et al. Recombinant human erythropoietin treatment improves platelet function in uremic patients. *Kidney Int* 1992;42: 668–672.

127. Fisher JW. Mechanism of the anemia of chronic renal failure. Editorial review. *Nephron* 1980;25:106–111.

128. Ohne Y, et al. Inhibitors of erythroid colony-forming cells (CFU-E and BFU-E) in sera of azotemic patients with anemia of renal disease. *J Lab Clin Med* 1978;92:916–923.

129. Moriyama Y, et al. Studies on an inhibitor of erythropoiesis II. Inhibitory effect of serum from uremic rabbits on heme synthesis in rabbit bone marrow cultures. *Proc Soc Exp Biol Med* 1975;148:94–97.

130. Wallner SF, et al. The effect of serum from patients with chronic renal failure on erythroid colony growth in vitro. *J Lab Clin Med* 1978; 92:370–375.

131. Radtke HW, et al. Identification of spermine as an inhibitor of erythropoiesis in patients with chronic renal failure. *J Clin Invest* 1980;67:1623–1629.

132. Zappacosta AR, et al. The normalization of hematocrit in end-stage renal disease patients on continuous ambulatory peritoneal dialysis: the role of erythropoietin. *Am J Med* 1982;72:53–57.

133. Wallner SF, et al. The anemia of chronic renal failure: studies of the affect of organic solvent extraction of the serum. *J Lab Clin Med* 1978;92:363–369.

134. Pershagen G, et al. Increased arsenic concentration in the bone marrow in chronic renal failure—a contribution to anemia? *Nephron* 1982;30:250–252.

135. Cambell RA. Anemia, uremia, and polyamines. *Nephron* 1985;41: 299–301.

136. Ono K, et al. Hypervitaminosis A: a contributing factor to anemia in regular dialysis patients. *Nephron* 1984;38:44–47.

137. Meytes D, et al. Effect of parathyroid hormone on erythropoiesis. *J Clin Invest* 1981;67:1263–1269.

138. Segal GM, et al. Spermine and spermidine are non-specific inhibitors of in vitro hematopoiesis. *Kidney Int* 1987;31:72–76.

139. Eschbach JW, et al. Physiologic studies in normal and uremic sheep. *Kidney Int* 1980;18:725–731.

140. Eschbach JW, et al. The anemia of chronic renal failure in sheep: the response to erythropoietin-rich plasma in vivo. *J Clin Invest* 1984;74: 434–441.

141. Eschbach JW, et al. A comparison of the responses to recombinant erythropoietin in normal and uremic subjects. *Kidney Int* 1992;42: 407–416.

142. Delwechi F, et al. High levels of the circulating form of parathyroid hormone do not inhibit in vivo erythropoiesis. *J Lab Clin Med* 1983; 102:613–620.

143. Rao DS, et al. Effect of serum parathyroid hormone and bone marrow fibrosis on the response to erythropoietin in uremia. *N Engl J Med* 1993;328:171–175.

144. Barbour GL. Effect of parathyroidectomy on anemia in chronic renal failure. *Arch Intern Med* 1979;139:889–891.

145. Niwa T, et al. Efficient removal of albumin-bound furancarboxylic acid, an inhibitor of erythropoiesis, by continuous ambulatory peritoneal dialysis. *Nephron* 1990;56:241–245.

146. Himmelfarber J, et al. Reactive oxygen species production by monocytes and polymorphonuclear leukocytes during dialysis. *Am J Kidney Dis* 1991;3:271–276.

147. Morra L, et al. Inadequate ability of T-lymphocytes from chronic uremic subjects to stimulate the in vivo growth of committed erythroid progenitors (BFU-E). *Acta Haematol* 1988;79:187–191.

148. Le Meur Y, et al. Plasma levels and metabolism of AcsSDKP in patients with chronic renal failure: relationship with erythropoietin requirements. *Am J Kidney Dis* 2001;38:510-517.

149. Whitehead VM, et al. Homeostasis of folic acid in patients undergoing maintenance hemodialysis. *N Engl J Med* 1968;279:970–974.

150. Wolfson M. Use of water-soluble vitamins in patients with chronic renal failure. *Semin Dial* 1988;1:28–32.

151. Eschbach JW, et al. Correction of the anemia of end-stage renal disease with recombinant human erythropoietin: results of combined phase I & II clinical trials. *N Engl J Med* 1987;316:73–78.

152. Winearls CG, et al. Effect of human erythropoietin derived from recombinant DNA on the anemia of patients maintained by chronic haemodialysis. *Lancet* 1986;2:1175–1177.

153. Eschbach JW, et al. Recombinant human erythropoietin in anemic patients with end-stage renal disease: results of a phase III multicenter clinical trial. *Ann Intern Med* 1989:111:992–1000.

154. Sabota JT. Recombinant human erythropoietin in patients with anemia due to end-stage renal disease. *Contrib Nephrol* 1989;76: 166–178.

155. United States Renal Data System 1996 Annual Report. *Am J Kidney Dis* 1996;28[Suppl 3]:S56.

156. End-stage renal disease second annual report to Congress 1980. U.S. Dept. of Health & Human Services, 1980.

157. Statistical summary. Health Care Financing Review, 1995:36.

158. Powe NR, et al. Early dosing practices and effectiveness of recombinant human erythropoietin. *Kidney Int* 1993;43:1125–1133.

159. Powe NR, et al. Cost implications to Medicare of recombinant erythropoietin therapy for the anemia of end-stage renal disease. *J Am Soc Nephrol* 1993;3:1660–1671.

160. Eggers PW, et al. The use of Health Care Financing Administration data for the development of a quality improvement project on the treatment of anemia (review). *Am J Kidney Dis* 1994;24:247–254.

161. McNamee P, et al. Benefits and costs of recombinant human erythropoietin for end-stage renal failure: a review. *Int J Technol Assess Health Care* 1993;9:490–504.

162. Sisk JE, et al. Medicare payment options for recombinant erythropoietin therapy. *Am J Kidney Dis* 1991;18[Suppl 1]:93–97.

163. Obrator GT, et al. Trends in anemia management at initiation of dialysis in the United States. *Kidney Int* 2001;60:1875-84.

164. Eschbach JW. The anemia of chronic renal failure: pathophysiology and the effects of recombinant erythropoietin (review). *Kidney Int* 1989;35:134–148.

165. McCarthy JT, et al. Transfusional iron overload in patients undergoing dialysis: treatment with erythropoietin and phlebotomy. *J Lab Clin Med* 1989;114:193–199.

166. Lazarus JM, et al. Recombinant human erythropoietin and phlebotomy in the treatment of iron overload in chronic hemodialysis patients. *Am J Kidney Dis* 1990;16:101–108.

167. El-Reshaid K, et al. Erythropoietin treatment in haemodialysis patients with iron overload. *Acta Haematol* 1994;91(3):130–135.

168. Chan PCK, et al. The use of nuclear magnetic resonance imaging in monitoring total body iron in hemodialysis patients with hemosiderosis treated with erythropoietin and phlebotomy. *Am J Kidney Dis* 1992;19:484–489.

169. Cecchin E, et al. Efficacy of hepatic computed tomography to detect iron overload in chronic hemodialysis. *Kidney Int* 1990;37:943–950.

170. Pitts TO, et al. Hemosiderosis secondary to chronic parenteral iron therapy in maintenance hemodialysis patients. *Nephron* 1978;22: 316–321.

171. Goldman M, et al. Multiple blood transfusions and iron overload in patients receiving haemodialysis. *Nephrol Dial Transplant* 1987;2: 316–321.

172. Fleming LW, et al. Hepatic iron in dialyzed patients given intravenous iron dextran. *J Clin Pathol* 1990;43:119–124.

173. Waterlot Y, et al. Impaired phagocytic activity of neutrophils in patients receiving hemodialysis: the critical role of iron overload. *BJM* 1985;291:501–504.

174. Boelaert JR, et al. Iron overload in haemodialysis patients increases the risk for bacteremia: a prospective study. *Nephrol Dial Transplant* 1990;5:130–134.

175. Gaughan W, et al. Serum bactericidal activity for *Yersinia* enterocolitis in hemodialysis patients. *Am J Kidney Dis* 1992;19:144–148.

176. Tielemans C, et al. Respective roles of haemosiderosis and desferrioxamine therapy in the infectious risk of haemodialyzed patients. *Q J Med* 1988;68:573–574.

177. Grimm PC, et al. Effects of recombinant human erythropoietin on HLA sensitization and cell mediated immunity. *Kidney Int* 1990;38: 12–18.

178. Barany P, et al. Long term effects on lymphocytotoxic antibodies and immune reactivity in hemodialysis patients treated with recombinant human erythropoietin. *Clin Nephrol* 1992;37:90–96.

179. Sanfilippo F, et al. Comparative effects of pregnancy, transfusion, and prior graft rejection on sensitization and renal transplant results. *Transplant* 1982;34:360–366.

180. Silverberg J, et al. Role of anemia in the pathogenesis of left ventricular hypertrophy in end-stage renal disease. *Am J Cardiol* 1989;64: 222–224.

181. Rostandt SG, et al. Cardiac disease in dialysis patients. In: Nissenson AR, et al., eds. *Clinical dialysis*, 2nd ed. Norwalk, CT: Appleton & Lange, 1990:409–446.

182. Parfrey PS, et al. Outcome and risk factors for left ventricular disorders in chronic uraemia. *Nephrol Dial Transplant* 1996;11: 1277–1285.

183. Foley RN, et al. Clinical and echocardiographic disease in patients starting end-stage renal disease. *Am J Kidney Dis* 1995;47:186–192.

184. Goldberg N, et al. Changes in left ventricular size, wall thickness, and function in anemic patients treated with recombinant human erythropoietin. *Am Heart J* 1992;124:424–427.

185. Pascal J, et al. Regression of left ventricular hypertrophy after partial correction of anemia with erythropoietin in patients on hemodialysis: a prospective study. *Clin Nephrol* 1991;35:280–287.

186. Neff MS, et al. Hemodynamics of uremic anemia. *Circulation* 1971; 43:876–883.

187. Silberberg J, et al. Regression of left ventricular hypertrophy in dialysis patients following correction of anemia with recombinant human erythropoietin. *Can J Cardiol* 1990;6:1–4.

188. Cannella G, et al. Reversal of left ventricular hypertrophy following recombinant human erythropoietin of anemic dialyzed uremic patients. *Nephrol Dial Transplant* 1991;6:31–37.

189. Rademacher J, et al. Treatment of renal anemia by erythropoietin substitution. *Clin Nephrol* 1995;44[Suppl 1];S56–S60.

190. Fellner SK, et al. Cardiovascular consequences of the correction of the anemia of renal failure with erythropoietin. *Kidney Int* 1993;44: 1309–1315.

191. Onoyama K, et al. Effects of human recombinant erythropoietin on anaemia, systemic haemodynamics and renal function in pre-dialysis renal failure patients. *Nephrol Dial Transplant* 1989;4:966–970.

192. Schwartz AB, et al. Cardiovascular hemodynamic effects of correction of anemia of chronic renal failure with recombinant erythropoietin. *Transplant Proc* 1991;23:1827–1830.

193. Duke M, et al. The hemodynamic response to chronic anemia. *Circulation* 1969;39:503–515.

194. Maschio G. Erythropoietin and systemic hypertension. *Nephrol Dial Transplant* 1995;10[Suppl 2]:4–79.

195. van de Borne P, et al. Effect of recombinant human erythropoietin therapy on ambulatory BP and heart rate in chronic hemodialysis patients. *Nephrol Dial Transplant* 1992;7:45–49.

196. Santleben W, et al. Blood pressure changes during treatment of with recombinant human erythropoietin. *Contrib Nephrol* 1988;66: 114–122.

197. Cannella G, et al. Renormalization of high cardiac output and of left ventricular size following long-term recombinant human erythropoietin treatment of anemic dialyzed uremic patients. *Clin Nephrol* 1990: 34:272–278.

198. Fernández A, et al. Effect of recombinant human erythropoietin on hemodynamic parameters in continuous ambulatory peritoneal and hemodialysis patients. *Am J Nephrol* 1992;12:207–211.

199. Abraham PA, et al. Blood pressure in hemodialysis patients during amelioration of anemia with erythropoietin. *J Am Soc Nephrol* 1991; 2:927–936.

200. Raine AEG, et al. Effect of erythropoietin on blood pressure. *Am J Kidney Dis* 1991;18[Suppl 1]:76–83.

201. Stephen HM, et al. Peripheral hemodynamics, blood viscosity, and the renin-angiotensin system in hemodialysis patients under therapy with recombinant human erythropoietin. *Contrib Nephrol* 1989;76: 292–298.

202. Eggena P, et al. Influence of recombinant human erythropoietin on blood pressure and renin-angiotensin systems. *Am J Physiol* 1991;261: E642–E646.

203. Torralbo A, et al. Effects of hematocrit and vasoactive substance levels on blood pressure of patients treated with erythropoietin (EPO). *Kidney Int* 1993;44:1478(abst).

204. Carlini R, et al. Intravenous erythropoietin (rHuEPO) administration increases plasma endothelin and blood pressure in hemodialysis patients. *Am J Hypertens* 1993;6:103–107.

205. Takayama K, et al. Changes in endothelial vasoactive substances under recombinant human erythropoietin in hemodialysis patients. *ASAIO Trans* 1991;37:M187–M188.

206. Carlini R, et al. Recombinant human erythropoietin (rHuEPO) increases endothelin-1 release by endothelial cells. *Kidney Int* 1993; 43:1010–1014.

207. Nagai T, et al. Effects of rHuEpo on cellular proliferation and endothelin-1 production in cultured endothelial cells. *Nephrol Dial Transplant* 1995;10:1814–1819.

208. Torralbo A, et al. Endothelin (ET) in chronic renal failure (CRF) and treatment with recombinant human erythropoietin (rHuEPO). *Kidney Int* 1993;44:1478(abst).

209. Leben M, et al. Plasma immunoreactive endothelin levels in hemodialysis and in CAPD patients with and without erythropoietin therapy (abst). Proceedings of the XIIth International Congress of Nephrology, Jerusalem, Israel, June 1993:358.

210. Brunet P, et al. Plasma endothelin in haemodialysis patients treated with recombinant human erythropoietin. *Nephrol Dial Transplant* 1994;9:650–665.

211. Lai KN, et al. Effect of subcutaneous and intraperitoneal administration of recombinant human erythropoietin on blood pressure and plasma vasoactive hormones in patients on continuous ambulatory peritoneal dialysis. *Nephron* 1991;57:394–400.

212. Heidenreich S, et al. Direct vasopressor effect of recombinant human erythropoietin on renal resistance vessels. *Kidney Int* 1991;39: 259–265.

213. Vaziri ND, et al. In vitro and in vivo pressor effects of erythropoietin. *Am J Physiol* 1995;38:F838–F845.

214. Vaziri ND, et al. Role of nitric oxide resistance in erythropoietin-induced hypertension in rats with chronic renal failure. *Am J Physiol* 1996;34:E113–E122.

215. Hon G, et al. Lack of a fast-acting effect of erythropoietin on arterial blood pressure and endothelin level. *Artif Organs* 1995;19:188–191.

216. Frencken LAM, et al. Evidence for renal vasodilatation in pre-dialysis patients during correction of anemia by erythropoietin. *Kidney Int* 1992;41:384–387.

217. Raine AEG. Hypertension, blood viscosity and cardiovascular morbidity in renal failure: implications for erythropoietin therapy. *Lancet* 1988;1:97–99.

218. Brown CD, et al. Treatment of azotemic, nonoliguric, anemic patients with human recombinant erythropoietin raises whole blood viscosity proportional to hematocrit. *Nephron* 1991;59:394–398.

219. Linde T, et al. Impaired erythrocyte fluidity during treatment of renal anaemia with erythropoietin. *J Intern Med* 1992;232:601–606.

220. Martin J, et al. Blood pressure, erythropoietin and nitric oxide. *Lancet* 1988;1:644.

221. Kaupke CJ, et al. Effect of erythrocyte mass on arterial blood pressure in dialysis patients receiving maintenance erythropoietin therapy. *J Am Soc Nephrol* 1994;4:1874–1878.

222. del Castillo D, et al. The pressor effect of recombinant human erythropoietin is not due to decreased activity of the endogenous nitric oxide system. *Nephrol Dial Transplant* 1995;10:505–508.

223. Edmunds M, et al. Blood pressure and erythropoietin. *Lancet* 1988;1: 351–352.

224. Abraham PA, et al. Body fluid spaces and blood pressure in hemodialysis patients during amelioration of anemia with erythropoietin. *Am J Kidney Dis* 1990;16:438–446.

225. Lim VS, et al. The safety and efficacy of maintenance therapy of recombinant human erythropoietin treatment in patients with renal insufficiency. *Am J Kidney Dis* 1989;14:496–506.

226. Anastassiades E, et al. Influence of blood volume on the blood pressure of predialysis and peritoneal dialysis patients treated with erythropoietin. *Nephrol Dial Transplant* 1993;8:621–625.

227. Cascinu S, et al. Recombinant human erythropoietin in chemotherapy-associated anemia (review). *Cancer Treatment Rev* 1996;21: 553–564.

228. Schreiber S, et al. Recombinant erythropoietin for the treatment of anemia in inflammatory bowel disease. *N Engl J Med* 1996;334: 619–623.

229. Harris SA, et al. Erythropoietin treatment of erythropoietin-deficient anemia without renal disease during pregnancy. *Obstet Gynecol* 1996; 87:812–814.

230. Poux JM, et al. Uraemia is necessary for erythropoietin-induced hypertension in rats. *Clin Exp Pharmacol Physiol* 1995;22:769–771.

231. Bassi S, et al. Cardiovascular function in a chronic peritoneal dialysis pediatric population on recombinant human erythropoietin treatment. *Perit Dial Int* 1993;13[Suppl 2]:S267–S269.

232. Martin GR, et al. Recombinant erythropoietin (Epogen) improves cardiac exercise performance in children with end-stage renal disease. *Pediatr Nephrol* 1993;7:276–280.

233. Harnett JD, et al. Cardiac function and hematocrit level. *Am J Kidney Dis* 1995;25:S3–S7.

234. Wizemann V, et al. Effect of erythropoietin on ischemic tolerance in anemic hemodialysis patients with confirmed coronary artery disease. *Nephron* 1992;62:161–165.

235. Macdougall IC, et al. Long-term cardiopulmonary effects of amelioration of renal anaemia by erythropoietin. *Lancet* 1990;1:489–493.

236. Yang CS, et al. Effects of increasing dialysis dose on serum albumin and mortality in hemodialysis patients. *Am J Kidney Dis* 1996;17: 380–386.

237. Lowrie EC, et al. The relative contributions of measured variables to death risk among hemodialysis patients. In: Friedman EA, ed. *Death on hemodialysis: preventable or inevitable?* Dordrecht, the Netherlands: Kluwer Academic, 1995:121–141.

238. Klinkmann H, et al. Adverse events of subcutaneous recombinant human erythropoietin. *Contrib Nephrol* 1992;100:127–138.

239. Sikole A, et al. Analysis of heart morphology and function following erythropoietin treatment of anemic dialysis patients. *Artif Organs* 1993;17:977–984.

240. Churchill DN, et al. Effect of recombinant human erythropoietin on hospitalization of hemodialysis patients. *Clin Nephrol* 1995;43: 184–188.

241. Xia H, et al. Hematocrit levels and hospitalization risks in hemodialysis patients. *J Am Soc Nephrol* 1999;10:1309.

242. Collins AJ, et al. Impact of hematocrit on morbidity and mortality. *Semin Nephrol* 2000;20:345.

243. Powe NR, et al. Effect of recombinant erythropoietin on hospital admissions, readmissions, length of stay, and costs of dialysis patients. *J Am Soc Nephrol* 1994;4:1455–1465.

244. Mayer G, et al. Anaemia and reduced exercise capacity in patients on chronic haemodialysis. *Clin Sci* 1989;76:265–268.

245. Davenport A. The effect of treatment with recombinant human erythropoietin on skeletal muscle function in patients with end-stage renal failure treated with regular hemodialysis. *Am J Kidney Dis* 1993; 22:685–690.

246. Davenport A, et al. Blood lactate is reduced following successful treatment of anaemia in haemodialysis patients with recombinant human

247. Park JS, et al. Effect of recombinant human erythropoietin on muscle energy metabolism in patients with end-stage renal disease: a P-nuclear magnetic resonance spectroscopic study. *Am J Kidney Dis* 1993;21:612–619.

248. Mitch WE, et al. Mechanisms of muscle wasting: the role of the ubiquitin-proteasome pathway. In: Epstein FH, ed. *Mechanisms of disease.* Atlanta: Emory University, 1996:1897.

249. Grützmacher P, et al. Beneficial and adverse effects of correction of anaemia by recombinant human erythropoietin in patients on maintenance hemodialysis. *Contrib Nephrol* 1988;66:104–113.

250. Canadian Erythropoietin Study Group. Association between recombinant human erythropoietin and quality of life and exercise capacity of patients receiving haemodialysis. *BMJ* 1990;300:573–578.

251. Metra M, et al. Improvement in exercise capacity after correction of anemia in patients with end-stage renal failure. *Am J Cardiol* 1991;68: 1060–1066.

252. Grunze M, et al. Mechanisms of improved physical performance of chronic hemodialysis patients after erythropoietin treatment. *Am J Nephrol* 1990;10[Suppl 2]:15–23.

253. McMahon LP, et al. Hemodynamic changes and physical performance at comparative levels of haemoglobin after long-term treatment with recombinant erythropoietin. *Nephrol Dial Transplant* 1992;7:1199–1206.

254. Horina JH, et al. Increased red cell 2,3-diphosphoglycerate levels in haemodialysis patients treated with erythropoietin. *Nephrol Dial Transplant* 1993;8:1219–1222.

255. Linde T, et al. Reduced oxygen affinity contributes to improved oxygen releasing capacity during erythropoietin treatment of renal anaemia. *Nephrol Dial Transplant* 1993;8:524–529.

256. Brunet P, et al. Effect of recombinant human erythropoietin treatment in uremic patients on oxygen affinity of hemoglobin. *Nephron* 1994;66:147–152.

257. Wirtz JJ, et al. Long-term effects of recombinant human erythropoietin on macro- and microcirculation in chronic hemodialysis patients. *Blood Purif* 1993;11:237–247.

258. Celsing F, et al. Effect of anaemia and step-wise induced polycythemia on maximal aerobic power in individuals with high and low haemoglobin concentrations. *Acta Physiol Scand* 1987;129:47–54.

259. Marrades RM, et al. Effects of erythropoietin on muscle O2 transport during exercise in patients with chronic renal failure. *J Clin Invest* 1996;97:2092–2100.

260. Moore GE, et al. ^{31}P-magnetic resonance spectroscopy assessment of subnormal oxidative metabolism in skeletal muscle of renal failure patients. *J Clin Invest* 1993;91:420–424.

261. Lim VS. Recombinant human erythropoietin in predialysis patients. *Am J Kid Dis* 1991;18[Suppl 1]:34–37.

262. Barany P, et al. Physiologic effects of correcting anemia in haemodialysis patients to a normal hemoglobin concentration. *Clin Invest* 1994;72:B23(abst).

263. Delano BG. Improvements in quality of life following treatment with r-HuEPO in anemic hemodialysis patients. *Am J Kidney Dis* 1989;14 [Suppl 1]:14–18.

264. Evans RW. Recombinant human erythropoietin and the quality of life of end-stage renal disease patients: a comparative analysis. *Am J Kidney Dis* 1991;18[Suppl 1]:S62–S70.

265. Evans RW, et al. The quality of life of hemodialysis patients treated with recombinant human erythropoietin. *JAMA* 1990;263:825–830.

266. Painter P. The importance of exercise training in rehabilitation of patients with end-stage renal disease. *Am J Kidney Dis* 1994;24: S31–32.

267. Paganni EP. In search of optimal hematocrit level in dialysis patients: rehabilitation and quality-of-life implications. *Am J Kidney Dis* 1994;24[Suppl 1]:S10–S16.

268. Blagg CR. The socioeconomic impact of rehabilitation. *Am J Kidney Dis* 1994;24[Suppl 1]:S17–S21.

269. Auer J, et al. Quality of life improvements in CAPD patients treated with subcutaneously administered erythropoietin for anemia. *Perit Dial Int* 1992;12:40–42.

270. U.S. Recombinant Human Erythropoietin Predialysis Group. Dou-

ble-blind, placebo-controlled study of the therapeutic use of recombinant human erythropoietin for anemia associated with chronic renal failure in predialysis patients. *Am J Kidney Dis* 1991;14:50–59.

271. Bennett WM. A multicenter clinical trial of epoetin beta for anemia of end-stage renal failure. *J Am Soc Nephrol* 1991;1:990–998.

272. Beusterien LM, et al. The effects of recombinant human erythropoietin on functional health and well-being in chronic dialysis patients. *J Am Soc Nephrol* 1996;7:763–773.

273. Moreno F, et al. Influence of hematocrit on the quality of life of hemodialysis patients. *Nephrol Dial Transplant* 1994;9:1034–1037.

274. Eschbach JW, et al. Normalizing the hematocrit in hemodialysis patients with EPO improves quality of life and is safe. *J Am Soc Nephrol* 1993;4:445(abst).

275. Temple RM, et al. Recombinant human erythropoietin improves cognitive function in chronic haemodialysis patients. *Nephrol Dial Transplant* 1992;7:240–245.

276. Nissenson AR. Epoetin and cognitive function. *Am J Kidney Dis* 1992;20[Suppl 1]:21–24.

277. Marsh JT, et al. RhUEPO treatment improves brain and cognitive function of anemic dialysis patients. *Kidney Int* 1991;39:155–163.

278. Sagales T, et al. Effects of rHuEPO on Q-EEG and event-related potentials in chronic renal failure. *Kidney Int* 1993;44:1109–1115.

279. Nissenson AR, et al. Brain function is better in hemodialyzed patients when hematocrit is normalized with erythropoietin. *J Am Soc Nephrol* 1996;7:1459(abst).

280. Kusunoki M, et al. Effects of hematocrit variations on cerebral blood flow and oxygen transport on ischemic cerebrovascular disease. *J Cerebral Blood Flow Metab* 1981;1:413–417.

281. Digicaylioglu M, et al. Localization of specific erythropoietin binding sites in defined areas of the mouse brain. *Proc Natl Acad Sci U S A* 1995;92:3717–3720.

282. Marti HH, et al. Detection of erythropoietin in human liquor: intrinsic erythropoietin production in the brain. *Kidney Int* 1997;51:416–418.

283. Schaefer RM, et al. Improved sexual function in hemodialysis patients on recombinant erythropoietin: a possible role for prolactin. *Clin Nephrol* 1989;33:1–5.

284. Steffensen G, et al. Does erythropoietin cause hormonal changes in haemodialysis patients? *Nephrol Dial Transplant* 1993;8:1215–1218.

285. Ramirez G, et al. Effect of haemoglobin and endogenous erythropoietin on hypothalamic-pituitary thyroidal and gonadal secretion: an analysis of anaemic (high EPO) and polycythaemic (low EPO) patients. *Clin Endocrinol* 1995;43:167–174.

286. Carlson HE, et al. Endocrine effects of erythropoietin. *Int J Artif Organs* 1995;18:309–314.

287. Schaefer R, et al. Changes in the kinetics and biopotency of luteinizing hormone in hemodialyzed men during treatment with recombinant human erythropoietin. *J Am Soc Nephrol* 1994;5:1208–1215.

288. Barany P, et al. Nutritional assessment in anemic hemodialysis patients treated with recombinant human erythropoietin. *Clin Nephrol* 1991;35:273–279.

289. Riedel E, et al. Correction of amino acid metabolism by recombinant human erythropoietin therapy in hemodialysis patients. *Kidney Int* 1989;36[Suppl 27]:S216–S221.

290. Garibotto G, et al. Erythropoietin treatment and amino acid metabolism in hemodialysis patients. *Nephron* 1993;65:533–536.

291. Pollock CA, et al. Effects of erythropoietin therapy on the lipid profile in end-stage renal failure. *Kidney Int* 1994;45:897–902.

292. Berman DH, et al. Partial absorption of hard exudates in patients with diabetic end-stage renal disease and severe anemia after treatment with erythropoietin. *Retina* 1994;14:1–5.

293. Friedman EA, et al. Erythropoietin in diabetic macular edema and renal insufficiency. *Am J Kidney Dis* 1995;26:202–208.

294. Mailloux LU, et al. Mortality in dialysis patients: analysis of the causes of death. *Am J Kidney Dis* 1991;3:326–335.

295. United States Renal Data System Report. VI. Causes of death. *Am J Kidney Dis* 1997;30[Suppl 1]:S107–S117.

296. Vanholder R, et al. Infectious morbidity and defects of phagocytic function in end-stage renal disease: a review. *J Am Soc Nephrol* 1993;3:1541–1554.

297. Baum J, et al. Chemotaxis of the polymorphonuclear leukocyte and delayed hypersensitivity in uremia. *Kidney Int* 1975;2[Suppl]:S147–S153.

298. Ilvento MC, et al. Hemodialysis decreases spontaneous migration of polymorphonuclears in chronic renal failure. *Dial Transplant* 1992;21:705–708.

299. Descamps-Latscha B, et al. Respective influence of uremia and hemodialysis on whole blood phagocyte oxidative metabolism and circulating interleukin-1 and tumor necrosis factor. *Adv Exp Med Biol* 1991;297:183–192.

300. Vanholder R, et al. Phagocytosis in uremic and hemodialysis patients: a prospective and cross-sectional study. *Kidney Int* 1991;39:320–327.

301. Himmelfarber J, et al. Modulation of granulocyte LAM-1 and MAC-1 during dialysis—a prospective, randomized controlled trial. *Kidney Int* 1992;41:388–395.

302. Roccatello D, et al. Functional changes of monocytes due to dialysis membranes. *Kidney Int* 1989;35:622–635.

303. Ruiz P, et al. Impaired function of macrophage Fc receptors in end-stage renal disease. *N Engl J Med* 1990;322:717–722.

304. Dumann H, et al. Hepatitis B vaccination and interleukin-2 receptor expression in chronic renal failure. *Kidney Int* 1990;38:1164–1168.

305. Levin NW, et al. Effect of membrane types on causes of death in hemodialysis patients. *J Am Soc Nephrol* 1991;2:335(abst).

306. Hornberger JC, et al. A multivariate analysis of mortality and hospital admissions with high-flux dialysis. *J Am Soc Nephrol* 1993;3:1227–1237.

307. Collart FE, et al. Effect of recombinant human erythropoietin on T-cell lymphocyte subsets in hemodialysis patients. *ASAIO Trans* 1990;36:M219–M223.

308. Schaefer RM, et al. Improved immunoglobulin production in dialysis patients treated with recombinant erythropoietin. *Int J Artif Organs* 1992;3:71–75.

309. Veys N, et al. Correction of deficient phagocytosis during erythropoietin treatment in maintenance dialysis patients. *Am J Kidney Dis* 1992;19:358–363.

310. Boulart JR, et al. Recombinant human erythropoietin reverses polymorphonuclear granulocyte dysfunction in iron-loaded dialysis patients. *Nephrol Dial Transplant* 1990;5:504–507.

311. Shieh S-D, et al. Effect of erythropoietin on neutrophil chemiluminescence in hemodialysis patients. *ASAIO Trans* 1991;37:M189–M191.

312. Sennasael JJ, et al. Treatment with recombinant human erythropoietin increases antibody titers after hepatitis B vaccination in dialysis patients. *Kidney Int* 1990;40:121–128.

313. Gafter U, et al. Anemia of uremia is associated with reduced in vitro cytokine secretion: immunopotentiating activity of red blood cells. *Kidney Int* 1994;45:224–231.

314. Hegbrant J, et al. Erythropoietin treatment and plasma levels of corticotropin-releasing hormone, delta sleep-inducing peptide and opioid peptides in hemodialysis patients. *Scand J Urol Nephrol* 1992;26:393–396.

315. Creutzig A, et al. Skin microcirculation and regional peripheral resistance in patients with chronic anaemia treated with recombinant human erythropoietin. *Eur J Clin Invest* 1990;20:219–223.

316. De Marchi S, et al. Relief of pruritus and decreases in plasma histamine concentrations during erythropoietin therapy in patients with uremia. *N Engl J Med* 1992;326:969–974.

317. Balaskas EV, et al. Erythropoietin treatment does not improve uremic pruritus. *Perit Dial Int* 1992;12:330–331.

318. Sherman RA, et al. The effect of red cell transfusion on hemodialysis-related hypotension. *Am J Kidney Dis* 1988;11:33–35.

319. Perera R, et al. Effect of recombinant erythropoietin on anemia and orthostatic hypotension in primary autonomic failure. *Clin Autonomic Res* 1995;5:211–213.

320. Steiner RW, et al. Bleeding time in uremia: a useful test to assess clinical bleeding. *Am J Hematol* 1979;7:107–117.

321. Salzman EW, et al. Adhesiveness of blood platelets in uremia. *Thromb Diath Haemorr* 1966;15:84–92.

322. Remuzzi G, et al. Reduced platelet thromboxane formation in uremia: evidence for a functional cyclooxygenase defect. *J Clin Invest* 1983;71:762–768.

323. Castillo R, et al. Defective platelet adhesion on vessel subendothelium in uremic patients. *Blood* 1986;68:337–342.

324. Remuzzi G, et al. Bleeding in renal failure: altered platelet function in chronic uraemia only partially corrected with hemodialysis. Nephron 1978;22:347–353.

325. Noris M, et al. Enhanced nitric oxide synthesis in uremia: implications for platelet dysfunction and dialysis hypotension. *Kidney Int* 1993;44:445–450.

326. Huraib S, et al. Effect of recombinant human erythropoietin (rHuEPO) on the hemostatic system in chronic hemodialysis patients. *Clin Nephrol* 1991;36:252–257.

327. Vigano G, et al. Recombinant human erythropoietin to correct uremic bleeding. *Am J Kidney Dis* 1991;18:44–49.

328. Kaupke CJ, et al. Effect of recombinant human erythropoietin on platelet production in dialysis patients. *J Am Soc Nephrol* 1993;3:1672–1679.

329. Akizawa T, et al. Effects of recombinant human erythropoietin and correction of anemia on platelet function in hemodialysis patients. *Nephron* 1991;58:400–406.

330. Taylor JE, et al. Erythropoietin does not increase whole-blood platelet aggregation. *Nephrol Dial Transplant* 1993;8:1291–1293.

331. Taylor JE, et al. Effect of erythropoietin therapy and withdrawal on blood coagulation and fibrinolysis in hemodialysis patients. *Kidney Int* 1993;44:182–190.

332. Fluck RJ, et al. Modulation of platelet cytosolic calcium during erythropoietin therapy in uraemia. *Nephrol Dial Transplant* 1994;9:1109–1114.

333. Gura V, et al. Elevated thrombocyte calcium in uremia and its correction by 1 alpha(OH) vitamin D treatment. *Nephron* 1982;30:237–239.

334. Lai K-N, et al. Effect of hemodialysis on protein C, protein S, and antithrombin III levels. *Am J Kidney Dis* 1991;27:38–42.

335. Lai K-N, et al. Protein C, protein S, and antithrombin III levels in patients on continuous ambulatory peritoneal dialysis and hemodialysis. *Nephron* 1990;56:271–276.

336. Clyne N, et al. Effects of hemodialysis and long-term erythropoietin treatment on protein C, and on free and total protein S. *Thromb Res* 1995;80:161–168.

337. Huraib S, et al. One-year experience of very low doses of subcutaneous erythropoietin in continuous ambulatory peritoneal dialysis and its effect on haemostasis. *Haemostasis* 1995;25:299–304.

338. Maurin N, et al. Influence of recombinant human erythropoietin on hematological and hemostatic parameters with special reference to microhemolysis. *Clin Nephrol* 1995;43:196–200.

339. Besarab A. Hematologic aspects of uremia. In: Nissenson AR, et al., eds. *Clinical dialysis,* 3rd ed. Norwalk, CT: Appleton & Lange, 1995:618–651.

340. Sundal E, et al. Correction of anaemia of chronic renal failure with recombinant human erythropoietin: safety and efficacy of one year's treatment in a European multicentre study of 150 haemodialysis-dependent patients. *Nephrol Dial Transplant* 1989;4:979–987.

341. Pollock M, et al. Effects of recombinant human erythropoietin in end-stage renal failure patients. *Contrib Nephrol* 1989;6:201–211.

342. Dy GR, et al. Effect of recombinant human erythropoietin on vascular access. *ASAIO Trans* 1991;37:M274–M275.

343. Muirhead N, et al. Erythropoietin for anaemia in haemodialysis patients: results of a maintenance study (the Canadian Erythropoietin Study Group). *Nephrol Dial Transplant* 1991;7:811–816.

344. Churchill DN, et al. Probability of thrombosis of vascular access among hemodialysis patients treated with recombinant human erythropoietin. *J Am Soc Nephrol* 1994;4:1809–1813.

345. Tang I, et al. Vascular access thrombosis during recombinant human erythropoietin therapy. *ASAIO Trans* 1992;38:M528–M531.

346. Eschbach JW. Erythropoietin is not a cause of access thrombosis. *Semin Dial* 1993;6:180–184.

347. Muirhead N. Erythropoietin is a cause of access thrombosis. *Semin Dial* 1993;6:184–188.

348. Besarab A, et al. Recombinant human erythropoietin does not increase clotting in vascular accesses. *ASAIO Trans* 1990;36:M749–M753.

349. Besarab A, et al. The relation of intraaccess pressure to flow. *J Am Soc Nephrol* 1995;7:483(abst).

350. Strauch BS, et al. Forecasting thromboses of vascular access with Doppler color flow imaging. *Am J Kidney Dis* 1992;19:554–557.

351. Krivitsky NM. Theory and validation of access flow measurements by dilution technique during hemodialysis. *Kidney Int* 1995;48:244–250.

352. Depner TA, et al. Clinical measurement of blood flow in hemodialysis access fistulae and grafts by ultrasound dilution. *ASAIO J* 1995;41:M745–M749.

353. Oudenhoven LFIJ, et al. Magnetic resonance, a new method for measuring blood flow in hemodialysis fistulae. *Kidney Int* 1994;45:884–889.

354. Shand BI, et al. Hemorheology and fistula function in home hemodialysis patients following erythropoietin treatment: a prospective placebo-controlled study. *Nephron* 1993;64:53–57.

355. Macdougall IC, et al. Coagulation studies and fistula blood flow during erythropoietin therapy in haemodialysis patients. *Nephrol Dial Transplant* 1991;6:862–867.

356. Besarab A, et al. Effect of normalizing hemoglobin (HGB) on intraaccess pressure and flow. *ASAIO J* 1997;43:69(abst).

357. Standage BA, et al. Does the use of erythropoietin in hemodialysis patients increase dialysis graft thrombosis rates? *Am J Surg* 1993;165:650–654.

358. Besarab A, et al. Prospective evaluation of vascular access function: the nephrologist's perspective. *Semin Dial* 1996;9[Suppl 1]:S21–S29.

359. Taylor JE, et al. Erythropoietin and spontaneous platelet aggregation in haemodialysis patients. *Lancet* 1991;338:1361–1362.

360. Kooistra MP, et al. Low-dose aspirin does not prevent thrombovascular accidents in low-risk haemodialysis patients during treatment with recombinant human erythropoietin. *Nephrol Dial Transplant* 1994;9:1115–1120.

361. Acchiardo SR, et al. Evaluation of hemodialysis patients treated with erythropoietin. *Am J Kidney Dis* 1991;17:290–294.

362. Paganni E, et al. Recombinant human erythropoietin correction of anemia: dialysis efficiency, waste retention, and chronic dose variables. *ASAIO Trans* 1989;35:513–515.

363. Spinowitz BS, et al. Impact of epoetin beta on dialyzer clearances and heparin requirements. *Am J Kidney Dis* 1991;18:668–673.

364. Baur T, et al. Secondary effects of erythropoietin treatment on metabolism and dialysis efficiency in stable hemodialysis patients. *Clin Nephrol* 1990;34:230–235.

365. Veys N, et al. Influence of erythropoietin on dialyzer re-use, heparin needs, and urea kinetics in maintenance hemodialysis patients. *Am J Kidney Dis* 1994;23:52–59.

366. Lippi A, et al. Recombinant human erythropoietin and high flux haemodiafiltration. *Nephrol Dial Transplant* 1995;10[Suppl 6]:51–54.

367. Ksiazek A, et al. Hematocrit influence on peritoneal dialysis effectiveness during recombinant human erythropoietin treatment in patients with chronic renal failure. *Perit Dial Int* 1993;13[Suppl 2]:S550–S552.

368. Frenken LA, et al. Identification of the component part in an epoetin alfa preparation that causes pain after subcutaneous injection. *Am J Kidney Dis* 1993;22:553–556.

369. Veys N, et al. Pain at the injection site of subcutaneously administered erythropoietin in maintenance hemodialysis patients: a comparison of two brands of erythropoietin. *Am J Nephrol* 1992;12:68–72.

370. Granolleras C, et al. Experience of pain after subcutaneous administration of different preparations of recombinant human erythropoietin: a randomized, double blind cross over study. *Clin Nephrol* 1991;36:294–296.

371. Casadevall N, et al. Pure red-cell aplasia and antierythropoietin antibodies in patients treated with recombinant erythropoietin. *N Engl J Med* 2002;346:469.

372. Gershon SK, et al. Pure red-cell aplasia and recombinant erythropoietin. *N Engl J Med* 2002;346:1584.

373. Bunn, HF. Drug-induced autoimmune red-cell aplasia. *N Engl J Med* 2002;346:522.

374. Weber G, et al. Allergic skin and systemic reactions in a patient with pure red cell aplasia and anti-erythropoietin antibodies challenged with different epoetins. *J Am Soc Nephrol* 2002;13:2381–2383.

375. Skibeli V, et al. Sugar profiling proves that human serum erythropoietin differs from recombinant human erythropoietin. *Blood* 2001; 98:3626.

376. Schlags W, et al. Two-dimensional electrophoresis of recombinant human erythropoietin. A future method for the European Pharmacopeia? *Proteonomic* 2002;2:679–682.

377. U.S. Renal Data System: *USRDS 1991 annual report.* Bethesda, MD: National Institutes of Diabetes, Digestive and Kidney Diseases, 1991.

378. Amann K, et al. Reduced cardiac ischaemia tolerance in uraemia—what is the role of structural abnormalities of the heart? *Nephrol Dial Transplant* 1996;11:1238–1241.

379. Sikole A, et al. Recurrence of left ventricular hypertrophy following cessation of erythropoietic therapy. *Artif Organs* 2002;26:98–102.

380. Moreno F, et al. Increasing the hematocrit has a beneficial effect on quality of life and is safe in selected hemodialysis patients. Spanish Cooperative Renal Patients Quality of Life Study Group of the Spanish Society of Nephrology. *J Am Soc Nephrol* 2000;11:335.

381. Besarab A, et al. The effects of normal versus anemic hematocrit on hemodialysis patients with cardiac disease. *N Engl J Med* 1998;339:584.

382. Khan SS, et al. Health care utilization among patients with chronic kidney disease. *Kidney Int* 2002;62:229–236.

383. de Lissovoy G, et al. The relationship of provider organizational status and erythropoietin dosing in end-stage renal disease patients. *Med Care* 1994;32:130–140.

384. Westman MA, et al. Options for dialysis providers in a global capitated environment. *Nephrol News Issues* 1996:10:26–31.

385. Scheingold S, et al. The impact of recombinant human erythropoietin on medical care costs for hemodialysis patients in Canada. *Soc Sci Med* 1992;34:983–991.

386. Stevens ME, et al. Cost benefits of low dose subcutaneous erythropoietin in patients with anaemia of end-stage renal disease. *BMJ* 1992;304:474–477.

387. Erslev AJ. Erythropoietin. *N Engl J Med* 1991;324:1339–1344.

388. Besarab A, et al. Clinical pharmacology and economics of recombinant human erythropoietin in end-stage renal disease: the case for subcutaneous administration. *J Am Soc Nephrol* 1992;2:1405–1416.

389. Walter J, et al. The beneficial effect of low initial dose and gradual increase of erythropoietin treatment in hemodialysis patients. *Artif Organs* 1995;19:76–80.

390. Muirhead N, et al. Evidence-based recommendations for the clinical use of recombinant human erythropoietin. *Am J Kidney Dis* 1995;26 [Suppl 1]:S1–S24.

391. Salmonson T. Pharmacokinetic and pharmacodynamic studies on recombinant human erythropoietin. *Scand J Urol Nephrol* 1990;129 [Suppl]:166.

392. Uehlenger DE, et al. A pharmacodynamic model of erythropoietin therapy for uremic anemia. *Clin Pharmacol Ther* 1992;51:76–89.

393. Chaplin H, et al. Red cell life-span in nephritis and in hepatic nephrosis. *Clin Sci* 1953;12:351–360.

394. Sutherland DA, et al. The anemia of uremia: hemolytic state measured by the radiochromium method. *Am J Med* 1955;19:153.

395. Erslev A, et al. The rate and control of baseline red cell production in hematologically stable uremic patients. *J Lab Clin Med* 1995;126:283–286.

396. Besarab A, et al. Pharmacodynamics of erythropoietin: can determinants of erythropoiesis predict dose-response? *J Am Soc Nephrol* 1994;5:322(abst).

397. Muirhead N, et al. Comparison of subcutaneous and intravenous recombinant human erythropoietin for anemia in hemodialysis patients with significant comorbid disease. *Am J Nephrol* 1992;12:303–310.

398. Ahn JH, et al. Bone marrow findings before and after treatment with recombinant human erythropoietin in chronic hemodialyzed patients. *Clin Nephrol* 1995;43:189–195.

399. Beguin Y, et al. Early prediction of response to recombinant human erythropoietin in patients with the anemia of renal failure by serum transferrin receptor and fibrinogen. *Blood* 1993;82:2010–2016.

400. Beguin Y, et al. Quantitative assessment of erythropoiesis in haemodialysis patients demonstrates gradual expansion of erythroblasts during constant treatment with recombinant human erythropoietin. *Br J Haematol* 1995;89:17–23.

401. Fogh J. The increased dose response of ESF after ESF stimulation. *Ann N Y Acad Sci* 1968;149:217–222.

402. Gurney CW, et al. Studies on erythropoiesis. XVII. Some quantitative aspects of the erythropoietic response to erythropoietin. *Blood* 1961;17:531–546.

403. Flaherty KK, et al. Pharmacokinetics and erythropoietic response to human recombinant erythropoietin in healthy men. *Clin Pharmacol Ther* 1990;47:557–564.

404. Gladziwa U, et al. Pharmacokinetics of epoetin (recombinant human erythropoietin) after long term therapy in patients undergoing haemodialysis and haemofiltration. *Clin Pharmacokinet* 1993;25:145–153.

405. Montini G, et al. Pharmacokinetics and hematologic response to subcutaneous administration of recombinant human erythropoietin in children undergoing long-term peritoneal dialysis: a multicenter study. *J Pediatr* 1993;122:297–302.

406. Veng-Pedersen P, et al. Kinetic evaluation of nonlinear drug elimination by a disposition decomposition analysis. Application to the analysis of the nonlinear elimination kinetics of erythropoietin in adult humans. *J Pharm Sci* 1995;84:760–767.

407. McMahon FG, et al. Pharmacokinetics and effects of recombinant human erythropoietin after intravenous and subcutaneous injections in healthy volunteers. *Blood* 1990;76:1718–1722.

408. Spivak JL, et al. The in vivo metabolism of recombinant human erythropoietin in the rat. *Blood* 1989;73:90–99.

409. Misaizu T, et al. Role of antennary structure of N-linked sugar chains in renal handling of recombinant human erythropoietin. *Blood* 1995;86:4097–4104.

410. Piroso E, et al. Erythropoietin half-life in rats with hypoplastic and hyperplastic bone marrows. *Blood* 1989;74:270(abst).

411. Naets JP, et al. Effect of erythroid hyperplasia on the disappearance rate of erythropoietin in the dog. *Acta Haematol* 1968;39:42–50.

412. Hughes RT, et al. Correction of anemia of chronic renal failure with erythropoietin: pharmacokinetic studies in patients on hemodialysis and CAPD. *Contrib Nephrol* 1989;76:122–130.

413. Besarab A, et al. Erythropoietin in patients prior to end-stage renal disease. *Curr Opinion Nephrol Hypertens* 1995;4:155–161.

414. Boelaert JR, et al. Comparative pharmacokinetics of recombinant erythropoietin administered by the intravenous, subcutaneous, and intraperitoneal routes in continuous ambulatory peritoneal dialysis (CAPD) patients. *Perit Dial Int* 1989;9:95–98.

415. Macdougall IC, et al. Clinical pharmacokinetics of epoetin (recombinant human erythropoietin). *Clin Pharmacokinet* 1991;20:99–113.

416. Brockmoller J, et al. The pharmacokinetics and pharmacodynamics or recombinant human erythropoietin in hemodialysis patients. *Br J Clin Pharmacol* 1992;34:449–508.

417. Albitar S, et al. Subcutaneous versus intravenous administration of erythropoietin improves its efficacy for the treatment of anaemia in haemodialysis patients. *Nephrol Dial Transplant* 1995;10:40–43.

418. Grannolleras C, et al. Experience with daily self-administered subcutaneous erythropoietin. *Contrib Nephrol* 1989;76:143–148.

419. Granneloras C, et al. Subcutaneous erythropoietin: a comparison of daily and thrice weekly administration. *Contrib Nephrol* 1991;88:144–151.

420. Kampf D, et al. Single dose kinetics or recombinant human erythropoietin after intravenous subcutaneous and intraperitoneal administration. *Contrib Nephrol* 1989;76:106–111.

421. Halstenson CE, et al. Comparative pharmacokinetics and pharmacodynamics of epoetin alfa and epoetin beta. *Clin Pharmacol Ther* 1991;50:702–712.

422. Macdougall IC, et al. Pharmacokinetics of intravenous, intraperitoneal, and subcutaneous recombinant erythropoietin in patients on CAPD. *Contrib Nephrol* 1989;76:121–126.

423. Neumayer H-H, et al. Pharmacokinetics or recombinant human erythropoietin after subcutaneous administration and in long-term IV treatments in patients on maintenance hemodialysis. *Contrib Nephrol* 1989;76:131–142.

424. Kampf D, et al. Pharmacokinetics of recombinant human erythro-

poietin in dialysis patients after single and multiple subcutaneous administrations. *Nephron* 1992;61:393–398.

425. Macdougall IC, et al. Subcutaneous erythropoietin therapy: comparison of three different sites of injection. *Contrib Nephrol* 1991;88: 152–156.

426. Horl WH. Optimal route of administration of erythropoietin in chronic renal failure patients: intravenous versus subcutaneous. *Acta Haematol* 1992;87[Suppl 1]:16–19.

427. Stockenhuber F, et al. Pharmacokinetic and dose response after intravenous and subcutaneous administration of recombinant erythropoietin in patients on regular haemodialysis treatment or continuous ambulatory peritoneal dialysis. *Nephron* 1991;59:399–402.

428. Paganini EP, et al. Intravenous versus subcutaneous dosing of epoetin alfa in hemodialysis patients. *Am J Kidney Dis* 1995;26:331–340.

429. Bommer J, et al. Subcutaneous erythropoietin. *Lancet* 1988;1:406.

430. Parker KP, et al. Weekly subcutaneous erythropoietin maintains hematocrit in chronic hemodialysis patients. *J Am Soc Nephrol* 1993; 3:1717(abst).

431. Taylor JE, et al. Erythropoietin response and route of administration. *Clin Nephrol* 1994;41:297–302.

432. Schaller R, et al. Differences in intravenous and subcutaneous application of recombinant human erythropoietin; a multicenter trial. *Artif Organs* 1994;18:552–558.

433. Ashai NI, et al. Intravenous versus subcutaneous dosing of epoetin: a review of the literature. *Am J Kidney Dis* 1993;22[Suppl 1]:23–31.

434. Kaufman JS, et al. Subcutaneous compared with intravenous epoetin in patients receiving hemodialysis. *N Engl J Med* 1998;339:578.

435. Besarab A, et al. Meta-analysis of subcutaneous versus intravenous epoetin in maintenance treatment of anemia in hemodialysis patients. *Am J Kidney Dis* 2002;40:439–446.

436. Peterson J, et al. Erythropoietin can be administered during dialysis: a kinetic analysis. *ASAIO J* 1996;42:27–33.

437. Grohskopf LA, et al. *Serratia liquefaciens* bloodstream infections from contamination of epoetin alfa at a hemodialysis center. *N Engl J Med* 2001;344:1491.

438. Bargman JM, et al. The pharmacokinetics of intraperitoneal erythropoietin administered undiluted or diluted in dialysate. *Perit Dial Int* 1992;12:369–372.

439. Faller B, et al. Daily subcutaneous administration of recombinant human erythropoietin (rhEPO) in peritoneal dialysis patients: a European dose-response study. *Clin Nephrol* 1993;40:168–175.

440. Zappacosta AR, et al. Weekly subcutaneous recombinant human erythropoietin corrects anemia of progressive renal failure. *Am J Med* 1991;91:229–232.

441. Lui SF, et al. Once weekly versus twice weekly subcutaneous administration of recombinant human erythropoietin in patients on continuous ambulatory peritoneal dialysis. *Clin Nephrol* 1991;36:246–251.

442. Nonnast-Daniel B, et al. Hemodynamics in hemodialysis patients treated with recombinant human erythropoietin. *Contrib Nephrol* 1989;76:283–291.

443. Movilli E, et al. Predialysis versus postdialysis hematocrit evaluation during erythropoietin therapy. *Am J Kidney Dis* 2002;39:850–853.

444. Tatsumi N, et al. Reticulocyte count used to assess recombinant human erythropoietin sensitivity in hemodialysis patients. *Contrib Nephrol* 1990;82:41–48.

445. Bommer J, et al. Recombinant human erythropoietin therapy in haemodialysis patients-dose determination and clinical experience. *Nephrol Dial Transplant* 1987;2:238–242.

446. Barosi G, et al. Variations in erythropoiesis and serum ferritin during erythropoietin therapy for anaemia of end-stage renal disease. *Acta Haematol* 1993;9013–9018.

447. Schwartz AB, et al. The effects of recombinant human erythropoietin on mean corpuscular volume in patients with the anemia of chronic renal failure. *Clin Nephrol* 1995;43:256–259.

448. Baime M, et al. Making the best use of the CBC. *Intern Med* 1993;14:23–32.

449. Egrie JC, et al. Development and characterization of novel erythropoiesis stimulating protein (NESP). *Br J Cancer* 2001;84[Suppl 1]:3–10.

450. Macdougall IC, et al. Pharmacokinetics of novel erythropoiesis stim-

ulating protein compared with epoetin alfa in dialysis patients. *J Am Soc Nephrol* 1999;10:2392–2395.

451. Locatelli F, et al. Novel erythropoiesis stimulating protein for treatment of anemia in chronic renal insufficiency. *Kidney Int* 2001;60: 741–747.

452. Nissenson AR, et al. Novel erythropoiesis stimulating protein (NESP) safely maintains hemoglobin concentration levels in hemodialysis patients as effectively as r-HuEPO when administered once-weekly. *J Am Soc Nephrol* 2000;11:A1326.

453. Vanrenterghem Y, et al. Novel erythropoiesis stimulating protein (NESP) maintains hemoglobin in ESRD patients when administered once-weekly or once every other week. *J Am Soc Nephrol* 1999;10: 270A(abst A1365).

454. Vanrenterghem Y, et al. Novel erythropoiesis stimulating protein (NESP) administered once every 3 weeks by the intravenous or subcutaneous route maintains hemoglobin (Hb) in dialysis patients. *J Am Soc Nephrol* 2001;12:abstract A1878.

455. Koch KM, et al. Occult blood loss and iron balance in chronic renal failure. *Proc EDTA* 1975;12:362–369.

456. Sawelson S, et al. Incidence and cause of gastrointestinal bleeding in uremic, hemodialysis (HD) and continuous ambulatory peritoneal dialysis (CAPD) patients. *Kidney Int* 1990;37:244(abst).

457. Smoller BR, et al. Phlebotomy for diagnostic laboratory tests in adults. *N Engl J Med* 1986;314:1233–1235.

458. Mirahmadi KS, et al. Serum ferritin level. Determinant of iron requirement in hemodialysis patients. *JAMA* 1977;238:601–603.

459. Wingard RL, et al. Efficacy of oral iron therapy in patients receiving recombinant human erythropoietin. *Am J Kidney Dis* 1995;25: 433–439.

460. U.S. Renal Data Systems. The USRDS Dialysis Morbidity and Mortality Study (Wave 1). In: *U.S. Renal Data Systems annual report 1996*. Bethesda, MD: National Institutes of Health, National Institutes of Diabetes and Digestive and Kidney Diseases, 1996:45–67.

461. Van Wyck DB, et al. Iron status in patients receiving erythropoietin for dialysis-associated anemia. *Kidney Int* 1989;35:165–170.

462. Fishbane S, et al. Reduction in recombinant human erythropoietin doses by the use of chronic intravenous iron supplementation. *Am J Kidney Dis* 1995;26:41–46.

463. Macdougall IC, et al. A randomized controlled study of iron supplementation in patients treated with erythropoietin. *Kidney Int* 1996;50:1694–1699.

464. Sepandj F, et al. Economic appraisal of maintenance parenteral iron administration in treatment of the anaemia in chronic haemodialysis patients. *Nephrol Dial Transplant* 1996;11:319–322.

465. Rosenlof K, et al. Iron availability is transiently improved by intravenous iron medication in patients on chronic hemodialysis. *Clin Nephrol* 1995;43:249–255.

466. Taylor JE, et al. Regular, low dose intravenous iron therapy improves response to erythropoietin in haemodialysis patients. *Nephrol Dial Transplant* 1996;11:1079–1083.

467. Silverberg DS, et al. Intravenous ferric saccharate as an iron supplement in dialysis patients. *Nephron* 1996;72:413–417.

468. SunderPlassmann G, et al. Importance of iron supply for erythropoietin therapy. *Nephrol Dial Transplant* 1995,10:2070–2076.

469. Besarab A, et al. A study of parenteral iron regimens in hemodialysis patients. *Am J Kidney Dis* 1999;34:21.

470. Besarab A, et al. Optimization of epoetin therapy with intravenous iron therapy in hemodialysis patients. *J Am Soc Nephrol* 2000;11:530.

471. Nissenson AR, et al. Sodium ferric gluconate complex in sucrose is safe and effective in hemodialysis patients: North American Clinical Trial. *Am J Kidney Dis* 1999;33:471.

472. Fishbane S, et al. Sodium ferric gluconate complex in the treatment of iron deficiency for patients on dialysis. *Am J Kidney Dis* 2001;37:879.

473. Bailie GR, et al. Parenteral iron use in the management of anemia in end-stage renal disease patients. *Am J Kidney Dis* 2000;35:1.

474. Silverberg DS, et al. Intravenous ferric saccarate as an iron supplement in dialysis patients. *Nephron* 1996;72:413.

475. Charytan C, et al. Efficacy and safety of iron sucrose for iron deficiency in patients with dialysis-associated anemia: North American clinical trial. *Am J Kidney Dis* 2001;37:300.

476. Van Wyck DB, et al. Safety and efficacy of iron sucrose in patients sensitive to iron dextran: North American Clinical Trial. *Am J Kidney Dis* 2000;36:88.

477. Bolanos L, et al. Continuous intravenous sodium ferric gluconate improves efficacy in the maintenance phase of EPOrHu administration in hemodialysis patients. *Am J Nephrol* 2992;22:67–72.

478. Gupta A, et al. Dialysate iron therapy: Infusion of soluble ferric pyrophosphate via the dialysate during hemodialysis. *Kidney Int* 1999;55:1891.

479. Silverberg DS, et al. Intravenous iron supplementation for the treatment of the anemia of moderate to severe chronic renal failure patients not receiving dialysis. *Am J Kidney Dis* 1996;27:234–238.

480. Tarng DC, et al. Iron metabolism indices for early prediction of the response and resistance to erythropoietin therapy in maintenance hemodialysis patients. *Am J Nephrol* 1995;15:230–237.

481. Fishbane S, et al. The evaluation of iron status in hemodialysis patients. *J Am Soc Nephrol* 1996;7:2654–2657.

482. Moreb J, et al. Evaluation of iron status in patients on chronic hemodialysis: relative usefulness of bone marrow hemosiderin, serum ferritin, transferrin saturation, mean corpuscular volume and red cell protoporphyrin. *Nephron* 1983;35:196–200.

483. Fishbane S, et al. The utility of zinc protoporphyrin for predicting the need for intravenous iron therapy in hemodialysis patients. *Am J Kidney Dis* 1995;25:426–432.

484. Schaefer RM, et al. The hypochromic red cell: a new parameter for monitoring of iron supplementation during rhEPO therapy. *J Perinatal Med* 1995;23:83–88.

485. Horl WH, et al. How to diagnose and correct iron deficiency during r-huEPO therapy—a consensus report (review). *Nephrol Dial Transplant* 1996;11:246–250.

486. Kalantar-Zadeh K, et al. Diagnosis of iron deficiency anemia in renal failure patients during the post-erythropoietin era. *Am J Kidney Dis* 1995;26:292–299.

487. Fishbane S, et al. Reticulocyte hemoglobin content in the evaluation of iron status of hemodialysis patients. *Kidney Int* 1997;52:217–222.

488. Fishbane S, et al. A randomized trial of iron deficiency testing strategies in hemodialysis patients. *Kidney Int* 2001;60:2406.

489. Hamstra RD, et al. Intravenous iron dextran in clinical medicine. *JAMA* 1980;243:1726–1731.

490. Fishbane S, et al. Safety of intravenous iron dextran in hemodialysis patients. *Am J Kidney Dis* 1996;28:529–534.

491. Gastaldello K, et al. Resistance to erythropoietin in iron-overloaded haemodialysis patients can be overcome by ascorbic acid administration. *Nephrol Dial Transplant* 1995;10[Suppl 6]:44–47.

492. Goch J, et al. Treatment of erythropoietin-resistant anaemia with desferrioxamine in patients on haemofiltration. *Eur J Haematol* 1995;55:73–77.

493. Hakim RM, et al. Iron overload and mobilization in long-term hemodialysis patients. *Am J Kidney Dis* 1987;10:293–299.

494. McCarthy JT, et al. Transfusional iron overload in patients undergoing dialysis: treatment with erythropoietin and phlebotomy. *J Lab Clin Med* 1989;114:193–199.

495. Eschbach JW, et al. Disorders of red blood cell production in uremia. *Arch Intern Med* 1970;126:812–815.

496. Summerfield GP, et al. Haemoglobin concentration and serum erythropoietin in renal dialysis and transplant patients. *Scand J Haematol* 1983;30:389–400.

497. Radtke HW, et al. Improving anemia by hemodialysis: effect on serum erythropoietin. *Kidney Int* 1980;17:382–387.

498. Santiago GC, et al. Effect of dialysis therapy on the hematopoietic system: the National Cooperative Dialysis Study. *Kidney Int* 1983;23 [Suppl 13]:S95–S100.

499. Ifudu O, et al. The intensity of hemodialysis and the response to erythropoietin in patients with end-stage renal disease. *N Engl J Med* 1996;334:420–425.

500. Ifudu O, et al. Adequacy of dialysis and differences in hematocrit among dialysis facilities. *Am J Kidney Dis* 2000;36:1166.

501. Lin CL, et al. Improved iron utilization and reduced erythropoietin resistance by on-line hemofiltration. *Blood Purif* 2002;20:349–356.

502. Bonforte G, et al. Improvement of anemia in hemodialysis patients treated by hemodiafiltration with high-volume on-line-prepared substitution fluid. *Blood Purif* 2002:20:357–363.

503. Fafugli RM, et al. Behavior of non- protein bound and protein bound uremic solutes during daily dialysis. *Am J Kidney Dis* 2002;40: 339–347.

504. Brox AG, et al. Subtherapeutic erythropoietin and insulin-like growth factor-1 correct the anemia of chronic renal failure in the mouse. *Kidney Int* 1996;50:937–943.

505. Adamson JW, et al. Why do some hemodialysis patients (HPD) need large doses of recombinant erythropoietin (rHuEPO)? *Kidney Int* 1990;37:235(abst).

506. Danielson B. R-HuEPO hyporesponsiveness—who and why? *Nephrol Dial Transplant* 1995;10[Suppl 2]:69–73.

507. Drüecke TB. Modulating factors in the hematopoietic response to erythropoietin. *Am J Kidney Dis* 1991;18[Suppl 1]:87–92.

508. Macdougall IC. Poor response to erythropoietin: practical guidelines on investigation and management. *Nephrol Dial Transplant* 1995;10: 607–614.

509. Jongen-Lavrencic M, et al. Interaction of inflammatory cytokines and erythropoietin in iron metabolism and erythropoiesis in anaemia of chronic disease (review). *Clin Rheumatol* 1995;4:519–525.

510. Ryan J, et al. Evaluation of in vitro production of tumor necrosis factor by monocytes in dialysis patients. *Blood Purif* 1991;9:142–147.

511. Muirhead N, et al. Occult infection and resistance of anemia to rHuEPO therapy in renal failure. *Nephrol Dial Transplant* 1990;5: 232–234.

512. Herbelin A, et al. Elevated circulating levels of interleukin-6 in patients with chronic renal failure. *Kidney Int* 1991;39:954–960.

513. Ryan J, et al. Evaluation of in vitro production of tumor necrosis factor by monocytes in dialysis patients. *Blood Purif* 1991;9:142–147.

514. Drüecke TB. RHuEPO hyporesponsiveness who and why? *Nephrol Dial Transplant* 1995;10:62–68.

515. Goicoechea M, et al. Role of cytokines in the response to erythropoietin in hemodialysis patients. *Kidney Int* 1998;54:1337.

516. Almond MK, et al. Increased erythropoietin requirements in patients with failed renal transplants returning to a dialysis program. *Nephrol Dial Transplant* 1994;9:270–273.

517. Hymes LC, et al. Impaired response to recombinant erythropoietin therapy in children with peritonitis. *Dial Transplant* 1994;23: 462–463.

518. Huang TP, et al. Intraperitoneal recombinant human erythropoietin therapy: influence of the duration of continuous ambulatory peritoneal dialysis treatment and peritonitis. *Am J Nephrol* 1995;15: 312–317.

519. Nassar GM, et al. Occult infection of old nonfunctioning arteriovenous grafts: a novel cause of erythropoietin resistance and chronic inflammation in hemodialysis patients. *Kidney Int* 2002;61[Suppl 80]:49.

520. Muirhead N, et al. The role of aluminum and parathyroid hormone in erythropoietin resistance in haemodialysis patients. *Nephrol Dial Transplant* 1991;6:342–345.

521. Bia MJ, et al. Aluminum induced anemia: pathogenesis and treatment in patients on chronic hemodialysis. *Kidney Int* 1989:36:852–858.

522. Grutzmacher P, et al. Effect of aluminum overload on the bone marrow response to recombinant human erythropoietin. *Contrib Nephrol* 1989;76:315–323.

523. Yaqoob M, et al. Resistance to recombinant human erythropoietin due to aluminium overload and its reversal by low dose desferrioxamine therapy. *Postgrad Med J* 1993;69(808):124–128.

524. Thuraisingham RC, et al. Improvement in anaemia following renal transplantation but not after erythropoietin therapy in a patient with sickle-cell disease. *Nephrol Dial Transplant* 1993;8:371–372.

525. Tomson CR, et al. Effect of recombinant human erythropoietin on erythropoiesis in homozygous sickle-cell anaemia and renal failure. *Nephrol Dial Transplant* 1992;7:817–821.

526. Cheng IKP, et al. Influence of thalassemia on the response to recombinant human erythropoietin in dialysis patients. *Am J Nephrol* 1993;13:142–148.

527. Lai KN, et al. Use of recombinant erythropoietin in thalassemic patients on dialysis. *Am J Kidney Dis* 1992;19:239–245.

528. Rachmilewitz EA, et al. Sustained increase in haemoglobin and RBC following long-term administration of recombinant human erythropoietin to patients with homozygous beta-thalassaemia. *Br J Haematol* 1995;90:341–345.

529. Shetty A, et al. Continuous ambulatory peritoneal dialysis in endstage renal disease due to multiple myeloma. *Perit Dial Int* 1995;15:236–240.

530. Ono K, et al. Is folate supplementation necessary in hemodialysis patients on erythropoietin therapy? *Clin Nephrol* 1992;38:290–292.

531. Pronai W, et al. Folic acid supplementation improves erythropoietin response. *Nephron* 1995;71:395–400.

532. Zachee P, et al. Erythropoietin resistance due to vitamin B12 deficiency: case report and retrospective analysis of B12 levels after erythropoietin treatment. *Am J Nephrol* 1992;12:188–191.

533. Ng YY, et al. Resistance to erythropoietin: immunohemolytic anemia induced by residual formaldehyde in dialyzers. *Am J Kidney Dis* 1993;21:213–216.

534. Evers J. Cardiac hemolysis and anemia refractory to erythropoietin: on anemia in dialysis patients [Letter]. *Nephron* 1995;71:108.

535. Casadevall N, et al. Brief report: autoantibodies against erythropoietin in a patient with pure red-cell aplasia. *N Engl J Med* 1996;334:630–633.

536. Madour F, et al. A population study of the interplay between iron, nutrition, and inflammation in erythropoiesis in hemodialysis patients. *J Am Soc Nephrol* 1996;7:1456(abst).

537. Gunnell J, et al. Acute-phase response predicts erythropoietin resistance in hemodialysis and peritoneal dialysis patients. *Am J Kidney Dis* 1999; 33:63.

538. De Paepe MBJ, et al. Influence of continuous ambulatory peritoneal dialysis on the anemia of endstage renal disease. *Kidney Int* 1983;23:744–748.

539. Mehta BR, et al. Changes in red cell mass, plasma volume and hematocrit in patients on CAPD. *Trans ASAIO* 1983;24:50–52.

540. Linblad AS, et al. Hematocrit values in the CAPD/CCPD population: a report of the National CAPD Registry. *Perit Dial Int* 1990;10:275–278.

541. Macdougall IC, et al. Subcutaneous recombinant erythropoietin in the treatment of renal anaemia in CAPD patients. *Contrib Nephrol* 1989;76:219–226.

542. Piraino B, et al. The use of subcutaneous erythropoietin in CAPD patients. *Clin Nephrol* 1990;33:200–202.

543. Besarab A, et al. Response of continuous peritoneal dialysis patients to subcutaneous rHuEPO differs from that of hemodialysis patients. *ASAIO Trans* 1991;37:M395–M396.

544. Stevens JM, et al. Stepwise correction of anaemia by subcutaneous administration of human recombinant erythropoietin in patients with chronic renal failure maintained by continuous ambulatory peritoneal dialysis. *Nephrol Dial Transplant* 1991;6:487–494.

545. Barany P, et al. Subcutaneous epoetin beta in renal anemia: an open multicenter dose titration study of patients on continuous peritoneal dialysis. *Perit Dial Int* 1995;15:54–60.

546. Ballel SH, et al. Androgens potentiate the effects of erythropoietin in the treatment of anemia of end-stage renal disease. *Am J Kidney Dis* 1991;17:29–33.

547. Berns JS, et al. A controlled trial of recombinant human erythropoietin and nandrolone decanoate in the treatment of anemia in patients on chronic hemodialysis. *Clin Nephrol* 1992;37:264–267.

548. Teruel JL, et al. Androgen versus erythropoietin for the treatment of anemia in hemodialyzed patients: a prospective study. *J Am Soc Nephrol* 1996;7:140–144.

549. Labonia WL. L-Carnitine effects on anemia in hemodialyzed patients treated with erythropoietin. Am J Kidney Dis 1995;26:757–764.

550. Berard E, et al. Effects of low doses of L-carnitine on the response to recombinant human erythropoietin in hemodialyzed children: about two cases. *Nephron* 1992;62:368–369.

551. Kooistra MP, et al. The response to recombinant human erythropoietin in patients with the anemia of endstage renal disease is correlated with serum carnitine levels [Letter]. *Nephron* 1991;57:127–128.

552. Audet AM, et al. Practice strategies for elective red blood cell transfusion. *Ann Intern Med* 1992;116:403–406.

553. Julian BA, et al. Erythropoiesis after withdrawal of enalapril in posttransplant erythrocytosis. *Kidney Int* 1994;46:1397–1403.

554. Perazella M, et al. Enalapril treatment of posttransplant erythrocytosis: efficacy independent of circulating erythropoietin levels. *Am J Kidney Dis* 1995;26:495–500.

555. Shand BI, et al. Effect of enalapril on erythrocytosis in hypertensive patients with renal disease. *Blood Press* 1995;4:238–240.

556. Hess E, et al. Do ACE inhibitors influence the dose of human recombinant erythropoietin in dialysis patients? [Letter]. *Nephrol Dial Transplant* 1997;11:749–751.

557. Walter J. Does captopril decrease the effect of human recombinant erythropoietin in haemodialysis patients? [Letter]. *Nephrol Dial Transplant* 1993;8:142.

558. Dhondt AW, et al. Angiotensin-converting enzyme inhibitors and higher erythropoietin requirement in chronic haemodialysis patients. *Nephrol Dial Transplant* 1995;10:2107–2109.

559. Erturk S, et al. Unresponsiveness to recombinant human erythropoietin in haemodialysis patients: possible implications of angiotensin converting enzyme inhibitors. *Nephrol Dial Transplant* 1996;11:393–397.

560. Erturk S, et al. The impact of withdrawing ACE inhibitors on erythropoietin responsiveness and left ventricular hypertrophy in haemodialysis patients. *Nephrol Dial Transplant* 1999;14:1912

561. Conlon PJ, et al. ACE inhibitors do not affect erythropoietin efficiency in hemodialysis patients [Letter]. *Nephrol Dial Transplant* 1994;9:1359–1360.

562. Sanchez JA. ACE inhibitors do not decrease rHuEPO response in patients with endstage renal failure [Letter]. *Nephrol Dial Transplant* 1995;10:1476–1477.

563. Shand BI, et al. Effect of losartan on haematology and haemorheology in elderly patients with essential hypertension: a pilot study. *J Hum Hypertens* 1995;9:233–235.

564. Abels RI. Use of recombinant human erythropoietin in the treatment of anemia in patients who have cancer. *Semin Oncol* 1992;19:29–35.

565. Bargman JM, et al. The pharmacokinetics of intraperitoneal erythropoietin administered undiluted or diluted in dialysate. *Perit Dial Int* 1992;12:369–372.

566. Reddingius RE, et al. Pharmacokinetics of recombinant human erythropoietin in children treated with continuous ambulatory peritoneal dialysis. *Eur J Pediatr* 1994;153:850–854.

567. Loo AV, et al. Recombinant human erythropoietin corrects anaemia after renal transplantation: a randomized prospective study. *Nephrol Dial Transplant* 1996;11:1815–1821.

NEUROLOGIC COMPLICATIONS ASSOCIATED WITH DIALYSIS AND CHRONIC RENAL INSUFFICIENCY

IMRAN I. ALI AND NOOR A. PIRZADA

Chronic renal insufficiency is associated with neurologic derangements that involve both the central and the peripheral nervous system (1–4). Several of these neurologic syndromes are well defined and their clinical characteristics are protean and nonspecific (2,3). The diagnosis of these disorders is usually straightforward, although a high index of suspicion is required to exclude other potentially serious and possibly reversible causes. Moreover, it is important to remember that some disorders that result in renal failure may also cause neurologic symptoms. For example, polyarteritis nodosa may present with renal failure and mononeuritis multiplex or central nervous system involvement.

The clinician must distinguish the neurologic symptoms and signs associated with the primary disease from those associated with uremia. This requires familiarity not only with the neurologic features of renal insufficiency but also with those of disorders that may present with neurologic and renal involvement (Table 33.1). A comprehensive neurologic evaluation is necessary for precise diagnosis and subsequent management of these disorders. The spectrum of neurologic disorders seen in association with chronic renal failure (CRF) is listed in Table 33.2.

This chapter is divided into two sections. The first discusses central nervous system disorders in patients with chronic kidney disease and dialysis patients, and the second addresses the peripheral nervous system in patients with chronic kidney disease and in dialysis patients.

CENTRAL NERVOUS SYSTEM ABNORMALITIES

Uremic Encephalopathy

Chronic kidney disease may result in cognitive impairment associated with clouding of consciousness, especially when the glomerular filtration rate falls below 10 mL/minute (4). The clinical features of uremic encephalopathy are nonspecific and include confusion, psychomotor agitation, alteration of sleep-wake cycle, disorientation, impaired memory, inattention, paranoid ideation, impaired abstraction, visual hallucinations, myoclonus, and seizures (4–8). The clinical course is usually insidious in onset with waxing and waning of intellectual function, a typical feature of most metabolic encephalopathies.

Progression of renal insufficiency may subsequently result in gradual obtundation followed by coma unless dialysis is performed. Dialysis initiation usually results in gradual clinical improvement (4).

TABLE 33.1. SYSTEMIC DISORDERS WITH RENAL AND NERVOUS SYSTEM INVOLVEMENT

Disease	Clinical Presentation
Polyarteritis nodosa	Mononeuritis multiplex, CNS vasculitis
Systemic lupus erythematosus	Neuropsychiatric disease, cerebral infarction, myelitis, neuropathy
Wegener's granulomatosis	Midline granulomatous inflammation, peripheral neuropathy
Thrombotic thrombocytopenic purpura	Cerebral edema, seizures, fluctuating focal deficits
Rheumatoid arthritis	CNS vasculitis, cervical myelopathy, neuropathy
Hypertensive encephalopathy	Headaches, seizures, altered sensorium, coma
Autosomal dominant polycystic kidney disease	Intracranial aneurysms

TABLE 33.2. NEUROLOGIC DISORDERS ASSOCIATED WITH RENAL FAILURE AND DIALYSIS

Central nervous system disorders
  Uremic encephalopathy
  Dialysis dysequilibrium syndrome
  Dialysis dementia
  Cerebrovascular disease
Peripheral nervous system disorders
  Uremic neuropathy
  Autonomic and cranial neuropathy
  Mononeuropathies
    Carpal tunnel syndrome
    Ischemic monomelic neuropathy
    Compressive neuropathies
Myopathy

There is no absolute correlation between neurologic impairment and the blood urea nitrogen level, although it has been suggested that the rate of rise of urea and creatinine may be related to the development of neurologic symptoms (6,8). Neurologic examination is usually nonlateralizing; impaired higher cortical functions, hyperreflexia, and asterixis may be present.

Asterixis, a sudden loss of muscle tone that results in a "flapping" tremor, is best assessed by having the patient hyperextend at the elbow and wrist with the fingers spread apart; the asterixis is then best seen at the metacarpophalangeal joints and the wrist. This phenomenon is also seen in hepatic and other metabolic encephalopathies, and, although a nonspecific finding, it may be useful in assessment of a patient with declining renal function (2).

Patients with uremic encephalopathy characteristically also manifest multifocal myoclonus. Myoclonus is a sudden rhythmic movement of muscle groups; it is asymmetric and usually not related to seizures. In addition focal neurologic findings such as extensor plantar response, grasp or snout reflexes have been described.

The presence of focal neurologic findings should be fully investigated to look for other causes of altered mentation. Neuroimaging studies such as computed tomography (CT) or magnetic resonance imaging (MRI) may show cortical atrophy (9,10). Rarely, changes suggestive of edema are seen involving the basal ganglia, cerebral cortex, and centrum semiovale (Fig. 33.1) (10). Interestingly, these changes are similar to those seen in hypertensive encephalopathy. The cause and significance of these changes are unknown, but they are thought to be related to transient ischemia. The possibility that these changes are related to uremic toxins or other metabolic derangement cannot be excluded, because these changes usually resolve after dialysis (10). In patients with sudden onset focal neurologic deficits, MRI with diffusion weighted imaging (DWI) will show corresponding abnormality within a few minutes of the onset of symptoms. MRI with DWI is a very useful and powerful tool for evaluation of ischemic cerebrovascular disease (11).

Cerebrospinal fluid (CSF) examination usually is normal, although mildly elevated protein is seen in greater than half of the patients with uremia and lymphocytic pleocytosis may be seen in up to 10% of patients (2,12). It is of critical importance that encephalitis, meningitis, and other causes of CSF abnormalities be excluded before attributing the CSF changes to uremia.

One of the most perplexing questions in uremia is the pathogenesis of uremic encephalopathy. The substance responsible for the encephalopathy is not known. There is no direct relationship

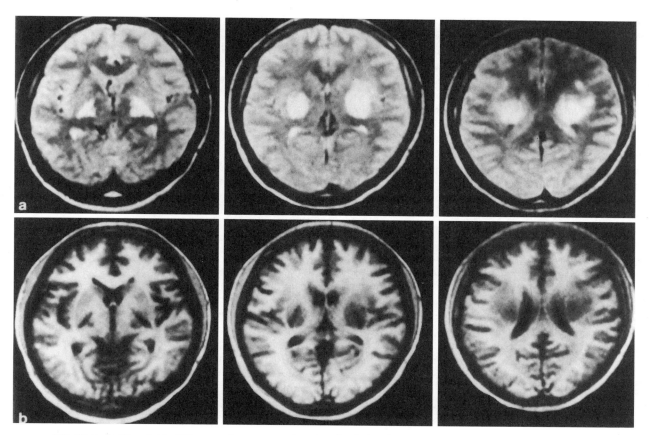

FIG. 33.1. A: T2-weighted SE magnetic resonance imaging (MRI) showing increased signal intensity involving basal ganglia, internal capsules, and periventricular white matter. **B:** T1-weighted IR MRI showing hypodensities in the same regions. (From Okada J, et al. Reversible MRI and CT findings in uremic encephalopathy. *Neuroradiology* 1991;33:524–526, with permission.)

between urea or creatinine levels and the level of encephalopathy (5–7). Most likely, uremic encephalopathy is a result of a combination of factors, including accumulation of various organic acids and substances such as myoinositol, purines, organic phosphates, oxalate, ascorbic acid, amino acid peptides, parathyroid hormone (PTH), β_2-microglobulin, methylguanidine, guanidosuccinic acid, hippuric acid, polyamines, phenoles, and indoles, in addition to urea and creatinine (6,7, 13–15). In animal models a number of these compounds of different molecular weights produce toxicity similar to that seen in uremic syndrome.

Urea and creatinine are considered low molecular weight compounds (<300 daltons), whereas myoglobulin is considered high molecular weight (>12,000 daltons). Similarly, compounds with molecular weight between 300 to 12,000 daltons are considered "middle molecules." Because the middle molecules are removed less efficiently than urea and creatinine during hemodialysis, these are considered likely candidates that contribute to uremic encephalopathy. These compounds include PTH, peptides, glucoronated conjugates, and β_2-microglobulin. Compounds such as methylguanidine, hippuric acid, polyamines, phenoles, and indoles have lower molecular weight, but their kinetics of removal during dialysis are similar to the "classic" middle molecules (14).

As stated previously, PTH has been implicated in the pathogenesis of uremic encephalopathy (15–17) because of secondary hyperparathyroidism and effect of PTH on neuronal function (16). Even in the absence of renal insufficiency, elevated levels of PTH can result in confusion and altered mental status. In animal models of uremia there is a marked increase in intracellular calcium (7,15), suggesting a possible link between PTH and neuronal dysfunction. In these animals, blockade of PTH function reverses the symptoms associated with uremic encephalopathy. Increased intracellular calcium results in impairment of energy metabolism with reduced adenosine triphosphate (ATP) levels because of abnormal mitochondrial function. There is also evidence to suggest abnormal phospholipid metabolism related to the previously mentioned events causes membrane instability and further neuronal injury (3,14,15).

Accumulation of various organic acids and the middle molecules described previously (6,7,13,14), either from increased permeability of the blood-brain barrier or impaired cellular transport mechanisms, may further compromise neuronal function. Biasioli et al. (8) describe an alteration in amino acid profile in serum and CSF of uremic patients that indicates an increase in glycine, dopamine, and serotonin and a decrease in gamma aminobutyric acid (GABA). Increased dopamine, serotonin, and glycine accumulation may result in increased irritability, sensorial clouding, tremors, and unsteadiness. Low GABA levels may lead to seizures and myoclonus and may exacerbate other uremic symptoms (8,15). However, no single abnormality fulfills all the criteria for being the putative neurotoxin, and uremic encephalopathy is most likely the result of derangements of neuronal function at multiple levels. Positron emission tomography (PET) scans in patients with CRF show reduced brain metabolism that correlates well with cognitive dysfunction and may be explained by the molecular events discussed previously (18).

Seizures

Seizures may occur during the course of uremic encephalopathy in as many as 10% to 20% of patients and are usually generalized tonic clonic, although simple or complex partial seizures may also be seen (2,6). It is important to exclude drug toxicity as a reversible cause of seizures, because a number of commonly used drugs are associated with seizures in renal failure. Drugs such as quinolones, penicillins, cephalosporins, acyclovir, and erythropoietin lower the seizure threshold and can lead to clinical seizure activity (19,20). The diagnosis is one of exclusion, and withdrawal of the presumed offending agent is enough to control the seizure activity.

Electroencephalography in patients with seizures usually shows marked slowing of the background with increased theta (4 to 7 Hz) and delta (1 to 3 Hz) activity, as well as bilateral frontal paroxysmal slowing and occasional frontal epileptiform activity in the form of spikes and sharp waves (6–8,21). It is important to note that these epileptiform abnormalities may be seen in patients with uremia and without a history of seizures as well. This finding in patients without seizures most likely represents evidence of cortical irritability and by themselves do not require any treatment. A characteristic electroencephalographic (EEG) finding in patients with uremic encephalopathy is triphasic waves, which are seen with advanced stages. However, this pattern may also be seen in other metabolic disorders such as hepatic encephalopathy, severe hyponatremia, and certain drug intoxications (e.g., lithium) (21).

The seizures should be treated the same as in other patients with metabolic encephalopathies. Long-term antiepileptic drug (AED) therapy is only required in patients with a high risk of recurrence, such as those with multiple seizures, history of recent status epilepticus, focal neurologic deficits, and seizures in the absence of any specific metabolic derangement. If long-term antiepileptic medication is indicated, the impact of renal insufficiency and dialysis on drug metabolism should be taken into account (Table 33.3) (22–24). Phenytoin, carbamazepine, and valproic acid are all reasonable first-line agents for the treatment of seizures. Phenytoin has the advantage of being available in intravenous (IV) form and can be given rapidly in an emergency. Because phenytoin is one of the most commonly used antiepileptic medications and its metabolism is significantly affected by uremia (2,25,26) the pharmacokinetics in renal failure must be well understood. Because of expanded volume of distribution there is a reduction in total level, although this is offset by a marked increase of the free fraction from 10% to 25% (25,26). This may result in clinical toxicity, even though the total level may be low; therefore, free phenytoin levels, which are easily available in most centers, should be used as a guide to dosing. The half-life of phenytoin is also reduced from 13 hours to approximately 8 hours; therefore, three times a day dosing is recommended.

Valproic acid is now also available in IV formulation, although there is very little data regarding its use in management of status epilepticus. Drugs that are metabolized by the cytochrome P-450 such as phenytoin, carbamazepine, oxarbazepine, and phenobarbital are enzyme inducers and may interfere with metabolism of a number of other drugs including

TABLE 33.3. ANTIEPILEPTIC DRUG THERAPY IN RENAL FAILURE

	Daily Dosage Range (mg/day)[a]	Plasma Concentration in CRF	Plasma Half Life	Dose Adjustment in CRF	Removal by Dialysis
Phenytoin	300–600 (IV load 10–15 mg/kg)	Total—decreased Unbound or free—increased	Decreased	Yes, follow free phenytoin levels	Negligible
Carbamazepine	600–1,800	No change	No change	No	Unknown
Phenobarbital	120–250	No change	Increased or no change	Yes, slight reduction	Significant
Gabapentin	1,800–3,600	Increased	Increased	Reduction based on GFR[b]	Significant
Lamotrigine	200–800	Increased?	Increased	Unknown	Moderate
Valproate	500–3,000 (IV dosing same as oral)	Decreased	No change	No	Negligible at therapeutic levels
Benzodiazepines		Decreased	No change	No	Negligible
Levetiracetam	1,000–4,000	Increased	Increased	No	Moderate
Oxcarbazepine	600–1,800	Increased	Increased	Yes	Unknown
Zonisamide	100–600	Increased	Increased	Yes—use with caution	Unknown
Topiramate	200–400	Increased	Increased	Yes—use with caution	Significant

[a]Dosages represent the range in patients without renal or hepatic disease.
[b]Gabapentin dosing in renal failure.

	Renal Failure	
Creatinine Clearance (mL/min)	Total Daily Dose (mg/day)	Dose Regimen (mg)
>60	1,200	400 TID
30–60	600	300 BID
15–30	300	300 QD
<15	150	300 QOD
Hemodialysis	—	300–300[b]

[a]Every other day.
[b]Loading dose of 300–400 mg in patients who have never received neurontin, then 200–300 mg. Neurontin following each 4 hours of hemodialysis. (Neurontin [package insert], Parke-Davis, 2001.)

cyclosporine; therefore, caution is advised when using these antiepileptic agents in medically complex patients. A number of new antiepileptic agents have been approved by the Food and Drug Administration (FDA) over the last few years and may be a reasonable alternative for these patients (Table 33.3). The choice of AED is based on the need for rapid dosing (phenytoin, valproic acid), side effect profile (renal toxicity with topiramate and zonisamide), and significant renal metabolism of the drug (gabapentin, levetirecetam, oxcarbazepine). We preferentially use phenytoin for rapid IV dosing in a patient with acute repetitive seizures or status epilepticus. However, in a patient with focal or secondary generalized seizures who is not in status epilepticus one may choose a drug like carbamazepine or oxcarbazepine. The newer AEDs such as lamotrigine and levetiracetam are additional exceedingly effective and safe options for add-on therapy if a single drug is ineffective at its maximally tolerable dose. A neurologic consultation may also be helpful in choosing the most appropriate AED.

Dosing adjustments for the commonly used antiepileptic medications are outlined in Table 33.3.

Cerebrovascular Disease in Chronic Renal Failure

Patients on chronic hemodialysis have a fivefold higher risk of cerebrovascular disease compared with the normal population (27–30). This may be related to the high prevalence of hypertension (27), underlying diabetes, hyperhomocystinemia, dyslipidemia, and atherosclerosis in hemodialysis patients (28). There are considerable data that suggest hyperhomocystinemia is an important risk factor in patients with ischemic cerebrovascular disease and chronic renal insufficiency (28). It is important to identify the cause of hyperhomocystinemia, which may be related to folate, cobalamin, or pyridoxine deficiency or because of a mutation of methylene tetrahydrofolate reductase (MTHFR) enzyme. Folic acid at 5 mg is recommended for most patients with MTHFR mutation, for folate deficiency, or when no other cause of hyperhomocystinemia is identified.

The management of ischemic cerebrovascular disease is the same as in patients without renal disease. Antiplatelet agents such as aspirin and clopidogrel are recommended for atherothrombotic disease, whereas patients with embolic infarction may need to be anticoagulated with warfarin. The decision to anticoagulate is based on the size of the infarct, the risk of recurrence, and the risk of systemic or intracranial bleeding in a particular patient.

Intracerebral hemorrhage is more common than cerebral infarct as the cause of stroke and most likely is related to hypertension (30). The actual incidence of intracerebral hemorrhage is 12.3 per 1,000 patient-years, and that of cerebral infarct is 3.9 per 1,000 patient-years (27). This is also associated with an overall 30-day stroke mortality that is 74.4%, compared with 12.3%

in the general population. This high mortality could be partly related to the disproportionately high incidence of intracerebral hemorrhage and associated systemic disease that was noted in this particular study.

Patients with autosomal dominant polycystic kidney disease (ADPKD) have a higher prevalence of intracranial aneurysms. These aneurysms are usually small, involve the anterior circulation, and are frequently multiple (29). The prevalence of these aneurysms is approximately 5%, depending on the screening method used. Cerebral angiography is the gold standard diagnostic method for locating these aneurysms (Fig. 33.2) (11). Magnetic resonance angiography (MRA) and high resolution CT scans are useful screening tests, but they may not detect very small aneurysms.

Screening is recommended for patients with a family history of aneurysms and intracranial hemorrhage, a previous history of aneurysms or subarachnoid hemorrhage, and clinical suspicion of aneurysm or for those patients who are undergoing surgery for unrelated reasons with significant perioperative risk of hypotension or hypertension. In addition, patients with symptoms suggestive of an aneurysm such as headaches, diplopia, or other focal neurologic signs should also be evaluated. Routine screening is of limited value for all patients with end-stage renal disease (ESRD) and polycystic kidney disease because of the reduced life expectancy of these individuals (29).

Clinical features may be related to mass effect in the case of a large aneurysm or because of a sudden rupture. Patients with subarachnoid hemorrhage usually present with sudden explosive headache that is frequently described as the "worst headache of their life." Nuchal rigidity and third cranial nerve palsy may also be present but are not seen in all patients. The initial evaluation must be rapid in patients with suspected subarachnoid hemor-

rhage, and urgent admission to an intensive care unit is warranted. The overall mortality of a ruptured aneurysm is approximately 30% to 50%, in patients with or without ADPKD (30, 31). Timely intervention can be life saving and most neurosurgeons perform early direct surgery *before* development of vasospasm, which usually occurs 3 to 4 days after rupture.

Management of asymptomatic aneurysms is somewhat controversial as there are limited data regarding the risk of rupture (32). Most neurosurgeons operate on large, asymptomatic aneurysms that are 10 mm or larger, because there is evidence that these aneurysms are often most likely to rupture. Unruptured intracranial aneurysms of less than 10 mm have a rupture rate of 0.05% per year as opposed to those greater than 10 mm with a rate of 1% per year. Giant aneurysms (greater than 25 mm) have the highest risk of bleeding (6% in the first year) (33). Aneurysms between 5 and 10 mm are followed with serial (every 6 months to 1 year) noninvasive studies. Aneurysm location does also affect management because those located in the posterior circulation such as the basilar artery or posterior communicating artery are more likely to rupture irrespective of size. Other factors that may have an impact on management of unruptured aneurysms include previous subarachnoid hemorrhage; age; family history; coexisting medical conditions; aneurysm characteristics such as size, location, and morphology; and neurosurgical expertise. Another approach to management of intracranial aneurysms is endovascular occlusion; this approach is attractive for patients with multiple medical problems or those who refuse direct surgery. The success rate appears to be lower than with direct surgery, although no comparative randomized trials have been performed as yet.

In our opinion, surgical decisions in an asymptomatic patient with intracranial aneurysms should be individualized after an informed discussion between the neurosurgeon, nephrologist, and the patient.

Approach to a Patient with Confusion and Renal Failure

In a patient who develops confusion associated with renal insufficiency, it is imperative to exclude other causes that may mimic uremic encephalopathy. A complete history and physical including a careful neurologic examination is mandatory. A systematic approach should be adopted to evaluate these patients. In these medically complex patients, systemic infections may result in profound confusion and should be looked for in addition to a complete neurologic evaluation. The differential diagnosis and the diagnostic workup for some of the neurologic diseases are listed in Table 33.4. It is important to exclude nonconvulsive status epilepticus as a cause of confusion in a uremic patient. It is a potentially life-threatening disorder that can be easily diagnosed by electroencephalogram and responds to antiepileptic therapy. If unrecognized and untreated nonconvulsive status epilepticus can lead to irreversible neurologic injury.

Dialysis Disequilibrium Syndrome

The dialysis disequilibrium syndrome is an unusual complication in current dialysis practice. It presents with a variety of con-

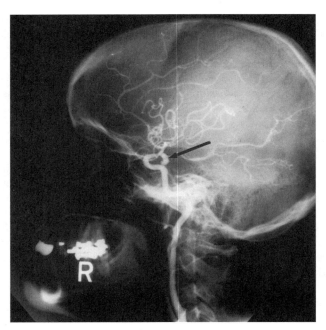

FIG. 33.2. A cerebral angiogram showing a posterior communicating artery aneurysm *(arrow)*. (Courtesy RA Brinker, MD, Department of Radiology, Medical College of Ohio, Toledo, Ohio.)

TABLE 33.4. APPROACH TO A PATIENT WITH CONFUSION IN RENAL FAILURE

Clinical Features	Diagnosis	Diagnostic Tests
Head trauma, headaches, falls	Subdural hematoma	CT or MRI
Focal neurologic findings (hemiparesis, homonymous hemianopsia, aphasia, etc.)	Infarct or intracerebral hemorrhage	CT or MRI
Fever, headaches, nuchal rigidity, seizures	Meningitis (bacterial, fungal, or mycobacterial)	CSF exam
Worst-ever headache, nuchal rigidity, subhyaloid hemorrhage on funduscopy	Subarachnoid hemorrhage	CT, cerebral angiography, neurosurgical evaluation
Altered sensorium, nonlateralizing examination	Hepatic encephalopathy, hyponatremia, hypoxia, hypercarbia gases	Liver function chemistries, arterial blood
Intermittent confusion, stereotypical behavior, automatisms	Nonconvulsive status epilepticus	EEG
Seizures with or without any other symptoms	Drug toxicity [penicillins, cephalosporins, carbapenams, acyclovir (58, 59), erythropoietin (60)]	History, drug withdrawal

stitutional and neurologic symptoms that include headache, fatigue, nausea, vomiting, hypertension, tremors, seizures, agitation, delirium, and subsequent coma (1–3,5,34–37). These symptoms usually appear within 24 hours of dialysis completion and last for a few hours (1). The syndrome is usually seen in severely uremic patients who are dialyzed aggressively. The electroencephalogram may show generalized and paroxysmal slowing during this period (3,21).

With regard to cause, some patients develop elevated intracranial pressure (ICP) during dialysis (14,37). This increase may be explained on the basis of reverse urea effect (34). Reverse urea effect results from more efficient removal of urea from plasma, as compared with the brain, with development of a reverse osmotic gradient. This intracellular accumulation of solutes such as urea favors movement of water to the intracellular space, leading to cerebral edema and the increase in ICP. The finding of more efficient removal of urea from the plasma compared with the brain during hemodialysis is disputed by some, but it is a plausible explanation for much of the clinical symptomatology seen.

Urea is, however, not the only compound responsible for the osmotic gradient and other compounds such as idiogenic osmoles may also be involved (1,34). Idiogenic osmoles are thought to be organic acids that are formed intracellularly in the brain and also contribute to the increased brain osmolality. Support for this comes from studies that show that the urea concentration in the brain can only account for 50% to 60% of the increase in brain osmolality; the rest is presumably related to these idiogenic osmoles (8).

Another somewhat controversial explanation for the development of cerebral edema is paradoxical intracellular acidosis (7,15), which may also be related to accumulation of organic acids. A fall in CSF pH is noted during dialysis in patients and in experimental animal models. This increase in the intracellular H^+ ion concentration in the brain results in increased osmolar content with a secondary increase in brain water. This would then result in cerebral edema and the symptoms of dialysis disequilibrium syndrome. This finding has, however, been refuted by other studies (8), which have not been able to demonstrate acidosis within the central nervous system. Similarly, the possible association of hemodynamic alterations and electrolyte shifts to the genesis of this syndrome is also unclear.

Dialysis Dementia or Dialysis Encephalopathy

Patients with chronic renal insufficiency on hemodialysis undergoing neuropsychologic testing show impaired performance on tests of short-term memory, attention, concentration span, and sequential information processing (4,38). This cognitive decline may or may not improve with therapy and is associated with diffuse cerebral atrophy, which may be seen on routine studies such as CT or MRI (9). Pathologically, there is neuronal cell loss and other nonspecific changes. The pathophysiology of these changes are unknown but are thought to be related to a combination of chronic aluminum toxicity, impaired cerebrovascular autoregulation, and breakdown of blood-brain barrier (9). Interestingly, patients undergoing peritoneal dialysis perform better on cognitive testing than those patients receiving hemodialysis (38).

Unlike the benign course described previously, some patients on hemodialysis for a period of greater than 2 years may develop a progressive dementia that is irreversible and invariably fatal (39–45). This form of dementia is exceedingly rare now, because of improved screening for aluminum in dialysate water (15). However, rare cases have been described in association with contamination of the dialysate water supply, such as when well water high in aluminum was used for home dialysis. The clinical features include aphasia, apraxia, myoclonus, seizures, progressive intellectual decline, confusion, auditory or visual hallucinations, and dysarthria (1–4). The symptoms are initially intermittent and may worsen immediately after dialysis (41).

As the disease progresses, there is persistent cognitive impairment, and an increase in seizures may also occur. These seizures are poorly responsive to AED therapy but may initially respond to benzodiazepines. Electroencephalogram may initially show paroxysmal slowing with predominant frontal spikes and sharp waves intermixed with normal background. As the disease progresses, the electroencephalogram may also show more severe background abnormalities (7,21,46). There is evidence that EEG changes may precede the clinical picture by months (4). Neuroimaging is usually unremarkable but may be useful in excluding tumors, subdural hematoma, or chronic infections.

The occurrence of dialysis dementia has been linked by a number of epidemiologic studies to aluminum intoxication

(39–46). These patients have a high serum aluminum level and may also show increased brain levels, especially in the gray matter (1,45). Removing aluminum from the dialysate and reducing intake of phosphate binding gels that have a high aluminum content have resulted in a dramatic decline in the incidence of this disease (2–4). However, there are patients who develop this disease with no evidence of exposure or evidence of aluminum intoxication (43). Children with CRF may develop this syndrome without ever undergoing dialysis or being exposed to aluminum. In such cases it is hypothesized that uremia may result in development of this syndrome through its effect on the developing brain (7).

Aluminum is normally absorbed in the gastrointestinal tract and is excreted through the kidneys. Increased absorption is probably the effect of PTH (16) on the gastrointestinal tract; in combination with reduced excretion, patients on dialysis have plasma levels that are six to eight times higher than normal (normal, 0 to 20 μg/L). At levels above 200 μg/L, chelating agents such as deferoxamine are recommended (2). To prevent the development of this complication, dialysate aluminum is kept below 20 μg/L by deionization (4,7). This process also removes other compounds such as cadmium, mercury, lead, manganese, copper, nickel, thallium, boron, and tin. The relationship of other substances including trace elements to dialysis dementia is not known (7).

PERIPHERAL NERVOUS SYSTEM INVOLVEMENT IN UREMIA

Involvement of the peripheral nervous system in CRF was described initially in the nineteenth century. Kussmaul (1864), Charcot (1870), and Osler (1892) wrote on various aspects of this condition. However, in the first half of the twentieth century descriptions of peripheral neuropathy in CRF virtually disappeared from the medical literature, which was instead dominated by central nervous system manifestations such as coma and seizures. After hemodialysis was introduced more than 30 years ago and patients began to live longer, peripheral neuropathy was reported more frequently and now is considered an integral part of the uremic syndrome.

Uremic Polyneuropathy

Uremic polyneuropathy is the most common type of peripheral nerve involvement, and typically occurs when the creatinine clearance is less than 10 mL/minute (Fig. 33.3). As determined by electrophysiologic studies and careful clinical examination, evidence of peripheral neuropathy is seen in 50% to 60% of patients with ESRD who require hemodialysis (47). It is more common in men than in women.

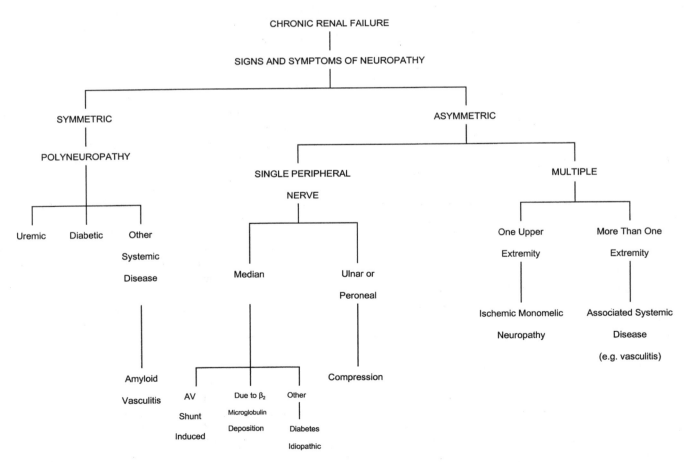

FIG. 33.3. Approach to the patient with chronic renal failure and neuropathy.

Usually the neuropathy has an insidious onset. Muscle cramps have been thought to herald peripheral nerve involvement, but many patients with similar complaints have no other manifestation of neuropathy. In such cases, the cramps probably are a nonspecific manifestation of uremia. Restless legs syndrome has also been thought to indicate early peripheral neuropathy in CRF and is seen in 40% of patients with varying degrees of renal failure (48). The syndrome of restless legs consists of creeping, crawling, prickling, and pruritic sensations deep within the legs that worsen in the evening and become particularly bothersome before the onset of sleep. The sensations disappear temporarily when the legs are moved, only to recur within a few seconds. The symptoms last from minutes to hours; they can significantly delay sleep onset and result in sleep deprivation. Other distal dysesthesias are described as painful tingling, aberrant sensation of swelling of fingers and toes, and a constrictive feeling around the feet and ankles. These prominent sensory manifestations may be accompanied by slowly progressive distal weakness and atrophy.

The earliest signs on examination are impaired vibration sense in the lower extremities associated with loss of deep tendon reflexes—first the Achilles reflex, then the patellar responses. Advanced cases display distal decrease in touch and position sense and may also show weakness and atrophy of distal muscles.

When fully developed, uremic polyneuropathy is a distal symmetric mixed motor and sensory polyneuropathy involving the legs more than the arms. The major factors correlating with the appearance of neuropathy are gender and degree and duration of CRF. No correlation has been demonstrated with other factors such as age, race, levels of specific uremic metabolites, or type of underlying renal disease. Although most commonly uremic polyneuropathy evolves over many months, there have been reports of severe fulminant motor neuropathies, sometimes associated with sepsis (49).

CSF protein levels are usually normal but may be elevated up to 100 to 200 mg/dL (normal 15 to 45 mg/dL) in patients with severe uremic polyneuropathy.

The most significant abnormality on electrophysiologic study is a reduction in the amplitude of the compound muscle and sensory action potential, a finding that is expected in an axonal neuropathy. Both motor and sensory conduction velocities are reduced and the late reflexes (H reflex and F wave) become abnormally prolonged, more commonly in the lower extremities. There is a high correlation between declining creatinine clearance and reduction in conduction velocities (Fig. 33.4) (50). However, the relationship between worsening conduction velocities and the clinical appearance of neuropathy is less clear. Specific predictors that herald the appearance of clinical symptoms and signs have not been identified. Quantitative sensory testing, especially the vibratory threshold, is a sensitive indicator of peripheral neuropathy in CRF and correlates well with severity (51). An early and unusual sign is the perception of heat in response to low temperature stimuli. This paradoxical heat sensation to cold can precede other signs of neuropathy (52).

Pathologically, uremic polyneuropathy represents a primary axonal disease with secondary segmental demyelination. All

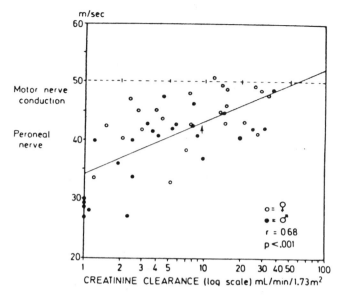

FIG. 33.4. Decrease in nerve conduction velocity with declining renal function in 56 patients. The arrow indicates the creatinine clearance at which 50% of patients will show abnormal values. The conduction velocities tended to be lower in males than females. (From Nielsen VK. The peripheral nerve function in chronic renal failure. *Acta Med Scand* 1973;194:455–462, with permission.)

fiber sizes, both myelinated and unmyelinated, are affected, although the largest and the most distal are especially vulnerable. The pathologic findings are not specific for uremia and cannot be distinguished from other causes of axonal degeneration such as alcoholic neuropathy.

The improvement of uremic neuropathy with dialysis led most observers to conclude that neuropathy results from accumulation of dialyzable metabolites. Initial reports of improvement of neuropathy with long-duration dialysis suggested that such metabolites or toxins had a molecular weight between 1,350 to 5,000 daltons (so-called middle molecules). Compounds of this size cross dialysis membrane more slowly than urea and creatinine, so increasing the dialysis time has a much greater effect on the removal of middle molecules and could account for the effectiveness of longer treatment in improving uremic neuropathy (53). In addition to middle molecules, the elevation of other putative neurotoxins in uremia such as myoinositol or PTH have also been purported to result in nerve damage.

In most patients on long-term dialysis, the neuropathy will stabilize, but improvement is less consistent. In a study of 14 patients, Nielsen (54) demonstrated clinical improvement and stabilization of nerve conduction studies. Cadilhac et al. (55), in a much larger series of 213 patients, reached the same conclusions, demonstrating stabilization of nerve conductions with some patients showing improvement (Fig. 33.5). Neuropathy occasionally appears or worsens during the initial weeks of dialysis, a development usually interpreted as a need to increase dialysis time. In recent years, the appearance of neuropathy in patients on chronic hemodialysis has become rare as a result of earlier treatment, more intensive dialysis, and, more impor-

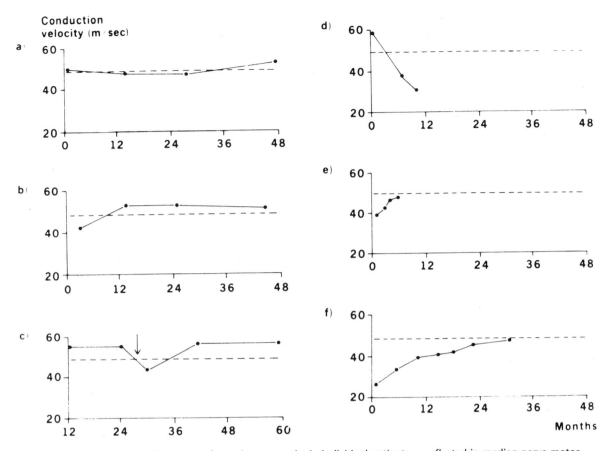

FIG. 33.5. Variations in the course of uremic neuropathy in individual patients as reflected in median nerve motor conduction velocity. (Dashed line = 2 SD below mean control value.) Other nerves tested showed similar results. **A:** A stable course in a 54-year-old man on regular home dialysis. **B:** Improvement in uremic neuropathy in a 55-year-old man on regular home dialysis. **C:** Transient worsening in uremic neuropathy in a 48-year-old woman during intercurrent illness (septicemia). **D:** Rapidly progressing neuropathy in a 21-year-old man on twice weekly hemodialysis with a Kolff twin coil unit. **E:** Rapid recovery of neuropathy after successful renal transplantation in a 43-year-old man. **F:** Gradual recovery after successful renal transplantation in a 21-year-old man with severe quadriplegic neuropathy. (From Bolton CF. Peripheral neuropathies associated with chronic renal failure. *Can J Neurol Sci* 1980;7:89–96, with permission.)

tantly, technical improvements in dialysis membranes. Earlier reports indicated that patients on peritoneal dialysis do not develop uremic polyneuropathy with the same frequency as patients on hemodialysis, but these observations have not been substantiated (56).

Successful renal transplantation has a more predictable and clear-cut beneficial effect on uremic polyneuropathy. Provided that the transplant is successful, progressive improvement has been the rule, with complete or near complete clinical recovery even in patients with severe neuropathy. Recovery often occurs in two phases, initial rapid improvement over days to weeks and then more protracted improvement over a period of months (57,58). Even in severe cases, walking is possible within 2 to 3 months, although some residual clinical signs such as absent ankle reflexes may persist. Serial electrophysiologic studies following transplantation have demonstrated rapid improvement in nerve conduction velocities (Fig. 33.5) (59). The restless legs syndrome responds poorly (if at all) to dialysis. Symptomatic relief can be provided by a number of medications, including clonazepam, carbamazepine, and L-dopa.

Autonomic and Cranial Neuropathies

Uremic neuropathy is not confined to motor and sensory nerves. Autonomic dysfunction is a well-known complication (60,61) (see Chapter 19). Patients with CRF demonstrate abnormal responses to the Valsalva maneuver, abnormal heart rate responses to atropine, and reduced baroreceptor sensitivity. Symptoms that indicate disordered autonomic function include orthostatic hypotension, impotence, diarrhea, and excessive perspiration. Reduced baroreceptor activity may be an important factor in producing hemodialysis-induced hypotension (see Chapter 19) (62). However, overt signs of autonomic dysfunction are very uncommon during the course of CRF.

Increased incidence of eighth cranial nerve (CN VIII) dysfunction, both auditory and vestibular, has been noted (63). The pathogenesis is obscure and is most likely multifactorial, potentially related to uremic toxins and prior exposure to ototoxic drugs such as aminoglycosides. There have been reports of esophageal dysfunction in patients with CRF, and uremic neuropathy of the vagus nerve (CN X) has been postulated (64).

Diabetes mellitus can also involve peripheral, cranial, and autonomic nerves. Because 40% to 45% of all ESRD patients have diabetes, it is important to distinguish diabetic from uremic neuropathy. The clinical picture in diabetic and uremic neuropathy can be similar, but there are some differences. In diabetic neuropathy overt autonomic dysfunction, cranial nerve involvement, and compressive neuropathies are more common. Diabetic neuropathy can be asymmetric and could present with a distinctive clinical picture, as in diabetic amyotrophy that manifests with painful proximal leg weakness. Electrophysiologic studies and nerve biopsy are not helpful in making this distinction, with both disorders showing evidence of axonal disease. Importantly, diabetic polyneuropathy will not respond to hemodialysis or transplantation.

Mononeuropathies

Carpal Tunnel Syndrome

Carpal tunnel syndrome is the most common mononeuropathy in patients with CRF, just as it is in patients without renal insufficiency. However, in certain situations renal failure patients are especially liable to develop median nerve entrapment. In patients with CRF, carpal tunnel syndrome has been associated with arteriovenous fistulas between the radial artery and the cephalic vein in the forearm (65). The symptoms of tingling dysesthesias in the median nerve distribution with nocturnal exacerbation are similar to those reported by nonuremic patients, although in uremic patients these symptoms may get worse during dialysis. This exacerbation is most likely related to a combination of compression and median nerve ischemia within the carpal tunnel because of venous congestion and edema. In refractory cases, treatment may ultimately require closure of the fistula.

Amyloidosis will develop in some patients on chronic hemodialysis because of β_2-microglobulin deposition and may produce carpal tunnel syndrome (this is discussed in detail in Chapter 23).

Ischemic Monomelic Neuropathy

Rarely, an arteriovenous fistula placed in the proximal upper arm can induce severe ischemia involving the median, ulnar, or radial nerve (see Chapter 4) (66,67). Pathologically, the shunting of blood in the arm and transient loss of blood flow produces acute multiple mononeuropathies, with axon loss that is most marked distally. Clinical manifestations consist of acute onset of limb pain associated with distal weakness and sensory loss. Nerve conduction studies demonstrate abnormalities in multiple distal nerves in the affected limb, and electromyography also shows distal greater than proximal abnormalities in muscles consistent with the clinical picture. Ischemic monomelic neuropathy is considered a medical emergency and requires prompt surgical closure of the fistula or shunt. Severe or permanent neurologic sequelae may occur even after the fistula or shunt has been closed.

Compressive Neuropathies

Compressive neuropathies involving the ulnar nerve at the elbow and the peroneal nerve at the fibular head occasionally occur during ESRD, particularly if the patient is malnourished and bedridden for any length of time. Uremic toxins make the nerves more susceptible to damage from focal compression. Successful renal transplantation restores the function of these nerves.

Myopathy

Myopathy can occur in CRF. It is probably multifactorial but especially important are abnormalities in the metabolism of calcium and phosphorus related to bone involvement and secondary hyperparathyroidism. The clinical features resemble those seen in association with hyperparathyroidism and osteomalacia and include proximal muscle weakness, bone pain, normal creatine kinase levels, and type 2 muscle fiber atrophy (68). CRF is, therefore, one of the causes of neuromyopathy in addition to drugs like colchicine, vincristine, and amiodarone. The myopathy of CRF may respond to high doses of vitamin D. Rarely CRF may be associated with widespread arterial calcification in small subcutaneous and intramuscular arteries with skin necrosis, painful myopathy, and myoglobinuria. The incidence of this complication has been greatly reduced by improvement in dialysis techniques (69). The differential diagnosis of chronic myopathy also includes the nonspecific cachexia associated with CRF. Acute myopathy can be caused by abnormalities of potassium metabolism, and muscle weakness resulting from defective transmission at the neuromuscular junction occurs as a complication of aminoglycoside antibiotics.

REFERENCES

1. De Deyn PP, et al. Clinical and pathophysiological aspects of neurological complications in renal failure. *Acta Neurol Belg* 1992;92: 191–206.
2. Raskin NH. Neurological aspects of renal failure. In: Aminoff MJ, ed. *Neurology and general medicine.* Churchill Livingstone, 1989:231–246.
3. Lockwood AH. Neurological complications of renal disease. In: Riggs JE, ed. Neurological manifestations of systemic disease. *Neurol Clin* 1989;7:617–627.
4. Fraser CL, et al. Nervous system complications in uremia. *Ann Intern Med* 1988;109:143–153.
5. Burn DJ, et al. Neurology and the kidney. *J Neurol Neurosurg Psychiatry* 1998;65:810–821.
6. Moe SM, et al. Uremic encephalopathy. *Clin Nephrol* 1994;42: 251–256.
7. Mahoney CA, et al. Uremic encephalopathies: clinical, biochemical and experimental features. *Am J Kidney Dis* 1982;2:324–336.
8. Biasioli S, et al. Uremic encephalopathy: an updating. *Clin Nephrol* 1986;25(2):57–63.
9. Savazzi GM. Pathogenesis of cerebral atrophy in uremia. *Nephron* 1988;49:94–103.
10. Okada J, et al. Reversible MRI and CT findings in uremic encephalopathy. *Neuroradiology* 1991;33:524–526.
11. Grunwald I, et al. Non-traumatic neurological emergencies: imaging of cerebral ischemia. *Eur Radiol* 2002;12:1632–1637.
12. Freeman RB, et al. The blood cerebrospinal fluid barrier in uremia. *Ann Intern Med* 1962;56:233–240.
13. Costigan MG, et al. Hypothesis: is accumulation of a furan dicarboxylic acid (3-carboxy-4-methyl-5-propyl-2-furanpropanoic acid) related to neurologic abnormalities in patients with renal failure? *Nephron* 1996;73:169–173.
14. Vanholder R, et al. Uremic toxicity: the middle molecule hypothesis revisited. *Semin Nephrol* 1994;14:205–218.

15. Smogorzewski MJ. Central nervous dysfunction in uremia. *Am J Kid Dis* 2001;38:S122–S128.
16. Parfitt AM. The hyperparathyroidism of chronic renal failure: a disorder of growth. *Kidney Int* 1997;52:3–9.
17. Cooper JD, et al. Neurodiagnostic abnormalities in patients with acute renal failure: evidence for neurotoxicity of parathyroid hormone. *J Clin Invest* 1978;61:1448–1455.
18. Kanai H, et al. Depressed cerebral oxygen metabolism in patients with chronic renal failure: a positron emission tomography study. *Am J Kidney Dis* 2001;38:S129–S133.
19. Norrby SR. Neurotoxicity of carbapenem antibacterials. *Drug Safety* 1996;15(2):87–90.
20. Massetini R, et al. Status epilepticus in chronically dialysed patients treated with erythropoietin. *Riv Neurol* 1991;61(6):215–218.
21. Vas GA, et al. Diffuse encephalopathies. In: Daly DD, et al., eds. *Current practice of clinical electroencephalography,* 2nd ed. New York: Raven Press, 1990:374–377.
22. Brewster D, et al. Valproate plasma protein binding in the uremic condition. *Clin Pharmacol Ther* 1980;27:76–82.
23. Boggs JG. Seizures in medically complex patients. *Epilepsia* 1997;38(S4):S55–S59.
24. Matzke GR, et al. Drug administration in patients with renal failure: minimising renal and extrarenal toxicity. *Drug Safety* 1997;16(3):205–231.
25. Letteri JM, et al. Diphenylhydantoin metabolism in uremia. *N Engl J Med* 1971;285:648–652.
26. Burgess ED, et al. Serum phenytoin concentrations in uremia. *Ann Intern Med* 1981;94:59–60.
27. Iseki K, et al. Predictors of stroke in patients receiving chronic hemodialysis. *Kidney Int* 1996;50:1672–1675.
28. Bostom A, et al. Hyperhomocysteinemia in ESRD: prevalence, etiology, and potential relationship to arteriosclerotic outcomes. *Kidney Int* 1997;52:10–20.
29. Perrone RD. Extrarenal manifestations of ADPKD. *Kidney Int* 1997;51:2022–2036.
30. Iseki K, et al. Evidence for high risk of intracerebral hemorrhage in chronic dialysis patients. *Kidney Int* 1993;44:1086–1090.
31. Selman WR, et al. Intracranial aneurysms. In: Bradley WG, et al., eds. *Neurology in clinical practice,* 3rd ed. Boston: Butterworth Heinemann, 2000:1185–1199.
32. AHA Scientific Statement. Recommendations for management of patients with unruptured intracranial aneurysms. *Stroke* 2000;31:2742–2750.
33. ISUIA Investigators. Unruptured intracranial aneurysms: risks of rupture and risks of surgical intervention. *N Engl J Med* 1998;339:1725–1733.
34. Silver SM, et al. Brain swelling after dialysis: old urea or new osmoles. *Am J Kidney Dis* 1996;28:1–13.
35. Schilling L, et al. Brain edema: pathogenesis and therapy. *Kidney Int* 1997;59:S69–S75.
36. Yoshida S, et al. Dialysis dysequilibrium syndrome in neurosurgical patients. *Neurosurgery* 1987;20:716–721.
37. Wolcott DL, et al. Relationship of dialysis modality and other factors to cognitive function in chronic dialysis patients. *Am J Kidney Dis* 1988;12:275–284.
38. Arieff AI, et al. Dementia, renal failure, and brain aluminum. *Ann Intern Med* 1979;90:741–747.
39. Alfrey A. Dialysis encephalopathy. *Kidney Int* 1986;29(S18):S53–S57.
40. Mayer G, et al. The metabolism of aluminum and aluminum related encephalopathy. *Semin Nephrol* 1986;6(4):1–4.
41. Platts MM, et al. Dialysis encephalopathy: precipitating factors and improvement in prognosis. *Clin Nephrol* 1981;15:223–228.
42. Russo LS, et al. Aluminum intoxication in undialyzed adults with chronic renal failure. *J Neurol Neurosurg Psychiatry* 1992;55:697–700.
43. Bates D, et al. Aluminum encephalopathy. *Contrib Nephrol* 1985;45:29–41.
44. Reusche E, et al. Correlation of drug related aluminum intake and dialysis treatment with deposition of argyrophilic aluminum-containing inclusions in CNS and in organ systems of patients with dialysis associated encephalopathy. *Clin Neuropathol* 1996;15:342–347.
45. La Greca G, et al. Dialytic encephalopathy. *Contrib Nephrol* 1985;45:9–28.
46. Noriega-Sanchez A, et al. Clinical and electroencephalographic changes in progressive uremic encephalopathy. *Neurology* 1978;28:667–669.
47. Asbury AK. Uremic polyneuropathy. In: Dyck PJ, et al., eds. *Peripheral neuropathy,* 2nd ed. Philadelphia: WB Saunders, 1994:1811–1825.
48. Nielsen VK. The peripheral nerve function in chronic renal failure. I: clinical symptoms and signs. *Acta Med Scand* 1971;190:105–111.
49. McGonigle RJS, et al. Progressive predominantly motor uremic neuropathy. *Acta Neurol Scand* 1985;71:379–384.
50. Nielsen VK. The peripheral nerve function in chronic renal failure. VI. The relationship between sensory and motor nerve conduction and kidney function, azotemia, age, sex, and clinical neuropathy. *Acta Med Scand* 1973;194:455–462.
51. Tegner R, et al. Vibratory perception threshold compared with nerve conduction velocity in the evaluation of uremic neuropathy. *Acta Neurol Scan* 1985;71:285–289.
52. Yosipovitch G, et al. Paradoxical heat sensation in uremic polyneuropathy. *Muscle Nerve* 1995;18:768–771.
53. Babb AL, et al. The middle molecule hypothesis in perspective. *Am J Kidney Dis* 1981;1:46–50.
54. Nielsen VK. The peripheral nerve function in chronic renal failure. VII. Longitudinal course during terminal renal failure and regular hemodialysis. *Acta Med Scand* 1974;195:155–162.
55. Cadilhac J, et al. Motor nerve conduction velocities as an index of maintenance dialysis in patients with end-stage renal failure. In: Canal N, et al., eds. *Peripheral neuropathies.* New York: Elsevier/Noan-Holland, 1978:372–380.
56. Tegner R, et al. Uremic polyneuropathy: different effects of hemodialysis and continuous ambulatory peritoneal dialysis. *Acta Med Scand* 1985;218:409–416.
57. Bolton CF, Baltzam MA. Effects of renal transplantation on uremic neuropathy. *N Engl J Med* 1971;284:1170–1174.
58. Nielsen VK. The peripheral nerve function in chronic renal failure. VIII. Recovery after renal transplantation. *Acta Med Scand* 1974;195:163–170.
59. Funck-Brentano JL, et al. Polyneuritis during the course of chronic renal failure: follow up after renal transplantation (10 personal observations). *Nephron* 1968;5:31–42.
60. Zuchelli P, et al. Dysfunction of the autonomic nervous system in patients with end-stage renal failure. *Contrib Nephrol* 1985;45:69–81.
61. Solders G, et al. Autonomic dysfunction in non-diabetic terminal uremia. *Acta Neurol Scand* 1985;71:321–327.
62. Kersh E, et al. Autonomic insufficiency as a cause of hemodialysis-induced hypotension. *N Engl J Med* 1974;290:650–653.
63. Kusakari J, et al. The inner ear dysfunction in hemodialysis patients. *Tohuku J Exp Med* 1981;135:359–369.
64. Siampolous KC, et al. Esophageal dysfunction in chronic hemodialysis patients. *Nephron* 1990;55:389–393.
65. Harding AE, et al. Carpal tunnel syndrome related to antebrachial Cimino-Brescia fistula. *J Neurol Neurosurg Psychiatry* 1977;40:511–513.
66. Wilbourn AJ, et al. Ischemic monomelic neuropathy. *Neurology* 1983;33:447–451.
67. Bolton CF, et al. Ischemic neuropathy in uremic patients caused by bovine arteriovenous shunt. *J Neurol Neurosurg Psychiatry* 1979;42:810–814.
68. Floyd M, et al. Myopathy in chronic renal failure. *Q J Med* 1974;43:509–524.
69. Goodhue WW, et al. Ischemic myopathy in uremic hyperparathyroidism. *JAMA* 1972;221:911–912.

34

ACQUIRED CYSTIC KIDNEY DISEASE IN DIALYSIS PATIENTS

RICHARD A. LAFAYETTE AND GEORGE LAI

The finding of multiple cysts in end-stage kidneys has been described for more than 100 years (1). However, the clinical significance of these cysts was not examined until Dunnill et al. (2) described adverse outcomes in a group of patients with acquired cystic kidney disease (ACKD) in 1977. Since that time, numerous studies have sought to define the incidence, pathogenesis, and complications of this condition and attempts have been made to establish diagnostic and therapeutic guidelines. This chapter reviews these findings and offers a possible approach to the diagnosis and management of ACKD.

DEFINITION AND DIFFERENTIAL DIAGNOSIS

ACKD is the development of any new cysts in the failing kidney. Previous reports of ACKD have included kidneys with few bilateral simple cysts and have extended to cysts numerous enough to replace the entire renal parenchyma. Gardner (3) has suggested that renal cysts be defined as any enclosed or communicating segment of nephron or duct that is dilated to a diameter of greater than 200 microns. He suggests that acquired renal cystic disease be defined as the spontaneous bilateral development of multiple cysts in previously noncystic kidneys. Because of the high prevalence of one or two renal cysts in the normal aging population, many authors have adopted an arbitrary definition of greater than four cysts per kidney (3–5).

It is generally easy to differentiate this process from other renal cystic diseases. Simple cysts associated with aging tend to be few in number and unassociated with renal dysfunction or other parenchymal abnormalities. Autosomal dominant polycystic kidney disease (ADPKD) is frequently diagnosed before significant azotemia. There is usually a strong family history of ADPKD (3). The kidneys remain large, often occupying a large part of the abdominal cavity. Patients with ADPKD also frequently have extrarenal cysts, particularly in the liver. In patients with ACKD, the cause of chronic renal failure is often known and the cysts usually occur in small, shrunken kidneys. However, the diagnosis can be difficult in patients who have not had prior medical care. Rarely, the kidneys in ACKD can enlarge, with reports of kidneys as large as 22 cm and kidney weights as great as 1,000 g (6,7). However, these large kidneys are generally found in patients with long-standing renal failure who have already been on renal replacement therapy for many years.

PATHOLOGY

Gross pathology of the kidney with ACKD usually demonstrates the small, contracted end-stage kidney with multiple small cysts, typically numbering in the hundreds (Fig. 34.1). These cysts predominate in the renal cortex but frequently involve the renal medulla as well (8). Most cysts are small, less than 0.5 cm., but they can become as large as 5.0 cm (9). Cysts larger than 3.0 cm are frequently the result of bleeding within a cyst or tumor involvement. The kidneys usually retain the appearance of the shrunken end-stage kidney with regular outlines.

Microscopically, the cysts are easily apparent against the background of tubular atrophy and interstitial fibrosis typically seen in the end-stage kidney. Glomerular obsolescence, vascular changes, and both hypertrophic and dilated proximal tubules are frequently seen (Fig. 34.2). The underlying glomerular pathology may still be discernible (10). Most cysts are lined with single layers of squamous, low cuboidal, or columnar epithelial cells, occasionally accompanied by surface or luminal crystalline oxalic acid and β_2-microglobulin accumulation (11,12). Microdissection studies have demonstrated that there is continuity between cysts and tubular segments, suggesting that the cysts start as simple dilatations of normal renal tubules (13). The epithelium may be derived from proximal, distal, or collecting tubule cells. These epithelial cells often demonstrate proliferation, with either hyperplasia or polypoid papillary projections into the cyst lumina (Fig. 34.3). Structural, functional, and cyst fluid characteristics suggest that most cysts are derived from proximal tubules (14,15).

Epithelial atypia is associated with the development of neoplasia in cysts (Fig. 34.4). There appears to be a histologic continuum from simple cysts with single-layered epithelium, to multilayered cysts, to renal cell carcinoma. The tumors range from the papillary type mentioned previously, to a tubular type with basophilic cytoplasm, to clear cell solid tumors that are pathologically identical to primary renal cell carcinoma (4). These tumors are often multiple and bilateral.

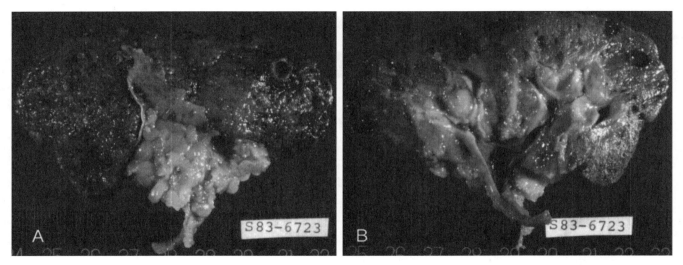

FIG. 34.1. Gross pathologic appearance of acquired cystic kidney disease. **A:** Whole kidney. **B:** Cut section.

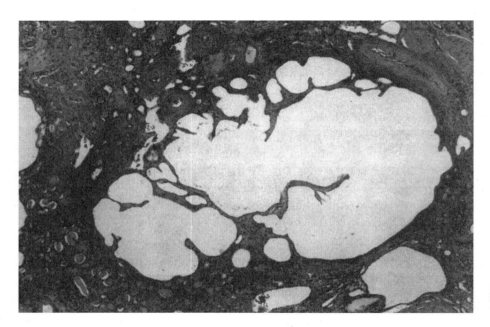

FIG. 34.2. Microscopic appearance of end-stage kidney affected by acquired cystic kidney disease.

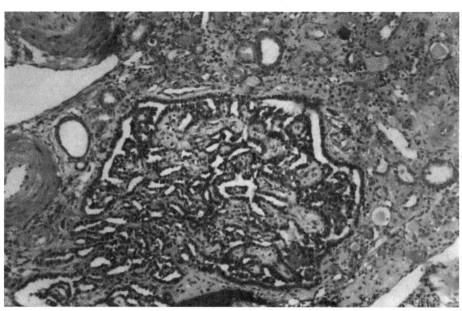

FIG. 34.3. Microscopic appearance of end-stage kidney affected by acquired cystic kidney disease with presence of papillary projections.

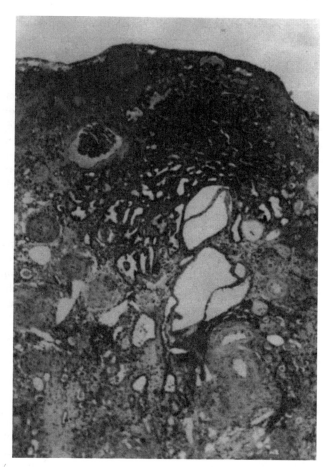

FIG. 34.4. Microscopic appearance of end-stage kidney affected by acquired cystic kidney disease with presence of island of hyperplasia, neoplasia.

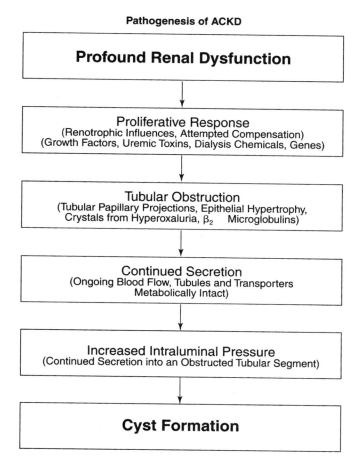

FIG. 34.5. Schema for the theoretical pathogenesis of acquired cystic kidney disease.

PATHOGENESIS

The manner in which the end-stage kidney becomes cystic and the causes of cyst growth are unknown. Nonetheless, the hypothesis illustrated in Fig. 34.5 is generally supported by the literature. A severe reduction in renal excretory function is the obligatory, initial step in cyst formation. The uremic state must allow for the production or retention of factors that lead to tubular proliferation, in turn leading to impingement of the tubular lumen. Continued tubular secretion into these proliferating tubules leads to cysts. Obstruction with crystals, fibrosis, or simply the further proliferation of epithelial cells (as described later) results in cyst growth under pressure. Genetic or environmental factors might then lead to dysplasia and the development of malignancy.

Proliferation of the epithelial cells lining the cysts is one of the hallmarks of ACKD. A 10-fold increase in proliferation of the tubular epithelium in end-stage kidneys has been reported, with a 30- to 40-fold increase in tubular epithelium actually comprising cyst walls (16). Proliferation of the cells outward toward the interstitium could result in cyst-like structures. On the other hand, proliferation of the cells into the lumina could cause luminal obstruction and cyst-like dilation of the tubules proximal to the obstruction. In experimental and human cystic diseases, pressures within the cysts are normal or elevated above normal tubular pressures. This suggests that luminal obstruction secondary to proliferation into the lumen is a more compatible explanation for cystogenesis. In addition, the frequent finding of papillary projections into the lumen also supports the hypothesis that epithelial proliferation becomes obstructive and leads to cyst formation.

Fluid accumulation is also necessary for cyst formation. Without fluid accumulation, tubular proliferation would lead directly to solid tumors, which are unusual in end-stage kidney disease. The accumulation of fluid within the cysts is unlikely to result from glomerular filtration. There is considerable glomerular obsolescence and sclerosis in end-stage kidneys and very little or no glomerular filtration. Based on cyst fluid analysis, fluid is more likely to accumulate because of continuing transepithelial secretion from proximal tubule cells (5).

Changes in the extracellular matrix, particularly the tubular basement membrane, could predispose to cyst formation in the absence of tubular obstruction. Abnormal compliance in the basement membrane has been implicated in ADPKD, accounting for cystic dilation of tubular structures (17). In ADPKD, abnormal compliance of the basement membrane is suggested by the presence of cystic changes in several other organs of the body including the liver, spleen, and pancreas. However, involvement of other organs is not seen in ACKD. Furthermore, the high or normal pressure of fluid collections within the cyst does not support the hypothesis of an abnormally compliant basement membrane (18).

Besides epithelial proliferation, several processes have been implicated in obstructing the tubules of chronically diseased kidneys. Stone formation commonly occurs in hemodialysis patients and has been ascribed to increased urine concentrations of oxalate (19). Hyperoxaluria and a lack of natural inhibitors of stone formation have been noted in hemodialysis, peritoneal dialysis, and chronic renal failure patients not yet on renal replacement (20,21). This results in an incidence of renal calculi that is 2- to 10-fold higher than reference populations with normal kidney function. Several investigators have implicated other substances as possible proliferating or obstructing agents. These include β_2-microglobulin, microfibrillar protein, silicon, and vanadium, but only limited evidence supports these hypotheses (18,21,22).

Regardless of the cause of tubular obstruction in ACKD, any pathogenetic scheme must account for the epithelial proliferation. Because ACKD was first detected in hemodialysis patients and the incidence of cystic disease increases with duration of dialysis, investigators postulated a role for the hemodialysis treatment in the pathogenesis of ACKD. Several chemicals can cause cysts in laboratory animals. These chemicals appear to cause renal epithelial damage followed by tubular dilation and cyst formation (23,24). Plasticizers used in hemodialysis (diethylexylphthalate) have been tested and found to have potential for tubular injury, as has formaldehyde (25). However, because the incidence of ACKD is similar in chronic ambulatory peritoneal dialysis (CAPD) and hemodialysis patients and has also been reported in some patients before renal replacement therapy, the hemodialysis treatment seems unlikely to be a major contributor to cyst formation (26–30).

More likely, the uremic state leads to cyst formation. Many naturally occurring factors have been implicated in the epithelial hyperplasia that occurs in ACKD. They include renotrophic hormones, an increased sensitivity to circulating growth factors, and polyamines (31). As an example of a renotrophic hormone, parathyroid hormone (PTH) has been implicated as a possible factor in cystogenesis through its effect of increasing cytosolic cyclic adenosine monophosphate (cAMP) (5). These factors make the uremic state a likely contributor to the initiation of cyst formation and to unchecked proliferation following the development of ACKD. Supporting this notion is the fact that ACKD does not occur in the presence of preserved kidney function, as in patients with unilateral renal disease. In addition, ACKD is unusual in the native kidneys of patients with a functioning transplant kidney (see later). Cysts may actually regress

with resumption of kidney function after renal transplantation (32).

Renal ischemia has also been postulated to play a role in cyst formation (2,33,34). Arterial disease is common in the end-stage kidney. Unilateral cysts have been noted in patients with unilateral atherosclerotic disease (34). One of the mechanisms by which ischemia could cause ACKD is through the generation of cellular acidosis, which has been shown to cause epithelial proliferation and cyst formation. Growth factors, such as angiotensin II, might also be directly liberated from ischemic nephron populations. However, conclusive experimental evidence of tubular ischemia leading to cyst formation is presently lacking.

A genetic susceptibility may either permit or predispose to the development of ACKD. The *c-myc* oncogene has been documented in several cases of renal cell cancer (35). *C-erb-b2*, a gene encoding a protein that shares homology with epidermal growth factor, has been shown to be overexpressed in tissue from patients with cystic disease (36). A better understanding of the pathogenesis of ACKD is crucial in finding treatments to limit the clinical consequences of this process.

DEMOGRAPHICS AND CLINICAL CHARACTERISTICS

Although not recognized as a clinical entity before 1977, ACKD is a common condition in patients with end-stage renal disease (ESRD). It is present in roughly half of all patients on dialysis. Twenty percent of patients are likely to have cystic changes before initiating renal replacement therapy. It appears there is an approximate 10% incidence of additional cases of ACKD per year after starting dialysis. Table 34.1 depicts the prevalence of cysts, tumors, and renal cell carcinoma in several radiologic studies of dialysis patients.

The prevalence of ACKD and its complications vary depending on definition and screening procedures. ACKD has been reported in hemodialysis patients, in peritoneal dialysis patients, and in patients who are chronically azotemic before starting dialysis. Unlike simple renal cysts, the disease is not a function of age but rather a function of the duration of renal failure. Thus, the incidence of ACKD ranges from 35% to 44% in patients dialyzed less than 3 years and to greater than 75% in patients dialyzed longer than 3 years. In one study of patients dialyzed more than 8 years, the incidence approached 100% (13).

There appears to be a predominance of men in reports of ACKD, with male to female ratios as high as 3:1 (10,37). However, not all series have shown a clear male predominance (38,39). Racial differences may alter the rate of cyst progression, with blacks reported to develop cysts faster. However, racial characteristics have only rarely been evaluated (36). The cause of the chronic renal failure does not seem to play any role in predisposing to ACKD. Patients with glomerulonephritis, diabetes, and hypertensive glomerulosclerosis all appear equally susceptible to ACKD (3,39,40).

TABLE 34.1. PREVALENCE OF ACQUIRED CYSTIC KIDNEY DISEASE (ACKD) AND RENAL TUMORS

Study (Reference)	Number of Patients	Method of Dialysis	Dialysis Duration (Months)	Method of Screening	Patients with ACKD (Total)	(With Tumor)	(With RCC)
1 (92)	41	HD, PD	>36	US, CT	24	NA	NA
2 (107)	31	HD, PD	NA	US	1	0	0
3 (108)	79	HD	>66	US	56	0	0
4 (108)	21	PD	>32	US	6	0	0
5 (39)	51	HD, PD	>58	US, CT	30	1	0
6 (39)	50	—	>0	US	4	0	0
7 (109)	43	HD	>22	US	21	0	0
8 (110)	26	HD	NA	US, CT	12	2	1
9 (111)	205	HD	>55	US	43	1	1
10 (80)	101	HD, PD	>58	US	63	0	0
11 (38)	43	HD, PD	NA	US	20	2	1
12 (112)	58	HD	>54	US	12	0	0
13 (113)	111	HD	NA	US	55	0	0
14 (114)	20	HD	NA	US	17	0	0
15 (37)	100	HD, PD	>36	US, CT	22	0	0
16 (37)	30	—	>0	US, CT	2	0	0
17 (80)	22	HD	>27	US, CT	11	1	1
18 (115)	21	PD	>13	US, CT	7	1	1
19 (97)	30	HD, PD	>49	CT	13	2	0
20 (13)	120	—	>0	US	31	0	0
21 (13)	117	HD	>74	US	70	1	1
22 (33, 78)	96	HD, PD	>96	CT	73	9	6
23 (33)	261	HD, PD	>69	US	152	5	5
24 (116)	24	—	>13	US	11	2	2
25 (117)	54	PD	>18	US, CT	16	0	0
26 (118)	206	—	>4	US, CT	63	7	7
TOTAL[a] (%) CI 95%	1961	HD or PD	>41	US, CT	835 (42%) [34%– 50%]	34 (4.7%) [0.9%– 7.2%]	26 (3.2%) [1.2%– 5.3%]

HD, hemodialysis; PD, peritoneal dialysis; RCC, renal cell carcinoma; NA, data not available.
[a]Total does not include nondialysis patients. CI 95%, 95% confidence interval for mean percentiles.
Modified from Glicklich D. Acquired cystic kidney disease and renal cell carcinoma: a review. *Semin Dial* 1991;4:273–283, with permission.

COMPLICATIONS

General

Although dramatic complications such as bleeding, erythrocytosis, and renal cell carcinoma may arise, ACKD is usually asymptomatic and not detected without screening or autopsy. Table 34.2 depicts the range of complications. Unlike ADPKD, infectious complications appear to be rare, with only scattered reports. Flank and abdominal pain is more frequently reported in ACKD, often associated with large kidney size. Renal stones appear to be more common in patients with ACKD. Calculi

TABLE 34.2. COMPLICATIONS OF ACQUIRED CYSTIC KIDNEY DISEASE

None
Flank pain
Nephrolithiasis
Infection
Erythrocytosis
Bleeding, hematuria, or retroperitoneal hemorrhage
Tumors, benign or malignant

likely arise from the hyperoxaluria present in patients with renal insufficiency, which causes supersaturation of calcium oxalate, then they are further exacerbated by the lack of flow within cystic segments of kidney. Additional reports of stones caused by β_2-amyloid (matrix stones) suggests that obstruction with this material may also lead to symptoms (41).

Bleeding

Bleeding complications are a frequent finding in patients with ACKD, ranging from mild hematuria or perirenal hematomas to massive retroperitoneal hemorrhage (42–44). In a prospective study of 30 patients, five developed hemorrhagic cysts and four developed large perinephric hematomas (45). Hemorrhagic complications in dialysis patients had been reported even before the clinical description of ACKD (42,46). The hemorrhage probably results from rupture of attenuated and/or inflamed blood vessels within the walls of cysts.

The severity of bleeding complications may be related to uremia-induced coagulopathies or the use of heparin during hemodialysis (44,47–49). Presenting symptoms are often gross hematuria, abdominal pain, or hypotension leading to shock

(46,50). Rarely, severe hypertension may occur secondary to a perirenal hematoma inducing renin secretion (51). Even fatal hemorrhages have been reported (47,52). Nephrectomy has been advocated for kidneys with significant bleeding, but both conservative management and vascular embolization have been suggested as alternatives in patients without evidence of malignancy (52,53). The administration of cryoprecipitate, desmopressin (DDAVP), or conjugated estrogens may help control the severity of bleeding in patients who suffer platelet dysfunction from their renal disease.

Bleeding is not necessarily related to the extent of cyst formation or to the presence of tumors or malignancy. Nonetheless, hematuria may be a clue to further complications from ACKD and it has been suggested that patients with bleeding be further evaluated for malignancy.

Erythrocytosis

End-stage kidney disease is nearly always complicated by anemia, requiring treatment by transfusion, erythropoietin, or other hematinic factors. Maintenance of a normal hematocrit or frank erythrocytosis often points to the presence of associated disease processes. Benign and malignant tumors, hydronephrosis, renal artery stenosis, ADPKD, and even acute hepatitis have been associated with enhanced erythropoiesis.

Changes in hematopoiesis have also frequently been attributed to the presence of ACKD. The association was first suggested in 1982. Two patients who had significant anemia at the initiation of dialysis were found to have significant increases in their hematocrit to levels as high as 52% and 54% several years later. These patients demonstrated significant cystic changes in their kidneys by computed tomography (CT) scan.

Early investigators hypothesized that the epithelial proliferation typical of ACKD may result in enhanced production of erythropoietin and higher hematocrits. Higher levels of erythropoietin were demonstrated in those patients with erythrocytosis (54). A recent study has also confirmed higher levels of erythropoietin in patients with ACKD (55). Other reports have suggested that the increase of hematocrit is a function of length of time on dialysis and thus not directly resulting from the presence of ACKD (56). Nonetheless, it does appear that patients with ACKD do have higher hematocrits than chronic renal failure patients without cystic disease (6,52). This complication of ACKD may be beneficial in limiting exogenous erythropoietin or transfusion requirements, but polycythemia has also been reported in some dialysis patients as an adverse response to increased erythropoietin production.

Renal Cell Carcinoma

The most worrisome complication of ACKD is renal cell carcinoma. The overall prevalence of all renal tumors approximates 3.5%, with a prevalence of renal cell cancer of 2.5%. As can be seen in Table 34.1, the reported prevalence varies greatly. This may be due to the definition or screening method employed to detect cancers. As in normal kidneys, complex cysts greater than 3 cm are considerably more likely to represent renal cell carcinoma and have a high potential for metastasis as compared with small, simple cysts (57).

In all reported series, renal tumors and cancers are predominantly found among those dialysis patients with ACKD. The risk of malignancy has been prospectively evaluated. In one 7-year prospective study, 2 of 30 dialysis patients (7%) developed renal cell carcinoma (45). In a separate study, 96 patients were followed for a 10-year period with annual CT scanning. Six patients (6%) were found to develop clear cell carcinoma. Five of the six were men from a population that included 61 men and 35 women. All cancers were associated with ACKD. Three additional cases of cystadenomas were also found (33). Thus, the risk of developing cancer associated with ACKD appears to be 0.5% to 1% per year of observation. Even though the incidence of ACKD is similar in CAPD and hemodialysis patients, the risk of malignant cystic transformation among these treatment groups is disputed. None of 353 CAPD patients developed renal cancer in a study by Katz et al. (27). However, patients with ESRD treated by CAPD are certainly not fully protected, if at all, by this modality because many case reports of malignancy exist (28). With the increasing survival of ESRD patients and the enhanced ability to detect renal cysts and tumors by radiologic techniques, the reported prevalence of cancer can be expected to rise.

The risk of several types of cancer is significantly higher in dialysis patients than in the general population. The incidence of renal cancer has long been reported to be excessive in patients with renal failure, with a relative risk as high as 41 to 100 times that of an otherwise healthy population (58–62). Furthermore, ACKD-associated renal cell cancer occurs approximately 20 years earlier than in the general population (45 ±18 years vs. 64 ±12 years) (63). Other malignancies, most notably uterine and prostate cancer, also appear in excess among dialysis patients (60). Thus, it has been suggested that defects in immune status associated with renal failure may predispose to this enhanced susceptibility to malignancy in many organs. However, the excess in malignancy is mainly due to cancers of the kidney, predominantly renal cell carcinoma. This points to some additional alteration in cell regulation within the kidney.

As discussed previously, the reported prevalence of renal carcinoma in patients with renal failure determined by careful screening or autopsy is 2.3% (4,61). This is in considerable excess of the 0.3% prevalence of renal cell carcinoma found in an autopsy series of patients without ACKD (64). Most cases of renal tumors in patients with renal failure arise in the setting of ACKD (10,50,61). Thus, many investigators have suggested that renal cancers follow directly from the epithelial hyperplasia that occurs in ACKD. In fact, many of the proliferative characteristics of tubular epithelium in ACKD are strikingly similar to those found in primary renal cell cancer (16).

However, the pathogenesis of malignancy in ACKD appears to be different than that seen with primary renal cell cancer. The histology is often different; papillary and chromophilic tumors are seen more frequently in ACKD-associated cancer than the usual histology of clear cell seen in primary renal cell cancer (65). Interestingly, patients who develop nonpapillary renal carcinoma tend to do so earlier than those who develop papillary renal cancers, suggesting a distinct genetic pathway (66). Indeed, genetic markers appear to be different among these tumors. Sporadic renal cell cancer is frequently associated with changes in chromosome 3 or with the von Hippel-Lindau tumor suppressor gene; this association is rare in patients with ACKD-associated tumor (65).

Despite these differences, the clinical and prognostic features of renal cell carcinoma occurring in patients with ACKD appear similar to those of patients with primary renal cell carcinoma. Presenting symptoms of primary renal cell carcinoma include bleeding, flank pain, abdominal mass, and polycythemia. Although patients with ACKD are also more likely to experience these symptoms if they have cancer, approximately 86% of ACKD-associated renal cell neoplasms are asymptomatic (67).

In addition, the risk of metastatic disease in ACKD-associated tumors is similar to that of primary renal cell carcinoma, with a high risk of metastasis with large tumor size (57,68). In primary renal cell carcinoma, the risk of metastasis with a tumor less than 3 cm is less than 5%. This risk increases to almost 30% when the tumor size exceeds 3 cm (68,69). In ACKD, the risk of metastasis has also been reported to be increased with tumor sizes greater than 3.0 cm (4,39). Indeed, several cases of metastatic disease have been reported in ACKD, including cases with complications ranging from hypercalcemia to death (70,71).

Metastatic disease in ACKD follows the same trends as primary renal cell carcinoma, with renal vein extension and metastasis to the lungs, bones, paraaortic lymph nodes, brain, and liver as common sites (10,39,72,73). Metastasis to the myocardium, mediastinum, and pancreas has also been reported (74). The overall incidence of metastasis in ACKD ranges from 16% to 27% (11).

Patient survival with renal cell carcinoma in ACKD appears similar to that in primary renal cell carcinoma. Primary renal cell carcinoma as a whole carries a 5-year survival of approximately 35% to 45% (75). Survival depends on the stage of cancer at diagnosis, with a 10-year survival of 66% in patients with disease limited to the kidney and a 10-year survival of less than 5% in patients with distant metastasis (76). In an analysis by Matson and Cohen (39), the life expectancy of patients with renal cell carcinoma associated with ACKD was similar, with an approximate 5-year survival of 35% to 40%.

Several independent risk factors have been noted for primary renal cell carcinoma. There is a striking male predominance both in primary renal cell carcinoma and in renal cell carcinoma associated with ACKD. Male to female ratios of 5:1 to 7:1 in ACKD-associated cancer are higher as compared with 2:1 in primary renal cell carcinoma. There may be racial factors as well, with a predominance of black patients developing renal cell carcinoma associated with ACKD. Genetic factors are likely to be important in the risk of cancer; oncogenes have been reported to be expressed more frequently in patients with primary renal cell carcinoma (35) and, as discussed before, in patients with ACKD. Environmental factors may also play a role. Obesity, cigarette smoking, and caffeine consumption have been reported to put patients at higher risk for primary renal cell carcinoma (77). Some of these factors are also thought to play a role in renal cell carcinoma associated with ACKD (5,36).

In addition, Ishikawa et al. (78) have correlated kidney volume with relative risk of tumors and malignancy, with progressive increases in kidney volume significantly associated with the development of cancer. A more recent study has demonstrated that kidney weight may strongly predict the presence of carcinoma in patients with ACKD. Kidney weights greater than 150g had a sixfold probability of harboring a malignancy, regardless of the radiologic features (7).

TRANSPLANTATION

The impact of renal transplantation on the incidence and complications of ACKD is not entirely clear. In principle, by reversing the uremic milieu, the factors predisposing to cyst growth may be halted. In some studies, progression of cystic kidney disease was seen in patients followed on dialysis and not in patients followed after successful renal transplantation (79). In fact, radiologic studies have shown isolated cases of actual cyst regression in the retained native kidneys of transplant recipients (32). Based on these studies, it has been suggested that renal transplantation may protect the native kidneys from the complications of ACKD (32,80).

However, it is clear that not all cystic disease regresses following transplantation, especially if the renal allograft only achieves poor function (32,81). In 2,372 renal transplant patients, Kliem et al. (82) reported 12 (0.5%) patients who developed renal cancer in native kidneys at a mean of 6 years posttransplant follow-up (0.5–15 years). Most of these patients had ACKD and 4 of the 12 died of metastatic disease. In another study of 385 patients examined after a mean interval of 58 months following successful transplantation, 96 (25%) of the patients exhibited ACKD by ultrasound. Seven of them had tumors, and six had renal cell cancer. One of these patients refused intervention and died 7 months after diagnosis (83). Several cases of renal adenocarcinoma originating from ACKD in the native kidneys, including widespread metastases, have been reported in patients long after successful transplantation (84,85). Indeed, renal cell cancer was reported to be responsible for 2% of the deaths in one transplant center (86).

Some have suggested that the routine use of cyclosporine may contribute to the maintenance and progression of ACKD through an uncertain mechanism (87). It is of great concern that transplant patients may have a more aggressive course of carcinoma because of immunosuppressive therapy. However, there does not appear to be any increase in the incidence or complications of renal cell carcinoma in the native kidney in patients after transplantation as compared with patients treated by dialysis (88). Moreover, it is unclear whether cancers detected after transplantation were already present at the time of transplantation or developed after transplantation. Regardless, if renal cancer is fully eradicated before immunosuppressive therapy, it is unlikely to recur after transplantation (89). Because native kidneys are no longer routinely removed in preparation for renal transplantation, further studies are needed to better establish the course of ACKD in patients following renal transplantation.

RADIOLOGIC EVALUATION

The evaluation of, or screening for, complications of ACKD starts with ascertaining if the patient has ACKD. Radiologic options for diagnosis of ACKD include all renal imaging procedures. Renal ultrasound, CT scanning, magnetic resonance imaging (MRI), intravenous (IV) pyelography, nuclear medicine scanning, and arteriography have all been advocated as means for diagnosis and evaluation of renal masses (90). However, the major methods for detection of multiple renal cysts remain renal ultrasound and CT scan (91).

Renal ultrasound, a noninvasive and relatively inexpensive procedure, has been the most advocated technique for initial diagnostic evaluation. It can be effective in detecting cysts as small as 0.5 cm in the small, dense kidneys of ESRD patients (92). A baseline ultrasound is helpful in comparing new ultrasound abnormalities and in their characterization (93). Ultrasound occasionally fails to visualize end-stage kidneys well because of their small size and increased echogenicity, and this can make ultrasound detection of small masses difficult (94). It has been suggested that ACKD is unlikely to be present in kidneys that cannot be well visualized, because one expects some enlargement and enhancing of echo differentiation with the presence of cysts (40). In addition, it has been suggested that lesions of interest such as tumors and hematomas occur in kidneys heavily involved with cystic disease, which would be easily detected by ultrasound (95). Although ultrasound is highly operator dependent, this technique is very effective when serial studies are available and the study is performed the same way each time. Thus, many authors have advocated ultrasound as the diagnostic or screening tool of choice (92–94).

Alternatively, others have advocated CT scanning for the evaluation of ACKD (33,39). It is clear that CT scanning provides enhanced visualization and can readily detect masses as small as 0.3 cm (45,91,96). In addition, the use of contrast allows better characterization of the mass. CT is the preferred procedure in the evaluation of primary renal cell carcinoma (97). In a comparative study of CT and ultrasound, the prevalence of ACKD in a dialysis population was found to be 59% by CT compared with only 18% as determined by ultrasound, suggesting higher sensitivity of CT scanning in detecting cysts (91). Contrast enhancement was found to be useful in separating out cysts and better defining their contour. CT scanning has been effective in longitudinal studies on the development of solid tumors in hemodialysis populations (33,45,74). Finally, bolus-enhanced spiral CT scanning may be a technique to better define the vascularity of a suspect lesion (98).

Still, it has been argued that differences in the sensitivity of ultrasound and CT may disappear with increased use of more sensitive machinery (99). A study using the most advanced ultrasound machines found that ultrasound detected all cases of ACKD found by CT (40). Therefore, some authors have advocated initial evaluation with ultrasound followed by CT only if cystic disease is present, to better characterize the lesions (40).

Finally, MRI with gadolinium contrast has become established as a safe and effective tool for characterizing renal cystic and solid tumors. Contrast enhancement is necessary to determine whether neovascularity is present (100). MRI was superior to ultrasound in differentiating simple from complex lesions of native kidneys in renal allograft recipients, but the advantages gained from MRI did not justify routine screening by this modality (100). Although preliminary data suggest that MRI is not better than CT scanning, even after gadolinium enhancement, it can replace contrast-enhanced CT scanning in ACKD patients with chronic kidney disease (CKD) before dialysis, in whom IV contrast may worsen renal function (67).

Ultimately, the diagnosis of renal cell cancer in ACKD requires surgical intervention with biopsy or nephrectomy. Cyst aspiration has proven unsuccessful as a diagnostic test in this setting (101). Thus, once patients are identified as being at high risk for renal cell cancer based on their radiologic studies, the next step is operative assessment for risks and benefits.

SCREENING

The excessive rate of cancer and other serious complications have led many reviewers of the subject to advocate careful screening of dialysis patients, to identify those patients who may benefit from nephrectomy. Indeed, it has been suggested that screening tests be employed in all dialysis patients to detect those with ACKD, with additional testing of those patients with ACKD to detect and remove tumors before they metastasize (102). No clinical trial has been carried out to attempt to validate these screening strategies.

Decision analysis has been used to examine the consequences of routine CT or ultrasound screening of asymptomatic patients for ACKD and cancer (103). Table 34.3 summarizes the data employed in the baseline and sensitivity analyses. Under the no-screening strategy, no screening for ACKD is performed. However, patients who develop symptomatic cysts and/or cancer undergo CT. Under the CT-screening strategy, CT screening occurs after 3 years of dialysis and patients found to have cysts undergo annual CT thereafter. Patients without cysts undergo repeat CT screening every 3 years. The ultrasound-screening strategy follows the same scheme, using ultrasound instead of CT. A tumor growth model represents the natural history of ACKD-related cancer. The model employs published data on renal cell carcinoma to estimate the relationship between tumor size, clinical stage, and patient survival.

The results of each strategy are calculated using a Markov state transition model (104). For each strategy, deaths occur at a rate determined by age and by the cause of renal failure, classified as either diabetes mellitus or other kidney disease. During each year, survivors may develop ACKD, the cysts may undergo malignant transformation, symptoms may make cancer clinically evident, and surgical treatment of localized cancer may result in death. Cancers that become clinically evident or are detected by screening are evaluated and treated within the same year. False-negative and false-positive results from the screening tests are taken into account. Patients in whom the evaluation suggests the presence of Robson stage I to III cancer undergo bilateral radical nephrectomy. Patients who have stage IV cancer receive no specific treatment for the malignancy. Surgical survivors who actually had cancer and all patients in stage IV are assigned a cancer-stage-specific excess mortality rate.

So as not to overlook any possible benefit of screening, the model was constructed with a consistent bias in favor of the screening strategies. Despite this bias, the model predicts only a very modest benefit from screening (Table 34.4). In a hypothet-

TABLE 34.3. RATES AND PROBABILITIES USED IN DECISION ANALYSIS OF SCREENING FOR ACKD AND MALIGNANCY

Variable	Baseline Value	Range Tested in Sensitivity Analysis
Annual rates (%/year)		
ACKD development		
Initial	13	15–70
Slope/year	7	
Cancer development	0.9	0.5–7
Renal cancer mortality		
Stage I	1	0.5–3
Stage II		4–10
Stage IIIA	10	9–27
Stage IIIB	28	25–35
Stage IV	50	35–60
Chronic dialysis mortality		
Nondiabetic		
Age 30	6	
Age 60	15	
Diabetic		
Age 30	21	
Age 60	33	
Probabilities (%)		
Perioperative mortality	2	0.5–6
Test characteristics		
Sensitivity		
Renal mass <3 cm (diameter)		
CT	94	80–100
Ultrasound	80	60–100
Renal mass >3 cm (diameter)		
CT	100	80–100
Ultrasound	100	80–100
Sensitivity		
Renal cysts		
CT	100	50–100
Ultrasound	60	30–100
Specificity (renal masses, all sizes)		
CT	100	90–100
Ultrasound	100	90–100
Specificity (cysts)		
CT	100	90–100
Ultrasound	100	90–100

ACKD, acquired cystic kidney disease.

ical cohort of 10,000 (20-year-old) nondiabetic dialysis patients, who have an average life expectancy of 25 years (105), both CT screening and ultrasound screening reduced the number of cancer deaths. However, the decrease in cancer deaths occurs at the cost of an increase in the number of surgical deaths. (The two surgical deaths in the no-screening strategy occur in patients whose cancers are discovered because of symptoms.) The overall effect for this hypothetical cohort of 20 year olds is a gain of life expectancy of approximately 1.6 years by either CT or ultrasound screening, an increase of 6%.

For a hypothetical cohort of 10,000 (58-year-old) nondiabetic dialysis patients, in whom the average life expectancy is only 5 years (105), CT screening or ultrasound screening still decreases the number of deaths from cancer and increases the number of surgical deaths. However, the gain in life expectancy in this cohort by either method of screening is only 4 or 5 days. For diabetic ESRD patients, life expectancy at age 20 is comparable to the life expectancy in nondiabetic ESRD patients at age 58; thus the benefit of screening diabetic patients is similarly limited.

This analysis shows that CT or ultrasound screening of asymptomatic patients for ACKD might prolong average patient survival. However, the gain is only meaningful among the healthiest and youngest patients, with a 1.6 year gain in life expectancy (106). In the presence of increased age and other comorbid conditions, the benefit is negligible. The most important variable in the decision whether to screen is cancer incidence. The true incidence of cancer in ACKD is not firmly established. If future studies find the cancer incidence to be substantially higher than estimated, reanalysis may show that screening offers a clinically important benefit in more subgroups. However, a compilation of current data does not show such a benefit or support a policy of routine screening among other than the healthiest ESRD subjects.

The prevalence of ACKD, malignancy rates, and the benefits of radiologic investigation is likely to be much higher among patients with symptoms or signs such as flank pain, hematuria, or relative erythrocytosis than among asymptomatic patients. The conclusion that the current evidence does not support routine screening should not deter evaluation of patients in whom clinical clues suggest the presence of disease.

CONCLUSION

ACKD is a common complication of chronic renal failure. As increasing numbers of patients start and remain on renal replacement therapy and as it is increasingly common for transplant patients to retain their native kidneys, the prevalence and complications of ACKD can be expected to increase.

TABLE 34.4. OUTCOMES OF DECISION ANALYSIS IN HYPOTHETICAL COHORTS OF 10,000 PATIENTS PER SCREENING STRATEGY

Patient Age (At Screening)	Screening Strategy	Cancer Deaths	Surgical Deaths	Average Life Expectancy (Remaining)
20 years	CT	705	33	26 years, 6 months
	US	785	30	26 years, 4 months
	None	1,337	2	25 years
58 years	CT	41	4	5 years, 5 days
	US	52	3	5 years, 4 days
	None	82	1	5 years

Although the present evidence does not support routine screening for cystic disease in most patients, it is clear that practitioners must be well informed about this disease. Bleeding, erythrocytosis, or signs of cancer in patients with long-standing renal failure should prompt an investigation for ACKD. Ultrasound appears to be a satisfactory initial diagnostic tool. CT scanning or MRI should be reserved for detailing cyst characteristics useful in the differentiation between simple cysts and potential cancer. Future research may allow for early intervention in preventing ACKD and its complications.

REFERENCES

1. Simon J. On sub-acute inflammation of the kidney. *Medicosurg Trans Soc Med Lond* 1847;30:141–164.
2. Dunnill MS, et al. Acquired cystic disease of the kidneys: a hazard of long-term intermittent maintenance haemodialysis. *J Clin Pathol* 1977;30:868–877.
3. Gardner KD. Cystic kidneys. *Kidney Int* 1988;33:610–621.
4. Glicklich D. Acquired cystic kidney disease and renal cell carcinoma: a review. *Semin Dial* 1991;4:273–283.
5. Grantham JJ. Acquired cystic kidney disease. *Kidney Int* 1991;40:143–152.
6. Gehrig JJ, et al. Acquired cystic disease of the end-stage kidney. *Am J Med* 1985;79:609–620.
7. MacDougall M, et al. Prediction of carcinoma in acquired cystic disease as a function of kidney weight. *J Am Soc Nephrol* 1990;1:828–831.
8. Grantham JJ, et al. Acquired cystic disease: replacing one kidney disease with another. *Kidney Int* 1985;28:99–105.
9. Lee M, et al. A case of acquired renal cystic disease with unusually large cysts. *Aust Radiol* 1995;39:84–85.
10. Hughson MD, et al. Renal neoplasia and acquired cystic disease in patients receiving long-term hemodialysis. *Arch Pathol Lab Med* 1986;110:592–601.
11. Ishikawa I. Uremic acquired renal cystic disease, natural history and complications. *Nephron* 1991;58:257–267.
12. Ishikawa I. Uremic acquired cystic disease of kidney. *Urology* 1985;26:101–108.
13. Mickisch O, et al. Multicystic transformation of kidneys in chronic renal failure. *Nephron* 1984;38:93–99.
14. Ishikawa I. Unusual composition of cyst fluid in acquired cystic disease of the end-stage kidney. *Nephron* 1985;41:373–374.
15. Ishikawa I, et al. Excretion of Hippuran into acquired renal cysts in chronic hemodialysis patients. *Nephron* 1989;52:110–111.
16. Nadasky T, et al. Proliferative activity of cyst epithelium in human renal cystic diseases. *J Am Soc Nephrol* 1995;5:1462–1468.
17. Wilson PD, et al. Abnormal extracellular matrix and excessive growth of human adult polycystic kidney disease epithelia. *J Cell Physiol* 1992;150:360–369.
18. Gardner KD. Pathogenesis of human cystic renal disease. *Ann Rev Med* 1988;39:185–191.
19. Caralps A, et al. Urinary calculi in chronic dialysis patients. *Lancet* 1979;2(8150):1024–1025.
20. Oren A, et al. Calcium oxalate kidney stones in patients on continuous ambulatory peritoneal dialysis. *Kidney Int* 1984;25:534–538.
21. Bommer J, et al. Urinary matrix calculi consisting of microfibrillar protein in patients on maintenance hemodialysis. *Kidney Int* 1979;16:722–728.
22. Marco-Franco JE, et al. Oxalate, silicon and vanadium in acquired cystic kidney disease. *Clin Nephrol* 1991;35:52–58.
23. Crocker JFS, et al. An animal model of hemodialysis induced polycystic kidney disease. *Kidney Int* 1984;25:183.
24. Carone FA, et al. The nature of a drug-induced concentrating defect in rats. *Lab Invest* 1975;31:658–664.
25. Council on Scientific Affairs. Formaldehyde. *JAMA* 1989;261:1183–1187.
26. Truong LD, et al. Acquired cystic kidney disease: occurrence in patients on chronic peritoneal dialysis. *Am J Kidney Dis* 1988;11:192–195.
27. Katz A, et al. Acquired cystic disease of the kidney in association with chronic ambulatory peritoneal dialysis. *Am J Kidney Dis* 1987;9:426–429.
28. Trabucco AF, et al. Neoplasia and acquired renal cystic disease in patients undergoing chronic ambulatory peritoneal dialysis. *Urology* 1990;35:1–4.
29. Chung-Park M, et al. Acquired cystic disease of the kidneys and renal cell carcinoma in chronic renal insufficiency without dialysis treatment. *Nephron* 1989;53:157–161.
30. Sasaki H, et al. Comparative study of cystic variations of the kidneys in haemodialysis and continuous ambulatory dialysis patients. *Int Urol Nephrol* 1996;28:247–254.
31. Fine L. The biology of renal hypertrophy. *Kidney Int* 1986;29:619–634.
32. Ishikawa I, et al. Regression of acquired cystic disease of the kidney after successful renal transplantation. *Am J Nephrol* 1983;3:310–314.
33. Ishikawa I, et al. Ten-year prospective study on the development of renal cell carcinoma in dialysis patients. *Am J Kidney Dis* 1990;16:452–458.
34. Cohen EP, et al. The role of ischemia in acquired cystic kidney disease. *Am J Kidney Dis* 1990;15:55–60.
35. Klein EA, et al. Cellular genetics of urologic tumors. *Am Urol Assoc Update Ser* 1989;8:113–120.
36. Herrera GA. C-erb B-2 amplification in cystic renal disease. *Kidney Int* 1991;40:509–513.
37. Narasimhan N, et al. Clinical characteristics and diagnostic considerations in acquired renal cystic disease. *Kidney Int* 1986;30:748–752.
38. Fallon B, et al. Renal cancer associated with acquired cystic disease of the kidney and chronic renal failure. *Semin Urol* 1989;7:228–236.
39. Matson MA, et al. Acquired cystic kidney disease: occurrence, prevalence, and renal cancers. *Medicine* 1990;69:217–226.
40. Manns RA, et al. Acquired cystic disease of the kidney; ultrasound as the primary screening procedure. *Clin Radiol* 1990;41:248–249.
41. Branten AJW, et al. Matrix stones and acquired renal cysts in a non-dialyzed patient with chronic renal failure. *Nephrol Dial Transplant* 1995;10:123–125.
42. Cabaluna C, et al. Gross hematuria as a manifestation of advanced glomerular disease. *Nephron* 1973;12:59–62.
43. Bhasin HK, et al. Spontaneous retroperitoneal bleeding in chronically hemodialyzed patients. *Nephron* 1978;22:322–327.
44. Kassirer JP. Case records of the Massachusetts General Hospital. *N Engl J Med* 1982;306:975–984.
45. Levine E, et al. Natural history of acquired renal cystic disease in dialysis patients: a prospective longitudinal CT Study. *Am J Radiol* 1991;156.
46. Tuttle RJ, et al. Spontaneous renal hemorrhage in chronic glomerular nephritis and dialysis. *Radiology* 1971;98:137–138.
47. Meyrier A, et al. Acute internal hemorrhage due to spontaneous visceral ruptures in hemodialysis patients. *Kidney Int* 1979;16:97.
48. Milutinovich J, et al. Spontaneous retroperitoneal bleeding in patients on chronic hemodialysis. *Ann Intern Med* 1977;86:189–192.
49. Tielemans CL, et al. Renal hematoma in a patient undergoing hemodialysis. *Arch Intern Med* 1983;143:1623–1625.
50. Brendler CB, et al. Acquired renal cystic disease in the end-stage kidney: urologic implications. *J Urol* 1984;132:548–552.
51. Bongu S, et al. Uncontrolled hypertension and hyperreninemia after hemorrhage in a patient with end-stage renal disease and acquired renal cysts. *J Am Soc Nephrol* 1994;5:22–26.
52. Ratcliffe PJ, et al. Clinical importance of acquired cystic disease of the kidney in patients undergoing dialysis. *BMJ* 1983;287:1855–1857.
53. Pak K, et al. Spontaneous renal subcapsular hematoma in a patient undergoing hemodialysis. *J Urol* 1986;135:117–119.
54. Shalhoub RJ, et al. Erythrocytosis in patients on long-term hemodialysis. *Ann Intern Med* 1982;97:686–690.
55. Edmunds ME, et al. Plasma erythropoietin levels and acquired cystic disease of the kidney in patients receiving regular hemodialysis treatment. *Br J Hematol* 1991;78:275–277.
56. Glickich D, et al. Time-related increase in hematocrit on chronic hemodialysis: uncertain role of renal cysts. *Am J Kidney Dis* 1990;15:46–54.

57. Brennan JF, et al. Acquired renal cystic disease: implications for the urologist. *Br J Urol* 1991;67:342–348.
58. Park JH, et al. Comparison of acquired cystic kidney disease between hemodialysis and continuous ambulatory peritoneal dialysis. *Korean J Intern Med* 2000;15(1):51–55.
59. Matas AJ, et al. Increased incidence of malignancy during chronic renal failure. *Lancet* 1975;1(7912):883–886.
60. Port FK, et al. Neoplasms in dialysis patients: a population-based study. *Am J Kidney Dis* 1989;14:119–123.
61. Miller LR, et al. Acquired renal cystic disease: an autopsy study of 155 cases. *Am J Nephrol* 1989;9:322–328.
62. Ishikawa I. Renal cell carcinoma in chronic hemodialysis patients: a 1990 questionnaire study in Japan. *Kidney Int* 1993;43:S167–S169.
63. Hughson MD, et al. Atypical cysts, acquired cystic disease, and renal cell tumors in end-stage dialysis kidneys. *Lab Invest* 1980;42:475–480.
64. Silverberg E. Statistical and epidemiologic data on urologic cancer. *Cancer* 1987;60:692–717.
65. Hughson MD, et al. Renal cell carcinoma of end-stage renal disease: a histopathologic and molecular genetic study. *J Am Soc Nephrol* 1996;7:2461–2468.
66. Ishikawa I, et al. High incidence of papillary renal cell carcinomas in patients on chronic hemodialysis. *Histopathology* 1993;22:135–139.
67. Truong LD, et al. Renal neoplasm in acquired cystic kidney disease. *AJKD* 1995;26:1–12.
68. Stenzl A, et al. The natural history of renal cell carcinoma. *Semin Urol* 1989;7:144–148.
69. Hermanek P, et al. Evaluation of the new tumor, nodes and metastases classification of renal cell carcinoma. *J Urol* 1990;144:238–242.
70. Almirall J, et al. Metastatic renal cell carcinoma in a hemodialysis patient with acquired renal cystic disease. *Nephron* 1989;52:96–97.
71. Thompson BJ, et al. Acquired cystic disease of kidney: metastatic renal adenocarcinoma and hypercalcemia. *Lancet* 1985;2(8453):502–503.
72. Morrison A. A new chest mass in a 49-year-old man with a transplant kidney (CPC). *Am J Med* 1988;84:121–128.
73. Lien YH, et al. Metastatic renal cell carcinoma associated with acquired cystic kidney disease 15 years after successful renal transplantation. *Am J Kidney Dis* 1991;18:711–715.
74. MacDougall ML. Renal adenocarcinoma and acquired cystic disease in chronic hemodialysis patients. *Am J Kidney Dis* 1987;9:166–171.
75. McNichols DW, et al. Renal cell carcinoma: long-term survival and late recurrence. *J Urol* 1981;126:17–23.
76. Golimbu M, et al. Renal cell carcinoma: survival and prognostic factors. *Urology* 1986;27:291–301.
77. Yu MC, et al. Cigarette smoking, obesity, diuretic use, and coffee consumption as risk factors for renal cell carcinoma. *Natl Cancer Inst* 1986;77:351–356.
78. Ishikawa I, et al. Development of acquired cystic disease and adenocarcinoma of the kidney in glomerulonephritic chronic hemodialysis patients. *Clin Nephrol* 1980;14:1–6.
79. Thompson BJ, et al. Acquired cystic disease of the kidney: an indication for renal transplantation? *BMJ* 1986;293:1209–1210.
80. Vaziri ND, et al. Acquired renal cystic disease in renal transplant recipients. *Nephron* 1984;37:203–205.
81. Ishikawa I, et al. Severity of acquired renal cysts in native kidneys and renal allograft with long-standing poor function. *Am J Kidney Dis* 1989;14:18–24.
82. Kliem V, et al. Risk of renal cell carcinoma after kidney transplantation. *Clin Transplant* 1997;11:255–258.
83. Heinz-Peer G, et al. Prevalence of acquired cystic kidney disease and tumors in native kidneys of renal transplant recipients: a prospective U.S. study. *Radiology* 1995;195:667–671.
84. Faber M, et al. Renal cell carcinoma and acquired cystic kidney disease after renal transplantation. *Lancet* 1987;1(8540):1030–1031.
85. Ng RCK, et al. Renal cell carcinoma occurring in a polycystic kidney of a transplant recipient. *J Urol* 1980;124:710–712.
86. Dlugosz BA, et al. Causes of death in kidney transplant recipients: 1970 to present. *Transplant Proc* 1989;21:2168–2170.
87. Lien YHH, et al. Association of cyclosporin A with acquired cystic kidney disease of the native kidneys in renal transplant recipients. *Kidney Int* 1993;44:613–616.
88. Penn I, et al. Malignant tumors rising de novo in immunosuppressed organ transplant recipients. *Transplantation* 1972;14:407–417.
89. Penn I. Transplantation in patients with primary renal malignancies. *Transplantation* 1977;24:424–434.
90. Fleischmann J, et al. Diagnostic approaches to the renal mass. *Semin Urol* 1989;7:153–157.
91. Taylor AJ, et al. Renal imaging in long-term dialysis patients: a comparison of CT and sonography. *Am J Radiol* 1989;153:765–767.
92. Endreny R, et al. Acquired cystic disease. *Nephron* 1990;55:222.
93. Kutcher R, et al. Uremic renal cystic disease: value of sonographic screening. *Radiology* 1983;147:833–835.
94. Mindell HJ. Pitfalls in sonography of renal masses. *Urol Radiol* 1989;11:215–216.
95. Anderson B, et al. Sonography of evolving renal cystic transformation associated with hemodialysis. *Am J Radiol* 1983;141:1003–1004.
96. Levine E, et al. CT of acquired cystic kidney disease and renal tumors in long-term dialysis patients. *Am J Radiol* 1984;142:125–131.
97. Amendola MA, et al. Small renal cell carcinomas: resolving a diagnostic dilemma. *Radiology* 1988;166:637–641.
98. Kauczor H-U, et al. Bolus-enhanced renal spiral CT: technique, diagnostic value and drawbacks. *Eur J Radiol* 1994;18:153–157.
99. Skolnick L. Renal imaging in long-term dialysis patients: a comparison of CT and sonography. *Am J Radiol* 1990;154:1125–1126.
100. Heinz-Peer G, et al. Role of magnetic resonance imaging in renal transplant recipients with acquired cystic kidney disease. *Urology* 1998;51:534–538.
101. Hayakawa M, et al. Patients with renal cysts associated with renal cell carcinoma and the clinical implications of cyst puncture: a study of 223 cases. *Urology* 1996;47:643–646.
102. Almirall J, et al. Acquired cystic disease and renal call carcinoma. *Nephron* 1991;59:165.
103. Sarasin FP, et al. Screening for acquired cystic kidney disease: a decision analytic perspective. *Kidney Int* 1995;48:207–219.
104. Beck JR, et al. The Markov model in medical prognosis. *Med Decis Making* 1983;3:419–458.
105. Eggers PW. Mortality rates among dialysis patients in Medicare's end-stage renal disease program. *Am J Kidney Dis* 1990;15:414–21.
106. Wilson P, et al. The pathology of human renal cystic disease. *Curr Top Pathol* 1995;88:1–50.
107. Sieniawska M, et al. Acquired cysts of the kidneys in children with chronic renal failure. *Pol Tyg Lek* 1989;44:217–219.
108. Thomson BJ, et al. Acquired cystic disease of the kidney in patients with end-stage chronic renal failure: a study of prevalence and aetiology. *Nephrol Dial Transplant* 1986;1:38–43.
109. Minar E, et al. Acquired cystic disease of the kidneys in chronic hemodialysis and renal transplant patients. *Eur Urol* 1984;10:245–248.
110. Cho C, et al. Acquired renal cyst disease and renal neoplasms in hemodialysis patients. *Urol Radiol* 1984;6:153–157.
111. Takeyabashi S. Sonographic evaluation of kidneys undergoing dialysis. *Urol Radiol* 1985;7:69–74.
112. Fayemi AO, et al. Acquired renal cysts and tumors superimposed on chronic primary kidney diseases: an autopsy study of 24 patients. *Pathol Res Pract* 1980;168:73–83.
113. Lie B, et al. Erworbene Nierenzysten bei daverdialyze patienten. *Urologe* 1986;25:109–112.
114. Goldsmith HJ, et al. Association between rising haemoglobin concentration and renal cyst formation in patients on long term regular haemodialysis treatment. *Proc Eur Dial Transplant Assoc* 1982;19:313–318.
115. Smith JW, et al. Acquired cystic disease of the kidney: two cases of associated adenocarcinoma and a renal ultrasound survey of a peritoneal dialysis population. *Am J Kidney Dis* 1987;10:41–46.
116. Matoo TK, et al. Acquired cystic disease in children and young adults on maintenance dialysis. *Pediatr Nephrol* 1997;11:447–450.
117. Kyushu Pediatric Nephrology Study Group. Acquired cystic kidney disease in children undergoing continuous ambulatory peritoneal dialysis. *Am J Kidney Dis* 1999;34:242–246.
118. Gulanikar AC, et al. Prospective pretransplant ultrasound screening in 206 patients for acquired renal cysts and renal cell carcinoma. *Transplant* 1998;66:1669–1672.

THE GERIATRIC DIALYSIS PATIENT

WENDY WEINSTOCK BROWN

DEMOGRAPHICS OF THE GERIATRIC END-STAGE RENAL DISEASE POPULATION

At least one major renal textbook notes "chronic renal failure is predominantly a disease of the elderly" (1). Patients older than 65 years represent the most rapidly growing segment of the end-stage renal disease (ESRD) population in North America, Europe, and Australia (1–4). In 1977, 15,832 new ESRD Medicare beneficiaries, representing 93% of new ESRD patients in the United States, began renal replacement therapy; 26.7% were aged 65 years or older; and 5.2 % were 75 years or older (5). In 1999, more than 88,000 patients entered the Medicare ESRD program; 47% were aged 65 years or older, and 23.4% were aged 75 years or older (6). Medicare ESRD enrollment for individuals aged 85 or older increased by 2051% between 1978 and 1989 (7). United States ESRD incidence and prevalence continue to demonstrate a striking increase with age (6). The median age at start of renal replacement therapy when dialysis is the first modality was 63 years in 1999. For patients older than 65 years, average annual change in incident rates in 1995 to 1999 increased considerably more than in the previous 5-year period (8.2% vs. 5.4% for those 65 to 74 years old; 12.5% vs. 7.6% for those 75 years and older), compared with a modest average annual increase for the hemodialysis population as a whole (7.3% vs. 6.3%) (6). ESRD incidence was 315 patients per million population (PMP) in 1999; the rate for individuals 75 years and older was 1,434 patients PMP (6). United States ESRD point prevalence was 1,217 PMP on December 31, 1999; it was 4,163 PMP for individuals 65 to 74 years old and 3,449 PMP for those 75 years and older (6). As with younger patients, there is a disproportionate representation of ethnic minorities in the U.S. ESRD population (6,8). At least one report speculates that elderly persons with chronic diseases and progressive kidney disease are living longer because of better disease management of nonrenal comorbidities and, therefore, contributing to the increasing incidence of ESRD (9).

The most common reported causes of ESRD in the elderly are diabetes and nephrosclerosis that is presumed secondary to hypertension (2,10,11), although the data may be misleading because of the reluctance of many nephrologists to biopsy elderly patients (3,10,12,13) even when the usual indications, such as nephrotic-range proteinuria or unexplained renal failure, are present. Elderly patients with atypical presentations of ESRD should be evaluated for treatable causes of renal failure just as younger patients are.

Care of the elderly patient with renal dysfunction is particularly challenging for the nephrologist and renal health care team, both because of the increased number of comorbid conditions that tend to be present in the elderly patient and because these conditions are superimposed on the anatomic and physiologic changes seen with normal aging (14,15). Most elderly patients do not tolerate rapid changes in volume or electrolytes and have an impaired response to medications; stress; illness; or changes in diet, mobility, or environment (11,15–21). Clearly, comorbidity has a strong influence on survival: Mallick et al. (22) note that diabetes mellitus as a comorbid condition effectively "ages" a dialysis patient by a decade. However, age alone should not be a contraindication to dialysis and/or renal transplantation (1,5,18,23). In addition, not all individuals age biologically at the same rate (24,25); some elderly individuals with significant renal disease are surprisingly resilient and cope physiologically as well as much younger patients.

With careful management, many elderly dialysis patients can accommodate well to ESRD with a reasonably good quality of life (26–28). In Italy, patients initiating dialysis at age 65 years or older (mean = 71.3 years) had a survival rate of 82.7% at 1 year and 62.3% at 2 years (29). In Spain, dialysis patients aged 65 to 85 years had the same mortality rate as the age-matched general population (30). A report of 83 German hemodialysis patients older than 80 years found a 1-year survival of 70.5%, 2-year survival of 50.3%, and 5-year survival of 18.5%. Five-year survival was 29% in those who began dialysis treatment after 1990 (31)! Röhrich et al. (32) note that in their practice, with improvements in dialysis techniques, diet, and erythropoietin therapy, there has been a progressive increase in mean survival time for patients who begin treatment when older than 80 years, from 22.7 months before 1990 to 28.3 months after 1990. However, in a survey of physicians in the United Kingdom, a previously healthy octogenarian would not be referred for dialysis by 68% of primary care physicians or accepted for dialysis by 28% of nephrologists (33).

Selection of ESRD Modality

Factors affecting the selection of ESRD treatment modality include patient or physician preference, availability of trained personnel, distance to nearest dialysis center, concurrent illness or comorbidity, specific contraindications to a particular modality, financial reimbursement, allocation of scarce resources, and age bias (34). Some nephrologists treat all patients with center hemodialysis, whereas others have a clear preference for home dialysis and/or transplantation.

Patients who tolerate hemodialysis poorly because of cardiovascular disease or difficulty with vascular access may do better with peritoneal dialysis (35,36). In addition, many patients find peritoneal dialysis more compatible with an independent lifestyle and have the willingness to participate actively in their treatment.

Hemodialysis is a better choice for patients with inguinal or abdominal hernias, diverticulitis, compromised peritoneal surface area secondary to abdominal surgery or adhesions, abdominal aortic aneurysm, morbid obesity, or physical or psychosocial inability to perform peritoneal dialysis (21).

Recent reports have shown that carefully selected older patients do well with renal transplantation (37–50). One-year recipient survival ranges from 83% to 98%, and graft survival is 68% to 93% in patients older than 60 years (47–51). An analysis comparing 3,000 patients aged 60 to 74 years who received a cadaveric transplant with 3,900 who were wait listed but not transplanted found the relative risk of death at 1½ years posttransplant was significantly less for those who were transplanted [relative risk (RR) 0.39; $p < 0.001$]. The relative risk of death for transplanted elderly diabetic patients was 0.46 ($p < 0.001$) (52). Selection of treatment modality should be made on an individual basis, independent of age (5,26,47–50,53). Some have advocated transplantation of older adults with grafts from older adults: an "old for old" program. The Eurotransplant Senior Program matches recipients and cadaver donors who are both older than 65 years. One-year patient survival was 86%; 1-year graft survival was 79%. When graft loss was censored for patient death with functioning graft, 1-year graft survival was 86% (54). There may also be patient and graft survival advantage with the use of living-related donor transplantation compared with cadaveric renal transplantation, even when the donor is also elderly (55,56).

In the United States, almost 65% of ESRD patients are treated with hemodialysis, about 30% have functioning transplants, and the remainder are treated with a form of peritoneal dialysis (6.6%) (6). In contrast to the general ESRD population, on December 31, 1999, 93% of patients aged 65 years or older were treated with hemodialysis, 6.4% were treated with peritoneal dialysis, and only 1% had a functioning transplant (6). This compares to 83%, 10.7%, and 5% six years previously (57). The distribution of dialysis patients is skewed toward the older age groups, whereas the transplant population exhibits a normal distribution (Fig. 35.1). With adjustment for comorbidity, survival rates for patients younger than 75 years are equivalent for hemodialysis or peritoneal dialysis (1,4,13,28,58,59). In the United States Renal Data System (USRDS) population, mortality rates have declined in all age groups except those 0 to 19 years of age, for both hemodialysis and peritoneal dialysis. However, the USRDS reports that first-year death rates are slightly higher for incident peritoneal dialysis patients 65 years or older compared with hemodialysis patients; this difference is accentuated in the second year (6). A recent multivariate analysis of hemodialysis and peritoneal dialysis first-year mortality rates for 2,503 patients older than 65 years in a single state confirmed an increased death rate for elderly peritoneal dialysis patients, particularly those with diabetes (60). In a second report of the same patients, after controlling for a large number of variables, they found higher mortality for patients initially treated with peritoneal dialysis in the first 90 days of treatment and after 180 days of treatment that was accentuated in those patients with diabetes. The differences persisted after controlling for center effect. There were similar mortality rates for the two modalities between days 90 and 180 of treatment (61).

Other studies have suggested that this excess mortality for elderly peritoneal dialysis patients is primarily for elderly female

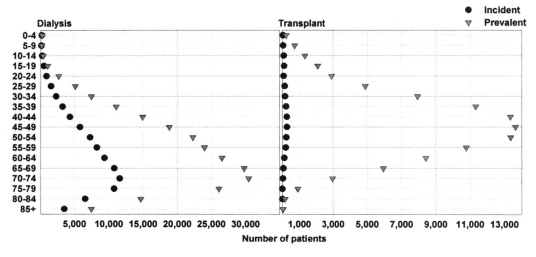

FIG. 35.1. Dialysis and transplant incidence and prevalence counts, by age and modality, 1999. (Adapted from U.S. Renal Data System annual data report. Bethesda, MD: National Institutes of Health, 2001.)

TABLE 35.1. PERCENTAGE OF ELDERLY PATIENTS TREATED WITH PERITONEAL DIALYSIS IN VARIOUS COUNTRIES

Country	Year	Patients Older Than 65 (%)
United Kingdom (1)	1981	58
Italy (58)	1987	9
Italy (65)	1998	12.5[a]
Europe (28)	1987	15
Japan (13)	1990	3.6[b]
France (59)	1992	28[b]
Australia (66)	2000	29
New Zealand (66)	2000	61.9
United States (67)	1989	10.4
United States USRDS (68)	1993	10.7
United States USRDS (6)	1999	6.4

[a]65–74 years of age.
[b]75 years and older.

diabetics (62,63). It has been suggested that poor nutritional status in diabetic peritoneal dialysis patients accounts for increased mortality (64). Excess mortality for elderly peritoneal dialysis patients is relevant in consideration of appropriate treatment modality and must be included in the equation along with considerations of comorbidity, quality of life, distance from center, and other issues.

There is great variability in selection of modality among countries (Table 35.1). A survey of nephrologists conducted in North Carolina, southern California, and Australia and New Zealand regarding the optimal treatment modality for patients older than 60 years showed a clear preference for home peritoneal dialysis over hemodialysis in North Carolina and in Australia and New Zealand. In southern California, a four-antigen match living-related donor transplant or center hemodialysis were both deemed preferable to peritoneal dialysis. Examination of actual practice patterns, however, revealed that in 1985, although 36% of Australian and New Zealand patients older than 60 years were treated with home peritoneal dialysis, the percentage was 4% in southern California and 17% in North Carolina, and only 3% to 5% of patients older than 60 years received a transplant (69). Another study confirmed that even in facilities in which the percentage of patients on peritoneal dialysis far exceeds the national average, fewer elderly patients are treated with peritoneal dialysis (70). The reason for this discrepancy is unclear. Interestingly, an analysis of United States National Continuous Ambulatory Peritoneal Dialysis (CAPD) Registry data revealed that fewer black patients older than 60 years are treated with peritoneal dialysis than white patients (71).

Hemodialysis

Elderly patients can do surprisingly well on hemodialysis. One of the earliest reports of long-term hemodialysis of the geriatric patient appeared in 1979. Chester et al. (27) compared 45 hemodialysis patients older than 70 years with 70 younger hemodialysis patients with a mean age of 42 years. Two-year survival was 42% for the elderly patients compared with 58% for

the younger patients. Interestingly, age did not correlate with survival for the elderly patients; nine patients older than 80 years had a 2-year survival of 41%! The authors noted that elderly dialysis patients had significantly lower prehemodialysis and posthemodialysis blood pressure compared with younger patients, and only 13% of the elderly patients required antihypertensive medication compared with 41% of the younger patients. The older patients had twice as many comorbid conditions as the younger patients (5 vs. 2.5) and had a mean survival of 22 months compared with 40 months for the younger patients (27). In 1995, Mignon et al. (59) observed that dialysis patients 45 years old had a 20-fold greater risk of death than age-matched nondialysis patients did, but for 75-year-old dialysis patients the increased risk of death for their age-matched cohort was less than threefold. An interesting recent 11-year multicenter cohort study showed that elderly hemodialysis patients who dialyzed in the morning survived significantly longer than those who dialyzed in the afternoon. These findings were independent of frequency of dialysis, length of treatment, months on dialysis before the study, age, race, gender, body mass index, functional status, cardiovascular disease, or diagnosis of diabetic nephropathy. The authors speculated that the effect might be related to sleep patterns or other as yet undetermined factors (72).

Peritoneal Dialysis

Peritoneal dialysis is considered the treatment of choice by many for the dialysis elderly, particularly those with cardiovascular disease or hemodynamic instability (69,73–76). Nicholls et al. (73) initiated CAPD in 38 patients older than 60 years who were considered unsuitable for hemodialysis because of age or coexisting disease. These patients had 1-year and 2-year actuarial survivals of 72% and 61%, respectively. Two patients eventually switched to hemodialysis. Twenty-one of the 23 surviving patients were considered fully rehabilitated (fully independent), and two remained partially disabled but could live at home. Of the nonsurvivors, two patients failed training because of previously unrecognized dementia. The authors noted that patient survival was similar to that of European hemodialysis patients older than 55 years, and patients either thrived or died soon after initiation of dialysis (73).

Nolph et al. (71) analyzed National CAPD Registry data for peritoneal dialysis patients older than 60 years and compared them with a baseline group of patients who were white, 20 to 50 years of age, male, nondiabetic, and on peritoneal dialysis as the first form of ESRD treatment. There was little difference in peritonitis rates, hospitalization, or transfer to other modality related to age alone (Table 35.2), but increased relative risk was shown if the elderly patient was also black and/or diabetic. Older patients had a greater risk of dying that increased if they were also black and/or diabetic (71).

An Italian study reported outcomes for 21 patients who began CAPD at 79 years or older. Although they did not do quite as well as younger patients, and required more frequent hospitalization, technique survival was similar to younger patients and the authors believed that peritoneal dialysis was a reasonable alternative for carefully selected older patients

TABLE 35.2. RELATIVE RISKS OF MORBIDITY AND MORTALITY

Characteristic	Relative Risks			
	Peritonitis	Hospitalization	Transfer	Death
Baseline patients[a]	1.00	1.00	1.00	1.00
Older than 60	1.12	1.10	1.00	3.23
Older than 60 + black	1.28	1.25	1.43	4.17
Older than 60 + diabetes	1.28	1.25	1.00	7.65
Older than 60 + black + diabetes	1.46	1.42	1.43	9.84

[a]Baseline patients: 20–59, nondiabetic, white, male, living without family, no prior dialysis treatment.
Adapted from Nolph KD, et al. Experiences with the elderly in the National CAPD Registry. *Adv Perit Dial* 1990;6[Suppl]:33–37, with permission.

because of inadequate local hemodialysis facilities (77). Jagose et al. (78) reported an 80% three-year survival rate for 18 patients beginning CAPD after the age of 80 years.

Sometimes peritoneal dialysis appears to be the most desirable ESRD treatment modality for medical reasons, but for various reasons the patient cannot perform CAPD. Assistance from a family member or paramedical staff may be appropriate (79). Nissenson (76) suggests the use of peritoneal dialysis adult day care centers, home-assisted peritoneal dialysis, or peritoneal dialysis in the nursing home setting. Continuous cyclic peritoneal dialysis (CCPD) or intermittent peritoneal dialysis (IPD) may be a good option for the elderly patient who needs some assistance (80,81). It is a particularly good option when the assisting spouse or children work during the day (82). A recent retrospective study evaluated CAPD and CCPD in institutionalized and noninstitutionalized patients 80 years and older with multiple nondialysis related comorbidities. Most of the noninstitutionalized patients required assistance from a home care nurse to perform dialysis. The peritonitis rate was low (1/28.6 patient-months), and 48% of these patients had no episodes of peritonitis. Technique survival was 91.5% at 1 year and 81.4% at 2½ years. One-year survival was 72%; almost half of the patients survived 2½ years, and almost 40% survived 30 months. It was noted that by the end of the follow-up period all patients required assistance for the performance of dialysis, and most required help with activities of daily living (83).

DIALYSIS TECHNICAL CONSIDERATIONS
Indications for Initiation of Dialysis

Porush et al. (2) evaluated the signs and symptoms present before initiation of maintenance dialysis in 118 elderly patients. The most common symptoms were anorexia and weight loss (61%), generalized weakness (58%), encephalopathy (49%), and nausea and vomiting (41%). The usual indicators of ESRD may be misleading in the elderly patient, however. Serum creatinine may not accurately estimate renal dysfunction in the geriatric patient. Population studies demonstrate a 10% decrease in glomerular filtration rate per decade after the age of 40 years, without a change in serum creatinine (84). Elderly patients frequently eat less protein and have less muscle mass. A serum creatinine of 4 or 5 mg/dL in an elderly patient can represent a profound decrease in renal function.

The Cockcroft and Gault formula (Table 35.3) for age-adjusted estimation of creatinine clearance may be helpful, but it is only an estimate and not a substitute for careful clinical evaluation (11,85). Gentric et al. (86) found that the Cockcroft and Gault formula underestimated glomerular filtration rate when compared with isotopic measurements in well-nourished patients with stable renal function who were 81 to 96 years old. A more recent study, using iothalamate clearance as the gold standard compared creatinine clearance, reciprocal creatinine plots, and the Cockcroft-Gault formula in 41 patients aged 65 to 85 years and found poor correlations with all of them (87). A newer equation, developed by Levey et al. (88) during the Modification of Diet in Renal Disease (MDRD) trials uses age, serum creatinine, gender, and race to estimate glomerular filtration rate and appears to provide better correlation than the Cockcroft and Gault formula (Table 35.3). Recent reports have examined serum cystatin C concentration as a marker of kidney function in the elderly but have not found it to be a better marker than serum creatinine, the Cockcroft & Gault Formula, or the MDRD Formula (89,90).

Ifudu et al. (91) found significantly greater late referral for black, Hispanic, and elderly patients than for white, Asian, and younger patients. All patients had health insurance. Mignon et al. (59) found that the increased mortality observed in the elderly in the first 3 months of dialysis correlated both with comorbidity and late referral. Fifty-seven percent of their elderly patients who died quickly had been referred less than 6 months before initiation of dialysis compared with 44% of elderly patients who survived longer. It has been suggested that earlier initiation of dialysis, particularly in those older than 80 years,

TABLE 35.3. AGE-ADJUSTED ESTIMATION OF CREATININE CLEARANCE

Cockcroft & Gault formula
Men: CrCl (mL/min) = 140 − age (years) × body weight (kg) ÷ 72 × sCr (mg/dL)
Women: multiply formula by 0.85
Modified MDRD equation
GFR (mL/min/1.73 m²) = 186 × sCr (mg/dL)$^{-1.145}$ × age (years)$^{-0.203}$
Blacks: multiply by 1.212
Females: multiply by 0.742

CrCl, creatinine clearance; sCr, serum creatinine; GFR, glomerular filtration rate; MDRD, Modification of Diet in Renal Disease.

TABLE 35.4. INDICATIONS FOR TRIAL OF DIALYSIS IN ELDERLY

Uremia
Potentially reversible acute renal failure
Unexplained dementia
Unexplained worsening of congestive heart failure
Personality change
Irritability, irascibility, or newly subdued demeanor
Adult failure to thrive
Change in sense of well-being

might reduce this excess early mortality (13). Some indications for a trial of dialysis in the elderly are listed in Table 35.4.

The effect of age as an independent risk factor for development, mortality, and prognosis in acute renal failure is controversial. Almost equal numbers of studies purport to show a positive correlation as those that deny it (92–99). An increased incidence of acute renal failure in the elderly has been demonstrated, however, particularly with the use of aminoglycoside antibiotics or after cardiovascular surgery and may be related to a higher incidence of multiple-organ disease in the elderly and to the progressive renal impairment seen with normal aging (93,94,97).

Prognosis and survival appear to be related to comorbid conditions (such as coma, hypotension, mechanical ventilation, pulmonary and cardiovascular complications, catabolic state, preexisting malignancy, presence of jaundice) and cause rather than age (92–94,97,99–101). Acute renal failure secondary to sepsis carries a particularly high mortality, approaching 90% in some studies (97). Oliguria, need for dialysis, and number of nephrotoxic events carry poor prognosis for all patients (93,97). At least one study demonstrated significantly higher mortality in elderly patients requiring dialysis than younger patients (102). Klouche et al. (103) studied 68 intensive care patients with acute renal failure who were older than 65 years; they found highest survival rates in those with nonoliguric acute renal failure, normal serum lactate levels, low catabolic rates, and failure of no more than two organ systems, suggesting that this subset of elderly patients with acute renal failure ought to be treated aggressively. There was not a comparison with younger acute renal failure patients, however.

There is frequently reluctance to initiate dialysis in an elderly individual with acute renal failure and multiple medical or psychosocial disorders because of the fear of committing the patient to chronic long-term dialysis or because of ethical concerns (104). However, although elderly survivors of acute renal failure seem to require more time for total recovery and recover function less completely, they can recover function and generally deserve a trial of dialysis (94,104,105). Also, shown in Table 35.4, the problems of failure to thrive (106) may trigger a formal geriatric assessment (107).

Vascular Access

Temporary Vascular Access

Until recently, some authors recommended subclavian catheterization as the access of choice for initiation of dialysis, particu-

larly in elderly patients (108). Cimochowski et al. (109), however, demonstrated that more than 50% of patients who received subclavian catheters had angiographically demonstrable subclavian strictures, whereas none of the patients with internal jugular catheters had strictures. These findings were independent of age (109). Femoral access is the preferred short-term approach for acute dialyses (84). When long-term central access is necessary, an internal jugular approach is preferred over a subclavian placement (110). Placement of central access lines can be facilitated and complications minimized with the use of portable ultrasound imaging systems to guide cannulation (111).

Permanent Vascular Access

Few studies have reviewed vascular access for hemodialysis in the elderly. Because of the high incidence of diabetes and atherosclerotic peripheral vascular disease in this age group, it is generally recommended that vascular access be placed early to allow time for maturation. A 1985 review of experience with vascular access in patients older than 65 years at a single center revealed that the three primary fistulas constructed had failed at 1 year but that 80% of polyethylene arteriovenous grafts were without thrombosis at 1 year in the 44 patients alive at 1 year. This compared favorably with 76% patency in 33 of 36 patients younger than 65 years who were alive at 1 year. In fact, all seven elderly patients who died before 1 year had functioning grafts at the time of death (112). Although another study noted that 25% of hospitalizations in elderly dialysis patients were related to vascular access (113), several recent papers quote the same figure for all dialysis patients (114–116). Woods et al. (117) found no difference in arteriovenous graft survival for patients younger or older than 65 years, although, for both groups of patients, arteriovenous graft survival was significantly lower than fistula survival (Fig. 35.2).

Arteriovenous fistula survival was better in patients younger than 65 years; however, such survival was better than arteriovenous graft survival for both younger and older patients (117). Ifudu et al. (118) found that vascular access accounted for 48%

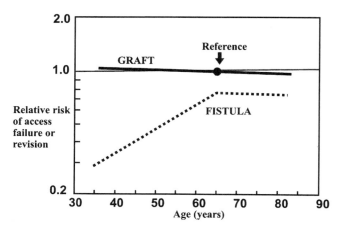

FIG. 35.2. Relative risk of failure or revision for arteriovenous (AV) fistula versus AV graft by patient age. (Adapted from Woods JD, et al. Vascular access survival among incident hemodialysis patients in the United States. *Am J Kidney Dis* 1997;30:50–57, with permission.)

of hospitalizations in 430 adult hemodialysis patients. Although diabetes and increased age were not independent risk factors for access-related hospitalization, they were associated with longer hospital stays. Ponce (119) noted that a prospective access registry in the Almada region of Portugal revealed that 69% of patients are dialyzed via a native arteriovenous fistula; however, 80% of all polytetrafluoroethylene (PTFE) grafts and 100% of tunneled catheters were placed in patients older than 65 years.

Primary Arteriovenous Fistulas

Primary arteriovenous Cimino fistulas are preferable to prosthetic grafts because of the decreased incidence of infection and thrombosis and other complications and better long-term patency (2,115,120–122); however, they require at least 6 to 8 weeks to mature. Atherosclerosis frequently precludes the construction of primary arteriovenous fistulas in elderly or diabetic patients (123). Leapman et al. (124) found poor patency rates for primary arteriovenous fistulas in both diabetic patients and patients 70 years or older and suggested that elderly diabetic patients preferentially receive prosthetic grafts or long-term indwelling catheters. Wing et al. (125), however, reported 80% one-year fistula survival in individuals older than 65 years. Berardinelli et al. (126) described their almost 30-year experience with creation of 494 new permanent accesses in 348 hemodialysis patients 65 years or older, using primary fistulas, various types of grafts, and a few external shunts. They examined their results by decade, using increasing numbers of primary fistulas and decreasing numbers of grafts and shunts with each decade. For the period 1990 to 1997, 58% of the accesses placed in 215 patients were primary fistulas, 87% of which were elbow fistulas. Elbow fistulas had 78% three-year patency compared with 57.2% for forearm fistulas. Their results are particularly impressive because all of the patients had been referred from other centers as "difficult patients" because multiple prior surgical attempts had not resulted in a reliable access. Konner et al. (127) describe excellent 1-year primary access survival of first arteriovenous fistulas for nondiabetic patients 65 years and older (73% for women, 77% for men) and diabetic patients 65 years and older (78% women, 81% men). Their approach included careful preoperative evaluation and an individualized surgical approach using three types of primary access: forearm arteriovenous fistulas, perforating vein fistulas at the elbow, or nonperforating fistulas at the elbow. Cante et al. (128), in a comparison of primary arteriovenous fistulas and prosthetic grafts in patients older than 65 years, concluded that the use of prosthetic grafts in the elderly was not justified because they were ultimately more costly because of a higher reoperation rate and poorer quality of life for the patient.

A study that evaluated blood flow in elderly patients with fistulas found that, although blood flow rates were lower compared with younger patients, more than 78% of elderly patients had a blood flow rate greater than 400 mL/minute and there was no difference in dialysis adequacy as measured by Kt/V (129). Barril et al. (130) recommend the use of a transonic flow monitor and Doppler studies to diagnose arteriovenous stenoses in the elderly before thrombosis.

About one quarter of primary arteriovenous fistula failures occur in the first month, generally secondary to inadequate venous size or poor development (121,131). After the first month, patency rates of arteriovenous fistulas and synthetic grafts are equal. Infections of Cimino fistulas are rare, usually occur at the needle site, and are responsive to antibiotics and local care (121,132). Several authors suggest that preoperative arterial and venous mapping by Doppler ultrasound can identify vessels with adequate lumina and veins with good compliance and thereby increase the number of fistulas placed in elderly patients (133,134).

Prosthetic Grafts

Prosthetic grafts have a higher complication rate and eventually deteriorate (see Chapter 4) (114,123,135). One study of prosthetic graft complications found a significant correlation between increased age and prosthetic graft complications in nondiabetic patients. Interestingly, there was no correlation between increased age and prosthetic fistula complications in diabetic patients, although these patients had earlier fistula loss and complications than nondiabetics (131).

The most common causes of graft loss in diabetics and nondiabetics are uncorrected stenoses with associated thrombosis and infection (131). This is probably not different in the elderly. As in younger patients, it is vital to look for underlying cause(s) of thrombosis and try to correct them (2,123,135,136). Elderly patients with peripheral vascular disease are particularly prone to complications. We have cared for an elderly patient who developed compromise of his distal circulation and a popliteal deep vein thrombosis following thrombosis of a loop graft in his thigh.

Long-term or Permanent Silastic Catheters

An indwelling central double-lumen silastic catheter with felt cuffs (Permacath) (137) or twin single-lumen tunneled catheters (Tesio access system) (138) may be the preferred intermediate or long-term access for patients with frequent access infections, thromboses, and revisions; for elderly patients who cannot tolerate arteriovenous fistulas or prosthetic grafts because of hemodynamic instability or extensive peripheral vascular disease; or for patients who have exhausted potential access sites. De Meester et al. (139) suggest that permanent in-dwelling catheters should be the access of first choice for elderly patients, and Canaud et al. (140) consider them a viable option for elderly patients who have failed surgical attempts and/or have limited life expectancy. Mean duration of use was 14.2 months; median catheter survival was 2.5 years, and technical survival (performance as measured by blood flow rate) and rates of complications were independent of age.

Subcutaneous Central Venous Access Systems

Two permanently implantable subcutaneous systems have been developed that allow transcutaneous access to the central venous system. The LifeSite hemodialysis access device consists of two subcutaneously implanted valves connected to catheters that are accessed via a buttonhole technique (141–143). The Dialok Hemodialysis System is a subcutaneous portlike device, also accessed percutaneously, that provides access to twin catheters (143,144). Both are protected between treatments with antimicrobial locking solution (144,145), and both are reported to have comparable or higher blood flow rates (145,146) and a decreased infection rate compared with other methods of central venous access (143,146,147). At least one multicenter study demonstrated increased device survival for the LifeSite compared with conventional central venous access (146). Although, none of the studies stratified patients by age group, these new devices may show promise as dialysis access for the elderly patient with comorbidities, poor vessels, and increased susceptibility to infection.

Dialysis Access in Geriatric Dialysis Patients

Successful vascular access in the elderly dialysis patient is complicated by physiologic changes that occur with aging. Elderly patients may have peripheral vascular calcification or narrowing caused by diabetes, hyperlipidemia, or hypertension. Placement of vascular access in calcified vessels is associated with greater risk of ischemia and greater potential for thrombosis. If there is significant distal calcification, it may be necessary to use larger, more proximal vessels (148). See Chapter 4 for a more detailed discussion of hemodialysis vascular access.

We favor early access placement and encouragement of exercise with a rubber ball to develop the fistula (132); we also encourage arteriovenous fistula placement as a first option (149). Obviously, avoidance of hypotension (2,148) (see Chapter 3), prompt replacement of blood loss, and adequate nutrition (150,151) (see Chapter 30) are important. If repeated access thrombosis is noted (114), enteric coated aspirin (325 mg) or other antiplatelet drugs may be helpful (116,152,153), and occasionally low-dose warfarin may be useful (115,148), although a recent multicenter, randomized, placebo-controlled trial questioned its efficacy and safety (154). Recently published clinical practice guidelines outline the management of oral anticoagulant therapy in the elderly (155). Our recommendations for vascular access in the elderly are outlined in Table 35.5.

Peritoneal Dialysis Access

Catheter Survival

In the early days of CAPD experience (1982), Ponce et al. (156) found decreased 2-year peritoneal catheter survival (67 vs. 78%)

TABLE 35.5. RECOMMENDATIONS FOR VASCULAR ACCESS IN ELDERLY PATIENTS

Place access early
Avoid venipuncture in designated extremity
Preoperative arterial and venous mapping by Doppler ultrasound
Primary arteriovenous fistula preferred
Consider elbow fistulas
Avoid hypotension and hypovolemia
Replace blood loss promptly
Liberalize dry weight
Ensure adequate nutrition
Titrate blood pressure
Antiplatelet drugs
Graft diagram or fistulogram on chart
Permanent indwelling catheter

and increased pericatheter dialysate leakage (42.3% vs. 26.9%) in patients older than 60 years compared with younger patients. They hypothesized that the difference was secondary to "loose abdominal walls." Because more than 90% of dialysate leaks occurred within the first week after insertion (catheters were used immediately) and leakage resolved if the catheter was not used for 1 to 2 weeks, catheters are usually inserted 2 to 3 weeks before use, with temporary hemodialysis if necessary, until the insertion site is completely healed (28). If it is necessary to use the catheter earlier, small frequent dialysate exchanges are employed, with a gradual increase in quantity once integrity has been established (1).

Recent studies support the fact that catheter survival is either equivalent or improved in old versus young patients (35,70,75). Kim et al. (157) in a retrospective multiyear comparison of peritoneal catheter survival with arteriovenous access found greater long-term patency of peritoneal access, particularly in diabetic patients and the elderly. Gentile et al. (70) observed fewer catheter-related complications in elderly patients than in younger patients.

Peritonitis

Several large studies reveal no differences in peritonitis rates between young and old peritoneal dialysis patients (1,35,70,71,75,158,159). Nissenson et al. (75), in a large two-center study, reported that after 1 year of CAPD 60% of patients younger than 60 years were free of peritonitis versus 65% of the patients older than 60 years. At 3 years the figures were 38% and 46%, respectively; at 5 years, 33% and 43%; and at 7 years, 30% and 38%. Williams et al. (15) found a CAPD peritonitis rate of one episode per 7.4 patient-treatment months in patients 65 years or older compared with one episode per 12.9 patient-treatment months for all CAPD patients. Nolph et al. (71) found an increased incidence of peritonitis in bedridden patients, although no increase in exit-site and tunnel infection rates or catheter replacements. See Chapter 41 for further discussion of peritonitis in CAPD patients.

Exit-site and Tunnel Infections

There is little difference in exit-site infection rates (1,71), tunnel infections (35,71), or dialysate drainage pain in young compared with elderly CAPD patients (1,160).

CLINICAL CONSIDERATIONS IN DIALYSIS

As with most generalizations, a hypothesis by Macias-Nuñez et al. (1) contains some truth. They describe two groups of elderly dialysis patients. The first group is compliant and stable, with few symptoms. The second group of patients has frequent cardiovascular complications and/or failure to thrive (1).

Compliance

Avram et al. (161) describe a positive correlation between age and lower intradialytic weight gain, lower serum creatinine, and lower urea generation rate for both hemodialysis and peritoneal dialysis patients. Another study of 84 patients aged 60 years and older found good compliance as measured by serum potassium levels, fair to good compliance for serum phosphorus, and fair to poor compliance with fluid restriction (162). These patients were less compliant than elderly patients studied in the same unit 5 years previously (163), but those patients were also significantly older, poorer, and less educated. There was a positive and significant correlation among improved fluid compliance and length of time on dialysis, the number of medical problems, and decreased functional capacity (Karnofsky score). The authors speculated that there was increased social support and supervision for more compromised patients (162). They and others have stressed the importance of individualized approaches to compliance and social support for the elderly dialysis patient, including evaluation of physiologic and psychosocial factors (107,162,164).

Infection and Immunity

Abnormalities of Immune Function in Uremia

Infection is a major cause of morbidity and mortality in the ESRD population. It has been known for a long time that uremic patients have abnormalities of immune function (165) with impaired cell-mediated (166) and humoral (167) immunity, absolute lymphopenia (168–170) with a decrease in circulating T and B lymphocytes (171), cutaneous anergy (172), impaired phagocytosis (173), delayed graft rejection (174), altered response to infection (175), and an increased incidence of malignancy (176–179).

Abnormalities of Immune Function with Aging

The altered immune status of uremia is complicated in many elderly patients by similar changes in the immune system that may occur with aging, including increased susceptibility to infection and malignancy (180), and abnormalities in lymphocyte function and cell-mediated and humoral immunity (181,182). Hilden et al. (183), for example, found that 30% of elderly patients with active tuberculosis had a negative purified protein derivative compared with 20% of the general population.

Recent studies of "successful" mentally and physical agile centenarians suggest that immunosenescence may be a variable phenomena, more dependent on genetics and environment than aging per se (180,184–186), but as expected there is a positive correlation between increased morbidity and mortality from infection in elderly patients (180,187). An Israeli study found that infection was the most common cause of death in patients beginning dialysis at age 80 years or older (188).

Nutrition and Immunity

Nutritional status can also affect the ability of patients to respond to immunization. Hemodialysis patients with high normal serum albumin concentrations were more than five times as likely to respond to hepatitis B vaccine than those with serum albumin concentrations of 3.01 to 3.5 g/dL (189).

Presentation of Infection in the Elderly

In addition to changes in immune responsiveness, the presentation of infection in elderly patients is frequently subtle. The elderly patient may not manifest fever or leukocytosis; the elderly patient with an intraabdominal catastrophe may never develop the classic acute abdomen (190). The elderly dialysis patient may manifest occult infection by new-onset anorexia, apparent depression, vague feelings of malaise, apparent development of dementia, or decreased ability to cope with the usual activities of daily living. Occasionally, the only indication of infection is an increase in predialysis blood urea nitrogen levels without any apparent change in clinical status or an increased erythrocyte sedimentation rate (191). A European consensus statement on nutritional status in dialysis patients suggests measurement of C reactive protein as a marker of inflammation because of the close relationship between malnutrition, comorbid conditions, and inflammation (192).

Investigation might reveal an infected vascular access site (central line or peripheral graft), dental abscess, subcutaneous wound infection in an apparently healed surgical site, or other infection. Urinary tract infections are particularly common in elderly patients (193,194) but may be overlooked as a source of infection in the geriatric dialysis population. Infections such as bronchitis or pneumonia may be more obvious. Successful treatment of infection is generally associated with a return to the previous level of function.

Enhancement of Immune Function in the Elderly

It has been suggested that pharmacologic therapy with vitamin C, interleukin 2, thymus-stimulating agents, and various experimental compounds might be used in the future to enhance immune function in the elderly (181). Oral pyridoxine supplements, 50 mg daily, have been recommended because cell-mediated and humoral immunity may be inhibited by pyridoxine deficiency (195) and small amounts of water-soluble vitamins are removed by dialysis. Interestingly, patients on peritoneal dialysis appear to have better T-cell function than patients on hemodialysis (35).

Nutrition and Infection

It is particularly important to emphasize adequate nutrition in the older dialysis patient. Kenny et al. (190) demonstrated a significant negative correlation of serum albumin levels with prognosis in elderly patients with significant infection, and another study showed that serum albumin and nutritional markers such as retinol binding protein, serum transferrin, and prealbumin were more likely to be lower in hospitalized patients of any age who later died (196). A more recent study correlated reduced serum albumin with increased 3-year mortality in healthy elderly persons (197), and it is well established that dialysis patients of any age have increased mortality in the presence of low serum albumin, low prealbumin, low serum cholesterol, and other markers of nutritional status (198–204). Kalantar-Zadeh et al. (205) postulate the existence of a "malnutrition inflammation complex syndrome" in maintenance dialysis patients with protein-energy malnutrition that predisposes to illness and infection and leads to poor quality of life and increased morbidity and mortality.

The problem of malnutrition in dialysis patients is discussed in detail in Chapter 30. It is important to remember that the elderly are predisposed to this problem, although it may not be obvious initially in many. Kutner et al. (206) found that higher body mass index was a predictor of long-term survival in black female, black male, and white male dialysis patients 60 years and older.

Strategies to Enhance Nutrition in Elderly Dialysis Patients

Some strategies to enhance good nutrition in elderly dialysis patients are listed in Table 35.6. Many of these strategies are self-explanatory.

Patients who are disabled or living alone may benefit from programs such as Meals-on-Wheels, which deliver one or two prepared meals per day to the patient's home. Many of these programs can accommodate a prescribed diet. Home assistance services that provide aides to prepare meals, shop for groceries, and/or provide companionship can be very helpful. Patients with nausea or gastropathy may benefit from metoclopramide (Reglan), 10 mg orally 30 minutes before meals. Zinc deficiency can occur in dialysis patients and may be associated with dysgeusia; supplementation may enhance the taste of food (207). Megestrol acetate can stimulate appetite in selected patients (208–211).

Good oral hygiene is also very important. It is difficult for elderly patients to eat properly if they have sore gums, poor dentition, or poorly fitting dentures. Depression and constipation, both of which inhibit appetite, must also be treated.

Finally, a thorough review of the patient's medication list may reveal a phenomenal number of prescribed pills. I have heard more than one patient complain of early satiety because of the sheer volume of medication. Consolidating and eliminating unnecessary medication may be associated with improved appetite.

TABLE 35.6. STRATEGIES TO ENHANCE NUTRITION IN ELDERLY DIALYSIS PATIENTS

Ensure adequacy of dialysis
Correction of metabolic acidosis
Dietary supplements
Vitamin and mineral supplements
Megestrol acetate
Minimal dietary restrictions
Meals on Wheels
Companionship
Home assistance services
Metoclopropamide
Adequate dental care
Treatment of depression
Treatment of constipation
Therapeutic nihilism
Consider intradialytic parenteral nutrition

DIALYSIS-ASSOCIATED MORBIDITY

Pruritus is a problem more common in the elderly dialysis patient, possibly because of skin changes seen with aging (2). Treatment consists of keeping the skin moist with baby oil and humectants, using oatmeal soap, bathing less frequently and with tepid rather than hot water, and increasing ambient humidity with vaporizers or humidifiers. Antihistamines such as diphenhydramine or hydroxyzine HCl may be used, but the sedative effects of these medications may cause confusion in elderly patients. Increased sun exposure has been recommended. Although Gilchrest et al. (212) found a decrease in uremic pruritus after treatment with ultraviolet light, another placebo-controlled study of the effect of ultraviolet light found a significant reduction in pruritus in both placebo and treatment groups (213). They suggested the benefit might actually be from blue light rather than ultraviolet.

The problems of anemia (Chapter 32), β_2-amyloid (Chapter 23), and renal osteodystrophy (Chapter 26) are discussed in detail elsewhere. It is worth noting, however, that at least one study has documented significantly better mobility in elderly nondialysis patients, adjusted for comorbidity, with even relatively small increases in hemoglobin level, for example, less than 12.0 g/dL versus 12 to 13 g/dL versus 13 to 14 g/dL (214). Silverberg et al. (215) found that correction of anemia in elderly patients with chronic kidney disease and severe resistant heart failure is associated with an increase in left ventricular ejection fraction, a decrease in fatigue, and a significant decrease in need for hospitalization. Bedani et al. (216) confirmed that increasing serum hemoglobin concentration with subcutaneous erythropoietin in elderly dialysis patients was associated with partial regression of left ventricular hypertrophy and subjective improvement in quality of life and ability to perform activities of daily living, and they suggested that there should also be improved exercise performance and better cognitive function (216,217). In addition, several recent studies have suggested that the use of nandrolone decanoate in elderly hemodialysis and peritoneal dialysis patients has a beneficial effect on anemia; results in better nutritional parameters (218–220); and has a beneficial effect on lymphocyte subsets, potentially enhancing immune responsiveness (221). It was noted, however, that there was a significant decrease in high-density lipoprotein (HDL) and apo-A1 levels and an increase in triglyceride levels.

Hemodialysis-Associated Morbidity

Advanced age is an independent risk factor for left ventricular hypertrophy, dilated cardiomyopathy, congestive heart failure (222,223), and coronary heart disease (224). Elderly hemodialysis patients clearly have more severe cardiovascular impairment than younger hemodialysis patients (36) and impaired autonomic function that can inhibit their ability to tolerate volume removal during dialysis (225). Zucchelli et al. (226) compared the incidence of intradialytic complications of acetate hemodialysis in patients older than 64 years with patients younger than 55 years and, not surprisingly, found a significantly higher incidence of hypotension, angina, and arrhythmia in the older patients. There was no difference in the incidence of headache, vomiting, or cramps.

TABLE 35.7. STRATEGIES TO MINIMIZE HYPOTENSION IN ELDERLY HEMODIALYSIS PATIENTS

Bicarbonate buffer
High dialysate sodium concentration
High dialysate calcium concentration
Biocompatible dialyzer membrane
Cool temperature dialysis
Dry ultrafiltration and volume expanders
Blood volume controlled hemodialysis
Blood pressure control
Correction of anemia
Avoid excessive weight gain
Avoid postprandial hypotension
Adequate nutrition
Adequate salt intake
Midodrine
Exercise
Consider peritoneal dialysis

Chapters 3 and 19 discuss particular problems with dialysis hypotension and selection of the proper dialysate. The elderly represent a dialysis group that is particularly fragile in this regard. Table 35.7 lists strategies for minimizing hypotension in elderly hemodialysis patients.

Peritoneal Dialysis-Associated Morbidity

There is a higher incidence of inguinal hernias, fluid leaks, and vascular ischemia of the lower extremities in older peritoneal dialysis patients as compared with younger patients (1,227).

Hernias

Inguinal or abdominal hernias may be aggravated by decreased abdominal muscle tone. Kyphosis in the elderly patient may be associated with widening of the diaphragm and subsequent development of a hiatal hernia (1). Hernias may be aggravated by the stress of carrying 2 L or more fluid in the abdominal cavity. They should be repaired, as in a younger patient. If surgical repair is not feasible, it may be possible to continue peritoneal dialysis by doing small volume exchanges with a cycler while the patient is recumbent.

Back Pain

Back pain and musculoskeletal disorders in elderly peritoneal dialysis patients may be related to decreased abdominal muscle tone, preexisting back pain or lumbar disk disease, obesity, or weight of dialysate in the abdominal cavity (228).

Patients may benefit from exercises to strengthen back and abdominal muscles that do not increase intraabdominal pressure and from training in body mechanics—for example, squatting to pick up an object rather than bending over. If back pain continues to be a problem, the patient can be trained to do low-volume exchanges with a cycler at night and keep the abdominal cavity empty during the day (229). If the problem persists despite these measures, the patient may need to switch to hemodialysis.

Hypotension

As in hemodialysis patients, volume status and fluid intake must be monitored in peritoneal dialysis patients, and patients must be educated about the importance of adjusting their peritoneal dialysis prescription to allow for fluid losses from sources such as diarrhea, vomiting, fever, or perspiration. If hypotension is secondary to poor cardiovascular status, performing small frequent exchanges with a cycler and keeping the abdominal cavity empty during the day may be considered. Meticulous attention to weight gain or loss and adequate salt intake are also important.

Peripheral Vascular Disease

There may be mechanical aggravation of ischemia in elderly peritoneal dialysis patients with compromise of iliac or femoral vessels (1) secondary to pressure of the dialysate or because of decreased perfusion secondary to hypotension. Cycler dialysis at night with the patient empty during the day may be tried, but it may be necessary to change modalities unless the vascular insufficiency can be relieved with vascular bypass procedures.

Diverticulosis

Diverticulosis is a relative contraindication to peritoneal dialysis in elderly patients because of their increased predisposition to diverticulitis and intestinal perforation. It is particularly important to avoid constipation in these patients, both because of the risk of perforation with attendant high mortality and because of the tendency for constipation to interfere with dialysate drainage.

Constipation

Constipation is generally more common in elderly patients but is a particular problem in elderly peritoneal dialysis patients because it may interfere mechanically with dialysate drainage. Recommendations include the use of sorbitol or other nonstimulant cathartics, adequate fluid intake, and avoidance of medications that interfere with bowel function.

Polyneuropathy

Moriwaki et al. (230) found that elderly peritoneal dialysis patients were more likely to complain of symptoms such as paresthesias, burning, and painful dysesthesias than younger patients and to have associated vitamin B_6 deficiency. Correction of vitamin B_6 levels with 30 mg of oral vitamin B_6 daily resulted in a decrease in symptoms in two thirds of their patients.

Comorbidity

Mailloux et al. (231) documented that comorbid risk factors with the greatest prognostic impact on survival for ESRD patients are hypertension, low serum albumin, and predialysis cardiac disease. Comorbid illnesses seen most commonly in elderly ESRD patients include ischemic heart disease, congestive heart failure and myocardial dysfunction, hypertension, pulmonary disease, gastrointestinal disorders, cerebrovascular disease, and cancer (15). These disorders are covered in Chapters 16–19 and 25.

Gastrointestinal bleeding is very common in elderly dialysis patients. Chester et al. (27) found evidence of gastrointestinal bleeding in 22% of elderly hemodialysis patients older than 70 years compared with 7% of younger controls. Porush et al. (2) found that gastrointestinal bleeding accounts for 18% of hospital admissions in elderly dialysis patients. The sources of gastrointestinal bleeding are often multiple in elderly patients. In addition to the usual causes of gastrointestinal blood loss, uremia and nonsteroidal antiinflammatory agents may be involved in the elderly dialysis patient. If the patient is uremic and has a prolonged bleeding time, dialysis time can be increased to restore platelet function. If nonsteroidal antiinflammatory agents are required, misoprostol (200 μg with meals and at bedtime) may be helpful.

According to Porush et al. (2), the second most common cause of gastrointestinal bleeding in elderly patients with ESRD is angiodysplasia. The lesions are usually multiple and may be treated with endoscopy and laser photocoagulation or electrocautery, surgery, heparin-free dialysis, or peritoneal dialysis. Patients with gastrointestinal blood loss and prolonged bleeding time may respond to treatment with desamino-D-arginine-8-vasopressin or conjugated estrogens.

In addition to the usual dementia evaluation of any patient with mental status changes, it is important to consider subdural hematoma or hemorrhage in the elderly dialysis patient. It may be desirable to use low-dose heparin or heparin-free dialysis in elderly patients. Functional compromise may occur secondary to intradialytic hypotension. The elderly patient may need a higher blood pressure to maintain adequate cerebral blood flow. Mental status changes may also be due to overmedication (sedatives, antihistamines for itching, soporifics, minor or major tranquilizers) that is iatrogenic, inadvertent secondary to patient confusion ("Did I take my pills yet or not?"), or related to poor eyesight (patients may mistake one medication for another with serious consequences). Some strategies for assisting elderly patients in taking their medication appropriately are listed in Table 35.8.

Mild dementia may respond to small amounts of medication such as haloperidol or thioridazine, although it should be stressed that it is easy to overmedicate these patients. Ultimately, the demented elderly dialysis patient becomes a social, moral,

TABLE 35.8. STRATEGIES FOR ASSISTING ELDERLY PATIENTS IN TAKING MEDICATION

Compartmented medication box labeled by day and time of day
Cardboard or file card with pill samples taped to card by time of day
Large print labels
Prefilled insulin syringes
Pill counts
Home nurse visits
Repetitive and frequent review of medication and dosage intervals by nurses, doctors, and others
Regular eye exams and refraction

and ethical dilemma for the renal team and the patient's family (26).

DIALYSIS IN A NURSING HOME

Very few authors address the topic of dialysis in the nursing home setting, although most practicing nephrologists must deal with this issue. As the dialysis population ages and becomes more debilitated, it is inevitable that some proportion of patients require skilled nursing care on a temporary or permanent basis. In 1984, Westlie et al. (232) noted a 6.0% prevalence of nursing home placement of ESRD patients, which is probably not different from that of the general population older than 65 years (233).

Anderson et al. (234) conducted a prospective survey of ESRD patients in Network 5 on dialysis and residing in nursing homes. The issues they addressed included demographic and social factors, comorbidity, functional capacity, mode of dialysis, and survival. The survey, which went to the 156 dialysis centers in Network 5, resulted in a remarkable contribution of information from 132 dialysis center social workers who represented 90% of patients on dialysis within the network (234); 87% of dialysis nursing home residents with ESRD were treated with hemodialysis and the remainder with peritoneal dialysis.

The nursing home ESRD patients were older and more likely to be white, female, and diabetic. Survival was 74%, 56%, and 42% at 3, 6, and 12 months, respectively, with worse survival for patients who were older than 75 years, who were less functional, or who were treated with peritoneal dialysis. Most of the peritoneal dialysis patients were treated at one center; the excess mortality for nursing home patients on peritoneal dialysis appeared to be from patients on peritoneal dialysis at other centers. This suggests that mortality may decrease with increased experience with peritoneal dialysis of the nursing home elderly.

A small number of patients could move to more independent living situations. Distressingly, the authors found a prevalence rate of nursing home residence of 2% for ESRD patients older than 65 years, less than half that of the general population. A previous study by the same authors of CAPD in a nursing home found peritonitis rates and acute hospitalization rates comparable with National CAPD Registry data for all patients. Not unexpectedly, patient survival was decreased for the nursing home patients (262).

Schleifer (235) found that almost half of 197 nursing homes contacted in the Philadelphia area accepted ESRD patients, 19% of whom were treated with peritoneal dialysis and the rest with hemodialysis; 18% of the nursing homes refused ESRD patients; and 34% had never been asked. Reasons given for not accepting ESRD patients included lack of nurse training, transportation problems, inadequate physician coverage, administrative objection, and financial concerns (235).

The National Kidney Foundation of Michigan has developed an educational curriculum for nursing home personnel to assist in the care of the ESRD nursing home patient (236).

Carey et al. (237) developed a highly structured educational program to train personnel in 10 community based extended care facilities to care for continuous peritoneal dialysis patients who required temporary or permanent placement following inpatient care for intercurrent medical or surgical illness. Over a 5-year period, 1-month, 6-month, and 1-year patient survival rates were 90%, 50%, and 40%, respectively, with short-term rehabilitation patients having significantly better survival than long-term patients as expected. Technique survival rates, censored for deaths, were 94%, 86% and 79%, respectively. Peritonitis rates were higher than in noninstitutionalized patients (1 episode/9.6 patient-months vs. 1 episode/13.5 patient-months), but considered acceptable. The authors stressed the importance of continuing education and support from the training team in the acceptance and success of the program. The study demonstrated the feasibility of continuous peritoneal dialysis in the extended care setting.

ETHICAL ISSUES AND ELDERLY ESRD PATIENTS

As the dialysis population becomes larger, older, and more disabled and the cost of the ESRD Medicare program continues to grow (238,239), many ethical dilemmas arise (Table 35.9).

Access to ESRD Treatment

Do elderly dialysis patients have equal access to treatment or is age an independent risk factor for denial of treatment (239–241)? Most essayists on the subject are fond of quoting Berlyne's letter regarding dialysis age discrimination in the United Kingdom (242), and other reports have noted ESRD treatment age inequality in other European countries (30,243). In a survey of French nephrologists, 90% refused patients 75 years and older if they were not independent and did not have a supportive family (13). A recent report from Brazil that examined factors associated with acceptance for maintenance dialysis treatment found that the adjusted odds ratio of not being accepted for dialysis was 2.94 for persons older than 65 years compared with younger persons (244).

Kjellstrand et al. (245) also found considerable age discrimination when analyzing the U.S. dialysis population in 1979, although it had somewhat lessened since 1977. However, Rosansky et al. (246) examined U.S. ESRD treatment incidence between 1978 and 1987 and established apparent increased selection for elderly and sicker patients. Moulton et al. (247) found great geographic variation in ESRD treatment of the elderly when examining regional U.S. incidence rates. Low referral rates were particularly striking in several southern states (246). It is unclear whether the regional differences observed were due to differences in true incidence or to differences in patient or physician bias or availability of ESRD services.

TABLE 35.9. ETHICAL ISSUES IN DIALYSIS OF ELDERLY

Access to ESRD treatment
Selection of ESRD modality
Quality of life/rehabilitation
Initiation and termination of treatment
Cardiopulmonary resuscitation

Difficult ethical questions relate to allocation of scarce financial resources, the increasing poverty among children, and the constant pressure to reduce health care costs and the national debt (239,248–252). Ethicists suggest that decisions must be morally based and must consider treatment goals, physiologic and chronologic age, and equitable access in addition to allocation of resources and cost (253). Solutions to these difficult ethical questions will never be easy, and they require the utmost respect for the individual, great compassion for the patient and family, and a considerate health care provider. Appropriateness of life-sustaining technology must be reevaluated with major changes in medical condition.

Quality of Life and Rehabilitation

Elderly ESRD patients seem to segregate into two populations. The first group of elderly patients adjusts to dialysis very well and seems satisfied with the lifestyle. Some of these patients appear to enjoy the increased social interaction of thrice weekly visits to the dialysis unit. Some investigators have found an unusually high level of life satisfaction among the dialysis elderly (232), and others note that older patients frequently appear satisfied with a lifestyle that might be unacceptable to a younger patient (27). A German study of dialysis patients older than 80 years found that 80% would advocate dialysis to others their age (31).

The second group of patients has more comorbidity and less functional capacity. These are the patients who have higher rates of depression. The functional status of some of these patients improves markedly with dialysis (254). Others deteriorate rapidly physically and/or emotionally and have a high rate of withdrawal from dialysis.

Quality of life assessment is very subjective, and the different outcomes reported in various studies may reflect differences in physician and patient-family treatment goals, patient selection, rehabilitation needs, support services, and attitude. Avram et al. (161) found no difference in Karnofsky score—a measure of functional capacity—between dialysis patients older than 70 years and younger patients. Disney (255) reported that 55% of ESRD patients aged between 75 and 84 years were "capable of normal activity," but 10% were considered disabled, 7% to 8% required frequent assistance, and 2% to 3% required constant care. Two studies comparing dialysis patients at least 60 years old with age-, race-, and gender-matched peers not on dialysis found more functional disability and a greater need for health care and other services among the dialysis elderly, but these comparisons suggested that increased attention to improving exercise tolerance, improving anemia, and maintaining a degree of independence and self-care contribute to improved psychologic and functional status (256,257).

Recent prospective studies and controlled trials suggest resistance training, muscle strengthening, and regular exercise result in improved functional status, physical fitness, and independence for elderly dialysis patients (258–260). Selected elderly dialysis patients also appear to benefit from intensive inpatient rehabilitation (261,262). The message for the practicing nephrologist is to individualize patient care decisions, encourage physical and psychologic independence and use of appropriate support services, encourage realistic treatment goals and decisions, and be prepared to redirect treatment goals as changes in medical condition warrant.

Initiation and Termination of Treatment

Most elderly dialysis patients die of cardiovascular disease (2,35, 53,106,263). The next most common cause in the United States is withdrawal from dialysis (264). Patients are more likely to withdraw if they are white, female, diabetic, older than 65 years (264), or living in nursing homes (265).

Singer et al. (266) surveyed nephrologists in six New England states regarding decisions to withhold or withdraw dialysis. Only 11% of nephrologists indicated they had not withheld dialysis in the previous years; 19% did not withdraw dialysis once it had been initiated. Eighty-eight percent of nephrologists indicated they stop dialysis at the request of a competent patient and 90% at the request of an incompetent patient's family when the patient's prior wishes were known. Only 63% would withdraw dialysis if the patient's wishes were unclear, and only 1% if an incompetent patient's wishes were unknown and the family wanted dialysis continued. Holley et al. (267) found that preexisting medical conditions and the wishes of the patient's family more commonly influenced practicing nephrologists in their decision to initiate or withdraw dialysis. Agraharkar et al. (268) suggest that staff-assisted home hemodialysis may be an appropriate short-term option for debilitated or terminally ill patients when the major barrier to continuing dialysis is the cost of ambulance transportation to the dialysis center or patient comfort issues. Financial analysis revealed that staff-assisted hemodialysis was much less costly than either in-hospital hemodialysis or outpatient hemodialysis with ambulance transportation. Although the difference between the Medicare capitated fee and the cost of staff assisted hemodialysis in this study was borne by third-party payers, which would not be an option for uninsured patients.

Although decisions to withhold or withdraw dialysis are very difficult and have generated a complex legal and ethical literature (269), consideration of established ethical principles may make decisions somewhat easier (Table 35.10). Recently developed resources for patients, family members, and the health care team regarding initiation and withdrawal of dialysis can assist with these issues (270–273).

Self-determination and Autonomy

The first issue to be considered is whether the patient is competent to make a decision to withdraw a life-sustaining technology, in this case dialysis. Is there evidence of dementia or psychiatric

TABLE 35.10. ETHICAL PRINCIPLES FOR WITHDRAWING AND/OR WITHHOLDING DIALYSIS

Self-determination/autonomy
Benefit versus burden
Futile therapy
Conflict between physician and family

disorder, or is the patient's judgment clouded by depression, pain, medication, or metabolic derangement? Can the patient understand the choices involved and consequences of any decision? If the patient is truly competent, then he or she has the right to make an informed decision regarding medical care (269,274), and several reports note that they do wish to participate (275,276). The *American College of Physicians Ethics Manual* (277) suggests that if the patient is not competent, the order of priority for decision making should be advance directives, substituted judgments, and the best interests of the patient.

Although there is general sentiment favoring the completion of advance directives by all patients and legislation is in place that patients must be asked if they have one or wish to complete one when admitted to a hospital (Patient Self-Determination Act of 1990), there appears to be reluctance among dialysis professionals to discuss advance directives with patients (278). Barriers to such discussion include lack of knowledge or training, conflicts with personal values, stress, inadequate time, and fear of upsetting the patient (278).

Physicians and other dialysis staff must be familiar with the concepts and legal ramifications of advance directives, durable powers of attorney, and living wills and be willing and able to discuss them when indicated. The patient's family or significant other may be asked to assist in the decision making and must know they are basing that decision on the patient's best interests, on prior advance directives made by the patient when competent, or on knowledge of what the patient would have wished given the circumstances (269,279).

Understanding the dynamics of the patient-family relationship may also be necessary. Decisions may be made for various reasons, including the best interest of the patient, financial interest, guilt because of the family member's limited contact with the patient, or a misunderstanding of role and process. If the caretaker or physician is uncomfortable with the decision to withhold or withdraw dialysis, he or she may wish to refer the patient to another physician.

Benefit versus Burden

Is the patient likely to benefit from dialysis? In this situation, age is not an appropriate independent criterion (269). Each patient must be evaluated individually for medical and psychologic suitability for dialysis and whether dialysis is technically possible.

A nephrologist is not ethically or legally obligated to offer dialysis if treatment would not benefit the patient. Hirsch et al. (280) suggest that dialysis is inappropriate for patients with poor prognoses, including those with multiple-organ system failure; nonuremic dementia; metastatic, refractory malignancy; or irreparable and debilitating neurologic disease. Ninety-five percent of dialysis unit medical directors surveyed by Kilner (269) considered medical benefit to be the most important criterion in the dialysis decision.

When dialysis is appropriate, the patient and/or family member may believe that dialysis poses a burden to the patient that outweighs potential benefit, either because of the process or because of its impact on quality of life (269,279). Understanding why the patient and/or family considers dialysis burdensome is important, because it may be possible to modify treatment or even initiate dialysis on a trial basis for a patient who fears dialysis but does not actually know what it is like. Also, the patient's environment or support system can perhaps be adjusted in a way that makes dialysis more tolerable or desirable.

Dialysis as Futile Therapy

Dialysis may be viewed as a futile therapy—prolonging death rather than sustaining life. For example, a patient may be facing imminent death from terminal cancer or may be comatose with irreversible brain damage. Removing a life support such as dialysis would not "cause" the patient's death but rather allow it to occur naturally. Kilner (269) refers to this as "passive facilitating."

Conflict between Physician and Family

When the physician and family cannot agree on the best course of action for a patient, several options are available. These options may include review by an ethics committee or the courts or transfer of the patient to another physician or hospital. It is generally preferable for these discussions to remain among medical staff, patient, and family rather than resorting to the courts. Ethics committees provide a forum for discussion rather than make medical decisions (277).

Adequate and clear communication is the most important factor in resolving conflicts regarding terminal care, not only between physician and family but also among all the health professionals involved in the care of the patient. Roberts et al. (281), in a study of the impact of withdrawal of dialysis on surviving relatives, noted that the relatives were most disappointed when physicians failed to tell the truth; were too optimistic; continued dialysis too long; and/or were unwilling to discuss withdrawal, alternatives, and implications.

Cardiopulmonary Resuscitation

A recent evaluation of outcomes of cardiopulmonary resuscitation in dialysis patients revealed poorer long-term survival compared with a control group of nondialysis patients receiving cardiopulmonary resuscitation (282). Holley et al. (283) surveyed dialysis patients of all ages regarding their attitudes toward cardiopulmonary resuscitation, ventilatory support, withdrawal from dialysis, and participation in the medical decision making. Dialysis patient responses were similar to those of ambulatory elderly patients. Age was not a factor in decisions to refuse respiratory support or dialysis, although older dialysis patients were more likely to have thought about it. Most dialysis patients wanted to take part in medical decision making and most never considered withdrawal from dialysis (215).

REFERENCES

1. Macias-Nunez JF, et al. Treatment of end-stage renal disease in the elderly. In: Cameron JS, et al., eds. *The Oxford textbook of clinical nephrology.* London: Oxford, 1992:1621–1635.
2. Porush JG, et al. Chronic renal failure. In: Porush JG, et al., eds. *Renal disease in the aged.* Boston: Little, Brown, 1991:285–313.
3. Barbanel C. Renal diseases and dialysis in elderly patients. *Contrib Nephrol* 1989;71:95–99.
4. Disney APS. Demography and survival of patients receiving treatment for chronic renal failure in Australia and New Zealand: report on dialysis and renal transplantation treatment from the Australia and New Zealand Dialysis and Transplant Registry. *Am J Kidney Dis* 1995; 25:165–175.
5. Brown WW. Dialysis and transplantation in the elderly. In: Morley JE, ed. *Geriatric care.* St. Louis: GW Manning (in press).
6. U.S. Renal Data System annual data report. Bethesda, MD: National Institutes of Health, 2001.
7. U.S. Renal Data System annual data report. Bethesda, MD: National Institutes of Health, 1991.
8. Obialo CI, et al. Kidney disease in elderly minorities. *J Natl Med Assoc* 2002;94[Suppl 8]:76S–82S.
9. Russell A, et al. Increasing incidence of end-stage renal disease in Wisconsin: an unintended consequence of increased survival? *Wis Med J* 2001;100:35–38.
10. Glickman JF, et al. Aetiology and diagnosis of chronic renal insufficiency in the aged: the role of renal biopsy. In: Macias-Nunez JF, et al., eds. *Renal function and disease in the elderly.* London: Butterworths, 1987:485–508.
11. Brown WW, et al. Aging and the kidney. *Arch Intern Med* 1986;146: 1790–1796.
12. Levison SP. Renal disease in the elderly: the role of renal biopsy. *Am J Kidney Dis* 1990;16:300–306.
13. Mignon F, et al. Worldwide demographics and future trends of the management of renal failure in the elderly. *Kidney Int* 1993;42[Suppl 41]:S18–S26.
14. Radecki S, et al. Dialysis for chronic renal failure: comorbidity and treatment differences by disease etiology. *Am J Nephrol* 1989;9: 115–123.
15. Williams AJ, et al. Continuous ambulatory peritoneal dialysis and haemodialysis in the elderly. *Q J Med* 1990;274:215–223.
16. Hutteri H, et al. Retirement to renal failure: the management of the elderly dialysis patient. *J Can Assoc Nephrol Nurses Technicians* 1992;2: 14–16.
17. Brown WW. Introduction. Proceedings from the International Conference: geriatric nephrology and urology: interdisciplinary perspectives. *Am J Kidney Dis* 1990;16:273–274.
18. Oreopoulos DG. Opinion: how can the care of elderly dialysis patients be improved? *Semin Dial* 1992;5:24–25.
19. Bower JD. Opinion: how can the care of elderly dialysis patients be improved? *Semin Dial* 1992;5:26–28.
20. Boag J, et al. The impact of aging on dialysis: human and technical considerations. *Dial Transplant* 1992;21(3):124–127.
21. Ross CJ, et al. Dialysis modality selection in the elderly patient with end-stage renal disease: advantages and disadvantages of peritoneal dialysis. *Adv Perit Dial* 1990;6[Suppl]:11–17.
22. Mallick NP, et al. The changing population on renal replacement therapy: its clinical and economic impact in Europe. *Nephrol Dial Transplant* 1996;11[Suppl 1]:2–5.
23. DeLuca L, et al. Opinion: how can the care of elderly dialysis patients be improved? *Semin Dial* 1992;5:28–29.
24. Mooradian AD. Biological and functional definition of the older patient: the role of biomarkers of aging. *Oncology* 1992;6[Suppl]: 39–44.
25. Oreopoulos DG. The aging kidney. *Adv Perit Dial* 1990;6[Suppl]:2–5.
26. Capelli JP. Haemodialysis and the elderly patient. In: Michelis MF, et al., eds. *Geriatric nephrology.* New York: Field, Rich and Associates, 1986:129–134.
27. Chester AC, et al. Hemodialysis in the eighth and ninth decades of life. *Arch Intern Med* 1979;139:1001–1005.
28. Ponticelli C, et al. Dialysis treatment of end-stage renal disease in the elderly. In: Macias-Nunez JF, et al., eds. *Renal function and disease in the elderly.* London: Butterworths, 1987:509–528.
29. Giuseppe P, et al. Elderly patients on dialysis: epidemiology of an epidemic. *Nephrol Dial Transplant* 1996;11[Suppl 9]:26–30.
30. Rotellar E, et al. Must patients over 65 be haemodialyzed? *Nephron* 1985;41:152–156.

31. Schaefer K, et al. The dilemma of renal replacement therapy in patients over 80 years of age: dialysis should not be with held. *Nephrol Dial Transplant* 1999;14:35–36.

32. Röhrich B, et al. The elderly dialysis patient: management of the hospital stay. *Nephrol Dial Transplant* 1998;13[Suppl 7]:69–72.

33. Parry RG, et al. Referral of elderly patients with severe renal failure: questionnaire survey of physicians. *BMJ* 1996;313:466.

34. Nissenson AR. Chronic peritoneal dialysis in the elderly. *Geriatr Nephrol Urol* 1991;1:3–12.

35. Maiorca R, et al. Modality selection for the elderly: medical factors. *Adv Perit Dial* 1990;6[Suppl]:18–25.

36. Capuano A, et al. Cardiovascular impairment, dialysis strategy and tolerance in elderly and young patients on maintenance haemodialysis. *Nephrol Dial Transplant* 1990;5:1023–1030.

37. Shah B, et al. Current experience with renal transplantation in older patients. *Am J Kidney Dis* 1988;12:516–523.

38. Roza AN. Renal transplantation in patients more than sixty-five years old. *Transplantation* 1989;48:689–690.

39. Lauffer G, et al. Renal transplantation in patients over 55 years old. *Br J Surg* 1988;75:984–987.

40. Kyllonen L, et al. Kidney transplantation in the elderly in Finland. *Transplant Proc* 1990;22:163–164.

41. Velez RL, et al. Renal transplantation with cyclosporine in the elderly population. *Transplant Proc* 1991;23:1749–1752.

42. Schulak JA, et al. Kidney transplantation in patients aged sixty years and older. *Surgery* 1990;108:726–733.

43. Schulak JA, et al. Kidney transplantation in the elderly. *Geriatr Nephrol Urol* 1991;1:105–112.

44. Pirsch JD, et al. Cadaveric renal transplantation with cyclosporine in patients more than 60 years of age. *Transplantation* 1989;47:259–261.

45. Cantatovich D, et al. Cadaveric renal transplantation in patients older than 60 year of age. *Geriatr Nephrol Urol* 1993;3:1–5.

46. Johnson DW, et al. A comparison of the effects of dialysis and renal transplantation on the survival of older uremic patients. *Transplantation* 2000; 69:794–799.

47. Doyle SE, et al. Predicting clinical outcome in the elderly renal transplant patient. *Kidney Int* 2000;57:2144–2150.

48. Saudan P, et al. Renal transplantation in the elderly: a long-term, single-centre experience. *Nephrol Dial Transplant* 2001;16:824–828.

49. Cameron JS. Renal transplantation in the elderly. *Int Urol Nephrol* 2000;32:193–201.

50. Basu A, et al. Renal transplantation in patients above 60 years of age in the modern era: a single center experience with a review of the literature. *Int Urol Nephrol* 2000;32:171–176.

51. Becker BN, et al. Renal transplantation in the older end-stage renal disease patient. *Semin Nephrol* 1996;16:353–362.

52. Wolfe RA, et al. Comparison of mortality in all patients on dialysis, patients on dialysis awaiting transplantation, and recipients of a first cadaveric transplant. *N Engl J Med* 1999;341:1725–1730.

53. Taube DH, et al. Successful treatment of middle aged and elderly patients with end-stage renal disease. *BMJ* 1983;286:2018–1020.

54. Smits JMA, et al. Evaluation of the Eurotransplant Senior Program: the results of the first year. *Am J Transplant* 2002;2:664–670.

55. Fauchald P, et al. The use of elderly living donors in renal transplantation. *Transplant Int* 1991;4:51–53.

56. Hayashi T, et al. Living-related renal transplantation from elderly donors (older than 66 years of age). *Transplant Proc* 1995;27:984–985.

57. U.S. Renal Data System Annual data report. Bethesda, MD: National Institutes of Health, 1996.

58. Zucchelli P. Hemodialysis-induced symptomatic hypotension: a review of pathophysiologic mechanism. *Int J Artif Organs* 1987;10:139–144.

59. Mignon F, et al. The management of uraemia in the elderly: treatment choices. *Nephrol Dial Transplant* 1995;10[Suppl 6]:55–59.

60. Winkelmayer WC, et al. Comparing mortality of elderly patients on hemodialysis versus peritoneal dialysis: a propensity score approach. *J Am Soc Nephrol* 2002;12:2353–2362.

61. Winkelmayer WC, et al. Comparing mortality of elderly patients on hemodialysis versus peritoneal dialysis: a propensity score approach. *J Am Soc Nephrol* 2002;13:2353–2362.

62. Vonash EF, et al. Mortality in end-stage renal disease: a reassessment of differences between patients treated with hemodialysis and peritoneal dialysis. *J Am Soc Nephrol* 1999;10:354–365.

63. Maitra S, et al. Increased mortality of elderly female peritoneal dialysis patients with diabetes—a descriptive analysis. *Adv Perit Dial* 2001;17:117–121.

64. Chung SH, et al. Influence of initial nutritional status on continuous ambulatory peritoneal dialysis patient survival. *Perit Dial Int* 2000;20:19–26.

65. Italian Registry of Dialysis and Transplantation, 1998 report. Available at www.sin-italia.org/registri/ridt/ridt98/ridt98.htm (accessed xx).

66. 2001 Australia and New Zealand Dialysis and Transplant Registry (ANZDATA) annual report. Available at www.anzdata.org.au/ (accessed xx).

67. U.S. Renal Data System annual data report. Bethesda, MD: National Institutes of Health, 1989.

68. U.S. Renal Data System annual data report. Bethesda, MD: National Institutes of Health, 1997.

69. Mattern WD, et al. Selection of ESRD treatment: an international study. *Am J Kidney Dis* 1989;13:457–464.

70. Gentile DE, Geriatric Advisory Committee. Peritoneal dialysis in geriatric patients: a survey of clinical practices. *Adv Perit Dial* 1990;6[Suppl]:29–32.

71. Nolph KD, et al. Experiences with the elderly in the National CAPD Registry. *Adv Perit Dial* 1990;6[Suppl]:33–37.

72. Bliwise DL, et al. Survival by time of day of hemodialysis in an elderly cohort. *JAMA* 2001;286:2690–2694.

73. Nicholls AJ, et al. Impact of continuous ambulatory peritoneal dialysis on treatment of renal failure in patients aged over 60. *BMJ* 1984;288:18–19.

74. Vlachojannis J, et al. CAPD in elderly patients with cardiovascular risk factors. *Clin Nephrol* 1988;30[Suppl 1]:S13–S17.

75. Nissenson AR, et al. Peritoneal dialysis in the elderly patient. *Am J Kidney Dis* 1990;16:335–338.

76. Nissenson AR. Opinion: how can the care of elderly dialysis patients be improved? *Semin Dial* 1992;5:25–26.

77. De Vecchi AF, et al. Peritoneal dialysis in the ninth decade of life experience in a single center. *Geriatr Nephrol Urol* 1996;6:75–80.

78. Jagose J, et al. Successful use of continuous ambulatory peritoneal dialysis in octogenarians. *Geriatr Nephrol Urol* 1995;5:135–141.

79. Michel C, et al. CAPD with private home nurses: an alternative treatment for elderly and disabled patients. In: Nissenson AR, ed. Peritoneal dialysis in the geriatric patient. *Adv Perit Dial* 1990;6[Suppl]:331–335.

80. Diaz-Buxo JA, et al. Experience with continuous cyclic peritoneal dialysis in the geriatric patient. *Adv Perit Dial* 1990;6[Suppl]:61–64.

81. Diaz-Buxo JA. The place for cycler-assisted peritoneal dialysis in geriatric patients: comparison with hemodialysis. *Geriatr Nephrol Urol* 1993;3:7–13.

82. Mattern WD, et al. A three-year experience with CCPD in a university-based dialysis and transplantation program. *Clin Nephrol* 1988;30[Suppl 1]:S49–S52.

83. Dimkovic NB, et al. Chronic peritoneal dialysis in octogenarians. *Nephrol Dial Transplant* 2001;16:2034–2040.

84. Rowe JW, et al. Age-adjusted normal standards for creatinine clearance in man. *Ann Intern Med* 1976;84:567–569.

85. Cockroft DW, et al. Prediction of creatinine clearance from serum creatinine. *Nephron* 1976;16:31–41.

86. Gentric A, et al. Validity of creatinine clearance from serum creatinine in subjects over 80 years old. *Geriatr Nephrol Urol* 1992;2:143–145.

87. Baracskay D, et al. Geriatric renal function: estimating glomerular filtration in an ambulatory elderly population. *Am J Kidney Dis* 1997;47:222–228.

88. Levey AS, et al. A simplified equation to predict glomerular filtration rate from serum creatinine. *J Am Soc Nephrol* 2000;11:155A.

89. Burkhardt H, et al. Creatinine clearance, Cockcroft-Gault formula and cystatin C: estimators of true glomerular filtration rate in the elderly? *Gerontology* 2002;48:140–146.

90. Van Den Noortgate NJ, et al. Serum cystatin C concentration compared with other markers of glomerular filtration rate in the old old. *J Am Geriatr Soc* 2002;50:1278–1282.

91. Ifudu O, et al. Delayed referral of black, Hispanic, and older patients with chronic renal failure. *Am J Kidney Dis* 1999;33:728–733.

92. Macias-Nunez JF, et al. Acute renal failure in old people. In: Macias-Nunez JF, et al., eds. *Renal functions and disease in the elderly.* London: Butterworths, 1987:461–484.

93. Pascual J, et al. Incidence and prognosis of acute renal failure in older patients. *J Am Geriatr Soc* 1990;38:25–30.

94. Pascual J, et al. Acute renal failure in the elderly. *Geriatr Nephrol Urol* 1992;2:51–61.

95. Lameire N, et al. A review of the pathophysiology, causes and prognosis of acute renal failure in the elderly. *Geriatr Nephrol Urol* 1991;1:77–91.

96. Turney JH, et al. The evolution of acute renal failure, 1956–1988. *Q J Med* 1990;273:83–104.

97. Corwin HL, et al. Factors influencing survival in acute renal failure. *Semin Dial* 1989;2:220–225.

98. Gentric A, et al. Immediate and long-term prognosis in acute renal failure in the elderly. *Nephrol Dial Transplant* 1991;6:86–90.

99. Groeneveld ABJ, et al. Acute renal failure in the medical intensive care unit: predisposing, complicating factors and outcome. *Nephron* 1991;59:602–610.

100. Sonnenblick M, et al. Acute renal failure in the elderly treated by one-time peritoneal dialysis. *J Am Geriatr Soc* 1988;36:1039–1044.

101. Spiegel DM, et al. Determinants of survival and recovery in acute renal failure patients dialyzed in intensive-care units. *Am J Nephrol* 1991;11:44–47.

102. Pascual J, et al. Prognosis of acute renal failure among elderly patients. *J Am Geriatr Soc* 1991;39:102–103.

103. Klouche K, et al. Prognosis of acute renal failure in the elderly. *Nephrol Dial Transplant* 1995;10:2240–2243.

104. Dahlberg PJ, et al. Acute renal failure in octogenarians. *Wis Med J* 1989;88:19–23.

105. Macias-Nunez JF, et al. Acute renal failure in the aged. *Semin Nephrol* 1996;16:330–338.

106. Henrich WL. Dialysis considerations in the elderly patient. *Am J Kidney Dis* 1990;16:339–341.

107. Kaiser FE. Principles of geriatric care. *Am J Kidney Dis* 1990;16:354–359.

108. Al-Mohaya S, et al. Percutaneous subclavian vein catheterization for hemodialysis: a report of 57 insertions. *Angiology* 1989;40:569–573.

109. Cimochowski GE, et al. Superiority of the internal jugular over the subclavian access for temporary dialysis. *Nephron* 1990;54:154–161.

110. Bander SJ, et al. Central venous angioaccess for hemodialysis and its complications. *Semin Dial* 1992;5:121–128.

111. Farrell J, et al. Ultrasound-guided cannulation versus the landmark-guided technique for acute haemodialysis access. *Nephrol Dial Transplant* 1997;12:1234–1237.

112. Hinsdale JG, et al. Vascular access for hemodialysis in the elderly: results and perspectives in a geriatric population. *Dial Transplant* 1985;14:560–565.

113. Schaefer K, et al. Optimum dialysis treatment for patients over 65 years with primary renal disease: survival data and clinical results from 242 patients treated either by haemodialysis or hemofiltration. *Proc Eur Dial Transplant Assoc ERA* 1984;21:510–523.

114. Fan P-Y, et al. Vascular access: concepts for the 1990s. Editorial review. *J Am Soc Nephrol* 1992;3:1–11.

115. Besarab A, et al. Opinion: what can be done to preserve vascular access for dialysis? *Semin Dial* 1991;4:155–156.

116. Kaufman JL. Opinion: what can be done to preserve vascular access for dialysis? *Semin Dial* 1991;4:160–162.

117. Woods JD, et al. Vascular access survival among incident hemodialysis patients in the United States. *Am J Kidney Dis* 1997;30:50–57.

118. Ifudu O, et al. Correlates of vascular access and nonvascular access-related hospitalizations in hemodialysis patients. *Am J Nephrol* 1996;16:118–123.

119. Ponce P. Vascular access for dialysis in the elderly. *Int Urol Nephrol* 2001;33:571–573.

120. Glanz S. Opinion: what can be done to preserve vascular access for dialysis? *Semin Dial* 1991;4:157–158.

121. Palder SB, et al. Vascular access for hemodialysis. *Ann Surg* 1985;202:235–239.

122. National Kidney Foundation-Dialysis Outcome Quality Initiative clinical practice guideline for vascular access. *Am J Kidney Dis* 1997;30[Suppl 3]:150–191.

123. Schwab SJ. Opinion: what can be done to preserve vascular access for dialysis? *Semin Dial* 1991;4:152–153.

124. Leapman SB, et al. The arteriovenous fistula for hemodialysis access: gold standard or archaic relic? *Am Surg* 1996;62:652–657.

125. Wing AJ, et al. Combined report on regular dialysis and transplantation in Europe, IX 1978. *Proc Eur Dial Trans Assoc* 1979;13:2–52.

126. Berardinelli L, et al. Lessons from 494 permanent accesses in 348 hemodialysis patients older than 65 years of age: 29 years of experience. *Nephrol Dial Transplant* 1998;13[Suppl 7]:73–77.

127. Konner K, et al. Tailoring the initial vascular access for dialysis patients. *Kidney Int* 2002;62:329–338.

128. Cante P, et al. Distal vascular access for chronic hemodialysis in patients over 65 years of age: surgical results. *Progres en Urologie* 1998;8:83–88.

129. Lin SL, et al. Effects of age and diabetes on blood flow rate and primary outcome of newly created hemodialysis arteriovenous fistulas. *Am J Nephrol* 1998;18:96–100.

130. Barril G, et al. Hemodialysis vascular assessment by an ultrasound dilution method (transonic) in patients older than 65 years. *Int Urol Nephrol* 2001;32:459–462.

131. Windus DW, et al. Prosthetic fistula survival and complications in hemodialysis patients: effects of diabetes and age. *Am J Kidney Dis* 1992;19:448–452.

132. Bennion RS, et al. The radiocephalic fistula. *Contemp Dial* 1982;3:12–16.

133. Silva M, et al. A strategy of increasing use of autogenous hemodialysis access procedures. *J Vasc Surg* 1998;27:302–308.

134. Robin M, et al. US vascular mapping before hemodialysis access placement. *Radiology* 2000;217:83–88.

135. Windus DW, et al. Opinion: what can be done to preserve vascular access for dialysis? *Semin Dial* 1991;4:153–154.

136. Valji K, et al. Pharmacomechanical thrombolysis and angioplasty in the management of clotted hemodialysis grafts: early and late clinical results. *Radiology* 1991;178:243–247.

137. Shusterman NH, et al. Successful use of double-lumen, silicone rubber catheters for permanent hemodialysis access. *Kidney Int* 1989;35:887–890.

138. Prabhu PN, et al. Long-term performance and complications of the Tesio twin catheter system for hemodialysis access. *Am J Kidney Dis* 1997;30:213–218.

139. De Meester J, et al. Factors and complications affecting catheter and technique survival with permanent single-lumen dialysis catheters. *Nephrol Dial Transplant* 1994;9:678–683.

140. Canaud B, et al. Permanent twin catheter: a vascular access option of choice for hemodialysis in elderly patients. *Nephrol Dial Transplant* 1988;13[Suppl 7]:82–88.

141. Beathard GA, et al. Initial clinical results with the LifeSite Hemodialysis Access system. *Kidney Int* 2000;58:2021–2227.

142. Schwab SJ, et al. Multicenter clinical trial results with the LifeSite hemodialysis access system. *Kidney Int* 2002;62:1026–1033.

143. Moran JF. Subcutaneous vascular access devices. *Semin Dial* 2001;14:452–457.

144. Megerman J, et al. Development of a new approach to vascular access. *Artif Organs* 1999;23:10–14.

145. Canaud B, et al. Dialock: a new vascular access device for extracorporeal renal replacement therapy. *Nephrol Dial Transplant* 1999;14:692–698.

146. Schwab, et al. The LifeSite hemodialysis access system: implications for the nephrology nurse. *J Am Nephrol Nurs Assoc* 2002;29:27–33.

147. Quarello F, et al. Prevention of hemodialysis catheter-related bloodstream infection using an antimicrobial lock. *Blood Purif* 2002;20:87–92.

148. Waltzer WC. The surgical approach to dialysis access and transplan-

tation in the elderly. In: Michelis MF, et al., eds. *Geriatric nephrology.* New York: Field, Rich and Associates, 1986:23–128.

149. Bennion RS, et al. The radiocephalic fistula. *Contemp Dial* 1982;3:12–16. The arteriovenous fistula for hemodialysis access: gold standard or archaic relic? *Am Surg* 1996;62:652–657.

150. Churchill DN, et al. Canadian hemodialysis morbidity study. *Am J Kidney Dis* 1992;19:214–234.

151. Kario K, et al. Heparin cofactor II deficiency in the elderly: comparison with antithrombin III. *Thromb Res* 1992;66:489–498.

152. Harter HR, et al. Prevention of thrombosis in patients on hemodialysis by low-dose aspirin. *N Engl J Med* 1979;301:577–579.

153. Domoto DT, et al. Combined aspirin and sulfinpyrazone in the prevention of recurrent hemodialysis vascular access thrombosis. *Thromb Res* 1991;62:737–743.

154. Crowther MA, et al. Low-intensity Warfarin is ineffective for the prevention of PRFE Graft Failure in patients on hemodialysis: a randomized controlled trial. *J Am Soc Nephrol* 2002;13:2331–2337.

155. The use of oral anticoagulants (Warfarin) in older people. *J Am Geriatr Soc* 2002;50:1439–1445.

156. Ponce SP, et al. Comparison of the survival and complications of three permanent peritoneal dialysis catheters. *Perit Dial Bull* 1982;2:82–86.

157. Kim YS, et al. Comparison of peritoneal catheter survival with fistula survival in hemodialysis. *Perit Dial Int* 1995;15:147–151.

158. Gokal R. CAPD in the elderly—European and U.K. experience. *Adv Perit Dial* 1990;6[Suppl]:38–40.

159. Segoloni GP, et al. CAPD in the elderly: Italian multicenter study experience. *Adv Perit Dial* 1990;6[Suppl]:41–46.

160. Holley JL, et al. Risk factors for tunnel infections in continuous peritoneal dialysis. *Am J Kidney Dis* 1991;18:344–348.

161. Avram MR, et al. Hemodialysis and the elderly patient: potential advantages as to quality of life, urea generation, serum creatinine and less interdialytic weight gain. *Am J Kidney Dis* 1990;16:342–345.

162. McKevitt PM, et al. The elderly on dialysis: some considerations in compliance. *Am J Kidney Dis* 1990;16:346–350.

163. McKevitt PM, et al. The elderly on dialysis: physical and psychosocial functioning. *Dial Transplant* 1986;15:130–137.

164. King K. Strategies for enhancing compliance in the dialysis elderly. *Am J Kidney Dis* 1990;16:351–353.

165. Kay NE, et al. Immune abnormalities in renal failure and hemodialysis. *Blood Purif* 1986;4:120–129.

166. Boulton-Jones JM, et al. Immune responses in uremia. *Clin Nephrol* 1973;1:351–360.

167. Pabico RC, et al. Influenza vaccination of patients with glomerular disease. *Ann Intern Med* 1974;81:171–174.

168. Jensson O. Observations on the leucocyte blood picture in acute uremia. *Br J Haematol* 1958;4:422–427.

169. Slavin RG, et al. Lymphocytopenia in acute experimental renal failure. *Int Arch Allergy Appl Immunol* 1974;47:80–86.

170. Hosking CS, et al. Immune and phagocytic functions in patients on maintenance dialysis and post-transplantation. *Clin Nephrol* 1976;6:501–504.

171. Reddy MM, et al. T and B lymphocytes in patients with chronic renal disease on hemodialysis. *Experientia* 1975;980–981.

172. Kirkpatrick CH, et al. Immunologic studies in human organ transplantation. I. Observation and characterization of suppressed cutaneous reactivity in uremia. *J Exp Med* 1964;119:727–742.

173. McIntosh J, et al. Defective immune and phagocytic functions in uremia and renal transplantation. *Int Arch Allergy Appl Immunol* 1976;51:544–559.

174. Dammin GJ, et al. Prolonged survival of skin hemografts in uremic patients. *Ann N Y Acad Sci* 1956/1957;64:967–976.

175. London WT, et al. Host responses to hepatitis B infection in patients in a chronic hemodialysis unit. *Kidney Int* 1977;12:51–58.

176. Matas AJ, et al. Increased incidence of malignancy during chronic renal failure. *Lancet* 1975;1:883–886.

177. Sutherland GA, et al. Increased incidence of malignancy in chronic renal failure. *Nephron* 1977;18:182–184.

178. Lindner A, et al. High incidence of neoplasia in uremic patients receiving long-term dialysis. *Nephron* 1981;27:292–296.

179. Inamoto H, et al. Incidence and mortality pattern of malignancy and factors affecting the risk of malignancy in dialysis patients. *Nephron* 1991;59:611–617.

180. Francheschi C, et al. Successful immunosenescence and the remodeling of immune responses with ageing. *Nephrol Dial Transplant* 1996;11[Suppl 9]:18–25.

181. Delafuente JC. Immunosenescence: clinical and pharmacologic considerations. *Med Clin North Am* 1985;69:475–486.

182. Gillis S, et al. Immunologic studies of aging: decreased production of and response to T cell growth factor by lymphocytes from aged humans. *J Clin Invest* 1981;67:937–942.

183. Hilden M, et al. Frequency of negative intermediate-strength tuberculin sensitivity in patients with active tuberculosis. *N Engl J Med* 1971;285:1506–1509.

184. Francheschi C, et al. Aging, longevity and cancer: studies in Down's syndrome and in centenarians. *Ann N Y Acad Sci* 1991;621:428–440.

185. Morellini M, et al. HLA antigens and aging. *Ann N Y Acad Sci* 1992;663:499–500.

186. Sansoni P, et al. Lymphocyte subsets and natural killer cell activity in healthy old people and centenarians. *Blood* 1993;80:2767–2773.

187. Levy SM, et al. Persistently low natural killer cell activity, age and environmental stress as predictors of infectious morbidity. *Nat Immun Cell Growth Regulat* 1991;10:389–407.

188. Morduchowicz GA, et al. Renal replacement therapy in the ninth decade of life. *Geriatr Nephrol Urol* 1992;2:147–149.

189. Fernandez E, et al. Response to the hepatitis B virus vaccine in hemodialysis patients: influence of malnutrition and its importance as a risk factor for morbidity and mortality. *Nephrol Dial Transplant* 1996;11:1559–1563.

190. Kenny RA, et al. Acute phase protein response to infection in elderly patients. *Age Ageing* 1984;13:89–94.

191. Tinetti ME, et al. Use of the erythrocyte sedimentation rate in chronically ill, elderly patients with a decline in health status. *Am J Med* 1986;80:844–848.

192. Locatelli F, et al. Nutritional status in dialysis patients: a European consensus. *Nephrol Dial Transplant* 2002;17:563–572.

193. Baldassare JS, et al. Special problems of urinary tract infection in the elderly. *Med Clin North Am* 1991;75:375–390.

194. Marketos SG, et al. Bacteriuria and nonobstructive renovascular disease in old age. *J Gerontol* 1969;24:33–35.

195. Beisel WR. Single nutrients and immunity. *Am J Clin Nutr* 1982;35 [Suppl]:417–468.

196. Kemm JR, et al. The distribution of supposed indicators of nutritional status in elderly patients. *Age Ageing* 1984;12:21–28.

197. Klonoff-Cohen H, et al. Albumin levels as a predictor of mortality in the health elderly. *J Clin Epidemiol* 1992;45:207–212.

198. Young GA, et al. Nutritional assessment of continuous ambulatory peritoneal dialysis patients: an international study. *Am J Kidney Dis* 1991;17:462–471.

199. Lindsay RM, et al. Is the lower serum albumin concentration in CAPD patients a reflection of nutritional status: the lower serum albumin does reflect nutritional status. *Semin Dial* 1992;5:215–218.

200. Lowrie EG, et al. Death risk in hemodialysis patients: the predictive value of commonly measured variables and an evaluation of death rate differences between facilities. *Am J Kidney Dis* 1990;15:458–482.

201. Held PJ, et al. Survival probabilities and causes of death. In: Agadoa LYC, et al., eds. *U.S. renal data system annual data report*, 2nd ed. Bethesda, MD: National Institutes of Health, 1991:31–40.

202. Steinman TI. Nutritional management of the chronic dialysis patient. *Semin Dial* 1992;5:155–158.

203. Owen WF Jr, et al. The urea reduction ratio and serum albumin concentration as predictors of mortality in patients undergoing hemodialysis. *N Engl J Med* 1993;329:1001–1006.

204. Lowrie EG. Conceptual for a core pathobiology of uremia with special reference to anemia, malnourishment, and mortality among dialysis patients. *Semin Dial* 1997;10:115–129.

205. Kalantar-Zadeh K, et al. Relative contributions of nutrition and inflammation to clinical outcomes in dialysis patients. *Am J Kidney Dis* 2001;38:1343–1350.

206. Kutner NG, et al. Body mass index as a predictor of continued survival in older chronic dialysis patients. *Int Urol Nephrol* 2001;32:441–448.

207. Jern NA, et al. The effects of zinc supplementation on serum zinc concentration and protein catabolic rate in hemodialysis patients. *J Ren Nutr* 2000;10:148–153.

208. Karcic E, et al. Treating malnutrition with megestrol acetate: literature review and review of our experience. *J Nutr Health Aging* 2002;6(3): 191–200.

209. Selgas R. Anorexia in end-stage renal disease: pathophysiology and treatment. *Exp Opin Pharmacother* 2001;2:1825–1838.

210. Kopple JD. Therapeutic approaches to malnutrition in chronic dialysis patients: the different modalities of nutritional support. *Am J Kidney Dis* [Online] 1999;33:180–185.

211. Lien YH, et al. Low dose megestrol increases serum albumin in malnourished dialysis patients. *Int J Artif Organs* 1996;19(3):147–150.

212. Gilchrest BA, et al. Relief of uremic pruritus with ultraviolet phototherapy. *N Engl J Med* 1977;297:136–138.

213. Taylor R, et al. A placebo-controlled trial of UV-A phototherapy for the treatment of uraemic pruritus. *Nephron* 1983;33:14–16.

214. Chaves PHM, et al. Looking at the relationship between hemoglobin concentration and prevalent mobility difficulty in older women: should the criteria currently used to define anemia in older people be reevaluated? *J Am Geriatr Soc* 2002;50:1257–1264.

215. Silverberg DS, et al. The correction of anemia in severe resistant heart failure with erythropoietin and intravenous iron prevents the progression of both the heart and renal failure and markedly reduces hospitalization. *Clin Nephrol* 2002;58[Suppl 1]:S37–S45.

216. Bedani PL, et al. Erythropoietin and cardiocirculatory condition in aged patients with chronic renal failure. *Nephron* 2001;89:350–353.

217. Pickett JL, et al. Normalizing hematocrit in dialysis patients improves brain function. *Am J Kidney Dis* 1999;33:1122–1130.

218. Gascon A, et al. Nandrolone decanoate is a good alternative for the treatment of anemia in elderly male patients on hemodialysis. *Geriatr Nephrol Urol* 1999;9:67–72.

219. Navarro JF, et al. Randomized prospective comparison between erythropoietin and androgens in CAPD Patients. *Kidney Int* 2002;61: 1537–1544.

220. Gascon A, et al. Androgens in the treatment of anemia in aged patients on hemodialysis: effects on nutritional parameters. *Kidney Int* 1997;52:1153(abst).

221. Gascon A, et al. Androgens in the treatment of anemia in elderly patients on hemodialysis: effects on lymphocyte subsets. *Kidney Int* 1997;52:1153–1154(abst).

222. Parfrey PS, et al. Congestive heart failure in dialysis patients. *Arch Intern Med* 1988;148:1519–1525.

223. Harnett JD, et al. Left ventricular hypertrophy in end-stage renal disease. *Nephron* 1988;48:107–115.

224. Levy D, et al. Left ventricular mass and incidence of coronary heart disease in an elderly cohort. *Ann Intern Med* 1989;110:101–107.

225. Cleroux J, et al. Effects of aging on the cardiopulmonary receptor reflex in normal humans. *J Hypertens* 1988;6:S141–S144.

226. Zucchelli P, et al. Hemodynamic alterations in aged patients during hemodialysis, other dialysis procedures and transplantation. In: Martinez-Maldonado M, ed. *Hypertension and renal disease in the elderly.* Boston: Blackwell Scientific, 1992.

227. Nissenson AR, et al. Peritoneal dialysis in the elderly. In: Oreopoulos DG, ed. *Geriatric nephrology.* Dordrecht, the Netherlands: Martinus Nijhof, 1986:147–156.

228. Homodraka-Mailis A. Pathogenesis and treatment of back pain in peritoneal dialysis patients. *Perit Dial Bull* 1983;3[Suppl 3]:S41–S43.

229. Twardowski ZJ, et al. Intraabdominal pressure during natural activities in patients treated with continuous ambulatory peritoneal dialysis. *Nephron* 1986;44:129–135.

230. Moriwaki K, et al. Vitamin B6 deficiency in elderly patients on chronic peritoneal dialysis. *Adv Peritoneal Dial* 2000;16:308–312.

231. Mailloux LU, et al. The impact of co-morbid risk factors at the start of dialysis on the survival of ESRD patients. *ASAIO J* 1996;42:164–169.

232. Westlie L, et al. Mortality, morbidity, and life satisfaction in the very old dialysis patient. *Trans Am Soc Artif Intern Organs* 1984;30:21–30.

233. Anderson JE, et al. Use of continuous ambulatory peritoneal dialysis in a nursing home: patient characteristics, technique success, and survival predictors. *Am J Kidney Dis* 1990;16:137–141.

234. Anderson JE, et al. Incidence, prevalence, and outcomes of end-stage renal disease patients placed in nursing homes. *Am J Kidney Dis* 1993; 21:619–627.

235. Schleifer CR. Peritoneal dialysis in nursing homes. *Adv Perit Dial* 1990;6[Suppl]:86–91.

236. National Kidney Foundation of Michigan and Michigan Council of Nephrology Social Workers. *Care of the dialysis patient in the nursing home. An educational curriculum for nursing home personnel.* Ann Arbor, MI: National Kidney Foundation of Michigan, 1987.

237. Carey HB, et al. Continuous peritoneal dialysis and the extended care facility. *Am J Kidney Dis* 2001;37:580–587.

238. Eggers PW. Health care policies economics of the geriatric renal population. *Am J Kidney Dis* 1990;16:384–391.

239. Fox RC, et al. Social and ethical problems in the treatment of end-stage renal disease patients. In: Narins EG, ed. *Controversies in nephrology and hypertension.* New York: Churchill Livingstone, 1984: 45–70.

240. Wetle T. Age as a risk factor for inadequate treatment. *JAMA* 1987; 258:516.

241. Rothenberg LS. Withholding and withdrawing dialysis from elderly ESRD patients: part 1. a historical review of the clinical experience. *Geriatr Nephrol Urol* 1992;2:109–117.

242. Berlyne GM. Over 50 and uremic. *Nephron* 1982;31:189–190.

243. Kjellstrand CM, et al. Inequalities in chronic dialysis and transplantation in Sweden. *Acta Med Scand* 1988;224:149–156.

244. Sesso R, et al. Factors associated with acceptance of patients for chronic dialysis. *Clin Nephrol* 2001;56:231–235.

245. Kjellstrand CM, et al. Racial, sexual and age inequalities in chronic dialysis. *Nephron* 1987;45:257–263.

246. Rosansky SJ, et al. Rate of change of end-stage renal disease treatment incidence, 1978–1987. Has there been selection? *J Am Soc Nephrol* 1992;1502–1506.

247. Moulton LH, et al. Patterns of low incidence of treated end-stage renal disease among the elderly. *Am J Kidney Dis* 1992;20:55–62.

248. Klahr S. Rationing of health care and the end-stage renal disease program. *Am J Kidney Dis* 1990;16:393–395.

249. Cassel CK. Issues of age and chronic care: another argument for health care reform. *J Am Geriatr Soc* 1992;40:404–409.

250. Pawlson LG, et al. An overview of allocation and rationing: implications for geriatrics. *J Am Geriatr Soc* 1992;40:628–634.

251. Cummings NB. Ethical issues in geriatric nephrology: overview. *Am J Kidney Dis* 1990;16:367–371.

252. Lamm RD. High technology health care. *Am J Kidney Dis* 1990; 16:378–383.

253. Brodeur D. Ethical issues in geriatric nephrology. *Am J Kidney Dis* 1990;16:372–373.

254. Horina JH, et al. Elderly patients and chronic hemodialysis. *Lancet* 1992;339:183.

255. Disney APS. Dialysis treatment in Australia, 1982 to 1988. *Am J Kidney Dis* 1990;15:402–409.

256. Kutner NG, et al. Assisted survival, aging, and rehabilitation needs: comparison of older dialysis patients and age-matched peers. *Arch Phys Med Rehabil* 1992;73:309–315.

257. Kutner NG, et al. Rehabilitation, aging, and chronic renal disease. *Am J Phys Med Rehabil* 1992;71:97–101.

258. Moore GE, et al. Determinants of VO2 peak in patients with end-stage renal disease: on and off dialysis. *Med Sci Sports Exerc* 1993;25 (1):18–23.

259. Asai K, et al. Hemodialysis and the elderly patient: retrospective analysis of morbidity and mortality. *Geriatr Nephrol Urol* 1993;3: 139–144.

260. Ota S, et al. Exercise rehabilitation for elderly patients on chronic hemodialysis. *Geriatr Nephrol Urol* 1995;5:157–165.

261. Chaplin ER, et al. Challenges facing dialysis patients requiring physical rehabilitation. *Nephrol News Issues* 1995;8:34–36.

262. Cowen TD, et al. Functional outcomes after inpatient rehabilitation

of patients with end-stage renal disease. *Arch Phys Med Rehabil* 1995;76:355–359.

263. Port FK. Mortality and causes of death in patients with end-stage renal failure. *Am J Kidney Dis* 1990;15:215–217.

264. U.S. Renal Data System annual data report. Bethesda, MD: National Institutes of Health, Aug 1992.

265. Husebye DG, et al. Old patients and uremia: rates of acceptance to and withdrawal from dialysis. *Int J Artif Organs* 1987;10:166–172.

266. Singer PA, End-Stage Renal Disease Network of New England. Nephrologists' experience with and attitudes towards decisions to forego dialysis. *J Am Soc Nephrol* 1992;2:1235–1240.

267. Holley JL, et al. Nephrologists' reported attitudes about factors influencing recommendations to initiate or withdraw dialysis. *J Am Soc Nephrol* 1991;1:1284–1288.

268. Agraharkar M, et al. Staff-assisted home hemodialysis in debilitated or terminally ill patients. *Int Urol Nephrol* 2002;33:139–144.

269. Kilner JF. Ethical issues in the initiation and termination of treatment. *Am J Kidney Dis* 1990;15:218–227.

270. *Initiation and withdrawal of dialysis in end-stage renal disease: guidelines for physicians and the care team.* New York: National Kidney Foundation, 1996.

271. The Kidney Foundation of Canada. *Living with kidney disease.* Montreal: The National Office of the Kidney Foundation of Canada, 1995.

272. Moss AH. To use dialysis appropriately: the emerging consensus on patient selection guidelines. *Adv Ren Replace Ther* 1995;2:175–183.

273. Clinical practice guidelines on shared decision-making in the appropriate initiation of and withdrawal from dialysis. Renal Physicians Association/American Society of Nephrology Working Group. *J Am Soc Nephrol* 2000;11:1340–1342.

274. Rodin GM, et al. Stopping life-sustaining medical treatment: psychiatric considerations in the termination of renal dialysis. *Can J Psychiatry* 1981;26:540–544.

275. Lo B, et al. Patient attitudes to discussing life-sustaining treatment. *Arch Intern Med* 1986;146:1613–1615.

276. Frankl D, et al. Attitudes of hospitalized patients towards life support: a survey of 200 medical in patients. *Am J Med* 1989;86:645–648.

277. American College of Physicians. American College of Physicians ethics manual, 3rd ed. *Ann Intern Med* 1992;117:947–960.

278. Perry E, et al. Why is it difficult for staff to discuss advance directives with chronic dialysis patients? *J Am Soc Nephrol* 1996;7:2160–2168.

279. Tobe SW, et al. Foregoing renal dialysis: a case study and review of ethical issues. *Am J Kid Dis* 1996;28:147–153.

280. Hirsch DJ, et al. Experience with not offering dialysis to patients with poor prognosis. *Am J Kidney Dis* 1994;23:463–466.

281. Roberts JC, et al. Withdrawing life support—the survivors. *Acta Med Scand* 1988;224:141–148.

282. Moss AH, et al. Outcomes of cardiopulmonary resuscitation in dialysis patients. *J Am Soc Nephrol* 1992;3:1238–1243.

283. Holley JL, et al. Dialysis patients' attitudes about cardiopulmonary resuscitation and stopping dialysis. *Am J Nephrol* 1989;9:245–251.

DIABETIC DIALYSIS PATIENTS

ANNE MARIE V. MILES AND ELI A. FRIEDMAN

IMPACT OF DIABETES ON RENAL REPLACEMENT THERAPY PROGRAMS

Diabetes mellitus leads the causes of end-stage renal disease (ESRD) in the United States (Fig. 36.1), Japan, and most nations in industrialized Europe. As tabulated in the *United States Renal Data System (USRDS) 2002 Report,* of 96,192 patients begun on therapy for ESRD during 2000, 41,772 (43.4%) had diabetes, an incidence rate of 145 per million population (1). Reflecting their relatively higher death rate compared with other causes of ESRD, the prevalence of U.S. diabetic ESRD patients on December 31, 2000 was only 34% (131,173 of 378,862 patients). Both chronic glomerulonephritis and hypertensive renal disease rank below diabetes in frequency of diagnosis among new ESRD patients, substantiating Mauer et al.'s (2) contention that "Diabetes is the most important cause of ESRD in the Western world (2)." This is due both to an increased prevalence of diabetes in the general population and to increased acceptance of diabetics into renal replacement programs.

According to the *National Diabetes Fact Sheet* of the Centers for Disease Control (3), more than 16 million people in the United States have diabetes—one third of whom are unaware of their diagnosis. During 2001, 798,000 people in the United States were diagnosed with diabetes, and 187,000 people died from diabetes. In 1996, diabetes was the fourth leading cause of death in black women 45 years and older and the eighth leading cause of death in white men 45 to 65 years old (4). Health care expenditures for diabetes in the United States amount to $98 to $150 billion annually. The full impact of diabetic complications is unmeasured but includes in addition to 34,874 new cases of ESRD, 56,000 lower limb amputations, and 24,000 cases of blindness.

Clinical nephrologists must, therefore, deal with diabetics and their multisystem complications on an increasing basis. Considered now are the options open to the diabetic ESRD

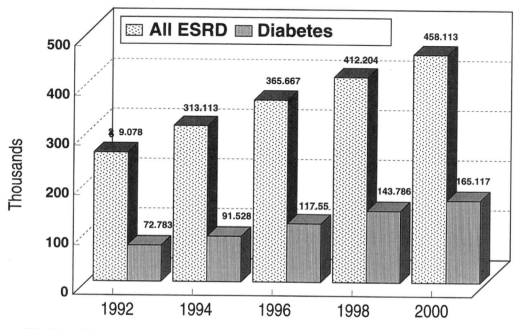

FIG. 36.1. Rising prevalence of diabetic ESRD in the United States. (U.S. Renal Data System, 2002[1].)

patient, their complications on dialysis, and the need for overall diabetic care during uremia therapy.

HISTORY OF RENAL REPLACEMENT THERAPY IN DIABETICS

Because of high morbidity and mortality rates attributed to coronary artery, cerebrovascular, and peripheral vascular disease, diabetics were excluded from many dialysis programs in the 1960s and early 1970s. In addition, facilities and funding for dialysis were limited. In 1966 in Brooklyn, no diabetic on maintenance hemodialysis (HD) lived for longer than 6 months (5). In another series reported in 1969, of 32 diabetics started on HD, only 8 survived as long as 3 months (6). Most early reports of diabetics (mainly insulin-dependent patients) on dialysis from the United States recounted a 2-year survival ranging from 25% to 40% (7–9). In Europe, only 34% of diabetics survived after 3 years of dialysis (10).

Pioneering work with HD (and renal transplantation) in uremic diabetics at the University of Minnesota helped widen acceptance of diabetics into programs for long-term uremia therapy. Since the late 1970s and early 1980s, less disappointing results have been reported for diabetics in renal replacement therapy programs. Although morbidity from coronary artery and peripheral vascular disease, blindness, and vascular access complications may be disabling, *an aggressive, preventive, and proactive management program spearheaded by the nephrologist (the physician who most often sees these patients) has the potential to significantly improve outcome.*

One-year mortality in diabetics (and nondiabetics) on HD ranges between 11% and 30% (1,11,12) compared with markedly lower 1-year mortality rates of 9.9% for cadaver and 2.1% for live-donor kidney transplants in diabetics (1). Ten-year mortality, however, is significantly greater in hemodialyzed diabetics than in nondiabetic HD patients (Fig. 36.2) and is due mainly to coronary artery and cerebrovascular disease.

DIABETIC RENAL DISEASE

Although in reports from two to three decades ago, 3% to 10% of patients with non-insulin-dependent diabetes mellitus (NIDDM) (type II) were believed to develop ESRD (13) compared with 30% to 45% of those with insulin-dependent diabetes mellitus (IDDM) (14), it is now recognized that kidney disease is as likely to develop in long-duration NIDDM as in IDDM (15,16). Because of their greater prevalence, patients with NIDDM, however, account for most diabetics on dialysis. In a study from Rochester, Minnesota (15), cohorts of 1,832 individuals with NIDDM and 136 with IDDM, followed for 30 years, had similar rates of renal failure (133/100,000 person-years in individuals with NIDDM and 170/100,000 person-years in those with IDDM). In Heidelberg, West Germany, cohorts of both major types of diabetes followed for 20 years developed renal impairment (defined as a serum creatinine level of >1.4 mg/dL) at nearly equal rates of 59% in IDDM and 63% in NIDDM (16). Studies of NIDDM in other populations [American Pima Indians (17), blacks and Hispanics (18)] also reveal much higher incidence rates of renal failure in the NIDDM population than have been previously reported.

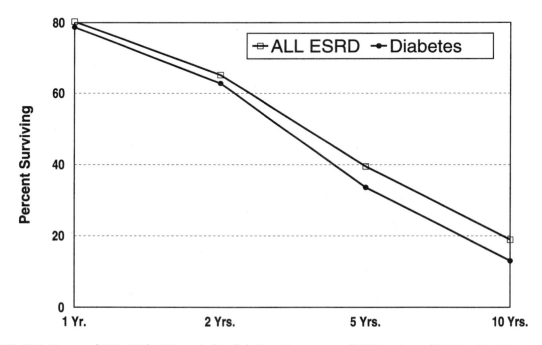

FIG. 36.2. Ten-year (1990–1999) ESRD survival in diabetic patients versus all ESRD patients. (U.S. Renal Data System, 2002[1].)

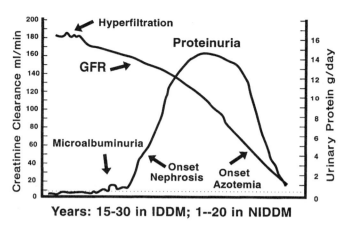

FIG. 36.3. Natural history of diabetic renal disease.

Non-insulin-dependent diabetics who develop nephropathy do so usually within 5 to 10 years of diagnosis of diabetes. If suboptimally managed, diabetic nephropathy follows a predictable and inexorable course starting with microalbuminuria, through proteinuria and azotemia, and culminating in ESRD. The older the diabetic at onset of nephropathy, the more rapid the progression to ESRD (19). Other risk factors for development of renal failure in diabetics include inadequate (>130/80 mm Hg) blood pressure control, the level of proteinuria at presentation, poor glycemic control (hemoglobin A_{1c} levels >7.5%), and hyperlipidemia. In insulin-dependent diabetics, nephropathy progresses through well-defined stages, as eluci-

dated by Mogensen et al. (20), and ESRD occurs some 15 to 30 years after diagnosis of diabetes, usually within 2 to 3 years of onset of the nephrotic syndrome (Fig. 36.3).

PREPARING FOR RENAL REPLACEMENT THERAPY

Which Mode of Therapy Is Best?

The 2002 USRDS reports that of 131,173 diabetic ESRD patients, 77% were treated with HD, 6% with some form of peritoneal dialysis (PD), and 16% with renal transplantation (Fig. 36.4) (1). The modality of ESRD therapy must be individualized depending on the patient's age; education; geographic location; family and social support systems; and extent of comorbid conditions, particularly cardiovascular disease. Other factors that may influence the choice of therapeutic modality (Table 36.1) include expected patient compliance and data related to the particular treatment modality, such as patient survival, degree of rehabilitation, and expected stabilization of extrarenal diabetic complications.

The consensus of workers in the field indicates that the best survival and rehabilitation for a uremic diabetic is achieved by living-related renal transplantation. The morbidity from blindness and neuropathy, but not coronary artery or peripheral vascular disease, is decreased in diabetic renal transplant recipients (21). Mortality from coronary artery disease (CAD) is the major cause of death in diabetics with all modalities of renal replacement therapy.

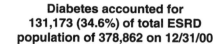

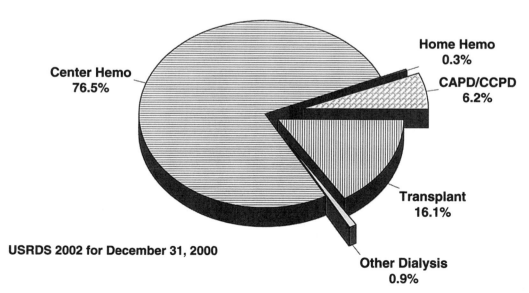

FIG. 36.4. Treatment modalities in diabetic ESRD patients. Hemo, hemodialysis; CCPD, continuous cyclic peritoneal dialysis. (U.S. Renal Data System, 2002[1].)

TABLE 36.1. FACTORS INVOLVED IN CHOICE OF THERAPY FOR UREMIC DIABETIC

Patient Related	Treatment Modality Related
Age	Degree of rehabilitation
Education level	Stability of extrarenal diabetic complications
Place of residence	
Availability of family and social support	Patient survival data
Expected patient compliance	
Presence of comorbid conditions (e.g., cardiovascular disease, blindness)	

The understandable tendency of transplant surgeons to select younger and healthier patients leaves a residual subset of diabetic ESRD patients managed by dialysis who are older and sicker. Because of ethical and logistic difficulties, there has been no randomized prospective trial of diabetics of similar age, sex, type of diabetes, and degree and type of comorbid conditions that compares results on HD with continuous ambulatory peritoneal dialysis (CAPD) and renal transplantation. Hence, although the best rehabilitation is effected by renal transplantation, there is no clearly superior method of treatment for the uremic diabetic, and assessment and treatment of diabetics with ESRD must be highly individualized.

Transition to Renal Replacement Therapy

The transition from conservative management of renal failure to renal replacement therapy is often an extremely difficult period for the diabetic patient faced with yet another in a series of multisystem complications. An angry, depressed, or noncompliant diabetic patient who refuses dialysis despite burgeoning uremic complications is a familiar problem to nephrologists in large urban dialysis units. The primary goal in managing diabetic nephropathy is to slow its progression while smoothing transition to the modality of renal replacement best suited to the patient. Assistance of a trained diabetes nurse educator is invaluable in attaining this objective.

Patient Education and Multidisciplinary Approach

Patient education should begin in the predialytic stage, and the importance of blood pressure control and dietary protein restriction in slowing disease progression must be stressed. To avert protein calorie malnutrition, we recommend only moderate protein restriction (80 to 100 g/day). Although glycemic control in advanced nephropathy has not been shown to retard the onset of ESRD, it too must be addressed, and home glucose monitoring must be routinely taught. Restriction of sodium, potassium, and fluid intake is also indicated as renal function declines.

A multidisciplinary approach to interdict the devastating microvascular and macrovascular complications of diabetes will often significantly improve rehabilitation after renal replacement therapy is initiated. Ophthalmologic evaluation should be obtained at least three to four times per year once proliferative retinopathy is discovered. Panretinal photocoagulation may preserve vision in patients with severe proliferative retinopathy. A foot care regimen with daily detailed inspection of the feet, use of heel booties in those confined to bed, and regular visits to a podiatrist and vascular surgeon if necessary reduces the high rate of limb amputations before and after dialysis is initiated.

When the creatinine clearance falls to about 20 to 30 mL/minute or the serum creatinine rises above 4 mg/dL, the therapeutic options for renal replacement therapy should be presented to the patient and a choice made based on patient preference and the previously mentioned factors. In actuality, physician bias is often a major factor in determining the type of renal replacement therapy chosen (22).

If HD is to be the chosen mode of therapy, planning for vascular access is of great importance. Forearm cutaneous veins should be preserved by avoiding long-dwelling intravenous catheters or venipunctures. Arteriovenous access should be constructed 3 to 6 months in advance of anticipated need for dialysis.

Creation of vascular access for diabetic HD patients poses a special challenge to vascular surgeons because of the presence of advanced atherosclerotic disease with or without medial arterial calcification of the vessels of the forearm and arm. An autologous radiocephalic arteriovenous fistula of the Cimino-Brescia type is preferable to the use of a Dacron or polytetrafluoroethylene graft, because the fistula has a longer lifespan and a very low risk of infection. Newer polytetrafluoroethylene grafts are reported to have equivalent survival to endogenous fistulas (23). The 3-year survival of an arteriovenous fistula in diabetics is 80%, whereas for arteriovenous grafts it is 47% (24). Unfortunately, nonmaturation rates for Cimino-Brescia fistulas in diabetic patients have been reported to be as high as 70% in some series. Alternatives are the forearm loop fistula where a U-shaped transposed loop of basilic or cephalic vein in the forearm is anastomosed to the brachial or proximal radial or ulnar artery distal to the antecubital fossa (25) or, more commonly, the upper arm transposed basilic vein fistula (26).

Many diabetics will ultimately require graft placement because of failure of maturation or early thrombosis of a fistula or lack of an adequate distal vein or artery at the outset, and some will remain with cuffed, tunneled catheters as the chronic mode of dialysis access with the attendant morbidity from sepsis and underdialysis resulting from catheter malfunction or thrombosis (27).

If PD is selected as long-term therapy, the peritoneal catheter should be inserted 2 to 4 weeks before starting therapy. Arrangements should be made with a nearby training facility that will thereafter support the PD-treated diabetic ESRD patient.

If living-related transplantation is to be the therapeutic modality, the goal should be to avoid an interim period on dialysis and to perform renal transplantation at the stage of early uremic symptoms. With cadaveric renal transplantation, the patient may be placed on a waiting list for transplantation when the creatinine clearance is approximately 10 to 15 mL/minute.

TABLE 36.2. CAUSES OF MORTALITY IN HEMODIALIZED DIABETICS

Coronary artery and cerebrovascular disease	61.5%
Uremic complications	16.3%
Infections	9.6%
Other	12.6%

Starting Dialysis in Diabetics

Diabetics develop symptomatic uremia and volume overload at creatinine clearances that are higher than those in the nondiabetic population. Although dialysis is usually initiated at creatinine clearances of 5 to 10 mL/minute or less in nondiabetics, in the diabetic, uremia therapy usually must be started at creatinine clearances of 10 to 20 mL/minute, with serum creatinines that may be as low as 3 to 5 mg/dL.

Further deterioration of renal function may be extremely rapid in this group of patients, and the aim of most nephrologists today is to initiate dialysis before the onset of symptoms of uremia or volume overload. At a serum creatinine concentration of 5 to 8 mg/dL, we most often begin renal replacement therapy. Although no randomized trial comparing early versus late initiation of dialysis in diabetics exists, we believe that earlier institution of therapy is one factor that has improved survival and reduced morbidity of diabetics in dialysis programs over the past 15 to 20 years. Retinopathy in diabetics may progress rapidly during the 1 to 2 years before initiation of dialysis (28). Early institution of dialysis may help retard progression of retinopathy by controlling hypertension and sodium and water retention and by correcting the bleeding diathesis that contributes to retinal edema, hemorrhage, and eventual retinal detachment. Early dialysis may also prevent the additional burden of uremic neuropathy in patients who already have severe autonomic and peripheral neuropathy related to diabetes.

Other factors improving the survival of dialyzed diabetics include better control of hypertension, reduction in volume overload, better nutrition, and advances in the field of vascular access surgery. Control of volume-dependent hypertension by dialysis decreases the cardiovascular complications related to hypertension such as myocardial infarction, congestive heart failure, and stroke.

Hemodialysis in Diabetics

Despite unfavorable initial reports in diabetics (5,7,9), HD has continued to be the most common means of treating diabetic renal failure (Fig. 36.4) (1). One-year mortality rate in diabetics has decreased from 27% in 1997 to 21% in 2000 (1), but long-term mortality rates remain two to three times higher than in nondiabetic patients.

High mortality in hemodialyzed diabetics is attributable primarily to coronary artery and cerebrovascular disease (Table 36.2). A 19.2% yearly incidence of myocardial infarction or congestive heart failure and a 10% incidence of cerebral hemorrhage or thrombosis in diabetics on dialysis have been reported (29). A retrospective study from West Germany of 200 age- and sex-matched diabetic and nondiabetic HD patients receiving treatment over a 10-year period found cardiovascular mortality to be 4.8 times higher in type I diabetics and 3.0 times higher in type II diabetics when compared with nondiabetic HD patients (Fig. 36.5) (30). Sudden death (80%), myocardial infarction (13%), and stroke (7%) were the main causes of cardiovascular death. Systolic blood pressure of greater than 60 mm Hg at the start of

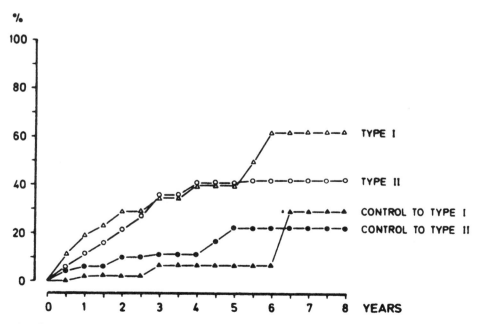

FIG. 36.5. Cardiovascular mortality in patients with type I or type II diabetes and their matched controls receiving maintenance hemodialysis. (From Ritz E, et al. Hypertension and cardiovascular risk factors in hemodialyzed diabetic patients. *Hypertension* 1985;7[Suppl 2]:118–124, with permission.)

dialysis and cardiomegaly on chest x-ray film (particularly in association with electrocardiographic evidence of left ventricular hypertrophy) were the strongest predictors of cardiovascular death in hemodialyzed diabetics. In addition to traditional risk factors for cardiovascular disease, elevated calcium and phosphate levels with high coronary calcification indices on electron beam computerized tomography of the heart (31), hypoalbuminemia (32), and a proinflammatory or prooxidative milieu related to uremia or its treatment (33) are other factors that may contribute to the excess cardiovascular death risk in diabetic and all ESRD patients (see Chapters 17 and 18). In addition, many diabetics starting ESRD therapy already have significant asymptomatic CAD: 11 of 17 consecutive unselected diabetics starting HD at a Japanese center had significant occlusive disease on coronary angiography despite absence of angina (34).

Reports of morbidity in diabetics on HD vary widely. Progression of neuropathy, retinopathy, and peripheral vascular disease is variably reported as being better with HD, PD, and renal transplantation. In general, morbidity from blindness and peripheral neuropathy tends to be less in diabetic ESRD patients treated with renal transplantation and CAPD than in those treated with HD. Coronary artery and peripheral vascular disease are significant problems with all three major modalities of renal replacement therapy.

HEMODIALYSIS-RELATED COMPLICATIONS

Complications Arising during Dialysis

Hypotension

Diabetics have a 20% increase in episodes of hypotension during HD and three times the number of episodes of nausea and vomiting compared with nondiabetics (35). Hypotension is usually accompanied or heralded by nausea and vomiting, and sometimes occurs in the face of obvious clinical volume overload and edema (see Chapter 19). Hypotensive episodes may precipitate angina pectoris and myocardial infarction or may be the result of silent myocardial infarction.

Major contributors to recurrent intradialytic hypotension in diabetics are reduced myocardial contractility related to ischemic heart disease (acute or chronic) (36) and diastolic dysfunction related to diabetic cardiomyopathy with resultant decreased left ventricular compliance and filling. Also contributing is autonomic neuropathy (diabetic ±uremic), which results in abolition of the reflex increase in heart rate and increased peripheral vascular resistance that usually occur to prevent hypotension before interstitial fluid is mobilized into the intravascular compartment. Hypoalbuminemia, resulting from nephrotic syndrome or malnutrition, may produce low colloid oncotic pressure, which reduces the plasma refilling rate and also contributes to hypotension (37).

Anemia also predisposes to hypotension on HD. Anemia reduces blood viscosity and peripheral vascular resistance and impairs the ability to maintain blood volume during ultrafiltration (37). Anemia may contribute to dialysis-related angina pectoris, so a recent fall in hematocrit should always be sought in the diabetic patient who develops chest pain on dialysis.

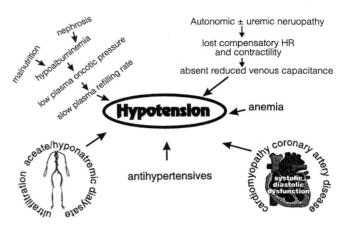

FIG. 36.6. Factors contributing to hemodialysis-associated hypotension in diabetics. HR, heart rate.

The theory of thermal amplification proposed by Gotch et al. (38) may provide another contributory factor to dialysis-associated hypotension. The slight buildup of core heat during HD, in association with a reduction in heat loss caused by cutaneous vasoconstriction in response to hypovolemia early in dialysis, results in reflex vasodilatation of the cutaneous blood vessels near the end of dialysis and sudden hypotension. Other factors contributing to dialysis-related hypotension are shown in Fig. 36.6.

Dialysis-related hypotension is usually improved by using the approaches listed in Table 36.3 (see Chapters 3 and 19). Nasal oxygen and sublingual nitroglycerin should be given to patients with angina precipitated by HD, and the ultrafiltration rate should be reduced. In patients with inoperable CAD, application of 2% nitroglycerin ointment to the chest wall 30 to 60 minutes before dialysis may prevent anginal episodes. In some cases, recurrent hypotension on HD may be severe enough to require change to another modality of treatment.

Hypertension

Hypertension is more common in diabetic than nondiabetic HD patients: 50% of hemodialyzed diabetics require antihypertensive medications compared with 27.7% of nondiabetics (30).

TABLE 36.3. MANAGING DIABETICS WITH HEMODIALYSIS-RELATED HYPOTENSION

Bicarbonate dialysate
High sodium (140–145 mmol/L) dialysate with linear sodium modeling (96)
Slow rate of ultrafiltration
Sequential ultrafiltration (if grossly edematous)
Prime dialysis circuit with hypertonic albumin
Maintain hematocrit at or above 30% with erythropoietin
No antihypertensive medications on morning of dialysis
Restrict meals immediately before or during hemodialysis
Leg-toning exercises to improve venous return
Decrease dialysate temperature (particularly near end of dialysis)
Medications: α-agonists (e.g., midodrine)

Although hypertension is largely volume dependent in most diabetics, improves as a HD session proceeds, and ameliorates or disappears as dry weight is attained, some patients continue to require antihypertensive medications after initiation of HD. Some may, in addition, paradoxically experience progressive elevation in blood pressure during HD sessions or at the end of treatment. This phenomenon may sometimes be due to acute activation of the renin-angiotensin system by reduction in intravascular volume produced by ultrafiltration, and respond to angiotensin-converting enzyme inhibitor (ACEI) therapy (see Chapter 16) or may occur as a result of clinically inapparent hypervolemia with amelioration with gradual challenge and reduction in the dry weight (39).

Use of ACEIs as part of an antihypertensive regimen, or at the start of or during dialysis, has effectively controlled this problem in most of our patients. Long-acting ACEIs with dominant cardiac and vascular endothelial effects (the "tissue" ACEIs: ramipril, trandolapril, quinapril, perindopril) may help to decrease cardiovascular morbidity and mortality (40) and may also decrease the incidence of arteriovenous graft thrombosis (41). As in the predialysis diabetic population, ACEIs or angiotensin receptor blockers are often the first line of therapy for hypertensive diabetic dialysis patients. Calcium channel blockers and central vasodilators such as clonidine are also efficacious, and, occasionally, patients with recalcitrant hypertension may need addition of minoxidil (along with a beta blocker to control reflex tachycardia) for blood pressure control.

High Interdialytic Weight Gain

The tendency for high interdialytic weight gain in diabetic HD patients is well recognized (35,42). Diabetics gain 30% to 50% more weight in interdialytic periods than nondiabetics (35). Increased interdialytic weight gain has not previously been shown to correlate with glycemic control, age, duration of ESRD, continuing urine output, dry weight, or duration of diabetes (35). A close relationship between degree of hyperglycemia and amount of interdialytic weight gain has been reported however (42).

High intracellular sodium content is proposed to produce increased thirst in diabetics (43). In many patients, noncompliance with sodium, fluid, and caloric restrictions contributes to large increments in weight (>5 to 10 lb) between dialysis sessions. Volume overload worsens hypertension and contributes to cardiovascular morbidity and mortality in diabetics. Dietary counseling, use of sodium modeling on dialysis, and sequential ultrafiltration may ameliorate the problem.

Problems Related to Vascular Access (See Chapter 4 for Complete Discussion)

Radial Steal Syndrome

When the radial artery is used for construction of a side to side arteriovenous fistula with the cephalic vein, the blood supply to the fingers may be compromised. Radial arterial blood no longer supplies the fingers, and in addition, the fistula provides a low pressure "run off" system that short circuits the ulnar and interosseous arterial blood supply of the fingers through the palmar arch, a system that may have been previously compromised from medial arterial calcification (44). Pain and numbness in the fingers may proceed to ischemia and gangrene, which might require amputation of one or more fingers or even below-elbow amputation. Nonhealing ulcers of the fingers may also be a manifestation of vascular steal. In cases of clinical uncertainty, noninvasive vascular studies documenting digital pressures less than 50 mm Hg provide useful confirmatory evidence (45).

A steal syndrome may be avoided or ameliorated by ligation of the distal radial artery segment to prevent retrograde flow of blood from the ulnar arterial system into the fistula or by primary creation of an *end*-artery to side- or end-vein fistula. Severe cases of vascular steal require ligation or removal of the access.

Venous Hypertension

Another complication of placement of arteriovenous access in diabetics and other ESRD patients is chronic swelling of the hand and especially of the thumb (sore thumb syndrome), related to the presence of the distal segment of the vein used for creation of the access. Venous hypertension occurs in association with venous stenosis of the access or a more proximal stenosis at the level of the subclavian vein, which may have been previously catheterized for temporary vascular access. Ligature of the distal venous limb of the fistula or graft will usually correct the problem.

Thrombosis and Infection

Seventy-five percent of diabetics with arteriovenous grafts for vascular access will require either revision or replacement of the access within 3 years, whereas only 20% of those with fistulas will require operative intervention (23). Vascular accesses in diabetics have similar 1-year patency rates when compared with nondiabetic patients (24). In a large series from Boston (24), 324 arteriovenous accesses were created in 256 patients between June 1979 and October 1983. Thirty-four of the patients were diabetic and had 22 Brescia-Cimino fistulas and 27 polytetrafluoroethylene grafts placed. When compared with similar vascular accesses in nondiabetics, there was no difference in the patency rates at 1 year in diabetics and nondiabetics.

Early failure of fistulas caused by poor maturation or failure of maturation is more common in diabetics than nondiabetics. In our experience, diabetic and nondiabetic HD patients have similar durations of hospital stay for problems related to vascular access (46). Nationally, however, diabetic HD patients have more frequent and longer hospitalizations than nondiabetic HD patients (1). Routine arterial and venous Doppler ultrasound with or without arteriography and venography of upper limb vessels and proximal veins before attempted vascular access is being practiced by an increasing number of vascular access surgeons, particularly for diabetic patients, and may make primary fistula placement in diabetics and nondiabetics similar (47).

Monitoring static venous pressures and feeling for a good thrill at the start of each dialysis will forewarn of impending thrombosis of the access related to venous outflow stenosis. Venous pressures in excess of 250 mm Hg and a prominent, tapping arterial pulse replacing the usual thrill and indicating high intraaccess pressures should prompt angiography of the access. Periodic access blood flow monitoring using a transcutaneous optical sensor device (CritlineIII, Hemametrics, Kaysville, Utah) is also useful in detecting the blood flow velocity reductions that herald access thrombosis. Balloon angioplasty of the stenosed segment of vein (usually just distal to the venous anastomosis where the jet of blood shunted across the access impinges) can be performed before thrombosis supervenes. Alternatively, a patch or jump graft may be inserted at surgery.

Infection of arteriovenous grafts is more common than with fistulas, may occur in association with graft thrombosis, and may be present even without overt external evidence of infection. Infection of a perigraft hematoma is a common initiating event. Strict attention to skin preparation before cannulation of the arteriovenous access is, therefore, of great importance.

Ischemic Monomelic Neuropathy

Multiple distal mononeuropathies may occur in the upper limbs of diabetics after placement of a brachiocephalic arteriovenous access (48). Acute painful weakness of the forearm and hand muscles occurs within hours of creation of the access and is related to ischemia of the peripheral nerves caused by sudden diversion of the blood supply by placement of the proximal access. Early closure of the fistula or removal of the graft may result in reversal of the syndrome.

Multisystem Complications

Metabolic Complications

Insulin requirements after beginning maintenance HD vary. Typically, diabetic patients with ESRD experience reduction in insulin needs caused by decreased renal excretion and catabolism of injected and endogenous insulin. With control of uremia by dialysis, improved appetite in some diabetics may result in increased insulin needs. Hemoglobin A_{1c} (HbA_{1c}) levels fairly accurately reflect blood glucose levels in diabetics with ESRD and should be maintained not greater than 7% to 8% (49).

Mild hypertriglyceridemia, seen in 30% to 50% of all patients with ESRD, is more frequent in diabetic than in nondiabetic patients. Dietary restriction of simple sugars and saturated fats in association with good glucose control is usually sufficient to control hypertriglyceridemia. Hypercholesterolemia should be treated according to National Cholesterol Education Program Guidelines. We recommend quarterly measurement of HbA_{1c} levels and lipid profiles for our diabetic dialysis patients.

Retinopathy

Diabetic retinopathy is the most common cause of new blindness among patients aged 20 to 74 years in the United States (49). About 97% of newly evaluated uremic diabetics have significant retinopathy (50), and 25% to 30% are blind. Visual loss is most commonly related to proliferative retinopathy with associated vitreous hemorrhage and retinal detachment, but it may also result from macular edema, glaucoma, cataracts, and corneal disease.

The presence of proliferative retinopathy is correlated with duration of diabetes, gender (women more often than men), and degree of blood pressure control. Visual loss was often relentlessly progressive in diabetic patients in early HD programs. Improved preservation of sight is attributed to better blood pressure control and more aggressive referral for ophthalmologic treatment. Heparinization during HD is no longer thought to contribute to visual loss in diabetics.

Focal or panretinal laser photocoagulation can reduce the incidence of serious visual loss in patients with proliferative retinopathy (51), and vitrectomy may restore vision in patients with vitreous hemorrhage but fairly intact retinas, as determined by electroretinography.

Peripheral Vascular Disease

Lower extremity amputation rates in diabetics on HD vary from 5% to 25% per year (11). Multiple progressively invaliding amputations, usually of the lower extremities, are sometimes required in the same patient. Poor blood glucose control, peripheral vascular disease, and peripheral neuropathy are the major risk factors for amputations in diabetics (52). The role of secondary hyperparathyroidism and poor phosphate control in producing vascular wall calcium and phosphate deposits that may contribute to peripheral vascular disease (and CAD) is being increasingly recognized in ESRD patients; tight control of calcium/phosphate product levels to around 55, with more widespread use of the non-calcium-containing phosphate binders such as sevelamer hydrochloride in patients with serum calcium levels greater than 9.0 mmol/L is now advocated by many nephrologists.

Preventive care is paramount. The patient must do the following:

- Wash, dry, and examine the nails, soles, and interdigital creases of the feet every day.
- Wear comfortable, nonconstricting shoes with socks or stockings.
- Use heel booties if confined to bed.
- Make regular visits to a podiatrist for nail and callus care and prescription of customized, contoured shoes if necessary.

Diabetic ESRD patients should not cut their own toenails. At intervals of about every 3 to 4 months, diabetic patients should be asked to remove their shoes and socks for inspection by the nurse, physician, or both during dialysis rounds. A simple test for loss of protective sensation on the soles—and the most practical measure of risk assessment for foot ulcers—is sensation testing with the Semmes-Weinstein 5.07 monofilament (53). At the first symptoms or signs of limb ischemia or ulceration, early referral to a podiatrist for corrective shoes or to a vascular surgeon may enable vascular bypass surgery or limb-preserving amputation.

There is no evidence that the amputation rate in diabetic ESRD patients is lower on CAPD or after a renal transplantation than on HD.

Peripheral Neuropathy

Sensorimotor and/or autonomic neuropathy related to diabetes, and probably to uremia as well, may become disabling in the hemodialyzed diabetic. The histopathology of diabetic and uremic neuropathy is similar, if not indistinguishable. Underdialyzed uremic diabetics may suffer paraplegia and quadriplegia. Peripheral neuropathy appears to progress less frequently in diabetic ESRD patients treated with renal transplantation (54): over 6 years, 53% of 43 insulin-dependent diabetics on maintenance HD who initially had mild or moderate neuropathy experienced worsening of neuropathy, whereas none of 15 patients with similar clinical severity of neuropathy treated by renal transplantation had worsening of neuropathy.

Neuropathy is also less frequently seen and is less severe in diabetics treated with CAPD. Thus, severe neuropathy on HD may be one reason to switch, if possible, to CAPD, in which the enhanced removal of middle molecular proteins (deemed responsible for uremic neuropathy) may help symptoms. Amelioration of symptoms may result from maintaining good glucose control with maintenance of glycosylated hemoglobin levels below 7.5% and from ensuring adequate HD. Amitriptyline at bedtimes in doses up to 100 mg and gabapentin 300 to 400 mg loading followed by 200 to 300 mg after each dialysis thrice weekly may also be useful in treating neuropathy.

Bone Disease

Adynamic bone disease, characterized by low rates of bone turnover without excess of unmineralized osteoid, is a form of renal osteodystrophy commonly seen in diabetics (see Chapter 26) (54). Decreased osteoblast proliferation and defective mineralization contribute to a low rate of bone formation in diabetic rats (55). Reduced bone formation may allow time for enhanced deposition of aluminum on the ossification front; within 1 year of HD, aluminum deposition (usually related to use of aluminum-containing phosphate binders) is observed on bone surfaces in diabetics. Symptoms of bone pain and fractures related to aluminum bone disease may start as early as 2 years after initiation of HD (56). Aluminum bone disease may also be unmasked or accelerated after parathyroidectomy.

Aluminum-containing phosphate binders should, therefore, be avoided in diabetics, and all diabetics with bone pain and/or fractures should have plasma aluminum levels measured before and after a single infusion of desferrioxamine. Aluminum-associated bone disease in hemodialyzed diabetics responds to a regimen of vitamin D, calcium, and desferrioxamine.

Malnutrition

Malnutrition is frequently seen in diabetic HD patients, particularly in the presence of intercurrent illnesses (see Chapter 30). Causes of malnutrition in diabetics on HD include the following:

1. Poor glycemic control leading to gluconeogenesis and catabolism of muscle
2. Gastroparesis leading to nausea and vomiting
3. Diabetic diarrhea
4. Underdialysis related to difficulties with vascular access or to repeated early termination of dialysis sessions caused by recurrent hypotension (see Chapter 17)

A diet of 25 to 30 kcal/kg/day, with 50% of the calories coming from complex carbohydrates, and protein content of 1.3 to 1.5 g/kg/day is recommended for hemodialyzed diabetics. In diabetic HD patients who develop intercurrent illnesses (e.g., sepsis), early and intensive nutritional support with enteral or peripheral parenteral nutrition is necessary. Dialysate fluid should contain at least 200 mg/dL glucose, because use of glucose-free dialysate results in rapid glucose loss, hypoglycemia, and production of acute starvation with acidosis and hyperkalemia.

Metoclopramide taken before meals in divided doses often improves gastroparesis. Severe cases of diabetic diarrhea may be treated with broad-spectrum antibiotics to decrease bacterial overgrowth in adynamic segments of bowel. Loperamide hydrochloride given in doses of 1 to 2 mg/day is useful in reducing the frequency of bowel movements.

Psychosocial Problems

Depression and denial are common in diabetics during the often turbulent period of initial adjustment to the need for ESRD therapy and may be contributed to by complications of failing vision and limb loss. Delayed initiation of dialysis and eventual need for emergent initiation are the sequelae. Noncompliance with dietary and fluid restrictions and missed or shortened HD treatments may also result from the psychosocial maladjustments commonly seen after diabetics start dialysis. Counseling, involvement in patient support groups, and antidepressant therapy in selected patients can assist in coping with the stress of ESRD therapy.

CONTINUOUS AMBULATORY PERITONEAL DIALYSIS IN DIABETICS

PD was first proposed for the treatment of diabetics with ESRD in 1978 (57). Some centers use PD as the method of choice for diabetics because of anticipated difficulty with vascular access, the convenience of intraperitoneal insulin, and hemodynamic instability from autonomic neuropathy or CAD. The convenience of a non-facility-based treatment regimen or limited national resources may also make PD preferable to HD in some instances.

Survival outcome of diabetics on PD and HD are similar when comorbidity and delivered dose of dialysis are adjusted (58). Many diabetics are switched from HD to PD in desperation after multiple failed vascular accesses or because of severe hemodynamic instability or intercurrent illness on HD; these patients, of course, often have continued high morbidity and mortality. Overall, diabetics on CAPD have a lower actuarial survival and technique success rate than nondiabetic patients of similar age (59).

Six percent of diabetics entering renal replacement programs in the United States are treated with some form of PD (1). In a report from Toronto (60), diabetic patient survival on CAPD was 86% at 1 year and 38% at 4 years. Technique survival (excluding death) was 87% at 1 year and 65% at 4 years. These figures are similar to those in other reports (61–63). Among diabetics, survival rates on CAPD are lower than those of non-diabetics (64). Adverse factors affecting survival of diabetics on CAPD include age older than 45 years, previous or current cardiovascular disease, and systolic blood pressure in excess of 160 mm Hg (65).

In CAPD, regular exchanges of hypertonic glucose solutions are initiated 7 to 10 days after insertion of a double-cuffed, usually curled, Tenchoff catheter into the peritoneal cavity. The Moncrieffe-Popovich catheter is buried in the subcutaneous tissue of the anterior abdominal wall for 6 weeks and then is externalized for use, but rates of leaks and peritonitis have been found not to be significantly lower with prolonged burial of the catheter. A new long subcutaneously tunneled catheter with the exit site in the anterior chest wall may result in reduction in infection rates. Four 2-L exchanges/day are usually performed at 6-hour intervals. A 1.5%, 2.5%, or 4.25% glucose-containing dialysate is used, depending on the amount of ultrafiltration required: 1.5% dialysate will provide an ultrafiltration rate of approximately 3 mL/minute, whereas a 4.25% solution provides an ultrafiltration rate of approximately 10 mL/minute.

Continuous cyclic PD performed nightly in the home or intermittent PD performed in the hospital 3 days/week using a cycler are other PD regimens that may prove less demanding for some patients. In addition, these methods reduce the risk of peritonitis, because they require fewer disconnect and connect procedures. Nightly cycling dialysis with or without one to two daytime exchanges is becoming increasingly popular; it affords more convenience and use of larger total dialysate volumes in patients who are receiving inadequate dialysis with CAPD.

Intraperitoneal Insulin

First introduced in 1979 (66), intraperitoneal regular insulin in dosages somewhat higher than those used with the subcutaneous route (averaging 60 to 130 U/day) may be conveniently added to each bag of dialysis solution or preferably injected through the connecting tubing (so that adsorption of insulin to the polyvinylchloride of the bag does not occur) just before each exchange. Insulin requirements increase during episodes of peritonitis.

Intraperitoneally instilled insulin is best absorbed when the abdominal cavity is free of fluid and is predominantly taken up by the portal circulation, to produce a more physiologic effect than subcutaneously administered insulin. The dosage of insulin is adjusted to achieve fasting and 2-hour postprandial glucose levels of 150 to 250 mg/dL. If insulin requirements are greater than 100 U/exchange, or if blood glucose control is erratic with intraperitoneal insulin, a subcutaneous long-acting insulin preparation may be added.

Intraperitoneal insulin provides better mean blood glucose control and reduces the amplitude of glycemic excursions (67,68).

Advantages of CAPD

The advantages of PD are listed in Table 36.4. PD may be the only lifeline available for some uremic diabetics: patients in whom vascular access sites have been exhausted or those with severe HD-associated hypotension or angina related to atherosclerotic heart disease. Slower rates of ultrafiltration and less rapid removal of urea resulting in smaller changes in serum osmolality account for the absence of significant hypotension on CAPD, although it should be recognized that hypotension may still be induced by repeated use of hypertonic (4.25%) exchanges.

Diabetic retinopathy may stabilize in many patients in PD programs (69), although no prospectively controlled studies exist. Better preservation and even improvement of vision are thought to be due to fewer rapid changes in intravascular volume with less potential for exacerbation of retinal ischemia. More effective blood pressure control and blood glucose control are also major factors in stabilizing retinopathy. Even if retinopathy progresses, however, successful PD may be performed. Once motivation and family support are present, blind diabetics can be successfully taught blind CAPD protocols.

Enhanced clearance of purportedly toxic middle molecules by the peritoneal membrane has been thought to underlie the variably reported improvement in peripheral neuropathy seen in some diabetics on CAPD.

Another well-known advantage of CAPD is the preservation of residual renal function, with concomitant maintenance of urine output that sometimes allows for only three dialysate exchanges per day. Absence of cytokine-mediated responses (with associated progressive glomerular damage) to the extracorporeal circuit and membranes used in HD is proposed as a major factor in the maintenance of residual renal function (70). Other possible explanations include stable and comparatively high blood urea nitrogen levels that promote osmotic diuresis and hemodynamic stability and prevention of glomerular ischemia. Eventually, however, patients will lose all endogenous renal function and, thus, will need more dialysis at that time.

Disadvantages of CAPD

Within the first year of starting CAPD, 49% of patients will switch to another modality of renal replacement therapy (71).

TABLE 36.4. ADVANTAGES OF PERITONEAL DIALYSIS

Home lifestyle and independence maintained
Fewer dietary restrictions
Freedom from daily insulin injections
Improved glycemic control with intraperitoneal insulin
No vascular access required; freedom from pain of repeated access cannulations
Better blood pressure control
Less cardiovascular stress
No systemic heparinization
Better preservation of residual renal function
Potential stabilization of retinopathy
Slower progression of neuropathy
Steady-state chemistries

By comparison, only 37% of HD patients change treatment modality during the first year (Table 36.5). It is much more likely that a CAPD or continuous cyclic PD patient will switch to HD (15.6%) than that a HD patient will switch to CAPD (4.4%) (60). The high technique failure rate on CAPD is due mainly to peritonitis (72).

Recurrent peritonitis, usually caused by *Staphylococcus epidermidis* or *Staphylococcus aureus* and often in association with exit-site infections, is the major disadvantage of CAPD. Fungal peritonitis is seen more commonly in diabetic than in nondiabetic CAPD patients and usually requires removal of the peritoneal catheter. Peritonitis in diabetic CAPD patients occurs at a rate of one episode per 11 to 21 patients per month (60,61,67). Diabetics on CAPD need twice the number of hospitalization days as nondiabetic CAPD patients do (73), and peritonitis accounts for 30% to 50% of the hospitalization days (74). There is, however, no overall increased risk of peritonitis in diabetics over nondiabetics (75).

Encouraging reports have come from Italy, where use of Y set dialysate drainage systems have resulted in very low rates of peritonitis and good technique survival rates (61). In this multicenter Italian study, 480 CAPD and 373 HD patients were studied. The 7-year patient survival rate was similar in CAPD patients and HD patients. When adjustments were made for peritonitis, there was no significant difference between CAPD and HD technique survival (61).

Patients on CAPD tend to have higher levels of blood urea nitrogen and creatinine than HD, and there is concern about the adequacy of CAPD as a long-term uremia therapy (76). Based on peritoneal equilibration testing, a minimum clearance of 6 to 7 L/day is recommended for patients on PD (77). Length of the dwell times and volume of each exchange are adjusted based on the transport characteristics of the individual's peritoneal membrane as determined by the peritoneal equilibration testing.

Urea kinetic modeling has been applied to PD (see Chapter 14) (78). To maintain the same level of blood urea nitrogen in a CAPD patient and a HD patient, the Kt/V (where K is dialyzer clearance, t is time on dialysis, V is volume of distribution of urea) in the CAPD patient must be maintained at a higher level. A Kt/V of 1.59 on HD is equivalent to a weekly CAPD dose of 2.1 to 2.2 (58). The amount of dialysis delivered on CAPD may have to be increased with time because residual renal function is lost and peritoneal clearance decreases because of advanced vascular disease or to recurrent episodes of peritonitis.

TABLE 36.5. DISADVANTAGES OF PERITONEAL DIALYSIS

Risk of peritonitis
Inferior solute extraction (compared with hemodialysis)
Progressively increasing dialysis time
Time and effort intensive
Obligate protein losses in dialysate
Hyperglycemia and hypertriglyceridemia caused by glucose-rich
  dialysate
Low clearances with advanced vascular disease of peritoneal vessels
Abdominal wall and inguinal hernias
Respiratory compromise or bradyarrhythmias during fluid instillation

Malnutrition may occur in long-term CAPD patients (65,79). In an international study of CAPD patients (63), 8% were severely malnourished, 33% were moderately malnourished, and 59% had no evidence of malnutrition. In another study of 43 insulin-dependent diabetics (26 on HD and 17 on CAPD) followed for a mean of 11.6 months, 26% of patients were below the eighty-fifth percentile of ideal body weight, and 41% had a serum albumin below 3.5 mg/dL (80). Malnutrition in CAPD-treated diabetics may occur because of (a) reduced appetite caused by the large glucose load in dialysate or by early satiety from increased intraabdominal pressure or (b) large protein losses (8 to 10 g/day) in the dialysate effluent that may lower serum albumin and total protein levels (81). Loss of protein through the peritoneal membrane is increased during episodes of peritonitis and may worsen with time as a result of a generalized increase in permeability related to diabetic microangiopathy involving the peritoneal vessels (82) or nausea and vomiting related to diabetic gastroparesis.

To maintain adequate nutrition, CAPD patients should ingest at least 1.5 g/kg protein each day and between 130 and 150 g of carbohydrate each day. Malnourished CAPD patients may benefit from intraperitoneal amino acids (see Chapter 30) (83). Blood glucose control may sometimes be difficult on CAPD because of the absorption of a mean of 182 ±61 g of glucose per day from the peritoneal cavity (84). A combination of subcutaneous and intraperitoneal insulin administration usually results in adequate glucose control, however.

RENAL TRANSPLANTATION IN PATIENTS WITH DIABETIC NEPHROPATHY

All uremic diabetics should be questioned about the availability of a living-related kidney donor, because rehabilitation is best after a kidney transplant. In addition, renal transplantation is the cheapest form of renal replacement therapy (after the initial 3 years). There is no absolute age cut-off for renal transplantation in diabetics (our oldest transplanted diabetic was a 72-year-old politician), but generally patients older than 65 years are not considered for transplantation. Other contraindications to renal transplantation in diabetics are listed in Table 36.6.

Patients with a history of angina pectoris, previous myocardial infarction, or heart failure should have preoperative coronary angiography with angioplasty or bypass grafting of significant occlusive lesions. Because diabetics often have clinically silent CAD, some form of preoperative cardiac assessment is necessary, even in diabetics with no symptoms of cardiac disease. We refer all diabetics older than 30 years and those with diabetes of longer

TABLE 36.6. CONTRAINDICATIONS TO RENAL TRANSPLANTATION IN DIABETICS

Age >65 years (relative)
Gangrene of extremity (present or incipient)
Severe (uncorrected or uncorrectable) coronary artery disease
Immobilization from peripheral neuropathy or peripheral vascular
  disease

than 15 years' duration for cardiologic evaluation. An exercise stress test and/or a dipyridamole thallium stress test is our current screening test, but dobutamine stress echocardiography is reported to afford greater sensitivity (95%) and may be the screening test of choice if available at your institution (85). Routine coronary angiography for patients without cardiac symptoms does not seem warranted because only 31 of 151 insulin-dependent diabetics screened with coronary angiography pretransplantation had angiographically significant lesions (86).

In diabetic patients who have been followed through their earlier stages of renal insufficiency, it may be possible to plan for preemptive renal transplantation, without an interim period on HD.

The comparative incidence and rate of progression of diabetic complications with renal transplantation, CAPD, and HD are difficult to assess, because a younger population of diabetic patients with fewer comorbid conditions (who have survived long enough on dialysis to get a transplant) is selected for renal transplantation programs. The prevalence of both blindness and amputations are less with chronic dialysis than with transplantation: 12.5% versus 23% and 13% versus 30%, respectively (87). After 10 years, 31% of transplanted diabetics have had lower extremity amputations (88). Correction of uremia does not prevent or retard progression of diabetic peripheral neuropathy (89). Some series, however, report no difference in late diabetic complications in patients on chronic dialysis versus transplantation (90).

CONCLUSION

Diabetics comprise the largest group of patients on dialysis today and are subject to increased morbidity and long-term mortality when compared with nondiabetic patients. An aggressive, preemptive approach to managing the multisystem complications that accrue from macrovascular and microvascular disease is necessary. HD-related complications and lack of vascular access may mandate change from HD to PD, but the best rehabilitation and longest survival for the uremic diabetic is afforded by successful renal transplantation.

REFERENCES

1. United States Renal Data System. USRDS 2002 Annual Data Report. Bethesda, MD: National Institutes of Health, National Institute of Diabetes and Digestive and Kidney Diseases, July 2002.
2. Mauer SM, et al. A comparison of kidney disease type I and type II diabetes. *Adv Exp Med Biol* 1985;189:299–303.
3. Centers for Disease Control and Prevention. National Diabetes Fact Sheet: National estimates and general information on diabetes in the United States. Revised edition. Atlanta, GA: U.S. Department of Health and Human Services, 1998.
4. National Center for Health Statistics. Health, United States, 1998. Hyattsville, MD: Public Health Service, 1999.
5. Avram MM. Use of special hemodialysis methods in diabetic uremia. Conference on dialysis as a practical workshop. New York: National Union Catalogue, 1966:15–16.
6. Chazran BI, et al. Dialysis in diabetics: a review of 44 patients. *JAMA* 1969;209:2026–2030.
7. Comty CM, et al. Management and prognosis of diabetic patients treated by chronic hemodialysis. *Am Soc Nephrol* 1971;5:15.
8. Comty CM, et al. A reassessment of the prognosis of diabetic patients treated by chronic hemodialysis. *Trans Am Soc Artif Intern Organs* 1976;22:404.
9. Ghavamian M, et al. The sad truth about hemodialysis in diabetic nephropathy. *JAMA* 1972;222:1386–1389.
10. Jacobs C, et al. Combined report on regular dialysis and transplantation in Europe, XI, 1980. 17th Congress of the European Dialysis and Transplantation Association, Paris, July 5–8, 1981.
11. Kjellstrand CM, et al. Dialysis in patients with diabetes mellitus nephropathy. *Diabet Nephropathy* 1983;2:15–17.
12. Whitley KY, et al. Hemodialysis for end-stage diabetic nephropathy. In: Friedman EA, et al., eds. *Diabetic renal retinal syndrome.* New York: Grune & Stratton, 1986:349–362.
13. Balodimus MC. Diabetic nephropathy. In: Marbel A, et al., eds. *Joslin's diabetes.* Philadelphia: Lea & Febiger, 1971:526–561.
14. Marks HH. Longevity and mortality of diabetics. *Am J Public Health* 1965;55:416–422.
15. Humphrey LL, et al. Chronic renal failure in non-insulin dependent diabetes mellitus. *Ann Intern Med* 1989;111:788–796.
16. Hasslacher CH, et al. Similar risks of nephropathy in patients with type I or type II diabetes mellitus. *Nephrol Dial Transplant* 1989;4:859–863.
17. Nelson RG, et al. Incidence of end-stage renal disease in type 2 (non-insulin dependent) diabetes mellitus in Pima Indians. *Diabetologia* 1988;31:730–736.
18. Cowie CC, et al. Disparities in incidence of diabetic end-stage renal disease according to race and type of diabetes. *N Engl J Med* 1989;321:1074–1079.
19. Nolph KD, et al. Current concepts: continuous ambulatory peritoneal dialysis. *N Engl J Med* 1988;318:1595–1600.
20. Mogensen CE, et al. The stages of diabetic renal disease with emphasis on the stage of incipient diabetic nephropathy. *Diabetes* 1983;32:64–78.
21. Legrain M, et al. Selecting the best uremia therapy. In: Friedman EA, et al., eds. *Diabetic renal retinal syndrome.* New York: Grune & Stratton, 1986:453–468.
22. Friedman EA. Physician bias in uremia therapy. *Kidney Int* 1985;17 [Suppl A]:S38–S40.
23. Ortega-Gayton M, et al. Angioaccess for maintenance hemodialysis in end-stage diabetic nephropathy. *Proc Clin Dial Transplant* 1979;9:99.
24. Palder SB, et al. Vascular access for hemodialysis: patency rates and results of revision. *Ann Surg* 1985;202:235–239.
25. Gefen JY, et al. The transposed forearm loop arteriovenous fistula: a valuable option for primary hemodialysis access in diabetic patients. *Ann Vasc Surg* 2002;16:89–94.
26. Dixon BS, et al. Hemodialysis vascular access survival: upper arm native arteriovenous fistula. *Am J Kidney Dis* 2002;39:92–101.
27. Little MA, et al. A prospective study of complications associated with cuffed, tunneled hemodialysis catheters. *Nephrol Dial Transplant* 2001;16:2194–2200.
28. Kjellstrand CM, et al. Mortality and morbidity in diabetic patients accepted for renal transplantation. *Proc Eur Dialysis Transplant Assoc* 1972;9:345–358.
29. Rubin JE, et al. Dialysis and transplantation of diabetics in the United States. *Nephron* 1977;18:309–315.
30. Ritz E, et al. Hypertension and cardiovascular risk factors in hemodialyzed diabetic patients. *Hypertension* 1985;7[Suppl 2]:118–124.
31. Goodman WG, et al. Coronary artery calcification in young adults with end-stage renal disease who are undergoing dialysis. *N Engl J Med* 2000;342:1478–1483.
32. Stack AG, et al. A cross-sectional study of the prevalence and clinical correlates of congestive heart failure among incident U.S. dialysis patients. *Am J Kidney Dis* 2001;38:992–1000.
33. Kim SB, et al. Persistent elevation of C-reactive protein and ischemic heart disease in patients with continuous ambulatory peritoneal dialysis. *Am J Kidney Dis* 2002;39:342–346.
34. Joki N, et al. Coronary artery disease as a definitive risk factor of short-term outcome after starting hemodialysis in diabetic renal failure patients. *Clin Nephrol* 2001;55:109–114.
35. Shideman JR, et al. Hemodialysis in diabetics. *Arch Intern Med* 1976;136:1126–1130.

36. Nakamoto M. The mechanism of intradialytic hypotension in diabetic patients. *Nippon Jinzo Gakkai Shi/Jpn J Nephrol* 1994;36:374–381.

37. Daugirdas JT. Dialysis hypotension: a hemodynamic analysis. *Kidney Int* 1991;39:223–246.

38. Gotch FA, et al. An analysis of thermal regulation in hemodialysis with one and three compartment models. *Trans Am Soc Artif Intern Organs* 1989;35:622–624.

39. Dorhout Mees EJ. Rise in blood pressure during hemodialysis ultrafiltration: a 'paradoxical' phenomenon? *Int J Artif Organs* 1996;569–570.

40. Yusuf S, et al. Effects of an angiotensin converting enzyme inhibitor, ramipril, on cardiovascular events in high risk patients. *N Engl J Med* 2000;342:145–153.

41. Gradzki R, et al. Use of ACE inhibitors is associated with prolonged survival of arteriovenous grafts. *Am J Kidney Dis* 2001;38:1240–1244.

42. Ifudu O, et al. Diabetics manifest excess weight gain on maintenance hemodialysis. *Am Soc Artif Organs* 1992;21:85.

43. Jones R, et al. Weight gain between dialysis in diabetics: possible significance of raised intracellular sodium content. *BMJ* 1980;1:153.

44. Tzamaloukas AH, et al. Hand gangrene in diabetic patients on chronic dialysis. *Trans Am Soc Intern Organs* 1991;37:638–643.

45. Redfern AB, et al. Neurologic and ischemic complications of upper extremity vascular access for dialysis. *J Hand Surg (US)* 1995;20:199–204.

46. Mayers JD, et al. Vascular access surgery for maintenance hemodialysis: variables in hospital stay. *Am Soc Artif Int Organ J* 1992;38:113–115.

47. Sedlacek M, et al. Hemodialysis access placement with preoperative non-invasive vascular mapping: comparison between patients with and without diabetes. *Am J Kidney Dis* 2001;38:560–564.

48. Riggs JE, et al. Upper extremity ischemic monomelic neuropathy: a complication of vascular access procedures in uremic diabetic patients. *Neurology* 1989;39:997–998.

49. Joy MS, et al. Long term glycemic control measurements in diabetic patients receiving hemodialysis. *Am J Kidney Dis* 2002;39:297–307.

50. Blagg CR. Visual and vascular problems in dialyzed diabetic patients. *Kidney Int* 1974;6[Suppl 1]:S27–S30.

51. Klein R, et al. Vision disorders in diabetes. Diabetes in America (NIH pub. no. 85-1468). Washington, DC: Government Printing Office, 1985;13:1–36.

52. Levin ME. Saving the diabetic foot. *Intern Med* 1997;20:90–103.

53. Lehto S, et al. Risk factors predicting lower extremity amputations in patients with NIDDM. *Diabet Care* 1996;19:607–613.

54. Khauli RB, et al. Comparison of renal transplantation and dialysis in rehabilitation of diabetic end-stage renal disease patients. *Urology* 1986;27:521–525.

55. Vincenti F, et al. Parathyroid and bone response of the diabetic patient to uremia. *Kidney Int* 1984;25:677–682.

56. Andress DL, et al. Early deposition of aluminum in bone in diabetic patients on hemodialysis. *N Engl J Med* 1987;316:292–296.

57. Amair P, et al. Continuous ambulatory peritoneal dialysis in diabetics with end-stage renal disease. *N Engl J Med* 1982;306:625–630.

58. Keshaviah P, et al. Survival comparison between hemodialysis and peritoneal dialysis based on matched doses of delivered therapy. *J Am Soc Nephrol* 2002;13[Suppl]:S48–S52.

59. Passadakis P, et al. Long-term survival with peritoneal dialysis in ESRD due to diabetes. *Clin Nephrol* 2001;56:257–270.

60. Yuan ZY, et al. Is CAPD or hemodialysis better for diabetic patients? CAPD is more advantageous. *Semin Dial* 1992;5:181–188.

61. Maiorca R, et al. A multicenter, selection-adjusted comparison of patient and technique survivals on CAPD and hemodialysis. *Perit Dial Int* 1991;11:118–127.

62. Cavalli PL, et al. CAPD versus hemodialysis: 7 years of experience. In: Khanna R, et al., eds. *Advances in peritoneal dialysis*. Toronto: University of Toronto Press, 1989;5:52–55.

63. Rotellar C, et al. Ten years' experience with continuous ambulatory peritoneal dialysis. *Am J Kidney Dis* 1991;17:158–164.

64. Chandran PKG, et al. Patient and technique survival for blind and sighted diabetics on continuous ambulatory peritoneal dialysis: a 10-year analysis. *Int J Artif Organs* 1991;14:262–268.

65. Kemperman FAW, et al. Continuous ambulatory peritoneal dialysis in patients with diabetic nephropathy. *Neth J Med* 1991;38:236–245.

66. Flynn CT, et al. Intraperitoneal insulin with CAPD—an artificial pancreas. *Trans Am Soc Artif Intern Organs* 1979;25:114–117.

67. Scarpioni LL, et al. Continuous ambulatory peritoneal dialysis in diabetic patients. *Contrib Nephrol* 1990;84:50–74.

68. Tzamaloukas AH, et al. Subcutaneous versus intraperitoneal insulin in the management of diabetics on CAPD: a review. *Adv Perit Dial* 1991;7:81–85.

69. Mitchell JC, et al. Chronic peritoneal dialysis in juvenile-onset diabetes mellitus: a comparison with hemodialysis. *Mayo Clin Proc* 1978;53:775–781.

70. Nolph KD. Is residual renal function preserved better with CAPD than with hemodialysis? *American Kidney Foundation Nephrol Lett* 1990;7:1–4.

71. Held PJ, et al. The United States renal data systems annual data report. *Am J Kidney Dis* 1990;16[Suppl 2]:34–43.

72. Nolph KD. Continuous ambulatory peritoneal dialysis as long term treatment for end-stage renal disease. *Am J Kidney Dis* 1991;17:154–157.

73. Khanna R, et al. Continuous ambulatory peritoneal dialysis in diabetics with end-stage renal disease: a combined experience of 2 North American centers. In: Friedman EA, et al., eds. *Diabetic renal retinal syndrome*. New York: Grune & Stratton, 1986:363–381.

74. Rottemburg J. Peritoneal dialysis in diabetics. In: Nolph KD, ed. *Peritoneal dialysis*. Boston: Martinus Nijhoff, 1985:365–379.

75. Rubin J, et al. Chronic peritoneal dialysis in the management of diabetics with terminal renal failure. *Nephron* 1977;19:265–270.

76. Diaz-Buxo JA. Is continuous ambulatory peritoneal dialysis adequate long-term therapy for end-stage renal disease? A critical assessment. *J Am Soc Nephrol* 1992;3:1039–1048.

77. Twardowski ZJ. PET—a simpler approach for determining prescriptions for adequate dialysis therapy. In: Khanna R, et al., eds. *Dialysis*. Toronto: University of Toronto Press, 1990;6:186–191.

78. Gotch F. The application of urea kinetic modelling to CAPD. In: LaGreca G, et al., eds. *Peritoneal dialysis*. Milan: Wichtig Editore, 1991:47–51.

79. Young GA, et al. Nutritional assessment of chronic ambulatory peritoneal dialysis patients: an international study. *Am J Kidney Dis* 1991;17:462–471.

80. Miller DG, et al. Diagnosis of protein calorie malnutrition in diabetic patients on hemodialysis and peritoneal dialysis. *Nephron* 1983;33:127–132.

81. Blumenkrantz MJ, et al. Protein losses during peritoneal dialysis. *Kidney Int* 1981;19:593–602.

82. Krediet RT, et al. Peritoneal permeability to protein in diabetic and non-diabetic continuous ambulatory dialysis patients. *Nephron* 1986;42:133–140.

83. Oreopoulos DG, et al. CAPD in diabetics. American Society of Nephrology Annual Meeting, Baltimore, November 1991.

84. Grodstein GP, et al. Glucose absorption during continuous ambulatory peritoneal dialysis. *Kidney Int* 1981;19:564–567.

85. Reis G, et al. Usefulness of dobutamine stress echocardiography in detecting coronary artery disease in end-stage renal disease. *Am J Cardiol* 1995;75:707–710.

86. Manske CL, et al. Coronary revascularization in insulin-dependent diabetic patients with chronic renal failure. *Lancet* 1992;340:998–1002.

87. Bentley FR, et al. The status of diabetic renal allograft recipients who survive for ten or more years after transplantation. *Transplant Proc* 1986;17:1573–1576.

88. Bentley F, et al. Status of diabetic renal allograft recipients who survive for 10 or more years after transplantation. *10th Int Cong Transplant Soc* 1984;219.

89. Najarian JS, et al. Long-term survival following kidney transplantation in 100 type I diabetic patients. *Transplantation* 1989;47:106–113.

90. Khauli RB, et al. Comparison of renal transplantation and dialysis in rehabilitation of diabetic end-stage renal disease patients. *Urology* 1986;27:521–525.

37

QUALITY OF LIFE AND REHABILITATION IN DIALYSIS PATIENTS

DANIEL J. SALZBERG AND DONNA S. HANES

DEFINITION OF QUALITY OF LIFE

The *American Heritage Dictionary* defines *life* as the physical, mental, and spiritual experiences that constitute existence (1). This chapter explores how we have come to define quality of life (QOL) and various methods by which QOL is assessed in patients with end-stage renal disease (ESRD). The World Health Organization defines QOL as "an individual's perception of their position in life in the context of the culture and value system where they live, and in relation to their goals, expectations, standards and concerns" (2). The measurement of QOL should incorporate the many factors that affect a subject's existence and satisfaction. It should include not just the physical aspect, but also the emotional, intellectual, social, cultural, and ethnic components that comprise daily life.

Terms that are sometimes equated with QOL include functional status, sense of well-being, life-satisfaction, and health status. Although health status is not synonymous with QOL, the two are interrelated, with health affecting QOL and QOL affecting health. Illustrative of this point is that survival appears to be greater in subjects with a higher measured QOL (3–5).

Given this foundation, one can define an aspect of QOL as being health-related. This health-related quality of life (HRQOL) represents the "physical, psychological, and social domains of health that are influenced by a person's experience, beliefs, expectations, and perceptions" (6). Within this context, health is defined as not only the absence of disease and infirmity, but also the presence of physical, mental and social well-being (2). HRQOL includes both an objective assessment of functional status and a subjective perception of one's health (6).

When approaching a chronic illness like ESRD, it is necessary to have a multidisciplinary approach. Given the number and complexity of stressors faced by patients with ESRD, it would be naïve to draw conclusions about their global health based solely on a single measurement, such as Kt/V or protein catabolic rate (PCR). Similarly, methodologic studies that evaluate only one primary endpoint, such as blood pressure control, may miss other significant aspects that affect health. It is with this global concept of health that HRQOL tools have been developed. The use of HRQOL instruments are even more

important in patients with ESRD, as compared with other chronic disease states, because this population has significant associated comorbid conditions.

An important concept that underscores the study of QOL is that a new procedure or drug may decrease mortality, but it may not necessarily improve QOL and, therefore, may not be of overall benefit to the patient. To further illustrate this paradigm, take the example of two patients with virtually identical medical conditions. Despite similar care and objective disease states, they may have vastly different perceived QOL, based on their social support systems, psychologic outlook, and coping mechanisms. HRQOL measurements allow for the assessment of these factors contributing to QOL.

Some of the practical applications of measuring HRQOL include assessment of therapeutic interventions and their impact on QOL, effect of different modalities of renal replacement therapy and affect on QOL, determination of change in QOL within the same population over the course of the disease, and assessment of the impact of interventions on cost and/or morbidity with relation to QOL.

MEASUREMENT OF QUALITY OF LIFE

Optimal HRQOL measurement instruments capture all the impact that disease and treatment have on the physical, emotional, social, and mental dimensions of an individual (7). Ideally, instruments should be comprehensive, valid, have test-retest reliability, and be responsive to change and yet be brief enough to allow for quick administration. They should allow for comparisons between groups of subjects with different illnesses and be sensitive enough to pick up subtle differences within a specific group. Lastly, for a HRQOL measure to be of value, the life experience must be converted into a quantitative, numerical value.

Unfortunately, there is no one ideal tool that measures HRQOL, and, therefore, multiple different instruments have been developed (Table 37.1). Most of these instruments use a psychometric approach, which is based on the item measure theory (8). This theory postulates that true QOL cannot be directly

TABLE 37.1. HEALTH-RELATED QUALITY OF LIFE INSTRUMENTS USED IN ASSESSMENT OF DIALYSIS PATIENTS

Generic Instruments
  Global assessment instruments
    Sickness Impact Profile (SIP)
    Medical Outcomes Study 36-Item Short Form Health Survey (MOS SF-36)
    Time Trade-Off approach (TTO)
  Domain specific tools
    Physical Health
      Karnofsky Performance Status (KPS) Scale, or the Karnofsky Index (KI)
      Symptoms and comorbidity checklist
      Sexual functioning scale
    Mental Health
      Index of General Affect, Index of Life Satisfaction and Index of Well-Being
      Affect Balance Score
      Beck Depression Inventory
      Rosenberg's Self Esteem Inventory
      Locus of control scales
    Social Health
      Illness intrusiveness
      Employment status measures
End Stage Renal Disease Targeted Instruments
  Parfrey et al. Health Questionnaire Specific for ESRD
  Kidney Disease Questionnaire (KDQ)
  Kidney Disease Quality-of-Life Instrument (KDQOL)
  Kidney Disease Quality-of-Life Instrument Short Form (KDQOL-SF)
  CHOICE Health Experience Questionnaire (CHEQ)
  Dialysis-Quality of Life Questionnaire (DIAQOL)
  Dialysis Discontinuation Quality of Dying (DDQOD)
  Dialysis Quality of Dying Apgar (DQODA)

Adapted from Edgell ET, et al. A review of health-related quality-of-life measures used in end-stage renal disease. *Clin Ther* 1996;18:887–938, with permission.

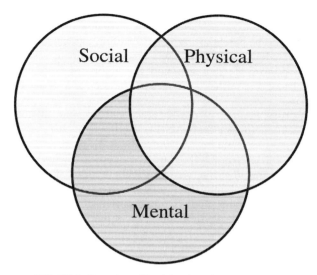

FIG. 37.1. Domains of health-related quality of life.

HRQOL instruments can be subdivided into categories based on whether the tool is global or domain specific. Three major domains comprise global HRQOL: the physical domain, the social domain, and the psychosocial or mental domain (12) (Fig. 37.1). Certain HRQOL instruments examine only one domain of HRQOL such as the Karnofsky Performance Status (KPS) Scale, which primarily assesses the dimension of physical health. Other instruments, such as the Sickness Impact Profile not only examine the physical domain but also give a global, overall measurement of HRQOL.

The types of HRQOL instruments can be further grouped into disease-targeted versus generic disease nonspecific tools (Table 37.1). The major advantage of disease-targeted tools is their ability to focus on the unique aspects and treatments of the disease being studied. However, extrapolation to other disease populations is severely limited. On the other hand, generic tools allow for comparisons of HRQOL across different populations and disease states but may not be specific or sensitive for subtle changes within a specific disease.

Generic Instruments

Generic instruments are designed to be applicable to a wide variety of populations. The major advantage of using a generic measure of HRQOL is that one can compare groups of subjects across different health and disease states. A number of these HRQOL instruments, however, have not been validated in the ESRD population, and these include Spitzer QL-index, Nottingham Health Profiles, Campbell Index of Well-Being, Cantril's Self-Anchoring Scale, and the Life Satisfaction Scale (12,13). Others have been demonstrated to be valid and will, therefore, be examined further.

Generic measures of HRQOL can be further subdivided into those that give a global assessment of HRQOL and those that focus on a specific domain, that is, physical health, mental health, or social health.

measured but can be assessed indirectly through a series of questions. These questions are defined as "items" (9). Each item is then given a numerical value, based on a predetermined scale. For example, in the RAND 36-Item Health Survey 1.0 Questionnaire (10), a subject is asked to rate his or her health on a scale from 1 (excellent) to 5 (poor).

When items are rated in this way, they are often referred to as Likert-type items. This rating presumes the existence of an underlying continuous variable whose value characterizes the respondents' attitudes and opinions. Each Likert-type item provides a discrete approximation of the variable being assessed (11). The advantage of this ordinal scale is its ability to rank order subjective responses that are otherwise difficult to quantify. When using these Likert-type items, there is no assumption that the difference between the possible responses is of the same magnitude. Said another way, the difference between responses 2 and 4 may not have the same meaning as the difference between responses 3 and 5.

The numerical score of each Likert-type item is then added together to obtain a sum score, which represents the overall global HRQOL score. It is the ability of these instruments to quantify QOL and produce a meaningful numerical score that allows for intragroup and intergroup comparisons.

Generic, global assessment instruments are designed to provide a comprehensive overview of the three domains included in HRQOL. The potential advantages of using a global assessment tool include the ability to use a single instrument instead of many domain-specific ones and the ability to combine the global tool with either a disease-specific tool or a domain-specific tool.

A classic example of these generic, global assessment tools is the Sickness Impact Profile (SIP), developed by Bergner et al. (14,15). As its name implies, the SIP was designed to assess the impact of sickness on QOL. The SIP contains 136 behavior-based items that are either interviewer or self-administered. These 136 items are divided into 12 health-related categories, including ambulation, mobility, body care and movement (these three categories comprise the physical dimension of the SIP), social interaction, alertness, emotional behavior, communication (these four categories comprise the psychosocial dimension), sleep and rest, eating, work, home management, and recreation and pastimes. Combining the score of all the items gives a global QOL score, which ranges from 0 to 100 points. A lower score indicates better QOL. The SIP has been proven to be reliable and valid in the ESRD population (7,12).

The Medical Outcomes Study Short Form 36-Item Health Survey (MOS SF-36, also abbreviated as SF-36) (16) is another widely used generic HRQOL measurement instrument. It was designed specifically to be a quick tool that would allow comparisons of HRQOL across different groups. As with the SIP, the SF-36 can be either interviewer or self-administered. Unlike the SIP, which contains 136 items, the SF-36 only contains 36 items, through which it evaluates eight health concepts of HRQOL. The eight health concepts are physical functioning (10 items), role limitations resulting from physical problems (4 items), role limitations caused by emotional or personal problems (3 items), social functioning (2 items), bodily pain (2 items), energy/fatigue (4 items), emotional well-being (5 items), and general health perceptions (5 items). In addition, there is one single item that provides an indication of perceived change, now versus 1 year ago. For example, the questions that are used to assess social functioning are "During the past 4 weeks, to what extent has your physical health or emotional problems interfered with your normal social activities with family, friends, neighbors, or groups?" ranked from 1 (not at all) to 5 (extremely); and "During the past 4 weeks, how much of the time has your physical health or emotional problems interfered with your social activities (like visiting with friends, relatives, etc.)?" ranked from 1 (all of the time) to 5 (none of the time) (10). Two additional components can be calculated from the SF-36 and they are the Physical Component Summary (PCS) and the Mental Component Summary (MCS). There are different methods for determining an overall score within each health concept, but the overall concept is that a higher score represents a more favorable health state. The SF-36 has been proven to be both reliable and valid in the ESRD population (7,12). Unlike the SIP and the SF-36, the Time-Trade Off (TTO) approach to HRQOL is not a psychometric item based instrument but rather uses a preference-based approach. The TTO approach makes use of modern utility theory, which postulates that, if presented with two alternatives with full disclosure of the risks and benefits involved, a person will choose the option that serves them best (17). In this model of decision making, subjects are first given a fixed amount of time that they will live in their current chronic disease state, defined as time (t). Next, they are presented with a theoretical question: "How many years of life would you be willing to give up in order to live the remaining years of your life in perfect health?" This variable time period is defined as (x) and is the amount of time that the subject would live in perfect health. If both t and x are equal, then the utility theory postulates that everyone should choose to live in perfect health. The subject is then asked if the amount of time they were to live in perfect health, that is, the variable x, were decreased, would they still choose perfect health? In this approach, t is a fixed number, and x is varied to achieve a point of indifference (h_i). The indifference point is defined as the point at which there is no preference between shorter life with perfect health and longer life with chronic disease. Mathematically, this is expressed as $h_i = x/t$, with a resultant single value, ranging between 0.0 and 1.0. For example, a subject who is willing to trade no more than 2 years of their life to achieve perfect health, when given 10 years to live with ESRD, has a h_i score of 0.8. In this example, t equals 10 years and x equals 8 years. The higher the h_i, the better the estimated HRQOL (7). Although the TTO approach appears to be reliable in the setting of ESRD (18), its validity has been questioned (19–22).

Generic domain-specific instruments are less comprehensive for measuring overall HRQOL, when compared with generic global tools. However, the domain-specific instruments may have the advantage of being more sensitive to changes within the assessed particular domain (Fig. 37.1).

The physical health domain encompasses the concept of performance status, which can be defined as the functional capacity of an individual. These instruments were originally tested in patients with cancer and demonstrated a significant positive correlation with survival (23,24). The prototypical example of a measure of performance status is the KPS Scale. The KPS scale has been used extensively in ESRD studies (7). Unlike the SIP and SF-36, it is clinician assessed and is not self-administered. There are 11 descriptive statements that rank performance status on an ordinate scale from normal (score of 100) to death (score of 0) (Table 37.2). In the ESRD population, as with cancer patients, the KPS appears to be a predictor of mortality (12).

The symptoms checklist and sexual functioning scales are other types of approaches used to assess physical health. These are typified by a list of physical symptoms, which are rated on a numerical scale. Examples of these instruments include the Index of Comorbidity (25), the Sexual Dysfunction Scale (26), the Index of Sexual Function (27), and the checklist created by Parfrey et al. (28). Unfortunately, most of these measures have not been established to be reliable and/or valid in the ESRD population (7).

Tools that measure the mental health domain primarily assess for depression, anxiety, and psychologic well-being. In ESRD, the most frequently used measures include Campbell's Indices of General Affect, Well-Being, and Life Satisfaction; the Affect Balance Scale (ABS); the Beck Depression Inventory; the Self-Esteem Inventory; and Locus of Control Scales (7).

Campbell's indices combine the Index of Life Satisfaction and the Index of General Affect to determine the Index of Well-

TABLE 37.2. THE KARNOFSKY PERFORMANCE STATUS SCALE

Description	Scale (%)
Normal, no complaints	100
Able to carry on normal activities; minor signs or symptoms of disease	90
Normal activity with effort	80
Cares for self; able to carry on normal activity or do active work	70
Requires occasional assistance but able to care for most needs	60
Requires considerable assistance and frequent medical care	50
Disabled; requires special care and assistance	40
Severely disabled; hospitalization indicated although death not imminent	30
Very sick: hospitalization necessary; active supportive treatment necessary	20
Moribund	10
Dead	0

TABLE 37.3. THE AFFECT BALANCE SCALE

During the past few weeks did you ever feel...	
Positive feelings:	Yes/No
■ Pleased about having accomplished something?	
■ That things were going your way?	
■ Proud because someone complimented you on something you had done?	
■ Particularly excited or interested in something?	
■ On top of the world?	
Negative feelings:	Yes/No
■ So restless that you couldn't sit long in a chair?	
■ Bored?	
■ Depressed or very unhappy?	
■ Very lonely or remote from other people?	
■ Upset because someone criticized you?	

Adapted from Bradburn N. *The structure of psychological well-being. Two dimensions of psychological well-being: positive and negative affect.* Chicago: Aldine, 1967, with permission.

Being (29,30). The Index of Life Satisfaction (ILS), as the name implies, explores the concept of life satisfaction. It consists of one global item, "How satisfied are you with your life as a whole these days?" rated on a 7-point scale from completely dissatisfied to completely satisfied (29). The Index of General Affect (IGA) consists of eight pairs of diametrically opposed items. These items are presented at either end of a 7-point scale. For example, in the pair of adjectives "discouraging to hopeful," discouraging would be 1 and hopeful would be 7. Respondents are asked to rank how they feel about their present life for each item. This technique is called a semantic differential scale developed by Osgood. The items that comprise the IGA are boring versus interesting, miserable versus enjoyable, useless versus worthwhile, lonely versus friendly, empty versus full, discouraging versus hopeful, disappointing versus rewarding, doesn't give me much chance versus brings out the best in me (29). The IGA score is obtained by averaging all eight items and ranges from 1 to 7. The Index of Well-Being (IWB) is then calculated from the ILS and the IGA. Mathematically, IWB = (ILS × 1.1) + IGA, with a resultant range of scores between 2.1 and 14.7, with a higher score indicating a better level of well-being. Campbell's indices are reliable and valid in the ESRD population (7), and can be either interviewer or self-administered.

Like Campbell's indices, the Affect Balance Scale (ABS) is also a composite of two scales, the Positive Feeling Scale (PFS) and the Negative Feeling Scale (NFS), each consisting of 5 items (Table 37.3) (31). The questions are presented in a yes or no format, with yes = 1 and no = 0. A composite score is calculated using the following formula: ABS = (PFS +5) − NFS. Scores range from 0 to 10, with 10 representing a better affect. It can be either interviewer or self-administered. The ABS is both reliable and valid (7).

Unlike the ABS and Campbell's indices, the Beck Depression Inventory (BDI) is used to measure the presence and intensity of depression (32,33). It consists of 21 items that deal with a specific behavioral manifestation of depression, ranked from 0 to 3. Overall scores range from 0 to 63, with higher scores cor-

relating with more severe depression. When compared with the *Diagnostic and Statistical Manual of Mental Disorders* (DSM-III) criteria for depression, the BDI was found to be valid in the ESRD population (31). Of note, there is a new edition of the BDI, the BDI-II, which revised the BDI to match the revamped criteria for depression in the DSM-IV. Both the BDI and the BDI-II take less than 10 minutes to complete and can be either interviewer or self-administered.

Other HRQOL instruments relating to mental health attempt to quantify one's self-esteem. Self-esteem, in this setting, is defined as an overall evaluation of one's worth or value (34). The most widely used tool for measuring self-esteem is the Rosenberg Self Esteem Inventory (SEI) scale. The SEI scale uses 10 Likert-like items, such as "On whole, I am satisfied with myself" and "At times I think I am no good at all," that are answered on a scale from strongly agree to strongly disagree. A higher score indicates a higher self-esteem (32). With regard to the ESRD population, the Rosenberg SEI scale has not been established as valid and reliable (7). These instruments are often used as a component of a battery of tests used to assess the mental domain of HRQOL.

Another type of mental health HRQOL instrument that has been used in ESRD patients is the locus of control scales. These tools attempt to measure the extent to which a subject believes that health is or is not determined by his or her own behavior, that is, that outcomes are the result of his or her own actions (internal) or the result of external forces (external). Examples of locus of control scales include the Health Locus Of Control (HLC) Scale developed by Wallston et al. (35), the Internal-External Locus of Control (IELC) Scale developed by Rotter (36,37), and the Locus of Control of Behaviour (LCB) scale developed by Craig et al. (38). The LCB consists of 17 items, rated in a Likert-type response scale from 0 (strongly agree) to 5 (strongly disagree). One example from Craig's scale is "People are victims of circumstance beyond their control." A higher score corresponds to a stronger external locus of control. Both of the IELC and the LCB have not been established as reliable or valid in the ESRD population (7). As with the assessment of self-esteem, these are often used as a component of a battery of tests used to assess the mental domain of HRQOL.

The social health domain of HRQOL is the least well characterized, and tools used to measure this domain focus mainly on illness intrusiveness and employment status. HRQOL tools that measure illness intrusiveness attempt to quantify the degree to which a chronic illness or treatment disrupts a patient's life. The Illness Intrusiveness Rating Scale (IIRS) was developed by Devins et al. (39) to assess perceived intrusiveness of ESRD on HRQOL. The IIRS is a self-administered scale that rates perceived intrusiveness on 11 to 13 life domains, including work, recreation, family and marital relations, sex, and diet. Each item is rated in a Likert-type response scale ranging from not very much (1) to very much (7). The IIRS is valid and reliable in the ESRD population (40–42).

Various approaches have been attempted to quantify vocational rehabilitation ranging from objective measure of working status (yes and no), to subjective determination of ability to work, to detailed self-reports such as the Psychosocial Adjustment to Physical Illness Scale (PAIS) (43). Despite the apparent ease of determining this variable, it appears that this measure may not be a valid measure of the social domain of HRQOL (44).

The other major category of HRQOL instruments are the disease-targeted instruments, which are applicable to a defined population of subjects. Examples of these include Parfrey's Health Questionnaire Specific for ESRD (28), Laupacis' Kidney Disease Questionnaire (45), Hays' Kidney Disease Quality of Life Instrument (46), and Wu's CHOICE Health Experience Questionnaire (47).

Parfrey et al. (28) developed the first published ESRD-targeted HRQOL instrument in 1989. The "Health Questionnaire Specific for ESRD" goal was to measure the effect of specific ESRD therapy on QOL. Parfrey et al. constructed two unique scales for the ESRD population exploring physical symptoms (the symptom scale) and examining emotional symptoms (the affect scale). The symptom scale consists of 12 items (tiredness, headache, sleep disturbance, joint pain, cramps, pruritus, dyspnea, angina, nausea/vomiting, abdominal pain, muscle weakness, and other) rated from 1 to 5, that is, from very severe to absent. Like the symptom scale, the affect scale also consists of 12 items (determination*, faith*, confused, different, angry, scared, helpless, alone, fed up, sad, desperate, and other) again rated from 1 to 5. They then combined these two indices with two subjective measures of HRQOL (Campbell's Indices of General Affect, Well-Being, and Life Satisfaction and the Spitzer Subjective Quality of Life Index) and two objective measures of HRQOL (KPS Scale and the Spitzer Concise QL-Index). Overall, this questionnaire has good reproducibility (except for the Spitzer Subjective QOL Index), is responsive to change, has construct validity, and allows for comparisons between ESRD and other disease states. The questionnaire takes between 15 to 20 minutes to complete but does require a trained interviewer to administer it.

In 1992 Laupacis developed the Kidney Disease Questionnaire (KDQ), a disease-specific HRQOL tool specifically for patients on chronic hemodialysis (HD) therapy (45). The KDQ contains 26 items in 5 dimensions, physical symptoms (6 items), fatigue (6 items), depression (5 items), relationships (6 items), and frustration (3 items) (45). Unlike other HRQOL questionnaires, the physical symptoms dimension of the KDQ is patient specific. The 6 physical symptoms that are most important to each subject are identified and used to assess that dimension. Items are ranked from 1 (all of the time) to 7 (none of the time). The KDQ has construct validity and reliability (45) and is more responsive to change than the SIP or TTO (45,48). The two major limitations of the KDQ are that it is designed for use only in ESRD subjects undergoing HD and that there is no single overall health rating.

Like the KDQ, Hays' Kidney Disease Quality of Life Instrument (KDQOL) was also developed for use in subjects with ESRD on HD. Unlike the KDQ, the KDQOL uses the SF-36 as its core and supplements this with 19 additional multiitem scales (46). The use of the global, generic assessment tool allows for comparisons of HRQOL across disease states. Major advantages of the KDQOL are its comprehensive scope and the inclusion of a single-item overall health rating. The major limitation of the KDQOL is its length, 134 items, which take approximately 30 minutes to complete. Rao et al. (49) have subsequently developed an 11 multiitem subscale from the KDQOL's Symptoms/Problems and Effects of Kidney Disease scales, which correlate with the SF-36 and number of disability days.

Because of its length, the KDQOL short form (KDQOL-SF) was created. It includes the core SF-36 scale, 43 kidney-disease-targeted items from the original KDQOL, and a single overall health-rating item, thus containing only 80 items. As with the KDQOL, the KDQOL-SF is self-administered but takes about half as long to complete. Both appear to be reliable and have construct validity (46,50). In addition to the KDQOL-SF, there is the KDQOL-36 that only contains 36 items. We recommend the 80-item KDQOL-SF in routine clinical practice. It incorporates the core SF-36 scale (a generic scale allowing comparisons across diseases), it has proven kidney disease targeted items, it takes a relatively short amount of time to administer, and it has a single overall health-rating item.

Like the KDQOL, the Choice for Health Outcomes in Caring for ESRD (CHOICE) Health Experience Questionnaire (CHEQ) also incorporates the SF-36 as its core (47). It consists of 83 items divided into 21 domains. It can be used for subjects on either peritoneal dialysis (PD) or HD and appears to be reliable and have construct validity (47).

Although not a direct measure of QOL, there have been a number of studies looking at the quality of dying in dialysis patients. ESRD offers a unique opportunity to quantify this process, because it is the only life-support therapy that is frequently discontinued. An estimated 17.8% of dialysis patients between 1990 and 1995 withdrew from dialysis before death (51). To better understand this aspect of QOL, Cohen et al. (52) developed a prototype tool to assess the quality of dying, the Dialysis Discontinuation Quality of Dying (DDQOD) instrument. The DDQOD is comprised of three domains: duration (of dying), pain and suffering, and psychosocial. Each domain is scored on a scale from 1 to 5. A summed score can range from 3 to 15 and is divided into three types of death: a very good

---

*Faith and determination are actually rated from 1 (absent) to (5) very strong.

death defined as greater than 12, a good death greater than 8 to 12, and a bad death ≤8. The major problem with this tool is that it is inapplicable to ESRD deaths that are not preceded by dialysis termination (52,53).

The Dialysis Quality of Dying Apgar (QODA) is another tool that attempts to quantify quality of dying. It is modeled after the original pediatric Apgar assessment and consists of five domains (pain, nonpain symptoms, advanced care planning, peace, and time). Each domain is scored from 0 to 2, with a range of scores between 0 and 10. At this time, QODA scores correlating to the three types of deaths (as in the DDQOD) have not been established (53).

QUALITY OF LIFE IN ESRD

As more and more patients advance to ESRD and require renal replacement therapy, HRQOL issues become more paramount. The ESRD medicare program has saved many lives, with annual expenditures exceeding $12.3 billion (54). However, several studies have raised concerns regarding the QOL of these patients, particularly those requiring long-term replacement therapy. A landmark study by Evans et al. (25) from the National Kidney Dialysis and Transplant Study rigorously examined the HRQOL of 859 patients undergoing dialysis or transplantation to determine major variables that affect patient outcomes. Using Campbell's indices (IGA, ILS, and IWB), Evans reported that 79% of the transplant recipients were able to function at nearly normal levels, compared with 59% on home HD, 44.7% on in-center HD, and 47.5% on PD. Overall, patients' functional scores were significantly lower than the general population, with subjective scores being only slightly lower. Nonetheless, the study suggested that patients with ESRD are able to adapt to very adverse life circumstances.

In a Canadian study, transplantation was associated with lower distress and greater well-being than dialysis (55). These findings have been confirmed and extended by others. Bremer et al. (56) found similar results among 957 patients using the Index of General Affect, Well Being, and Life Satisfaction. In this trial, transplant patients with working allografts fared the best. However, those subjects whose allograft failed requiring reinitiation on dialytic therapy had the greatest measured loss of HRQOL. Similarly, DeOreo (3) demonstrated that the most severe loss of HRQOL in dialysis patients was in physical function. In the DIA-QOL Project, 304 patients were administered the SF-36. Important factors influencing HRQOL included age and presence of diabetes (57). There were no significant associations with the *Kt/V*, hemoglobin (Hb) levels, body mass index, parathyroid levels, or type of dialysis. There was, however, a strong association between the serum albumin level and the physical functioning measure on the SF-36.

In the Spanish Quality of Life Study, over 1,000 patients were assessed using the KI and SIP; most patients were on HD (58). All patients reported a reduced HRQOL, and the most severely affected factors were work, activities, and sleep. There was no significant affect predicted by mode of dialysis, dialysis membrane, *Kt/V*, or PCR. Higher Hb levels and greater education and socioeconomic levels predicted positive measures of HRQOL. Patients with diabetes, peripheral vascular disease (PVD), multiple comorbidities, and female gender scored lower. Unfortunately, there were variations in QOL between the different centers, thus increasing the complexity and applicability of these results (59).

There is consistent data that patients with chronic kidney disease (CKD) and ESRD have an impaired HRQOL and that mortality and outcome measures alone do not provide a comprehensive understanding of overall patient care. Molzahn et al. (60) demonstrated that nurses' ratings of a patient's QOL are lower than patients, and physician's ratings were higher. Given that there are perceptual differences between a subject's QOL and the physician's assessment of that subject's QOL, confounded by different HRQOL instruments, it is important to understand the complexity when using these HRQOL measures (61).

IMPACT OF QOL

The importance of assessing the HRQOL cannot be overemphasized, because it not only reflects our patients' satisfaction but also has been independently correlated with hospital use, morbidity, and survival. In DeOreo's study (3), significant predictors of survival included not only PCR and *Kt/V* but also the PCS score of the SF-36. The survival rate increased 10% for each 5-point increment in the PCS score. Preliminary data from more than 7,000 patients in the Dialysis Outcomes and Practice Patterns Study (DOPPS), currently underway, reveal that a higher physical component score, mental component score, and kidney disease burden score (as measured by the KDQOL) are associated with a 5% to 8% and 9% to 23% reduction in the risk of hospitalization and mortality, respectively (62). Higher HRQOL physical functioning and provider-reported functional performance also correlates with survival (63). In a prospective study, baseline comorbidity, low serum albumin, and physical and mental scores greater than two standard deviations lower than the general population (as measured on the SF-36) predict poor outcomes such as malnutrition, prolonged hospitalization, and death (64).

EARLY REFERRAL

Because of the substantial effect that kidney disease can have on a patient's functional status, social functioning, and overall well-being, it is important to consider HRQOL measures early in the course of renal failure. Numerous studies have demonstrated the importance of early referral to a nephrologist (65,66) (Table 37.4). The National Institutes of Health recommend that patients with CKD be referred to a multidisciplinary predialysis team to optimize morbidity and ease the transition to renal replacement therapy (67). Early referral affords (a) the benefit of improved patient involvement and compliance; (b) greater participation in the selection and initiation of a dialysis modality; (c) better patient education; (d) time for access maturation and avoidance of unnecessary central catheters; (e) broader employment opportunities; (f) improved ability to delay the progres-

TABLE 37.4. PROGNOSTIC FACTORS ASSOCIATED WITH THE QUALITY OF LIFE (QOL) IN DIALYSIS PATIENTS

Improved QOL	Reduced QOL
Early referral to nephrologist	Younger age
Higher hematocrit	Diabetes
Black race	Intermittent claudication
Socioeconomic level	Female sex
Educational level	Depression
Adequate dialysis	Multiple comorbidities
Exercise	Malnutrition
Social support	Sleep disorders

Adapted from Valderrabano F, et al. Quality of life in end-stage renal disease patients. *Am J Kidney Dis* 2001;38:443–464, with permission.

sion of ESRD; (g) delayed development of associated comorbidities such as anemia and malnourishment; (h) improved QOL with less frustration, dissatisfaction, and depression; and (i) improved mortality rate (65,68–73) (Table 37.5). Patients with established predialysis care also require fewer emergency starts and in-hospital days compared with standard care (74). Although Dialysis Outcomes Quality Initiative (DOQI) guidelines advocate an early start of dialysis, the evidence is not convincing (see Chapter 9 for discussion) (75). Korevaar et al. (76) studied 275 new dialysis patients, all of whom showed marked improvement in HRQOL during the first 6 months. Compared with the 38% of the patients who had a late start, patients who started dialysis in time according to the DOQI guidelines had significantly higher HRQOL immediately after initiation of dialysis, but the effect was not significant after 12 months. Insofar as initiation of dialysis is accompanied by a high cost and many personal restrictions, the advantage of early initiation is questionable and should be individualized. Multidisciplinary approaches and predialysis care can help to optimize this decision and improve patient-oriented QOL assessments.

Using the SF-36 measure, White et al. (65) compared 74 incident dialysis patients who had attended predialysis clinics with 46 who had not. Adjusting for age, sex, residual renal function, and other comorbidities, predialysis clinic attendance was an independent predictor of higher HRQOL scores for physical function, emotional role limitation, social function, and general health. Such patients generally show improved compliance and less depression and difficulties with interpersonal relationships.

TABLE 37.5. POTENTIAL BENEFITS OF EARLY NEPHROLOGY REFERRAL

Better patient involvement
Improved compliance
Greater participation in one's care
Time for access maturation
Avoidance of unnecessary catheters
Better patient education
Improved employment opportunities
Delayed progression to ESRD
Delayed development of anemia
Delayed development of malnutrition
Improved quality of life
Improved mortality

These findings are exaggerated in the elderly population, who may require more intensive medical education and support in the setting of already compromised physical function. The finding that predialysis patients initiated on continuous ambulatory peritoneal dialysis (CAPD) therapy have a greater HRQOL as compared with HD, may be related to the fact that they often receive more intensive, individualized predialysis training (77).

SLEEP DISTURBANCES

Sleep disturbances are one of the most common problems encountered by dialysis patients. Recent studies reveal that the prevalence of primary dyssomnias, defined as disturbances in the amount, quality, or timing of sleep, exceeds 60% in dialysis patients, in comparison to 15% to 25% in the general population (78). In diabetic HD patients, the prevalence of sleep disturbances is 68% (79). Many individuals experience significant distress or impairment resulting in a compromised HRQOL as measured by physical and emotional problems, reduced general health and vitality, increased pain and social isolation, and possibly increased mortality (79).

The most commonly encountered sleep disorders in dialysis patients include insomnia, sleep apnea and related breathing disorders, and the restless legs syndrome. In the Kidney Outcomes Prediction and Evaluation (KOPE) Study, significant numbers of patients report waking during the night (57%), waking too early (55%), trouble falling asleep (41%), and excessive daytime sleepiness (31%) (80). Risk factors for sleep disturbances in patients on HD with diabetes include advanced age, depression, and compromised nutritional status (79). Increased perception of pain and greater depressive symptoms are more likely to be related to difficulty falling asleep and excessive daytime sleepiness. Patients with reduced functional status are more likely to wake during the night or too early. Women are more than twice as likely to wake too early and experience restless sleep. Patients encounter more frequent sleep disturbances if they have bone pain, pruritus, or inadequate dialysis; if they smoke; or if they have been on dialysis a long time (78,81–83). This is in contrast to patients with a higher level of functional status who report fewer sleep disturbances (80). Interestingly, nutritional status and the dose of dialysis as measured by Kt/V do not correlate with sleep disturbances; the effect of increasing Hb concentration is controversial (80,82,84–86).

Measures to improve successful sleep habits include limitation of smoking and alcohol, relaxation and biofeedback techniques, avoiding daytime and intradialytic naps, and changes in the sleep environment. When necessary, benzodiazepines that are converted into inactive metabolites, such as clonazepam, lorazepam, oxazepam, temazepam, or the hypnotic agent, zolpidem, can be used for sedation with appropriate dose adjustments for renal failure (87). Initial doses should be reduced by 25%.

Sleep-related breathing disorders and pathologic breathing patterns affect up to 70% of dialysis patients and frequently present as excessive sleepiness (88). In addition to impairing normal cognitive function, patients with sleep-related breathing disorders are at greater risk for cardiovascular morbidity and mortality (89). Sanner et al. (90) reported clinically significant increases in the number of apnea and hypopnea episodes that exceeded 13 per hour in most dialysis patients, with normal defined as less than 10/hour. Such abnormalities were associated with a median oxygen saturation of 92.5%. The severity of the breathing disorder was significantly correlated with impairments in physical functioning, social functioning, role limitation, and general health and vitality, as measured on the SF-36. It was also correlated with pain, sleep, social isolation, and emotional reactions. The etiology of sleep apnea remains unclear but may be related to alterations in acid-base balance, favoring periodic hyperventilation/hypoventilation cycles (91,92). Because of the high prevalence of sleep apnea, clinicians should maintain a high clinical suspicion in hypersomnolent patients.

Another common cause of sleep disturbances in patients on dialysis is the periodic limb movement/restless legs syndrome. Twenty percent to 30% of patients with ESRD report lower extremity symptoms of ascending and migratory paresthesias or cramps so severe as to interfere with sleep (81,93). Patients typically experience prolonged muscle contractions preceded by sensory discomfort (94). These are associated with sudden jerking movements that occur two to three times per minute and can lead to sudden waking. Although fluid and electrolyte imbalances may contribute to the pathophysiology, many patients have hyperactivity of the motor neurons (95). Anecdotal reports of improvement in the cramping symptoms have been reported with quinine sulfate, which appears to interfere with the excitability of the motor end plate and subsequent contractility of the muscles. Although the Food and Drug Administration has withdrawn its use for cramps because of hypersensitivity and adverse reactions, it is probably safe in doses not exceeding 300 mg per day. Levodopa 100 to 200 mg/day or moderate doses of carbamazepine or gabapentin 300 mg three times weekly have also been successful with widely variable efficacy (96–98).

SOCIAL SUPPORT AND THE QUALITY OF LIFE FOR CAREGIVERS

The interplay between patients and their social support is multidimensional. In dialysis patients, social support scores correlate with depression, psychosocial measures, and compliance (99,100). Patients' perceptions of increased social support correlate with lower depression scores, lower perceptions of illness burden, and higher marital and life satisfaction scores independent of age and severity of illness. Higher socioeconomic, education, and employment levels generally are associated with a greater QOL, except perhaps in blacks (58,101). Perception of social support and living with family in ESRD are predictors of survival (63,99,102,103).

Loss of employment also affects QOL. Unemployed ESRD patients score significantly lower in the SF-36 measure than those employed (in physical function, role physical, bodily pain, general health, vitality, and emotional scales) (104). Multiple comorbidities, a physical occupation before the onset of CKD, and poor physical function are independent predictors of unemployment in ESRD. Patients who are employed or do housework also tend to be more compliant (105).

An equally important but frequently ignored component of a dialysis patient's well-being is the QOL of the caregivers. Healthy, well-balanced relationships can provide the support many dialysis patients need to maintain compliance with medications, diet, and treatments; reduce the severity or occurrence of depression; and improve the overall care that patients receive. Social support from family members improves compliance with interdialytic fluid restrictions (106). It is well documented that families that live with chronically ill patients have a greater frequency of physical and mental disturbances (107,108). The burden and QOL of the caregivers for HD patients can be substantial. In a study by Belasco et al. (109), most caregivers were women (84%), married (66%), and had a low socioeconomic level. The health and vitality of the caregivers, as measured by the SF-36, were the most frequently affected variables and varied inversely with the burden of the caregiver, the illness of the patient, and perceived pain of the caregiver. Other studies support this finding. Lindqvist et al. (110) reported that optimistic and palliative coping strategies and less confrontational and emotional behaviors resulted in improved health related QOL of the caregivers. Spouses who were female more frequently used these skills (110). Interestingly, caregiver race and mode of dialysis does not significantly affect their perceived QOL (111). Highly functioning patients and families report the least burden and best coping strategies. To circumvent the stress associated with the ubiquitous uncertainty about the patient's health and life expectancy, frequent dialytic treatments, and potential for transplant, families and caregivers rely heavily on their support groups and religious beliefs, living one day at a time (112). Such family and interpersonal dynamics should be explored for all patients to optimize overall well-being.

ANEMIA

The impact of anemia on the HRQOL is well described and spans the continuum from early renal insufficiency to CKD to ESRD. Symptoms associated with uncorrected anemia in patients with kidney disease include fatigue, sexual dysfunction, cognitive dysfunction, cold intolerance, angina, dyspnea, and an impaired HRQOL. The introduction of human recombinant erythropoietin (rhEPO) therapy into clinical practice to increase the Hb has had a dramatic affect on these parameters, particularly HRQOL measures. In patients on HD or PD, correction of anemia consistently results in improvement in functional status, exercise ability, cognitive function, sexual function, and somatic complaints (48,113–117). In the cross-sectional Spanish Cooperative Study, Hb concentrations correlated significantly with physical and global scores on the SIP (58). Large clinical studies confirm improvements in fatigue, perceived strength, and global scores on the SIP, KI and SF-36, even with only modest increases in hematocrit (Hct) to 30.1% (118,119). In these trials, patients on HD who were not receiving rhEPO had significantly lower scores on the SF-36 than those who were receiving rhEPO. The gap in the scores progressively diminished as the patients were initiated on rhEPO therapy. In a similar trial, Moreno et al. (120) observed significant improvement in all three dimensions of the SIP when dialysis patients were started on rhEPO. Health-related QOL had a positive correlation with HCT between the levels of 29% and 35%, as assessed using the KI and SIP. Evans (113) showed that the perceived

HRQOL of dialysis patients treated with rhEPO, using the KI and objective measures of employment status, actually exceeded that of untreated, diabetic and nondiabetic, anemic transplant patients after 10 months.

Anemic predialysis patients also gain substantial improvements in HRQOL when started on rhEPO (121,122). In a randomized prospective trial, Revicki et al. (70) compared pre-ESRD patients treated with rhEPO to achieve an Hct of 35% with comparable untreated cohort whose mean Hct was 26.8%. Treated patients reported improvements in physical function, energy, role function, health distress, sexual dysfunction, depression, and satisfaction with life using various measures; results correlated with the improvement in Hct. It has also been suggested that early correction of anemia may prevent some of the complications of CKD. Correction of anemia can regress left ventricular hypertrophy, improve myocardial contractility and increase left ventricular ejection fraction. Early treatment of anemia instituted when the Hct falls below 35% may prevent cardiovascular deterioration, reduce overall morbidity and mortality, and is essential in maintaining HRQOL (123–126).

Unfortunately, the target Hct that optimizes HRQOL remains controversial. Both the DOQI guidelines and the European Best Practice Guidelines for the Management of Anemia recommend a target Hb concentration greater than 11 g/dL (127). Whether HRQOL measures are improved by further increasing the Hct is uncertain. In the Canadian Erythropoietin Study, the increase in HRQOL effects plateaued at an Hb concentration of 11.7 g/dL (21,48). The KI and SIP scores obtained by Moreno et al. (128) showed a positive correlation with Hct between 29% and 35%; the benefits are most evident at higher levels of Hct. Eschbach et al. (129) showed continued improvement in HRQOL with increasing Hct up to 42%. In another trial by Moreno et al. (130), the Hct of patients on dialysis was increased five points above their baseline Hct. Baseline Hct ranged between 28% and 35%. The increase in Hct was associated with a significant improvement in both the KI and SIP scores. Although this trial was not associated with other problems, it should be noted that the cohort tested did not have significant comorbidities.

In contrast, in patients on HD with ischemic heart disease or congestive heart failure, normalization of the Hct may be detrimental. In the North American Multicenter Study, Besarab et al. (131) prospectively randomized 1,233 patients with known heart disease to target Hct levels of either 42%, that is, a normal Hct, or 30%. Concern regarding the risk to the higher Hct group prompted an independent data monitoring committee to terminate the study early. After 29 months, there were 183 deaths and 19 nonfatal myocardial infarctions (MIs) in the normal Hct group as compared with 150 deaths and 14 MIs in the low Hct group. Of note, the mortality of both groups decreased with increasing Hct, and HRQOL, as measured by the SF-36, increased 0.6 points for each percentage increase in the Hct. Recent studies have demonstrated that patients with higher Hct also experience less morbidity (130). Currently, national guidelines do not recommend use of rhEPO to obtain Hct greater than 36% in subjects with renal disease and ischemic heart disease. However, because the HRQOL improves more the closer the Hct is to normal, more emphasis must be placed on at least achieving currently recommended levels of Hb and Hct.

DEPRESSION

Depression appears to be the most common psychologic problem experienced by patients on HD, affecting 20% to 70% of subjects (12,132,133). Estimates of the prevalence of depression vary widely based on the instruments used to detect it and differing diagnostic criteria. In subjects on dialysis, depression clearly correlates with a compromised HRQOL (134), is more common in women, is unrelated to satisfaction with the dialysis staff or the nephrologist, and is most common in HD as compared with PD and transplantation (135,136). The etiology of depression in dialysis patients is multifactorial. Impaired physical status; complex medical regimens; and the loss of time, finances, sexual function, and control contribute to depressive symptoms. As in other chronic illnesses, the extent of depression over time in patients with ESRD predicts patient mortality (133,135,137). Kovac et al. (135) investigated whether the risk of mortality and rate of hospitalization can be predicted from physician-diagnosed depression and patients' self-reports of depressive symptoms. In their cohort of over 5,000 HD patients, the prevalence of depression was 20%. The relative risk of mortality and hospitalization among depressed patients, as measured by medical records and the KDQOL-SF, was 23% higher than in nondepressed patients. Consequently, patients should be periodically evaluated for depression using sensitive tools such as the BDI and treated accordingly (33).

DEMOGRAPHIC VARIABLES

Age

As the age of the dialysis and transplant population increases, it is critical to explore the impact of age on the HRQOL. Unfortunately, studies have shown variable results. Early studies indicated that age has a negative impact on the HRQOL (25,64,138). These studies compared the HRQOL of patients with CKD younger than 65 years with those older than 65 and found that HRQOL was worse in the older cohort. In the Spanish Quality of Life study, deterioration in the physical dimension of the SIP was strongly correlated to age (12,58,128). However, Rebollo et al. (139) studied 485 patients on HD or posttransplant using the SIP and SF-36 to evaluate their HRQOL; the scores of the elderly patients were significantly higher than those of the younger subset. Elderly renal transplant patients had even higher scores than in the general population. This data suggest that ESRD has less of an impact in the elderly and that transplantation in this group offers a reasonable alternative to dialysis. As measured by the SF-36, elderly dialysis patients had better physical functioning, lower levels of pain, and better general health perceptions than their younger counterparts. Interestingly, these elderly patients on dialysis were also less likely to be hospitalized, and, when they were, they had shorter lengths of stay. A higher economic level, higher educational level, higher KI score, and lower number of comorbid conditions were associated with higher HRQOL (140). Elderly patients tend to be more satisfied with their life while on dialysis and appear to accept their limitations better than younger patients. This may be due, in part, to the fact that older individuals expect some degree of deterioration in their HRQOL and are more grateful for the extension of life provided by renal replacement therapy (4,141,142).

Among elderly patients on PD, despite having worse appetites and moods than their younger counterparts, there is no significant difference in their HRQOL (143). In addition, clinical outcomes and HRQOL, as measured by the SF-36 and KDQOL in elderly patients, do not differ significantly among patients treated with PD or HD (144). Therefore, based on HRQOL alone, subjects should not be excluded from a treatment modality simply on the basis of age.

Sex

Studies consistently demonstrate that women have a lower HRQOL than men, regardless of the renal replacement modality, and this exists even among predialysis subjects (58,61,140,145, 146). It has been suggested that much of the measured decrement in HRQOL may be related more to psychologic and social factors and depression, particularly the change in women's social role, rather than because of physical factors (12). However, when compared with men, women appear less effective at coping with the physical aspects of ESRD (147). In the Swedish trial, women treated with PD had lower scores on the SWED-QUAL index (developed from the MOS), as compared with HD.

Race

Despite the overrepresentation of racial and ethnic minorities among dialysis patients and underrepresentation among transplant patients, the adjusted mortality and HRQOL for minority participants in the ESRD program are better than for the majority population (148). Welch et al. (149) evaluated the HRQOL among 79 inner-city dialysis patients using the Wisconsin Quality of Life Index. The HRQOL was fairly high among the patients and similar to that of whites. In this cohort, psychologic and spiritual health ranked higher than physical functioning. Younger age, more education, and a lower HCT were associated with worse HRQOL. Elderly African-American patients on dialysis report better HRQOL than elderly whites (101). In Kutner's trial, the elderly whites, who had a mean age of 72, more frequently complained of nausea, fatigue, and post-dialysis inertia. They were also more likely to perceive dialysis as an intrusion to their health and diets and to be dissatisfied with their health and life, despite a lower incidence of diabetes.

When compared with whites, Asian subjects reported significantly lower HRQOL both while on dialysis and after successful transplantation (150). Analysis of the KDQOL-SF scores indicates that Asian patients, in particular, perceive kidney disease as a social burden. Of concern, minorities typically have longer waiting times for transplantation, limited referral for home dialysis, fewer native fistulas, and inadequate dialysis prescriptions. Correction of these inequities may affect positively on their HRQOL.

COMORBID CONDITIONS

As renal function declines, many patients experience fatigue, lethargy, cramps, loss of appetite, and a sense of loss of self-con-

trol. This physical deterioration is accompanied by a decline in the HRQOL (145). In the MDRD trial, the severity of symptoms correlated with a decline in HRQOL that paralleled the loss of renal function. Some patients experience an improvement in HRQOL after the initiation of dialysis, but the improvement is variable and depends on coexisting medical problems. In subjects both before and after initiation of dialysis, comorbidity strongly correlates with physical function and worse scores on the SIP (12,58). Specifically, the presence of intermittent claudication because of PVD, uncontrolled hypertension, and physical symptoms are important determinants of a poor HRQOL (57,151). Having diabetes is strongly associated with a poor HRQOL (138). Subjects who are diabetic consistently score lower in all variables of HRQOL measures, independent of age. This may be related to the multisystem involvement of diabetes mellitus (DM) and, in particular, to the neuropathy associated with DM (152). Importantly, intensive education seems to improve the HRQOL in these subjects. McMurray et al. (153) randomized 83 diabetic dialysis patients to either intensive versus standard education. The control group's risk of foot disease and amputation increased over the course of a year but was unchanged in the study group. The group receiving intensive education reported significant improvement in HRQOL indices when compared with the controls, highlighting the important benefits of intensive education and support.

DIALYSIS-RELATED FACTORS

Studies examining the effect of dialysis modality on HRQOL have yielded inconsistent results. Some trials demonstrated better satisfaction in patients on HD as compared with PD (25,55,56). In Cameron's study (55), patients on PD were less distressed and enjoyed a greater sense of well-being than patients on HD. However, criticism of this study includes significant variation in the case mix and differences in medical complications, effective dialysis, and lifestyles. Mittal et al. (154) compared 177 dialysis patients using the PCS and MCS summaries of the SF-36 over 15 months. Subjects on PD had a significantly lower PCS score than subjects on HD, despite having similar MCS scores and prevalence of depression. However, the serum albumin level was lower in subjects on PD, which may explain the decrease in PCS. In this study, the HRQOL remained stable over time. Other investigators have found that although patients on PD have a greater degree of independence, they appear to be more anxious and insecure than patients on HD (12,155).

In the NECOSAD study, the physical dimension decreased more over time in patients on PD as compared with HD. The mental dimension remained stable (156). Bakewell et al. (157) found similar results. Using the KDQOL instrument, 88 patients on PD were studied in a longitudinal manner. Male gender, Asian ethnicity, and poor nutritional status were independently associated with worse physical and mental scores. The HRQOL declined over the 2-year study period, and increased hospitalizations were associated with worse outcomes. Icodextrin has been reported to improve the HRQOL in patients on PD, but further studies are needed to substantiate this finding (158).

Other studies have evaluated the impact of Kt/V and innovative approaches to dialysis on the HRQOL. Manns et al. (159) found that patients on HD with an average Kt/V value greater than or equal to 1.3 had better HRQOL using the KDQOL-SF, SF-36, and EuroQol EQ-5D. The adjusted EQ-5D scores increased 0.036 points for each 0.1 increment in Kt/V. Patients on PD with adequate total solute clearance based on Kt/V_{urea} had a better HRQOL. This study found no significant correlation between health-related quality of life and weekly creatinine clearance (160). Uremic patients on PD with poor residual renal function may show increased HRQOL with once weekly HD added to their PD treatment (161). However, this combination requires further study. No long-term studies have demonstrated the effect of type of dialysis membrane or dialysate buffer on an individual's HRQOL. However, other methods to improve the dose of delivered dialysis have been reported to improve HRQOL. Daily dialysis and nightly home HD show promise in reducing dialysis-related symptoms and hospitalizations and in improving physical and mental well-being (162–164). Because of substantial cost and the technical support needed for these interventions, further cost-benefit analysis is needed.

NUTRITION AND PHYSICAL ACTIVITY

The importance of maintaining adequate nutrition in ESRD has been well established (see Chapter 30 for discussion). Multiple studies, although not examining nutrition directly, report an association between low albumin levels and a low HRQOL. In general, there is a significant inverse relationship between SF-36 scores and serum albumin and anemia, and negative correlation with obesity (165,166). Low albumin levels are independently associated with decreased physical function, social function, and burden of kidney disease, as assessed by the SF-36. Low protein catabolic rate is associated with decreased physical function scores and disability, as measured by the KI (167).

Many authors describe the advantages of physical exercise in improving the HRQOL. This is true both at the initiation of dialysis, when muscle deterioration begins, and throughout the course of dialytic therapy (168,169). Exercise activity independently predicts performance measures of gait speed and chair rising and perceived physical functioning (170). Interventions to improve exercise may include in-center cycling, home regimens, and rehabilitation (171,172) and should be explored for all patients.

CONCLUSION

Recognition that a patient's HRQOL is as important as morbidity and mortality has been an important advancement in caring for patients with renal disease. Measurement of HRQOL using various tools can be helpful to assess the impact of interventions on outcomes, increase patients' participation in their own care, and increase patient satisfaction (173). Improvement of anemia, malnutrition, inactivity, predialysis care, and social support systems enhance the HRQOL of dialysis patients and are associated with improved survival. Strategies aimed at these

components and in controlling blood pressure, preserving residual renal function, and assuring adequacy of dialysis will further reduce the risk of poor outcomes. In the future, telemedicine and other technologic advances may provide additional mechanisms to improve the HRQOL (174). Presently, care providers should focus on HRQOL issues and consistently measure life satisfaction at periodic intervals.

REFERENCES

1. *The American Heritage dictionary of the English language,* 3rd ed. Boston: Houghton Mifflin, 1992.
2. Constitution of the World Health Organization. *World Health Organization. Handbook of basic documents,* 5th ed. Geneva: Palais des Nations, 1952:3–20. (www.who.int/msa/qol/ql1.htm).
3. DeOreo PB. Hemodialysis patient-assessed functional health status predicts continued survival, hospitalization, and dialysis-attendance compliance. *Am J Kidney Dis* 1997;30:204–212 (UI 9261030).
4. Ifudu O, et al. Predictive value of functional status for mortality in patients on maintenance hemodialysis. *Am J Nephrol* 1998;18:109–116 (UI 9569952).
5. McClellan WM, et al. Functional status and quality of life: predictors of early mortality among patients entering treatment for end-stage renal disease. *J Clin Epidemiol* 1991;44:83–89 (UI 1986062).
6. Testa MA, et al. Assessment of quality-of-life outcomes. *N Engl J Med* 1996;334:835–840 (UI 8596551).
7. Edgell ET, et al. A review of health-related quality-of-life measures used in end-stage renal disease. *Clin Ther* 1996;18:887–938 (UI 8930432).
8. Lord FM. *Applications of item response theory to practical testing problems.* Hillsdale, NJ: Lawrence Erlbaum Associates, 1980.
9. Kimmel PL. Just whose quality of life is it anyway? Controversies and consistencies in measurement of quality of life. *Kidney Int* 2000;57:S113–S120.
10. Ware JE, et al. The RAND MOS 36-Item Short Form Health Survey (SF-36) 1.0, developed at RAND for the Medical Outcomes Study, Santa Monica, CA: RAND, 1986, 1992 (www.rand.org/health/surveys/sf36item/).
11. Clason D, et al. Analyzing data measured by individual Likert-type items. *J Agri Ed* 1994;35(4):31–35.
12. Valderrabano F, et al. Quality of life in end-stage renal disease patients. *Am J Kidney Dis* 2001;38:443–464 (UI 11532675).
13. Cagney KA, et al. Formal literature review of quality-of-life instruments used in end-stage renal disease. *Am J Kidney Dis* 2000;36:327–336 (UI 10922311).
14. Bergner M, et al. The sickness impact profile: conceptual formulation and methodology for the development of a health status measure. *Int J Health Serv* 1976;6:393–415 (UI 955750).
15. Bergner M, et al. The Sickness Impact Profile: development and final revision of a health status measure. *Med Care* 1981;19:787–805 (UI 7278416).
16. Ware JE Jr, et al. The MOS 36-item short-form health survey (SF-36). I. Conceptual framework and item selection. *Med Care* 1992;30:473–483 (UI 1593914).
17. Torrance GW. Utility approach to measuring health-related quality of life. *J Chronic Dis* 1987;40:593–603 (UI 3298297).
18. Churchill DN, et al. Measurement of quality of life in end-stage renal disease: the time trade-off approach. *Clin Invest Med* 1987;10:14–20 (UI 3545580).
19. Maor Y, et al. A comparison of three measures: the time trade-off technique, global health-related quality of life and the SF-36 in dialysis patients. *J Clin Epidemiol* 2001;54:565–570 (UI 11377116).
20. Churchill DN, et al. A comparison of evaluative indices of quality of life and cognitive function in hemodialysis patients. *Control Clin Trials* 1991;12[4 Suppl]:159S–167S (UI 1663852).
21. Keown PA. Quality of life in end-stage renal disease patients during recombinant human erythropoietin therapy. The Canadian Erythro-

poietin Study Group. *Contrib Nephrol* 1991;88:81–86; discussion 87–89 (UI 2040199).

22. Laupacis A, et al. The use of generic and specific quality-of-life measures in hemodialysis patients treated with erythropoietin. The Canadian Erythropoietin Study Group. *Control Clin Trials* 1991;12[4 Suppl]:168S–179S (UI 1663853).

23. Maltoni M, et al. Prediction of survival of patients terminally ill with cancer: results of an Italian prospective multicentric study. *Cancer* 1995;75:2613–2622 (UI 7537625).

24. Llobera J, et al. Terminal cancer: duration and prediction of survival time. *Eur J Cancer* 2000;36:2036–2043(UI 11044639).

25. Evans RW, et al. The quality of life of patients with end-stage renal disease. *N Engl J Med* 1985;312:553–559 (UI 3918267).

26. Revicki DA. Relationship between health utility and psychometric health status measures. *Med Care* 1992;30[5 Suppl]:MS274–MS282 (UI 1583939).

27. Berkman AH, et al. Sexuality and the life-style of home dialysis patients. *Arch Phys Med Rehabil* 1982;63:272–275 (UI 7082154).

28. Parfrey PS, et al. Development of a health questionnaire specific for end-stage renal disease. *Nephron* 1989;52:20–28 (UI 2651947).

29. Campbell A, et al. *The quality of American life.* New York: Russell Sage Foundation, 1976:32–60.

30. Campbell A. Subjective measures of well-being. *Am Psychol* 1976;31: 117–124 (UI 1267244).

31. Bradburn N. *The structure of psychological well-being. Two dimensions of psychological well-being: positive and negative affect.*Chicago: Aldine Publishing, 1969.

32. Beck AT, et al. An inventory for measuring depression. *Arch Gen Psychiatry* 1961;4:561–571.

33. Craven JL, et al. The Beck Depression Inventory as a screening device for major depression in renal dialysis patients. *Int J Psychiatry Med* 1988;18:365–374 (UI 3235282).

34. Silber E, et al. Self-esteem: clinical assessment and measurement validation. *Psychol Rep* 1965;16:1017–1071.

35. Wallston BS, et al. Development and validation of the health locus of control (HLC) scale. *J Consult Clin Psychol* 1976;44:580–585 (UI 939841).

36. Rotter JB. Generalized expectancies for internal versus external control of reinforcement. *Psychol Monogr* 1966;80:1–28 (UI 5340840).

37. Rotter JB. *The development and applications of social learning theory.* New York: Praeger, 1982.

38. Craig AR, et al. A scale to measure locus of control of behaviour. *Br J Med Psychol* 1984;57(Pt 2):173–180 (UI 6743598).

39. Devins GM, et al. The emotional impact of end-stage renal disease: importance of patients' perception of intrusiveness and control. *Int J Psychiatry Med* 1983–84;13:327–343 (UI 6671863).

40. Devins GM, et al. Psychosocial impact of illness intrusiveness moderated by self-concept and age in end-stage renal disease. *Health Psychol* 1997;16:529–538 (UI 9386998).

41. Devins GM, et al. Structure of lifestyle disruptions in chronic disease: a confirmatory factor analysis of the Illness Intrusiveness Ratings Scale. *Med Care* 2001;39:1097–1104 (UI 11567172).

42. Devins GM, et al. Illness intrusiveness and quality of life in end-stage renal disease: comparison and stability across treatment modalities. *Health Psychol* 1990;9:117–142 (UI 2331973).

43. Kaplan De-Nour A. Psychosocial adjustment To Illness Scale (PAIS): a study of chronic hemodialysis patients. *J Psychosom Res* 1982;26: 11–22 (7038108).

44. Kaplan De-Nour A. Renal replacement therapies. In: Spilker B, ed. *Quality of life assessments in clinical trials.* New York: Raven Press, 1990:381–389.

45. Laupacis A, et al. A disease-specific questionnaire for assessing quality of life in patients on hemodialysis. *Nephron* 1992;60:302–306 (UI 1565182).

46. Hays RD, et al. Development of the kidney disease quality of life (KDQOL) instrument. *Qual Life Res* 1994;3:329–338 (UI 7841967).

47. Wu AW, et al. Developing a health-related quality-of-life measure for end-stage renal disease: the CHOICE Health Experience Questionnaire. *Am J Kidney Dis* 2001;37:11–21. (UI 11136162).

48. Canadian Erythropoietin Study Group. Association between recombinant human erythropoietin and quality of life and exercise capacity of patients receiving haemodialysis. Canadian Erythropoietin Study Group. *BMJ* 1990;300:573–578 (UI 2108751).

49. Rao S, et al. Development of subscales from the symptoms/problems and effects of kidney disease scales of the kidney disease quality of life instrument. *Clin Ther* 2000;22:1099–1111 (UI 11048907).

50. Korevaar JC, et al. Validation of the KDQOL-SF: a dialysis-targeted health measure. *Qual Life Res* 2002;11:437–447 (UI 12113391).

51. Neff MS. To be or not to be: the decision to withdraw or be withdrawn from dialysis. *Am J Kidney Dis* 1999;33:601–606 (UI 10070928).

52. Cohen LM, et al. Dying well after discontinuing the life-support treatment of dialysis. *Arch Intern Med* 2000;160:2513–2518 (UI 10979064).

53. Cohen LM, et al. A very good death: measuring quality of dying in end-stage renal disease. *J Palliat Med* 2001;4:167–172 (UI 11441625).

54. Health Care Financing Review/Fall 2000;22(1):55–60.

55. Cameron JI, et al. Differences in quality of life across renal replacement therapies: a meta-analytic comparison. *Am J Kidney Dis* 2000;35:629–637 (10739783).

56. Bremer BA, et al. Quality of life in end-stage renal disease: a reexamination. *Am J Kidney Dis* 1989;13:200–209 (2493190).

57. Mingardi G, et al. Health-related quality of life in dialysis patients: a report from an Italian study using the SF-36 Health Survey. DIA-QOL Group. *Nephrol Dial Transplant* 1999;14:1503–1510 (10383015).

58. Moreno F, et al. Quality of life in dialysis patients: a Spanish multicentre study. *Nephrol Dial Transplant* 1996;[Suppl 2]:11:S125–S129 (UI 8804012).

59. Mozes B, et al. Differences in quality of life among patients receiving dialysis replacement therapy at seven medical centers. *J Clin Epidemiol* 1997;50:1035–1043 (9363038).

60. Molzahn AE, et al. Quality of life of individuals with end-stage renal disease: perceptions of patients, nurses, and physicians. *ANNA J* 1997;24:325–333 ,discussion 334–335 (9238904).

61. Mingardi G. Quality of life and end-stage renal disease therapeutic programs. DIA-QOL Group. Dialysis quality of life. *Int J Artif Organs* 1998;21:741–747 (9894753).

62. Mapes DL, et al. Quality of life predicts mortality and hospitalization for hemodialysis patients in the U.S. and Europe. *J Am Soc Nephrol* 1999;10:249(abstr).

63. Parkerson GR Jr, et al. Health-related quality of life predictors of survival and hospital utilization. *Health Care Financ Rev* 2000;21(3): 171–184 (11481754).

64. Merkus MP, et al. Quality of life in patients on dialysis: self-assessment 3 months after the start of treatment. *Am J Kidney Dis* 1997; 29:584–592.

65. White CA, et al. Pre-dialysis clinic attendance improves quality of life among hemodialysis patients. *BMC Nephrol* 2002;3:3.

66. Binik YM, et al. Live and learn: patient education delays the need to initiate renal replacement therapy in end-stage renal disease. *J Nerv Ment Dis* 1993;181:371–376.

67. NIH consensus statement: Morbidity and mortality of dialysis. *Ann Intern Med* 1994;121:62–70.

68. Klang B, et al. Predialysis education helps patients choose dialysis modality and increases disease-specific knowledge. *J Adv Nurs* 1999, 29:869–876.

69. Ahlem J, et al. Well-informed patients with end-stage renal disease prefer peritoneal dialysis to hemodialysis. *Perit Dial Int* 1993;12 [Suppl 2]:S196–S198.

70. Revicki DA, et al. Health-related quality of life associated with recombinant human erythropoietin therapy for pre-dialysis chronic renal disease patients. *Am J Kidney Dis* 1995,25:548–554.

71. Sesso R, et al. Time of diagnosis of chronic renal failure and assessment of quality of life in hemodialysis patients. *Nephrol Dial Transplant* 1997;12:2111–2115.

72. Arora P, et al. Prevalence, predictors and consequences of late nephrology referral at a tertiary care center. *J Am Soc Nephrol* 1999;10: 1281–1286.

73. Obrador GT, et al. Early referral to the nephrologist and timely initiation on renal replacement therapy: a paradigm shift in the management of patients with chronic renal failure. *Am J Kidney Dis* 1998; 31:398–417.

74. Holland DC, et al. Sub-optimal dialysis initiation in a retrospective cohort of predialysis patients. *Scand J Urol Nephrol* 2000;34:341–347.

75. Eknoyan G, et al. Clinical practice guidelines: final guideline summaries from the work groups of the National Kidney Foundation–Dialysis Outcomes Quality Initiative. New York: National Kidney Foundation, 1997.

76. Korevaar JC, et al. Evaluation of DOQI guidelines: early start of dialysis treatment is not associated with better health-related quality of life. National Kidney Foundation–Dialysis Outcomes Quality Initiative. *Am J Kidney Dis* 2002;39:108–115 (11774109).

77. Korevaar JC, et al. Quality of life in pre-dialysis end-stage renal disease patients at the initiation of dialysis therapy. The NECOSAD Study Group. *Perit Dial Int* 2000;20:69–75.

78. *Diagnostic and statistical manual of mental disorders,* 4th ed. Washington, DC: American Psychiatric Association, 2000.

79. Han SY, et al. Insomnia in diabetic hemodialysis patients: prevalence and risk factors by a multicenter study. *Nephron* 2002;92:127–132.

80. Williams SW, et al. Correlates of sleep behavior among hemodialysis patients: the kidney outcomes prediction and evaluation (KOPE) study. *Am J Nephrol* 2002;22:18–28 (11919399).

81. Walker S, et al. Sleep complaints are common in a dialysis unit. *Am J Kidney Dis* 1995;26:751–756.

82. Holley JL, et al. A comparison of reported sleep disturbances in patients on chronic hemodialysis and continuous peritoneal dialysis. *Am J Kidney Dis* 1992;19:156–161.

83. Soldatos C, et al. Cigarette smoking associated with sleep difficulty. *Science* 1980;207:551–553.

84. Evans RW. The quality of life of hemodialysis recipients treated with recombinant human erythropoietin. *JAMA* 1990;263:825–830.

85. Levin NW. Quality of life and hematocrit level. *Am J Kid Dis* 1992;[Suppl 1]:16–20.

86. Benz RL, et al. A preliminary study of the effects of correction of anemia with recombinant human erythropoietin therapy on sleep, sleep disorders, and daytime sleepiness in hemodialysis patients (The SLEEPO Study). *Am J Kidney Dis* 1999;34:1089–1095.

87. Salva P, et al. Clinical pharmacokinetics and pharmacodynamics of zolpidem: therapeutic implications. *Clin Pharmacokinetics* 1995;29: 142–153.

88. Kimmel PL, et al. Sleep apnea syndrome in chronic renal dialysis. *Am J Med* 1989;86:308–314.

89. Partinen M, et al. Long-term outcome for obstructive sleep apnea syndrome patients. *Chest* 1988;94:1200–1204.

90. Sanner BM, et al. Sleep-related breathing disorders impair quality of life in haemodialysis recipients. *Nephrol Dial Transplant* 2002;17: 1260–1265 (12105250).

91. Fletcher EC. Obstructive sleep apnea and the kidney. *J Am Soc Nephrol* 1993;4:1111–1121.

92. Hallett MD, et al. Sleep apnea in end-stage renal disease patients on hemodialysis and continuous ambulatory peritoneal dialysis. *ASAIO J* 1995;41:M435–M441.

93. Winkelman JW, et al. Restless legs syndrome in end-stage renal disease. *Am J Kidney Dis* 1996;28:372–378.

94. Trenkwalder C, et al. Electrophysiologic pattern of involuntary limb movements in the restless leg syndrome. *Muscle Nerve* 1996;19:155.

95. McGee SR. Muscle cramps. *Arch Intern Med* 1990;150:511.

96. Trenkwalder C, et al. L-dopa therapy of uremic and idiopathic restless legs syndrome: a double blind, cross over trial. *Sleep* 1995;18: 681–688.

97. Serrao M, et al. Gabapentin treatment for muscle cramps: an open-label trial. *Clin Neuropharmacol* 2000;23:45.

98. Thorp ML, et al. A crossover study of gabapentin in the treatment of restless legs syndrome among hemodialysis patients. *Am J Kidney Dis* 2001;38:104–108.

99. Kimmel PL. Psychosocial factors in adult end-stage renal disease patients treated with hemodialysis: correlates and outcomes. *Am J Kidney Dis* 2000;35[4 Suppl 1]:S132–S140 (10766011).

100. Boyer CB, et al. Social support and demographic factors influencing compliance of hemodialysis patients. *J Appl Soc Psychol* 1990;20: 1902–1918.

101. Kutner NG, et al. A comparison of the quality of life reported by elderly whites and elderly blacks on dialysis. *Geriatr Nephrol Urol* 1998;8:77–83.

102. Christensen AJ, et al. Predictors of survival among hemodialysis patients: effect of perceived family support. *Health Psychol* 1994;13: 521–525.

103. McClellan WM, et al. Social support and subsequent mortality among patients with end-stage renal disease. *J Am Soc Nephrol* 1993;4:1028–1034.

104. Blake C, et al. Physical function, employment and quality of life in end-stage renal disease. *J Nephrol* 2000;13:142–149.

105. Lamping DL, et al. Hemodialysis compliance: assessment, prediction and intervention: part II. *Semin Dial* 1990;3:105–111.

106. Brown J, et al. Factors influencing compliance with dietary restrictions in dialysis patients. *J Psychosom Res* 1988;32:191–196.

107. Cantor MH. Strain among caregivers: a study of the experiences in the United States. *Gerontologist* 1983;23:597–618.

108. Schultz R, et al. Psychiatric and physical morbidity effects of dementia caregiving: prevalence, correlates, and causes. *Gerontologist* 1995; 35:771–775.

109. Belasco AG, et al. Burden and quality of life of caregivers for hemodialysis patients. *Am J Kidney Dis* 2002;39:805–812.

110. Lindqvist R, et al. Coping strategies and health-related quality of life among spouses of continuous ambulatory peritoneal dialysis, haemodialysis, and transplant patients. *J Adv Nurs* 2000;31: 1398–1408 (10849152).

111. Wicks MN, et al. Subjective burden and quality of life in family caregivers of patients with end-stage renal disease. *ANNA J* 1997;24: 531–538.

112. Pelletier-Hibbert M, et al. Sources of uncertainty and coping strategies used by family members of individuals living with end-stage renal disease. *Nephrol Nurs J* 2001;28:4117–4417.

113. Evans RW. Recombinant human erythropoietin and the quality of life of end-stage renal disease patients: a comparative analysis. *Am J Kidney Dis* 1991;18[4 Suppl 1]:62–70 (1928082).

114. Delano BG. Improvements in quality of life following treatment with r-HuEPO in anemic hemodialysis patients. *Am J Kidney Dis* 1989; 14:14–18.

115. Auer J, et al. Quality of life improvements in CAPD patients treated with subcutaneously administered erythropoietin for anemia. *Perit Dial Int* 1992;12:40–42.

116. Guthrie M, et al. Effects of erythropoietin on strength and functional status of patients on hemodialysis. *Clin Nephrol* 1993;39:97–102 (8448925).

117. Mayer G, et al. Working capacity is increased following recombinant human erythropoietin treatment. *Kidney Int* 1988;34:525-528 (3199672).

118. Bennet WM. A multicenter clinical trial of epoetin beta for anemia of end-stage renal failure. *J Am Soc Nephrol* 1991;1:1990–1998.

119. Beusterein LM, et al. The effects of recombinant human erythropoietin on functional health and well being in chronic dialysis patients. *J Am Soc Nephrol* 1996;7:763–773.

120. Moreno E, et al. Influence of hematocrit on the quality of life of hemodialysis patients. *Nephrol Dial Transplant* 1994;9:1034–1037.

121. Lim VS. Recombinant human erythropoietin in predialysis patients. *Am J Kidney Dis* 1991;18[Suppl]:34–37.

122. U.S. Recombinant Human Erythropoietin Predialysis Group. Double-blind, placebo controlled study of the therapeutic use of recombinant human erythropoietin for anemia associated with chronic renal failure in predialysis patients. *Am J Kidney Dis* 1991;14:50–59.

123. Drueke TB, et al. Does early anemia correction prevent complications of chronic renal failure? *Clin Nephrol* 1999;51:1–11 (9988140).

124. Bedani PL, et al. Erythropoietin and cardiocirculatory condition in aged patients with chronic renal failure. *Nephron* 2001;89:350–353.

125. McMahon LP, et al. Effects of haemoglobin normalization on quality of life and cardiovascular parameters in end-stage renal failure. *Nephrol Dial Transplant* 2000;15:1425–1430 (10978402).

126. Valderrabano F. Quality of life benefits of early anaemia treatment. *Nephrol Dial Transplant* 2000;15[Suppl 3]:23–28 (11032354).

127. Valderrabano F, et al. European Best Practice Guidelines 1-4. Evaluating anaemia and initiating treatment. *Nephrol Dial Transplant* 2000;15:S8–S14.

128. Moreno F, et al. Controlled study on the improvement of quality of life in elderly hemodialysis patients after correcting end-stage related anemia with erythropoietin. *Am J Kidney Dis* 1996;27:548–556.

129. Eschbach JW, et al. Normalizing the hematocrit in hemodialysis patients improves quality of life and is safe. *J Am Soc Nephrol* 1993;4:445(abst).

130. Moreno F, et al. Increasing the hematocrit has a beneficial effect on quality of life and is safe in selected hemodialysis patients. Spanish Cooperative Renal Patients Quality of Life Study Group of the Spanish Society of Nephrology. *J Am Soc Nephrol* 2000;11:335-342 (10665941).

131. Besarab A, et al. The effects of normal as compared with low hematocrit values in patients with cardiac disease who are receiving hemodialysis and epoetin. *N Engl J Med* 1998;339:584–590 (9718377).

132. Finkelstein FO, et al. Depression in chronic dialysis patients: assessment and treatment. *Nephrol Dial Transplant* 2000;15:1911–1913.

133. Kimmel PL, et al. Multiple measurements of depression predict mortality in a longitudinal study of urban hemodialysis patients. *Kidney Int* 2000;57:2093–2098.

134. Tsay SL, et al. Self-care-efficacy, depression, and the quality of life among patients receiving hemodialysis in Taiwan. *Int J Nurs Stud* 2002;39:245–251.

135. Kovac JA, et al. Patient satisfaction with care and behavioral compliance in end-stage renal disease patients treated with hemodialysis. *Am J Kidney Dis* 2002;39:1236–1244 (12046037).

136. Zimmermann PR, et al. Depression, anxiety and adjustment in renal replacement therapy: a quality of life assessment. *Clin Nephrol* 2001; 56:387–390.

137. Kimmel PL. Psychosocial factors in dialysis patients. *Kidney Int* 2001;59:1599–1613.

138. Baiardi F, et al. Effects of clinical and individual variables on quality of life in chronic renal failure patients. *J Nephrol* 2002;15:61–67.

139. Rebollo P, et al. Is the loss of health-related quality of life during renal replacement therapy lower in elderly patients than in younger patients? *Nephrol Dial Transplant* 2001;16:1675–1680 (11477173).

140. Rebollo P, et al. Health-related quality of life in end-stage renal disease (ESRD) patients over 65 years. *Geriatr Nephrol Urol* 1998;8: 85–94.

141. Lamping DL, et al. Clinical outcomes, quality of life, and costs in the North Thames Dialysis Study of elderly people on dialysis: a prospective cohort study. *Lancet* 2000;356:1543–1550 (1075766).

142. Kutner NG, et al. Quality of life and rehabilitation of elderly dialysis patients. *Semin Dial* 2002;15:107–112.

143. Trbojevic JB, et al. Quality of life of elderly patients undergoing continuous ambulatory peritoneal dialysis. *Perit Dial Int* 2001;21 [Suppl]3:S300–S303.

144. Harris SA, et al. Clinical outcomes and quality of life in elderly patients on peritoneal dialysis versus hemodialysis. *Perit Dial Int* 2002;22:463–470.

145. Rocco MV, et al. Cross-sectional study of quality of life and symptoms in chronic renal disease patients. The Modification of Diet in Renal Disease Study. *Am J Kidney Dis* 1997;32:557–566.

146. Simmons RG, et al. Quality of life issues for end-stage renal disease patients. *Am J Kidney Dis* 1990;15:201–208.

147. Lindqvist R, et al. Coping strategies and quality of life among patients on hemodialysis and continuous ambulatory peritoneal dialysis. *Scand J Caring Sci* 1998;12:223–230.

148. Redden DN, et al. Racial inequities in America's ESRD program. *Semin Dial* 2000;13:399–403.

149. Welch JL, et al. Quality of life in black hemodialysis patients. *Adv Ren Replace Ther* 1999;6:351–357.

150. Bakewell AB, et al. Does ethnicity influence perceived quality of life of patients on dialysis and following renal transplant? *Nephrol Dial Transplant* 2001;16:1395–1401 (11427631).

151. Merkus MP, et al. Physical symptoms and quality of life in patients on chronic dialysis: results of the Netherlands Cooperative Study on Adequacy of Dialysis (NECOSAD). *Nephrol Dial Transplant* 1999; 14:1163–1170.

152. Apostolou T, et al. Neuropathy and quality of life in diabetic continuous ambulatory peritoneal dialysis patients. *Perit Dial Int* 1999;19:S242–S247.

153. McMurray SD, et al. Diabetes education and care management significantly improve patient outcomes in the dialysis unit. *Am J Kidney Dis* 2002;40:566–575.

154. Mittal SK, et al. Self-assessed quality of life in peritoneal dialysis patients. *Am J Nephrol* 2001;21:215–220 (11423691).

155. Maiorca R, et al. Psychological and social problems of dialysis. *Nephrol Dial Transplant* 1997;13:S89–S95.

156. Merkus MP, et al. Quality of life over time in dialysis: The Netherlands Cooperative Study on the Adequacy of Dialysis. NECOSAD Study. *Kidney Int* 1999;56:720–728.

157. Bakewell AB, et al. Quality of life in peritoneal dialysis patients: decline over time and association with clinical outcomes. *Kidney Int* 2002;61:239-248 (11786106).

158. Guo A, et al. Early quality of life benefits of icodextrin in peritoneal dialysis. *Kidney Int Suppl* 2002;81:72–79.

159. Manns BJ, et al. Dialysis adequacy and health related quality of life in hemodialysis patients. *ASAIO* 2002;48:565–569.

160. Chen YC, et al. Relationship between dialysis adequacy and quality of life in long-term peritoneal dialysis patients. *Perit Dial Int* 2000; 20:534–540.

161. Hashimoto Y, et al. Combined peritoneal dialysis and hemodialysis therapy improves quality of life in end-stage renal disease patients. *Adv Perit Dial* 2000;16:108–112.

162. Mohr PE, et al. The case for daily dialysis: its impact on costs and quality of life *Am J Kidney Dis* 2001;37:777–789 (11273878).

163. McPhatter LL, et al. Nightly home hemodialysis: improvement in nutrition and quality of life. *Adv Ren Replace Ther* 1999;6:358–365.

164. Kooistra MP, et al. Daily home hemodialysis in The Netherlands: Effects on metabolic control, hemodynamics and quality of life. *Nephrol Dial Transplant* 1998;13:2853–2860.

165. Kalantar-Zadeh L, et al. Association among SF36 quality of life measures and nutrition, hospitalization, and mortality in hemodialysis. *J Am Soc Nephrol* 2001;12:2979–2806.

166. Shield CH. The impact of nutrition and fitness on quality of life. *Nephrol News Issues* 2002;16:52–55.

167. Ohri-Vachaspati P, et al. Quality of life implications of inadequate protein nutrition among hemodialysis patients. *J Ren Nutr* 1999;9:9–13.

168. Iborra MC, et al. Quality of life and exercise in renal disease. *EDTNA ERCA J* 2000;26:38–40.

169. Brodin E, et al. Physical activity, muscle performance and quality of life in patients treated with chronic peritoneal dialysis. *Scand J Urol Nephrol* 2001;35:71–78.

170. Kutner NG, et al. Patient-reported quality of life early in dialysis treatment: effects associated with usual exercise activity. *Nephrol Nurs J* 2000;27:357–367.

171. Painter P, et al. Physical functioning and health related quality of life changes with exercise training in hemodialysis patients. *Am J Kidney Dis* 2000;35:482–492.

172. Curtin RB, et al. Renal rehabilitation and improved patient outcomes in Texas dialysis facilities. *Am J Kidney Dis* 2002;40:331–338.

173. Callahan MB. Using quality of life measurement to enhance interdisciplinary collaboration. *Adv Ren Replace Ther* 2001;8:148–151.

174. Stroemann KA, et al. Improving quality of life for dialysis patients through telecare. *J Telemed Telecare* 2000;6:S80–S83.

EXTRACORPOREAL METHODS IN THE TREATMENT OF POISONING

SRIVASA B. CHEBROLU, TODD S. ING, AND SERAFINO GARELLA

EXTRACORPOREAL METHODS IN THE TREATMENT OF POISONING

In 2001, the Toxic Exposure Surveillance System (TESS) data compiled by the American Association of Poison Control Centers (AAPCC) revealed that there were 2,267,979 reported human poison exposure cases and 1,074 deaths in the United States (1). Because most poisoning fatalities occur before the patients reach a health care facility, it is probable that the total number of fatalities resulting from poisoning is higher than that gathered by the AAPCC report.

In this chapter we do not propose to review the entire topic of what constitutes appropriate treatment of the patient with poisoning or overdose. It is now well recognized that the most important advance in such treatment lies in providing attentive supportive care—ensuring adequate respiration; supporting hemodynamic status; and promoting maintenance of fluid, electrolyte, and acid-base balance—which by itself has been shown to reduce mortality and morbidity to very low levels (2–4). The recognition of the predominant role of supportive care in the treatment of poisoning has led to the abandonment of the use of stimulants (when the intoxicant is a sedative) and has reduced the emphasis on the use of antidotes, except in a few special types of intoxications for which specific antidotes are available (Table 38.1). Even the use of "forced diuresis" requiring the administration of large fluid loads coupled with a diuretic agent, which enjoyed some popularity because of the belief that it would accelerate the elimination of most intoxicants, is now recognized to be helpful only when the poisoning is due to agents that can be rapidly excreted unchanged by the kidney (e.g., amphetamines, long-acting barbiturates, bromide salts). Gastric lavage, once a mainstay of therapy, has been questioned as an inappropriate technique that may increase rather than reduce absorption at times and must be used selectively (5–7).

Other maneuvers such as alkalinization of the extracellular fluid and/or of the urine are also employed in special circumstances. For example, alkalinization of the extracellular fluid is carried out in tricyclic antidepressant poisoning (to diminish cardiac arrhythmias) (8). Alkalinization of the urine (should there be any urinary output) is useful in poisonings resulting from weakly acidic substances (whose anions include salicylates and long-acting barbiturates) that are eliminated in the urine and whose excretion is enhanced by increased ionization within the tubular lumen as a result of an alkaline urine pH.

One maneuver that has survived the test of time is the administration by mouth or by nasogastric intubation of substances that can nonspecifically adsorb toxins present in the gastrointestinal tract. Activated charcoal is the best known of these sorbents (9). This agent is often administered even before the identity of the intoxicating agent is known because of its capacity to bind a wide variety of toxins. One exception to this practice is when considering the use of N-acetylcysteine for acetaminophen poisoning, in which case activated charcoal may bind the N-acetylcysteine and render the administration of charcoal useless. In general, however, by virtue of interrupting the toxin's enterohepatic circulation, activated charcoal is effective even when the toxin is no longer present in the stomach or, as in the case of theophylline, when the toxin has been given parenterally.

Another means of enhancing toxin elimination that has received substantial attention in the last 30 years involves techniques of extracting intoxicating substances directly from the bloodstream. The rationale for the application of such techniques in the treatment of acute intoxication and the review of those relatively few intoxications that have been shown to be positively affected by extracorporeal means to enhance toxin elimination are the focus of this chapter.

EXTRACORPOREAL METHODS OF DETOXIFICATION

The development of techniques that made access to high blood flow rates feasible spawned the notion that active removal of toxins from the circulating blood would markedly reduce the duration, morbidity, and mortality associated with poisoning and overdose. This notion has obvious intrinsic appeal; consequently, a large body of work has emerged in this area since the late 1940s, work consisting of theoretical considerations, in vitro and in vivo laboratory studies, and clinical observations ranging from large case series to anecdotal reports. An array of methods has been proposed and studied, both singly and in combination: hemodialysis with aqueous dialysate, hemodialysis with lipid dialysate, hemofiltration, hemodiafiltration, peritoneal dialysis, continuous renal replacement therapies

TABLE 38.1. COMMON EMERGENCY ANTIDOTES[a]

Poison	Antidote	Adult Dosage	Mechanism/Comment
Acetaminophen	N-acetylcysteine	140 mg/kg initial oral dose, followed by 70 mg/kg q 4 hr for 17 doses	Most effective within 16 hr; may be useful up to 24 hr; IV N-acetylcysteine protocols available
Atropine	Physostigmine	Initial dose: 0.5–2 mg (IV); children: 0.02 mg/kg	Cholinesterase inhibitor that antagonizes central and peripheral nervous system effects; may cause convulsions, bradycardia, and asystole
Benzodiazepines	Flumazenil	0.2 mg (2 mL) (IV) over 15 sec repeat 0.2 mg (IV) every minute as necessary; initial dose not to exceed 1 mg	Recommended only for reversal of pure benzodiazepine sedation
β-Blockers	Glucagon	1 mg/mL ampoule; 5–10 mL (IV) initially	Stimulates cyclic adenosine monophosphate synthesis; increases myocardial contractility
Calcium channel blockers	Calcium	Calcium chloride 10% 1 g (10 mL) (IV) over 5 min as initial dose; repeat as necessary in critical patients	Each syringe contains 1 g or 10 mL of 10% calcium chloride; each milliliter contains 100 mg of calcium chloride or 1.4 mEq of calcium; used for hypotension, bradyarrhythmias
Carbon monoxide	Oxygen	Hyperbaric oxygen in critical patients	
Cyanide	Amyl nitrate	Pearls every 2 min	
	Sodium thiosulfate	25% solution 50 mL (IV) over 10 min; 1.65 mL/kg for children	Forms harmless sodium thiocyanate
	Sodium nitrite	10 mL of 3% solution over 3 min (IV); 0.33 mL (10 mL 3% solution)/kg initially for children	Methemoglobin-cyanide complex causes hypotension; dosage assumes normal hemoglobin
Digitalis	Digibind FAB antibodies (antigen-binding fragments)	IV dose of Digibind in critical patients with unknown ingestion; 800 mg (20 vials); dosage if serum digoxin and patient's weight (in kg) are known: the number of vials to administer = [concentration (in ng/mL) × 5.6 × kg]/600	IV dose of Digibind should be equimolar to total body load of digoxin; one vial of Digibind contains 40 mg of FAB fragments, which neutralize 0.6 mg of digoxin; the number of mg of digoxin ingested divided by 0.6 is the number of vials required; indicated for life-threatening cardiac arrhythmias, hyperkalemia, serum digoxin level >10 ng/mL in adults or 4 ng/mL in children
Hydrofluoric acid	Calcium	Calcium gluconate gel or calcium carbonate paste; 10% calcium gluconate 10 mL in 40 mL D5W via intraarterial infusion over 4 hr may be indicated for significant digital hydrofluoric acid burns	An intraarterial infusion of 10 mL 10% calcium gluconate (1 syringe) provides 4.65 mEq (84 mg) of elemental calcium to bind fluoride ion, preventing cellular injury and tissue necrosis
Iron	Deferoxamine	Initial dose: 40–90 mg/kg (IM), not to exceed 1 g; 15 mg/kg/hr (IV)	Deferoxamine mesylate forms renally excretable ferrioxamine complex; IV route to be used in patients with shock
Lead	Dimercaptosuccinic acid (succimer)	5-day course of 30 mg/kg/d in 3 divided doses; then 14-day course of 20 mg/kg/d divided in 2 doses	Succimer 100-mg capsule; oral congener of chelator dimercaprol, indicated for blood lead levels >45 μg/dL
Mercury, arsenic, gold	Dimercaprol	5 mg/kg (IM) as soon as possible	Each mL of dimercaprol-in-oil has dimercaprol, 100 mg, in 210 mg (21%) benzyl benzoate and 680 mg peanut oil; forms stable, nontoxic, excretable cyclic compound
Methyl alcohol, ethylene glycol	Ethyl alcohol, fomepizole	See text	See text
Nitrites	Methylene blue	0.2 mL/kg of 1% solution (IV) over 5 min	Accelerates methemoglobin reductase system; often, exchange transfusion is needed for severe methemoblobinemia
Opiates, propoxyphene, diphenoxylate	Naloxone	2.0 mg (IV); 0.1 mg/kg (IV) for children; repeat as needed	Antagonizes opiates via its higher affinity for some receptors; naloxone has no respiratory depression (0.4 mg/1 mL amp)
Organophosphates	Pralidoxime [2-PAM], (protopam chloride)	Initial dose: 1 g (IV); children: 25–50 mg/kg (IV)	Breaks alkyl phosphate-cholinesterase bond and reactivates cholinesterase; up to 500 mg every hour may be necessary in the critical adult patient
Tricyclic antidepressants	Sodium bicarbonate	Sodium bicarbonate 1–2 ampules (IV); (1 mEq/kg) (IV) bolus for initial dose: (IV) drip to maintain arterial pH of 7.5	One ampule of 50 mL sodium bicarbonate contains 50 mEq NaHCO3, in 50 mL or 1 molar sodium bicarbonate; IV bolus for life-threatening cardiac arrhythmias

[a]Note that in most cases the use of a specific antidote is at best only *partial* therapy, because it may antagonize only one or some toxic effects of poison. Adjunctive therapy and usual supportive measures must be employed with antidotal treatment. Modified and adapted from Haddad LM. Acute poisoning. In: Goldman L, Bennett JC, eds. *Cecil textbook of medicine,* 21st ed. Philadelphia: WB Saunders, 2000:515–524.

(CRRTs), charcoal hemoperfusion, resin hemoperfusion, plasma exchange, and exchange blood transfusion:

- Hemodialysis. This technique is based mainly on the principle of diffusion. Because small solutes exhibit random molecular motion to a greater extent than larger solutes, the former solutes can diffuse through the semipermeable membrane more readily than the latter. Hence, the efficiency of dialysis in drug removal is inversely related, other things being equal, to the molecular size of the drug involved.

- Hemofiltration. This process involves the removal of an ultrafiltrate from the blood through the semipermeable membrane of a dialyzer/ultrafilter accompanied by the simultaneous, appropriate replacement (usually volume for volume; but appropriate adjustments must be made in the face of dehydration or overhydration) of a plasma-resembling fluid. The efficiency of the procedure is related to the total volume so exchanged. Ultrafiltration is based on the principle of convection, and ultrafiltrates are obtained by the application of a transmembrane pressure gradient. For all solutes that manage to pass through the pores of a semipermeable membrane, the relatively larger solutes and their smaller counterparts all pass through the membrane at the same rate (10).

- Hemodiafiltration. This technique consists of the performance of hemodialysis and hemofiltration at the same time using the same dialyzer/ultrafilter. The procedure is more efficient than either hemodialysis or hemofiltration alone in the removal of poisons that are small enough to pass through a semipermeable membrane (10,11).

- CRRTs (see Chapter 13). (a) Continuous arteriovenous hemodialysis (CAVHD) or continuous venovenous hemodialysis (CVVHD), (b) continuous arteriovenous hemofiltration (CAVH) or continuous venovenous hemofiltration (CVVH), and (c) continuous arteriovenous hemodiafiltration (CAVHDF) or continuous venovenous hemodiafiltration (CVVHDF). These continuous therapies can serve as adjunctive therapeutic measures to augment toxin removal or as primary therapeutic modalities when hemodynamic instability militates against the use of conventional hemodialysis, hemofiltration, or hemodiafiltration (12). CRRT has been proposed as effective in the removal of tissue-bound substances such as paraquat, in which the offending agent is released slowly from its reservoir and associated with the occurrence of a "rebound phenomenon" (13,14). However, in most circumstances, the amount of drug removed is hampered by the slowness of conventional slow CRRT therapies. In this regard, it should be noted that high-efficiency CRRTs have also recently been described.

- Peritoneal dialysis. Peritoneal dialysis does not result in a noticeable enhancement of drug removal over and above that provided by the native kidneys and is, therefore, employed in the poisoned patient only in the presence of significant renal functional impairment. Because of its slow efficiency per unit time, peritoneal dialysis is seldom used in the treatment of poisoning except in circumstances under which other more efficient extracorporeal therapies are not available or cannot be performed. Peritoneal dialysis can, however, be used as an adjunctive therapy to other extracorporeal modalities.

- Plasma exchange, exchange blood transfusion. These procedures are not usually effective in the treatment of poisoning, because of the limitations on the amount of plasma or of blood that can be exchanged, especially in the case of toxins with large volumes of distribution (15).

- Hemoperfusion. This method involves the use of a cartridge packed with activated charcoal (coated with a thin, relatively porous semipermeable membrane) through which blood is passed. Adsorption occurs because of the hydrophobic properties of charcoal. Hemoperfusion using nonionic resins [e.g., polystyrene copolymer resin (Amberlite XAD-2)] were developed in an effort to increase the removal of lipid-soluble intoxicants (16). The total amount of drug removed is usually small and is not of great clinical consequence. Hemoperfusion devices using resin as the sorbent are no longer available in the United States but are still being used in many other parts of the world.

- Albumin dialysis. Selective removal of albumin-bound substances can be achieved in a high-flux dialysis setting by the enrichment of dialysate with human albumin that functions as a molecular adsorbent. The albumin-enriched dialysate is then recirculated over sorbents (molecular adsorbent recirculating system). This novel dialytic approach enables removal of excess water and water-soluble substances as well (17). Holding promise for removal of protein-bound toxins, this technique has been used successfully in anecdotal reports for the treatment of poisoning resulting from acetaminophen and cytotoxic mushrooms in the presence or absence of concomitant renal insufficiency (18,19).

- Sustained low-efficiency dialysis (SLED). This is a new technique that allows the use of conventional machines to perform slow, low-efficiency hemodialysis (20). Conventional hemodialyzers are used with a slower than normal dialyzer blood-flow rate of 200 mL/min and a slower than normal dialysate flow rate of 100 mL/min. Each treatment can last up to 10 to 12 hours everyday. The relatively long treatment duration compensates for the low efficiency of the procedure. Because of the slow blood and dialysate flow rates, it is better tolerated by critically ill patients with hemodynamic instability (21). The procedure can be carried out during the daytime when problems with the dialysis run can be handled by the more readily available daytime health care personnel. It is conceivable that this method may serve as an adjunctive approach to conventional extracorporeal measures in the treatment of poisoning.

According to the AAPCC report for 2001 (1), hemodialysis was employed in 1,280 instances and hemoperfusion in 45 instances of poisoning, demonstrating the continued, although relatively infrequent, clinical use of these extracorporeal means of toxin removal.

Hemodialysis versus Hemoperfusion in Drug Removal

Table 38.2 lists the factors to be weighed when considering hemodialysis versus hemoperfusion as a treatment modality. At present, insufficient data are available to compare the results of hemoperfusion with those of the other extracorporeal modalities using either high-flux or low-flux membranes.

TABLE 38.2. FACTORS TO BE CONSIDERED WHEN CHOOSING BETWEEN HEMODIALYSIS (HD) AND HEMOPERFUSION (HP)

Toxin characteristics	
Low molecular weight	HD
High molecular weight	HP
Water solubility	HD
Lipid solubility	HP
Low protein-binding	HD
High protein-binding	HP
Patient characteristics	
Presence of renal failure	HD
Acid-base, electrolyte, volume problems	HD
Hypotension, hemodynamic instability	HP
Low platelet count	HD

Hemodialysis

The principles governing solute removal by hemodialysis are reviewed extensively in Chapter 7 (22–25) and will not be commented on in detail except in areas that are related to drug removal. Certain drugs present in the circulation can be removed to various extents by dialysis in accordance with a variety of factors. These include the rate of blood flow and that of dialysate flow through the dialyzer; the physical and biologic characteristics of the offending agent (such as degree and affinity of protein binding, water or lipid solubility, state of ionization, molecular size and shape, and the manner of compartmentalization in the body fluids); the physical characteristics of the dialyzing membrane [such as surface area, mass transfer area coefficient (KoA), porosity, electric charge, ability to adsorb the offending substance]; rate of ultrafiltration; and concentration gradient between blood and dialysate.

For a solute that has a low molecular weight, is not ionized, is water-soluble, and is not protein-bound, plasma dialyzer clearance can even exceed plasma flow rate and approximate blood-flow rate if that particular solute is readily equilibrated across the red cell membrane. Methanol is a drug that approaches this model. Thus, it would follow that, from the purely technical viewpoint, hemodialysis should be considered for poisoning resulting from those intoxicants that have the appropriate favorable physical characteristics but not for poisoning resulting from those intoxicants that are lipid-soluble, are protein-bound, or possess high molecular weights. In addition, hemodialysis should be employed whenever the intoxicated patient suffers concurrently from renal failure or has developed acid-base, electrolyte, or volume abnormalities that can be readily rectified by dialysis also. Table 38.3 lists the various drugs that can be removed by hemodialysis.

Most poisoned subjects are not commonly overhydrated to begin with. Consequently, should their blood pressures happen to be low during dialysis, physiologic saline can be readily administered when compared with the case of the frequently fluid-overloaded maintenance hemodialysis patient. Bicarbonate-based dialysate, cool (e.g., 35°C) dialysate, and the use of vasoconstrictors such as midodrine can all help to promote hemodynamic stability (see Chapter 19). In addition, dialysate composition should be adjusted to tailor to each patient's indi-

TABLE 38.3. REPRESENTATIVE DRUGS REMOVED BY DIALYSIS

Alcohols	***Sedatives-anticonvulsants***
Ethanol	Butabarbital
Ethylene glycol	Pentobarbital
Isopropanol	Phenobarbital
Methanol	Carbamazine
Analgesics	Chloral hydrate
Acetaminophen	Ethchlorvynol
Colchicine	Glutethimide
Salicylates	Meprobamate
Antibiotics and	Primidone
chemotherapeutic agents	(Valproic acid)
Amoxicillin	***Cardiovascular drugs***
Clavulanic acid	Atenolol
Penicillin	Captopril
Ticarcillin	Enalapril
Cefixime	Metoprolol
Cefuroxime	Methyldopa
Cephalexin	Nadolol
Amikacin	Procainamide
Gentamicin	Propanolol
Kanamycin	Sotalol
Neomycin	Tocainide
Streptomycin	***Solvents***
Tobramycin	Acetone
Metronidazole	Camphor
Nitrofurantoin	Thiols
Sulfisoxazole	Toluene
Sulfonamides	Trichloroethylene
Tetracycline	***Miscellaneous***
Imipenem	Lithium
Ciprofloxacin	Theophylline
Acyclovir	Paraquat
Isoniazid	Aniline
Ethambutol	Boric acid
Didanosine	Chromic acid
Zidovudine	Chlorates
Foscarnet	Diquat
Ganciclovir	Thiocyanate
Cyclophosphamide	
5-Flurouracil	

() Not well removed.
Reprinted from Winchester JF. Active methods for detoxification. In: Haddad LM, et al., eds. *Clinical management of poisoning and drug overdose*, 3rd ed. Philadelphia: WB Saunders, 1998, with permission.

vidual needs. For example, if hyperkalemia or hypokalemia is absent, dialysate potassium level in the order of 4 mEq/L or so should be used. Noteworthy also is the fact that conventional hemodialysate geared for use in maintenance hemodialysis patients commonly contains 35 to 39 mEq/L of bicarbonate. This dialysate bicarbonate level should be lowered in the face of metabolic alkalosis and maintained at a high value in instances of severe metabolic acidosis.

Hemoperfusion

The hemoperfusion technique is based on percolating blood through a cartridge packed with activated charcoal or other sorbents coated with a very thin and relatively porous semipermeable membrane. Removal of many toxins is influenced by the affinity of the charcoal for the toxin and by the avidity of the toxin to bind plasma proteins. Table 38.4 lists the various drugs and chemicals that can be removed with hemoperfusion. Clinical use of this technique has been restricted to the treatment of theophylline poisoning in recent times.

In hemoperfusion cartridges, the function of the semipermeable membrane is not to withstand pressure differences but to impede the release of the particulate matter constituting the sorbent into the circulation and to prevent or reduce the adherence, onto the sorbents, of platelets and other formed elements of the blood. Consequently, the membrane coating of the activated

TABLE 38.4. DRUGS AND CHEMICALS REMOVED WITH HEMOPERFUSION

Barbiturates	Thiabendazole
Amobarbital	(5-Fluorouracil)
Butabarbital	*Antidepressants*
Hexabarbital	(Amitriptyline)
Pentobarbital	(Imipramine)
Quinalbital	(Tricyclics)
Secobarbital	*Plant and animal toxins, herbicides,*
Thiopental	*insecticides*
Vinalbital	Amanitin
Nonbarbiturate hypnotics,	Chordane
sedatives and tranquilizers	Demeton sulfoxide
Carbromal	Dimethoate
Chloral hydrate	Diquat
Chlorpromazine	Methylparathion
(Diazepam)	Nitrostigmine
Diphenhydramine	(Organophosphate)
Ethchlorvynol	Phalloidin
Glutethimide	Polychlorinated-biphenyls
Meprobamate	Paraquat
Methaqualone	Parathion
Methsuximide	*Cardiovascular*
Methyprylon	Digoxin
Promazine	Diltiazem
Promethazine	(Disopyramide)
(Valproic acid)	Flecainide
Analgesics, antirheumatic	Metoprolol
Acetaminophen	N-Acetylprocainamide
Acetylsalicylic acid	Procainamide
Colchicine	Quinidine
D-Propoxyphene	*Miscellaneous*
Methylsalicylate	Aminophylline
Phenylbutazone	Cimetidine
Salicylic acid	(Fluoroacetamide)
Antimicrobials/anticancer	(Phencyclidine)
(Adriamycin)	Phenols
Ampicillin	(Podophyllin)
Carmustine	Theophylline
Chloramphenicol	*Solvents, gases*
Chloroquine	Carbon tetrachloride
Clindamycin	Ethylene oxide
Dapsone	Trichlorethane
Doxorubicin	Xylene
Gentamicin	*Metals*
Isoniazid	(Aluminium)*
(Methotrexate)	(Iron)*

() Not well removed.
()* Removed with chelation.
Reprinted from Winchester JF. Active methods for detoxification. In: Haddad LM, et al., eds. *Clinical management of poisoning and drug overdose*, 3rd ed. Philadelphia: WB Saunders, 1998, with permission.

charcoal is extremely thin (0.05 μm) and does not significantly restrict solute diffusion.

The process of activation of the charcoal sorbent has the effect of enormously increasing the total available surface area of the sorbent. Activated charcoal is capable of adsorbing and, therefore, extracting lipid-soluble substances much more efficiently than hemodialysis. For example, glutethimide is extracted poorly by hemodialysis but to a greater extent by charcoal hemoperfusion (16). On the other hand, hemoperfusion does not contribute to the overall treatment of the patients with renal failure and/or with acid-base, electrolyte, and fluid problems.

Other potential disadvantages of this technique are (a) hemoperfusion may cause a fall in the blood platelet count and (b) despite the large adsorbent area, hemoperfusion cartridges do become saturated and lose their efficiency over time, so that they may need to be replaced or employed in conjunction with other measures. It should be noted that both hemodialysis and hemoperfusion require the establishment of a vascular access and the administration of anticoagulants [exception: anticoagulant-free hemodialysis (e.g., performed by infusing 250 mL of physiologic saline into the dialyzer blood inlet every 15 minutes) can effectively be used for short-duration hemodialysis].

Clearance versus Drug Removal, or Technical Efficiency versus Clinical Effectiveness

A number of methods have been used to measure the efficiency of dialysis, hemofiltration, hemodiafiltration, or hemoperfusion in achieving drug removal. For ease of explanation, the case of dialysis is used here as an example. The dialyzer clearance of a substance is defined as the volume of blood (or plasma, as the case may be) from which the substance is completely removed per unit time. Given the drug concentrations in the blood entering and exiting the dialyzer and the rate of dialyzer blood flow, the dialyzer clearance of the drug can be calculated as

$$C = QB (A - V)/A$$

where C is dialyzer clearance, QB is blood-flow rate through the dialyzer, A is the blood concentration of the drug at the blood inlet of the dialyzer, and V is the blood concentration of the drug at the blood outlet of the dialyzer.

Another method of calculating clearance involves the accurate collection of spent dialysate from the dialysate outlet of a dialyzer (say for 1 minute) accompanied by the prompt obtainment of arterial blood (or plasma) at the blood inlet at 30 seconds (26). In this example, then, dialyzer clearance of a substance (in mL of blood or plasma/minute) = amount of substance in mg collected in dialysate/arterial blood (or plasma) concentration of the substance in mg/mL.

Using either of the two methods, it can be shown that, given the proper drug characteristics and the use of appropriate dialyzers/ultrafilters or hemoperfusion apparatus, drugs can be extracted from circulating blood with startling efficiency. In this example, the clearance of many intoxicants approximates the rate of blood flow, which can easily be in the range of 400 mL/min, and the extraction ratio can approach 100%, with drug concentrations at the dialyzer/ultrafilter outlet being close to 0.

Although these data can be interpreted to signify that drugs are being eliminated efficiently, thereby supporting the use of extracorporeal measures in a large variety of intoxications (22–25), such an interpretation is not often warranted. An efficient extracorporeal procedure does not imply that a clinically significant amount of intoxicant is being removed from the patient. To appreciate the total amount of drug removed relative to the total amount present in the body, one must evaluate the efficiency in the context of the apparent volume of distribution (Vd) of the intoxicant. A drug with a large Vd indicates that the substance is sequestered somewhere other than the vascular compartment (being present in the interstitial or intracellular fluid or being bound to cellular proteins, cellular lipids or cellular membranes, etc.). As a result, under many circumstances, the apparent extravascular distribution volume of a substance is multicompartmental in nature, allowing the release of the substance into the vascular compartment only slowly. Such a scenario means that only a small fraction of the total amount present in the body is accessible to withdrawal by the extracorporeal method during a particular time period.

Intoxication with digoxin or tricyclic antidepressants demonstrates this phenomenon admirably. With these drugs, the largest amount of the ingested toxin is not circulating but rather is bound to intracellular components; thus, the total quantity of drug available for extraction from the blood is minimal. Even when the entire circulating drug is extracted in one treatment session through the extracorporeal device, only a trivial fraction of the body poison store is removed. Thus, the potential complications, the expense resulting from the use of extracorporeal devices, and, above all, the fact that this use detracts from paying due attention to the all important supportive therapy vastly outstrip the possible minimal gain derived from the procedure (27–32).

CRITERIA FOR THE USE OF EXTRACORPOREAL TECHNIQUES IN THE TREATMENT OF EXOGENOUS INTOXICATIONS

We propose that extracorporeal means of detoxification be considered when the following clinical and toxicologic characteristics are present:

- The drug has been shown to be sufficiently toxic to cause severe morbidity and mortality.
- Clinical data, including but not limited to blood levels, indicate that the quantity of ingested drug is in the range capable of causing severe morbidity or mortality and/or that the patient suffers concomitantly from conditions that may impair disposal of the drug, such as the following:
  -Renal failure or liver failure for drugs eliminated by the kidney or the liver respectively.
  -Ingestion or administration of "slow-release" drugs.
  -Nausea or vomiting that prevents the administration of charcoal to effect drug removal from the gastrointestinal tract, especially in theophylline intoxication.
- The patient is available for treatment before extensive and irreversible complications have become manifest.

- The mechanism of action of the drug does not result in immediate irreversible damage (e.g., in contrast to the case of cyanide poisoning in which extensive and irreversible damage is promptly inflicted).
- The drug has been shown to be removed efficiently by the currently available extracorporeal measures. This feature indicates that the drug is not importantly bound to proteins or lipids and that its molecular size, shape, and charge permit removal through dialyzer/ultrafilter membranes or by adsorption to sorbents.
- The Vd, volume of distribution of the drug, is relatively small, implying that a large fraction of the drug is present in body water, from which it can be removed more readily.
- No effective and specific antidotes are available to reverse the effects of the toxin [e.g., in contrast to the case of digoxin poisoning in which digoxin-specific antibody Fab fragment (Digibind) can be used].

When these criteria are applied, it becomes apparent that only a handful of toxins have the toxicologic characteristics conducive to potential effective treatment by extracorporeal means. Unfortunately, many of the drugs or toxins that account for a substantial fraction of total morbidity and mortality are not amenable to removal by extracorporeal techniques, despite the demonstration for some offending agents that such techniques can bring about a high clearance rate. These drugs and/or toxins include the following:

Tricyclic antidepressants. The tricyclic antidepressant class of drugs is typified by a high Vd because of high lipid solubility. The fraction of drug available for extraction from the circulation is minuscule (31,32).

Barbiturates. The short-acting barbiturates are highly lipid bound and poorly dialyzable. The longer acting barbiturates, especially phenobarbital, are more water-soluble and are efficiently removed by renal excretion and hemodialysis. Alkalinization of the urine and the induction of high urine flow rates have been used to increase the rate of excretion. Hemoperfusion, although effective in removing circulating long-acting barbiturates, has not been proven to provide clinical benefits (33). Hemodialysis is indicated in the patient intoxicated with long-acting barbiturates and possessing poor renal function.

Acetaminophen. Acetaminophen, one of the most common agents leading to lethal events, is not efficiently extracted. Early and prolonged use of *N*-acetylcysteine is the therapy of choice (34).

Narcotics and "street" drugs. A common cause of overdose and death, narcotics and other street drugs are not amenable to extraction by extracorporeal techniques. Opium antagonists and supportive therapy are the mainstays of treatment.

Nonbarbiturate hypnotics, sedatives, and tranquilizers. Many of these types of drugs cause little morbidity and mortality, even in apparently severely intoxicated patients. Furthermore, they all display a high apparent volume of distribution and lipid solubility (31).

Other miscellaneous toxins. This group includes paraquat, amanita mushroom toxin, and methotrexate. Despite some contrary opinion and anecdotal reports, there is little evidence that extracorporeal techniques are clinically effective or needed for the treatment of poisonings resulting from these toxins.

TABLE 38.5. INTOXICANTS FOR WHICH EXTRACORPOREAL METHODS HAVE BEEN SHOWN TO HAVE CLINICAL EFFECTIVENESS AND THEIR MAIN PHARMACOLOGIC CHARACTERISTICS[a]

Intoxicant	Molecular Weight	Protein Binding (%)	Vd (L/kg)	Severe Toxic Levels[b]
Ethylene glycol	62		0.6	?
Methanol	32		0.6	50 mg/dL
Isopropanol	60		0.6	400 mg/dL
Ethanol	46		0.6	450–1500 mg/dL
Salicylate	138	50–90[c]	0.2	800 mg/dL
Lithium	7		0.8	2.5 mEq/L
Theophylline	180	40–60	0.5	60 μg/mL

[a]Please note that comments on the effectiveness of hemodialysis are not necessarily applicable to sorbent-based dialysate regeneration systems; these systems are not effective and not recommended for the treatment of ethylene glycol, methanol, or isopropyl alcohol poisonings. Furthermore, whereas the characteristics of the cartridges and/or some anecdotal reports suggest that they may be effective in the treatment of salicylate, lithium, and theophylline intoxication, no specific definitive studies documenting their effectiveness are available.
[b]Commonly accepted potentially lethal concentrations. These should be considered only as approximate guidelines, because toxicity is determined by a variety of clinical characteristics in combination with the serum concentration.
[c]Salicylate protein binding is highest at low (therapeutic) values and progressively lower with increasing (toxic) levels.
Modified from Garella S. Extracorporeal techniques in the treatment of exogenous intoxications. *Kidney Int* 1988;33:735–740, with permission.

Because paraquat and *N*-acetyl procainamide (NAPA) are tightly tissue-bound and released slowly, it has been proposed that CRRT, which can be employed continuously for many hours, may be efficacious (8,31,35). Although clinical case reports have suggested that patients suffering from life-threatening NAPA intoxication could be helped with the various extracorporeal measures, the issue of their effectiveness is still debatable (36).

As a consequence of these considerations, we believe that extracorporeal methods should be considered in the treatment of acute intoxications resulting from the agents or conditions listed in Table 38.5. The remainder of this chapter outlines the clinical syndromes resulting from these intoxicants and proposes clinical guidelines for the use of extracorporeal techniques in their management.

Sorbent Cartridge Systems

Comments regarding the effectiveness of dialytic therapy are not necessarily applicable to those dialysis systems that employ sorbent cartridges to regenerate dialysate. These systems employ small volumes of dialysate, and the cartridge used does not effectively bind alcohols; therefore, such systems are not indicated in the treatment of ethylene glycol, methanol, or isopropyl alcohol poisoning. Although the cartridge may adsorb salicylate or lithium, there are, to our knowledge, no published studies documenting the effectiveness of sorbent systems in these intoxications. Finally, sorbent-based systems are said to be efficacious in the treatment of theophylline intoxication, but again no quantitative published reports are available.

ETHYLENE GLYCOL

The TESS data for the year 2001 indicate a total of 5,833 reported toxic exposures to ethylene glycol resulting in 34 deaths and 222 life-threatening poisonings (1). Most of the poisonings are unintentional and seen usually in the pediatric population. Intentional use is secondary to its employment as an inexpensive substitute/inebriant for ethanol. Ethylene glycol, also referred to as "sweet killer," is an organic solvent commonly found in antifreeze preparations, deicers, coolants, brake and hydraulic fluids, and household cleaners. Ethylene glycol is a sweet-tasting, viscous, colorless liquid with a molecular formula of $C_2H_6O_2$ [molecular weight (MW) = 62 Dalton] (37,38).

Pharmacokinetics

Ethylene glycol, an alcohol, is rapidly absorbed from the gastrointestinal tract with peak serum concentrations appearing 1 to 4 hours after ingestion. Being highly soluble and non-protein bound, it diffuses promptly through the total body water; its volume of distribution is approximately 0.5 to 0.8 L/kg (39). The liver metabolizes 80% of the absorbed ethylene glycol in a stepwise NAD-dependent fashion (37,38). Alcohol dehydrogenase, the first enzyme in the pathway, oxidizes ethylene glycol to glycoaldehyde and is competitively inhibited by both ethanol and fomepizole (Fig. 38.1). Glycoaldehyde is then rapidly converted to glycolic acid. The next step involving the conversion of glycolic acid to glyoxylic acid is the rate-limiting step resulting in the accumulation of glycolic acid in massive poisonings. Along with lactic acid, glycolic acid is the main contributor to the accompanying metabolic acidosis (40,41). Glyoxylic acid is converted further to oxalic acid that can precipitate with calcium to form calcium oxalate crystals. The latter are deposited in tissues and may appear in the urine. Minor pathways involving thiamine and pyridoxine as cofactors can also bring about the conversion of glyoxylic acid to glycine and benzoic acid. However, these pathways are clinically insignificant and there are no data to support the use of these cofactors in the treatment of ethylene glycol intoxication (42).

The average elimination half-life of ethylene glycol is approximately 3 hours. Ethanol, at serum concentrations of 22 to 44 mmol/L (100 to 200 mg/dL), can adequately inhibit alcohol dehydrogenase and prolong the half-life of ethylene glycol in the realm of 18 hours (43). Fomepizole at serum concentrations greater than 9.8 μmol/L (0.08 mg/dL) can bring about similar prolongation of the half-life of ethylene glycol to the order of 20 hours (44,45).

Clinical and Pathologic Effects of Ethylene Glycol

Classically, three different stages of ethylene glycol intoxication are described based on the predominant systemic effects (31,46). The stage and its severity depend on the amount of ethylene glycol ingested, the possible coingestion of ethanol or other chemicals, and the timing of medical interventions (37,38,46). The presence of severe acidosis, hyperkalemia, seizures, and coma on admission indicates severe intoxication (47).

Stage I is marked by the predominance of central nervous system (CNS) involvement; it begins shortly after ingestion and may last for 12 hours. Initially, the patient appears inebriated, sometimes with sustained nausea and vomiting, but there is no odor of ethanol (if no ethanol has been ingested concomitantly); these symptoms are probably related to the direct effects of ethylene glycol. Then hyporeflexia, coma, and generalized or focal seizures appear, often accompanied by ophthalmoplegia, nystagmus, and papilledema. These manifestations are most likely to reach their peak between 6 and 12 hours after ingestion and have been attributed to the toxic effects of the glycoaldehyde metabolites. Cerebral edema and diffuse petechiae are found in patients who die during this stage; focal deposition of calcium oxalate crystals is also seen.

In the second stage, 12 to 24 hours after ingestion, cardiorespiratory problems become apparent, consisting of tachycardia and hypertension when mild but progressing to pulmonary edema and cardiovascular collapse when severe. Patients who survive beyond the second stage develop renal failure, with oliguria, flank pain, and often the presence of calcium oxalate crystals in the urine approximately 24 hours after ingestion (Table 38.6). The mechanism responsible for the cardiopulmonary and renal manifestations is not known with precision but is likely due to the toxic effects of the metabolic products of ethylene glycol. The role of calcium oxalate deposits in causing the renal failure is debated but probably not prominent. Given proper supportive therapy, the renal failure can be reversible.

Diagnosis

A history of ingestion of substances containing ethylene glycol is useful in arriving at the proper diagnosis. The diagnosis of ethylene glycol poisoning should be considered in every inebriated patient without the odor of ethanol. The presence of severe metabolic acidosis with a large anion gap and a large osmolal gap (greater than 10 mOsm/kg) helps further. As mentioned previously, metabolic acidosis develops as a result of the production of glycolic acid and other acidic metabolites secondary to ethylene glycol breakdown. The plasma anion gap, representing unmeasured anions, is elevated as a result of the accumulation of the anions of the acid metabolites.

The presence of an osmolal gap is supportive of the diagnosis of ethylene glycol poisoning. Osmolal gap is the difference between the serum osmolality level determined by freezing point depression and that calculated from the measured serum levels of sodium, glucose, and urea nitrogen (same as blood urea nitrogen) (48).

$$\text{Calculated serum osmolality (mOsm/kg)} = 2 \times \text{Na (mEq/L)} + \text{Glucose (mg/dL)}/18 + \text{BUN (mg/dL)}/2.8$$

The normal osmolal gap should be between 5 to 10 mOsm/kg. Each 100 mg/dL of ethylene glycol will produce an osmolal gap of 16 mOsm/kg. Because the half-life of ethylene glycol is about 3 hours, the increase in osmolal gap as a result of the presence of ethylene glycol in the blood may only be transient. Hence, a normal osmolal gap does not rule out ethylene glycol intoxication. However, under such circumstances, the presence of the resultant acid metabolites will still engender metabolic acidosis and an elevated anion gap. [These acid metabolites cannot bring about an increase in osmolal gap. This is because the hydrogen ions of these acids are neutralized by serum bicarbonate ions to form water. The decrease in bicarbonate ions is balanced by a rise in the unmeasured anions of these acids (e.g., glycolate, glyoxylate, and oxalate). As a result, the total number of osmoles in the serum remains unchanged.]

The finding of urinary calcium oxalate crystals, present in nearly 50% of the patients with ethylene glycol intoxication, and the associated occurrence of hypocalcemia are also highly suggestive of ethylene glycol poisoning. Urinary calcium oxalate crystals usually appear after a latent period of 4 to 8 hours; consequently, repeat urinalysis should be carried out after this period (49). These crystals can have the classic appearance of "envelopes" (a square or rectangle with the vertices connected by an X) if they consist of calcium oxalate dihydrate or more commonly the appearance of needles or prisms if they consist of calcium oxalate monohydrate (50). Occasionally, Wood's lamp may be of assistance in the diagnosis because antifreeze, one of the most common sources for ethylene glycol poisoning, contains sodium fluorescein, a marker geared for the detection of radiator leaks in motor vehicles (51,52). Gas chromatographic demonstration of the presence of ethylene glycol is required to make a definitive diagnosis. Although determination of serum ethylene glycol levels remains the method of choice for confirming the presence of intoxication, this method is unavailable in many hospital laboratories. The measurement by referral laboratories adds a considerable delay in making a diagnosis. In

TABLE 38.6. CLINICAL AND LABORATORY MANIFESTATIONS OF ETHYLENE GLYCOL INTOXICATION

Stage	Clinical Manifestations	Laboratory Findings[a]
I. Neurologic (30 min–12 hr)	Inebriation, nausea, vomiting Hyporeflexia, generalized or focal seizures, coma Ophthalmoplegia, nystagmus, papilledema	Nonspecific findings: • Leukocytosis (10,000–40,000/μL) • Xanthochromia, pleocytosis ↑ protein in CSF • Hypocalcemia
II. Cardiopulmonary (12–24 hr)	Tachycardia, hypertension Pulmonary edema, then shock if severe	Highly suggestive findings: • Hypocalcemia • Metabolic acidosis with a high anion gap • Osmolal gap (16 mOsml/kg for every 100 mg/dL of ethylene glycol) • Calcium oxalate crystals in urinary sediment
III. Renal (>24 hr)	Flank pain, oliguria progressing to anuria, renal failure	

[a]CSF, cerebrospinal fluid.

addition, as stated previously, the presence of low levels of ethylene glycol does not necessarily imply a less severe poisoning.

Treatment

1. Supportive maneuvers in all cases
2. Inhibition of oxidative metabolism
3. Extracorporeal methods to remove ethylene glycol and its toxic metabolites

In addition to taking care of the airway, breathing, and circulation via advanced cardiac life support (ACLS) protocols, severe metabolic acidosis may need to be treated with intravenous sodium bicarbonate therapy. Seizures, if present, can be treated with benzodiazepines and by correction of the severe hypocalcemia. Aggressive treatment of acidosis and induction of an alkaline diuresis increase the renal elimination of glycolate and decrease the likelihood of renal failure (53). Induction of emesis is usually not employed because of the risk of aspiration and the rapid absorption of ethylene glycol from the gastrointestinal tract.

Oxidative metabolism of ethylene glycol can be inhibited by the use of alcohol dehydrogenase inhibitors, namely ethanol and fomepizole, and indications for their use are listed in Table 38.7. Fomepizole is approved for the treatment of ethylene glycol poisoning by the U.S. Food and Drug Administration. The Methylpyrazole For Toxic Alcohols (META) study group documented that fomepizole, if administered early in the course of intoxication, can prevent renal injury (45). The drug is given as an intravenous loading dose of 15 mg/kg followed by an intravenous injection of 10 mg/kg every 12 hours for 4 doses. Furthermore, the administration is continued at the rate of 15 mg/kg every 12 hours until the serum ethylene glycol concentration is undetectable or less than 3.2 mmol/L (20 mg/dL). Fomepizole is given every 4 hours if the patient is placed on hemodialysis (42). Adverse effects are minimal and include dizziness, headache, and nausea (54).

Ethanol also competitively inhibits the metabolism of ethylene glycol to its toxic metabolites by alcohol dehydrogenase and has been used as an antidote successfully for many years. Serum ethanol concentration of 22 to 44 mmol/L (100 to 200

mg/dL) can saturate receptor sites of the enzyme, thus inhibiting the breakdown of ethylene glycol (43). Ethanol can be administered (a) orally or through a nasogastric tube as a 20% solution, (b) intravenously as a 10% solution and (c) via an ethanol-enriched hemodialysate. Because the pharmacokinetics of ethanol depend on a multitude of factors such as age, sex, chronic use of alcohol, and conditions that prolong gastric emptying, serum levels of ethanol need to be monitored frequently and dosing modified accordingly to achieve and maintain serum levels of 22 to 44 mmol/L (100 to 200 mg/dL). An intravenous loading dose of 0.6 to 1.0 mg/kg followed by an intravenous maintenance dose of 100 to 150 mg/kg/hour usually suffices to achieve the target therapeutic level. Ethanol is commonly administered until ethylene glycol can no longer be detected in the serum or until the patient is asymptomatic with a normal arterial pH and a serum ethylene glycol concentration of less than 3.2 mmol/L (20 mg/dL). Ethanol is readily available and conveniently inexpensive when compared with the availability and cost of fomepizole. Ethanol therapy can, however, be associated with CNS depression especially in patients who have ingested other CNS depressants. Hypoglycemia has been noted when used in pediatric and malnourished patients. Clinical signs and symptoms of ethanol intoxication can be produced by the dosages quoted previously. Consequently, patients should be monitored closely and, if necessary, assisted appropriately. Finally, it should be noted that fomepizole and ethanol can only inhibit the breakdown of ethylene glycol. The elimination of ethylene glycol from the body, however, still requires either adequate renal function or effective extracorporeal measures.

Hemodialysis, but not hemoperfusion, is an effective treatment option in the management of ethylene glycol poisoning by removing both ethylene glycol and its metabolites (41,55). It should be considered whenever patients with ethylene glycol poisoning have deteriorating vital signs despite intensive supportive care, significant metabolic acidosis (pH <7.25 to 7.30), and renal failure or electrolyte abnormalities refractory to conventional therapy (31,42). Previously, a serum ethylene glycol concentration of greater than 11 mmol/L (50 mg/dL) was used as a criterion for hemodialysis. This approach is not supported by scientific data, however, and patients with such blood levels can be adequately managed with fomepizole or ethanol alone (42,56), when the criteria listed previously are absent and provided that adequate renal function exists. Hemodialysis should be performed with a bicarbonate bath and the concentration of bicarbonate in the dialysate should be in accordance with the degree of acidosis. For example, in the face of severe metabolic acidosis, a dialysate bicarbonate value of 40 mmol/L or higher can be used. Administered fomepizole and ethanol, given either before or during dialysis, are removed by hemodialysis and should be replaced appropriately. In patients who have received an intravenous loading dose of ethanol and are being given an intravenous maintenance dose of the alcohol to maintain a serum level of 22 to 44 mmol/L (100 to 200 mg/dL), the maintenance dose can be discontinued during dialysis provided the dialysate is enriched with 22 to 33 mmol/L (100 to 150 mg/dL) of 95% ethanol. Such a dialysate concentration would allow serum ethanol levels higher than 33 mmol/L to fall and those

TABLE 38.7. INDICATIONS FOR TREATMENT OF ETHYLENE GLYCOL POISONING WITH AN ANTIDOTE

1. History or strong clinical suspicion of ethylene glycol poisoning and at least 2 of the following criteria:
   A. Arterial pH <7.3
   B. Serum bicarbonate <20 mEq/L
   C. Osmolal gap >10 mOsm/kg
   D. Presence of urinary calcium oxalate crystals

OR

2. Documentation of a recent (hours) history of ingestion of ethylene glycol and osmolal gap >10 mOsm/kg

OR

3. Documentation of serum ethylene glycol concentration >3.2 mmol/L (20 mg/dL)

Adapted from the American Academy of Clinical Toxicology practice guidelines in the treatment of ethylene glycol poisoning. *Clin Toxicol* 1999;37:537–560, with permission.

lower than 22 mmol/L to rise, so that the final serum level can approach that in the dialysate (57).

Hemodialysis should be continued until serum ethylene glycol is undetectable or until it is less than 3.2 mmol/L (20 mg/dL), along with the disappearance of acid-base and electrolyte abnormalities and of signs of systemic toxicity. In patients with severe intoxication, it cannot be overemphasized that prolonged and intensive dialysis is often needed. In normophosphatemic patients, such aggressive dialysis may engender hypophosphatemia. Phosphate-enriched dialysates containing 1.3 mmol/L phosphorus or thereabouts, prepared by the addition of sodium phosphate salts to sodium bicarbonate-containing "dialysate base concentrate," have been used successfully to prevent such dialysis-induced hypophosphatemia (58,59). Hirsch et al. (60) have proposed a simple formula to estimate the required dialysis time (hours) to reach a serum ethylene glycol concentration of 5 mmol/L. Required dialysis time (hours) =[-V In (5/A)]/0.06K where V (liter) is the Watson's estimate of total body water, A is the initial ethylene glycol concentration in mmol/L, and K is 80% of the manufacturer's specified dialyzer urea clearance (mL/minute) at the properly observed blood-flow rate (60).

Being slower, peritoneal dialysis remains a less effective treatment option when hemodialysis is unavailable (37). Slow CRRT in the form of hemofiltration has also been used and is an alter-native in patients with circulatory instability (61). Sorbent-based dialysate regeneration systems are not effective in the treatment of this intoxication and should not be used.

METHANOL

Methanol (CH_3OH; MW = 32 Dalton), also known as wood alcohol because it was originally obtained from the destructive distillation of hardwood, is widely used as an industrial solvent, antifreeze fluid, windshield wiper fluid, and windshield deicer as well as an alternate fuel (62,63). Because it possesses inebriating qualities similar to those of ethanol and because it is inexpensive, tax-free, and widely available, it has been responsible for many intoxication epidemics and outbreaks of poisoning (62). In the United States, most of the exposures that have been recently recorded are primarily due to unintentional exposures to windshield wiper fluid and other automotive products with nearly a third of these occurring among children younger than 12 years old (64).

Methanol is rapidly and completely absorbed from the gastrointestinal tract. It does not bind to protein and has an apparent volume of distribution of approximately 0.6 to 0.7 L/kg. Only about 5% of ingested methanol is excreted unchanged in the urine; the remainder is oxidized in the liver (Fig. 38.1), first

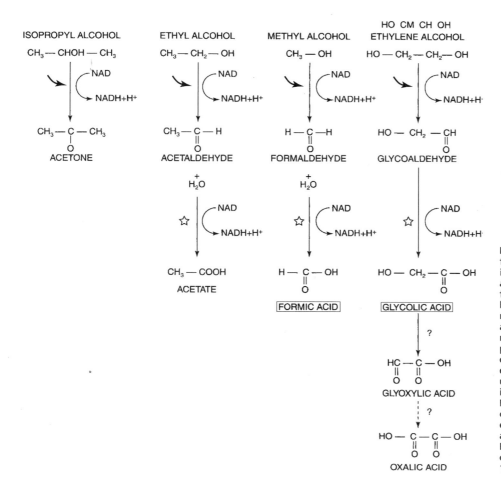

FIG. 38.1. Pathways of metabolism of the four alcohols that most commonly cause intoxication. Alcohol dehydrogenase *(bold arrow)* is the cytosolic enzyme responsible for the first oxidative step in all four alcohols. Aldehyde dehydrogenase *(star)* is the mitochondrial enzyme responsible for catalyzing the second oxidative step in ethanol, methanol, and ethylene glycol. The main products of metabolism responsible for toxicity are enclosed in boxes. Question marks denote metabolic steps where there is uncertainty on the specific enzyme(s) involved and on the generation of NAD^+H^+. Note that oxalic acid represents only a small fraction of the metabolites of ethylene glycol, and that other metabolites are not shown in the figure. (From Garella S. Extracorporeal techniques in the treatment of exogenous intoxications. *Kidney Int* 1988;33:735–740, with permission.)

to formaldehyde (which does not accumulate in measurable amounts because of its extremely short half-life) and then to formic acid. The latter compound, together with lactic acid, is responsible for the acidosis and presumably also for most of the toxicity of this poisoning (65), although formaldehyde appears to be involved in bringing about blindness (66). The first oxidative step of methanol depends on the enzymatic action of alcohol dehydrogenase, which has a tenfold greater affinity for either ethanol or fomepizole than for methanol. This phenomenon is the basis for the use of ethanol and fomepizole as antidotes in the therapy of methanol poisoning (67–70), and explains the prolongation of the half-life of methanol to more than 30 hours (compared with the normal of 12 to 20 hours) in certain patients who had ingested both methanol and ethanol at the same sitting (38). Oxidation of methanol, like that of ethanol, proceeds independently of the serum concentration but at a rate of only 15% of that of ethanol, accounting for the fact that the complete oxidation and excretion of methanol ordinarily requires several days, thus delaying the onset of toxic symptoms (62).

Clinical Picture and Laboratory Data

The variable and relatively slow metabolism of methanol, which can be further delayed by the frequent concurrent ingestion of ethanol, coupled with toxicity resulting from its breakdown products, results in two distinctive traits of methanol intoxication (38,62). An initial and fairly brief period of confusion and mild inebriation is often followed by a "free interval" of 6 to 30 hours before the appearance of toxic manifestations (Table 38.8). The asymptomatic free interval is followed by a clinical picture characterized by vertigo, vomiting, abdominal pain (probably as a result of gastritis and/or pancreatitis), dyspnea and Kussmaul's respiration, blurred vision progressing to blindness, restlessness, seizures, opisthotonus, and eventually coma and death (62,63). Physical examination is largely nonspecific but for papilledema and hyperemia of the optic disc. A helpful diagnostic clue that develops several hours after ingestion is the presence of a visual disturbance variously described as difficulty in seeing as if being in the midst of a snowstorm or fogginess

(62). However, this visual abnormality is not uniformly noted. Death is commonly from respiratory failure.

The quantity of ingested methanol required to engender serious morbidity and mortality is highly variable. Some patients develop severe complications following the ingestion of a few milliliters; others survive the ingestion of several hundred milliliters. The serum concentrations of methanol do not correlate well with the severity of the clinical picture and with prognosis, which seem to be better correlated with serum levels of formate and with the degree of metabolic acidosis (38,65).

Laboratory findings include increased serum amylase value, metabolic acidosis with an increased anion gap, and elevated serum formate and lactate levels. The increased lactate values are, as in the case of ethylene glycol intoxication, most likely the result of both an increased NADH/NAD ratio and a reduction in tissue perfusion. A high osmolal gap may be apparent. Methanol contributes 31 mOsm/kg for each 100 mg/dL; therefore, a sizable osmolal gap is more likely to be present in the initial stages of the intoxication before the alcohol is metabolized. After the latency period, the serum methanol value alone is not a reliable prognostic indicator because toxicity is mainly mediated by the metabolites. Other abnormal laboratory tests include an increased erythrocyte mean corpuscular volume, attributed to a toxic effect of formaldehyde on cellular ion transport. In 10% to 20% of cases, hemorrhagic and nonhemorrhagic necrosis of the putamen can occur (71). Permanent blindness and parkinsonism are common sequelae among survivors (62,63). Severe metabolic acidosis with initial arterial pH less than 7 and coma or seizure on presentation are poor prognostic indicators in methanol poisoning and are associated with a higher mortality (72).

Indications for and Mode of Treatment

As in the case of ethylene glycol intoxication, treatment must be aggressive and must be started promptly when there is a reasonable suspicion of methanol intoxication. Metabolic acidosis when present should be treated with intravenous infusions of sodium bicarbonate (38,62). Following drainage of stomach contents—especially necessary if the ingestion is recent—

TABLE 38.8. CLINICAL AND LABORATORY MANIFESTATIONS OF METHANOL INTOXICATION

Symptoms	Physical Findings	Laboratory Findings
Early stage, <6 hr Mild and transient Inebriation and drowsiness	Nonspecific	May have high methanol level Osmolal gap (31 mOsm/100 mg/dL)
Delayed stage, 6–30 hr Vertigo Vomiting Abdominal pain Restlessness Dyspnea Blurred vision → blindness Seizures, opisthotonus Coma → death	± Kussmaul respiration, papilledema, hyperemia of discs	Metabolic acidosis High anion gap High formate levels High lactate levels ↑ Amylase ↑ Mean corpuscular volume

ethanol or fomepizole should be administered (38,67–69). The prompt administration of ethanol or fomepizole is very effective in preventing the development of metabolic acidosis by markedly decreasing the oxidative metabolism of methanol. This is exemplified by the description of a patient with documented high ethanol levels and toxic methanol levels but without the development of either acidosis or visual problems (73). Indications for starting intravenous ethanol or fomepizole administration include (a) a serum methanol level greater than 6 mmol/L (20 mg/dL); (b) a history of ingesting more than 0.4 mL/kg body weight of methanol; and (c) any ingestion history with delayed access to toxicologic testing and metabolic acidosis with otherwise unexplained elevated anion and osmolal gaps (the latter being greater than 10 mOsm/kg), especially if other symptoms are present (38,62,74). The doses of ethanol or of fomepizole used are similar to those recommended for ethylene glycol poisoning (42,74).

Hemodialysis is the most effective means of removal of both methanol and formate (62,63). It is indicated when (a) severe acidosis unresponsive to intravenous bicarbonate therapy is present; (b) visual, funduscopic, or mental status changes are present; (c) deteriorating vital signs despite intensive supportive care are present; (c) the patient has consumed more than 30 mL of pure methanol or its equivalent; or (d) serum methanol levels are greater than 16 mmol/L (50 mg/dL) (62,74–76). Hemodialysis is best performed with the help of a bicarbonate bath because the alkali requirement may be massive due to the presence of severe metabolic acidosis associated with the intoxication (31). Elimination kinetics may be complicated by redistribution or a slow equilibration across cellular membranes, especially with regard to formate necessitating prolonged hemodialysis as a therapeutic measure (77). Hypophosphatemia may occur in those patients who require prolonged and intensive dialysis sessions, especially in individuals who are normophosphatemic to begin with. Enrichment of dialysate with sodium phosphate salts (1.3 mmol/L of phosphorus in the dialysate) has been used successfully to prevent hypophosphatemia in such patients (78,79). Hemodialysis must be continued until the serum methanol level is less than 9.4 mmol/L (30 mg/dL), the osmolal gap becomes normal, and metabolic acidosis is rectified (38,62,74). Ethanol-enriched dialysate has been used in patients in an attempt to maintain stable levels of ethanol during dialysis (78–80). Because of the possibility of intracerebral hemorrhage in methanol poisoning (71), an effort should be made to perform anticoagulant-free or citrate dialysis (81). In patients with cardiovascular instability, the use of blood transfusion and/or vasoconstrictors to maintain adequate blood pressure levels for the purpose of hemodialysis should be initiated. In the face of gastrointestinal bleeding, the previously described measures to avoid systemic anticoagulation should also be applied.

Peritoneal dialysis and slow CRRTs are less efficient than hemodialysis but have a place as adjunctive therapeutic measures (62). Only when conventional hemodialysis cannot be performed should these less effective techniques be practiced (ideally peritoneal dialysis in combination with one of the CRRTs). Hemoperfusion using activated charcoal is ineffective.

Administration of folic acid and folinic acid have been used empirically in methanol poisoning because animal data have demonstrated that these agents can stimulate folate-mediated oxidative metabolism of formate to carbon dioxide and water. Such therapy may be efficacious in folate-deficient patients (68,74,82).

ISOPROPANOL (ISOPROPYL ALCOHOL)

In the home, isopropanol (C_3H_7OH; MW = 60 Dalton), is a compound found in highest concentrations in rubbing alcohol. It is also used in deicing products, solvents, cements, and cleaning products. It is a clear, colorless, bitter liquid with a characteristic odor. Isopropanol is readily absorbed by the gastrointestinal tract but may cause intoxication even via absorption by inhalation, especially in small children (38,83).

Isopropanol has effects on the CNS that resemble those of ethanol (83,84). It is, however, metabolized more slowly than ethanol, displaying a half-life of approximately 3 hours normally and a much more protracted half-life occasionally. It is excreted in part by the kidney and in part by the lung; approximately 80% is oxidized to acetone via the action of alcohol dehydrogenase (Fig. 38.1) (85). In contrast to ethylene glycol and methanol, the toxic effects of isopropanol appear to be mostly caused by the parent compound rather than by its metabolites. Thus, no therapeutic attempts to slow its metabolism are in order (38,86).

Clinical Picture and Laboratory Data

Initially, the symptoms and signs of isopropanol intoxication resemble those of ethanol intoxication: dizziness, incoordination, and confusion. However, these manifestations are more prolonged and more severe, often progressing to ataxia and coma and, in some instances, death by respiratory arrest. CNS depression is generally considered to be 2 to 2.5 times as severe as that produced by an equal amount of ethanol (83). The patient may smell of acetone, a helpful aid in arriving at the diagnosis. Vomiting and hematemesis resulting from hemorrhagic gastritis are frequent. Tachyarrhythmias and, in severe cases, hypotension can occur. Evidence of hepatocellular damage has been described, as have acute renal failure, myoglobinuria, hypothermia, and hemolytic anemia (83–85).

Laboratory tests reveal the presence of an elevated osmolal gap and a normal anion gap, although in severe cases some degree of high anion-gap metabolic acidosis may be seen. The latter is due to lactic acidosis, which occurs in severe cases and is probably secondary to hypotension and tissue hypoperfusion. The high osmolal gap results from the combination of two components: (a) isopropanol contributes 17 mOsm/kg per 100 mg/dL and (b) acetone contributes 18 mOsm/kg per 100 mg/dL. Serum and urine tests for acetone (e.g., the sodium nitroprusside test) are positive in the absence of hyperglycemia and glycosuria (83–85).

Indications for and Mode of Treatment

Lethal doses of isopropanol have ranged from 150 to 240 mL (84). Death has been reported to take place in 45% of patients who suffered from both coma and hypotension. Coma by itself in the absence of hypotension was not associated with a high mortality (85). Severe intoxication along with a higher mortality is seen in patients with a serum isopropanol level in excess of 67 mmol/L (400 mg/dL).

The usual recommended therapy is supportive, including gastrointestinal lavage. No specific antidote is available. Ethanol is not indicated as inhibition of isopropanol metabolism would lead to continued toxicity and would diminish its excretion in the form of its major breakdown product, namely acetone. Hemodialysis is indicated in patients with an isopropanol concentration of 67 mmol/L (400 mg/dL) or higher and in the presence of coma or hemodynamic instability (83–85). We believe that it is prudent to perform hemodialysis in poorly arousable or comatose patients when good presumptive evidence of isopropanol ingestion is available, even before cardiovascular instability becomes manifest. Studies on the kinetics of isopropanol elimination by hemodialysis have shown that the procedure is highly efficient, in view of the low molecular weight, the absence of protein binding, and the low volume of distribution (83,86–88).

The previous general statements pertaining to methanol poisoning in the areas of gastrointestinal bleeding, cardiovascular instability, peritoneal dialysis, and CRRTs (14) are also applicable to isopropanol poisoning. Sorbent-based dialysate regeneration systems are not effective.

SALICYLATES

The salicylate class of drugs causes the highest number of chronic or acute poisonings, either as a single toxic agent or as the main intoxicant when several toxic compounds are ingested together (89,90). Aspirin (acetylsalicylic acid, $C_9H_8O_4$; MW = 180 Dalton), the most commonly prescribed and available preparation, is associated with the largest number of poisonings (1).

All salicylates are readily and almost completely absorbed from the gastrointestinal tract. Methyl salicylate (oil of wintergreen) can also cause intoxication through skin absorption, but this intoxicant is seldom used nowadays. Although absorption of therapeutic doses is rapid, absorption may be considerably delayed when large quantities are ingested; furthermore, variability in the rate of dissolution of different pharmaceutical preparations, the presence of food in the stomach, or the use of enteric-coated formulations may delay the onset of symptoms or the attainment of peak serum levels to 12 hours or more after ingestion.

Used mainly for their capacity to inhibit cyclooxygenase and diminish the formation of prostaglandins—with the resultant effects of antipyresis, analgesia, and antiinflammatory activity—salicylates display a variety of toxic effects as a result of their interference with a number of metabolic processes (91). Prominent among these processes is uncoupling of oxidative phosphorylation, similar to that induced by 2,4-dinitrophenol. This uncoupling, along with direct stimulation of the respiratory center, accounts for the characteristic hyperpnea and, at least in part, for the increased production of organic acids, which participates in the genesis of metabolic acidosis observed particu-

larly among children (92). In addition, salicylates inhibit a variety of oxidases, stimulate the release of epinephrine (with resultant hyperglycemia and depletion of hepatic glycogen) and of glucocorticoids, induce aminoaciduria and a negative nitrogen balance, and reduce urate excretion at therapeutic doses and raise such excretion at toxic doses (91).

Aspirin is hydrolyzed to salicylic acid, which is largely glycinated to salicyluric acid. The latter is then excreted via the kidney. At therapeutic doses, only approximately 10% of the ingested drug is excreted as salicylate in the urine. When therapeutic doses and therapeutic serum levels are exceeded, two events occur which tend to aggravate markedly the likelihood of toxicity. First, the capacity of serum proteins to bind salicylates is exceeded; as a result, the ratio between the "free" and the total serum salicylate levels rises. At therapeutic concentrations, only 10% of the drug is free (not bound to protein), but at concentrations of 5.8 mmol/L (80 mg/dL) up to 50% is free (91,93). Second, the biotransformation to salicyluric acid is retarded because of saturation of the responsible metabolic pathways and because of glycine depletion. This phenomenon results in a relatively higher proportion of the drug being present as salicylate, which is less efficiently excreted by the kidney than salicyluric acid. The combination of these two events engenders a greater and more prolonged toxicity. The higher proportion of the drug circulating in its free form also facilitates its entry into the cerebrospinal fluid and the intracellular compartment, thus expanding the apparent volume of distribution to approximately 50% of the body weight from the 20% or so encountered at therapeutic serum levels (91,93).

The renal excretion of salicylate and its metabolites depends, of course, on the glomerular filtration rate but is also markedly augmented by high urine flow rates and especially by an alkaline urine pH. In view of the acidic pK_a values of these compounds, a urine pH higher than 7.0 can greatly enhance renal excretion because of the fact that these compounds cannot be reabsorbed by the renal tubules in their ionized forms. For the same reason, cellular entry of salicylate and its metabolites is facilitated by acidosis and hindered by alkalosis, an observation highlighting the deleterious effect of salicylate-induced acidosis and emphasizing the need for the prompt rectification of this acid-base abnormality (94).

Clinical Picture and Laboratory Data

Despite the frequency of this intoxication and its plethora of symptoms and signs, a large percentage of affected patients remains undiagnosed. Moderate and chronic intoxications usually manifest as salicylism in the form of headaches, tinnitus, impaired auditory acuity, dizziness, and weakness progressing to nausea, vomiting, confusion, and hyperventilation. In addition to these symptoms, more severe and acute intoxications can also result in hyperpyrexia, seizures, coma, and metabolic acidosis (95,96).

The typical acid-base disturbance encountered is characterized by having two phases: (1) a respiratory alkalosis resulting from stimulation of respiration and (2) the resulting hyperpnea followed by a metabolic acidosis with an elevated anion gap. The metabolic acidosis is seen primarily in small children. This acidosis is secondary to the loss of bicarbonate in the urine (the result of the initial primary respiratory alkalosis) and to the accumulation of a variety of organic acids, with salicylic acid contributing to the lowering of only a few mEq/L of the initial serum bicarbonate concentration (95–98).

Other serum abnormalities include hypouricemia, hypokalemia, a prolongation of the prothrombin time, a positive ferric chloride test, and a positive Phenistix test (99,100). The Phenistix reagent strips are impregnated with ferric and magnesium salts that will impart a purple color if the salicylate concentration is more than 5 mmol/L (70 mg/dL), providing immediate confirmation in instances of suspected salicylate intoxication (99,101).

Increasingly severe seizures, deepening coma, and cardiovascular collapse are terminal events. In some patients, especially older ones who are smokers and take salicylates chronically, noncardiogenic pulmonary edema has also been described (102–105).

Indications for and Mode of Treatment

Doses of 10 to 30 g of aspirin or of sodium salicylate have resulted in fatalities, although much larger doses have been associated with recovery. The calculation of lethal doses is complicated by the frequent combination of "acute-on-chronic" intoxication. Symptoms of salicylism are usually present at serum levels of 2.2 mmol/L (30 mg/dL) or higher, but the correlation between serum values and the severity of intoxication is not strong (106). This poor correlation may be related to acute versus chronic ingestion, the variability of underlying or confounding factors, and the presence of delayed absorption. A widely available nomogram has been proposed to estimate the severity of intoxication on the basis of serum concentrations, taking into account the time transpired between ingestion and blood sampling (107). However, it might not be useful when sustained-release or enteric-coated preparations have been consumed (108,109).

There is no specific antidote to treat salicylate intoxication. The mainstay of therapy is supportive, including gastric emptying in patients up to 24 hours following ingestion; the administration of activated charcoal; and the intravenous administration of appropriate amounts of fluids, electrolytes, and other agents to repair volume, electrolyte, and acid-base abnormalities if necessary, in particular the use of potassium chloride supplements to combat hypokalemia. Such maneuvers may be adequate for patients with moderate salicylism and serum levels less than 3.6 mmol/L (50 mg/dL).

For patients with higher serum levels or with more pronounced symptoms, especially if metabolic acidosis is present, measures to bring about the elimination of salicylates are warranted. These maneuvers include the repeated administration of activated charcoal (89,110), despite some recent data that cast doubt on the effectiveness of this technique (111,112), and the induction of an alkaline diuresis (113,114). Salicylate excretion is greatly accelerated in the face of a highly alkaline urine (pH greater than 7.5). The use of carbonic anhydrase inhibitors to alkalinize the urine is no longer recommended, especially in the face of metabolic acidosis, when such therapy is usually ineffec-

tive [if carbonic anhydrase inhibitors were effective, they would lower serum bicarbonate level and increase the degree of metabolic acidosis, thus further facilitating the cellular entry of salicylate (94)]. Similarly, the use of forced diuresis appears to be no better at augmenting salicylate excretion than alkalinization of the urine. As a matter of fact, forced diuresis may be deleterious, exacerbating the tendency of salicylates to induce pulmonary edema if a patient has been overhydrated already. Consequently, the administration of isotonic sodium bicarbonate at a rate sufficient to repair acidemia and induce the passage of an alkaline urine is now preferred (109,113). The total amount of isotonic sodium bicarbonate (supplemented as required with potassium salts) necessary to achieve these ends may reach several liters a day. If a diuresis is not established after appropriate amounts of fluid administration (and depending on hemodynamic parameters), a "loop" diuretic may be added to control volume overload (113).

In view of the relatively low molecular weight, the low apparent volume of distribution, and the small degree of protein binding, it is not surprising that hemodialysis has been proposed as a method to combat salicylate intoxication (89,110,115). This method should be employed in patients with high serum levels [usually 5.8 mmol/L (80 mg/dL) or higher], who display major symptomatology such as seizures or coma and/or who have developed metabolic acidosis and other electrolyte disturbances, especially in the presence of renal functional impairment. Factors that are associated with the development of noncardiogenic pulmonary edema also should be considered in deciding whether dialysis (with the ability to remove fluid from the body also) should be employed, including older age, a history of smoking and acute-on-chronic salicylate intoxication, and difficulty in establishing a diuresis (89,102–105,110,115).

Hemoperfusion has also been used in the treatment of salicylate poisoning. However, the procedure is less effective than hemodialysis as the latter offers the additional advantage of correcting the associated acid-base, electrolyte and fluid abnormalities (89,116,117). Because salicylate interferes with coagulation pathways thus making bleeding more likely and a hemoperfusion device can trap platelets, the modality of hemoperfusion may not be an ideal therapy, at least theoretically. Peritoneal dialysis is less efficient and should be reserved for children in whom hemodialysis may be more difficult to perform (89).

LITHIUM

Lithium (MW 7=Dalton) is the lightest alkali metal known and has been successfully used in modern medicine for the treatment of mania and bipolar affective disorders (118–120). However, lithium has a narrow therapeutic index and is a potentially toxic substance. Most commonly, its intoxication occurs in patients who have been receiving chronic lithium therapy. Acute toxic effects may be superimposed on those of chronic toxicity. Also, instances of acute accidental or suicidal ingestions do occur (118–121).

Usually supplied as the carbonate salt in tablets or capsules, lithium is also available in slow-release formulations or as the citrate salt in liquid preparations. It is completely absorbed by the gastrointestinal tract within 8 hours of ingestion with peak serum levels occurring 2 to 4 hours after ingestion. Use of sustained-release preparations delays the onset of peak serum levels. Unbound to proteins, lithium distributes promptly in the extracellular fluid and has a distribution volume of 0.7 to 0.9 L/kg. The cation then slowly enters the intracellular fluid and reaches higher concentrations preferentially in certain tissues, such as the white matter of the brain, the thyroid, the skeleton, and the distal tubular cells of the kidney (118–121). Although a specific lithium pump does not appear to exist, the cation is not passively distributed throughout the body fluids. It is actively transported out of cells by a Na^+/Li^+ exchanger; however, because of the negative intracellular potential prevailing in certain cells, intracellular lithium concentrations may be twice as high as those in the plasma (122). Within cells, lithium is capable of inhibiting adenyl cyclase and inositol-1-phosphate, both being important intracellular messengers (118–121). Whether this mechanism is the one through which lithium exerts its therapeutic or toxic effects is unclear. However, observations that the rate of equilibration of lithium across cellular membranes is slow and that the effects of lithium occur intracellularly help explain the clinical findings that, at comparable serum lithium levels, chronic intoxication is more likely to be accompanied by toxic untoward effects than its acute counterpart (123,124).

Lithium is almost entirely eliminated via the kidney: it is freely filtered by the glomerulus and largely reabsorbed (80%) by the proximal tubule (123). The rate of excretion of lithium is profoundly affected by factors that alter renal tubular sodium handling in that any factor that tends to increase sodium reabsorption, such as volume depletion or dietary sodium restriction, also markedly enhances lithium reabsorption. This phenomenon is responsible for the frequent occurrence of toxicity in patients receiving stable doses of lithium if they happen to develop volume depletion (from any cause such as vomiting, diarrhea, and thiazide diuretic therapy) with its associated heightened sodium (and hence lithium) reabsorption (125). Angiotensin-converting enzyme inhibitors and nonsteroidal antiinflammatory drugs also increase the reabsorption of lithium and result in higher serum lithium concentrations (126,127). However, factors that augment sodium excretion enhance lithium excretion only to a minor extent (118–120).

Clinical Picture and Laboratory Data

The therapeutic index of lithium is low, only 2 or 3, with therapeutic serum levels being 0.4 to 1.3 mEq/L. Toxic manifestations appear at serum levels of 1.5 mEq/L or at even lower values in the elderly. Many patients receiving lithium therapy manifest, at least intermittently, some collateral effects, such as polyuria and nephrogenic diabetes insipidus, renal acidification defects, evidence of chronic interstitial nephritis, leukocytosis, and enlargement of the thyroid gland without clinical evidence of hypothyroidism (118–122,128). Acute intoxication is manifested by vomiting, diarrhea, neuromuscular irritability, coarse tremor, confusion, delirium, ataxia, hyperpyrexia, stupor, coma, and cardiovascular collapse (124,128–130). Toxicity is thought to be correlated primarily with intracellular lithium concentrations. Thus, at comparable serum levels, the clinical picture of

the chronically intoxicated patient (with higher intracellular levels) may be more alarming than that of the acutely intoxicated counterpart (128,129). When serum level of lithium is inordinately elevated, a lower-than-normal serum anion gap, (when calculated as $Na-Cl-CO_2$) can be observed (131,132).

Indications for and Mode of Treatment

Lithium intoxication is always a serious problem in that even when manifestations of toxicity appear relatively minor, seizures and other CNS complications may occur unexpectedly. A serum level of 2.5 mEq/L or greater typically is associated with significant morbidity and mortality and must be treated aggressively (119–121,124), although some reports have stressed that recovery may occur with conservative therapy even in the face of higher levels (129).

When clinical manifestations are mild and the serum lithium level is less than 2.5 mEq/L, aggressive supportive treatment along with discontinuation of lithium therapy may well suffice. In patients with accidental or suicidal ingestion, gastric lavage should be employed; this therapy is not recommended in patients with chronic intoxication. Administration of activated charcoal is not useful, because this agent does not bind lithium ions (133). Whole bowel irrigation can enhance the elimination of sustained-release preparations of lithium and should be considered in patients with acute toxic ingestion, especially in the face of rising serial serum lithium concentrations (134). In vivo studies have documented the ability of orally administered sodium polystyrene sulfonate resin to reduce serum lithium values but this therapy may be limited by the quantity of the resin that must be given and by the resultant development of hypokalemia (135,136).

Lithium-intoxicated patients often present with a certain degree of renal dysfunction; this finding is due to the collateral effects of lithium on the kidney, which include chronic interstitial nephritis (119–122). Most importantly, a state of volume depletion can occur because of a renal defect in concentrating mechanisms, and the frequent concurrence of mental status deterioration may prevent patients from securing an adequate fluid intake. Diuretic therapy and other conditions that aggravate volume depletion, such as vomiting or diarrhea, are also common occurrences. Consequently, ensuring an adequate fluid volume by vigorously replacing preexisting volume losses is of prime importance in reestablishing a desirable level of renal lithium excretion. Any attempt to raise lithium excretion to supranormal levels by the infusion of large quantities of saline solutions is not effective and not recommended. Such infusions are likely to make matters worse by causing volume overload and/or hypernatremia (119–124).

Hemodialysis is highly effective in the removal of lithium. Because of its low atomic weight and its lack of protein binding, lithium is readily diffusible through dialyzer membranes. The extraction ratio for lithium is in the range of 0.7 for plasma and 0.5 for whole blood, the discrepancy resulting from the low extraction of lithium from red blood cells (137). In view of these characteristics and of the relatively low V_d, dialysis can engender a rapid fall in total body lithium burden. Hemodialysis can reduce the half-life of lithium from 12 to 27 hours to

3.6 to 5.7 hours and can raise its clearance rate from 10 to 40 mL/min (via the patient's own kidneys) to 70 to 170 mL/min (119,124,138).

Hemodialysis is indicated in any lithium-intoxicated patient presenting with coma, convulsions, deteriorating mental status, severe cardiac toxicity, respiratory failure, or renal failure. The procedure must be considered in any patient placed on chronic lithium therapy with serum lithium levels exceeding 4 mEq/L. Hemodialysis should also be performed if serum lithium levels fail to fall despite conservative therapy (whether the failure to fall is due to continued gastrointestinal absorption or to diffusion from cells). It is rarely indicated in patients with serum concentrations less than 2.5 mEq/L unless these individuals have end-stage renal disease (ESRD), exhibit continuous increase in serum levels after admission, or fail to achieve a concentration less than 1 mEq/L over 30 hours (119–121, 137–141).

Several factors complicate hemodialysis treatments, largely related to the relatively slow equilibration of lithium across cellular membranes. Following dialysis and a rapid lowering of extracellular lithium concentration, the patient may not improve until reequilibration has occurred. Indeed, the slow exit of lithium from cells often results in a rebound of serum lithium values following dialysis. Therefore, the procedure must be continued beyond the point when apparently safe serum lithium levels are achieved (124,137–140). Prompt determination of serum lithium levels may not be readily available in many healthcare settings. Under such circumstances, it would seem prudent to offer patients more intensive and prolonged dialytic therapy (e.g., 8 or more hours of dialysis right away) during the initial dialysis session (rather than offering a short 3- to 4-hour dialysis session and waiting for the postdialysis lithium level to be determined). Hemodialysis catheters should be preferably left in place for subsequent dialyses (128). Rebound also may occur in cases of poisoning resulting from the ingestion of sustained-release preparations as a result of continued gastrointestinal absorption.

The use of a bicarbonate bath is preferred to that of an acetate bath as lithium clearance from intracellular stores has been suggested to be reduced when the latter bath is used. Acetate bath, in contrast to bicarbonate bath, is thought to activate the sodium-hydrogen antiporter on the cell membrane, allowing lithium (substituting for sodium) to be driven into the cells (142). Hypophosphatemia is a concern with prolonged and recurrent dialysis sessions. Phosphorus-enriched hemodialysis has been used successfully in the prevention of dialysis-induced hypophosphatemia in the lithium-intoxicated patient (143).

High-performance CRRTs (CAVHDF and CVVHDF) have been used successfully in lithium intoxication, achieving lithium clearance rates of 60 to 85 L/day (144). Because of their continuous nature, these therapies create a persistent concentration gradient between the intracellular and extracellular compartments over longer periods, allowing a gradual and more complete elimination of lithium from all intracellular compartments thereby avoiding significant rebound (14,144). In addition, these procedures may be specifically applicable to patients with hemodynamic instability who are unable to tolerate intermittent hemodialysis (145).

Dialysis using sorbent-based dialysate regeneration cartridges would be expected to be effective in extracting lithium, which, because of its polarity, is probably avidly adsorbed to the zirconium phosphate cation exchanger layer. However, we are not aware of published data attesting to the effectiveness and saturability of these cartridges. Hence, we do not recommend their clinical use.

THEOPHYLLINE

Theophylline, chemically known as 1,3-dimethyl xanthine ($C_7H_8N_4O_2$; MW = 180 Dalton), a member of the methylxanthine family of pharmacologic agents, is used in the treatment of respiratory ailments (146). Theophylline intoxication is most commonly seen as the inadvertent consequence of chronic theophylline therapy for asthma and other chronic obstructive pulmonary diseases. Intoxication can occur as a therapeutic mishap or because of intentional overdose (146–148).

When taken orally, theophylline is promptly and efficiently absorbed, with peak serum levels occurring at approximately 2 hours. However, many delayed-release preparations are available, and, when these agents are responsible for the intoxication, peak serum levels may be delayed to 12 to 17 hours after ingestion (149). In the circulation, theophylline is loosely bound to albumin: the fraction bound is highest (approximately 60%) at relatively low therapeutic serum concentrations and is lower at higher toxic serum levels, in adults with liver disease, and in infants (150,151). Able to traverse cellular membranes easily, the unbound fraction equilibrates readily in all fluid compartments, with the drug's V_d amounting to 0.4 to 0.6 L/Kg. In adults, only 10% to 15% of theophylline is excreted unchanged in the urine, the remainder is metabolized in the liver by the cytochrome P-450 pathway. The rate of endogenous hepatic clearance of theophylline is relatively slow—in the order of 0.7 mL/min/kg in adult nonsmokers, in whom the half-life is approximately 8 hours.

The metabolic clearance of theophylline, however, can be profoundly modified by several factors. In infants, hepatic metabolism is slower, resulting in a longer half-life and in a higher renal excretion (50% excreted via this route). Fever, severe chronic liver disease, congestive heart failure, and antibiotic therapy with macrolides and quinolones prolong theophylline half-life, whereas smoking; hyperthyroidism; or the previous administration of barbiturates, phenytoin, rifampin, carbamazepine, and oral contraceptives reduce the half-life of the drug. Theophylline exhibits Michaelis-Menten (saturable) kinetics at therapeutic levels and in cases of supratherapeutic levels follows zero-order (dose-dependent kinetics). In the latter situation, metabolic pathways may become saturated, with reduction in endogenous clearance and a consequent increment in half-life (146–148,151). It is usually these kinetics in addition to the drug-drug and drug-disease interactions that are often responsible for inadvertent theophylline intoxications (152,153).

The mode of action of theophylline has been thought to be due to its capacity to inhibit cyclic nucleotide phosphodiesterase (146). More recent evidence indicates that both the therapeutic and toxic effects of theophylline may be mediated by its action as a competitive antagonist at adenosine receptor sites (154,155). In addition, theophylline results in a release of catecholamines and in positive inotropic and chronotropic effects on the heart (150). Furthermore, its effects on the intracellular calcium transport could also play a role in its various pharmacologic actions.

Clinical Picture and Laboratory Data

Some therapeutic effects of theophylline are observed at serum levels as low as 27.5 μmol/L (5 mg/L), and most benefits of therapy are achieved at serum concentrations in the realm of 55 μmol/L (10 mg/L). Toxic effects become manifest in some patients at concentrations as low as 82.5 μmol/L (15 mg/L), and most patients manifest toxicity at levels greater than 138 μmol/L (25 mg/L) (156). Symptoms of toxicity include gastrointestinal (nausea, vomiting, diarrhea, hematemesis, abdominal pain), neurologic (tachypnea secondary to stimulation of the respiratory centers, anxiety, restlessness, agitation, and muscular tremors progressing to confusion and eventually to seizures), and cardiovascular (supraventricular tachycardia, multifocal atrial tachycardia, ventricular premature beats, ventricular tachycardia, and vasodilatation with hypotension) manifestations. Patients with chronic theophylline toxicity are at an increased risk of developing serious cardiac dysrhythmias (157). Hyperthermia occurs in conjunction with repeated seizures. Hypokalemia and hyperglycemia, secondary to catecholamine-induced β_2-adrenergic stimulation, are commonly observed laboratory manifestations (158). Hypercalcemia, hypomagnesemia, and hypophosphatemia are the other reported abnormalities. In severe and advanced cases, lactic acidosis (most likely secondary to hypotension) and rhabdomyolysis (the consequence of muscular hyperactivity, hyperthermia, and hypokalemia) are observed (153,156–159).

The development of seizures implies a poor prognosis, because this manifestation portends a high mortality or the sequelae of permanent neurologic damage (160,161). Although there is a generic correlation between serum levels and the likelihood of seizures, several factors modify this relationship. Seizures tend to occur at lower concentrations in patients receiving chronic theophylline therapy than in those with acute intoxication. In patients on chronic theophylline therapy, the probability of seizures was 50% in patients with a theophylline concentration of 220 μmol/L (40 mg/L), whereas the same probability was not reached until a theophylline concentration of 660 μmol/L (120 mg/L) was obtained in patients with acute intoxication (152,157). This observation may well be related to the fact that patients receiving chronic theophylline therapy often suffer from other concomitant diseases or receive concurrent medications that lower the seizure threshold (148,156–159). A prior history of neurologic abnormalities does appear to increase the likelihood of seizures (162,163).

Indications for and Mode of Treatment

Because of the serious consequences that follow the onset of seizures, the critical concept underlying the treatment of theophylline toxicity revolves around eliminating the effects of the

toxin or the toxin itself before seizures appear—or at the very least, stopping the recurrence of seizures if this complication has already arisen (147,148). This issue is complicated by many factors: seizures may occur several hours after peak theophylline levels have been achieved, patients are not uncommonly intoxicated with slow-release preparations of the drug (with consequent prolongation of half-life), many endogenous and exogenous factors can alter the expected duration of the intoxication, and patients with chronic versus acute overdosing may have different severities of intoxication at the same serum levels (152,156–161).

In addition to the usual supportive measures, the treatment of theophylline intoxication includes close monitoring of serum potassium and phosphorus concentrations with aggressive replacement of any deficits as indicated and the use of β-blocking agents to control cardiac arrhythmias. Although noncardioelective agents such as propranolol may offer some advantage because of their capacity to counteract theophylline-induced vasodilatation and hypokalemia (164), cardioselective β-blockers are usually required in patients with bronchial asthma (165). Serial monitoring of theophylline levels should be done every 2 to 4 hours until peak levels are reached.

Benzodiazepines are agents of choice to control theophylline-induced seizures. Barbiturates such as phenobarbital are second-line agents. Phenytoin is relatively contraindicated as animal data have suggested that it may increase the risk of theophylline-induced seizures (166). If these seizure-afflicted patients do not respond to anticonvulsant therapy, general anesthesia and neuromuscular paralysis may become necessary (167).

The oral administration of repeated doses of activated charcoal has been proven to shorten theophylline half-life markedly, even in patients who have received theophylline by the intravenous route. Charcoal binds the fraction of ingested theophylline that has not yet been absorbed as well as that which diffuses into the intestine from the circulation, the latter phenomenon being referred to as enterocapillary exsorption (168,169). Activated charcoal is administered depending on body size in the form of a slurry of 15 to 20 g every 1 to 2 hours in adults, or in doses of 2.5 to 10 g hourly in children until serum concentrations of theophylline are less than 110 μmol/L (20 mg/L) along with resolution of manifestations of toxicity (168–170). Such maneuvers should be employed routinely in all theophylline-intoxicated patients except for those with minimal signs and symptoms of toxicity. The charcoal slurry may be administered by mouth or, in uncooperative or comatose patients, via nasogastric intubation. Should the latter become necessary, to avoid aspiration, nasogastric intubation should be carried out only after the patient has been placed in the Trendelenburg position with the head turned to one side (if awake) or after endotracheal intubation (if the patient is uncooperative or unconscious). Unfortunately, the concomitant nausea and vomiting may make the use of multiple-dose activated charcoal difficult in many afflicted patients. Under such circumstances, antiemetics such as metoclopramide and ondansetron may be used liberally. Because prochlorperazine may lower seizure threshold, its use is contraindicated (171). Use of cathartics with activated charcoal may hasten the evacuation of charcoal-theophylline complex (172). Forced diuresis is not recommended.

Hemoperfusion with either resin cartridges (such as Amberlite XAD-4) or activated charcoal cartridges is very effective in eliminating the toxin, reaching extraction ratios of close to 1 (173–176). Indeed, because of the ease of transmembrane movement of theophylline, the drug is efficiently removed not only from the plasma phase but also from the erythrocytes. The total amount of drug removed can be calculated using blood, rather than plasma flow rates through the hemoperfusion cartridge (177). Unfortunately, the capacity of hemoperfusion cartridges to extract theophylline is not limitless, and the efficiency of theophylline elimination falls with time as the cartridge becomes saturated. Consequently, a cartridge must be replaced every 2 hours (174–176,178).

Hemodialysis, as expected from the pharmacologic characteristics of theophylline, has been shown to be effective in the drug's removal (179,180). Using modern, high-efficiency hemodialyzers [with a high mass-transfer area coefficient (KoA)] for urea as well as high blood and dialysate flow rates, extraction ratios greater than 0.5 to 0.6 can be expected and clearance rates similar to those of hemoperfusion can be achieved, especially if dialysis is prolonged (148). Substantial amounts of the drug may be removed in a relatively short time—for example, up to 40% of the total body burden in 3 hours. Intensive and prolonged hemodialysis sessions may be required to obtain results equivalent to those achieved by hemoperfusion. As previously stated, hypophosphatemia is an occasional concern in patients with theophylline intoxication. If intensive and prolonged dialytic sessions are employed, the use of a phosphorus-enriched hemodialysate should be considered. Finally, hemodialysis has been suggested to be comparable to hemoperfusion in its ability to reduce morbidity and mortality from theophylline poisoning and may be associated with fewer procedural complications (181).

The "in series" use of simultaneous hemodialysis and charcoal hemoperfusion (HD/HP) can remove several hundred milligrams of theophylline per hour at a time when correction of fluid, acid-base, and electrolyte disturbances can also be carried out by dialysis. This combined procedure also delays the saturation of the charcoal cartridge and is, therefore, a favorable treatment option for patients with very advanced theophylline intoxication, in centers where such a combined procedure is available (178,179).

In patients who already had seizures or those who are clinically unstable, hemodialysis or hemoperfusion should be started as soon as possible (147,180). In those who appear clinically stable, the administration of charcoal may suffice until serum theophylline levels become available. If the level is close to 330 μmol/L (60 mg/L) in patients receiving theophylline chronically or close to 550 μmol/L (100 mg/L) in patients with acute intoxication and if the patient is tolerating the administration of charcoal well, then hemodialysis or hemoperfusion may be delayed further (while making preparations for either procedure's implementation) until the next theophylline level becomes available to gauge if the charcoal therapy has been effective. All patients who have higher serum levels, even without major toxic manifestations, and those who do not tolerate charcoal well should be treated with hemodialysis or hemoperfusion. In the presence of concomitant renal failure, hepatic failure, cardiac failure, or

advanced age, either of the previously mentioned extracorporeal measures should be considered even sooner (148,179). Because hemodialysis can remove waste products and rectify electrolyte, acid-base, and fluid abnormalities, the procedure is the treatment of choice in many of the patients suffering from various comorbid conditions.

The question of whether sorbent-based dialysate regeneration systems are effective in the treatment of theophylline intoxication has not been studied exhaustively. The REDY machine using Sorb cartridges is presently the only hemodialysis apparatus readily available at certain community hospitals. The Sorb cartridge contains a layer of activated charcoal that can adsorb up to 5 g of the drug (182). However, to reach the cartridge, theophylline must first be dialyzed into the system's bath; consequently, the extraction ratio and total amount removed would at best be equal to that achieved via hemodialysis alone. Finally, the bicarbonate ion used in a sorbent-based dialysate regeneration system originates from the conversion of dialyzed urea to ammonium carbonate. The ammonium ion generated is subsequently removed by another layer in the cartridge that contains zirconium phosphate. Thus, in patients who do not have sufficiently high blood urea concentrations, such a system not only may fail to repair but also may indeed induce metabolic acidosis (183). Nonetheless, anecdotal reports indicate that these sorbent systems are effective in the treatment of theophylline intoxication. In light of these considerations, it is suggested that sorbent-based dialysate regeneration systems be used only if single-pass hemodialysis is not available and then only with close monitoring of acid-base parameters and of theophylline levels. Should metabolic acidosis develop, intravenous infusions of bicarbonate or conversion of the machine to a "single pass" mode, which requires frequent (every 30 minute) dialysate bath changes, should be employed (183).

CVVHF has also been used successfully in the treatment of theophylline intoxication with a nearly fourfold increase in the removal of theophylline and may be a practical alternative therapy in patients with hemodynamic instability (184,185).

Plasmapheresis removes both the free and the protein-bound fractions of theophylline and has been used successfully in one instance of theophylline poisoning (186). No significant difference in the elimination rate between charcoal hemoperfusion and venovenous plasmapheresis was found. Consequently, plasmapheresis may be an effective alternative therapy (171,186). Peritoneal dialysis is not effective in the treatment of theophylline poisoning (187).

ETHANOL

Ethanol (C_2H_5OH; MW = 46 Dalton), is one of the most frequently encountered toxins in the emergency departments in the United States (188). The detailed description of its pharmacokinetics, clinical effects, and management of withdrawal syndromes is beyond the purview of this chapter. Acute alcoholic intoxication is responsible for a number of deaths annually, most notably among young college students with binge drinking patterns (189). Most of the deaths are caused by respiratory depression, aspiration-induced asphyxia, or traumatic injuries in severely inebriated subjects. Acute intoxication can also engender severe hypotension and cardiac arrhythmias at lethal concentrations. Lethal level is at the realm of 98 mM (450 mg/dL) for half of the non-ethanol-dependent population, although individuals with serum concentrations as high as 326 mM (1,500 mg/dL) have survived (190,191). Most patients can be treated adequately with proper supportive care consisting of the administration of fluids, electrolytes, thiamine, folate, and other vitamins in addition to the prevention of hypoglycemia (with its attendant damaging effects on the brain) and hypoxia. Gastric emptying may be ineffective in view of the rapid absorption of ethanol. Charcoal may be administered if circumstances suggest the coingestion of other toxins (188). The vast majority of inebriated individuals recover on their own with the previously mentioned symptomatic and supportive care (188,192). However, in severely intoxicated patients with lethal serum ethanol levels and at risk of respiratory depression and circulatory failure, extracorporeal techniques such as hemodialysis, hemofiltration, and hemodiafiltration can be employed (192–194). Because of its small molecular weight and the absence of protein-binding, ethanol is readily removed by these techniques. Hemodialysis increases the plasma elimination rate of alcohol from a physiologic one of 15 mg/dL/hour to one of nearly 100 mg/dL/hour (192).

REFERENCES

1. Lebowitz T, et al. 2001 Annual report of American Association of Poison Control Centers Toxic Exposure Surveillance System. *Am J Emer Med* 2002;20:391–452.
2. Clemmesen C, et al. Therapeutic trends in the treatment of barbiturate poisoning: the Scandinavian method. *Clin Pharmacol Ther* 1961; 2:220–229.
3. Lorch JA, et al. Hemoperfusion to treat intoxications. *Ann Intern Med* 1979;91:301–304.
4. Kirk M, et al. Pearls, pitfalls, and updates in toxicology. *Emerg Med Clin North Am* 1997;15:427–449.
5. Shrestha M, et al. A comparison of three gastric lavage methods using the radionuclide gastric emptying study. *J Emerg Med* 1996;14: 413–418.
6. Pond SM, et al. Gastric emptying in acute overdose: a prospective randomised controlled trial. *Med J Aust* 1995;163:345–349.
7. Smilkstein MJ. Techniques used to prevent gastrointestinal absorption of toxic compounds. In: Goldfrank LR, et al., eds. *Goldfrank's toxicologic emergencies,* 6th ed. Stamford, CT: Appleton & Lange, 1998:35–51.
8. Benowitz NL, et al. Cardiac disturbances. In: Haddad LM, et al., eds. *Clinical management of poisoning and drug overdose,* 3rd ed. Philadelphia: WB Saunders, 1998:90–119.
9. McFarland AK III, et al. Selection of activated charcoal products for the treatment of poisonings. *Ann Pharmacother* 1993;27:358–361.
10. Ledebo I. Principles and practice of hemofiltration and hemodiafiltration. *Artif Organs* 1998;22:20–25.
11. Wizemann V, et al. Efficacy of haemodiafiltration. *Nephrol Dial Transplant* 2001;16[Suppl]:27–30.
12. Ronco C, et al. Continuous renal replacement therapy: evolution in technology and current nomenclature. *Kidney Int* 1998;53:S125–S128.
13. Bohler J, et al. Continuous arteriovenous haemoperfusion (CAVHP) for the treatment of paraquat poisoning. *Nephrol Dial Transplant* 1992;7:875–878.
14. Riegel W. Use of continuous renal replacement therapy for detoxification. *Int J Artif Organs* 1996;19:111–112.
15. Jones JS, et al. Current status of plasmapheresis in toxicology. *Ann Emerg Med* 1986;15:474–482.
16. Rosenbaum JL. Hemoperfusion for acute drug intoxication. *Kidney Int* 1980;18[Suppl 10]:S106–S108.
17. Mitzner SR, et al. Albumin dialysis using the molecular adsorbent recirculating system. *Curr Opin Nephrol Hypertens* 2001;10:777–783.
18. McIntyre CW, et al. Use of albumin dialysis in the treatment of hepatic and renal dysfunction due to paracetamol intoxication. *Nephrol Dial Transplant* 2002;17:316–317.
19. Shi Y, et al. MARS: optimistic therapy method in fulminant hepatic failure secondary to cytotoxic mushroom poisoning—a case report. *Liver* 2002;22[Suppl]:78–80.
20. Marshall MR, et al. Sustained low-efficiency dialysis for critically ill patients requiring renal replacement therapy. *Kidney Int* 2001;60: 777–785.
21. Marshall MR, et al. Urea kinetics during sustained low-efficiency dialysis in critically ill patients requiring renal replacement therapy. *Am J Kidney Dis* 2002;39:556–570.
22. Schreiner GE, et al. Dialysis of poisons and drugs—annual review. *Trans Am Soc Artif Intern Organs* 1972;18:563–599.
23. Winchester JF, et al. Dialysis and hemoperfusion of poisons and drugs—update. *Trans Am Soc Artif Intern Organs* 1977;23:762–842.
24. Maher JF. Principles of dialysis and dialysis of drugs. *Am J Med* 1977; 62:475–481.
25. Winchester JF. Active methods for detoxification. In: Haddad LM, et al., eds. *Clinical management of poisoning and drug overdose,* 3rd ed. Philadelphia: WB Saunders, 1998:175–188.
26. Sam R, et al. Removal of foscarnet by hemodialysis using dialysate-side values. *Int J Artif Organs* 2000;23:165–167.
27. Gibson TP, et al. Effect of changes in intercompartment rate constants on drug removal during hemoperfusion. *J Pharm Sci* 1978;67: 1178–1179.
28. Haapanen EJ. Hemoperfusion in acute intoxication: clinical experience with 48 cases. *Acta Med Scand Suppl* 1982;668:76–81.
29. Blye E, et al. Extracorporeal therapy in the treatment of intoxication. *Am J Kidney Dis* 1984;3:321–338.
30. Peterson RG, et al. Cleansing the blood: hemodialysis, peritoneal dialysis, exchange transfusion, charcoal hemoperfusion, forced diuresis. *Ped Clin North Am* 1986;33:675–689.
31. Garella S. Extracorporeal techniques in the treatment of exogenous intoxications. *Kidney Int* 1988;33:735–740.
32. Pentel PR, et al. Tricyclic and newer antidepressants. In: Haddad LM, et al., eds. *Clinical management of poisoning and drug overdose,* 3rd ed. Philadelphia: WB Saunders, 1998:636–655.
33. Keusch G. Sekundare dekontamination: wann sind hamodialyse oder hamoperfusion indiziert? *Ther Umschau* 1992;49:113–117.
34. McBride PV, et al. Acetaminophen intoxication. *Semin Dial* 1992;5: 292–298.
35. Okonek S. Hemoperfusion in toxicology: basic considerations of its effectiveness. *Clin Toxicol* 1981;18:1185–1198.
36. Kar PM, et al. Combined high efficiency hemodialysis and charcoal hemoperfusion in severe N-acetyl procainamide intoxication. *Am J Kidney Dis* 1992;20:403–406.
37. Seyffart G. Ethylene glycol. In: Seyffart G, ed. *Poison index—the treatment of acute intoxication.* Lengerich, Germany: Pabst Science Publishers, 1997:318–328.
38. Winchester JF. Methanol, isopropyl alcohol, higher alcohols, ethylene glycol, cellosolves, acetone, and oxalate. In: Haddad LM, et al., eds. *Clinical management of poisoning and drug overdose,* 3rd ed. Philadelphia: WB Saunders, 1998:491–504.
39. Eder AF, et al. Ethylene glycol poisoning: toxicokinetic and analytical factors affecting laboratory diagnosis. *Clin Chem* 1998;44:168–177.
40. Gabow PA, et al. Organic acids in ethylene glycol intoxication. *Ann Intern Med* 1986;105:16.
41. Jacobsen D, et al. Glycolate causes the acidoses in ethylene glycol poisoning and is effectively removed by hemodialysis. *Acta Med Scand* 1984;216:409–416.
42. Barceloux DG, et al. American Academy of Clinical Toxicology practice guidelines in the treatment of the ethylene glycol poisoning. *Clin Toxicol* 1999;37:537–560.
43. Peterson CD, et al. Ethylene glycol poisoning: pharmacokinetics during therapy with ethanol and hemodialysis. *N Engl J Med* 1981;304: 21–23.

44. McMartin KE, et al. Studies on the metabolic interactions between 4-methylpyrazole and methanol using the monkey as an animal model. *Arch Biochem Biophys* 1980;199:606–614.

45. Brent J, et al. Fomepizole for the treatment of ethylene glycol poisoning. *N Engl J Med* 1999;340:832–838.

46. Kahn HS, et al. A recovery from ethylene glycol (antifreeze) intoxication: a case of survival and two fatalities from ethylene glycol including autopsy findings. *Ann Intern Med* 1950;32:284–294.

47. Hylander B, et al. Prognostic factors and treatment of severe ethylene glycol intoxication. *Intensive Care Med* 1996;22:546–552.

48. Gennari FJ. Serum osmolality: uses and limitations. *N Engl J Med* 1984;310:102–105.

49. Jacobsen D, et al. Urinary calcium monohydrate crystals in ethylene glycol poisoning. *Scand J Clin Lab Invest* 1982;42:231–234.

50. Terlinsky AS, et al. Identification of atypical calcium oxalate crystalluria following ethylene glycol ingestion. *Am J Clin Pathol* 1981;76:223–226.

51. Winter ML, et al. Urine fluorescence using a Wood's lamp to detect the antifreeze additive sodium fluorescein: a qualitative adjunctive test in suspected ethylene glycol ingestions. *Ann Emerg Med* 1990;19:663–667.

52. Wallace K, et al. Accuracy and reliability of urine fluorescence by Wood's lamp examination for antifreeze ingestion. *J Toxicol Clin Toxicol* 1997;37:711–719.

53. Underwood F, et al. Ethylene glycol intoxication: prevention of renal failure by aggressive management. *JAMA* 1973;226:1453–1454.

54. Jacobsen D, et al. Effects of 4-methylpyrazole, methanol/ethylene glycol antidote, in healthy humans. *J Emerg Med* 1990;8:455–461.

55. Cheng JT, et al. Clearance of ethylene glycol by kidneys and hemodialysis. *Clin Toxicol* 1987;27:95–108.

56. Watson W. Ethylene glycol toxicity: closing in a rational evidence-based treatment. *Ann Emerg Med* 2000;36:139–141.

57. Noghnogh AA, et al. Preparation of ethanol-enriched, bicarbonate-based hemodialysis. *Artif Organs* 1999;23:208–216.

58. Chow MT, et al. Use of a phosphorus-enriched dialysate to hemodialyze patients with ethylene glycol intoxication. *Int J Artif Organs* 1997;20:101–104.

59. Chow MT, et al. Hemodialysis-induced hypophosphatemia in a normophosphatemic patient dialyzed for ethylene glycol poisoning: treatment with phosphorus-enriched hemodialysis. *Artif Organs* 1998;22:905–913.

60. Hirsch DJ, et al. A simple method to estimate the required dialysis time for cases of alcohol poisoning. *Kidney Int* 2001;60:2021–2024.

61. Christiansson LK, et al. Treatment of severe ethylene glycol intoxication with continuous arterio-venous hemofiltration dialysis. *Clin Toxicol* 1995;33:267–270.

62. Seyffart G. Methyl alcohol. In: Seyffart G, ed. *Poison index—the treatment of acute intoxication.* Lengerich, Germany: Pabst Science Publishers, 1997:457–464.

63. Agency for toxic substances and disease registry (ATSDR). Methanol toxicity. *Am Fam Physician* 1993;47:163–171.

64. Davis LE, et al. Methanol poisoning exposures in the United States: 1993–98. *Clin Toxicol* 2002;40:499–505.

65. McMartin KE, et al. Methanol poisoning in human subjects: role for formic acid accumulation in the metabolic acidosis. *Am J Med* 1980;68:414–418.

66. Martin-Amat G, et al. Methanol poisoning: ocular toxicity produced by formate. *Toxicol Appl Pharmacol* 1978;45:201–208.

67. Burns MJ, et al. Treatment of methanol poisoning with intravenous 4-methylpyrazole. *Ann Emerg Med* 1997;30:829–832.

68. Jacobsen D, et al. Antidotes for methanol and ethylene glycol poisoning. *Clin Toxicol* 1997;35:127–143.

69. Brent J, et al. Fomepizole for the treatment of methanol poisoning. *N Engl J Med* 2001;344:424–429.

70. Pappas SC, et al. Treatment of methanol poisoning with ethanol and hemodialysis. *Can Med Assoc J* 1982;126:1391.

71. Phang PT, et al. Brain hemorrhage associated with methanol poisoning. *Crit Care Med* 1988;16:137–140.

72. Liu JL, et al. Prognostic factors in patients with methanol poisoning. *Clin Toxicol* 1998;36:175–181.

73. Palmisano J, et al. Absence of anion gap metabolic acidosis in severe methanol poisoning: a case report and review of the literature. *Am J Kidney Dis* 1987;9:441–444.

74. Barceloux DG, et al. American academy of clinical toxicology practice guidelines on the treatment of methanol poisoning. *Clin Toxicol* 2002;40:415–446.

75. Gonda A, et al. Hemodialysis for methanol intoxication. *Am J Med* 1978;64:749–758.

76. Alvarez R, et al. Effectiveness of hemodialysis with high flux polysulfone membrane in the treatment of life-threatening methanol intoxication. *Nephron* 2002;90:216–218.

77. Burgess E. Prolonged hemodialysis in methanol intoxication. *Pharmacotherapy* 1992;12:238–239.

78. Dorval M, et al. The use of an ethanol and phosphate enriched dialysate to maintain stable serum ethanol levels during hemodialysis for methanol intoxication. *Nephrol Dial Transplant* 1999;14:1274–1277.

79. Chow MT, et al. Treatment of acute methanol intoxication with hemodialysis using an ethanol-enriched, bicarbonate-based dialysate. *Am J Kidney Dis* 1997;30:568–570.

80. Wadgymar A, et al. Treatment of acute methanol intoxication with hemodialysis. *Am J Kidney Dis* 1998;5:897.

81. Carauna RJ, et al. Heparin-free dialysis: comparative data and results in high-risk patients. *Kidney Int* 1987;6:1351–1355.

82. Noker PE, et al. Methanol toxicity: treatment with folic acid and 5-formyl-tetrahydrofolic acid. *Alcohol Clin Exp Res* 1980;4:378–383.

83. Seyffart G. Isopropyl alcohol. In Seyffart G, ed. *Poison index—the treatment of acute intoxication.* Lengerich, Germany: Pabst Science Publishers, 1997:385–389.

84. Lehman AJ, et al. The acute and chronic toxicity of isopropyl alcohol. *J Lab Clin Med* 1944;29:561–567.

85. Lacouture PG, et al. Acute isopropyl alcohol intoxication: diagnosis and management. *Am J Med* 1983;75:680–686.

86. Abramson S, et al. Treatment of the alcohol intoxications: ethylene glycol, methanol and isopropanol. *Curr Opin Nephrol Hypertens* 2000;9:695–701.

87. Rosansky SJ. Isopropyl alcohol poisoning treated with hemodialysis: kinetics of isopropyl alcohol and acetone removal. *J Toxicol Clin Toxicol* 1982;19:265–271.

88. Pappas AA, et al. Isopropanol ingestion: a report of six episodes with isopropanol and acetone serum concentration time data. *J Toxicol Clin Toxicol* 1991;29:11–21.

89. Seyffart G. Salicylates. In: Seyffart G, ed. *Poison index—the treatment of acute intoxication.* Lengerich, Germany: Pabst Science Publishers, 1997:606–612.

90. McGuigan MA. A two-year review of salicylate deaths in Ontario. *Arch Intern Med* 1987;147:510–512.

91. Roberts LJ, et al. Analgesic-antipyretics and anti-inflammatory agents and drugs employed in the treatment of gout. In: Hardman JG, et al., eds. *Goodman and Gilman's the pharmacological basis of therapeutics,* 10th ed. New York: McGraw-Hill, 2001:687–731.

92. Harrington JT, et al. Metabolic acidosis. In: Cohen JJ, et al., eds. *Acid/base.* Boston: Little, Brown and Company, 1982:121–225.

93. Wosilait WD. Theoretical analysis of the binding of salicylate by human serum albumin: the relationship between free and bound drug and therapeutic levels. *Eur J Clin Pharmacol* 1976;9:285–290.

94. Rubin GM, et al. Concentration-dependence of salicylate distribution. *J Pharm Pharmacol* 1983;35:115–117.

95. Hill JB. Salicylate intoxication. *N Engl J Med* 1973;288:1110–1113.

96. Proudfoot AT. Toxicity of salicylates. *Am J Med* 1983;75:88–103.

97. Winters RW, et al. Disturbances of acid-base equilibrium in salicylate intoxication. *Pediatrics* 1959;23:260–285.

98. Gabow PA, et al. Acid-base disturbances in the salicylate-intoxicated adult. *Arch Intern Med* 1978;138:1481–1484.

99. Clarkson AR. Phenistix in screening. *Aust Fam Physician* 1978;7:1324–1328.

100. Brenner BE, et al. Management of salicylate intoxication. *Drugs* 1982;24:335–340

101. Johnston PK, et al. A simplified urine and serum screening test for salicylate intoxication. *J Pediatr* 1963;63:949–953.

102. Bowers RE, et al. Salicylate pulmonary edema: the mechanism in sheep and review of the literature. *Am Rev Resp Dis* 1977;115:261–268.

103. Hormaechea E, et al. Hypovolemia, pulmonary edema, and protein changes in severe salicylate poisoning. *Am J Med* 1979;66: 1046–1050.

104. Heffner JE, et al. Salicylate-induced pulmonary edema. *Ann Intern Med* 1981;95:405–409.

105. Walters JS, et al. Salicylate-induced pulmonary edema. *Radiology* 1983;146:289–293.

106. Chapman J, et al. Adult salicylate poisoning: deaths and outcome in patients with high plasma salicylate concentration. *Q J Med* 1989;268:699–707.

107. Done AK. Aspirin overdosage: incidence, diagnosis, and management. *Pediatrics* 1978;62(part 2 Suppl):890–897.

108. Kwong TC, et al. Self-poisoning with enteric-coated aspirin. *Am J Clin Path* 1983;80:888–890.

109. Notarianni L. A reassessment of the treatment of salicylate poisoning. *Drug Safety* 1992;7:292–303.

110. Krenzelok EP, et al. Salicylate toxicity. In: Haddad LM, et al., eds. *Clinical management of poisoning and drug overdose*, 3rd ed. Philadelphia: WB Saunders, 1998:675–687.

111. Filippone GA, et al. Reversible adsorption (desorption) of aspirin from activated charcoal. *Arch Intern Med* 1987;147:1390–1392.

112. Mayer AL, et al. Multiple-dose charcoal and whole-bowel irrigation do not increase clearance of absorbed salicylate. *Arch Intern Med* 1992;152:393–396.

113. Prescott LF, et al. Diuresis or alkalinisation for salicylate poisoning? *BMJ* 1982;285:1383–1386.

114. Gordon IJ, et al. Algorithm for modified alkaline diuresis in salicylate poisoning. *BMJ* 1984;289:1039–1040.

115. Richlie DG, et al. Contemporary management of salicylate poisoning: when should hemodialysis and hemoperfusion be used? *Semin Dial* 1996;9:257–264.

116. Winchester JF, et al. Extracorporeal treatment of salicylate or acetaminophen poisoning—is there a role? *Arch Intern Med* 1981;141: 370–374.

117. Jacobsen D, et al. Hemodialysis or hemoperfusion in severe salicylate poisoning. *Hum Toxicol* 1988;7:161–163.

118. Baldessarini RJ, et al. Drugs and the treatment of psychiatric disorders: psychosis and mania. In: Hardman JG, et al., eds. *Goodman and Gilman's the pharmacological basis of therapeutics*, 10th ed. New York: McGraw-Hill, 2001:485–520.

119. Seyffart G. Lithium. In: Seyffart G, ed. *Poison index—the treatment of acute intoxication*. Lengerich, Germany: Pabst Science Publishers, 1997:402–410.

120. Winchester JF. Lithium. In: Haddad LM, et al., eds. *Clinical management of poisoning and drug overdose*, 3rd ed. Philadelphia: WB Saunders, 1998:467–474.

121. Goddard J, et al. Hammersmith staff rounds. Lithium intoxication. *BMJ* 1991;302:1267–1269.

122. Holstein-Rathlou NH. Lithium transport across biological membranes. *Kidney Int* 1990;37[Suppl 28]:S4–S9.

123. Godinich MJ, et al. Renal tubular effects of lithium. *Kidney Int* 1990;37[Suppl 28]:S52–S57.

124. Hansen HE, et al. Lithium intoxication. *Q J Med* 1978;17:123–144.

125. Bennet WM. Drug interactions and consequences of sodium restriction. *Am J Clin Nutr* 1997;65:678–815.

126. Finley PR, et al. Clinical relevance of drug interactions with lithium. *Clin Pharmacokinet* 1995;29:172–191.

127. Finley PR, et al. Lithium and angiotensin-converting enzyme inhibitors: evaluation of a potential interaction. *J Clin Psychopharmacol* 1996;16:68–71.

128. Timmer RT, et al. Lithium intoxication. *J Am Soc Nephrol* 1999;10: 666–674.

129. Gadallah MF, et al. Lithium intoxication: clinical course and therapeutic considerations. *Miner Electrolyte Metab* 1988;14:146–149.

130. Sheehan GL. Lithium neurotoxicity. *Clin Exp Neurol* 1991;28: 112–127.

131. Jurado RL, et al. Low anion gap. *South Med J* 1998;91:624–629.

132. Kelleher SP, et al. Reduced or absent serum anion gap as a marker of severe lithium intoxication. *Arch Intern Med* 1986;146:1839–1840.

133. Favin F, et al. In-vitro study of lithium carbonate adsorption by activated charcoal. *J Toxicol Clin Toxicol* 1988;26:443–450.

134. Smith SW, et al. Whole-bowel irrigation as a treatment for acute lithium overdose. *Ann Emerg Med* 1991;20:536–539.

135. Gehrke JC, et al. In-vivo binding of lithium using the cation exchange resin sodium polystyrene sulfonate. *Am J Emerg Med* 1996;14:37–38.

136. Scharman EJ. Methods used to decrease lithium absorption or enhance elimination. *Clin Toxicol* 1997;35:601–608.

137. Clendeninn NJ, et al. Potential pitfalls in the evaluation of the usefulness of hemodialysis for the removal of lithium. *J Toxicol Clin Toxicol* 1982;19:341–352.

138. Jaeger A, et al. When should dialysis be performed in lithium poisoning? A kinetic study in 14 cases of lithium poisoning. *Clin Toxicol* 1993;31:429–447.

139. Okusa MD, et al. Clinical manifestations and management of lithium intoxication. *Am J Med* 1994;97:383–389.

140. Hauger RI, et al. Lithium toxicity: when is hemodialysis necessary? *Acta Psychiatr Scand* 1990;81:515–517.

141. Bailey B, et al. Comparison of patients hemodialyzed for lithium poisoning and those for whom dialysis was recommended by PCC but not done: what lesson can we learn? *Clin Nephrol* 2000;54:388–392.

142. Szerlip HM, et al. Comparison between acetate and bicarbonate dialysis for the treatment of lithium intoxication. *Am J Nephrol* 1992; 12:116–120.

143. Zabaneh RI, et al. Use of a phosphorus-enriched dialysis solution to hemodialyze a patient with lithium intoxication. *Artif Organs* 1995; 19:94–112.

144. Leblanc M, et al. Lithium poisoning treated by high-performance continuous arteriovenous and venovenous hemodiafiltration. *Am J Kidney Dis* 1996;27:365–372.

145. Beckman U, et al. Efficacy of continuous venovenous hemodialysis in the treatment of severe lithium toxicity. *Clin Toxicol* 2001;39:393–397.

146. Undem BJ, et al. Drugs used in the treatment of asthma. In: Goodman Gilman A, et al., eds. *Goodman and Gilman's the pharmacological basis of therapeutics,* 10th ed. New York: Pergamon Press, 1990: 733–754.

147. Seyffart G. Theophylline. In: Seyffart G, ed. *Poison index—the treatment of acute intoxication.* Lengerich, Germany: Pabst Science Publishers, 1997:638–646.

148. Shannon MW. Theophylline. In: Haddad LM, et al., eds. *Clinical management of poisoning and drug overdose,* 3rd ed. Philadelphia: WB Saunders, 1998:1093–1106.

149. Clayton D, et al. Delayed toxicity with slow-release theophylline. *Med J Aust* 1986;144:386–387.

150. Bukowskyj M, et al. Theophylline reassessed. *Ann Intern Med* 1984; 101:63–73.

151. Hendeles L, et al. Theophylline. In: Evans WE, et al., eds. *Applied pharmacokinetics: principles of therapeutics drug monitoring,* 2nd ed. Philadelphia: Lippincott, 1986:1105–1188

152. Shannon MW. Predictors of major toxicity after theophylline overdose. *Ann Intern Med* 1993;119:1161–1167.

153. Sessler CN. Theophylline toxicity: clinical features of 116 consecutive cases. *Am J Med* 1990;88:567–576.

154. Feoktistov I, et al. Adenosine A2B receptors: a novel therapeutic target in asthma? *Trends Pharmacol Sci* 1998;19:148–153.

155. Fredholm BB, et al. Xanthine derivatives as adenosine receptor antagonists. *Eur J Pharmacol* 1982;81:673–676.

156. Jacobs MH, et al. Clinical experience with theophylline—relationships between dosage, serum concentration, and toxicity. *JAMA* 1976; 235:1983–1986.

157. Olson KR, et al. Theophylline overdose: acute single ingestion versus chronic repeated overmedication. *Am J Emerg Med* 1985;3:386–394.

158. Kearney TE, et al. Theophylline toxicity and the beta-adrenergic system. *Ann Intern Med* 1985;102:766–769.

159. Cooling DS. Theophlline toxicity. *J Emerg Med* 1993;11:415–425.

160. Zwillich CW, et al. Theophylline-induced seizures in adults: correlation with serum concentration. *Ann Intern Med* 1975;82:784–787.

161. Aitken ML, et al. Life-threatening theophylline toxicity is not predictable by serum levels. *Chest* 1987;91:10–14.

162. Covelli HD, et al. Predisposing factors to apparent theophylline-induced seizures. *Ann Allerg* 1985;54:411–415.

163. Singer EP, et al. Seizures due to theophylline overdose. *Chest* 1985;87: 755–757.

164. Biberstein MP, et al. Use of beta-blockade and hemoperfusion for acute theophylline poisoning. *West J Med* 1984;141:485–490.

165. Seneff M, et al. Acute theophylline toxicity and the use of esmolol to reverse cardiovascular instability. *Ann Emerg Med* 1990;19: 671–673.

166. Blake KV, et al. Relative efficacy of phenytoin and phenobarbital for the prevention of theophylline-induced seizures in mice. *Ann Emerg Med* 1988;17:1024–1028.

167. Gaudreault P, et al. Theophylline poisoning—pharmacological considerations and clinical management. *Med Toxicol* 1986;1:161–191.

168. Amitai Y, et al. Repetitive oral activated charcoal and control of emesis in severe theophylline toxicity. *Ann Intern Med* 1986;105:386–387.

169. Park GD, et al. Effects of size and frequency of oral doses of charcoal on theophylline clearance. *Clin Pharmacol Ther* 1983;34:663–666.

170. Goldberg MJ, et al. Treatment of theophylline toxicity. *J Allergy Clin Immunol* 1986;78:811–817.

171. Byrd RP, et al. Clinical theophylline toxicity: acute and chronic. *J Ky Med Assoc* 1993;91:198–202.

172. Goldberg MJ, et al. The effect of sorbitol and activated charcoal on serum theophyline concentrations after slow-release theophylline. *Clin Pharmacol Ther* 1987;41:108–111.

173. Lawyer C, et al. Treatment of theophylline neurotoxicity with resin hemoperfusion. *Ann Intern Med* 1978;88:515–516.

174. Ehlers SM, et al. Massive theophylline overdose: rapid elimination by charcoal hemoperfusion. *JAMA* 1978;240:474–475.

175. Russo ME. Management of theophylline intoxication with charcoal-column hemoperfusion. *N Engl J Med* 1979;300:24–26.

176. Park GD, et al. Use of hemoperfusion for treatment of theophylline intoxication. *Am J Med* 1983;74:961–966.

177. Van Kesteren RG, et al. Massive theophylline intoxication: effects of charcoal haemoperfusion on plasma and erythrocyte theophylline concentrations. *Hum Toxicol* 1985;4:127–134.

178. Hootkins R, et al. Sequential and simultaneous "in series" hemodialysis and hemoperfusion in the management of theophylline intoxication. *J Am Soc Nephrol* 1990;1:923–926.

179. Benowitz NL, et al. The use of hemodialysis and hemoperfusion in the treatment of theophylline intoxication. *Semin Dial* 1993;6: 243–252.

180. Lee CS, et al. Hemodialysis of theophylline in uremic patients. *J Clin Pharmacol* 1979;19:219–226.

181. Shannon MW. Comparative efficacy of hemodialysis and hemoperfusion in severe theophylline intoxication. *Acad Emerg Med* 1997;4: 674–678.

182. Guide to custom dialysis. Lakewood, CO: The RedyB Company (a division of Cobe Renal Care), Revision E, 1992:43–48.

183. Brezis M, et al. An unsuspected cause for metabolic acidosis in chronic renal failure: sorbent system hemodialysis. *Am J Kidney Dis* 1985;6:425–427.

184. Henderson JH, et al. Continuous venovenous haemofiltration for the treatment of theophylline toxicity. *Thorax* 2001;56:242–243.

185. Urquhart R, et al. Increased theophylline clearance during hemofiltration. *Ann Pharmacother* 1995;29:787–788.

186. Lawssen P, et al. Use of plasmapheresis in acute theophylline toxicity. *Crit Care Med* 1991;19:288–290.

187. Miceli JN, et al. Peritoneal dialysis of theophylline. *Clin Toxicol* 1979; 14:539–544.

188. Kleinschmidt KC, et al. Ethanol. In: Haddad LM, et al., eds. *Clinical management of poisoning and drug overdose,* 3rd ed. Philadelphia: WB Saunders, 1998:475–491.

189. Hingson R, et al. Magnitude of alcohol-related mortality and morbidity among U.S. college students ages 18–24. *J Stud Alcohol* 2002;63:136–144.

190. Adinoff B, et al. Acute ethanol poisoning and the ethanol withdrawal syndrome. *Med Toxicol* 1988;3:172–196.

191. O'Neill S, et al. Survival after high blood alcohol levels. *Arch Intern Med* 1984;144:641–642.

192. Seyffart G. Ethyl alcohol. In: Seyffart G, ed. *Poison index—the treatment of acute intoxication.* Lengerich, Germany: Pabst Science Publishers, 1997:311–317.

193. Elliot RW, et al. Acute ethanol poisoning treated by haemodialysis. *Postgrad Med J* 1974;50:515–517.

194. Atassi WA, et al. Hemodialysis as a treatment of severe ethanol poisoning. *Int J Artif Organs* 1999;22:18–20.

CHRONIC DIALYSIS IN CHILDREN

BRADLEY A. WARADY, KATHY L. JABS, AND STUART L. GOLDSTEIN

This chapter reviews current approaches to the clinical application of hemodialysis (HD) and peritoneal dialysis (PD) in children. Although successful dialysis is more difficult to achieve in children, both technically and psychosocially, substantial progress has been made in recent years that has dramatically improved the outlook for children requiring renal replacement therapy (RRT). Much of the information contained in this chapter reflects current practice in the authors' pediatric dialysis centers. We have tried to focus on those areas of care in which the pediatric patient differs most from the adult patient, and we have tried to keep the nephrologist who does not routinely care for pediatric patients in mind. Although we do not encourage those who rarely treat children to embrace this difficult patient group when referral to a pediatric dialysis center is an option, we recognize that referral is not always possible.

This chapter deals primarily with maintenance HD and PD in children and has been substantially updated from the last edition; selected aspects of acute HD in children are also covered. Acute dialysis in children is covered in Chapter 40.

EPIDEMIOLOGIC ISSUES

Incidence and Prevalence of End-Stage Renal Disease in Children

End-stage renal disease (ESRD) is not a common pediatric disorder. In the United States there are about 15 new pediatric ESRD cases per million children of similar age reported each year (1). It is noteworthy that a higher incidence of ESRD with older age is found within the pediatric and adult cohorts when adjusting for differences in gender and race. In 1999, the incidence rate for children 15 to 19 years (29 per million) was nearly three times higher than the rate for children 0 to 4 years (10 per million) (1). However, this data contrasts sharply with the incidence of other chronic childhood disorders such as congenital heart disease (8,000 per million) and leukemia (40 per million) (2,3). The incidence of ESRD in children is also substantially lower than the ESRD incidence among adults, as is shown by data from the United States Renal Data System (USRDS) (Table 39.1) (1). Although the pediatric incidence data has remained fairly stable over the past decade in contrast to the adult experience, an apparent increase in the incidence of ESRD did occur among younger pediatric patients between

1977 and 1987 (4). This was most likely due to improvements in RRT for smaller patients introduced during this period, notably continuous peritoneal dialysis (CPD). These improvements allowed for successful treatment of the youngest pediatric ESRD patients who previously had been considered too small to survive (5).

Children account for only a small fraction of the total dialysis patient population. On December 31, 1999, the USRDS counted a total of 243,320 dialysis patients in the United States (1). Of these, only 1,857 (0.76%) were younger than 20 years. Absolute pediatric dialysis patient counts increased from 1,587 to 1,857 between 1990 and 1999, compared with an adult dialysis patient count increase from 126,911 to 241,463 during the same period (1). Low pediatric dialysis patient counts are due both to the relatively low incidence of ESRD in children and to the extensive use of renal transplantation among pediatric ESRD patients. For almost 20 years, it has been widely accepted that renal transplantation is the optimal treatment for children with irreversible renal failure. Recent USRDS data show that 70% of children with ESRD in the United States are maintained by a functioning renal transplant, compared with 40% of adults (1).

Causes of ESRD in Children

Approximately one half of pediatric ESRD patients have a congenital or hereditary disorder and one half have an acquired renal lesion (6). This is in contrast to the adult ESRD population in which more than 80% of patients have an acquired renal disease (1). Table 39.2 lists the primary renal disease diagnoses of 4,546 pediatric dialysis patients reported between 1992 and 2001 to the dialysis patient database of the North American Pediatric Renal Transplant Cooperative Study (NAPRTCS) (7). The most frequently identified primary renal disease diagnoses were aplastic/hypoplastic/dysplastic kidneys (14.8%), focal and segmental glomerulosclerosis (14.2%), and obstructive uropathy (12.6%). Note that no single diagnosis accounted for more than 15% of all cases and that more than 20 different conditions each contributed from 1% to 8% of the total. This is again contrasted with adult ESRD patients in whom more than 79% of prevalent cases are accounted for by only three primary renal diseases: diabetic nephropathy, hypertensive nephropathy, and chronic glomerulonephritis (1).

TABLE 39.1. ESRD INCIDENCE IN THE UNITED STATES (PER MILLION POPULATION, ADJUSTED FOR AGE, GENDER, AND RACE)

Age Group (yrs)	1991	1993	1996	1999
0–4	8	8	9	10
5–9	7	7	7	8
10–14	13	12	14	15
15–19	25	26	29	29
0–19	13	13	15	15
20–44	102	105	120	122
45–64	426	462	567	620
65–74	933	1049	1229	1354
+75	777	889	1176	1474

U.S. Renal Data System. USRDS 2002 annual data report: atlas of end-stage renal disease in the United States. Bethesda, MD: National Institutes of Health, National Institute of Diabetes and Digestive and Kidney Diseases, 2002, with permission.

PRINCIPLES OF DIALYSIS IN CHILDREN: PERITONEAL DIALYSIS

Peritoneal Membrane Function in Children: Physiologic Concepts

It has long been held that the peritoneal membrane of the child is functionally different from that of the adult and that peritoneal transport kinetics change as a consequence of normal growth and development (8). This concept can be traced to

TABLE 39.2. PRIMARY RENAL DISEASE DIAGNOSIS IN PEDIATRIC DIALYSIS PATIENTS

Diagnosis	N	Percent
Aplastic/hypoplastic/dysplastic kidneys	725	14.8
Focal segmental glomerulosclerosis	691	14.1
Obstructive uropathy	630	12.9
Systemic immunologic disease	360	7.4
Chronic glomerulonephritis	167	3.4
Reflux nephropathy	167	3.4
Hemolytic uremic syndrome	157	3.2
Polycystic kidney disease	143	2.9
Congenital nephrotic syndrome	123	2.5
Idiopathic crescentic glomerulonephritis	105	2.1
Medullary cystic disease/juvenile nephronophthisis	104	2.1
Syndrome of agenesis of abdominal musculature	100	2.0
Membranoproliferative glomerulonephritis type I	98	2.0
Familial nephritis	85	1.7
Pyelonephritis/interstitial nephritis	80	1.6
Cystinosis	77	1.6
Renal infarct	76	1.6
Membranoproliferative glomerulonephritis type II	47	1.0
Wilms' tumor	35	0.7
Drash syndrome	33	0.7
Oxalosis	26	0.5
Membranous nephropathy	22	0.5
Sickle cell nephropathy	18	0.4
Diabetic glomerulonephritis	5	0.1
Other	455	9.3
Unknown	357	7.3

Neu AM, et al. Chronic dialysis in children and adolescents: the 2001 NAPRTCS annual report. *Pediatr Nephrol* 2002;17:656–663, with permission.

comparative measurements of peritoneal surface area performed more than 100 years ago. In 1884, in a paper read before the Siberian Branch of the Russian Geographic Society, Putiloff presented comparative data on the peritoneal membrane surface areas of infants and adults (9). Using direct oiled paper tracings of peritoneal contents, Putiloff found that the peritoneal surface area of an infant weighing 2.9 kg was 0.15 m², compared with 2.08 m² for an adult of unspecified weight. If a weight of 70 kg is assumed for Putiloff's adult subjects, the infant's peritoneal surface area is found to be almost twice that of the adult when scaled for body weight (522 cm²/kg vs. 285 cm²/kg). Earlier studies by Wegner (10) had suggested that the peritoneal surface area closely approximated the body surface area (BSA) of an adult.

The clinical implications of these anatomic relationships were explored in 1966 by Esperanca et al. (11). Direct measurements of peritoneal surface areas were made during autopsies performed on six neonates and six adults. The mean peritoneal surface area to body weight ratio in the infants was found to be roughly twice that of the adults, confirming Putiloff's measurements made 80 years earlier. Esperanca et al. assumed that the peritoneal surface area and peritoneal membrane function were directly correlated, postulating that "peritoneal dialysis should be twice as efficient in the infant." Peritoneal urea clearance studies in puppies and adult dogs performed by these same investigators seemed to support their hypothesis (11). When scaled for body weight, peritoneal urea clearance measured in puppies was two to three times greater than clearances measured in adult animals. However, these clearance studies were seriously flawed. Widely different dialysate delivery rates were used in the puppies and adult animals (128 vs. 42 mL/kg/hour, respectively). In this range, urea clearance is directly proportional to dialysate flow rate, providing ample explanation for the observed differences in urea clearances between the two study groups.

The report by Esperanca et al. provides an early example of the pitfalls associated with the use of variable dialysis mechanics when studying peritoneal membrane function. These pitfalls can be avoided if peritoneal transport studies are performed in accordance with the following principles, as defined by Gruskin et al. in 1987 (12):

1. Constant inflow, dwell, and outflow times must be used for all study exchanges.
2. Identical dialysate composition must be used in all study subjects.
3. Exchange volumes must be identically scaled per unit body size. Gruskin allows the use of body weight, height, or surface area as the scaling factor, but other work has shown BSA to be the most reliable scaling factor in pediatric patients (13).
4. Results must be reported according to the body size scaling factor used to determine the exchange volume.

Subsequent peritoneal kinetic studies performed in accordance with these principles have more clearly defined the relative performance characteristics of the peritoneal membrane in children of different ages and in adults (see later). It is also now evident that the total membrane size is likely less relevant than the total membrane pore area involved in the exchanges (see later) (14,15).

Principles of Peritoneal Membrane Solute and Fluid Transfer

The peritoneal transfer of solutes reflects two simultaneous and interrelated transport mechanisms: diffusion and convection (16). Diffusion refers to the movement of solute across a semipermeable membrane in response to differing concentrations of that solute on either side of the membrane. The solute moves from the side with higher to the side with lower concentration, down an electrochemical gradient and in accordance with basic thermodynamic principles. Convection refers to the movement of solutes swept across the membrane within the flux of fluid that arises as a consequence of ultrafiltration. Convective transport is determined by the ultrafiltration rate. Studies of peritoneal membrane function have classically characterized membrane transport properties in terms of effective membrane surface area and solute permeability, fluid transfer (ultrafiltration), and peritoneal lymphatic absorption (17,18). Recently, characterization of the three-pore model has helped to better explain the movement of solute and water across the peritoneal membrane. This model postulates three types of pores: (a) ultrasmall transcellular water pores, which account for 1% to 2% of total pore area and account for 40% of water flow; (b) small pores, accounting for 90% of total pore area and subject to both concentration gradients (diffusive forces) and osmotic gradients (convective forces); and (c) large pores, accounting for 5% to 7% of total pore area and allowing for movement of large molecules such as albumin. The three-pore model has been applied to studies of PD in infants and children (14,15).

Effective Membrane Surface Area and Solute Permeability: Diffusive Transport

In the absence of an osmotic gradient between blood and dialysate, the rate of diffusive transfer of a solute is directly related to the product of the mass transfer area coefficient (MTAC) and the concentration gradient of the solute across the peritoneal membrane. The MTAC reflects the rate of solute removal that would be achieved in the absence of ultrafiltration or solute accumulation in the dialysate. The MTAC, as applied to the current three-pore model of transperitoneal solute and water flux, is in turn equal to the product of the free diffusion coefficient for the solute, the fractional area available for diffusion, and the term A_0/Δ_x, the diffusion distance (19).

In an early study, Morgenstern et al. (20) found that the MTACs for urea, creatinine, uric acid, and glucose in eight children, 1.5 to 18 years of age, were similar to adult reference values. In contrast, Geary et al. (21) determined MTACs in 28 children and suggested that solute transport capacity varies with age and does not approach adult values until late childhood. Warady et al. (22) determined MTACs for various solutes in 83 children younger than 1 to 18 years of age. This study had the advantage of standardized dialysis mechanics, including a con-

sistent test exchange volume scaled to BSA at 1,100 mL/m². Mean MTACs (normalized to BSA) for creatinine, glucose, and potassium significantly decreased with age, in support of the notion that peritoneal permeability and/or effective membrane surface area relative to BSA is greater in children than in adults. More recently, MTAC studies by Bouts et al. (23), based on the three-pore model, have found that the values for children, when scaled to BSA, are similar to those of adults.

Diffusive transfer, as noted previously, is dependent on the MTAC and the transmembrane concentration gradient, which dissipates during exchanges. Recognition of the fact that the capacity with which a transmembrane concentration gradient dissipates is in part related to the dialysate exchange volume (e.g., geometry of diffusion) and the subsequent use of a consistent test exchange volume scaled to BSA represent important advances in methodology that are essential to the proper performance of another measure of peritoneal membrane function in children, the peritoneal equilibration test (PET) (see later) (24).

Ultrafiltration

Ultrafiltration, the movement of fluid from blood to dialysate, is a complex process that is incompletely understood and reflects the interaction of a number of factors including the hydraulic permeability of the peritoneal membrane, the permeability of the peritoneum to the osmotically active solutes on either side of the membrane, the absorption of fluid into peritoneal tissue, and lymphatic absorption. Convective mass transfer occurs as a consequence of ultrafiltration. When considered in the context of total solute removal during PD, convective mass transfer contributes little to the movement of small solutes but is responsible for most large solute removal (16). For example, during a 4-hour continuous ambulatory peritoneal dialysis (CAPD) exchange with 4.25% dextrose solution, the contributions of convection to total transport have been estimated by Pyle (25) to be 12% for urea, 45% for inulin, and 86% for total protein.

Early studies and much clinical experience suggested that adequate ultrafiltration could be difficult to achieve in infants and younger children. Initial studies found a more rapid decline in dialysate dextrose concentration and osmolality in younger children (26,27). Subsequent work by Kohaut et al. (28) has shown that apparent age-related differences in ultrafiltration capacity disappear when the test exchange volume is scaled to BSA rather than body weight. As mentioned previously, proper scaling of the exchange volume is an important determinant of the rate of dissipation of the osmotic gradient that determines ultrafiltration. Other aspects of solute flux and convection have been far more difficult to solve, and these difficulties reconciling theory with clinical findings have been critical to the development of the three-pore model of fluid and solute transfer (29).

Peritoneal Lymphatic Absorption

To some extent, studies of ultrafiltration in children have been hindered by the absence of information on the contribution of lymphatic absorption to net ultrafiltration. Mactier et al. (30)

studied lymphatic absorption in six children, 2 to 13 years of age. Peritoneal lymphatic drainage was reported to reduce mean ultrafiltration by 27%. When lymphatic absorption rates were scaled to body weight, higher values were obtained for pediatric patients when compared with adult reference values. When scaled to BSA, these differences were no longer seen. More recently, fluid absorption has been felt to primarily move directly into the tissues surrounding the peritoneal cavity. Lymphatic absorption is only thought to account for 20% of fluid absorption. The limited data on lymphatic absorption in children are conflicting (30,31).

PRINCIPLES OF DIALYSIS IN CHILDREN: HEMODIALYSIS

The principles of HD governing extracorporeal perfusion, solute clearance, ultrafiltration, and mass balance are basically the same when applied in children as in adult patients (see Chapters 7 and 8). Certain characteristics of dialyzers when used in children require comment.

Characteristics of Dialyzers

For many years, the flat-plate dialyzer was the only type of dialyzer that was specifically manufactured for the treatment of infants and small children. The flat-plate dialyzer had the advantage of a manufacturing process that was easily modified so that dialyzers of many different sizes could be produced. However, hollow-fiber dialyzers have now supplanted the flat-plate dialyzers in virtually all pediatric centers. Improvements in the manufacturing process of hollow-fiber dialyzers have led to decreased dialyzer volumes, making them more useful for the treatment of infants and small children in whom a small extracorporeal volume is desirable. Hollow-fiber dialyzers also have more predictable clearance characteristics and can be easily cleaned and reprocessed. There are several characteristics of dialyzers that should be considered before their clinical use: clearance, ultrafiltration, and biocompatibility.

Clearance

In the clinical setting, the clearance achieved by a dialyzer is a function of its KoA (see Chapter 7) and the blood and dialysate flow rates (Q_B, Q_D). The relationship between blood-flow rates and clearance for two different dialyzers is shown in Fig. 39.1. In that representation, dialyzer 2 has a larger KoA (urea) than does dialyzer 1. Several important conclusions can be drawn from the shape of the curves. First, at low blood-flow rates, the small solute clearance is equivalent to the blood-flow rate and is the same for both dialyzer 1 and 2, and for virtually all dialyzers. Second, for each dialyzer, a maximum clearance will be achieved at a certain blood-flow rate, after which increasing the blood flow will not increase clearance. The difference between larger and smaller dialyzers is principally the blood-flow rate at which the maximum urea clearance is achieved. For a large child, therefore, a large dialyzer would be preferable, because a

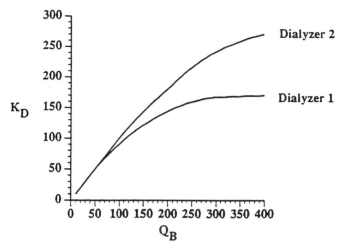

FIG. 39.1. Relationship between blood flow (Q_B) and dialyzer clearance (K_D) for two different dialyzers. Dialyzer 2 has a KoA for this solute that is twice that of dialyzer 1.

higher clearance could be achieved, whereas for a small child the difference in clearance rates at low blood-flow rates would be negligible and other considerations would be more appropriate, such as dialyzer volume.

A dialyzer has different clearances for different solutes, which are generally inversely related to molecular weight. Although generally not considered in the dialysis prescription for young infants, the relatively low blood-flow rates at which clearance of higher molecular weight solutes reach their maximum levels actually means that infants and young children have always been receiving high-efficiency dialysis (32). That is, they received an equivalent overall clearance of these solutes compared with adults, but, because their volumes of distribution are significantly less, the overall mass transfer has been much greater. A practical example in which this may have clinical relevance is the clearance of vancomycin. Dosing intervals for vancomycin in infants receiving HD are much shorter than in adults (33), probably because of this phenomenon.

Ultrafiltration

The ultrafiltration coefficient of the dialyzer should be sufficient to allow the desired ultrafiltration during the planned duration of a dialysis procedure. Concern has been raised in the past about the ultrafiltration coefficient of dialyzers used for pediatric patients because excessive ultrafiltration could lead to hypotension and shock (34). Theoretically, this could be a particular problem with the now standard high-efficiency dialysis. However, the routine use of ultrafiltration controlling dialysis machines has greatly reduced these concerns.

Biocompatibility

Biocompatibility of HD membranes is reviewed in Chapter 1. Although there is debate concerning the use of specific membranes for the chronic treatment of adults (35), there is evidence that the use of certain membranes can affect long-term leukocyte function, protein catabolism, and perhaps overall mass transfer of β_2-microglobulins (36). There have, however, not been any studies of the long-term use of specific membranes in children, and at the present time there are no clear-cut advantages to any type of membrane for pediatric patients.

DIALYSIS FOR ACUTE RENAL FAILURE IN CHILDREN

Indications and Contraindications

The conservative management of acute renal failure in pediatric patients requires meticulous attention to fluid and electrolyte balance. Minor errors can have grave consequences. Dietary restriction, phosphate binders, diuretics, sodium bicarbonate, calcium salts, antihypertensive medications, and sodium-potassium exchange resins can all play important roles in delaying or evading dialysis in some children, although such tactics are not likely to be successful for very long in children who are oligoanuric. Several factors are at work in the pediatric patient that tend to defeat even the most carefully conceived conservative management plans. Children with acute renal failure are profoundly catabolic, resulting in the rapid accumulation of potassium, phosphate, and other solutes. In the oliguric child, it is also difficult to meet energy requirements while abiding by stringent limitations on allowable fluid intake. As a result, dialysis and hemofiltration tend to be promptly used in children with acute renal failure.

Widely accepted clinical indications for RRT in children with acute renal failure are listed in Table 39.3. Such lists may not adequately portray the need to consider the rate at which conditions are deteriorating in the individual child. A marginal clinical situation should not be tolerated in any child when the prompt institution of RRT will reliably control fluid and solute imbalances and allow the patient to meet nutritional needs.

Historically, PD has been the most widely used RRT modality for children with acute renal failure because of its convenience, simplicity, relative safety, and the ease with which it could be adapted for use in pediatric patients of all ages and sizes (37–39). The popularity of PD over HD for the most seriously ill pediatric patients had traditionally rested on two important features: ready access to the peritoneal cavity and better tolerance of PD by hemodynamically unstable children. Advances in vascular access techniques and equipment, along with improve-

ments in HD (bicarbonate-based dialysate and ultrafiltration control modules), have narrowed the choice between dialysis modalities in many centers. Moreover, continuous renal replacement therapies (CRRTs) for children are replacing either dialysis modality for the most critically ill pediatric patients (40–42). Clear indications for one RRT modality over the others are now rarely present, and often it is the experience of the center that determines which RRT modality is selected. A survey of pediatric nephrologists in North America and Europe, designed to determine what is anticipated to be the most frequently used dialysis modality for acute renal failure in 2003, revealed that CRRT will be used most frequently in 53% of centers, PD in 20%, and HD in 25% (43).

There are few absolute contraindications to any dialysis modality. PD is contraindicated in patients with an omphalocele, diaphragmatic hernia, gastroschisis, bladder extrophy, and peritoneal membrane failure. Recent abdominal surgery is not an absolute contraindication to PD as long as there are no draining abdominal wounds; however, most centers prefer to treat such patients with HD or CRRT. Extensive intraabdominal adhesions will prevent PD in some patients. Surgical lysis of extensive adhesions frequently results in prolonged intraperitoneal bleeding in uremic children. PD may not be preferred in hydrocephalic children with ventriculoperitoneal shunts unless there is no alternative RRT modality possible. Finally, HD and CRRT are contraindicated in children who do not have adequate vascular access and in some hypercoagulable states.

A discussion of the use of CRRT and PD to treat acute renal failure in pediatric patients may be found in Chapter 40. Selected aspects of acute HD in children will be reviewed in the following sections.

Vascular Access and Dialyzers for Acute Hemodialysis

Catheters for temporary HD are usually placed percutaneously (44); those used for longer term dialysis should be placed using surgical techniques (45). Double-lumen dialysis catheters have replaced single-lumen catheters in most pediatric centers (44,45). There are currently sufficient catheters of various designs, diameters, and lengths to permit either temporary or permanent HD in infants and children of all sizes. A partial listing of HD catheters and their available sizes is presented in Table 39.4. The HD equipment used for acute dialysis is the same as that used for chronic dialysis and will be discussed in detail in that section of this chapter.

TABLE 39.3. INDICATIONS FOR DIALYSIS IN CHILDREN WITH ACUTE RENAL FAILURE[a]

Hyperkalemia (serum K^+ concentration >7.0 mEq/L)
Intractable acidosis
Fluid overload, often with hypertension, congestive heart failure, or pulmonary edema
Severe azotemia (BUN >150 mg/dL)
Symptomatic uremia (encephalopathy, pericarditis, intractable vomiting, hemorrhage)
Hyponatremia, hypernatremia, hypocalcemia, hyperphosphatemia (severe, symptomatic)
Fluid removal for optimal nutrition, transfusions, infusions of medications, and so forth

[a]These are general guidelines. Each case must be individualized.

TABLE 39.4. CUFFED HEMODIALYSIS CATHETER AND PATIENT SIZE GUIDELINE

Patient Size (kg)	Catheter Options
Less than 20 kg	8 French dual lumen
20 to 25 kg	7 French twin Tesio
	10 French dual lumen
25 to 40 kg	10 French Ash Split
	10 French twin Tesio
>40 kg	10 French twin Tesio
	11.5 or 12.5 French dual lumen

The Acute Hemodialysis Prescription

Rapid osmolar changes of large magnitude can be associated with cerebral edema, disequilibrium syndrome, and seizures, especially during the first few HD treatments (46). The intravenous infusion of mannitol at a dose of 0.25 to 0.50 g/kg has been proposed as a method by which these symptoms can be avoided or ameliorated in children by maintaining a relatively high extracellular fluid osmolality as urea is removed from the patient, although the clinical utility of this procedure has never been clearly established (47). Furthermore, accumulation of mannitol after repeated infusions may be harmful. A more satisfactory method to prevent large osmolar shifts during initial HD treatments is to limit the amount of urea clearance delivered at each treatment. Practically, this can be achieved by limiting the decrease in the blood urea nitrogen (BUN) to only 30 to 40 mg/dL at each of the first few dialysis treatments. The proportional fall in urea can be estimated by calculations using the following mass transfer equation.

$$C_t/C_0 = e^{-Kt/V}$$

where C_t is the concentration of BUN after t minutes of dialysis, C_0 is the initial concentration, K is the urea clearance (mL/minute), t is the duration of dialysis (minutes), and V is the urea volume of distribution (mL).

The urea volume of distribution is equivalent to the total body water (TBW), which is approximately 60% of the patient's weight.

For example, if a 10-kg child is to begin HD and has a BUN of 100 mg/dL, the following calculations could be used. At a blood-flow rate of 25 mL/min, a dialyzer will achieve a urea clearance of 25 mL/min. If the desired fall in BUN is 30 mg/dL, then C_t = 70 mg/dL at the conclusion of the dialysis treatment. Assuming an average body composition, the TBW is approximately 6,000 mL. Therefore

$C_t/C_0 = 70/100 = 0.7$ and $0.7 = e^{-25 \text{ mL/min} \times t \text{ minutes}/6,000 \text{ mL}}$

$Ln(0.7) = -0.36$ $-0.36 = -25$ mL/min $\times$ t minutes/6,000 mL or

$t = 0.36 \times 6,000/25$ or $t = 86$ minutes

The time of dialysis could be further shortened if a higher blood-flow rate, and thus a higher clearance can be tolerated. Conversely, when lower blood-flow rates are required, proportionately longer dialysis times are necessary to achieve the same outcome.

DIALYSIS FOR ESRD IN CHILDREN

Choice of Hemodialysis or Peritoneal Dialysis as a Chronic RRT in Children

HD, PD, and renal transplantation are all successful long-term treatments for ESRD in children. Renal transplantation has been widely recognized as the treatment of choice for children with ESRD, because it can relieve the burden of continuous and repetitive treatments while restoring the child to virtually normal metabolic homeostasis and permitting near normal growth and development (48). Unfortunately, because tolerance has not yet been achieved in humans after organ transplantation, virtually all grafts are eventually lost to chronic rejection (49). Renal transplantation should, thus, be considered a treatment rather than a cure for renal failure. Despite the preference for renal transplantation and the fact that up to 25% of children may receive a preemptive transplant without prior dialysis, large-scale registry data indicate that a large proportion of children with ESRD require a prolonged period of treatment with chronic dialysis either before or between renal transplants, making chronic dialysis a significant component of the treatment for all children with ESRD (6).

In the United States, more than 80% of all dialysis patients are currently receiving HD (1). However, the predominant form of dialysis for pediatric patients with ESRD is CPD (50). Before 1982, fewer than 100 pediatric patients had been treated with CPD worldwide (51). By the end of 1989, CPD accounted for 50% of pediatric chronic dialysis patients (younger than 15 years) in the United States, 65% in Canada, and 75% in Australia and New Zealand (5). In contrast to centers that provide dialysis for adults and children, CPD is more frequently used in children treated in pediatric centers, 45% versus 65% (52). Sixty-four percent of the children initiating dialysis at 140 North American Pediatric Renal Transplant Cooperative Study (NAPRTCS) dialysis centers from 1995 to 2000 were treated with CPD (7). The use of CPD varies from 88% of children younger than 6 years to 53% of those older than 12 years (7).

There are few studies directly comparing the efficacy of chronic HD and PD in pediatric patients. The proposed advantages of HD include its track record, minimal technical assistance required of the patient and family, and decreased treatment times. The proposed advantages of PD include decreased dependence on the treatment center, increased flexibility of the treatment schedule with improved school attendance, somewhat decreased dietary restrictions, and a decreased need for repeated venipunctures. In one comparison of the two chronic dialysis modalities in children from a single center, PD appeared to be associated with lower transfusion rates, improved rehabilitation and better metabolic control (50).

In addition to patient age, factors that play a role in the selection of a dialysis modality include lifestyle choice, parental preference, assessment of whether individual patients and families can be "compliant" with the dialysis regimen, and center bias (50,52). Factors related to the success of dialysis may be involved in the selection of a dialysis modality for an individual child (e.g., children with greater social support are more likely to be treated with CPD and more likely to attend school full time). Comparison of the children in NAPRTCS showed more full-time school attendance in those treated with CPD versus those receiving HD (e.g., 77% vs. 51% for children 6 to 18 years of age) (7).

At present, it is virtually impossible to find convincing evidence that either form of dialysis is clearly preferable for most children with ESRD, although clear preferences exist in individual cases. The choice of dialysis treatment may be influenced by the preference of the center or by its technical capabilities. In these circumstances, it is important that patient and family choice be preserved and not subverted by the overt or subtle influence of the unit's personnel (52).

CHRONIC PERITONEAL DIALYSIS FOR CHILDREN

Although successful as treatment for acute renal failure, PD historically appeared to have much less to offer to the child with ESRD. Initial chronic PD techniques required reinsertion of the dialysis catheter for each treatment, making prolonged use in small patients difficult. The development of a permanent peritoneal catheter, first proposed by Palmer et al. (53,54) and later refined by Tenckhoff et al. (55), made long-term PD an accessible form of RRT for pediatric patients. When Boen et al. (56) and then Tenckhoff et al. (57) devised an automated dialysate delivery system that could be used in the home, chronic intermittent peritoneal dialysis (IPD) became a practical alternative to chronic HD for children. Largely as a result of the pioneering efforts of the pediatric ESRD treatment team in Seattle (58,59), pediatric chronic IPD programs were established in a few prominent pediatric dialysis centers (60–63). However, enthusiasm for chronic IPD among pediatric nephrologists during this period was limited, perhaps because chronic IPD for children included many of the least desirable features of chronic HD (e.g., substantial dietary restrictions, fluid intake limits, immobility during treatments, and complex machinery), without providing the one great advantage of HD: efficiency.

A new era in the history of PD as a RRT modality for children with ESRD was heralded by the description of CAPD in 1976 by Popovich et al. (64). CAPD appeared particularly well-suited for use in children. Potential advantages of CAPD over HD of special importance to children included near steady-state biochemical control, reduced dietary restrictions and fluid limits, and freedom from repeated dialysis needle punctures. CAPD also allowed children of all ages to receive dialysis in the home, offering them the opportunity to experience more normal childhoods. Finally, CAPD made possible the routine treatment of very young infants, thereby extending the option of RRT to an entire population of patients previously considered too young for chronic dialysis.

CAPD was first used in a child in 1978 in Toronto (65,66). Subsequent experience was soon reported from growing pediatric CAPD programs in North America and western Europe (67–72). Continuous cycling peritoneal dialysis (CCPD) was first used in a child by Price et al. in 1981 (73). Cycler dialysis has since grown in popularity among many pediatric PD programs throughout North America and the world (74).

Permanent Peritoneal Dialysis Catheters for Children

A reliable peritoneal catheter is the cornerstone of successful CPD, well worth the attention and effort required to "perfect" the procedure in each center that proposes to treat children with long-term PD. There are multiple types of PD catheters presently available, with a variety of configurations. In general, most long-term PD catheters are constructed of soft material, such as silicone rubber or polyurethane. The catheters can be thought of as having two separate regions, the intraperitoneal portion and the extraperitoneal portion. The intraperitoneal portion contains holes or slots to allow passage of peritoneal fluid. The shape of the intraperitoneal portion typically is straight or curled, the latter configuration often associated with less patient pain with dialysate inflow and a decreased predisposition to omental wrapping of the catheter. The most common catheters with these characteristics used by pediatric patients have been the straight and curled Tenckhoff catheters. The extraperitoneal portion of each of these catheters has one or two Dacron cuffs to prevent fluid leaks and bacterial migration and to fix the catheter's position. The shape of this portion of the catheter is variable and may be straight or have a preformed angle (e.g., swan neck) to help create a downward directed catheter exit site (75).

In general, it is believed that infants and young children with vesicostomies, ureterostomies, or colostomies require placement of the catheter exit site as far from the stoma as possible to prevent contamination and infection. Placement of the exit site on the chest wall has successfully limited the number of infections in such high-risk situations in a small number of children and adults (75–77). The primary reason for catheter revision is catheter malfunction, often caused by omental wrapping of the catheter (7,78). However, the decision to perform an omentectomy in conjunction with catheter placement is not universal (79). Catheter occlusion by fibrin may also occur but can usually be successfully relieved by the installation of fibrinolytic agents into the catheter (80,81).

In a 1995 report from the 18 centers of the Pediatric Peritoneal Dialysis Study Consortium (PPDSC), most preferred a curled Tenckhoff catheter (88%), with fewer centers using a catheter with a straight intraperitoneal segment (79). The most common extraperitoneal design consisted of a straight tunnel with a single cuff (69%). Fewer centers used dual-cuff catheters with angled extraperitoneal regions. In most of the centers, the peritoneal catheter was placed by a surgeon, and, in 53% of the centers, an omentectomy was performed. Finally, the exit site was directed downward in 69% of the centers, and 25% of centers indicated an upward exit site. Although no correlation between catheter characteristics and infection rate was provided, this small experience confirmed a significant variation in PD catheter choice and implantation strategies.

Daschner et al. (82), have reported on the laparoscopic placement of 25 two-cuff Tenckhoff catheters in 22 pediatric patients. Postoperative leakage occurred in only 2 patients, and the procedure facilitated the performance of adhesiolysis and inguinal hernia repair at the time of catheter placement.

In the most recent report of the NAPRTCS, catheter characteristics were reported from 2,971 independent courses of PD accumulated from 1992 to 2001 (7). As was shown in previous reports, the annualized peritonitis rate decreased with increasing age and was best in association with Tenckhoff catheters with straight intraperitoneal segments, double-cuffs, swan-neck tunnels, and downward pointed exit sites (6,78,83). In addition, time to first peritonitis episode was longer for catheters with two cuffs compared with one, with swan-neck tunnels compared with straight tunnels, and with downward exit sites compared with lateral exit sites or exit sites directed upward. These results confirm findings from the adult PD population (84).

The Pediatric Chronic Peritoneal Dialysis Team

As noted earlier in this chapter, CPD can be attempted in any child whose peritoneal cavity is intact and will admit a sufficient volume of dialysate. Experience has shown that patient age, primary renal disease, and renal transplant status have no influence on outcome. Ideally, a treating facility should be able to provide the necessary multidisciplinary services required by the child and family. Successful chronic PD for children is a team effort, with the team consisting of PD nurse specialists, pediatric nephrologists, pediatric urologists, pediatric surgeons, renal nutritionists, renal social workers, child psychologists, child psychiatrists, child development specialists, child life therapists, speech pathologists, and chaplains—all of whom are specialists in pediatric care. Children require an investment of time and resources from the entire PD team that can be daunting. The effort involved is usually several orders of magnitude greater than that required to care for the typical adult PD patient (85).

Role of PET in Prescribing Peritoneal Dialysis for Children

PET was developed by Twardowski et al. (86) as a simple means of characterizing solute transport rates across the peritoneum that could have direct clinical applications. The construction of reference curves based on the kinetics of solute equilibration between dialysate and plasma (D to P ratio) after a 2-L exchange volume made possible the categorization of adult patients into those with high, high-average, low-average, and low peritoneal membrane solute transport rates and served as the basis for the dialysis prescription process (see later).

Twardowski et al.'s adult PET reference curves have not enjoyed widespread application in the pediatric PD population for two reasons. First, there has been the widely acknowledged but unproved perception that the solute transport function of the pediatric peritoneal membrane is different from that of the adult (9,26). The second reason is the uniform 2-L test exchange volume that is provided to all study patients, regardless of their size, in the Twardowski scheme. Obviously, this approach does not allow for modification of the exchange volume to reflect differences in body size (e.g., pediatric patient, small adult, large adult) and has contributed to the limited usefulness of this approach in children.

Application of a standardized PET procedure for children has resulted from an appreciation of the previously mentioned age-independent relationship between BSA and peritoneal membrane surface area and the recommended use of an exchange volume scaled to BSA whenever one conducts studies of peritoneal transport kinetics (22,28,87–89). In the largest pediatric study to date, the PPDSC evaluated 95 children using a test exchange volume of 1,100 mL/m^2 BSA to develop reference kinetic data (e.g., D to P and D to Do ratios), which can be used to categorize an individual pediatric patient's peritoneal membrane solute transport capacity (22). Similar reference data has been generated from pediatric studies in Europe with a test exchange volume of 1,000 mL/m^2 BSA (89).

Because the transport capacity of a patient's peritoneal membrane is such an important factor to consider when determining the dialysis prescription, a PET evaluation should be conducted soon after the initiation of dialysis (90,91). However, there is evidence that a PET performed within the first week after the initiation of PD may yield higher transport results than a PET performed several weeks later (92). Accordingly, whereas it may be most convenient to perform the initial PET at the conclusion of PD training, the results after 1 month of PD may more accurately reflect peritoneal transport properties (92,93). The PET evaluation should be repeated when knowledge of the patient's current membrane transport capacity is necessary for determination of the patient's PD prescription, especially when clinical events have occurred (e.g., repeated peritonitis) that may have altered transport characteristics. In addition, knowledge of a patient's transport capacity may have a profound impact on their overall care because of the important relationships that exist between transport status and patient outcome in children and adults (94–97).

Chronic Peritoneal Dialysis Prescription

In general, the PD prescription for children has evolved empirically from guidelines that adapted adult CAPD for pediatric patients. A CAPD regimen of four to five exchanges per day with an exchange volume of 900 to 1,100 mL/m^2 BSA (35 to 45 mL/kg) of 2.5% dextrose dialysis solution has routinely yielded net ultrafiltration volumes of up to 1,100 mL/m^2 per day. Using similar exchange volumes, the greatest percentage of children receiving PD receive cycler dialysis with a regimen consisting of 6 to 10 exchanges over 8 to 10 hours per night.

The current goal of achieving dialysis adequacy in the most cost-effective manner has highlighted the need to be cognizant of a patient's BSA, peritoneal membrane solute transport capacity, and residual renal function when designing the dialysis prescription (22,91,98,99). In most patients (except for the rapid transporter), the most effective way to increase solute clearance is to initially increase the exchange volume followed by an increase in dialysis duration by prolonging the dwell time. Ideally, the prescription for all children should include an exchange volume of 1,100 to 1,400 mL/m^2 BSA as tolerated by the patient. Measurement of the intraperitoneal pressure generated by escalating exchange volumes can be useful in determining the optimal dialysis prescription (100–102). In the case of the rapid transporter, an increase in the number of exchanges and a reduction of the dwell time per cycle can result in improved solute clearance.

As mentioned previously, the categorization of a patient's peritoneal membrane transport capacity can best be determined by the performance of a PET and comparison of the individual patient data to reference values (22). In turn, this information makes it possible to optimize the dialysis prescription in terms of dwell time. Recognizing that it is often impractical to consider the provision of a dialysis prescription based solely on kinetic data without reference to social constraints (e.g., school attendance, working parent), the use of the results of a PET evaluation can be particularly helpful in determining a cost-effective approach to PD modality selection (e.g., high transporter: cycling PD; high-average to low-average transporter: CAPD or cycling PD with the option of additional daytime exchange). Often, this can be most easily achieved with the use of one of several computer modeling programs that have been validated in pediatric patients and that can provide accurate estimates of solute clearance (14,103,104). It must be emphasized that in pediatric patients, as well as in adults, predicted values are only estimates and do not substitute for actual measurements of solute clearance (see later).

The residual renal function, a characteristic that appears to be better preserved by PD versus HD, is calculated as the average of urea and creatinine clearance and assumes greatest importance in the patient who does not attain target clearances with dialysis alone (93,105). Whereas the contribution of residual renal function toward a target goal may be significant early in the course of dialysis, a progressive loss of residual renal function usually occurs and mandates an associated enhancement of the dialysis prescription if target clearances are to be maintained (106–108).

Peritoneal Dialysis Adequacy

Most studies with adult PD patients, in which clinical outcome parameters (e.g., frequency of hospitalization, patient mortality) have been monitored, have characterized dialysis adequacy in terms of small solute clearance as a total (residual renal + PD) weekly Kt/V_{urea} greater than or equal to 2.0 and a total weekly creatinine clearance greater than or equal to 60 L/1.73 m^2 for the patient receiving CAPD (93). Slightly higher targets are recommended for the cycler dialysis patient. Recently, an analysis by Churchill et al. (96), of data generated in the CANUSA study has, however, revealed superior patient and technique survival in the adult CAPD population with low or low-average transport capacity and lower total creatinine clearance values than in patients who are high transporters. This has resulted in a change of the target clearance recommendation to 50 L/1.73m^2/week for the former group of patients in the guidelines of the National Kidney Foundation/Kidney Disease Outcome Quality Initiative (K/DOQI) and the Canadian Society of Nephrology (93,109).

Current clinical experience supports the use of similar (or greater) target clearances for children. Reports by Höltta et al. (110), McCauley et al. (111), Champoux et al. (112), and Chadha et al. (113) have all presented data suggestive of a correlation between patient outcome and solute clearance. The experience of Chadha et al. (113) was also significant for

demonstrating the influence that residual renal function has on patient outcome and the apparent contradiction of the presumed equivalence of PD and native solute clearance. The contribution of residual renal function is most apparent with respect to total creatinine clearance, as well as middle molecule clearance (114).

Can the solute clearance targets be achieved by children on PD without introducing a prescription that has a significant negative impact on their quality of life? Whereas data by van der Voort et al. (115), suggest otherwise, the clinical experiences of Höltta et al. (110) and Chadha et al. (116) provide good evidence that if the dialysis exchange volume is maximized and if the frequency of the exchanges is individualized and adjusted according to the peritoneal membrane transport characteristics, it should be possible to achieve the current K/DOQI clearance targets, at least for Kt/V_{urea}, in most children receiving PD.

The ability to accurately estimate a patient's TBW (or V) is integral to the determination of Kt/V_{urea} as an adequacy measure. The K/DOQI guidelines have recommended the use of the gender specific formulas of Mellits-Cheek for TBW assessment in pediatric patients, despite the fact that the formulas were derived from studies of healthy children (117). Recently, more accurate estimates of V have at last become feasible following the analysis of additional body water data in the literature and after the study of pediatric dialysis patients by bioelectrical impedance analysis as well as with the use of D$_2$0 or water labeled with radioactive oxygen (^{18}O) (118–121). It is noteworthy, however, that there are few data to support the preference of one solute clearance measure (Kt/V_{urea} vs. creatinine clearance) over another and that discrepancies in the results may occur in as many as 20% of patients. This has prompted the recommendation that the evaluation of adequacy be based on the results of both clearance measures and an ongoing assessment of the patient's clinical condition (122,123). If there is discordance in achieving these targets, it has been suggested that the Kt/V_{urea} be the immediate determinant of adequacy because it directly reflects protein metabolism and is less affected by extreme variations in residual renal function (93).

Implicit in the approach to achieve and maintain dialysis adequacy is the need to repeatedly measure total solute clearance. Ideally, 24-hour collections of urine and dialysate fluid should be obtained three times per year or when there have been significant changes in the patient's clinical status that may influence dialysis performance (e.g., severe or repeated peritonitis). In children with enuresis, we have elected to use a timed daytime urine collection and then extrapolate to a full 24-hour residual renal clearance value. For infants incontinent day and night, we currently attempt to achieve total clearance targets using dialysis clearances alone, rather than use indwelling urinary catheters for these patients.

In summary, current knowledge supports the clinical use of a target total weekly Kt/V_{urea} of greater than or equal to 2.0 and a total weekly creatinine clearance of greater than or equal to 60 L/1.73 m^2 to achieve dialysis adequacy in most children receiving CAPD (93). Patients receiving automated peritoneal dialysis (APD) likely require slightly greater clearances, and low transporters may do well with lower clearances if the pediatric experience is comparable to that of the adults. The continued accumulation of patient outcome data is critical to the ongoing assessment of these criteria.

Nutritional Management of Children on CPD

A normal nutritional status is uncommon among children treated with CPD, despite access to an essentially unlimited diet (124,125). Compared with healthy children, those on CPD have a significantly lower energy intake and diminished height, weight, triceps skin-fold thickness, and midarm muscle circumference (124). Hypoalbuminemia and hyperlipidemia are commonly seen (125,126). Anorexia and dysgeusia are often accompanied by gastroesophageal reflux and other feeding disorders (127). As part of the K/DOQI process, pediatric guidelines have been developed for the assessment of a patient's nutritional status and for the provision of optimal nutrition (128). In the opinion of the working group, the most valid measures of protein and energy nutrition status in children on maintenance dialysis include dietary interview/diary, estimated dry weight and height or length, weight/height index, midarm circumference and muscle circumference, skin-fold thickness, head circumference (children younger than 3 years), height standard deviation score, and serum albumin (128). Growth and nutritional parameters should be measured at the initiation of dialysis and at regular intervals. The K/DOQI guidelines recommend that the initial prescribed energy intake be 100% of the recommended dietary allowance (RDA) for children of the same gender and chronologic age. Total energy intake will be augmented by an additional 8 to 20 kcal/kg/day derived from dialysate dextrose absorption (129).

The members of the K/DOQI working group were unable to recommend with evidence the optimal protein intake for each child receiving CPD, and an initial dietary protein intake equal to the RDA for chronologic age plus an increment for anticipated peritoneal losses across the peritoneum is recommended (128). The efficacy of the prescribed intake must be assessed regularly to ensure that it is adequate. Dialysate protein losses are proportionately greater in children than in adults (130), and children often begin CPD with evidence of protein wasting (125,131). Therefore, the current recommendations are for daily protein intakes of 2.3 to 3.0 g/kg for infants, 1.7 to 2.0 g/kg for children 1 to 10 years of age, and 1.4 to 1.8 g/kg for adolescents 11 to 18 years of age (128). Supplementation of dietary protein intake with intraperitoneally administered amino acids has been performed on occasion (132).

Although there are no data on the levels of water-soluble vitamins in children undergoing dialysis without vitamin supplementation, supplements of water-soluble vitamins are generally recommended for all children receiving CPD (128). Insufficient dietary intakes of vitamins B_6 and B_2 have been reported (128,133). Supplements of the fat-soluble vitamin A should be avoided. In the absence of renal clearance of vitamin A metabolites, children with renal failure are at risk for hypervitaminosis A, and elevated circulating levels of vitamin A have been reported in children on CPD (134). Because acidemia has a negative effect on growth and nutritional status, serum bicarbonate levels below 22 mmol/L should be corrected with alkali supplementation (128).

Infants receiving CPD require aggressive nutritional support. Ad lib food intake frequently falls below recommended levels, requiring forced feeding via nasogastric or gastrostomy tubes (131,135–137). Infants also frequently require aggressive supplementation of sodium, potassium, and phosphorus. Sodium losses into the dialysate are compounded in polyuric infants by urinary sodium losses. Standard infant formulas do not contain sufficient sodium to replace these losses. Both hypophosphatemia and hypokalemia can occur in the vigorously growing infant who is maintained on a low-phosphorus, low-potassium formula (138).

The complexity of the nutritional management of pediatric CPD patients is compounded by the critical importance of proper nutrition to the growing and developing child. The crucial role of the pediatric renal dietitian in the care of these fragile patients has been emphasized (128,139).

COMPLICATIONS OF CHRONIC PERITONEAL DIALYSIS IN CHILDREN

Peritonitis

The single most common complication that occurs in children maintained on CPD is peritonitis (83,140–144). Unfortunately, present data make it clear that children have a significantly greater rate of peritonitis than adults with a substantial number of children experiencing an episode of peritonitis during their first year of CPD treatment. Reductions in observed peritonitis rates have been reported in both adults and children in association with treatment of *Staphylococcus aureus* nasal carriage, use of a two-cuff catheter as well as recent technical developments such as newer disconnect systems and the flush-before-fill technique (139,140,145–149). The important contribution of prolonged dialysis training has also been demonstrated in children (150).

Recent evaluation of the NAPRTCS database has revealed a total of 2,965 reported episodes of peritonitis in 3,621 years of follow-up, resulting in an annualized peritonitis rate of 0.82 or 1 infection every 14.7 patient months (7). The rate of peritonitis was highest in the youngest patients (0 to 1 year) who had an annualized peritonitis rate of 1.02 or 1 infection every 11.8 months versus an annualized rate of 0.75 or 1 episode every 16.1 patient-months in children older than 12 years. In this same report, gram-positive infections comprised slightly more than 50% of the episodes of peritonitis and gram-negative infections slightly more than 20%. Fungal peritonitis represented 2.3% of peritonitis episodes.

The current approach to the treatment of peritonitis relies primarily on the intraperitoneal administration of antibiotics. A key development has been the recent publication of the *Consensus Guidelines for the Treatment of Peritonitis in Pediatric Patients Receiving Peritoneal Dialysis* by an international committee of physicians and nurses under the auspices of the International Society of Peritoneal Dialysis (148). This set of 15 guidelines includes recommendations for empiric antibiotic therapy; treatment of gram-positive, gram-negative, and fungal peritonitis; and indications for catheter removal and replacement (Figs. 39.2–39.4). The concern that has arisen regarding the develop-

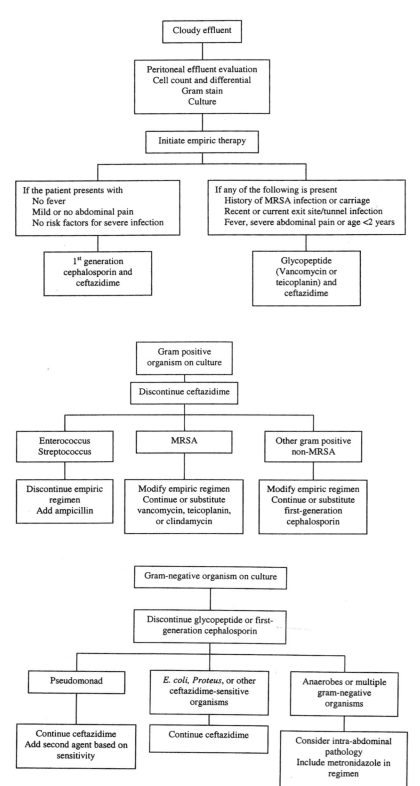

FIG. 39.2. Treatment algorithm for empiric therapy of peritonitis. MRSA, methicillin-resistant *Staphylococcus aureus.* (Reprinted from Warady BA, et al. Consensus guidelines for the treatment of peritonitis in pediatric patients receiving peritoneal dialysis. *Perit Dial Int* 2000;20:610–624, with permission.)

FIG. 39.3. Treatment algorithm for gram-positive peritonitis. (Reprinted from Warady BA, et al. Consensus guidelines for the treatment of peritonitis in pediatric patients receiving peritoneal dialysis. *Perit Dial Int* 2000;20:610–624, with permission.)

FIG. 39.4. Treatment algorithm for gram-negative peritonitis. (Reprinted from Warady BA, et al. Consensus guidelines for the treatment of peritonitis in pediatric patients receiving peritoneal dialysis. *Perit Dial Int* 2000;20:610–624, with permission.)

ment of vancomycin-resistant organisms and the vestibular, renal, and audiologic complications of aminoglycosides has influenced the content of several of the recommendations (151–153). An international registry is currently accumulating data regarding the application of these guidelines into clinical care.

Finally, sclerosing encapsulating peritonitis (SEP) is a rare but extremely serious clinical entity characterized by the presence of continuous, intermittent, or recurrent bowel obstruction associated with gross thickening of the peritoneum (154). Although primarily diagnosed in adults, it may also occur in children, typically those who have received PD for more than 5 years (155,156). The presence of peritoneal calcifications on abdominal computed tomography (CT) scan in association with ultrafiltration failure is highly suggestive of the diagnosis and may be an indication to discontinue PD.

Renal Anemia in Children on CPD

Before the widespread availability of recombinant human erythropoietin (rhEPO), a child receiving CPD typically required a red blood cell transfusion every 1.5 to 5 months to maintain a hematocrit of 22% to 25% (157). With rhEPO therapy, the need for transfusions has essentially been eliminated, and hematocrits can be maintained at near normal levels. rhEPO is used by more than 90% of children receiving CPD within 1 year of dialysis initiation (7).

Although rhEPO requirements vary, most children will respond to 80 to 120 U/kg/week given subcutaneously once or twice weekly. However, infants may require twice that amount to achieve and maintain a hemoglobin level of 11 to 12 g/dL. In one multicenter European trial of rhEPO in HD patients 2 to 21 years of age, the median weekly maintenance rhEPO dose varied from 136 U/kg in those older than 15 years to 321 U/kg in children younger than 5 years (158). The higher rhEPO requirement in infants may be related to the relative impact of blood loss, to the rate of expansion of the blood volume with somatic growth, or to a decrease in response to a given dose of rhEPO. The current treatment regimen of anemia can be anticipated to change with the availability of new erythropoiesis-stimulating proteins with longer terminal half-lives than rhEPO, (e.g., Darbepoetin alfa) (159).

Most CPD patients receive rhEPO by the subcutaneous (SC) route; however, a small number (<3% in NAPRTCS registry) receive intraperitoneal rhEPO (7). rhEPO is well absorbed from the peritoneal cavity when administered in a small volume (e.g., 50 mL) of dialysate for a prolonged dwell (160,161). In one study, nine children were changed from SC to intraperitoneal rhEPO administration and maintained their hematocrit levels with a rhEPO dose that was not significantly greater than the SC dose (160). In an evaluation of the pharmacokinetics of intraperitoneal dosing, a history of multiple episodes of peritonitis was associated with lower intraperitoneal absorption (162).

The erythropoietic response to rhEPO is blunted or eliminated in the presence of significant infection or inflammation. The most frequent form of infection in children undergoing CPD is peritonitis. The effect of a peritonitis episode on erythropoiesis persists beyond the period of evident infection. In one center, hematocrits remained at least 20% below baseline 4 weeks following the infection in association with 50% of peri-

tonitis episodes. Whereas the hematocrit had returned to baseline by 8 weeks, some patients required an increased rhEPO dose (163). The blunting of erythropoiesis by peritonitis or other inflammatory processes results from decreased erythropoietin levels, the inhibitory effects of circulating cytokines on marrow activity, and a decreased ability to mobilize iron from the reticuloendothelial system (164,165).

In order for rhEPO to be effective, sufficient iron stores are necessary. (See the discussion of erythropoietin later in chapter.) Correction of anemia with rhEPO may be associated with the exacerbation or initiation of hypertension, making careful monitoring of blood pressure (BP) and aggressive treatment of hypertension mandatory.

Growth Retardation

Before the use of recombinant human growth hormone (rhGH), severe growth retardation was almost universally present in children with chronic renal failure. The impact of growth retardation on adult height is greatest for those children with chronic renal failure during infancy and puberty, the periods of most rapid growth. Several factors may contribute to the poor growth of children with chronic renal failure, including protein and calorie malnutrition, metabolic acidosis, renal osteodystrophy, endocrine abnormalities, and the accumulation of uremic toxins. Although some of these factors are improved by dialysis, many persist despite aggressive dialytic therapy.

A number of endocrine abnormalities are present in chronic renal failure that may contribute to poor growth. These endocrine alterations include abnormalities of vitamin D metabolism, alterations of the growth hormone axis, hypothyroidism, and peripheral insulin resistance. Alterations in growth hormone secretion and the activity of insulin-like growth factor 1 (IGF-1) have been described in children with chronic renal failure (166,167). IGF-1 stimulates the clonal expansion of chondrocytes and collagen formation in the long-bone growth plates. The bioactivity of IGF-1 is limited in uremic children through an increase in IGF-1 binding proteins. Treatment with rhGH may accelerate growth by increasing IGF-1 levels to supraphysiologic levels with a resultant increase in its bioactivity.

The treatment of children who have developed ESRD with rhGH has been extensively reviewed elsewhere (168). Although rhGH improves the growth of children undergoing peritoneal and HD, the response may be blunted after the initial year of treatment (168–171). The basis for the diminishing response is not yet clear but may respond in part to an increased rhGH dose. When all other factors associated with growth retardation in children receiving HD or PD (i.e., acidosis, hyperphosphatemia, secondary hyperparathyroidism, sodium losses, and poor nutrition) are being aggressively treated and poor growth persists, rhGH therapy is indicated. The recent K/DOQI nutrition guidelines recommend the initiation of rhGH treatment in children with a height standard deviation score (SDS) more negative than −2.0 or a growth velocity more negative than −2.0 SDS (128). In the 2001 NAPRTCS annual report, the mean height SDS at CPD initiation was −1.75; nevertheless, only 19% of patients were treated with rhGH at 1 year and 25% at 2 years post dialysis initiation (7).

Renal Bone Disease

Children on CPD can experience progression of renal bone disease. Aggressive medical management with vitamin D analogues, calcium supplements, oral dietary phosphate binders, and diets with reduced phosphate content are all essential components of the effective management and prevention of renal bone disease in children. (See the discussion of calcium and phosphorus homeostasis later in the chapter.) Oral calcitriol has been shown to be effective in controlling renal bone disease in children receiving CPD (172). The optimal serum parathyroid hormone (PTH) level to avoid suppressing growth with adynamic bone disease or worsening renal osteodystrophy during rhGH treatment has been debated; however, at this time intact assay values of 100 pg/mL to less than 400 pg/mL are recommended (172). Calcium-containing phosphate binders have replaced aluminum-based binders in pediatric patients. When high doses of calcium-containing phosphate binders are required to maintain serum phosphate within normal limits, hypercalcemia is often seen, especially in the setting of adynamic bone disease. Low-calcium dialysate will help control hypercalcemia in these patients, and reduced doses of calcitriol are also often needed (173). In addition to adversely affecting bone, the role of an elevated calcium or an elevated calcium-phosphate product in the progression of vascular calcification has been recently demonstrated and may be a factor in the cardiovascular mortality recently described in children (174–176). It has been suggested that non-calcium-containing phosphate binders such as sevelamer may decrease the development of vascular calcification in adult HD patients (177). Their role in children is still being evaluated.

Mortality

In the most recent annual report of NAPRTCS, an overall mortality rate of 8.5% was noted for the pediatric PD population (7). An assessment related to age revealed a mortality rate of 14.9% for patients younger than 5 years at dialysis initiation, which was significantly greater than the mortality rate of 5.7% and 4.5% for patients in the 6 to 12 and older than 13 year age groups. The mortality rate for patients 0 to 1 year and 2 to 5 years was 18.9% and 8.3%, with 1- and 3-year postinitiation mortality rates of 15.3% and 32.5% for the youngest patients and 5.8% and 13.7% for the 2- to 5-year age group. These data confirm the high-risk status of the infant and young child with ESRD and are similar to data collected from children in Italy and Japan (178,179). The primary reported causes of death for all PD patients were infection (27.9%) and cardiopulmonary disease (20.9%). The primary causes of death for patients 0 to 5 years of age were the same, with infection accounting for 27.1% of deaths and cardiopulmonary disease 19.8%. Although the specific reasons for the higher death rates seen in infants receiving PD have not been well delineated, recent work has suggested that the presence of extrarenal disease, particularly pulmonary disease/hypoplasia and oliguria or anuria, are important risk factors (180,181).

CHRONIC HEMODIALYSIS FOR CHILDREN

Characteristics of a Pediatric Hemodialysis Center

Provision of optimal chronic pediatric HD requires a program philosophy that is geared to the particular needs of infants, children, adolescents and young adults. Although the equipment used for delivering pediatric HD is similar to that found in adult dialysis units, specialized personnel, in addition to physicians and nurses, with expertise in pediatric care are necessary to ensure that children receiving HD can receive developmentally appropriate care in the setting of a never-ending cycle of dialysis and renal transplantation (85). Child life specialists lend critical expertise to provide developmentally appropriate evaluations and assistance to children and their families during procedures and can serve as liaisons to help educate school personnel with respect to the particular medical and psychosocial needs of children with ESRD. Pediatric-trained ESRD social work personnel are essential to assess the psychosocial development of children with ESRD and to assist families with the complex socioeconomic challenges and barriers associated with ESRD. Dietitians expert in the nutritional requirements and restrictions imposed by ESRD are vital to the development of palatable menus for children with ESRD; work with school lunch programs; and closely monitor a multitude of nutrition status markers including weight, growth, body mass index, head circumference, normalized protein catabolic rate (nPCR), mid-arm circumference, triceps skin-fold thickness, and bioimpedance analysis (128).

Vascular Access

Adequate HD delivery depends on a functional vascular access. Current HD access options are divided into two categories: permanent access in the form of an arteriovenous fistula (AVF) or arteriovenous graft (AVG) and semipermanent access in the form of catheters with a SC cuff for chronic dialysis.

AVFs are comprised of a connection between a patient's native artery and vein. The most common sites for AVFs are the wrist (radiocephalic or Brescia-Cimino) and the antecubital fossa (brachial artery to cephalic vein). AVFs require at least 4 to 12 weeks for enough venous segment dilatation or maturation to allow for successful needle placement (182,183). The most common complications of AVFs include aneurysm formation from repeated puncture at the same site, arterial inflow stenosis with resultant poststenotic vessel dilatation, and collateral vessel development.

Young patients weighing less than 20 to 30 kg have relatively small vessels, which may not be able to support AVF placement and maturation. If native blood vessels are inadequate for an AVF, artificial materials can be used to create an AVG. Currently the most commonly used material is polytetrafluoroethylene/Teflon (PTFE). The advantage of AVGs over AVFs include an expanded variety of anatomic placement sites (distal arm, upper arm, thigh) and configurations (loop or straight). The major disadvantage associated with AVGs is the development of intimal hyperplasia and venous outflow stenosis, which can lead to decreased intraaccess flow and thrombosis. Recent pediatric data demonstrate that proactive noninvasive monitoring of AVG blood flow coupled to rapid referral for balloon angioplasty for a low AVG blood-flow reading leads to a significant decrease in thrombosis rates (184,185). A recent pediatric study showed 1-, 3- and 5-year pediatric AVF and AVG survival of 90%, 60%, and 40%, respectively (186). These data also demonstrated that although 5-year AVG and AVF survival rates are not significantly different, AVGs do exhibit higher thrombosis and surgical intervention rates.

Cuffed indwelling catheters serve as the most common form of access for children receiving chronic HD (7), which is unfortunate given catheters' higher complication rates and shorter survival times compared with AVFs or AVGs. Before 1998, dual-lumen configurations were the only options for pediatric HD catheters. Newer catheter configurations include dual-lumen catheters with split distal venous and arterial lumens to allow for free tip movement within the vein (Ash split catheter) and twin separate single-lumen catheter systems inserted into the same vein with different exit-sites or in different veins altogether (Tesio catheter system). Recent pediatric data demonstrate that Tesio catheters enjoy a longer survival and provide superior clearance more consistently than dual lumen catheters of similar size (187,188). There are currently sufficient catheters of various designs, diameters, and lengths to permit chronic HD in infants and children of all sizes (Table 39.4).

Equipment for Pediatric Hemodialysis

Hemodialysis Circuit

The HD circuit is comprised of the patient's vascular access, blood tubing that connects the access to the hemodialyzer, and the hemodialyzer itself. Blood tubing is produced in a variety of sizes and should be matched to allow for optimal blood flow while minimizing the volume of the extracorporeal circuit, which is the sum of the blood tubing volume and the hollow-fiber dialyzer volume. To prevent excessive repeated blood loss in the circuit and hemodynamic instability, the extracorporeal circuit should not exceed 10% of the patient's calculated blood volume. Neonatal lines with a volume of 40 mL are available for use in children less than 15 kg. A wide variety of dialyzers with different blood volumes is available from various manufacturers that can be matched to pediatric patient sizes. In some infants, for whom even the smallest blood tubing and dialyzer volumes exceed 10% of patient blood volume, the circuit should be primed with colloid [5% albumin or packed red blood cells (PRBCs) diluted with albumin to a measured hematocrit of 35%] instead of crystalloid.

Hemodialysis Machine

Provision of safe pediatric HD requires machines that have accurate blood pump flow rates and volumetric control of ultrafiltration. For infants, blood flows as low as 20 mL/min are often required. Clearance for pediatric HD is generally controlled by blood-flow rates, which should typically not exceed 400 mL/min/1.73m^2 of patient BSA to minimize the risk of cardiovascular compromise. The dialysate flow rate should be at least 1.5 times the blood-flow rate to prevent dialysate saturation from limiting solute clearance. Volumetric ultrafiltration controllers are critical to prevent rapid and excessive ultrafiltration rates in infants and young children receiving HD. Neonates receiving HD (e.g., for rapid serum ammonia reduction in patients with urea cycle defects) may require the use of accurate bed scales that can detect changes of less than 10 g, because many HD machines do not have resolution of ultrafiltration volumes of less than 100 g.

Pediatric Dialyzers

The ideal pediatric hemodialyzer would have a very small blood volume, a safe ultrafiltration coefficient, a low resistance blood circuit, a high degree of biocompatibility, and a predictable relationship between clearance and blood-flow rates. Current dialyzers are manufactured with a hollow-fiber design to minimize blood volume and provide reliable and predictable solute clearance and ultrafiltration coefficients. Activation of proinflammatory cytokines, leukocytes, and other mediators can occur when blood comes into contact with an inorganic surface. Although little pediatric data exist currently, numerous adult studies have suggested that repeated exposure to certain dialysis membranes may result in prolonged immune system activation, protein catabolism, and alteration of host proteins, which may have long-term adverse clinical consequences (189–196). Newer generation dialysis membranes constructed from materials such as polysulfone and polymethylmethacrylate (PMMA) cause less proinflammatory cytokine activation compared with older generation membranes made from cellulose or cuprophane (197,198). Whereas there are no data available on changes in patient outcomes with polysulfone or PMMA membrane, the incidence of anaphylactoid, complement-mediated immediate membrane reactions are far less common with biocompatible membranes.

Chronic Hemodialysis Prescription

Initiation of Dialysis

The approach to the initial HD treatments is the same as that used for acute HD described earlier in this chapter.

Hemodialysis Adequacy

Adequate HD is usually defined as a minimum level of toxic substance clearance (usually using BUN clearance as a surrogate) below which a clinically unacceptable rate of poor outcome occurs. A more complete definition of HD adequacy recognizes both HD treatment urea clearance and the patient's metabolic state as manifested by urea generation in between HD treatments. Significant research over the past 20 years has focused on refinement of complex mathematical models to more accurately quantify the total urea mass removed during a dialysis treatment (199–213).

The ideal parameter to use when prescribing an individual dialysis treatment should recognize the individual patient's size and metabolic state. It should be simultaneously informative of the overall production and removal of toxic substances. The conceptual basis of urea kinetic modeling is based on the analysis of the rates of accumulation and removal of urea. Urea is generated at a constant rate that is proportional to the patient's protein catabolic rate. At the beginning of dialysis, urea is distributed in a single body pool that is equivalent to the TBW, and thus the concentration of urea can be described by a sigle-pool mathematical model. The rate of removal of urea is depicted by the term Kt/V [dialyzer urea clearance at a particular blood-flow rate (K; mL/min), HD treatment duration (t; minutes) and the patient pretreatment and posttreatment weight (kg)]. The interdialytic accumulation of urea reflects the amount of protein catabolized during the time between dialysis treatments (214). In a steady state, this protein catabolic rate (g/day) reflects the amount of protein ingested by the patient and, hence, is a marker of nutritional status (215–221).

The validity of the urea kinetic model was demonstrated in the National Cooperative Dialysis Study (200), which demonstrated a higher probability of "patient failure" (i.e., patient death or hospitalization) in adult patients who received lower doses of HD and/or who were in a poor state of nutrition. In adults, the individual dialysis treatment should be such that the Kt/V is greater than 1.2 (213). Corresponding target Kt/V values for children have not been defined, although it is presumed that pediatric patients should receive dialysis that is at least equivalent to that provided for adults. Some initial pediatric outcome data have shown the utility of Kt/V in controlling for HD dose and nPCR in the assessment of nutrition status in malnourished patients receiving HD (219,220).

Recent pediatric data demonstrate that simplified algebraic equations reliably approximate Kt/V and nPCR (201,207). Some formulas further refine urea clearance measurement to account for the double-pool distribution of urea during dialysis and the resultant BUN rebound seen in the first hour after HD ends as urea reequilibrates between the intracellular and extracellular compartments (199,202,203,205). HD outcome study validity requires a control for HD dose, so the application of simpler, more accessible HD adequacy measurement methods should lead to an increase in pediatric HD outcome study research. Initial single-center and multicenter pediatric studies are starting to assess the impact of dialysis dose on outcome (220,221).

METHODS TO PREVENT ULTRAFILTRATION-ASSOCIATED SYMPTOMS

Sodium Modeling

Most sodium modeling programs create a hyperosmolar dialysate sodium concentration at the beginning of the dialysis treatment, which is followed by a progressive decrease in the sodium concentration. The increased sodium concentration early in the dialysis treatment leads to an increase in serum osmolality and thereby offsets a decline of serum osmolality caused by urea clearance. The decrease of the dialysate sodium throughout the treatment can be configured in an exponential, linear, or stepwise pattern. Sodium modeling has been shown to reduce dialysis morbidity in both adolescent and adult HD patients (222,223).

Noninvasive Monitoring of Hematocrit (NIVM)

Because red cell volume remains constant during dialysis, changes in hematocrit will be inversely proportional to changes in intravascular volume. Continuous optical methods of NIVM of the hematocrit take advantage of this relationship to demonstrate a real-time association between fluctuating hematocrit and intravascular volume during the HD treatment. In turn, optical methods of NIVM continuously monitor changes in intravascular volume and can help decrease symptomatology during a dialysis treatment (224–226). NIVM has been studied in pediatric patients receiving HD, and ultrafiltration-associated event rates (defined as hypotension, headache, or cramping that required a nursing intervention such as a saline bolus, Trendelenburg position, slow/stop ultrafiltration) were lower, especially for patients less than 35 kg, when NIVM was performed (227,228). Analysis of the timing of events at different blood volume changes using NIVM has led to NIVM-guided ultrafiltration modeling algorithms that optimize fluid removal during dialysis, lessen the need for antihypertensive medications, and minimize intradialytic and interdialytic patient symptoms (228).

Nutritional Management of the Child on Hemodialysis

The nutritional goal for children undergoing chronic HD is to optimize their growth and development, while avoiding exacerbation of their underlying fluid and electrolyte disturbances and uremia. An individual child's prescribed intake is based on an analysis of residual renal function and nutritional needs. Malnutrition, which plays a role in the poor growth of children with chronic renal failure, may result from inadequate dietary intake resulting from uremic anorexia and dysgeusia and prescribed nutrient restrictions (229–231). As a result, children will often require dietary supplementation above their spontaneous intake, as mentioned in the previously referred to K/DOQI pediatric nutrition guidelines. The dietary protein and caloric intake of each child should be sufficient to allow a positive nitrogen balance associated with an increase in lean body mass and stature (229,231,232). An increase in dietary energy intake without sufficient protein intake may result in obesity without increasing a child's lean body mass. In contrast, an increase in dietary protein intake without sufficient energy intake will increase the amount of protein used for energy needs rather than increasing lean body mass and, therefore, will increase the urea generation rate.

The dietary needs of children with chronic renal failure are not the same as the National Research Council's Food and Nutrition Board's RDA, because these recommendations are for populations of normal children. For example, the needs of children on HD are affected by the catabolic effects of HD, including the loss of amino acids in the dialysate. Protein intake must be sufficient to allow an increase in muscle mass and maximize growth while minimizing urea generation (233). An ongoing assessment of the balance of dietary protein intake and urea removal can be gained through the use of urea kinetic modeling (215,233).

The usual dietary requirements for protein and calories may be most accurately estimated in terms of stature, because this measure is independent of fluid balance or the amount of body fat. In one report, a positive nitrogen balance was attained in children receiving a diet that provided 0.3 g of protein per 1 cm of statural height with an energy intake of 10 kcal/cm (215). An increase in protein intake above this amount resulted in an increased urea generation rate and an increase in dialysis requirements without improving the nitrogen balance status. An alternative recommended intake is contained within the K/DOQI guidelines (128).

Children on HD have a pattern of lipid abnormalities similar to that seen in familial endogenous hypertriglyceridemia or type IV hyperlipidemia (234–236). The lipid profile consists of elevated triglyceride and very low density lipoprotein (VLDL) levels with decreased high-density lipoprotein (HDL) levels. The significance of lipid abnormalities in children with chronic renal failure is unclear, but such abnormalities may increase their risk of atherosclerosis. Although the basis for the lipid abnormalities has not been completely ascertained, possible contributing factors include a high proportion of fat in the diet and decreased lipoprotein lipase and hepatic triglyceride lipase activities (234–236). In addition, carnitine levels are decreased in children treated with HD as compared with healthy controls (237,238). Carnitine, a low-molecular-weight molecule that transports fatty acids from the cytoplasm to the mitochondria for oxidation, may be lost in the dialysate.

Treatment of lipid abnormalities is first directed at dietary restrictions. The role of pharmacologic lipid-lowering agents, such as lovastatin, in children on HD has not been determined. However, supplementation with L-carnitine has been suggested as a potential treatment. Although one short-term trial of intravenous L-carnitine (5 mg/kg during dialysis) resulted in a marked decrease in triglyceride levels and an increase in HDL cholesterol concentration (237), a more recent study failed to confirm these findings (239).

Water-soluble vitamins are removed during HD making supplementation with these vitamins, especially vitamins B_6, C, and folate necessary. Restriction of water intake is necessary to prevent interdialytic volume overload. A child's fluid restriction is generally the sum of insensible losses, residual urine output, and an amount that can be safely accumulated and ultrafiltered after a 2- to 3-day interdialytic period. The sodium intake of most children is restricted to help maintain the desired fluid restriction and avoid hypertension. In contrast to older children, infants with minimal urine output or with large urinary sodium losses from dysplastic renal syndromes receiving low-sodium formulas are at risk for hyponatremia. The accumulation of water over an interdialytic period coupled with a very low sodium content in the formula may result in dilutional hyponatremia.

Finally, intradialytic parenteral nutrition (IDPN) may have a role in treatment of severe protein-energy malnutrition in children receiving HD (219,240). IDPN is comprised of a 70% dextrose solution and a 15% amino acid solution. In addition, patients may receive intravenous lipids. IDPN is characteristically prescribed to provide 1.2 to 1.4 g protein per kilogram of patient weight each treatment (241).

Calcium and Phosphorus Homeostasis

The metabolic abnormalities that may arise in children treated with HD are common to all children with chronic renal failure and include elevated body phosphate stores, insufficient 1-alpha-hydroxylation of 25-hydroxy-cholecalciferol, and resultant inadequate intestinal absorption of calcium. As a consequence of decreased 1,25-dihydroxy-cholecalciferol and depressed serum ionized calcium concentrations, there is an increase in PTH levels. The resultant renal osteodystrophy may impede growth and lead to long-term bony abnormalities. In addition, the hyperphosphatemia may lead to extraskeletal metastatic calcifications. Prevention requires dietary phosphate restriction, administration of intestinal phosphate binders, and supplementation with calcium and vitamin D analogues.

Calcium carbonate and aluminum hydroxide have been shown to bind dietary phosphate at equivalent doses in both adult and pediatric dialysis patients (242–245). Thus, calcium carbonate use effectively decreases hyperphosphatemia without incurring the long-term sequelae of aluminum toxicity associated with aluminum-based binders. The amount of calcium carbonate required correlates with a child's phosphate intake (244). When calcium carbonate is used as a phosphate binder, 20% to 30% of the ingested calcium load is absorbed, which can result in hypercalcemia. Hypercalcemia may be averted in this situation by using different forms of calcium such as calcium acetate, decreasing the dialysate calcium content, and adding or replacing with polymeric forms of phosphate binders such as sevelamer (246,247). Calcium acetate has a greater affinity for intestinal phosphate than calcium carbonate, so a lower dose should be as effective (246). To date, no pediatric data exist that describe the efficacy of sevelamer in children receiving dialysis, but adult data demonstrate that sevelamer is effective either alone or in combination with calcium-based binders (247–249).

Traditionally, the dialysate calcium concentration has been 3.0 to 3.5 mEq/L to produce a positive calcium balance during a HD treatment. The use of physiologic, low-calcium (2.0 to 2.5 mEq/L) dialysate in place of the standard dialysate will produce a negative calcium balance during the dialysis treatment (242,245).

Finally, vitamin D supplementation is an essential component of the treatment of children with chronic renal failure. All forms of vitamin D stimulate intestinal calcium absorption. The active 1,25-dihydroxlyated form (calcitriol) has the added advantage of directly suppressing parathyroid gland growth and PTH synthesis (250,251). Intravenous forms of the Vitamin D analogs calcitriol and paricalcitol are currently available to treat the secondary hyperparathyroidism associated with renal failure (252,253); pediatric dosing and efficacy trials are underway in the United States.

Erythropoietin

The factors contributing to the anemia associated with chronic HD in adults and children include erythropoietin deficiency, decreased erythrocyte survival, inhibition of erythropoiesis, and increased blood loss (254–257). In comparison to children with nonrenal causes of anemia, children with chronic renal failure have markedly reduced erythropoietin levels for their degree of anemia (255). The average red cell life span is reduced from a normal value of 120 days to a mean of 80 days in uremic individuals. This shortened life span is due to dialytic and intestinal losses and low-level hemolysis resulting from oxidative stresses and erythrocyte rigidity in uremia (256,257). Anticoagulation for HD and uremic coagulopathy also contribute to blood loss in children on HD. Intestinal blood loss in 12 children undergoing chronic HD was 11.1 ±2.3 mL/m²/day. Extraintestinal blood losses were 8.3 ±5.1 mL/m² per dialysis treatment (258). In this same group of children, the erythrocyte life span was 80% normal.

The availability of rhEPO has had a major positive effect on children treated with chronic HD. Before the introduction of rhEPO, essentially all children on HD were transfusion dependent. An initial rhEPO dose of 80 to 120 U/kg/week administered intravenously (IV) three times weekly eliminates transfusion requirements in virtually all children. Although the optimal hemoglobin level is not yet known, the current hemoglobin target is 11 to 12 g/dL (259). In a selected group of adolescent HD patients in the United States, only 55% had a hemoglobin greater than 11 g/dL (260). This result may have been in part related to variable rhEPO dose requirements or rhEPO hyporesponsiveness. The most important cause of rhEPO hyporesponsiveness is insufficient iron stores (see later). Additional causes include infection or inflammation, latent blood loss, and hyperparathyroidism. Patients with severe hyperparathyroidism have been shown to be hyporesponsive to rhEPO (261). This poor response may be due to inhibition of erythropoiesis by circulating PTH or to osteitis fibrosa resulting in decreased marrow space for erythropoiesis.

The efficiency and cost effectiveness of subcutaneously administered rhEPO have been demonstrated in adult HD patients (262). A SC dose is more slowly absorbed than an intravenous dose, with a lower peak level but a longer half-life (263). It has been suggested that the sustained lower level is more physiologic and has a greater erythropoietic effect. Another approach to increasing the duration of the erythropoietic effect has been the modification of rhEPO to make a new protein with a longer half-life. Darbepoetin alfa (Aranesp) administered IV once a week has been shown to be as effective as rhEPO administered three times a week in adult HD patients (159). Preliminary pharmacokinetic studies in children suggest a similar profile to that in adults (264). Therefore, the treatment of anemia in children with chronic kidney disease can be expected to change over the next few years.

The benefits of rhEPO treatment are the result of the elimination of transfusions and the amelioration of anemia. In children who had been repeatedly transfused, levels of previously formed panel-reactive antibodies and cytotoxic antibodies to a T-cell panel decreased after the initiation of rhEPO and the cessation of transfusions (265). During rhEPO treatment, improvements in appetite, school attendance, physical activity, cognition, and overall well-being have been described (266–268). Improvements in exercise tolerance and regression of ventricular hypertrophy have also been demonstrated (266,267,269,270). Montini et al. (266) evaluated brainstem auditory-evoked responses and peripheral nerve conduction

velocity in children at baseline and during rhEPO treatment. At baseline, five of nine children evaluated had abnormal auditory-evoked responses. Four of the five abnormal children studied normalized their results after the hematocrit increased during rhEPO treatment. In contrast, there was no improvement in the peripheral nerve conduction velocity (266). The initial trials of rhEPO in adults described improvements in appetite, so the potential for improvements in nutritional status and growth were anticipated in children (271). Although increases in appetite and body weight have been described in some reports, there has not, however, been consistent improvement in nutrition or growth during rhEPO treatment in most pediatric studies (158,272–274).

The most significant adverse effect of rhEPO treatment is the development or exacerbation of hypertension. Reports of pediatric HD patients treated with rhEPO have noted that up to 36% of children develop new onset hypertension or experience an exacerbation of previously well-controlled hypertension (266–268). Seizures were initially described as a possible adverse effect of rhEPO therapy; however, most have been associated with hypertensive encephalopathy (275). There was an initial report of an increase in vascular access thrombosis with rhEPO; however, subsequent larger studies have not borne this out (271,276,277).

The goal of iron supplementation during rhEPO treatment is to maintain sufficient iron stores for optimal erythropoiesis without the development of hemosiderosis. In the past, children on HD were multiply transfused and eventually became iron overloaded. Because of the current elimination of transfusions, the blood and iron losses associated with chronic renal failure and dialysis are not replaced, and children have a net iron loss.

Iron stores are assessed indirectly by the measurement of iron, total iron-binding capacity (TIBC), and ferritin. The TIBC, which is an indirect measure of transferrin, increases in iron deficiency and decreases in inflammation. The serum ferritin level reflects iron stores and inflammation, whereas the transferrin saturation (TSAT) (iron/TIBC) indicates the amount of iron that is readily available for erythropoiesis. Therefore, the serum ferritin, TSAT, or a combination of the two do not optimally define iron stores. A number of other assessments have been proposed to measure iron availability for erythropoiesis. The most promising is measurement of the reticulocyte hemoglobin content (278). The hemoglobin content of reticulocytes reflects the iron content of newly formed red cells and serves as a sensitive early measure of iron deficiency erythropoiesis (278). This assay is available as part of an automated blood count in some laboratories but is not yet in widespread use. Iron stores should be assessed before the initiation of rhEPO therapy and on a monthly basis during therapy. A TSAT of at least 20% is recommended to ensure that sufficient iron is available for erythropoiesis (259). However, a TSAT of 25% to 35% may be optimal for many patients.

It is difficult to maintain iron stores in HD patients by oral iron supplementation alone. There is limited gastrointestinal iron absorption in patients with renal failure who have relative but not absolute iron deficiency. Intestinal iron absorption is inversely related to the body's iron stores (279). There are a number of oral iron preparations including ferrous gluconate, ferrous sulfate, ferrous fumarate, and polysaccharide-iron complexes. The absorption and the gastrointestinal toxicity of the iron in these preparations are related to the availability of ionic iron in the intestinal lumen. The absorption of oral iron is best if taken 1 hour before or 2 hours after a meal. Iron absorption is impaired by food containing phytates (green leafy vegetables) and tannins (tea, coffee, red wine). In addition, medications that decrease gastric acidity such as phosphate binders can lower iron absorption.

It is now recognized that most HD patients and many CPD patients require intravenous iron on a regular or maintenance basis. Current recommendations (based on data in adult patients) are to treat patients with a course of intravenous iron for a TSAT less than 20% and/or a ferritin less than 100 ng/mL. Once iron replete, one can consider the administration of intravenous iron on a regular schedule (259). In the NAPRTCS registry, 87% of children 24 months after the initiation of CPD were receiving oral iron supplementation, whereas only 2% had received intravenous iron. In contrast, 20% of those on HD were receiving intravenous iron (7). Three types of intravenous iron are currently in use: iron dextran, ferric sodium gluconate, and ferric saccharate (or iron sucrose). Ferric sodium gluconate and ferric saccharate have been used extensively in Europe for years, whereas iron dextran has been more extensively used in the United States.

Iron dextran was effectively used for years in adult and pediatric dialysis patients with multiple descriptions of its relative safety (280,281). However, anaphylactic-like reactions do occur. Such reactions may consist of dyspnea, wheezing, abdominal cramps, and hypotension, which usually respond to treatment with intravenous epinephrine, diphenhydramine, and/or corticosteroids. Idiosyncratic reactions may occur in patients who have previously received intravenous iron dextran without incident. Therefore, before the administration of a course of iron dextran, a test dose should be given. Anaphylactic-like reactions are more common in patients with a history of multiple drug allergies (282). Whereas data on the incidence of anaphylactic-like reactions in children is sparse, in one multicenter evaluation of adult dialysis patients, 4.7% experienced adverse events that were attributable to iron dextran (283,284). Serious reactions including the need for hospitalization occurred in 0.7% of patients.

The other forms of intravenous iron, iron sucrose and ferric gluconate, are associated with fewer serious adverse effects. Both have been shown to be safe and effective in adult dialysis patients (285,286). Of note, ferric gluconate has even been safely administered to iron dextran-sensitive patients and has been shown to be safe in children when administered at doses of 1 to 2 mg/kg (287–289). The safe use of iron sucrose, 2 mg/kg given daily for 18 days, has been reported in premature infants (290). In a recent publication, it has also been shown to be efficacious in pediatric HD patients (291).

Hypertension Control

The main factors that contribute to hypertension in children and adults undergoing chronic HD are expanded intravascular volume, increased sympathetic tone, renin-mediated hyperten-

sion, and an elevated serum calcium level with resultant increased peripheral vascular resistance (292–294). Regardless of the presence of native or transplanted kidneys, hypertension in these patients is most often due to or exacerbated by an expanded intravascular volume. Ambulatory blood pressure monitoring (ABPM) reveals that the normal nocturnal BP dip is attenuated, and sleep BP loads are elevated (295). The relative contributions of sympathetic nervous system or renin-mediated hypertension and volume overload can be determined in part by the BP response to ultrafiltration. The BP should improve with ultrafiltration when hypertension is primarily due to volume overload (293). One caveat is that the BP may increase during dialysis in those patients controlled with antihypertensive medications that are cleared by the dialysis treatment. In patients with primarily sympathetic overactivity or renin-mediated hypertension, the BP will not decrease and may actually increase with ultrafiltration during the dialysis treatment (292–294). Children with chronic renal failure as a result of glomerular disease, chronic or recurrent pyelonephritis, or reflux nephropathy are most likely to have renin-mediated hypertension.

The first approach to hypertension should always be a reassessment of the patient's dry weight. Correction of overhydration will ameliorate hypertension for most patients (293). However, ultrafiltration of large volumes of fluid during dialysis may result in increased dialytic morbidity, including cramps, nausea, vomiting, and fatigue. These symptoms may be decreased with the use of sodium modeling techniques and NIVM (see section earlier in this chapter). The initial approach to management in children with suspected renin-mediated hypertension is the use of angiotensin-converting enzyme (ACE) inhibitors and angiotensin II (A-II) receptor blockers, although in some cases nephrectomies are needed to achieve BP control. Aside from ACE-inhibitors/A-II blockers in those patients with renin-mediated hypertension, there is no single ideal or recommended type of antihypertensive medication for children receiving HD. It should be recognized that the use of a vasodilator will increase the incidence of intradialytic symptoms of intravascular depletion such as hypotension and cramps and, therefore, will limit ultrafiltration.

Educational Needs

School attendance is an important part of the development of children, because they acquire skill in interacting with peers in addition to developing their academic skills. Therefore, a goal of any pediatric HD program is to ensure that children attend school regularly. Because there may be some school absence as a result of the timing of HD sessions and intercurrent illnesses, school work should be supplemented with individualized tutoring. Young children may benefit from placement in an early intervention program. In one center, 88% of children receiving chronic HD attended school regularly, and 71% were at grade level (296). However, in a registry analysis, only 51% of children were attending school full time at dialysis initiation (78). An additional 28% attended school part-time with additional tutoring during dialysis and 8% received home schooling.

Neurophysiologic and Cognitive Deficits

A number of neurologic complications have been described in children treated with HD, including seizure disorders, dialysis dementia, cerebral atrophy, developmental delay, and the dialysis disequilibrium syndrome (297–299). Intradialytic seizures have been described in 7% to 16% of children receiving chronic HD treatment (297,298). Intradialytic seizures are more common in children with a prior history of seizures (298).

HD treatments are associated with repetitive osmolar shifts in the brain and alterations in brain cell volume (300). An increase in brain cell volume is known to cause the release of glutamate and aspartate, which are potent neuronal excitatory amino acids (301). The inappropriate release of the neurotransmitter amino acids could directly alter neural activity and lead to cytotoxic cell swelling and neuronal death (302). Cell swelling and shrinkage resulting from rapid osmolar shifts during dialysis may give rise to dialysis disequilibrium syndrome as a result of changes in the concentrations of these excitatory amino acids. The dialysis disequilibrium syndrome, which may consist of headache, nausea, and dizziness and more severe symptoms of disorientation, seizures, and coma, is most frequently seen with the initiation of dialysis or during rapid dialysis of small children (46,300,301,303).

Long-Term Outcomes

Renal transplantation is the treatment of choice for most children with ESRD. However, because of long waiting times for cadaver allografts, high levels of preformed anti-human leukocyte antigen (HLA) antibodies, or personal choice, many children require long-term dialysis treatment. Data from the USRDS 2002 annual report indicated that 19% of patients younger than 20 years received a transplant as their first treatment for ESRD and that 61% of males and 49% of females received a renal transplant within 2 years of initiating RRT (1). The median time to living-donor transplant from the start of ESRD for children younger than 18 years in 1999 was 106 days, which has not changed over the past 5 years. However, the median time to cadaveric donor transplant has increased from 185 days in 1990 to 322 days in 1994 and 359 days in 1999 reflecting the increased number of patients on the cadaver waiting list.

Over the last 10 years, the 5-year survival probabilities for incident ESRD patients younger than 20 years has increased from 84.1% in 1985 to 89.5% in 1995 (1). The survival of children with ESRD remains markedly better than the survival of older patients in the USRDS database (e.g., 68.1% for those 20 to 44 years at presentation). However, the 5-year patient survival remains best for those who receive a renal transplant: 82% for those who remain on dialysis, 95.5% for recipients of a first living-donor transplant, and 93.5% for recipients of a cadaver donor transplant.

HEMODIALYSIS FOR NEONATES AND INFANTS

Indications

In facilities with adequately trained nursing and technical support staff, HD is the most appropriate modality for the acute treatment of infants with hyperammonemia, azotemia, and hyperkalemia and in situations in which there is a need for rapid fluid removal, such as pulmonary edema. HD is also an alternative to PD in clinical settings of abdominal surgery, compromised mesenteric blood flow, or pulmonary disease when compression of the diaphragm might be harmful.

Vascular Access in Infants

In neonates, HD access can be readily attained though the use of standard umbilical catheters. Adequate blood flow for dialysis (25 to 50 mL/min) requires the use of an 8-Fr umbilical venous catheter and a 5-Fr umbilical artery catheter. The venous catheter can be placed safely above or below the liver. Also, 7-Fr double-lumen HD catheters can be placed in subclavian, internal jugular, or femoral veins of infants without accessible umbilical vessels, so a single-needle technique is rarely necessary. The subclavian or internal jugular location is preferred for infants requiring multiple days of dialysis.

Special Techniques

The HD of neonates and infants requires specialized dialysis and nursing techniques (304). Intensive nursing assessment and frequent interventions are required during the HD treatment. Therefore, a 1:1 or a 2:1 nurse-to-patient ratio is needed. To avoid an extracorporeal circulation of greater than 10% of the infant's estimated blood volume, the dialysis lines should be primed with albumin or a blood-albumin combination. This prime is not reinfused at the end of the treatment. Ultrafiltration-controlled dialysis machines are essential for safe HD in infants (304).

Outcome

In experienced hands, HD can be a successful treatment for infants with metabolic abnormalities or acute or chronic renal failure. As noted in a single-center review by Sadowski et al. (305), hypotension occurred in 64% of their infants but did not curtail the treatment in most of them. Of six infants who had seizures, five were due to underlying medical problems such as hyperammonemia. Overall survival was 52%. The survival rate was better for infants with hyperammonemia and primary renal disorders than for those with multisystem failure and acute renal failure. A similar survival rate (39%) has been reported for neonates treated with acute PD (306).

In most infants, PD will be the preferable chronic dialysis modality. However, technical problems may necessitate the interruption of PD in some infants. These situations include fungal peritonitis, catheter dysfunction, tunnel infections, and decreased ultrafiltration and clearance capabilities of the peritoneal membrane. The long-term outcome of 20 infants treated with chronic HD at a single center over a 14-year period demonstrated an overall patient survival rate of 60%, with 11 of 20 infants subsequently receiving renal allografts (304). Survival was better for those infants weighing more than 5 kg at the time of first dialysis treatment (73%) than for those weighing less than 5 kg (20%).

REFERENCES

1. U.S.Renal Data System. USRDS 2002 annual data report: atlas of end-stage renal disease in the United States. Bethesda, MD: National Institutes of Health, National Institute of Diabetes and Digestive and Kidney Diseases, 2002.
2. Hoffman JIE. Congenital heart disease. *Pediatr Clin North Am* 1990; 37:25–44.
3. Poplack DG. Acute lymphoblastic leukemia. In: Pizzo PA, et al., eds. *Principles and practice of pediatric oncology.* New York: Lippincott-Raven, 1989:323.
4. U.S. Renal Data System. USRDS 1996 annual data report. Bethesda, MD: National Institutes of Health, National Institute of Diabetes and Digestive and Kidney Diseases, 1996.
5. Alexander SR, et al. Continuous peritoneal dialysis for children: a decade of worldwide growth and development. *Kidney Int* 1993;43 [Suppl 40]:S65–S74.
6. Warady BA, et al. Renal transplantation, chronic dialysis, and chronic renal insufficiency in children and adolescents: the 1995 annual report of the North American pediatric renal transplant cooperative study. *Pediatr Nephrol* 1997;11:49–64.
7. Neu AM, et al. Chronic dialysis in children and adolescents: the 2001 NAPRTCS annual report. *Pediatr Nephrol* 2002;17:656–663.
8. Wiggelinkhuizen J. Peritoneal dialysis in children. *S Afr Med J* 1971; 45:1047–1054.
9. Putiloff PV. Materials for the study of the laws of growth of the human body in relation to the surface areas of different systems: the trial on Russian subjects of planigraphic anatomy as a means for exact anthropometry; one of the problems of anthropology. Report of Dr. P.V. Putiloff at the meeting of the Siberian Branch of the Russian Geographic Society, 1884.
10. Wegner G. Chirurgische Bemerkungen umlautuber die peritoneal Humlautohle, mit besonder Berucksichtigung der Ovariotomie. *Arch Klin Chir* 1887;20:51.
11. Esperanca MJ, et al. Peritoneal dialysis efficiency in relation to body weight. *J Pediatr Surg* 1966;1:162–169.
12. Gruskin AB, et al. Developmental aspects of peritoneal dialysis kinetics. In: Fine RN, ed. *Chronic ambulatory peritoneal dialysis (CAPD) and chronic cycling peritoneal dialysis (CCPD) in children.* Boston: Martinus Nijhoff, 1987:33–46.
13. Kohaut EC. Effects of dialysate volume on ultrafiltration in young patients treated with CAPD. *Int J Pediatr Nephrol* 1986;7:13–16.
14. Schaefer F, et al. Estimation of peritoneal mass transport by three-pore model in children. *Kidney Int* 1998;54:1372–1379.
15. Fischbach M, et al. Dynamic changes of the total pore area available for peritoneal exchange in children. *J Am Soc Nephrol* 2001;12: 1524–1529.
16. Rippe B, et al. Simulations of peritoneal transport during CAPD: application of two-pore formalism. *Kidney Int* 1989;35:1234–1244.
17. Nolph KD. Peritoneal anatomy and transport physiology. In: Drukker W, et al., eds. *Replacement of renal function by dialysis.* Boston: Martinus Nijhoff, 1983:440–456.
18. Mactier RA, et al. Role of peritoneal cavity lymphatic absorption in peritoneal dialysis. *Kidney Int* 1987;32:65–72.
19. Haraldsson B. Assessing the peritoneal dialysis capacities of individual patients. *Kidney Int* 1995;47:1187–1198.
20. Morgenstern BZ, et al. Transport characteristics of the pediatric peritoneal membrane. *Kidney Int* 1984;25:259–264.
21. Geary DF, et al. Mass transfer area coefficients in children. *Perit Dial Int* 1994;14:30–33.
22. Warady BA, et al. Peritoneal membrane transport function in children receiving long-term dialysis. *J Am Soc Nephrol* 1996;7: 2385–2391.
23. Bouts AH, et al. Standard peritoneal permeability analysis in children. *J Am Soc Nephrol* 2000;11:943–950.
24. Morgenstern BZ. Equilibration testing: close, but not quite right. *Pediatr Nephrol* 1993;7:290–291.
25. Pyle WK. *Mass transfer in peritoneal dialysis* (PhD dissertation). Austin: University of Texas, 1987.
26. Kohaut EC, et al. Ultrafiltration in the young patient on CAPD. In: Moncrief JW, et al., eds. *CAPD update.* New York: Masson, 1981: 221–226.
27. Balfe JW, et al. A comparison of peritoneal water and solute movement in younger and older children on CAPD. In: Fine RN, et al., eds. *CAPD in children.* New York: Springer-Verlag, 1985:14–19.
28. Kohaut EC, et al. The effect of changes in dialysate volume on glucose and urea equilibration. *Perit Dial Int* 1994;14:236–239.
29. Leypoldt JK. Solute transport across the peritoneal membrane. *J Am Soc Nephrol* 2002;13[Suppl 1]:S84–S91.
30. Mactier RA, et al. Kinetics of peritoneal dialysis in children: role of lymphatics. *Kidney Int* 1988;34:82–88.
31. Schroder CH, et al. Transcapillary ultrafiltration and lymphatic absorption during childhood continuous ambulatory peritoneal dialysis. *Nephrol Dial Transplant* 1991;6:571–573.
32. Kaiser VA, et al. Acid base changes and acetate metabolism during routine and high-efficiency hemodialysis in children. *Kidney Int* 1981;19:70–79.
33. Schroacher R, et al. Enhanced clearance of vancomycin by hemodialysis in a child. *Pediatr Nephrol* 1989;3:83–85.
34. Nevins TE, et al. Infant hemodialysis. In: Nissenson AR, et al., eds. *Dialysis therapy.* Philadelphia: Hanley & Belfus, 1992:349–352.
35. Hakim RM, et al. Biocompatibility of dialysis membranes: effects of chronic complement activation. *Kidney Int* 1984;26:194–200.
36. Zaoui PM, et al. Effects of dialysis membranes on beta 2-microglobulin production and cellular expression. *Kidney Int* 1990;38:962–968.
37. Day RE, et al. Peritoneal dialysis in children: review of 8 years' experience. *Arch Dis Child* 1977;52:56–61.
38. Manley GL, et al. Renal failure in the newborn: treatment with peritoneal dialysis. *Am J Dis Child* 1968;115:107–110.
39. Gianantonio CA, et al. Acute renal failure in infancy and childhood. *J Pediatr* 1962;61:660–678.
40. Leone MR, et al. Early experience with continuous arteriovenous hemofiltration in critically ill pediatric patients. *Crit Care Med* 1986;14:1058–1063.
41. Ronco C, et al. Treatment of acute renal failure in newborns by continuous arteriovenous hemofiltration. *Kidney Int* 1986;29:908–915.
42. Alexander SR. Continuous arteriovenous hemofiltration. In: Levin DL, et al., eds. *Essentials of pediatric intensive care.* St. Louis: Quality Medical, 1990:1022–1048.
43. Warady BA, et al. Dialysis therapy for children with acute renal failure: survey results. *Pediatr Nephrol* 2000;15:11–13.
44. Raja R, et al. Comparison of double lumen subclavian with single lumen catheter. *Am Soc Artif Organs* 1984;30:508–509.
45. Shusterman NH, et al. Successful use of double-lumen silicone rubber catheters for permanent hemodialysis access. *Kidney Int* 1989;35: 887–890.
46. Mahoney CA, et al. Uremic encephalopathies: clinical, biochemical and experimental features. *Am J Kidney Dis* 1982;2:324–336.
47. Borgess HF, et al. Mannitol intoxication in patients with renal failure. *Arch Intern Med* 1982;142:63–66.
48. Fine RN. Renal transplantation for children—the only realistic choice. *Kidney Int* 1985;17:S15–S17.
49. Ware M, et al. The goal of specific immunologic unresponsiveness in clinical kidney transplantation. *Semin Nephrol* 1992;12:325–331.
50. Baum M, et al. Continuous ambulatory peritoneal dialysis in children: comparison with hemodialysis. *N Engl J Med* 1982;307: 1537–1542.
51. Alexander SR. Pediatric CAPD update. *Perit Dial Bull* 1983;[Suppl 3]4:S15–S22.
52. Furth SL, et al. Relationship between pediatric experience and treatment recommendations for children and adolescents with kidney failure. *JAMA* 2001;285:1027–1033.
53. Palmer RA, et al. Prolonged peritoneal dialysis for chronic renal failure. *Lancet* 1964;15:700–702.
54. Palmer RA, et al. Treatment of chronic renal failure by prolonged peritoneal dialysis. *N Engl J Med* 1966;274:248–254.
55. Tenckhoff H, et al. A bacteriologically safe peritoneal access device. *Trans Am Soc Artif Intern Organs* 1966;14:181–186.
56. Boen ST, et al. Periodic peritoneal dialysis using the repeated punc-

ture technique and an automated cycling machine. *Trans Am Soc Artif Intern Organs* 1964;10:409–414.

57. Tenckhoff H, et al. A simplified automatic peritoneal dialysis system. *Trans Am Soc Artif Intern Organs* 1972;18:436–440.

58. Counts S, et al. Chronic home peritoneal dialysis in children. *Trans Am Soc Artif Intern Organs* 1973;19:157–167.

59. Hickman RO. Nine years' experience with chronic peritoneal dialysis in childhood. *Dial Transplant* 1978;7:803.

60. Brouhard BH, et al. Home peritoneal dialysis in children. *Trans Am Soc Artif Intern Organs* 1979;25:90–94.

61. Baluarte HJ, et al. Experience with intermittent home peritoneal dialysis (IHPD) in children. *Pediatr Res* 1980;14:994(abst).

62. Lorentz WB, et al. Home peritoneal dialysis during infancy. *Clin Nephrol* 1981;15:194–197.

63. Potter DE, et al. Peritoneal dialysis in children. In: Atkins RC, et al., eds. *Peritoneal dialysis.* New York: Churchill Livingstone, 1981: 356–361.

64. Popovich RP, et al. The definition of a novel wearable/portable equilibrium peritoneal dialysis technique. *Trans Am Soc Artif Intern Organs* 1976;5:64.

65. Balfe JW, et al. Continuous ambulatory peritoneal dialysis in children. In: Legrain M, ed. *Continuous ambulatory peritoneal dialysis.* Amsterdam: Excerpta Medica, 1980:131–136.

66. Oreopoulos DG, et al. Dialysis and transplantation in young children [Letter]. *Br Med J* 1979;1:1628–1629.

67. Alexander SR, et al. Clinical parameters in continuous ambulatory peritoneal dialysis for infants and young children. In: Moncrief JW, et al., eds. *CAPD update.* New York: Masson, 1981:195–209.

68. Kohaut EC. Continuous ambulatory peritoneal dialysis: a preliminary pediatric experience. *Am J Dis Child* 1981;135:270–271.

69. Potter DE, et al. Continuous ambulatory peritoneal dialysis (CAPD) in children. *Trans Am Soc Artif Intern Organs* 1981;72:64–67.

70. Salusky IB, et al. Continuous ambulatory peritoneal dialysis in children. *Pediatr Clin North Am* 1982;29:1005–1012.

71. Gullot M, et al. In: Gahl GM, et al., eds. *Advances in peritoneal dialysis.* Amsterdam: Excerpta Medica, 1981:203–207.

72. Eastham EJ, et al. Pediatric continuous ambulatory peritoneal dialysis. *Arch Dis Child* 1982;57:677–680.

73. Price CG, et al. New modification of peritoneal dialysis: options in the treatment of patients with renal failure. *Am J Nephrol* 1981;1: 97–104.

74. VonLilien T, et al. Five years' experience with continuous ambulatory or continuous cycling peritoneal dialysis in children. *J Pediatr* 1987; 111:513–518.

75. Sieniawska M, et al. Preliminary results with the swan neck presternal catheter for CAPD in children. *Adv Perit Dial* 1993;9:321–324.

76. Twardowski ZJ, et al. Four-year experience with swan neck presternal peritoneal dialysis catheter. *Am J Kidney Dis* 1996;27:99–105.

77. Chadha V, et al. Chest wall peritoneal dialysis catheter placement in infants with a colostomy. *Adv Perit Dial* 2000;16:318–320.

78. Lerner GR, et al. Chronic dialysis in children and adolescents. The 1996 annual report of the North American pediatric renal transplant cooperative study. *Pediatr Nephrol* 1999;13:404–417.

79. Neu AM, et al. Current approach to peritoneal access in North American children: a report of the pediatric peritoneal dialysis study consortium. *Adv Perit Dial* 1995;11:289–292.

80. Stadermann MB, et al. Local fibrinolytic therapy with urokinase for peritoneal dialysis catheter obstruction in children. *Perit Dial Int* 2002;22:84–86.

81. Shea M, et al. Use of tissue plasminogen activator for thrombolysis in occluded peritoneal dialysis catheters in children. *Adv Perit Dial* 2001;17:249–252.

82. Daschner M, et al. Laparoscopic Tenckhoff catheter implantation in children. *Perit Dial Int* 2002;22:22–26.

83. Warady BA, et al. Lessons from the peritoneal dialysis patient database: a report of the North American Pediatric Renal Transplant Cooperative Study. *Kidney Int* 1996;49[Suppl 53]:S68–S71.

84. Golper TA, et al. Risk factors for peritonitis in long-term peritoneal dialysis: the Network 9 peritonitis and catheter survival studies. *Am J Kidney Dis* 1996;28:428–436.

85. Warady BA, et al. Optimal care of the pediatric end-stage renal disease patient on dialysis. *Am J Kidney Dis* 1999;33:567–583.

86. Twardowski ZJ, et al. Peritoneal equilibration test. *Perit Dial Bull* 1987;7:378–383.

87. Sliman GA, et al. Peritoneal equilibration test curves and adequacy of dialysis in children on automated peritoneal dialysis. *Am J Kidney Dis* 1994;24:813–818.

88. de Boer AW, et al. The necessity of adjusting dialysate volume to body surface area in pediatric peritoneal equilibration tests. *Perit Dial Int* 1997;17:199–202.

89. Schaefer F, et al. Evaluation of peritoneal solute transfer by the peritoneal equilibration test in children. *Adv Perit Dial* 1992;8:410–415.

90. Warady BA. The peritoneal equilibration test (PET) in pediatrics. *Contemp Dial Nephrol* 1994;March:21–41.

91. Blake P, et al. Recommended clinical practices for maximizing peritoneal dialysis clearances. *Perit Dial Int* 1996;16:448–456.

92. Rocco MV, et al. Changes in peritoneal transport during the first month of peritoneal dialysis. *Perit Dial Int* 1995;15:12–17.

93. *NKF-K/DOQI clinical practice guidelines for peritoneal dialysis adequacy.* New York: National Kidney Foundation, 2001.

94. Schaefer F, et al. Peritoneal transport properties and dialysis dose affect growth and nutritional status in children on chronic peritoneal dialysis. *J Am Soc Nephrol* 1999;10:1786–1792.

95. Fried L. Higher membrane permeability predicts poorer patient survival. *Perit Dial Int* 1997;17:387–388.

96. Churchill DN, et al. Increased peritoneal membrane transport is associated with decreased patient and technique survival for continuous peritoneal dialysis patients: the Canada-USA (CANUSA) Peritoneal Dialysis Study Group. *J Am Soc Nephrol* 1998;9:1285–1292.

97. Kagan A, et al. Role of peritoneal loss of albumin in the hypoalbuminemia of continuous ambulatory peritoneal dialysis patients: relationship to peritoneal transport of solutes. *Nephrology* 1995;71: 314–320.

98. Burkart JM, et al. Solute clearance approach to adequacy of peritoneal dialysis. *Perit Dial Int* 1996;16:457–470.

99. Rocco MV. Body surface area limitations in achieving adequate therapy in peritoneal dialysis patients. *Perit Dial Int* 1996;16:617–622.

100. Fischbach M, et al. Relationship between intraperitoneal hydrostatic pressure and dialysate volume in children on PD. *Adv Perit Dial* 1996;12:330–334.

101. Fischbach M, et al. Impact of fill volume changes on peritoneal dialysis tolerance and effectiveness in children. *Adv Perit Dial* 2000;16: 321–323.

102. Fischbach M, et al. Optimal volume prescription for children on peritoneal dialysis. *Perit Dial Int* 2000;20:603–606.

103. Warady BA, et al. Validation of PD Adequest 2.0 for pediatric dialysis patients. *Pediatr Nephrol* 2001;16:205–211.

104. Verrina E, et al. The use of the PD Adequest mathematical model in pediatric patients on chronic peritoneal dialysis. *Perit Dial Int* 1998; 18:322–828.

105. Fischbach M, et al. Effects of automated peritoneal dialysis on residual daily urinary volume in children. *Adv Perit Dial* 2001;17: 269–273.

106. Ferber J, et al. Residual renal function in children on haemodialysis and peritoneal dialysis therapy. *Pediatr Nephrol* 1994;8:579–583.

107. Canada-USA (CANUSA) Peritoneal Dialysis Study Group. Adequacy of dialysis and nutrition in continuous peritoneal dialysis: association with clinical outcomes. *J Am Soc Nephrol* 1996;7:198–207.

108. Lutes R, et al. Loss of residual renal function in patients on peritoneal dialysis. *Adv Perit Dial* 1993;9:165–168.

109. Churchill DN, et al. Clinical practice guideline for initiation of dialysis. *J Am Soc Nephrol* 1999;10[Suppl 13]:S289–S291.

110. Höltta T, et al. Clinical outcome of pediatric patients on peritoneal dialysis under adequacy control. *Pediatr Nephrol* 2000;14:889–897.

111. McCauley L, et al. Enhanced growth in children on peritoneal dialysis (PD): dialysis dose, nutrition, and metabolic control. *Perit Dial Int* 2000;20[Suppl 1]:S89.

112. Champoux S, et al. Enhanced response to growth hormone in children on peritoneal dialysis. *Perit Dial Int* 2001;21[Suppl 1]:S86.

113. Chadha V, et al. Is growth a valid outcome measure of dialysis clear-

ance in children undergoing peritoneal dialysis? *Perit Dial Int* 2001; 21(3):S179–S184.

114. Montini G, et al. Middle molecule and small protein removal in children on peritoneal dialysis. *Kidney Int* 2002;61:1153–1159.

115. van der Voort JH, et al. Can the DOQI guidelines be met by peritoneal dialysis alone in pediatric patients? *Pediatr Nephrol* 2000;14: 717–719.

116. Chadha V, et al. What are the clinical correlates of adequate peritoneal dialysis? *Semin Nephrol* 2001;21:480–489.

117. Mellits ED, et al. The assessment of body water and fatness from infancy to adulthood. *Monogr Soc Res Child Dev* 1970;35:12–26.

118. Morgenstern B, et al. Impact of total body water errors on Kt/V estimates in children on peritoneal dialysis. *Adv Perit Dial* 2001;17: 260–263.

119. Wühl E, et al. Assessment of total body water error in paediatric patients on dialysis. *Nephrol Dial Transplant* 1996;11:75–80.

120. Morgenstern B, et al. Estimating total body water in children based upon height and weight: a reevaluation of the formulas of Mellits and Cheek. *J Am Soc Nephrol* 2002;13:1884–1888.

121. Morgenstern BZ, et al. Total body water (TBW) in children on peritoneal dialysis. *J Am Soc Nephrol* 2002;13:2A.

122. Chen HH, et al. Discrepancy between weekly Kt/V and weekly creatinine clearance in patients on CAPD. *Adv Perit Dial* 1995;11:83–87.

123. Twardowski ZJ. Relationship between creatinine clearance and Kt/V in peritoneal dialysis: a response to the defense of the DOQI document. *Perit Dial Int* 1999;19:199–203.

124. Canepa A, et al. Nutritional status in children receiving chronic peritoneal dialysis. *Perit Dial Int* 1996;16[Suppl 1]:S526–S531.

125. Salusky IB, et al. Nutritional status of children undergoing continuous peritoneal dialysis. *Am J Clin Nutr* 1983;38:599–614.

126. Scolnik D, et al. Initial hypoalbuminemia and hyperlipidemia persist during chronic peritoneal dialysis in children. *Perit Dial Int* 1993;13: 136–139.

127. Ruley EJ, et al. Feeding disorders and gastroesophageal reflux in infants with chronic renal failure. *Pediatr Nephrol* 1989;3: 424–429.

128. Clinical Practice Guidelines for Nutrition in Chronic Renal Failure: II. pediatric guidelines. K/DOQI, National Kidney Foundation. *Am J Kidney Dis* 2000;35[Suppl 2]:S105–S136.

129. Balfe JW, et al. The use of CAPD in the treatment of children with end-stage renal disease. *Perit Dial Bull* 1981;1:35–38.

130. Drachman R, et al. Protein losses during peritoneal dialysis in children. In: Fine RN, et al., eds. *CAPD in children.* New York: Springer-Verlag, 1985:78–83.

131. Wassner SJ, et al. Nutritional requirement for infants with renal failure. *Am J Kidney Dis* 1986;7:300–305.

132. Balfe JW. Intraperitoneal amino acids in children receiving chronic peritoneal dialysis. *Perit Dial Int* 1996;16[Suppl 1]:S515–S516.

133. Warady BA, et al. Vitamin status of infants receiving long-term peritoneal dialysis. *Pediatr Nephrol* 1994;8:354–356.

134. Parrott KA, et al. Plasma vitamin A levels in children on CAPD. *Perit Dial Bull* 1987;7:90–92.

135. Warady BA, et al. Nasogastric tube feeding in infants on peritoneal dialysis. *Perit Dial Int* 1996;16[Suppl 1]:S521–S525.

136. Geary DF, et al. Tube feeding in infants on peritoneal dialysis. *Perit Dial Int* 1996;16[Suppl 1]:S517–S520.

137. Coleman JE, et al. The optimal route for nutritional support of children with chronic renal failure. *Perit Dial Int* 1996;16[Suppl 1]: S517–S520.

138. Roodhooft AM, et al. Hypophosphatemia in infants on continuous ambulatory peritoneal dialysis. *Clin Nephrol* 1990;34:131–135.

139. Harvey E, et al. The team approach to the management of children on chronic peritoneal dialysis. *Adv Ren Replace Ther* 1996;3:3–13.

140. Verrina E, et al. Prevention of peritonitis in children on peritoneal dialysis. *Perit Dial Int* 2000;20:625–630.

141. Hisano S, et al. Immune status of children on continuous ambulatory peritoneal dialysis. *Pediatr Nephrol* 1992;6:179–181.

142. Warady BA, et al. Peritonitis with continuous ambulatory peritoneal dialysis and continuous cycling peritoneal dialysis. *J Pediatr* 1984; 105:726–730.

143. Watson AR, et al. Peritonitis during continuous ambulatory peritoneal dialysis in children. *Can Med Assoc J* 1986;134:1019–1022.

144. Levy M, et al. Optimal approach to the prevention and treatment of peritonitis in children undergoing continuous ambulatory and continuous cycling peritoneal dialysis. *Semin Dial* 1994;7:442–449.

145. Watkins S, et al. Impact of flush-before-fill methodology on peritonitis rates in patients receiving automated peritoneal dialysis. *J Am Soc Nephrol* 1998;9:716A.

146. Kingwatanakul P, et al. *Staphylococcus aureus* nasal carriage in children receiving long-term peritoneal dialysis. *Adv Perit Dial* 1997;13: 280–283.

147. Oh J, et al. Nasal carriage of *Staphylococcus aureus* in families of children on peritoneal dialysis. *Adv Perit Dial* 2000;16:324–327.

148. Warady BA, et al. Consensus guidelines for the treatment of peritonitis in pediatric patients receiving peritoneal dialysis. *Perit Dial Int* 2000;20:610–624.

149. Oh J, et al. Nasal mupirocin prophylaxis reduces the incidence of PD-related *S. aureus* infections in children: results of a double-blind, placebo-controlled multicenter trial. *Perit Dial Int* 2002;22[Suppl 1]:S74.

150. Holloway M, et al. Pediatric peritoneal dialysis training: characteristics and impact on peritonitis rates. *Perit Dial Int* 2001;21:401–404.

151. Troidle L, et al. Nine episodes of CPD-associated peritonitis with vancomycin-resistant enterococci. *Kidney Int* 1996;50:1368–1372.

152. Warady BA, et al. Aminoglycoside ototoxicity in pediatric patients receiving long-term peritoneal dialysis. *Pediatr Nephrol* 1993;7: 178–181.

153. Von Baum H, et al. Prevalence of Vancomycin-resistant enterococci among children with end-stage renal failure. *Clin Infec Dis* 1999; 29:912–916.

154. Warady BA. Sclerosing encapsulating peritonitis: what approach should be taken with children? *Perit Dial Int* 2000;20:390–391.

155. Araki Y, et al. Long-term peritoneal dialysis is a risk factor of sclerosing encapsulating peritonitis for children. *Perit Dial Int* 2000;20: 445–451.

156. Hoshii S, et al. Sclerosing encapsulating peritonitis in pediatric dialysis patients. *Pediatr Nephrol* 2000;14:275–279.

157. Alexander SR. Pediatric uses of recombinant human erythropoietin: the outlook in 1991. *Am J Kidney Dis* 1991;18[Suppl 1]:42–53.

158. Scigalla P. Effect of recombinant human erythropoietin treatment on renal anemia and body growth of children with end-stage renal disease. In: Gurland HJ, et al., eds. *Erythropoietin in renal and non-renal anemias.* Basel: Karger, 1991:201–211.

159. Nissenson AR, et al. Randomized, controlled trial of darepoetin alfa for the treatment of anemia in hemodialysis patients. *Kidney Dis* 2002;40:110–118.

160. Kausz AT, et al. Intraperitoneal erythropoietin in children on peritoneal dialysis. *Am J Kidney Dis* 1999;34:651–656.

161. Reddingius RE, et al. Intraperitoneal administration of recombinant human erythropoietin in children on continuous peritoneal dialysis. *Eur J Pediatr* 1992;151:540–542.

162. Huang TP, et al. Intraperitoneal recombinant human erythropoietin therapy: Influence of the duration of continuous ambulatory dialysis treatment and peritonitis. *Am J Nephrol* 1995;15:312–317.

163. Hymes LC, et al. Impaired response to recombinant human erythropoietin therapy in children with peritonitis. *Dial Transplant* 1994;23: 462–463.

164. Bargman JM, et al. The effect of in vivo erythropoietin on cytokine mRNA in CAPD patients. *Adv Perit Dial* 1994;10:129–134.

165. Stevens JM, et al. Serum from continuous ambulatory peritoneal dialysis patients with acute bacterial peritonitis inhibits in vitro erythroid colony formation. *Am J Kidney Dis* 1994;24:569–574.

166. Warady BA, et al. New hormones in the therapeutic arsenal of chronic renal failure: growth hormone and erythropoietin. *Pediatr Clin North Am* 1995;42:1551–1577.

167. Warady BA. Growth retardation in children with chronic renal insufficiency. *J Am Soc Nephrol* 1998;9[Suppl 12]:S85–S89.

168. Fine RN. Growth hormone treatment of children with chronic renal insufficiency, end-stage renal disease and following renal transplantation—update 1997. *Pediatr Endocrinol* 1997;10:361–370.

169. Tonshoff B, et al. Growth-stimulating effects of recombinant human growth hormone in children with end-stage renal disease. *J Pediatr* 1990;116:561–566.

170. Schaefer F, et al. Stimulation of growth by recombinant human growth hormone in children undergoing peritoneal or hemodialysis treatment. German Study Group for Growth Hormone Treatment in Chronic Renal Failure. *Adv Perit Dial* 1994;10:321–326.

171. Haffner D, et al. Effect of growth hormone treatment on the adult height of children with chronic renal failure. German Study Group for Growth Hormone Treatment in Chronic Renal Failure. *N Engl J Med* 2000;343:923–930.

172. Salusky IB, et al. Bone disease in pediatric patients undergoing dialysis with CAPD or CCPD. *Kidney Int* 1988;33:975–982.

173. Osorio A, et al. Hypercalcemia and pancreatitis in a child with adynamic bone disease. *Pediatr Nephrol* 1997;11:223–225.

174. Salusky IB, et al. Coronary-artery calcification in young adults with end-stage renal disease who are undergoing dialysis. *N Engl J Med* 2000;342:1478–1483.

175. Parekh RS, et al. Cardiovascular mortality in children and young adults with end-stage kidney disease. *J Pediatr* 2002;141:191–197.

176. Chavers BM, et al. Cardiovascular disease in pediatric chronic dialysis patients. *Kidney Int* 2002;62:648–653.

177. Chertow GM, et al. Sevelamer attenuates the progression of coronary and aortic calcification in hemodialysis patients. *Kidney Int* 2002;62:245–252.

178. Honda M, et al. The Japanese national registry data on pediatric CAPD patients: a ten-year experience—a report of the study group of pediatric PD conference. *Perit Dial Int* 1996;16:269–275.

179. Verrina E, et al. Clinical experience in the treatment of infants with chronic peritoneal dialysis. *Adv Perit Dial* 1995;11:281–284.

180. Ellis EN, et al. Outcome of infants on chronic peritoneal dialysis. *Adv Perit Dial* 1995;11:266–269.

181. Wood EG, et al. Risk factors for mortality in infants and young children on dialysis: a report of the North American Pediatric Renal Transplant Cooperative Study (NAPRTCS). *Am J Kidney Dis* 2001;37:573–579.

182. Clinical practice guidelines for vascular access: update 2000. *Am J Kidney Dis* 2001;37[Suppl 1]:S137–S181.

183. Bourquelot P, et al. Microsurgical creation and follow-up of arteriovenous fistulae for chronic hemodialysis in children. *Pediatr Nephrol* 1990;4:156–159.

184. Goldstein SL, et al. Ultrasound dilution evaluation of pediatric hemodialysis vascular access. *Kidney Int* 2001;59:2357–2360.

185. Goldstein SL, et al. Ultrasound dilution monitoring of pediatric hemodialysis vascular access: effects of a proactive monitoring program on thrombosis rates. *Kidney Int* 2002;62:272–275.

186. Sheth RD, et al. Permanent hemodialysis vascular access survival in children and adolescents with ESRD. *Kidney Int* 2002;62:1864–1869.

187. Sheth RD, et al. Successful use of Tesio catheters in pediatric patients receiving chronic hemodialysis. *Am J Kidney Dis* 2001;38:553–559.

188. Sharma A, et al. Survival and complications of cuffed catheters in children on chronic hemodialysis. *Pediatr Nephrol* 1997;13:245–248.

189. Horl WH. Interleukins, biocompatibility, and middle molecules. *J Am Soc Nephrol* 2002;13[Suppl 1]:S62–S71.

190. Dinarello CA. Pro-inflammatory cytokines. *Chest* 2000;118:503–508.

191. Kim PK, et al. Inflammatory responses and mediators. *Surg Clin North Am* 2000;80:885–894.

192. Brivet FG, et al. Pro- and anti-inflammatory cytokines during acute severe pancreatitis: an early and sustained response, although unpredictable of death. *Crit Care Med* 1999;27:749–755.

193. Gloor B, et al. Hydrocortisone treatment of early SIRS in acute experimental pancreatitis. *Dig Dis Sci* 2001;456:2154–2161.

194. Herbelin A, et al. Influence of uremia and hemodialysis on circulating interleukin-1 and tumor necrosis factor alpha. *Kidney Int* 1990;37:116–125.

195. Herbelin A, et al. Elevated circulating levels of interleukin-6 in patients with chronic renal failure. *Kidney Int* 1991;39:954–960.

196. Zwolinska D, et al. Serum concentration of IL-2, IL-6, TNF-alpha and their soluble receptors in children on maintenance hemodialysis. *Nephron* 2000;86:441–446.

197. Memoli B, et al. Hemodialysis-related lymphomononuclear release of interleukin-12 in patients with end-stage renal disease. *J Am Soc Nephrol* 1999;10:2171–2176.

198. Memoli B, et al. Role of different dialysis membranes in the release of interleukin-6-soluble receptor in uremic patients. *Kidney Int* 2000;58:417–424.

199. Evans JHC, et al. Mathematical modeling of hemodialysis in children. *Pediatr Nephrol* 1992;6:349–353.

200. Gotch FA, et al. A mechanistic analysis of the National Cooperative Dialysis Study (NCDS). *Kidney Int* 1985;28:526–534.

201. Goldstein SL, et al. Natural logarithmic estimates of Kt/V in the pediatric hemodialysis population. *Am J Kidney Dis* 1999;37[Suppl 1]:S7–S64.

202. Goldstein SL, et al. Evaluation and prediction of urea rebound and equilibrated Kt/V in the pediatric hemodialysis population. *Am J Kidney Dis* 1999;34:49–54.

203. Goldstein SL, et al. Logarithmic extrapolation of a 15-minute postdialysis BUN to predict equilibrated BUN and calculate double-pool Kt/V in the pediatric hemodialysis population. *Am J Kidney Dis* 2000;36:98–104.

204. Marsenic OD, et al. Prediction of equilibrated urea in children on chronic hemodialysis. *ASAIO J* 2000;46:283–287.

205. Sharma A, et al. Multicompartment urea kinetics in well-dialyzed children. *Kidney Int* 2000;58:2138–2146.

206. Daugirdas JT. Second generation logarithmic estimates of single-pool variable volume Kt/V: an analysis of error. *J Am Soc Nephrol* 1993;4:1205–1213.

207. Goldstein SL. Pediatric hemodialysis—state-of-the-art. *Adv Ren Replace Ther* 2001;8:173–179.

208. Pedrini LA, et al. Causes, kinetics, and clinical implications of posthemodialysis urea rebound. *Kidney Int* 1998;34:817–824.

209. Daugirdas JT, et al. Overestimation of hemodialysis dose depends on dialysis efficiency by regional blood flow but not by conventional two pool urea kinetic analysis. *ASAIO J* 1995;41:M719–M724.

210. Daugirdas JT, et al. Comparison of methods to predict equilibrated Kt/V in the HEMO Pilot Study. *Kidney Int* 1997;52:1395–1405.

211. Tattersall J, et al. The post-hemodialysis rebound: predicting and quantifying its effect on Kt/V. *Kidney Int* 1996;50:2094–2102.

212. Maduell F, et al. Validation of different methods to calculate Kt/V considering postdialysis rebound. *Nephrol Dial Transplant* 1997;12:1928–1933.

213. NKF-K/DOQI Clinical Practice Guidelines for Hemodialysis Adequacy: update 2000. *Am J Kidney Dis* 2001;37[Suppl 1]:S7–S64.

214. Borah MF, et al. Nitrogen balance during intermittent dialysis therapy of uremia. *Kidney Int* 1978;12:1928–1933.

215. Grupe WE, et al. Protein and energy requirements in children receiving chronic hemodialysis. *Kidney Int* 1983;24:S6–S10.

216. Sobh MA, et al. Study of effect of optimization of dialysis and protein intake on neuromuscular function in patients under maintenance hemodialysis treatment. *Am J Nephrol* 1998;18:399–403.

217. Maggiore Q, et al. Nutritional and prognostic correlates of bioimpedance indexes in hemodialysis patients. *Kidney Int* 1996;50:2103–2108.

218. Harmon WE, et al. Determination of protein catabolic rate (PCR) in children on hemodialysis by urea kinetic modeling. *Pediatr Res* 1979;13:513.

219. Goldstein SL, et al. nPCR assessment and IDPN treatment of malnutrition in pediatric hemodialysis patients. *Pediatr Nephrol* 2002;17:531–534.

220. Tom A, et al. Growth during maintenance hemodialysis: Impact of enhanced nutrition and clearance. *J Pediatr* 1999;134:464–471.

221. Brem AS, et al. Outcome data on pediatric dialysis patients from the end-stage renal disease clinical indicators project. *Am J Kidney Dis* 2000;36:310–317.

222. Sadowski RH, et al. Sodium modeling ameliorates intradialytic and interdialytic symptoms in young hemodialysis patients. *J Am Soc Nephrol* 1993;4:1192–1198.

223. Sang GL, et al. Sodium ramping in hemodialysis: a study of beneficial and adverse effects. *Am J Kidney Dis* 1997;29:669–677.

224. Steuer RR, et al. Hematocrit is an indicator of blood volume and a predictor of intradialytic morbid events. *ASAIO J* 1994;40:M691–M696.

225. Swartz RD, et al. Preservation of plasma volume during hemodialysis depends on the dialysate osmolality. *Am J Nephrol* 1982;2:189–194.

226. Steuer RR, et al. Reducing symptoms during hemodialysis by continuously monitoring the hematocrit. *Am J Kidney Dis* 1996;27:525–532.

227. Jain SR, et al. Non-invasive intravascular monitoring in the pediatric hemodialysis population. *Pediatr Nephrol* 2001;16:15–18.

228. Michael M, et al. Non-invasive monitoring of hematocrit (NIVM) optimizes achievement of target weight (wt) without increasing intra- or interdialytic symptoms (sx) in children and adolescents receiving hemodialysis (HD). *J Am Soc Nephrol* 2001;12:398(abst).

229. Simmons JM, et al. Relation of calorie deficiency to growth failure in children on hemodialysis and the growth response to calorie supplementation. *N Engl J Med* 1991;285:653.

230. Spinozzi NS, et al. Altered taste acuity in children with end-stage renal disease (ESRD). *Pediatr Res* 1971;12:442(abst).

231. Conley SB, et al. Effect of dietary intake and hemodialysis on protein turnover in uremic children. *Kidney Int* 1980;17:837–846.

232. Wassner SJ. The role of nutrition in the care of children with renal insufficiency. *Pediatr Clin North Am* 1982;29:973.

233. Harmon WE, et al. Use of protein catabolic rate to monitor pediatric hemodialysis. *Dial Transplant* 1981;10:324–330.

234. Asayama J, et al. Lipid profiles and lipase activities in children and adolescents with chronic renal failure treated conservatively or with hemodialysis or transplantation. *Pediatr Res* 1984;18:783–788.

235. Van Gool S, et al. Lipid and lipoprotein abnormalities in children on hemodialysis and after renal transplantation. *Transplant Proc* 1991;23:1375–1377.

236. Pennisi AJ, et al. Hyperlipidemia in pediatric hemodialysis and renal transplant patients associated with coronary artery disease. *Am J Dis Child* 1976;130:957–961.

237. Goggler A, et al. Effect of low dose supplementation of -carnitine on lipid metabolism in hemodialyzed children. *Kidney Int* 1989;27[Suppl]:S256–S258.

238. Gusmano R, et al. Plasma carnitine concentrations and dyslipidemia in children on maintenance hemodialysis. *Pediatrics* 1981;99:429–432.

239. Zachwieja J, et al. Amino acid and carnitine supplementation in haemodialysed children. *Pediatr Nephrol* 1994;8:739–743.

240. Krause I, et al. Intradialytic parenteral nutrition in malnourished children treated with hemodialysis. *J Ren Nutr* 2002;12:55–59.

241. National Kidney Foundation. Council of Renal Nutrition of New England. *Renal nutrition handbook for renal dietitians*. Dedham: Massachusetts-NKF, 1993.

242. Slatopolsky E, et al. Calcium carbonate as a phosphate binder in patients with chronic renal failure undergoing dialysis. *N Engl J Med* 1986;315:157–161.

243. Andreoli SP. Calcium carbonate is an effective phosphorus binder in children with chronic renal failure. *Am J Kidney Dis* 1987;9:206–210.

244. Salusky IB, et al. Effects of oral calcium carbonate on control of serum phosphorus and changes in plasma aluminum levels after discontinuation of aluminum containing gels in children receiving dialysis. *J Pediatr* 1986;108:767–770.

245. Mactier RA, et al. Calcium carbonate is an effective phosphate binder when dialysate calcium concentration is adjusted to control hypercalcemia. *Clin Nephrol* 1987;28:222–226.

246. Mai ML, et al. Calcium acetate, an effective phosphorus binder in patients with renal failure. *Kidney Int* 1989;36:690–695.

247. Amin N. The impact of improved phosphorus control: use of sevelamer hydrochloride in patients with chronic renal failure. *Nephrol Dial Transplant* 2002;17:340–345.

248. Malluche HH, et al. Management of hyperphosphataemia of chronic kidney disease: lessons from the past and future directions. *Nephrol Dial Transplant* 2002;17:1170–1175.

249. McIntyre CW, et al. A prospective study of combination therapy for hyperphosphataemia with calcium-containing phosphate binders and sevelamer in hypercalcaemic haemodialysis patients. *Nephrol Dial Transplant* 2002;17:1643–1648.

250. Delmez JA, et al. Parathyroid hormone suppression by intravenous 1-25-dihydroxyvitamin D: a role for increased sensitivity to calcium. *J Clin Invest* 1989;83:1349–1355.

251. Szabo A, et al. 1,25 (OH)2 vitamin D3 inhibits parathyroid cell proliferation in experimental uremia. *Kidney Int* 1998;35:1049–1056.

252. Sprague SM, et al. Suppression of parathyroid hormone secretion in hemodialysis patients: comparison of paricalcitol with calcitriol. *Am J Kidney Dis* 2001;38[Suppl 1]:S51–S56.

253. Andress DL. Intravenous versus oral vitamin D therapy in dialysis patients: what is the question? *Am J Kidney Dis* 2001;38[Suppl 5]:S41–S44.

254. Eschbach JW. The anemia chronic renal failure: pathophysiology and the effects of recombinant erythropoietin. *Kidney Int* 1989;35:134–148.

255. McGonigle RJS, et al. Erythropoietin and inhibitors of in vitro erythropoiesis in the development of anemia in children with renal disease. *J Lab Clin Med* 1985;105:449–458.

256. Meytes D, et al. Effects of parathyroid hormone on erythropoiesis. *J Clin Invest* 1981;67:1263–1269.

257. Eschbach JW, et al. 14C cyanate as a tag for red cell survival in normal and uremic man. *J Lab Clin Med* 1977;89:823–828.

258. Muller-Wiefel DE, et al. Hemolysis and blood loss in children with chronic renal failure. *Clin Nephrol* 1977;8:841–846.

259. National Kidney Foundation Dialysis Outcomes Quality Initiative. NKF-DOQI clinical practice guidelines for the treatment of anemia of chronic renal failure. *Am J Kidney Dis* 1997;30[Suppl 3]S192–S240.

260. Frankenfield DL, et al. Adolescent hemodialysis: results of the 2000 ESRD Clinical Performance Measures Project. *Pediatr Nephrol* 2002;17:10–15.

261. Rao DS, et al. Effect of serum parathyroid hormone and bone marrow fibrosis on the response to erythropoietin in uremia. *N Engl J Med* 1993;328:171–175.

262. Besarab A, et al. Meta-analysis of subcutaneous versus intravenous epoetin in maintenance treatment of anemia in hemodialysis patients. *Am J Kidney Dis* 2002;40:439–446.

263. Granolleras C, et al. Experience with daily self-administered subcutaneous erythropoietin. *Contrib Nephrol* 1989;76:143–148.

264. Lerner GR, et al. The pharmacokinetics of novel erythropoiesis stimulating protein (NESP) in pediatric patients with chronic renal failure (CRF) or end-stage renal disease. *J Am Soc Nephrol* 2000;11:282A.

265. Grimm PC, et al. Effects of recombinant human erythropoietin on HLA sensitization and cell mediated immunity. *Kidney Int* 1990;38:12–18.

266. Montini G, et al. Benefits and risks of anemia correction with recombinant human erythropoietin in children maintained by hemodialysis. *J Pediatr* 1990;117:556–560.

267. Rigden SP, et al. Recombinant human erythropoietin therapy in children maintained by haemodialysis. *Pediatr Nephrol* 1990;4:618–622.

268. Campos A, et al. Therapy of renal anemia in children and adolescents with recombinant human erythropoietin (rHuEPO). *Clin Pediatr (Phila)* 1992;31(2):94–99.

269. Baraldi E, et al. Exercise to tolerance after anemia correction with recombinant human erythropoietin in end-stage renal disease. *Pediatr Nephrol* 1990;4:623–626.

270. Warady BA, et al. Recombinant human erythropoietin therapy in pediatric patients receiving long-term peritoneal dialysis. *Pediatr Nephrol* 1991;5:718–723.

271. Eschbach JW, et al. Recombinant human erythropoietin in anemic patients with end-stage renal disease: results of a phase III multicenter clinical trial. *Nephrol Dial Transplant* 1989;111:992–1000.

272. Sinai-Trieman L, et al. Use of subcutaneous recombinant human erythropoietin in children undergoing continuous cycling peritoneal dialysis. *J Pediatr* 1989;114:550–554.

273. Morris KP, et al. Non-cardiac benefits of human recombinant erythropoietin in end-stage renal failure and anaemia. *Arch Dis Child* 1993;69:580–586.

274. Stefanidis CJ, et al. Effect of the correction of anemia with recombinant human erythropoietin on growth of children treated with CAPD. *Adv Perit Dial* 1992;8:460–463.

275. Edmunds ME, et al. Seizures in haemodialysis patients treated with recombinant human erythropoietin. *Nephrol Dial Transplant* 1989;4:1065–1069.

276. Tang IY, et al. Vascular access thrombosis during recombinant human erythropoietin therapy. *ASAIO J* 1992;38:M528–M531.

277. Besarb A, et al. Recombinant human erythropoietin does not increase clotting in vascular access. *ASAIO Trans* 1990;36:M749–M753.

278. Fishbane S, et al. Reticulocyte hemoglobin content in the evaluation of iron status of hemodialysis patients. *Kidney Int* 1997;52:217–222.

279. Milman N. Iron absorption measured by whole body counting and the relation to marrow iron stores in chronic uremia. *Clin Nephrol* 1982;17:77–81.

280. Van Wyck DB. Iron management during recombinant human erythropoietin therapy. *Am J Kidney Dis* 1989;14[Suppl]:9–13.

281. Greenbaum LA, et al. Intravenous iron dextran and erythropoietin use in pediatric hemodialysis patients. *Pediatr Nephrol* 2000;14:908–911.

282. Hamstra RD, et al. Intravenous iron dextran in clinical medicine. *JAMA* 1980;243:1726–1731.

283. Warady BA, et al. A comparison of intravenous and oral iron therapy in children receiving hemodialysis. *J Am Soc Nephrol* 2002;13:221A.

284. Fishbane S, et al. The safety of intravenous iron dextran in hemodialysis patients. *Am J Kidney Dis* 1996;28:529–534.

285. Charytan C, et al. Efficacy and safety of iron sucrose for iron deficiency in patients with dialysis-associated anemia: North American clinical trial. *Am J Kidney Dis* 2001;37:300–307.

286. Fudin R, et al. Correction of uremic iron deficiency anemia in hemodialyzed patients: a prospective study. *Nephron* 1998;79:299–305.

287. Tenbrock K, et al. Intravenous iron treatment of renal anemia in children on hemodialysis. *Pediatr Nephrol* 1999;13:580–582.

288. Yorgin PD, et al. Sodium ferric gluconate therapy in renal transplant and renal failure patients. *Pediatr Nephrol* 2000;15:171–175.

289. Nissenson AR, et al. Sodium ferric gluconate complex in sucrose is safe and effective in hemodialysis patients: North American clinical trial. *Am J Kidney Dis* 1999;33:471–482.

290. Pollak A, et al. Effect of intravenous iron supplementation on erythropoiesis in erythropoietin-treated premature infants. *Pediatrics* 2001;107:78–85.

291. Morgan HE, et al. Maintenance intravenous iron therapy in pediatric hemodialysis patients. *Pediatr Nephrol* 2001;16:779–783.

292. Zucchelli P, et al. Control of blood pressure in patients on haemodialysis. In: Cameron S, et al., eds. *Oxford textbook of clinical nephrology.* Oxford: Oxford University Press, 1992:1458–1467.

293. Zucchelli P, et al. Genesis and control of hypertension in hemodialysis patients. *Semin Nephrol* 1988;8:163–168.

294. Converse RL, et al. Sympathetic overactivity in patients with chronic renal failure. *N Engl J Med* 1992;327:1912–1918.

295. Sorof JM, et al. Ambulatory blood pressure monitoring and interdialytic weight gain in children receiving chronic hemodialysis. *Am J Kidney Dis* 1999;33:667–674.

296. Trachtman H, et al. Pediatric hemodialysis: a decade's (1974–1984) perspective. *Kidney Int* 1986;19[Suppl]:S15–S22.

297. Glenn CM, et al. Dialysis-associated seizures in children and adolescents. *Pediatr Nephrol* 1992;6:182–186.

298. Chan JC. Late complications of long-term hemodialysis in children: clinical aspects and some measurable variables concerning parathyroid hormone, divalent ions, acid-base metabolism, anemia, nutrition, growth and survival data. *J Urol* 1978;120:578–585.

299. Ford DM, et al. Unexpected seizures during hemodialysis: effect of dialysate prescription. *Pediatr Nephrol* 1987;1:597–601.

300. Arieff AI, et al. Brain water and electrolyte metabolism in uremia: effects of slow and rapid hemodialysis. *Kidney Int* 1973;4:177–187.

301. Kimelberg HK, et al. Swelling-induced release of glutamate, aspartate and taurine from astrocyte cultures. *J Neurosci* 1990;10:1583–1591.

302. Fraser CL. Nervous system complications in uremia. *Ann Intern Med* 1988;109:143–153.

303. Pollock AS, et al. Abnormalities of cell volume regulation and their functional consequences. *Am J Physiol* 1980;239:F195–F205.

304. Knight F, et al. Hemodialysis of the infant or small child with chronic renal failure. *ANNA J* 1993;20:315–323.

305. Sadowski RH, et al. Acute hemodialysis of infants weighing less than five kilograms. *Kidney Int* 1994;45:903–906.

306. Matthews DE, et al. Peritoneal dialysis in the first 60 days of life. *J Pediatr Surg* 1990;25:110–116.

ACUTE DIALYSIS IN CHILDREN

AYESA N. MIAN AND SUSAN R. MENDLEY

Renal replacement therapy options for the pediatric patient include the full spectrum of modalities available for adults—peritoneal dialysis (PD), intermittent hemodialysis, and continuous forms of renal replacement therapy [continuous renal replacement therapy (CRRT)] (1,2). Historically, PD has been preferred because peritoneal access is easier to achieve than vascular access and the technique is simpler to perform, not requiring specialized equipment or a need for highly trained personnel. In recent years, however, there have been several advances in vascular access placement techniques, availability of pediatric-sized catheters, and improvements in manufactured hemodialysis and CRRT machines and associated equipment (dialyzers and blood lines) such that the use of CRRT for management of pediatric acute renal failure is increasing in frequency (3,4). However, PD remains the most commonly used modality in pediatric acute renal failure. In addition, because outcome studies comparing the use of each of the three treatment modalities for management of pediatric acute renal failure are lacking, the choice of renal replacement therapy continues to be strongly influenced by the physician's experience and the technical expertise available at each hospital.

ACUTE RENAL FAILURE IN CHILDREN

It is important to recognize that the causes of acute renal failure in children differ from those in adults. Several comprehensive reviews on pediatric acute renal failure are available (5–8). Primary renal disease and genitourinary tract anomalies account for the most common causes of childhood acute renal failure. Table 40.1 summarizes and compares the causes of pediatric acute renal failure in industrialized and nonindustrialized countries. Secondary causes of acute renal failure such as sepsis or multiorgan system failure are more commonly seen in tertiary care centers. Finally, when evaluating the child with acute renal failure, one must also consider an acute presentation of previously unrecognized end-stage renal disease (ESRD).

Conservative management of the child with acute renal failure includes careful fluid resuscitation, if intravascular volume depletion is present. Once euvolemia has been restored, if oligoanuria is present, maintenance of fluid balance is attempted through use of diuretics and fluid restriction. Additional measures include diet modification (restriction of protein, potassium, and phosphorus) to minimize development of metabolic disturbances and the use of medications (sodium polystyrene, sodium bicarbonate, and phosphate binders) to correct electrolyte disturbances that may also be present. Conservative measures, however, are not always sufficient to allow optimal management particularly with prolonged and severe acute renal failure when fluid restriction often compromises the ability to provide appropriate nutrition, which is essential for recovery. In such cases, some form of renal replacement therapy is warranted.

INDICATIONS FOR RENAL REPLACEMENT THERAPY

The indications for initiation of renal replacement therapy in pediatric acute renal failure are well established and similar to those in adults. The indications include (a) oligoanuria requiring fluid and/or electrolyte removal to optimize nutritional and medical support; (b) hypervolemia complicated by congestive heart failure, pulmonary edema, or severe hypertension despite diuretic therapy and fluid restriction; (c) hyperkalemia refractory to medical management or associated with cardiac involvement as evidenced by electrocardiogram changes; (d) metabolic acidosis refractory to medical management with sodium bicarbonate or limited by sodium overload; (e) symptomatic uremia with pericarditis, neuropathy, or encephalopathy; and (f) tumor lysis syndrome or severe hyperuricemia. In pediatrics, there is also a role for renal replacement therapy in certain nonrenal failure settings such as toxic ingestions, hyperammonemia, and other inborn errors of metabolism.

PERITONEAL DIALYSIS

PD offers several advantages for the care of the pediatric patient with acute renal failure. Technically, it is a simple procedure that does not require specialized personnel. Nurses in pediatric intensive care units can be trained to perform the procedure with an acceptably low infection rate. Currently available automated cycler devices permit frequent dialysis exchanges without repeatedly opening the circuit, further lowering the infection

TABLE 40.1. CAUSES OF ACUTE RENAL FAILURE IN CHILDREN

Etiologies of Acute Renal Failure	Referral Center in Developing Country N (%)	Tertiary Center in Industrialized Country N (%)
Hemolytic uremic syndrome	25 (31)	5 (3)
Glomerulonephritis	18 (23)	—
Intrinsic renal disease	—	64 (44)
Urinary obstruction	7 (9)	—
Postoperative sepsis	14 (18)	49 (34)
Ischemic and prerenal	14 (18)	—
Organ and bone marrow transplant	—	19 (13)
Miscellaneous	2 (3)	9 (6)
Total	80	146

Adapted from Flynn JT. Causes, management approaches, and outcome of acute renal failure in children. *Curr Opin Pediatr* 1998;10:184–189, with permission.

risk. Fluid and solute removal occur gradually making the procedure well tolerated in the hemodynamically compromised child and eliminating the risk of hypotension or dialysis disequilibrium (9,10). From a practical standpoint, placement of a PD catheter is technically easier than placement of vascular access, which can be particularly challenging in the small infant (11,12).

PD provides particularly efficient solute and fluid removal in the youngest patients. Peritoneal membrane surface area correlates with body surface area rather than with body mass; this ratio is most favorable in infants and young children who can thus achieve large peritoneal clearance (13,14). Use of PD also avoids the need for anticoagulation and for blood exposure through priming of a blood circuit. Because PD is the preferred mode of dialysis for children with chronic renal failure, initiating the therapy in the acute setting can facilitate the transition to chronic dialysis. Finally, this form of dialysis is less expensive to perform and requires a smaller initial capital investment than other CRRTs (see later) (15).

PD, however, is not appropriate for all patients. It is contraindicated in those with abdominal wall defects (e.g., bladder extrophy, omphalocele, and gastroschisis) and diaphragmatic lesions (e.g., diaphragmatic hernia and surgical defects). It cannot be used immediately after abdominal surgery. The presence of a ventriculoperitoneal shunt is a relative contraindication because of the risk of ascending infection should peritonitis develop; most pediatric nephrologists choose another modality in that setting. PD may not be successful after extensive abdominal surgery because adhesions can cause failure of dialysate drainage, which is manifested as slow outflow rates or poor ultrafiltration.

In clinical situations in which rapid removal of solute (e.g., hyperkalemia), toxin (ingestion), or metabolite (e.g., ammonia) is required, PD often does not provide an adequate response. The gradual nature of the treatment, which is advantageous in uremia, will limit the rapid response those emergencies require. Furthermore, in states of acute volume overload with pulmonary edema or congestive heart failure, the ultrafiltration provided by PD may not be rapid enough to prevent clinical deterioration or the need for intubation.

Peritoneal Dialysis Catheters

Neonatal and pediatric sizes of most adult catheter configurations are available. These include acute "temporary" catheters such as the Trocath (McGaw, Irvine, California; stylet type catheter) and Cook catheter (Cook Critical Care, Bloomington, Indiana; over-the-wire type catheter) and chronic catheters appropriate for operative placement. Acute catheters can be placed percutaneously at the bedside after filling the abdomen with dialysate, as is done in adults (12). This permits dialysis therapy to be initiated quickly even in patients too unstable for surgery. Before placement of the dialysis catheter, a Foley catheter should be inserted to empty the bladder and decrease the risk of bladder perforation.

However, temporary catheters have several disadvantages. Percutaneous placement can result in injury to an abdominal viscus; bowel and bladder perforation are recognized complications (16). The catheters are stiff and even after successful placement they can cause bowel injury; this often necessitates immobilizing the child while the catheter is in place. In addition, they are uncuffed catheters and, therefore, carry a much greater risk of dialysate leakage at the exit site and subsequent infection. The risk of peritonitis increases significantly after 3 days of use, and it is usually impossible to predict renal recovery at the initiation of PD (17). Therefore, many nephrologists prefer an operatively placed catheter that is used immediately.

The Tenckhoff catheter, although designed as a chronic catheter, is often used in the acute setting (18). If the patient is stable and time permits, surgical placement under direct visualization is preferred. However, the catheter can be placed in the intensive care unit. This catheter is made of soft silicone rubber; therefore, the risk of bowel injury is decreased and the patient need not be immobilized. There is an increased risk of leakage at the exit site when the catheter is used immediately after placement and strategies to limit that complication are described later. Other chronic catheters can also be placed surgically and used acutely. The Toronto Western Hospital catheter (column disk catheter) has been used successfully in chronic pediatric dialysis (19). Although fewer problems with catheter obstruction have been noted with the Toronto Western Hospital catheter, bowel entrapment/adhesion to the catheter is a potential complication (20).

Data from the North American Pediatric Renal Transplant Cooperative Study (NAPRTCS) do not suggest that one type of chronic catheter design is superior to the others. However, data do suggest a downward (caudally) oriented exit site is preferable because this has been associated with a reduced risk of peritonitis in chronic dialysis (21,22). In infants, it is preferable to position the exit site above the diaper area to reduce the risk of fecal contamination. Similarly, in children with ostomies, it is preferred that the dialysis catheter be positioned on the contralateral side to maximize the distance between the ostomy and the catheter exit site, thereby minimizing the risk of exit-site contamination and infection. Omental obstruction resulting in poor outflow is common especially in small children; therefore, many advocate performing an omentectomy at the time of the original surgery to avoid outflow obstruction (23–25). This issue, however, remains controversial because other authors do not believe that it is necessary (11,26). Intraoperatively, should any hernial defects be noted, they should be repaired to minimize this potential complication of PD.

Peritoneal Dialysis Solutions

Acute pediatric PD is performed using the commercially available lactate-based dialysis solution, which is available in three dextrose concentrations (1.5%, 2.5%, and 4.25%) depending on ultrafiltration needs, and two calcium concentrations (1.25 and 1.75 mM) depending on the need for calcium-based phosphorus binders and vitamin D supplements. Lactate-based dextrose solutions have the disadvantages of low pH and glucose absorption with prolonged dwells. Low pH can contribute to pain on inflow and impaired phagocytic activity resulting in increased risk for infection (27). In recent years, there has been emphasis on developing more biocompatible PD solutions. "Custom-made" bicarbonate-based dialysis solution prepared in the hospital pharmacy has been used in acute dialysis, but it is labor-intensive to produce and carries the very real risk of formulation error.

Because peritoneal surface area in children is large relative to body surface area, glucose absorption during PD can, unfortunately, prove to be too efficient (28). Such glucose absorption during prolonged dwells dissipates the osmotic gradient between plasma water and dialysate leading to suboptimal ultrafiltration, hyperglycemia, hyperinsulinemia, and hyperlipidemia (29,30). Short dwells are used to limit glucose absorption. Alternative osmotic agents such as amino acids (Nutrineal, Baxter Healthcare, Deerfield, Illinois) may prove useful, at least permitting nutritional benefit from the enhanced absorption. There are reports of amino-acid-based dialysate used in children receiving chronic PD, but no role for this has yet been defined in acute PD (31,32). Icodextrin (Extraneal, Baxter Healthcare, Deerfield, Illinois) has been available in Europe for several years and has recently received Food and Drug Administration (FDA) approval. Only limited data on its use in pediatrics have been published (33). There are no data on icodextrin in acute therapy in children.

Dialysis Prescription Considerations

Acute PD is usually initiated with small volumes to limit leakage around a new catheter. Small fill volumes of approximately 15 to 30 mL/kg are often the starting range, although poor drainage, slow clearance, and inadequate ultrafiltration may limit the effectiveness of low-volume therapy. Fill volumes are gradually increased over several days to a goal of 40 to 50 mL/kg, as tolerated. Short exchange times (60 to 90 minutes) may be used to overcome the limitations of low fill volume and to facilitate ultrafiltration by limiting glucose absorption (34). Even shorter dwell times are possible; however, they are less efficient because a larger proportion of time is spent filling and draining leaving less time for actual dialysis (35).

Although efficient peritoneal glucose absorption may necessitate high dextrose concentrations for infants and small children to achieve ultrafiltration with long dwell times, short exchanges usually provide acceptable or even excessive ultrafiltration using 1.5% dextrose. Thus, frequent dialysis exchanges for adequate clearance may result in unpredictable fluid removal in small children; careful reassessment of volume status and supplemental fluid, either enteral or parenteral, must be provided to prevent intravascular volume depletion that, in turn, may impair renal recovery.

PD can be performed manually or with an automated cycler. Manual PD exchanges use a Y-type connector, one limb of which is attached to the inflow line and dialysate bag and the other limb is attached to the drain line and bag. A continuous cycling machine can be programmed for short dwell treatments appropriate for acute PD; this method permits only opening the catheter circuit once a day, which decreases the risk of contamination. Currently available cyclers that permit very low volume exchanges (beginning at 60 mL) and low-volume tubing (to decrease the dead space or recirculation volume) facilitate therapy in infants and small children. When a low-volume cycler is not available for acute PD in an infant, a graduated measuring device can be inserted between the dialysate bag and inflow tubing to allow more precise measurement of fill volumes. A commercially available product (Gesco Dialy-Nate Set, Gesco, San Antonio, Texas) is available as a closed system. This also permits repeated dialysis exchanges with infrequent opening of the dialysis circuit to limit potential contamination.

Complications of Peritoneal Dialysis

The most common complications of acute PD are catheter malfunction and infection. Catheter malfunction includes dialysate leakage, inflow problems, and outflow problems. Leakage can be external, occurring around the exit site or the incision used to insert the catheter, or internal, resulting in a hernia. Risk factors for external leaks include use of a stiff temporary catheter, frequent catheter manipulation, malnourishment, and initiation of PD with large fill volumes immediately after catheter placement. Strategies to minimize the risk of leakage include use of small fill volumes, minimal catheter manipulation, and two purse-string sutures to seal the peritoneum around the catheter and to seal the posterior rectus sheath opening (36). Temporary discontinuation of PD and use of smaller fill volumes is the initial approach to catheter leaks, but surgical repair is sometimes required. Three retrospective reviews of pediatric acute PD found an increased rate of complications with temporary catheters compared with Tenckhoff catheters (10,37,38).

Obstruction to dialysate flow or excessively slow flow are frequent catheter complications. Inflow obstruction is usually due to a mechanical blockage: a kink in the catheter, clamp on the catheter, or the presence of blood clot or fibrin. Addition of heparin to the dialysate at a concentration of 500 to 1,000 units/L may diminish fibrin and blood clots. Outflow obstruction is more common and is usually a greater impediment to successful therapy. Catheter entrapment or occlusion by omentum can limit flow and may require reoperation for omentectomy; many surgeons, therefore, perform this at the time of catheter placement. Intraabdominal adhesions may prevent free flow of dialysate throughout the abdomen and poor outflow will be noted. Catheter migration can occur and result in painful inflow of dialysate and poor outflow; this may be correctable using a stylet under fluoroscopy or it may require surgical repositioning. Constipation and intestinal distention often limit outflow and should be managed with stool softeners, enemas, or laxatives (avoiding magnesium and phosphorus) (39).

Infectious complications may involve the exit site, tunnel, and/or peritoneum. In the acute setting, an exit-site infection is essentially a surgical wound infection and should be managed as such with parenteral antibiotics. The risk for dialysate leakage and contamination of the peritoneal space is high. Peritonitis is a serious complication of acute PD. It presents a large inflammatory burden to already debilitated, catabolic patients. Resistant organisms and fungi are a greater risk in the intensive care setting where patients are often already receiving antibiotic therapy. Frequent surveillance cell counts and cultures are advisable in this setting because the typical features of fever, abdominal pain, and cloudy effluent may be difficult to discern. Empiric broad-spectrum antibiotic therapy is often required until culture results are available. Intravenous or intraperitoneal therapy are appropriate, depending on the severity of the infection; combined therapy has been used in debilitated patients. Risk factors for developing peritonitis include use of a temporary catheter for longer than 3 days, leakage around the exit site, age younger than 2 years, and poor dialysis technique (16,17).

Hernias are typically a complication of chronic PD, resulting from upright posture and increased intraabdominal pressure. However, a diaphragmatic defect (pleuroperitoneal fistula) can result in hydrothorax even at initiation of dialysis, compromising ventilation and preventing adequate dialysis drainage. A patent processus vaginalis can cause a hydrocele or genital edema. Although these hernias could be corrected surgically, in the acute setting one is more likely to turn to an alternate modality of dialysis.

Acute PD can cause metabolic complications, most often resulting from glucose absorption. Hyperglycemia may occur and require insulin therapy. Hypertriglyceridemia can result from glucose absorption and be difficult to distinguish from the effects of hyperalimentation. There is spontaneous loss of albumin into dialysate, which can cause hypoalbuminemia; this loss is dramatically increased if peritonitis complicates therapy (16). Lactic acidosis secondary to lactate absorption from the dialysate

is an uncommon problem; most patients see an improvement in acidosis with initiation of PD. Hyponatremia is common, particularly in very young patients. It is exacerbated by the administration of hypotonic fluids; hypernatremia can develop with excessive ultrafiltration and insufficient free water intake.

HEMODIALYSIS

Acute hemodialysis can be safely and effectively performed in infants and children of all sizes (40–42). It requires highly trained personnel, special equipment, and a well-functioning vascular access. Acute hemodialysis is often preferred in situations requiring rapid removal of fluid, solute, or toxins (e.g., hyperammonemic coma or other inborn errors of metabolism, ingestion, or hyperkalemia) (43–45). In fact, hemodialysis treatments in small children can be strikingly efficient because body water space (V) is small relative to the potential clearance that one can provide with standard or high-flux dialyzers and typical blood flows (Q_B) (46). Furthermore, clinical situations in which PD is mechanically problematic (e.g., abdominal wall defects, recent abdominal surgery, respiratory compromise) will mandate use of hemodialysis. Recent improvements in hemodialysis machinery and availability of size appropriate equipment (blood lines, dialyzers, and vascular access) have facilitated the use of hemodialysis in infants and small children. However, the ability to perform hemodialysis successfully is contingent on vascular access, which remains a continuing challenge in infants and small children.

Technical Considerations

Although the principles of hemodialysis are the same in children as in adults, there are several technical aspects unique to children.

Personnel

Skilled dialysis nurses, preferably with pediatric experience, are required for pediatric acute hemodialysis. A nurse-to-patient ratio of 1:1 is needed to provide focused continuous attention to small patients. Keen observation skills and an awareness of age-dependent norms for vital signs are necessary to assess pediatric hemodialysis patients and intervene appropriately. Ill children are often unable to communicate their distress verbally. Warning signs of decompensation such as agitation or poor perfusion must be recognized quickly; hypotension may develop precipitously without warning (47).

Hemodialysis Machines

Technologic improvements in the design of hemodialysis machines that have benefited children include the incorporation of volumetric ultrafiltration controllers and blood pumps capable of being calibrated for neonatal, infant, and pediatric blood lines. The blood pump must be able to accurately deliver blood-flow rates within the range 20 to 300 mL/min, appropriate for neonates through older adolescents. The presence of an accurate volumetric ultrafiltration controller is also essential because even small errors in ultrafiltration volume of a few hundred milliliters can result in symptomatic fluid overload or intravascular volume depletion and hypotension.

Extracorporeal Circuit—Blood Lines

In infants and small children, the extracorporeal circuit volume may represent a significant fraction of total blood volume and severe hypotension can occur at initiation of the treatment. The typical extracorporeal circuit for adult patients exceeds 150 mL, and neonatal, infant, and pediatric blood lines are available to limit the circuit volume. The blood pump must be calibrated for the chosen blood line for accurate blood flow. Neonatal lines may not be compatible with available volumetric dialysis machines. However, even using low-volume blood lines and dialyzers, the total circuit volume cannot always be reduced to less than 10% of the patient's blood volume, particularly in the case of newborns and small infants. When the circuit volume exceeds 10% of the patient's blood volume or when the patient is severely anemic, the circuit can be primed with blood to maintain hemodynamic stability (40). Packed red blood cells are generally diluted 1:1 with normal saline to decrease the hematocrit to approximately 40%, thereby decreasing the viscosity and risk for clotting. Blood priming carries its own particular risks. The greatest concern is that of potential antigen exposure, which will complicate future renal transplantation in patients who do not regain renal function. The risk of sensitization to antigens is multiplied by the number of hemodialysis treatments required, because each will require a separate blood prime. In addition, a blood prime is a potential infectious exposure, and young children may acquire cytomegalovirus infection as a result. Furthermore, even if the primed blood circuit is infused at a low blood-flow rate (20 to 50 mL/min), it represents a rather rapid rate of blood transfusion. This may result in a transfusion reaction or hypocalcemia from citrate infusion. Lastly, the potassium load associated with transfusion of packed red blood cells may produce sudden hyperkalemia with cardiac arrhythmias, which may not be corrected quickly enough by hemodialysis. This risk is diminished by washing packed red blood cells before the procedure. At the end of the hemodialysis treatment that began with a blood prime, the blood circuit is generally not returned to the patient unless it was intended for the patient to receive a blood transfusion.

Dialyzers

A wide variety of dialyzers have been used in children; no pediatric data suggest an advantage with one type of membrane, although studies in adults suggest a benefit of biocompatible membranes on survival and recovery of acute renal failure (48–50). Choices in dialyzers with surface area less than 0.4 m^2 are limited, and availability changes often. Small priming volume is an advantage when dialyzing infants because it may allow one to avoid priming the circuit with blood. Dialyzers with relatively large surface area may be advantageous when rapid clearance is needed. In most cases, clearance will be determined by the blood flow that one can achieve throughout the treatment, rather than the surface area or KoA of the dialyzer. In practice, all standard and high-flux dialyzers have a higher ultrafiltration coefficient (Kuf) than is needed for adequate ultrafiltration. Previously, this was a great concern because small errors in setting the dialysis machine transmembrane pressure (TMP) could result in large ultrafiltration errors and hypotension. In addition, because pediatric vascular access is generally of small caliber one finds high venous pressures that, in turn, result in greater TMP. This concern has been alleviated by the widespread use of machines with volumetric ultrafiltration controllers. However, during isovolemic hemodialysis (or even during modest ultrafiltration) with a high-flux dialyzer, backfiltration of dialysate is to be anticipated; this can be avoided by increasing the ultrafiltration rate sufficient to reverse negative TMP and infusing saline through the treatment.

Vascular Access

Obtaining a well-functioning vascular access remains a challenge in small patients. Vascular access for acute hemodialysis is usually established by percutaneous placement of a double-lumen catheter. Whether a temporary or permanent (tunneled) dialysis catheter is chosen depends on one's estimate of the duration of dialysis therapy needed. This is often merely an approximation; patients typically begin urgent dialysis therapy with a temporary catheter, and a tunneled catheter is placed electively. Catheters are available in sizes from 7 Fr to 12 Fr and come in various lengths; manufacturers and availability of the smallest catheters change frequently. Table 40.2 provides guidelines for catheter

TABLE 40.2. VASCULAR ACCESS RECOMMENDATIONS FOR THE PEDIATRIC PATIENT

Patient Size	Catheter Size	Access Site
Neonate	Umbilical artery catheter 3.5–5.0 Fr or	Umbilical vessels
	Umbilical vein catheter 5.0–8.5 Fr or	
	5.0 Fr single lumen or	Femoral vein
	7.0 Fr dual lumen	
5–15 kg	7.0 Fr dual lumen	Femoral/subclavian/internal jugular vein
16–30 kg	9.0 Fr dual lumen	Internal jugular/femoral/subclavian vein
>30 kg	11.0 Fr dual lumen	Internal jugular/femoral/subclavian vein

Adapted from Bunchman TE, et al. Continuous arterial-venous diahemofiltration and continuous veno-venous diahemofiltration in infants and children. *Pediatr Nephrol* 1994;8:96–102, with permission.

selection based on patient size. Ideally, the catheter should offer low resistance to blood flow and, therefore, should be a stiff catheter with a short length but large internal diameter (51). Broviac catheters, often already placed in oncology patients, are inappropriate because of their flexibility, length, and small lumen size. Acute dialysis catheters can be placed in the femoral vein, subclavian vein, or internal jugular vein; the choice depends on the size of the patient and the availability of central venous sites. Femoral catheters are technically easier to insert and are not associated with the risks of pneumothorax and pneumomediastinum or hemothorax and hemomediastinum. However, there is an increased risk of infection when left in place for more than a few days and patients are confined to bed. Catheters placed in the subclavian vein or internal jugular vein should have their tips positioned at the junction of the superior vena cava and right atrium to allow adequate blood flow and minimize recirculation. They may be left in place for several weeks, although a tunneled catheter would be a better choice for such a duration of dialysis.

In an infant, vessel size may make placement of even a small-caliber double-lumen catheter impossible, and one may be obliged to place single-lumen catheters in two sites. Single-needle, single-pathway dialysis is rarely possible because most machines are not capable of performing this treatment and practical experience has waned. In the newborn, hemodialysis can be performed through small-caliber single-lumen catheters placed in the umbilical artery and vein.

Dialysis Prescription

There are no prospective trials to assist clinicians in determining the adequacy of acute hemodialysis therapy in children with acute renal failure. Because the spectrum of diseases causing acute renal failure is different from that in adults, extrapolation from that literature may be difficult. Thus, the duration, frequency, and efficiency of the hemodialysis treatments are a matter of judgment, aided by an understanding of kinetic modeling and of the modifiable variables (blood flow, dialysate flow). Often a single metabolic derangement (e.g., intoxication, hyperammonemia) defines the length and efficiency of the treatment. Nonetheless, when children are dialyzed for advanced uremia with standard dialyzers, the urea clearances that are achieved may be sufficient to cause true disequilibrium or seizures (which are considered a more common complication in children than in adults) (52,53). Blood-flow rate for the first few treatments may be decreased to target urea clearance of 2 to 3 mL/kg/min, and treatment length will usually be shortened to $1\frac{1}{2}$ to 2 hours to avoid precipitous falls in blood urea nitrogen (BUN) (2,52). Single-pool Kt/V for a first treatment in a uremic child should probably not exceed 0.6. Short daily treatments are often the most appropriate way to initiate hemodialysis therapy without patient discomfort or instability. Subsequent treatments are lengthened to 3 to 4 hours or longer if needed, and higher urea clearance rates can be targeted (blood-flow rates of 4 to 5 mL/kg/min). Smaller blood vessels and catheters cause higher venous resistance than in adults and this will eventually limit blood flow, perhaps as low as 25 to 100 mL/min.

Acute hemodialysis treatments in children should only be performed with bicarbonate-based dialysate. Otherwise, small patients will be presented with a disproportionately large acetate load, and their small muscle mass will be inadequate to metabolize it. Dialysate flow rates range from 300 and 900 mL/min, as in adults. For treatments using low blood flows and dialyzers of low KoA, dialysate flow rates are not rate limiting for clearance and the lower range will be sufficient.

Ultrafiltration is targeted to the patient's clinical situation. If severe volume overload is present, rapid ultrafiltration may be appropriate. Otherwise, one attempts to limit total fluid removal per session to 5% of the patient's body weight (40). Critically ill patients in intensive care units often require large volumes of medications, feedings, and blood products resulting in ongoing fluid overload and hemodynamic instability with hemodialysis treatments. Close monitoring of blood pressure, ideally by an arterial line, is required. If isolated ultrafiltration without dialysate is planned in an infant or small child, hypothermia may develop because the dialysis circuit acts as a radiator that is relatively large for the patient's total blood volume.

Some form of anticoagulation is generally needed when performing hemodialysis in children particularly because the blood-flow rates are often slow, increasing the risk of clotting. Systemic heparinization is used most commonly with doses scaled to body size and then adjusted according to activated clotting times (ACTs). A loading dose of 10 to 30 units/kg is given at the start followed by a maintenance dose of 10 to 20 units/kg/hour. ACTs are followed at the bedside when machines and trained personnel are available, and the heparin dose is titrated to keep the ACT between 150 to 200 seconds (54).

There are alternative strategies for maintaining circuit patency in children at high risk for bleeding complications including (a) saline flushes without other anticoagulation, (b) regional heparinization with protamine reversal, (c) low-dose heparin, and (d) regional citrate anticoagulation. There is little published experience on the use of these other anticoagulation strategies in pediatric hemodialysis patients, and most nephrologists rely on saline flushes and avoid the use of anticoagulation (54). Heparin-induced thrombocytopenia appears to be an infrequent occurrence in pediatrics but has been reported, including two children requiring chronic hemodialysis. Danaparoid has been used successfully for anticoagulation in this setting (55). Hirudin and argatroban also are potentially useful in this setting. Please refer to Chapter 6 for further details regarding anticoagulation on hemodialysis.

Dialysis Prescription for Nonrenal Failure Indication—Hyperammonemia and Inborn Errors of Metabolism

Prescription considerations are somewhat different when children are being dialyzed for nonrenal failure indications such as intoxications, hyperammonemia, or other inborn errors of metabolism. In this situation, rapid clearance from the blood is paramount; therefore, it is essential to have a well-functioning vascular access because blood-flow rates as high as 10 to 15 mL/kg/min may be needed (43,45). Dialysis disequilibrium is not a concern in this situation because patients are not uremic. These children are critically ill and may be intravascularly volume depleted because there is often a preceding history of lethargy, poor intake, and vomiting. In addition, because their kidney function is normal, they continue to produce urine. Extremely careful monitoring of intravascular volume status and electrolyte balance is, therefore, required. Supplemental intravenous fluids should be provided as needed. Dialysate potassium and bicarbonate must be adjusted to avoid creating hypokalemia and metabolic alkalosis, and one should avoid high-calcium dialysate. Phosphorus levels can be expected to fall and supplementation may be required (44,45). Metabolite levels are monitored and dictate the duration, efficiency, and frequency of hemodialysis sessions. Rebound and ongoing production of metabolites following hemodialysis should be anticipated. CRRTs have also been used successfully alone and in conjunction with hemodialysis to control the hyperammonemia and other inborn errors of metabolism (56–58).

Hemodialysis for Management of Toxic Ingestions

Initial management of toxic ingestions involves gastric decontamination measures, administration of antidotes if available, and supportive care (59). Certain drugs and toxins have been shown to be effectively removed by extracorporeal therapies. Hemodialysis may be beneficial for removal of small molecular weight compounds (e.g., lithium, salicylates) that are not highly protein bound and that have a small volume of distribution. In addition, hemodialysis allows correction of metabolic disturbances that may result from the ingestion. For toxins with a large volume of distribution in which one anticipates a rebound following acute hemodialysis, addition of continuous hemofiltration or continuous hemodialysis has been reported to be effective (60). For toxins that are highly protein bound, hemofiltration may still be of benefit to remove free drug once the protein is saturated (61). Charcoal hemoperfusion has also been shown to be effective in removing certain drugs that are protein bound (e.g., phenytoin, phenobarbital, theophylline, carbamazepine). Published reports on the use of hemoperfusion in pediatrics are limited but suggest that the procedure can be safely performed in children (62–64). As with hemodialysis, the volume of the extracorporeal circuit is of concern and should not exceed 10% of the child's blood volume to ensure hemodynamic stability. Please refer to Chapter 38 for further detail regarding hemoperfusion and its indications. Recent case reports suggest that high-efficiency hemodialysis may be an effective alternative therapy to charcoal hemoperfusion for removal of certain drugs (e.g., vancomycin, carbamazepine) (65,66). Potential complications associated with charcoal hemoperfusion such as thrombocytopenia, coagulopathy, hypocalcemia, and hypothermia can also be avoided using high-efficiency hemodialysis.

Selected Complications of Hemodialysis

Hemodynamic instability is one of the most common complications occurring on dialysis. Risk factors in the pediatric patient include (a) excessive ultrafiltration, (b) extracorporeal circuit volume exceeding 10% of the patient's blood volume in the absence of a blood prime, and (c) increased volume of distribution because of extracorporeal circuit without concomitant increase in dose of pressor support. Under normal conditions, children have lower blood pressures than adults and a narrower margin to development of hypotension. Intradialytic hypotension may develop abruptly; therefore, volume removal must be closely monitored during treatments.

As mentioned previously, overly rapid urea clearance is more likely to occur in small children and in those with high BUN or prolonged azotemia. It may precipitate osmolar shifts and symptomatic disequilibrium with nausea, vomiting, headache, and even seizures and coma. Strategies to limit clearance (as mentioned previously) for the first few treatments in children with longstanding uremia are usually advisable.

Dialyzer reactions are infrequent but potentially fatal when they occur; therefore, prompt recognition and management are essential. Mild forms include itching, urticaria, wheezing, flushing, cough, and emesis and severe reactions include dyspnea and hypotension. Various inciting agents have been implicated including ethylene oxide, bradykinin (with the AN69 membrane), contaminated dialysate, and heparin (67–69). If suspected, dialysis should immediately be terminated and the blood not returned to the patient.

Additional potential complications include bleeding, infection, air embolus, and thrombosis. Those with a catheter in the subclavian or internal jugular vein are also at risk for developing the superior vena cava syndrome given the placement of a relatively large diameter catheter into a small vessel.

CONTINUOUS RENAL REPLACEMENT THERAPIES (SEE ALSO CHAPTER 13)

CRRT offers several advantages over the other forms of renal replacement therapy including more gradual and predictable, yet more efficient, correction of hypervolemia and uremia. However, as with hemodialysis, a well-functioning vascular access is mandatory and some form of anticoagulation is typically needed. Within the past decade industry has developed more sophisticated CRRT machines that are capable of providing precise ultrafiltration control, thermal control, and a variety of blood-flow rates appropriate for infants through adolescents. The machines offer a wide range of therapeutic options: slow continuous ultrafiltration (SCUF), continuous venovenous hemofiltration (CVVH), continuous venovenous hemodialysis (CVVHD), or continuous venovenous hemodiafiltration (CVVHDF), with some machines having the added flexibility for use in conventional hemodialysis (70). Additional improvements have included the development of pediatric blood lines and hemofilters and hemodialyzers. CRRT can now be safely and effectively performed in infants and children, and its use in the management of pediatric acute renal failure is increasing (4).

The use of CRRT in pediatrics now extends beyond therapy for acute renal failure and includes the management of diuretic resistant hypervolemia, tumor lysis syndrome, toxic ingestions, hyperammonemia, and inborn errors of metabolism (often in conjunction with hemodialysis) (56–58,60,71–75). In addition, it is used as an adjunctive therapy with extracorporeal membrane oxygenation (ECMO) (76,77).

Slow Continuous Ultrafiltration

Although used infrequently in pediatrics, SCUF has been beneficial in clinical situations such as postoperative congenital heart repair in which isolated fluid removal is required (78). Because the ultrafiltrate is isotonic and neither dialysate nor replacement fluid is provided, small children are at risk for significant solute loss if large volumes of fluid are removed (2). Therefore, ultrafiltration volumes must be carefully monitored to prevent both excessive fluid and solute loss. Furthermore, hypothermia may occur if warmed dialysate or replacement fluid is not used. Inline blood warmers are usually available, but they add significantly to the volume of the extracorporeal circuit.

Continuous Arteriovenous Hemofiltration (CAVH)

CAVH has been used successfully in the management of pediatric acute renal failure and in the management of fluid overload and azotemia in oliguric children following surgical repair of congenital heart disease (78–83). It is tolerated well in hemodynamically unstable children and offers the advantages of technical simplicity, low priming volume, and gentle fluid removal. However, it requires both arterial and venous vascular access. In the neonate, this may be accomplished by cannulating the umbilical vessels or the femoral vessels, whereas in an older child, arterial access can be obtained through the radial artery. Reasonable blood-flow rates have been reported with mean arterial pressures greater than 40 mm Hg (84). However, because the circuit is driven by the patient's arterial blood pressure, the blood-flow rate and ultrafiltration rate may vary as the blood pressure fluctuates, which in turn increases the risk for clotting. Some form of anticoagulation is, therefore, necessary to maintain circuit patency. Incorporation of a pump into the circuit to provide more consistent blood flow (pump-assisted CAVH) has been reported to be beneficial in patients with low blood pressures (85,86). If needed, dialysis can be added for better metabolic control (continuous arteriovenous hemodialysis or hemodiafiltration).

Continuous Venovenous Hemofiltration/Hemodialysis/Hemodiafiltration

The recent development of more sophisticated CRRT machines that are suitable for use in infants and small children makes CVVH, CVVHD, and CVVHDF more appealing for the management of pediatric acute renal failure; venovenous forms of CRRT are the most common of the continuous modalities used in children. With the venovenous forms of CRRT, one avoids the need for arterial catheter placement and its associated risks of bleeding, thrombosis, and limb ischemia with potential impaired future limb growth. Incorporation of a blood pump into the circuit increases the extracorporeal circuit volume and complexity of the procedure, but it also allows greater consis-

tency in blood-flow rate delivery (87). The addition of fluid or blood warmers provides better thermal control and the addition of integrated balances allows for greater ease in monitoring ultrafiltration (84,88). Newer machines are also equipped with software programs to assist in troubleshooting problems at the bedside, a particularly beneficial feature for the intensive care unit staff providing therapy.

Vascular Access and Extracorporeal Circuit

As with hemodialysis, a well functioning venous vascular access is critical. Please refer to the hemodialysis section of this chapter for a review of issues related to pediatric vascular access.

As in hemodialysis, whenever possible, the blood lines and hemofilter or hemodialyzer should be selected to keep the extracorporeal circuit volume less than 10% of the patient's blood volume or a blood prime may be necessary. Some systems currently available offer flexibility in choosing blood lines and hemofilters. However, even with this flexibility, the circuit volume may still exceed 10% of the patient's blood volume and a blood prime may be necessary (84). Risks associated with use of a blood prime are reviewed in detail in the section on hemodialysis and include potential antigen exposure, potential infectious exposure, transfusion reaction, and hyperkalemia. Use of a blood prime in conjunction with an AN-69 membrane may result in the bradykinin release syndrome, another potential complication. Brophy et al. (89) recently described this potentially fatal syndrome in two children beginning CRRT with an AN-69 hemofilter. Symptoms of hypotension, tachycardia, vasodilatation, and anaphylaxis typically begin within minutes of CRRT initiation and resolve with discontinuation of CRRT. It is important to be cognizant of this potential complication as it is potentially preventable. Based on the theory that exposure of blood to the AN-69 hemofilter in an acidotic milieu results in the generation of bradykinin, Brophy et al. propose two prevention strategies. One involves buffering the packed red cells with Tromethamine (THAM) and bicarbonate to correct the pH closer to physiologic (7.3–7.6) before priming the circuit, and the other involves use of a normal saline prime and direct transfusion of blood into the patient (89).

Anticoagulation

Most often, anticoagulation of the extracorporeal circuit is accomplished using systemic heparinization. Heparin doses are adjusted for body weight as for hemodialysis and then titrated as per the ACT or activated partial thromboplastin time (aPTT). A loading dose of 10 to 30 units/kg is administered at the start, followed by a maintenance dose of 10 to 20 units/kg/hour. ACT levels are monitored postfilter and the heparin dose adjusted to keep the ACT between 150 to 220 seconds or the aPTT 1.5–2 × control (84). Potential complications associated with heparin use include risk of bleeding, heparin-induced thrombocytopenia, and allergic reactions.

Alternative strategies for maintaining patency of the CRRT circuit are similar to those used in hemodialysis and include (a) use of saline flushes and no anticoagulation, (b) hemodilution by administration of replacement fluid prefilter, (c) regional heparinization with protamine reversal postfilter, (d) regional citrate anticoagulation, (e) low molecular weight heparin, (f) prostacyclin, and (g) use of other anticoagulants such as hirudin and argatroban. Regional heparinization with protamine reversal has been problematic because of difficulty achieving good control over the degree of anticoagulation and because of the potential risk of hypotension and anaphylaxis associated with protamine (84). Regional citrate anticoagulation, on the other hand, has been successfully used in adults for several years; recently its use in pediatrics has been increasing (90,91). There are no published data regarding the use of low molecular weight heparin or hirudin in children on CRRT. However, the successful use of argatroban in two neonates undergoing ECMO has been reported (92).

Regional citrate anticoagulation offers the major advantage of anticoagulating the extracorporeal circuit but not the patient and, therefore, reduces the risk of hemorrhage. Citrate exhibits its effect by chelating calcium, a necessary cofactor for the coagulation cascade. Citrate is infused into the arterial limb of the circuit at a rate that results in a postfilter ionized calcium level of 0.35 to 0.45 mmol/L. To prevent life-threatening hypocalcemia in the patient, a systemic calcium infusion must be administered postfilter or directly into the patient via a separate vascular access at a rate that maintains a systemic ionized calcium level of 1.1 to 1.3 mmol/L (91). Placement of a triple-lumen dialysis catheter can be advantageous when citrate anticoagulation is used because the third port can be used for calcium infusion. Calcium-free dialysate is preferable because calcium present in dialysate may chelate with citrate on the surface of the hemofilter membrane resulting in a higher citrate requirement to achieve adequate anticoagulation. Monitoring is much easier than with heparin and consists of following the postfilter ionized calcium and systemic ionized calcium. Citrate use can, however, result in several metabolic complications; therefore, close monitoring of serum electrolytes is also required. Generally, these metabolic derangements can be anticipated, allowing appropriate interventions to be made in a timely fashion. Metabolic alkalosis is the major disturbance that arises as citrate is metabolized into bicarbonate. Children are particularly prone to the development of metabolic alkalosis because the rate of citrate infusion is proportional to the blood-flow rate, which, in turn, relative to body mass is higher in smaller children as compared with adults. Management requires adjustment of the bicarbonate concentration in the dialysate (91). In one pediatric series, metabolic alkalosis was noted in every patient who required more than 7 days of CRRT (91). Additional metabolic complications include hypomagnesemia resulting from citrate chelation of magnesium and hypernatremia resulting from the sodium content of the citrate solution. Two citrate preparations are currently available: trisodium citrate (sodium citrate) and anticoagulant citrate dextrose-A (ACD-A; sodium citrate, anhydrous citrate, and dextrose) that differ in their sodium and dextrose content. ACD-A contains 2.45% dextrose and can result in hyperglycemia particularly in infants. "Citrate lock," another potential risk, manifests by a rising total serum calcium associated with a falling ionized calcium and results from citrate accumulation when the rate of infusion exceeds the clearance and metabolism. Caution with the use of citrate is, therefore,

required in the presence of liver disease and frequent blood transfusions. Bunchman et al. (91) have recently reported their success using regional citrate anticoagulation in pediatrics. Although no significant difference in circuit life was noted, they did note a significant decrease in nursing time compared with the use of heparin.

Solutions

Dialysate solutions specifically designed for use with CRRT are now commercially available with a choice of lactate (Hemofiltration Solution, Baxter Healthcare, Deerfield, Illinois; Hemosol LO, Gambro Inc., Quebec, Canada) or bicarbonate (Normocarb, Dialysis Solutions Inc., Ontario, Canada; Hemosol BO, Gambro Inc., Quebec, Canada) buffer. However, only Normocarb and Hemofiltration Solution are FDA approved and available in the United States. PD fluid is no longer a standard or desirable choice for dialysate with CRRT; pharmacy-based custom-made dialysate solutions are still used but are less desirable because industry-manufactured bicarbonate solutions are readily available and cheaper and are not associated with the risk of formulation errors. No data demonstrate improved survival with bicarbonate solution when compared with lactate in children with acute renal failure. However, studies in adults and children have shown improved hemodynamic stability and lower lactate levels when a bicarbonate-based solution is used (93,94). Normocarb is currently the only calcium-free dialysate solution commercially available and is, therefore, preferable when citrate anticoagulation is used.

Although progress has been made in developing industry-made CRRT dialysate solutions, currently, there are still no commercially manufactured replacement solutions in the United States. Many centers use Normocarb in this manner (91). Intravenous fluids such as lactated Ringer's and normal saline with or without other supplemental electrolytes are sometimes used. However, these are suboptimal because of the non-physiologic pH and electrolyte composition. Custom-made solutions are also used and have the advantage of tailoring the electrolyte replacement to the individual needs, but they lack regulated quality control standards, are time consuming for pharmacists to prepare, and carry the risk of formulation error. Replacement fluid can be administered either prefilter or postfilter. Prefilter replacement offers the advantage of hemodilution, which can be advantageous and may decrease the risk of filter clotting particularly in children requiring slow blood-flow rates.

Prescription Considerations

No data are available regarding the optimal blood-flow rate (Q_B), dialysate flow rate (Q_D), and ultrafiltration rates for pediatric patients receiving CRRT. In addition, data regarding the adequacy of CRRT do not exist. Prescription guidelines are, therefore, based on experience and extrapolation from the adult literature. Although the blood-flow rate for adults receiving CRRT is significantly lower than that required for hemodialysis, the blood-flow rate required for small children on CRRT is comparable to that required for hemodialysis in order to maintain circuit patency and typically ranges from 3 to 10 mL/kg/min (84,88). Dialysate flow rate, on the other hand, generally ranges from 10 to 20 mL/min/m² and is similar to the rate of 2 L/1.73 m²/hour used for adults. Data regarding a safe rate of fluid removal on CRRT are lacking.

There are no prospective pediatric data indicating that one modality (CVVH vs. CVVHD vs. CVVHDF) is superior to another. Small molecular weight solutes are removed equally well with continuous hemofiltration and continuous hemodialysis. However, larger molecular weight solutes are cleared better with hemofiltration than hemodialysis.

Selected Complications

Although CRRT is hemodynamically better tolerated than intermittent hemodialysis, hypotension still occurs particularly at the initiation of therapy if the extracorporeal circuit volume is large relative to the patient's circulating blood volume or when excessive fluid is removed. Unpredictable and excessive fluid removal was a concern in the past when pediatric CRRT was performed using adaptive machinery; the infusion pumps used to measure dialysate flow and ultrafiltration were often inaccurate especially at high volumes (84,88,95). Newer, more sophisticated CRRT machines contain integrated, precise scales or pumps that reduce errors in fluid balance.

Although a blood prime can reduce hemodynamic instability, the use of a blood prime in association with an AN-69 hemofilter membrane may result in the potentially fatal yet potentially preventable bradykinin release syndrome discussed in the section on vascular access and extracorporeal circuit (89). Other risks of blood priming were also discussed previously.

Dialysis disequilibrium, a serious metabolic complication that is present with intermittent hemodialysis generally does not occur with continuous therapies because solute removal occurs more slowly thereby avoiding the development of rapid osmolar shifts and risk for the disequilibrium syndrome. Nonetheless, at high Q_B and Q_D in a small child with prolonged azotemia such a syndrome could, in theory, occur.

Other metabolic complications, however, can be anticipated with CRRT and tend to be more frequent when hemofiltration is performed without simultaneous dialysis. Fluid loss with hemofiltration is isotonic with plasma, and, therefore, electrolyte losses can be substantial. Large clearance of phosphate may be desired in clinical situations associated with hyperphosphatemia, such as tumor lysis syndrome. Otherwise it will require replacement through other intravenous fluid sources. When commercial solutions are incorporated into the continuous therapy (CVVHD or CVVHDF), hyperglycemia may result. In such circumstances, one may switch to a hemofiltration solution containing less dextrose or may institute insulin therapy. In addition to solute and electrolyte losses on CRRT, recent data in children and neonates indicate that amino acid losses on CRRT can also be significant, contributing to negative nitrogen balance (96). Therefore, to maintain a positive nitrogen balance, nutritional supplementation adjusted to provide higher protein intake (up to 3 to 4 g/kg/day) may be required. The potential catabolic complications of pediatric CRRT require further research.

Hypothermia, another potential complication of CRRT, occurred more commonly when adaptive machinery was used for pediatric CRRT. Newer machines are available with an integrated fluid warmer or a blood warmer.

Additional risks associated with CRRT relate to the need for anticoagulation to maintain circuit patency and include (a) hemorrhage if heparin is used, (b) metabolic alkalosis if regional citrate is used (see section on anticoagulation for more complete discussion on potential complications associated with citrate use), and (c) blood loss through circuit clotting if anticoagulation therapy is not administered.

Finally, there are also risks associated with placing and maintaining vascular access. This is reviewed in the subsection regarding complications of pediatric hemodialysis.

CRRT and Extracorporeal Life Support Therapy (ECMO)

The use of ECMO for management of cardiac and respiratory failure has become more widespread. Hypervolemia and acute renal failure are well recognized complications during ECMO (97). CRRT has become an important adjunctive therapy in this setting when diuretic therapy alone is insufficient for fluid removal. A hemofilter can be incorporated into the ECMO circuit without the need for additional vascular access or the need for additional anticoagulation (76,77). Careful consideration must be given to positioning of the hemofilter within the ECMO circuit to minimize blood recirculation and shunting away from the oxygenator (98). If indicated, dialysate can be added to the system to allow continuous hemodialysis and/or hemodiafiltration.

CRRT and Cardiopulmonary Bypass

Hemofiltration has also been beneficial for fluid removal in children receiving cardiopulmonary bypass (99). In a novel extension of hemofiltration in this setting, Journois et al. reported initial experience with high-volume zero-balanced hemofiltration (5 L/m²) in ten children during the rewarming phase of cardiopulmonary bypass in an attempt to decrease the inflammatory response to cardiopulmonary bypass (100). The authors attributed the improved outcome (less blood loss, fever, and ventilatory support) to removal of proinflammatory mediators during the rewarming phase.

SUMMARY

Significant technologic advances in the past two decades have permitted nephrologists to provide all forms of renal replacement therapy to infants and children. However, despite these advances, the mortality rate from acute renal failure remains high, likely in part the result of the severity of the underlying disease process (101–105). Unfortunately, no prospective data exist comparing the three treatment modalities for management of pediatric acute renal failure, and data regarding the optimal dose of renal replacement therapy in acute renal failure are not available. Furthermore, the lack of standardized practice when prescribing renal replacement therapy makes it even more difficult to conduct outcomes research. Recent initiatives designed to begin addressing these issues include the organization of the Acute Dialysis Quality Initiative (ADQI). In addition, a Pediatric CRRT Registry was created to gather data on pediatric experience with CRRT from which better prescription guidelines and data on outcomes may emerge. At present, however, the choice of modality for renal replacement therapy in children continues to be made at the bedside.

REFERENCES

1. Flynn JT. Choice of dialysis modality for management of pediatric acute renal failure. *Pediatr Nephrol* 2001;17:61–69.
2. Parekh RS, et al. Dialysis support in the pediatric intensive care unit. *Adv Ren Replace Ther* 1996;3:326–336.
3. Belsha CW, et al. Dialytic management of childhood acute renal failure: a survey of North American pediatric nephrologists. *Pediatr Nephrol* 1995;9:361–363.
4. Warady BA, et al. Dialysis therapy for children with acute renal failure: survey results. *Pediatr Nephrol* 2000;15:11–13.
5. Mendley SR, et al. Acute renal failure in the pediatric patient. *Adv Ren Replace Ther* 1997;4[Suppl 1]:S93–S101.
6. Flynn JT. Causes, management approaches, and outcome of acute renal failure in children. *Curr Opin Pediatr* 1998;10:184–189.
7. Gouyon JB, et al. Management of acute renal failure in newborns. *Pediatr Nephrol* 2000;14:1037–1044.
8. Karlowicz MG, et al. Acute renal failure in the neonate. *Clin Perinatol* 1992;19:139–158.
9. Reznik VM, et al. Peritoneal dialysis for acute renal failure in children. *Pediatr Nephrol* 1991;5:715–717.
10. Flynn JT, et al. Peritoneal dialysis for management of pediatric acute renal failure. *Perit Dial Int* 2001;21:390–394.
11. Matthews DE, et al. Peritoneal dialysis in the first 60 days of life. *J Pediatr Surg* 1990;25:110–115.
12. Bunchman TE. Acute peritoneal dialysis access in infant renal failure. *Perit Dial Int* 1996;16[Suppl 1]:S509–S511.
13. Esperanca MJ, et al. Peritoneal dialysis efficiency in relation to body weight. *J Pediatr Surg* 1966;1:162–169.
14. Schaefer F, et al. Evaluation of peritoneal solute transfer by peritoneal equilibration test in children. *Adv Perit Dial* 1992;8:410–415.
15. Reznik VM, et al. Cost analysis of dialysis modalities for pediatric acute renal failure. *Perit Dial Int* 1993;13:311–313.
16. Day RE, et al. Peritoneal dialysis in children: review of 8 years' experience. *Arch Dis Child* 1977;52:56–61.
17. Stewart JH, et al. Peritoneal and haemodialysis: a comparison of their morbidity, and of the mortality suffered by dialysed patients. *Q J Med* 1966;35:407–420.
18. Lewis MA, et al. Practical peritoneal dialysis—the Tenckhoff catheter in acute renal failure. *Pediatr Nephrol* 1992;6:470–475.
19. Hogg RJ, et al. The Toronto Western Hospital catheter in a pediatric dialysis program. *Am J Kidney Dis* 1983;3:219–223.
20. Grefberg N, et al. Comparison of two catheters for peritoneal access in patients undergoing continuous ambulatory peritoneal dialysis (CAPD). *Scand J Urol Nephrol* 1983;17:343–346.
21. Furth SL, et al. Peritoneal dialysis catheter infections and peritonitis in children: a report of the North American Pediatric Renal Transplant Cooperative Study. *Pediatr Nephrol* 2000;15:179–182.
22. Warady BA, et al. Lessons from the peritoneal dialysis patient database: a report of the North American Pediatric Renal Transplant Cooperative Study. *Kidney Int* 1996;49[Suppl 53]:S68–S71.
23. Clark KR, et al. Surgical aspects of chronic peritoneal dialysis in the neonate and infant under 1 year of age. *J Pediatr Surg* 1992;27:780–783.
24. Orkin BA, et al. Continuous ambulatory peritoneal dialysis catheters in children. *Arch Surg* 1983;118:1398–1402.
25. Conlin MJ, et al. Minimizing surgical problems of peritoneal dialysis in children. *J Urol* 1995;154:917–919.
26. Lewis M, et al. Routine omentectomy is not required in children undergoing chronic peritoneal dialysis. *Adv Perit Dial* 1995;11:293–295.
27. Liberek T, et al. Peritoneal dialysis fluid inhibition of phagocytic functions: effects of osmolality and glucose concentration. *J Am Soc Nephrol* 1993;3:1508–1515.
28. Mendley SR, et al. Peritoneal equilibration test results are different in infants, children, and adults. *J Am Soc Nephrol* 1995;6:1309–1312.
29. Mak RH, et al. Glucose and insulin metabolism in uremia. *Nephron* 1992;61:377–382.
30. Ramos JM, et al. Sequential changes in serum lipids and their subfractions in patients receiving CAPD. *Nephron* 1983;35:20–23.
31. Canepa A, et al. Long-term effect of amino-acid dialysis solution in children on continuous ambulatory peritoneal dialysis. *Pediatr Nephrol* 1991;5:215–219.
32. Qamar IU, et al. Effects of amino acid dialysis compared to dextrose dialysis in children on continuous cycling peritoneal dialysis. *Perit Dial Int* 1999;19:237–247.
33. de Boer AW, et al. Clinical experience with icodextrin in children: ultrafiltration profiles and metabolism. *Pediatr Nephrol* 2000;15:21–24.
34. Wood EG, et al. Ultrafiltration using low volume peritoneal dialysis in critically ill infants and children. *Adv Perit Dial* 1991;7:266–268.
35. Fischbach M. Peritoneal dialysis prescription for neonates. *Perit Dial Int* 1996;16[Suppl 1]:S512–S514.
36. Alexander SR, et al. Surgical aspects of continuous ambulatory peritoneal dialysis in infants, children, and adolescents. *J Urol* 1982;127:501–504.
37. Wong SN, et al. Comparison of temporary and permanent catheters for acute peritoneal dialysis. *Arch Dis Child* 1988;63:827–831.
38. Chadha V, et al. Tenckhoff catheters prove superior to Cook catheters in pediatric acute peritoneal dialysis. *Am J Kidney Dis* 2000;35:1111–1116.
39. Stonehill WH, et al. Radiographically documented fecal impaction causing peritoneal dialysis catheter malfunction. *J Urol* 1995;153:445–446.
40. Donckerwolcke RA, et al. Hemodialysis in infants and small children. *Pediatr Nephrol* 1994;8:103–106.
41. Sadowski RH, et al. Acute hemodialysis of infants weighing less than five kilograms. *Kidney Int* 1994;45:903–906.
42. Bock GH, et al. Hemodialysis in the premature infant. *Am J Dis Child* 1981;135:178–180.
43. Rutledge SL, et al. Neonatal hemodialysis: effective therapy for the encephalopathy of inborn errors of metabolism. *J Pediatr* 1990;116:125–128.
44. Wiegand C, et al. The management of life-threatening hyperammonemia: a comparison of several therapeutic modalities. *J Pediatr* 1980;96:142–144.
45. Donn SM, et al. Comparison of exchange transfusion, peritoneal dialysis, and hemodialysis for the treatment of hyperammonemia in an anuric newborn infant. *J Pediatr* 1979;95:67–70.
46. Sargent JA, et al. Mathematic modeling of dialysis therapy. *Kidney Int* 1980;18[Suppl 10]:S2–S10.
47. Knight F, et al. Hemodialysis of the infant or small child with chronic renal failure. *ANNA J* 1993;20:315–323.
48. Hakim RM, et al. Effect of the dialysis membrane in the treatment of patients with acute renal failure. *N Engl J Med* 1994;331:1338–1342.
49. Himmelfarb J, et al. A multicenter comparison of dialysis membranes in the treatment of acute renal failure requiring dialysis. *J Am Soc Nephrol* 1998;9:257–266.
50. Schiffl H, et al. Biocompatible membranes in acute renal failure: prospective case-controlled study. *Lancet* 1994;344:570–572.
51. Jenkins RD, et al. Clinical implications of catheter variability on neonatal continuous arteriovenous hemofiltration. *ASAIO Trans* 1988;34:108–111.
52. Arieff AI. Dialysis disequilibrium syndrome: current concepts on pathogenesis and prevention. *Kidney Int* 1994;45:629–635.

53. Grushkin CM, et al. Hemodialysis in small children. *JAMA* 1972;221:869–873.

54. Geary DF, et al. Low-dose and heparin-free hemodialysis in children. *Pediatr Nephrol* 1991;5:220–224.

55. Neuhaus TJ, et al. Heparin-induced thrombocytopenia type II on hemodialysis: switch to danaparoid. *Pediatr Nephrol* 2000;14:713–716.

56. Falk MC, et al. Continuous venovenous haemofiltration in the acute treatment of inborn errors of metabolism. *Pediatr Nephrol* 1994;8:330–333.

57. Schaefer F, et al. Dialysis in neonates with inborn errors of metabolism. *Nephrol Dial Transplant* 1999;14:910–918.

58. Picca S, et al. Extracorporeal dialysis in neonatal hyperammonemia: modalities and prognostic indicators. *Pediatr Nephrol* 2001;16:862–867.

59. Tenenbein M. Recent advancements in pediatric toxicology. *Pediatr Clin North Am* 1999;46:1179–1188.

60. Meyer RJ, et al. Hemodialysis followed by continuous hemofiltration for treatment of lithium intoxication in children. *Am J Kidney Dis* 2001;37:1044–1047.

61. Dharnidharka VR, et al. Extracorporeal removal of toxic valproic acid levels in children. *Pediatr Nephrol* 2002;17:312–315.

62. Papadopoulou ZL, et al. The use of hemoperfusion in children—past, present, and future. *Pediatr Clin North Am* 1982;29:1039–1052.

63. O'Regan S, et al. Charcoal hemoperfusion for drug and poison intoxication in pediatric patients. *Dial Transplant* 1985;14:609–611.

64. Chavers BM, et al. Techniques for use of charcoal hemoperfusion in infants: experience in two patients. *Kidney Int* 1980;18:386–389.

65. Bunchman TE, et al. Treatment of vancomycin overdose using high efficiency dialysis membranes. *Pediatr Nephrol* 1999;13:773–774.

66. Schuerer DJ, et al. High-efficiency dialysis for carbamazepine overdose. *Clin Toxicol* 2000;38:321–323.

67. Pearson F, et al. Ethylene oxide sensitivity in hemodialysis patients. *Artif Organs* 1987;11:100–103.

68. Bommer J, et al. Anaphylactoid reactions in dialysis patients: role of ethylene-oxide. *Lancet* 1985;2:1382–1385.

69. Verresen L, et al. Bradykinin is a mediator of anaphylactoid reactions during hemodialysis with AN69 membranes. *Kidney Int* 1994;45:1497–1503.

70. Abdeen O, et al. Dialysis modalities in the intensive care unit. *Crit Care Clin* 2002;18:223–247.

71. Shah M, et al. Rapid removal of vancomycin by continuous venovenous hemofiltration. *Pediatr Nephrol* 2000;14:912–915.

72. Wong KY, et al. Ammonia clearance by peritoneal dialysis and continuous arteriovenous hemodiafiltration. *Pediatr Nephrol* 1998;12:589–591.

73. Castillo F, et al. Treatment of hydrops fetalis with hemofiltration. *Pediatr Nephrol* 2000;15:14–16.

74. Sakarcan A, et al. Hyperphosphatemia in tumor lysis syndrome: the role of hemodialysis and continuous veno-venous hemofiltration. *Pediatr Nephrol* 1994;8:351–353.

75. Saccente SL, et al. Prevention of tumor lysis syndrome using continuous veno-venous hemofiltration. *Pediatr Nephrol* 1995;9:569–573.

76. Sell LL, et al. Experience with renal failure during extracorporeal membrane oxygenation: treatment with continuous hemofiltration. *J Pediatr Surg* 1987;22:600–602.

77. Heiss KF, et al. Renal insufficiency and volume overload in neonatal ECMO managed by continuous ultrafiltration. *Trans Am Soc Artif Intern Organs* 1987;33:557–560.

78. Zobel G, et al. Continuous extracorporeal fluid removal in children with low cardiac output after cardiac operations. *J Thorac Cardiovasc Surg* 1991;101:593–597.

79. Ronco C, et al. Acute renal failure in infancy: treatment by continuous renal replacement therapy. *Intensive Care Med* 1995;21:490–499.

80. Paret G, et al. Continuous arteriovenous hemofiltration after cardiac operations in infants and children. *J Thorac Cardiovasc Surg* 1992;104:1225–1230.

81. Fleming F, et al. Renal replacement therapy after repair of congenital heart disease in children: a comparison of hemofiltration and peritoneal dialysis. *J Thorac Cardiovasc Surg* 1995;109:322–331.

82. Zobel G, et al. Continuous renal replacement therapy in critically ill neonates. *Kidney Int* 1998;53[Suppl 66]:S169–S173.

83. Latta K, et al. Continuous arteriovenous haemofiltration in critically ill children. *Pediatr Nephrol* 1994;8:334–337.

84. Bunchman TE, et al. Continuous arterial-venous diahemofiltration and continuous veno-venous diahemofiltration in infants and children. *Pediatr Nephrol* 1994;8:96–102.

85. Ellis EN, et al. Use of pump-assisted hemofiltration in children with acute renal failure. *Pediatr Nephrol* 1997;11:196–200.

86. Chanard J, et al. Ultrafiltration-pump assisted arteriovenous hemofiltration. (CAVH). *Kidney Int* 1988;33[Suppl 24]:S157–S158.

87. Yorgin PD, et al. Continuous venovenous hemofiltration. *Pediatr Nephrol* 1990;4:640–642.

88. Bunchman TE, et al. Continuous venovenous hemodiafiltration in infants and children. *Am J Kidney Dis* 1995;25:17–21.

89. Brophy PD, et al. AN-69 membrane reactions are pH-dependent and preventable. *Am J Kidney Dis* 2001;38:173–178.

90. Mehta RL, et al. Regional citrate anticoagulation for continuous arteriovenous hemodialysis in critically ill patients. *Kidney Int* 1990;38:976–981.

91. Bunchman TE, et al. Pediatric hemofiltration: normocarb dialysate solution with citrate anticoagulation. *Pediatr Nephrol* 2002;17:150–154.

92. Kawada T, et al. Clinical application of argatroban as an alternative anticoagulant for extracorporeal circulation. *Hematol Oncol Clin North Am* 2000;14:445–457.

93. Maxvold NJ, et al. Prospective, crossover comparison of bicarbonate versus lactate-based dialysate for pediatric CVVHD. *Blood Purif* 1999;17(abst 27).

94. Barenbrock M, et al. Effects of bicarbonate- and lactate-buffered replacement fluids on cardiovascular outcome in CVVH patients. *Kidney Int* 2000;58:1751–1757.

95. Jenkins R, et al. Accuracy of intravenous infusion pumps in continuous renal replacement therapies. *ASAIO J* 1992;38:808–810.

96. Maxvold NJ, et al. Amino acid loss and nitrogen balance in critically ill children with acute renal failure: a prospective comparison between classic hemofiltration and hemofiltration with dialysis. *Crit Care Med* 2000;28:1161–1165.

97. Roy BJ, et al. Venovenous extracorporeal membrane oxygenation affects renal function. *Pediatrics* 1995;95:573–578.

98. Yorgin PD, et al. Where should the hemofiltration circuit be placed in relation to the extracorporeal membrane oxygenation circuit? *ASAIO J* 1992;38:801–803.

99. Journois D. Hemofiltration during cardiopulmonary bypass. *Kidney Int* 1998;53[Suppl 66]:S174–S177.

100. Journois D, et al. High-volume, zero-balanced hemofiltration to reduce delayed inflammatory response to cardiopulmonary bypass in children. *Anesthesiology* 1996;85:965–976.

101. Zobel G, et al. Five years experience with continuous extracorporeal renal support in paediatric intensive care. *Intensive Care Med* 1991;17:315–319.

102. Lowrie LH. Renal replacement therapies in pediatric multiorgan dysfunction syndrome. *Pediatr Nephrol* 2000;14:6–12.

103. Maxvold NJ, et al. Management of acute renal failure in the pediatric patient: hemofiltration versus hemodialysis. *Am J Kidney Dis* 1997;5[Suppl 4]:S84–S88.

104. Gong W, et al. Eighteen years experience in pediatric acute dialysis: analysis of predictors of outcome. *Pediatr Nephrol* 2001;16:212–215.

105. Bunchman TE, et al. Pediatric acute renal failure: outcome by modality and disease. *Pediatr Nephrol* 2001;16:1067–1071.

INFECTIONS IN PATIENTS ON PERITONEAL DIALYSIS

ANTONIOS H. TZAMALOUKAS AND LUCY FOX

Peritonitis and catheter-related soft tissue infections remain significant problems for patients on peritoneal dialysis (PD). Although usually responsive to antimicrobial therapy, PD-associated peritonitis and exit-site and tunnel infections have tremendous significance because of costs associated with diagnosis, hospitalization, and therapy; loss of productivity; malnutrition; failure of PD in a subset of patients requiring transfer to hemodialysis; and increased mortality.

PD PERITONITIS

PD-associated peritonitis is different from that seen in postsurgical patients and should be regarded as a unique disease process, perhaps more closely resembling the spontaneous bacterial peritonitis occurring in patients with cirrhosis of the liver, ascites, and portal hypertension (1).

Etiology, Pathogenesis, and Predisposing Factors

Etiology

Table 41.1 shows the agents responsible for PD peritonitis. Typically, but not invariably, this peritonitis is caused by skin-dwelling Gram-positive organisms rather than Gram-negative fecal flora. The causative organism is frequently identical in terms of phage type for *Staphylococcus aureus* and biotype for *Staphylococcus epidermidis* to staphylococci isolated from surveillance cultures of catheter exit site, throat, and hands (2–4). Gram-negative infections are most frequently caused by *Escherichia coli* and *Pseudomonas* sp., most likely originating in the intestinal tract.

Routes of Peritoneal Infection

Five different routes of infection can be distinguished: intraluminal or transluminal, periluminal, transmural, hematogenous, and ascending—the first three types occurring most frequently and the first two directly involving the catheter. Table 41.2 lists the relative frequency of these routes and the usual bacterial species involved.

Intraluminal infections occur when bacteria enter the catheter via fluid traveling within it or through cracks. Dialysate may become infected when additives such as antibiotics, insulin, or heparin are instilled carelessly. Most commonly, intraluminal infections result from accidental inoculation of the open connection by touch contamination or from tubing disconnection. Two thirds of *S. epidermidis* infections occur by the intraluminal route, whereas only half of *S. aureus* infections are believed to develop in this manner. This discrepancy probably reflects the different mechanisms of adherence and pathogenicity exhibited by these staphylococci (2).

Intraluminal entry of bacteria in the absence of clinical peritonitis has been described. *Propionibacteria* are most commonly involved, usually in small numbers and requiring a long growth period of 8 to 12 days (5). Thus, surveillance dialysate cultures in asymptomatic patients are likely to be misleading and are generally not useful in patient management (6).

Periluminal infections result from entry of bacteria around the catheter exit site, initially causing an exit-site or tunnel infection. In the absence of exit-site or tunnel infection, bacterial penetration periluminally with resultant peritonitis has not been documented.

Transmural or intestinal infections are caused by enteric organisms, most often *E. coli* and *Pseudomonas* sp. Hematogenously transmitted infection in PD patients is uncommon. Occasional patients with antecedent respiratory infections and blood cultures positive for *Streptococcus viridans* have eventually developed peritonitis involving that organism, that were presumably seeded hematogenously (2). Mycobacterial infections, including *Mycobacterium tuberculosis*, are believed to reach the peritoneum by hematogenous spread (7).

Rare routes of infection include vaginal-peritoneal communication (8), intrauterine devices (which, for this reason, are not recommended for use by women on PD), and environmental sources such as tap water and swimming pools.

Predisposing Factors

Risk factors for the development of peritonitis include age younger than 20 years, substance abuse, poverty, and African American or native Canadian ethnicity (9–11). Diabetes melli-

TABLE 41.1. MICROORGANISMS CAUSING CAPD PERITONITIS

Cause	Incidence (%)
Gram-positive bacteria	
Coagulase-negative staphylococci	30–40
Staphylococcus aureus	10–20
Streptococcus species	10–15
Enterococcus	3–6
Neisseria species	1–2
Diphtheroid species	1–2
Gram-negative bacteria	
Escherichia coli	5–10
Pseudomonas species	5–10
Proteus species	3–6
Acinetobacter species	2–5
Klebsiella species	1–3
Serratia species	<1
Fungi	2–10
Other (mycobacteria, protozoa, etc.)	2–5
Culture negative	0–30

CAPD, continuous ambulatory peritoneal dialysis.
Modified from Vas SI. In: Nolph, KD, ed. *Peritoneal dialysis,* 3rd ed. Dordrecht, the Netherlands: Kluwer Academic, 1989, with permission.

tus appears to be a risk factor in some studies (9) but not in others (10). Gender is not a risk factor for peritonitis (9). Systemic diseases causing immunosuppression, such as systemic lupus erythematosus (12) and particularly acquired immunodeficiency syndrome (AIDS), are associated with a high risk for infection. Hypoalbuminemia has been reported to be associated with a high rate of peritonitis in some studies but not in others (13).

In children, risk factors for peritonitis include African-American ethnicity, single-cuffed PD catheters, upward pointing exit sites, and exit-site or tunnel infections (14)

Peritoneal Defense Mechanisms

Discussion of the uremic defects in the defense mechanisms against infections is beyond the scope of this chapter (see Chapter 21). We discuss here only the relationship between abnormalities in peritoneal defense mechanisms and frequency of

TABLE 41.2. ROUTES OF INFECTION IN CAPD PATIENTS

Route	Percent	Organism
Transluminal	30–40	*Staphylococcus epidermidis*
		Staphylococcus aureus
		Acinetobacter
Periluminal	20–30	*S. epidermidis*
		S. aureus
		Pseudomonas
		Yeast
Transmural	25–30	Enteric organisms
		Anaerobes
Hematogenous	5–10	*Streptococcus*
		Mycobacterium tuberculosis
Ascending	2–5	Yeast
		Lactobacillus

CAPD, continuous ambulatory peritoneal dialysis.
Reprinted from Vas SI. In: Nolph, KD, ed. *Peritoneal dialysis,* 3rd ed. Dordrecht, the Netherlands: Kluwer Academic, 1989, with permission.

peritonitis and the effect of dialysate on peritoneal defense mechanisms (15–17).

Both humoral and cellular factors participate in host defense processes (16–18). Individual variation in humoral immunity does not appear to explain patient-to-patient variation in the incidence of infections (19). Bacteria entering the peritoneal cavity undergo phagocytosis and are killed by peritoneal macrophages and neutrophils. Fig. 41.1 shows the sequence of events leading to bacterial killing.

Humoral Immunity

Opsonization of bacteria takes place when immunoglobulin G (IgG) molecules bind to specific epitopes on bacterial surface antigens via the antigen-specific site located close to the amino terminus of the IgG molecule. Both IgG and C3b are important opsonins with different affinities for Gram-negative and Gram-positive organisms. The Fc region of the IgG molecule interacts, through changes in its configuration, with the Fc receptor of the phagocytic cell. The opsonized microbe is ingested via receptor-mediated phagocytosis (16).

Phagocytosis is amplified by the complement cascade and by fibronectin. Complement is activated either through the classical pathway, via interaction with IgG or IgM bound to bacteria, or through the alternate pathway via interaction with microbial polysaccharides. C3b formed during C3 cleavage by either pathway is deposited on the bacterial surface and augments phagocytosis. Other activated complement compounds contribute to recruitment of neutrophils by chemotaxis. Fibronectin has binding sites for both macrophages and bacteria and augments *S. aureus* phagocytosis (16). Defensins are endogenous antimicrobial peptides contributing to the defense against peritoneal infection (19,20).

The concentrations of IgG, complement, and fibronectin in normal peritoneal fluid are similar to those in the normal serum. In peritoneal dialysate, however, these values are reduced by one to three orders of magnitude (21,22), even after several hours of dwell time. This dilutional effect blunts the humoral prevention of peritonitis. By analogy, low levels of proteins, including IgG and complement, in cirrhotic ascitic fluid are associated with a high incidence of subacute bacterial peritonitis (23).

An inverse relationship between either peritoneal opsonic activity or IgG concentration and frequency of PD peritonitis has been reported (24), but others could not confirm this finding (16). Furthermore, peritoneal IgG levels failed to prospectively predict the risk for peritonitis (25). In addition, IgG levels in spent dialysate vary over time in a given patient (23), and the opsonic activity in a given sample of spent dialysate against different strains of *S. epidermidis* is also inconsistent (26).

The opsonic activity of spent dialysate against Gram-negative bacteria is substantially lower than that against Gram-positive bacteria (27). This may account, at least in part, for the greater severity of the Gram-negative infections. Fibronectin has opsonic activity against Gram-positive organisms. Whether the concentration of fibronectin in the dialysate affects the rate of peritonitis or not has been disputed. Fibrinogen polymerizes to fibrin in the spent dialysate during episodes of peritonitis. The addition of urokinase enhances opsonic activity of spent

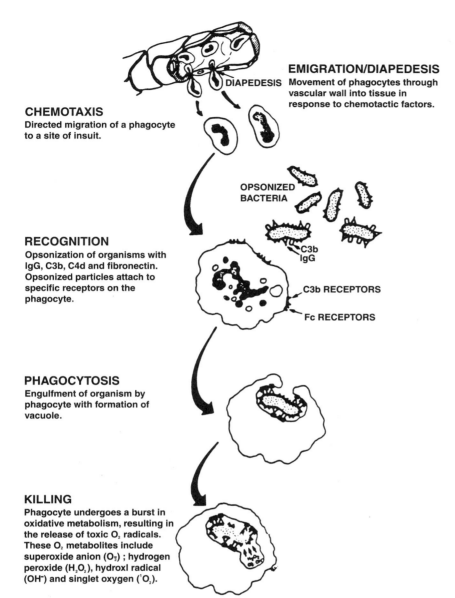

CHEMOTAXIS
Directed migration of a phagocyte to a site of insuit.

DIAPEDESIS

EMIGRATION/DIAPEDESIS
Movement of phagocytes through vascular wall into tissue in response to chemotactic factors.

OPSONIZED BACTERIA

RECOGNITION
Opsonization of organisms with IgG, C3b, C4d and fibronectin. Opsonized particles attach to specific receptors on the phagocyte.

C3b
IgG

C3b RECEPTORS

Fc RECEPTORS

PHAGOCYTOSIS
Engulfment of organism by phagocyte with formation of vacuole.

KILLING
Phagocyte undergoes a burst in oxidative metabolism, resulting in the release of toxic O_2 radicals. These O_2 metabolites include superoxide anion (O_2^-); hydrogen peroxide (H_2O_2), hydroxl radical (OH^-) and singlet oxygen ($^1O_2$).

FIG. 41.1. Phagocytosis and killing of bacteria by white blood cells. (Reprinted from Lewis S, et al. Host defense mechanisms in the peritoneal cavity of continuous ambulatory peritoneal dialysis patients. First of two parts. *Perit Dial Int* 1991;11:14–21, with permission.)

dialysate against *S. aureus* (28), probably because of splitting of the fibrin strands.

Cellular Immunity

The concentration of leukocytes in peritoneal dialysate is 100-fold to 1,000-fold less than in normal peritoneal fluid (15). Baseline peritoneal leukocyte counts do not predict peritonitis frequency, and differential counts in uninfected spent dialysate vary greatly among patients but remain stable over time in a given individual (29). Macrophages predominate, lymphocyte percentages may vary between 2% and 84%, and neutrophils are usually 5% to 10% (29).

Peritoneal macrophages, believed to originate from blood monocytes, constitute the first line of defense against bacterial invasion of the peritoneal cavity. These cells migrate intraperi-

toneally from the peritoneal membrane in the early stages of peritonitis (along with polymorphonuclear cells). In PD patients, phagocytic capacity of peritoneal macrophages incubated in usual media (not dialysate) is normal (18). Bacterial killing capacity of peritoneal macrophages studied in dialysate-free media has been reported as either normal (18) or slightly decreased (30).

The oxidative metabolism of macrophages from noninfected spent dialysate is less than that of macrophages from normal peritoneal fluid (15) but higher than that of peripheral blood monocytes (30). The oxidative metabolism of peritoneal macrophages is impaired in PD patients with frequent peritonitis (22). In comparison to blood monocytes, peritoneal macrophages exhibit increased Fc receptors, binding of C5a (a chemotactic factor), and certain surface transplantation antigens such as HLA-DR (Ia) antigens and CD14 antigens (monocyte growth or differentiation antigens. These findings suggest that peritoneal macrophages are activated in CAPD patients (31). However, long-term PD may have adverse effects on Fc-receptor-mediated phagocytosis and adhesion of polymorphonuclear cells and macrophages to endothelial walls (32).

Peritoneal T lymphocytes, both helper and suppressor, seem to be similarly activated (22). An increased percentage of blood and peritoneal T-suppressor cells has been associated with frequent peritonitis in isolated case reports (33). Compared with cells from normal individuals, blood neutrophils from PD patients exhibit decreased binding of C5a, decreased chemotaxis, and impaired opsonic activity (15). The oxidative metabolism of blood polymorphonuclear cells is adversely affected by low serum albumin levels (34).

Mesothelial cells lining the serosal surface of the peritoneal membrane represent another important cell line in the defense against peritonitis and containment of infection within the peritoneal cavity (35). The vital interaction of mesothelial cells and peritoneal macrophages early in the course of peritonitis occurs via cell-to-cell interaction, secretion of cytokines (both proinflammatory and antiinflammatory), prostaglandins, growth factors and fibrinolytic factors, and expression of adhesion proteins affecting leukocyte traffic (35). Fig. 41.2 shows the identified products of the mesothelium.

Cytokines

Cytokines released from peritoneal macrophages, mesothelial cells, and lymphocytes are important in the defense against peritonitis. Activated macrophages release tumor necrosis factor alpha (TNF-α) early in the course of peritonitis (35), whereas other cytokines including interleukin (IL)-1b, IL-8 and IL-6 peak later (17). Both IL-8 and IL-6, synthesized by mesothelial cells, are stimulated by IL-1b and TNF-α. IL-8 plays a role in the recruitment of leukocytes, whereas IL-6 may modulate the inflammatory response by inhibiting the transcription of other cytokines (35,36).

Lymphocytes activated by IL-1b and TNF-α release IL-2 and gamma-interferon (γ-IF). The latter enhances macrophage bactericidal activity, whereas IL-1b stimulates prostaglandin E$_2$ (PGE$_2$) release from macrophages and mesothelial cells. PGE$_2$ has a negative feedback effect on IL-1b production. In addition, IL-6, IL-8, and PGE$_2$ modulate the synthesis of IL-1a and IL-1b.

Effects of PD Solutions on Peritoneal Defense Mechanisms

The effects of PD solutions on peritoneal defense mechanisms are expressed via dilution, high osmolality, low pH, lactate, and heat sterilization of the dialysate. In addition to the effects of dilution on humoral defense mechanisms, decreased density of peritoneal macrophages reduces the probability of phagocyte-bacterium encounter and, thus, bacterial killing (15). Both sustained high dialysate osmolality and low dialysate pH suppress peritoneal leukocyte functions (37). Dialysate pH rises rapidly after intraperitoneal infusion, reaching blood pH by 30 minutes. However, the dialysate infusion period carries a high risk of bacterial entry at the same time that peritoneal host defenses are compromised by low dialysate pH.

Lactate in commercial dialysate preparations appears to have independent adverse effects on peritoneal inflammatory cell function, specifically affecting macrophages, polymorphonuclear cells, mesothelial cells, and fibroblasts (38). Heat sterilization of the dialysate causes a decrease in the adhesion of leukocytes to endothelial cells (39).

The development of PD solutions containing nonlactate buffers may augment peritoneal defense mechanisms. The cytotoxicity of bicarbonate-based dialysate appears to be less than that of lactate-based dialysate. However, polymorphonuclear cell function studied in vitro after incubation in bicarbonate-based dialysate remains deficient (40). Pyruvate-based dialysate has fewer adverse effects on macrophage and polymorphonuclear cell function than does lactate-based dialysate (41).

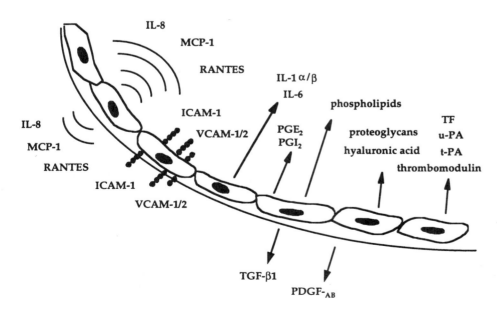

FIG. 41.2. Products of the mesothelial cell. (Reprinted from Topley N. The cytokine network controlling peritoneal inflammation. *Perit Dial Int* 1995;15[Suppl]:S35–S39, with permission.)

Clinical Picture

Incubation Period

Anecdotal information places the incubation period between 24 and 48 hours for peritonitis caused by touch contamination (2). However, incubation periods as short as 6 hours with rapid appearance of symptoms have been reported. The incubation period for slower growing organisms (fungi, mycobacteria) may be as long as weeks to months.

Clinical Features

Table 41.3 shows the clinical features of PD peritonitis from one study (42). Different studies have reported similar frequencies of symptoms and signs (43). Cloudy dialysate is the most common presenting complaint followed by abdominal pain and signs of peritoneal irritation. Occasionally, patients present with abdominal pain and diffuse tenderness with clear dialysate containing less than 100 cells/mm^3, and the dialysate becomes turbid after several days (42). The first sign of peritonitis in children may be fever (44). Coagulase-negative staphylococci and other low-virulence organisms often cause mild symptoms and signs. Severe pain accompanied by shock can signify infection with *S. aureus* or *Pseudomonas* species or may indicate fecal peritonitis. Nausea, vomiting, constipation, and diarrhea are nonspecific and less common. Fever, typically low grade, was present in 53% of the patients studied by Vas.

Laboratory Findings

Laboratory diagnosis of peritonitis includes a dialysate leukocyte count and differential based on a Wright's stain of the cytospin preparation, Gram stain of dialysate, and dialysate cultures (both aerobic and anaerobic). Typically, dialysate white blood cell (WBC) count exceeds 100 cells/mm^3 with a predominance of polymorphonuclear neutrophils (PMNs). The initial dialysate WBC count is lower than 100/mm^3 in less than 10% of cases

(45). Neither the magnitude of the leukocytosis nor the differential is useful in predicting the causative microorganism. However, a lymphocytic predominance suggests a mycobacterial or viral cause. Gram stain will reveal an organism in only 9% to 40% of cases (46) but is predictive of the type of organism present on culture in 68% of Gram-positive infections and 95% of Gram-negative infections (47); it is particularly useful in the early recognition of fungal peritonitis (48).

PD-associated peritonitis is a low inoculum infection. Thus, false-negative cultures can occur if a too small volume of dialysate is cultured (2). To enhance the likelihood of a positive result, the first cloudy bag should be saved for culture and a large volume of dialysate should be cultured. Overnight storage of dialysate before setting up the culture will not reduce the sensitivity. Several methods of enriching the yield of the culture have been described. The frequency of negative cultures varies considerably among the different methods. Most cultures become positive by 24 hours, and 75% by 3 days. Fast-growing mycobacteria require 7 to 10 days to grow in culture.

Culture-negative peritonitis is seen with higher frequency in patients who are older than 70 years or in those who have different substances added to the dialysate (49). On repeated culture, an organism will be identified in approximately one third of the cases of initially culture-negative peritonitis (49). The outcomes of culture-positive and culture-negative peritonitis are similar (49).

Peripheral blood leukocytosis, usually in the range of 10,000 to 15,000/mm^3 with a shift to the left, is a common finding in continuous ambulatory peritoneal dialysis (CAPD) peritonitis. Although blood cultures are uniformly negative for organisms and unnecessary in uncomplicated cases, bacteremia may occur in the presence of coexistent intraabdominal or extraabdominal septic foci, including catheter tunnel infection. Blood cultures are indicated when this complication is suspected, because the principles governing treatment are modified.

A practical or working definition of peritonitis in CAPD, which is characterized by long-dwell exchanges, requires that two of the three criteria listed in Table 41.4 be fulfilled. Increasing numbers of PD patients receive automated peritoneal dialysis (APD), which is characterized by short-dwell exchanges and often one very long-dwell exchange at daytime [continuous cycling peritoneal dialysis (CCPD)]. The daytime long-dwell exchange during CCPD may produce cloudy dialysate in noninfected patients. Dialysate WBC count may exceed 100/mm^3 in these patients with a predominance of mononuclear cells. Symptoms and signs of peritonitis are absent, and the short-dwell exchanges following the cloudy long-dwell exchange produce clear effluent.

TABLE 41.3. CLINICAL MANIFESTATIONS OF CAPD PERITONITIS

Symptoms and Signs	Percent
Symptoms	
Cloudy dialysis effluent	98
Diffuse abdominal pain	78
Fever	35
Nausea	29
Vomiting	25
Chills	18
Poor outflow	15
Constipation	10
Diarrhea	7
Signs	
Abdominal tenderness	76
Temperature >37.5°C	50

CAPD, continuous ambulatory peritoneal dialysis.
Modified from Peterson DK, et al. Current concepts in the management of peritonitis in continuous ambulatory peritoneal dialysis patients. *Rev Infect Dis* 1987;9:604–612, with permission.

TABLE 41.4. DIAGNOSTIC CRITERIA FOR CAPD PERITONITIS

100 or more WBC/mm^3 of dialysate
Presence of clinical manifestations of CAPD peritonitis
Positive dialysate culture

CAPD, continuous ambulatory peritoneal dialysis; WBC, white blood cell.

Differential Diagnosis

Table 41.5 shows the differential diagnosis of CAPD-related peritonitis. Most of the conditions listed in this table can develop during the course of peritonitis. The reader is referred to other texts for detailed discussion of these syndromes. Here we discuss only chemical peritonitis, eosinophilic peritonitis, and peritonitis associated with intraabdominal pathology.

Chemical Peritonitis

Chemical peritonitis results from either usual components of the dialysate or additives, such as vancomycin. Heat sterilization of the dialysate causes the accumulation of several glucose degradation products (GDPs), which have multiple toxic effects on the peritoneal membrane. Acetaldehyde is one GDP that was identified as the cause of an epidemic of chemical peritonitis (50).

Eosinophilic Peritonitis

Eosinophilic peritonitis is diagnosed by the presence of ≥100 eosinophils per mm^3 of dialysate and can occur early after initiation of PD without evidence of infection (51), probably secondary to an allergic reaction to air accidentally introduced in the peritoneal cavity or to constituents of the peritoneal catheter such as plasticizer. Corticosteroids have been advocated for patients with abdominal pain (51).

Eosinophilic peritonitis can also develop during certain types of fungal peritonitis, such as those caused by *Alternaria, Aspergillus, Paecilomyces,* and *Fusarium.*

The use of intraperitoneal additives such as vancomycin (52) and streptokinase (53) can also result in eosinophilic peritonitis. These two situations create diagnostic difficulties, because they occur during infectious peritonitis. Clinicians should suspect this process if intraabdominal administration of either of these two agents leads to increased dialysate turbidity, WBCs, and eosinophilia in blood and dialysate effluent.

Finally, peritoneal eosinophilia may be associated with symptomatic peripheral blood eosinophilia, such as during asthma.

Peritonitis Associated with Intraabdominal Pathology

It is important to distinguish CAPD-associated peritonitis from peritonitis secondary to intraabdominal sepsis, although this distinction may be difficult to make. The two entities often have similar clinical presentation, but the courses and management are different. Neither severity nor localization of findings at presentation helps in making the distinction (54,55). Food or fecal material in the dialysate and dialysate diarrhea are very specific but insensitive for intraabdominal sepsis (55). As a result of employing faulty CAPD technique, pneumoperitoneum may be visible on plain abdominal roentgenograms in asymptomatic patients (56). However, large or increasing amounts of air in a patient with peritonitis should raise the suspicion of hollow viscus perforation. Dialysate and blood leukocyte counts tend to be higher in patients with intraabdominal septic events than in those with PD-associated peritonitis (57).

When intraabdominal catastrophe occurs, dialysate culture commonly yields multiple enteric organisms or less frequently one unusual enteric species. However, polymicrobial peritonitis may also result from contamination with skin bacterial species (58,59).

Enteric peritonitis can result from passage of bacteria through a more or less intact bowel wall, or severely compromised bowel integrity can result in wall perforation or necrosis. The passage of bacteria through a viable bowel wall may be promoted by otherwise silent diverticulosis or bowel ischemia. In susceptible individuals, relatively innocuous events such as treatment of constipation may facilitate the transmural passage of bacteria.

Peritonitis associated with severe compromise of the bowel wall integrity carries a high mortality risk (42,54,55,60). When this type of enteric peritonitis is suspected, prompt exploratory laparotomy should be considered because delays in corrective surgical intervention are associated with mortality (55).

In contrast, peritonitis not associated with hollow viscus gangrene or perforation can be treated medically (58,59,61). Most patients with this type of enteric peritonitis are able to continue PD, often with the same peritoneal catheter (59).

Management

The principles governing management of PD peritonitis include early initiation of antibiotics, use of bactericidal and safe agents delivered in therapeutic concentrations with the choice guided by culture results, and close monitoring for prevention of sequelae.

Patients should be educated about early manifestations of peritonitis and the importance of immediate consultation with a medical practitioner. The practice of providing PD patients living far from the dialysis center with antibiotics for home use has its uses. This practice can lead, however, to erratic or inappropriate treatment of peritonitis. We, therefore, suggest that the patients be evaluated and treated at a dialysis center or, if this is not possible, in the closest clinic or emergency room, which can then communicate with the nephrologist in charge. Most patients can be evaluated and treated in the clinic setting and will not require hospital admission. However, patients with hypotension, refractory nausea and vomiting precluding oral intake, severe abdominal pain, or toxic appearance warrant inpatient observation and care.

Patients with cloudy dialysate and abdominal symptoms should be given antibiotics immediately, even if results of the dialysate examinations are not yet completed. When available,

TABLE 41.5. DIFFERENTIAL DIAGNOSIS OF PERITONEAL DIALYSIS-RELATED PERITONITIS

Fibrin strands in the dialysate
Chylous ascites
Chemical peritonitis
Eosinophilic peritonitis
Pancreatitis
Abdominal lymphoma
Peritonitis associated with intraabdominal septic condition

the dialysate cell count and Gram stain can direct the initial choice of antibiotics. Three rapid exchanges, each containing 500 to 1,000 units of heparin, can be used in patients with poor catheter draining because of fibrin deposition and in those with severe abdominal discomfort. Thrombolytic agents (urokinase or streptokinase) can be instilled intraperitoneally in cases of fibrinous catheter obstruction.

Table 41.6 presents pharmacokinetics and dosing of antibiotics for PD peritonitis. Several types of antibiotic regimens for use in treating PD peritonitis have been published. We suggest that the scheme proposed by the ad hoc committees on peritonitis management provide good frameworks for the management of PD peritonitis in adults (62) and children (63).

TABLE 41.6. ANTIBIOTIC DOSING RECOMMENDATIONS FOR CAPD (ONLY) PATIENTS WITH AND WITHOUT RESIDUAL RENAL FUNCTION[a]

Drug	CAPD Intermittent Dosing (once/day)		CAPD Continuous Dosing (Per Liter Exchange)	
	Anuric	Nonanuric	Anuric	Nonanuric
Aminoglycosides				
Amikacin	2 mg/kg	Increase all doses by 25%	MD 24 mg	Increase all MD by 25%
Gentamicin	0.6 mg/kg		MD 8 mg	
Netilmicin	0.6 mg/kg		MD 8 mg	
Tobramycin	0.6 mg/kg		MD 8 mg	
Cephaloaporins				All LD same as anuric MD increase by 25%
Cefazolin	15 mg/kg	20 mg/kg	LD 500 mg, MD 125 mg	
Cephalothin	15 mg/kg	ND	LD 500 mg, MD 125 mg	MD, ND
Cephradine	15 mg/kg	ND	LD 500 mg, MD 125 mg	MD, ND
Cephalexin	500 mg po, qid	ND	As intermittent	MD, ND
Cefuroxime	400 mg po/IV, qd	ND	LD 200 mg, MD 100–200 mg	MD, ND
Ceftazidime	1000–1500 mg	ND	LD 250 mg, MD 125 mg	MD, ND
Ceftizoxime	1000 mg	ND	LD 250 mg, MD 125 mg	MD, ND
Penicillins				All LD same as anuric
Piperacillin	4000 mg IV, bid	ND	LD 4 g IV, MD 250 mg	MD, ND
Ampicillin	250–500 mg po, bid	ND	MD 125 or 250–500 mg po, bid	MD, ND
Dicloxacillin	250–500 mg po, qid	ND	250–500 mg po, qid	MD, ND
Oxacillin	ND	ND	MD 125 mg	MD, ND
Nafcillin	ND	No change	MD 125 mg	MD, no change
Amoxicillin	ND	ND	LD 250–500 mg, MD 50 mg	MD, ND
Penicillin G	ND	ND	LD 50,000 U, MD 25,000 U	MD, ND
Quinolones				
Ciprofloxacin	500 mg po, bid	ND	LD 50 mg, MD 25 mg	ND
Ofloxacin	400 mg po, then 200 mg po, qd	ND	As intermittent	ND
Others				
Vancomycin	15–30 mg/kg q 5–7 d	Increase doses by 25%	MD 30–50 mg/L	Increase MD by 25%
Teicoplanin	400 mg IP, bid	ND	LD 400 mg, MD 40 mg[b]	ND
Aztreonam	ND	ND	LD 1000 mg, MD 250 mg	ND
Clindamycin	ND	ND	LD 300 mg, MD 150 mg	ND
Metronidazole	250 mg po, bid	ND	As intermittent	ND
Rifampin	300 mg po, bid	ND	As intermittent	ND
Antifungals				All LD same as anuric
Amphotericin	NA	NA	MD 1.5 mg	NA
Flucytosine	2 g LD, then 1 g qd, po	ND	As intermittent	ND
Fluconazole	200 mg qd	ND	As intermittent	ND
Itraconazole	100 mg q 12 hr	100 mg q 12 hr	100 mg q 12 hr	100 mg q 12 hr
Antituberculars	Isoniazid 300 mg po, qd + rifampin 600 mg po, qd + pyrazinamide 1.5 g po, qd + pyridoxine 100 mg/d	ND	As intermittent	ND
Combinations				All LD same as anuric
Ampicillin/sulbactam	2 g q 12 hr	ND	LD 1000 mg, MD 100 mg	ND
Trimeth/sulfamethox	320/1600 mg po, q 1–2 days	ND	LD 320/1600 mg po, MD 80/400 mg po	ND

bid, twice per day; CAPD, continuous ambulatory peritoneal dialysis; IP, intraperitoneally; LD, loading dose; MD, maintenance dose; NA, not applicable; ND, no data; po, oral; qd, once per day; qid, four times per day.
CAPD patients with residual renal function may require increased doses or more frequent dosing, especially when using intermittent regimens. For penicillins: No change is for those predominantly hepatically metabolized or hepatically metabolized and renally excreted; ND means no data but these are predominantly renally excreted, therefore probably an increase in dose by 25% is warranted; NA, not applicable, that is, drug is extensively metabolized and therefore there should be no difference in dosing between anuric and nonanuric patients. Anuric is <100 mL urine/24 hours; nonanuric is >100 mL/24 hours. These data for CAPD only.
[a]The route of administration is IIP unless otherwise specified. The pharmacokinetic data and proposed dosage regimens presented here are based on published literature reviewed through January 2000 or established clinical practice. There is no evidence that mixing different antibiotics in dialysis fluid (except for aminoglycosides and penicillins) is deleterious to the drugs or patients. Do not use the same syringe to mix antibiotics.
[b]This is in each bag × 7 days, then in 2 bags/day × 7 days, and then in 1 bag/day × 7 days.
Reprinted from Keane WF, et al. Adult peritoneal dialysis-related peritonitis treatment recommendations: 2000 update. *Perit Dial Int* 2000;20:396–411, with permission.

TABLE 41.7. EMPIRIC INITIAL THERAPY FOR PERITONEAL DIALYSIS-RELATED PERITONITIS, STRATIFIED FOR RESIDUAL URINE VOLUME

Antibiotic	Residual Urine Output	
	<100 mL/day	>100 mL/day
Cefazolin or cephalothin	1 g/bag, qd or 15 mg/kg BW/bag, qd	20 mg/kg BW/bag, qd
Ceftazidime	1 g/bag, qd	20 mg/kg BW/bag, qd
Gentamicin, tobramycin, netilmycin	0.6 mg/kg BW/bag, qd	Not recommended
Amikacin	2 mg/kg BW/bag, qd	Not recommended

BW, body weight; qd, once per day.
Reprinted from Keane WF, et al. Adult peritoneal dialysis-related peritonitis treatment recommendations: 2000 update. *Perit Dial Int* 2000;20:396–411, with permission.

Table 41.7 shows the recommended initial empiric treatment of peritonitis when there is no indication of the type of causative agent in a Gram stain. The treatment consists of a combination of a first-generation cephalosporin with either ceftazidime or an aminoglycoside, depending on whether there is substantial residual renal function or not. The medications are infused intraperitoneally once every day.

Gram-positive Peritonitis

Vancomycin was the antibiotic of choice for the treatment of Gram-positive peritonitis for more than a decade. The emergence of vancomycin-resistant enterococci (VRE), which are also resistant to penicillin and aminoglycosides, has necessitated that vancomycin use be limited to certain infections, including those caused by methicillin-resistant *S. aureus,* beta-lactam-resistant organisms, Gram-positive organisms in patients allergic to alternative antibiotics, and *Clostridium difficile* enterocolitis not responding to metronidazole (62). VRE appears to be uncommon in dialysis outpatients requiring vancomycin. However, VRE peritonitis follows a particularly severe course with mortality exceeding 40% (64).

The results of the culture of the dialysate should guide the use of antibiotics. Table 41.8 shows the recommended treatment for Gram-positive peritonitis in adult patients on CAPD (62). Ampicillin plus aminoglycosides is the regimen of choice for *Enterococcus* peritonitis. Cephalosporin alone is continued for all Gram-positive infections, except those caused by *S. aureus* for which rifampin is added to the cephalosporin while the aminoglycoside is discontinued. Treatment is continued for 21 days for *S. aureus* infections and 14 days for all other Gram-positive infections.

Gram-negative Peritonitis

Table 41.9 shows the treatment of Gram-negative peritonitis. With the exception of the *Pseudomonas* and *Stenotrophomonas* group, all Gram-negative infections can be treated with one drug only. Two antibiotics are recommended for infections caused by *Pseudomonas* or *Stenotrophomonas,* but the semisynthetic penicillins inactivate aminoglycosides in solution and should not be administered by the same route. Duration of treatment is 21 days for infections caused by *Pseudomonas* and *Stenotrophomonas* or multiple Gram-negative bacteria and 14 days for infections by a single Gram-negative species.

TABLE 41.8. TREATMENT STRATEGIES AFTER IDENTIFICATION OF GRAM-POSITIVE ORGANISM ON CULTURE

Enterococcus	Staphylococcus aureus	Other Gram-Positive Organism (Coagulase-Negative Staphylococcus)
At 24 to 48 hours		
Stop cephalosporins	Stop ceftazidime or aminoglycoside	Stop ceftazidime or aminoglycoside
Start ampicillin 125 mg/L/bag	Continue cephalosporin	Continue cephalosporin
Consider adding aminoglycoside	Add rifampin 600 mg/day, oral	
If ampicillin-resistant, start vancomycin or clindamycin	If MRSA, start vancomycin or clindamycin	If MRSE and clinically not responding, start vancomycin or clindamycin
If VRE, consider quinupristin/dalfopristin		
Duration of therapy		
14 days	21 days	14 days
At 96 hours		
If no improvement, reculture and evaluate for exit-site or tunnel infection, catheter colonization, etc.		
Choice of final therapy should always be guided by antibiotic sensitivities		

MRSA, methicillin-resistant *S. aureus;* MRSE, methicillin-resistant enterococcus; VRE, vancomycin-resistant enterococcus.
Reprinted from Keane WF, et al. Adult peritoneal dialysis-related peritonitis treatment recommendations: 2000 update. *Perit Dial Int* 2000;20:396–411, with permission.

TABLE 41.9. TREATMENT RECOMMENDATIONS IF A GRAM-NEGATIVE ORGANISM IS IDENTIFIED ON CULTURE AT 24 TO 48 HOURS

Organism	Treatment	Duration of Therapy
Single Gram-negative organism	Adjust antibiotics to sensitivity <100 mL urine, aminoglycoside >100 mL urine, ceftazidime	14 days
Pseudomonas/Stenotrophomonas	Continue ceftazidime and add <100 mL urine, aminoglycoside >100 mL urine, ciprofloxacin 500 mg, po bid or piperacillin 4 g IV q 12 hours or sulfamethoxazole/trimethoprim 1–2 DS/day or aztreonam load 1 g/L; maintenance dose 250 mg/L IP/bag	21 days
Multiple Gram-negatives and/or anaerobes	Continue cefazolin and ceftazidime and add metronidazole, 500 mg q 8 hours, po, IV, or rectally If no change in clinical status, consider surgical intervention	21 days

DS, double strength; IP, intraperitoneally.
Reprinted from Keane WF, et al. Adult peritoneal dialysis-related peritonitis treatment recommendations: 2000 update. *Perit Dial Int* 2000;20:396–411, with permission.

Aminoglycosides are effective but carry a high risk of ototoxicity, particularly when used continuously. Intermittent administration, once daily in a 6-hour exchange, appears to be less ototoxic and has prolonged effect on bacteria after the blood levels of the aminoglycosides have decreased below the minimum inhibitory concentration (MIC). Residual renal function, which has been shown to be of great importance in the survival of PD patients, is adversely affected by the use of aminoglycosides (65,66). Isolation of a Gram-negative anaerobe should raise concern for possible bowel perforation. In addition to the other antibiotics, the patient growing anaerobes should receive metronidazole intravenously, orally, or per rectum in a dose of 500 mg three times daily and should be thoroughly investigated for other signs of intraabdominal pathology.

Culture-negative Peritonitis

Table 41.10 shows the treatment of culture-negative peritonitis. The course and management will depend on the response to initial antibiotic therapy and the results of repeated cultures. The peritoneal catheter should be removed within 5 to 10 days if the cultures remain negative and peritonitis is not resolving.

Fungal Peritonitis

Candida species account for three fourths of fungal infections. *Candida* (especially *Candida albicans*) peritonitis can be treated conservatively in some instances. Prior use of antibiotics (67–70) and the immunosuppressed state (67) are risk factors for fungal peritonitis. A high level of suspicion is required to make the diagnosis of fungal peritonitis. Although *Candida* species can grow in fewer than 5 days, some of the fungi, particularly molds, may require several weeks. Thus, in culture-negative peritonitis, this diagnosis should be kept in mind. Noncandidal fungal infections are more difficult to eradicate.

Table 41.11 shows the current recommendations for treatment of fungal peritonitis. A trial of an imidazole or thiazole is warranted, with careful daily follow-up of the patients. A decision to remove the catheter or continue with the conservative treatment should be made within a week of treatment initiation (62). If the catheter is removed, the patient requires an additional 10 days' therapy with fluconazole or flucytosine. If the catheter is not removed, treatment should continue for 4 to 6 weeks. A small number of peritoneal catheters have been salvaged using this strategy, but the typical catheter loss rate is 85% to 96% (67–70). The optimal waiting period before new catheter insertion has not been established, but common practice involves a 6-week period of hemodialysis. Primary (early)

TABLE 41.10. TREATMENT STRATEGIES IF PERITONEAL DIALYSIS FLUID CULTURES ARE NEGATIVE AT 24 TO 48 HOURS OR NOT PERFORMED

		Duration of Therapy
Continue initial therapy		
If clinical improvement	Discontinue ceftazidime or aminoglycoside Continue cephalosporin	14 days
If no clinical improvement at 96 hours	Repeat cell count, Gram stain, and culture	
If culture positive, adjust therapy accordingly		14 days
If culture negative, continue antibiotics, consider infrequent pathogens and/or catheter removal		14 days

Reprinted from Keane WF, et al. Adult peritoneal dialysis-related peritonitis treatment recommendations: 2000 update. *Perit Dial Int* 2000;20:396–411, with permission.

TABLE 41.11. TREATMENT RECOMMENDATIONS IF YEAST OR OTHER FUNGUS IDENTIFIED ON GRAM STAIN OR CULTURE

At 24 to 48 hours	
Flucytosine	Loading dose 2 g po; maintenance dose 1 g po
and	
Fluconazole	200 mg, po, or intraperitoneally, daily
If organism is resistant, consider itraconozole	
At 4 to 7 days	
If clinical improvement, duration of therapy 4–6 weeks	
If no clinical improvement, remove catheter and continue therapy for 7 days after catheter removal	

Reprinted from Keane WF, et al. Adult peritoneal dialysis-related peritonitis treatment recommendations: 2000 update. *Perit Dial Int* 2000;20:396–411, with permission.

catheter loss in fungal peritonitis is approximately 70%, with an additional 20% requiring transfer to hemodialysis following antifungal drug failure. Mortality, at 15% to 20% (69,70) is much higher than in other types of PD-associated peritonitis.

Mycobacterial Peritonitis

M. tuberculosis and other mycobacteria including fast-growing species *(Mycobacterium chelonae, Mycobacterium fortuitum)* are rare causes of PD-associated peritonitis. Isolation of mycobacteria from the dialysate requires special culture media and long periods of incubation of the cultures (7 to 10 days for fast-growing species, 6 weeks for other mycobacterial species). Rapid detection of mycobacterial peritonitis may be achieved by peritoneal or omental biopsy or by amplification of mycobacterial ribonucleic acid (RNA) using polymerase chain reaction.

PD-related *M. tuberculosis* peritonitis typically arises by hematogenous spread in patients with an inadequately treated primary infection. Clinical presentation resembles that seen with more common forms of peritonitis, although dialysate mononuclear cells may predominate. Acid-fast stains are often negative, and mycobacterial cultures usually require 6 weeks. Extraction of mycobacterial deoxyribonucleic acid (DNA) from the dialysate and subsequent amplification by polymerase chain reaction can be used for early detection. The catheter must be removed in most instances. Drug treatment requires three agents, for example, 1 year of daily isoniazid 300 mg, rifampin 600 mg, and pyrazinamide 1.5 g (62).

Peritonitis caused by fast-growing mycobacteria is thought to result from water contamination. These organisms can be detected by dialysate acid-fast stain and culture. Management consists of both catheter removal and prolonged (6 month) administration of antibiotics guided by sensitivities, with macrolides and aminoglycosides the mainstay of treatment. *Mycobacterium avium complex* (MAC) peritonitis, often fatal in patients with AIDS, is otherwise treatable, but it poses diagnostic difficulties because dialysate WBC count may be low for months.

Viral Peritonitis

There are few documented cases of CAPD peritonitis caused by viruses (71). Much more important are the reports of peritonitis in human immunodeficiency virus (HIV)-positive patients.

Both a higher incidence of CAPD peritonitis (72) and a greater frequency of severe infections (73) have been reported in these individuals. Thus, prevention and successful management of CAPD peritonitis in this population is of paramount importance.

Of equal concern is the need to properly dispose of potentially infectious spent dialysate from which the virus has been isolated (74). Strict observation of universal precautions is essential, including use of gowns, goggles, and gloves when handling the dialysate, disposal of the dialysate in the sewer, and disposal of tubing and dialysate bags in separate plastic bags. Patients and close contacts should be trained in the application of these measures (74).

APD Peritonitis and PD-associated Peritonitis in Children

The doses of antibiotics discussed so far refer to patients on CAPD. The pharmacokinetics of antibiotics differ, in general, between CAPD and APD (75). Table 41.12 shows antibiotic doses for patients on APD (62). The schemes and doses of antibiotics presented here are those for adult patients with peritonitis. The reader is referred to the pediatric guidelines (63) for schemes and doses for treatment of PD-associated peritonitis in children (also, see Chapter 40).

Outcomes

Table 41.13 describes the major outcomes of CAPD peritonitis. The frequency of each outcome was computed from the series of Tranaeus et al. (45) and from our series of 167 peritonitis episodes (unpublished observation). The death rate was derived from the series of Digenis et al. (76), Krishnan et al. (77), and our own study (78).

Routine Peritonitis

Peritonitis caused by non-*S. aureus* Gram-positive bacteria is cleared by 96 hours in more than 80% of cases (79). *S. aureus* peritonitis, however, is more often persistent (79). Some non-*Pseudomonas* Gram-negative infections can follow a routine course (79), typified by rapid resolution of abdominal pain, defervescence, and clearing of the dialysate within 48 hours, although occasionally symptoms may persist for up to 96 hours.

TABLE 41.12. DOSING OF ANTIBIOTICS, BY IP INTERMITTENT ROUTE, IN AUTOMATED PD

Drug	Dose
Piperacillin[a]	4000 mg IV, bid
Vancomycin[a]	Loading dose 35 mg/kg
	Maintenance dose 15 mg/kg IP qd
Cefazolin[b]	20 mg/kg qd, in first or second ambulatory dwell
Tobramycin[b]	Loading dose 1.5 mg/kg day 1
	Maintenance dose 0.5 mg/kg qd, in first or second ambulatory dwell
Fluconazole	200 mg IP, q 24–48 hr

These data for automated peritoneal dialysis only.
bid, two times daily; IP, intraperitoneal; PD, peritoneal dialysis; qd, every day.
Unless otherwise specified, IP doses to be added to the 1st ambulatory dwell after the automated exchanges.
[a]Unpublished data.
[b]*J Am Soc Nephrol* 2000;11:1310–16.
Reprinted from Keane WF, et al. Adult peritoneal dialysis-related peritonitis treatment recommendations: 2000 update. *Perit Dial Int* 2000;20:396–411, with permission.

Persistent Peritonitis

If symptoms and dialysate leukocytosis fail to improve after 5 days of appropriate therapy, the disease is termed persistent (or refractory). Patients with persistent infection should be evaluated with repeated examination of the effluent dialysate, with attention to fungal or mycobacterial cause, and be carefully examined for intraabdominal pathology (62). Certain causative agents are strongly associated with persistence of CAPD peritonitis. *Pseudomonas* peritonitis virtually always follows a persistent course (79). A similar natural history is seen for peritonitis caused by fungi, *M. tuberculosis,* and fast-growing mycobacteria. Host factors such as advanced age (80), diabetes (45), or long duration of PD (77) may predispose patients to persistence of the infection.

The management of persistent peritonitis depends on the causative agent. For both *S. aureus* and coagulase-negative staphylococcal infections, rifampin in an oral dose of 300 mg twice daily is added to the first-generation cephalosporins. Van-

comycin may have a use also in these cases. If after 2 to 3 days of combined antibiotic management the infection fails to abate, the peritoneal catheter should be removed.

Peritonitis caused by *Pseudomonas* species is notoriously resistant to treatment (81–83), because this organism is highly adherent to Tenckhoff catheter material (84) and has a propensity to cause tunnel infections (85). Catheter infections caused by *Pseudomonas aeruginosa* with or without associated peritonitis result in catheter loss more frequently than do catheter infections caused by other organisms (81) and necessitate permanent transfer to hemodialysis (82). A high percentage of patients with *Pseudomonas* peritonitis also have exit-site and tunnel infection with the same organism (82,83). Even when *Pseudomonas* peritonitis responds to medical therapy, the treatment should be prolonged for at least 3 to 4 weeks. Early removal of the peritoneal catheter should be considered in cases that fail to improve within 96 hours.

Even when antibiotic treatment is prolonged to salvage the peritoneal catheter, removal becomes necessary in at least 60%

TABLE 41.13. OUTCOMES OF PD PERITONITIS

Outcome	Characteristic Features	Associated Features	Percent
Routine course	Cure within 96 hours of initiation of appropriate treatment	Gram-positive bacteria other than *Staphylococcus aureus*	54–66
Persistence	Persistence of symptoms and signs, positive cultures, and elevated dialysate WBC beyond 96 hours of appropriate antibiotic treatment	*Pseudomonas, Aeromonas,* fungi, mycobacteria Advanced age Diabetes	13–39
Relapse	Recurrence of peritonitis with the same organism within 30 days of treatment cessation	*Staphylococcus* species Peritoneal catheter biofilm Tunnel or intraabdominal abscess	8–16
Catheter loss	Removal of peritoneal catheter	Mycobacteria, fungi, *Pseudomonas* Persistence, relapse severity Simultaneous tunnel infection Intraabdominal pathology	15–20
Discontinuation of peritoneal dialysis (permanent)	Permanent transfer to hemodialysis	Ultrafiltration loss Extensive adhesions Solute clearance loss Patient choice	5–6
Death	Death from sepsis caused by peritonitis	None	1–3

PD, peritoneal dialysis; WBC, white blood count.

of the cases with persistent peritonitis (65). Adverse effects of prolonged peritoneal inflammation on anatomic and functional peritoneal membrane integrity and on patient nutrition (79) dictate early (after 120 hours) peritoneal catheter removal in poorly responsive patients.

Relapsing Peritonitis

Relapsing peritonitis is diagnosed when infection with the same organism recurs within 1 month of completion of appropriate antimicrobial treatment. Until culture results are obtained, the patients should be treated for Gram-positive and Gram-negative organisms, while the possibility of fungal infection is also entertained. Relapsing peritonitis typically occurs in episodes involving *S. aureus* and *S. epidermidis* (86), but *Pseudomonas* peritonitis may also relapse. Viable bacteria are sequestered in sites where antibiotic penetration is difficult, such as intraabdominal abscesses, fibrin aggregations (87), and exit sites and subcutaneous tunnels. An important reservoir of viable bacteria, particularly exopolysaccharide (slime) producing coagulase-negative staphylococci, is the biofilm coating the catheter wall (88,89). Incomplete drainage of the peritoneal cavity also favors bacterial survival. Residual volumes of 800 mL or greater facilitate the persistence of *S. epidermidis,* whereas volumes as small as 200 mL appear to favor the survival of *S. aureus* (90). Low trough levels of antibiotics may also be associated with relapse.

The evaluation of relapsing peritonitis should include a careful clinical examination, sonogram, computerized tomographic scan, and indium-labeled leukocyte scan to exclude intraabdominal or catheter tunnel abscess (53,91). Rifampin should be added to vancomycin, as in cases of persistent peritonitis. If these measures fail, the intraperitoneal infusion of a thrombolytic agent may yield positive results in 30% to 50% of instances (53,92). Urokinase is associated with fewer systemic side effects (e.g., fever, chills) and local reactions (e.g., bleeding, allergic or chemical peritonitis) than streptokinase (53).

Relapsing peritonitis leads to catheter loss in as many as 78% of cases (86). Following catheter removal, the traditional approach dictates a 2-week waiting period before insertion of a new catheter. However, infected catheter removal and new catheter insertion can safely take place in the same setting as long as antibiotics are continued (92,93). Another approach is to leave the infected catheter in situ but unused, while temporary hemodialysis is performed and antibiotics are continued for 2 to 3 weeks, at which time CAPD is resumed (94).

We generally favor catheter removal followed by a waiting period, unless hemodialysis is contraindicated on medical, geographic, or other logistical grounds. Particularly for malnourished patients, a short course of hemodialysis with attention to nutrition may be beneficial.

Septic Death

Septic death during CAPD peritonitis is associated with delays in therapy, (particularly in catheter removal in refractory cases), abscess formation, advanced age, and malnutrition (76).

Sequelae

CAPD peritonitis may lead to temporary or permanent sequelae, of which the most common are listed in Table 41.14.

Peritoneal Adhesions

Extensive peritoneal adhesions caused by intraperitoneal fibrin accumulation (95) may develop after severe episodes of peritonitis, especially those involving *P. aeruginosa* and *S. aureus.* Damage to both the visceral and the parietal peritoneal layers is necessary for adhesion development.

Peritoneal mesothelial cells produce tissue plasminogen activator (tPA), which may play a role in preventing adhesion development in association with CAPD peritonitis. Adhesions may, thus, be a consequence of an absolute or relative decrease in peritoneal tPA activity.

Some CAPD patients display high plasma levels of plasminogen activation inhibitor-I (96); they may be at increased risk for adhesion formation after peritonitis. The synthesis of hyaluronic acid by mesothelial cells, enhanced by IL-1b during peritonitis, may also decrease adhesion formation.

The use of frequent exchanges containing antibiotics (97) and several experimental compounds have been proposed as means of reducing adhesion formation.

Peritoneal Fibrosing Syndromes

Several degrees of peritoneal fibrosis have been recognized in CAPD (98). Fibrosis of the serosa and the outer longitudinal muscle layer, with fibrous bands encasing bowel loops (see Chapter 15), is called sclerosing encapsulating peritonitis and is clinically manifested by repeated bouts of intestinal obstruction with progressive malnutrition, associated with a mortality rate of 20% to 70% (98).

Sclerosing encapsulating peritonitis has been statistically associated with a high frequency of severe peritonitis (99). In animal models of CAPD, infection is clearly associated with fibrosis (100). Mesothelial cells prevent fibrosis by the release of tPA, prostacyclin, and surfactant, and they also control peritoneal inflammation through cytokine release (36). Destruction of mesothelial cells during peritonitis has been proposed as the initiating event in fibrosis (98). Stimulation of peritoneal fibroblasts may amplify fibrosis via cytokine release. Severe peritonitis episodes can denude the peritoneal membrane, with the resultant inability to lyse fibrin. Consequently, fibroblasts are able to invade the organized fibrin.

TABLE 41.14. SEQUELAE OF CAPD PERITONITIS

Intraperitoneal adhesions
Diffuse peritoneal fibrosis
Sclerosing encapsulating peritonitis
Loss of ultrafiltration
Malnutrition
Septic events
Increased mortality from nonseptic (cardiac) causes

CAPD, continuous ambulatory peritoneal dialysis.

Imbalance between fibrin formation and removal in the extravascular spaces may lead to progressive peritoneal fibrosis (101). Serum cancer antigen 125 (CA 125) levels reflect the number and metabolic activity of peritoneal mesothelial cells. An increase in serum CA 125 levels during peritonitis is seen with increased turnover in mesothelial cells, whereas low CA 125 levels indicate a denuded fibrosed peritoneal membrane (102).

Cytokines released during peritonitis, such as IL-1 and γ-interferon, may stimulate fibroblastic activity. Growth factors, such as transforming factor beta (103) or hepatocyte growth factor (104) promote peritoneal fibrosis during episodes of peritonitis. Increased levels of metalloproteinase in the peritoneal fluid during episodes of peritonitis lead to remodeling of the peritoneal extracellular matrix and may contribute to the development of fibrosis (105). Early removal of the peritoneal catheter in severe peritonitis, minimal use of hypertonic dialysate during peritonitis episodes, and resting of the peritoneum when feasible are measures proposed to prevent peritoneal fibrosis syndromes.

Loss of Ultrafiltration and Loss of Peritoneal Solute Clearance

Peritonitis-associated peritoneal inflammation and increased peritoneal capillary blood flow lead to greater permeability to solutes, with accelerated loss of serum proteins and a rapid decrease in dialysate glucose concentration. Elevated levels of TNF-α and IL-6 precede these transport changes (106), which accompany peritoneal vasodilation mediated by vasodilators such as nitric oxide (NO) formed intraperitoneally from macrophages and other cell lines. The increases in solute permeability and peritoneal blood flow cause a decrease in net ultrafiltration.

In most cases, peritoneal and solute transport characteristics revert to baseline within 6 weeks of successful treatment. However, frequent episodes of peritonitis may lead to permanent increases in peritoneal transport (107,108), with irreversible loss of ultrafiltration capability linked to peritoneal fibrosis (109).

Metabolic Sequelae of CAPD Peritonitis

CAPD peritonitis adversely affects metabolism in various ways. Daily baseline transperitoneal protein losses in CAPD patients, typically ranging from 5 to 15 g, include the entire spectrum of proteins found in serum and intestinal lymph (110,111). With the development of peritonitis, protein losses in peritoneal dialysate increase by 50% to 100% (111,112). The problem is compounded by poor protein and calorie intake because of nausea, vomiting, anorexia, and abdominal pain. Hepatic albumin synthesis is decreased by effects of inflammatory cytokines.

Stated simply, peritonitis worsens malnutrition. In routine episodes, malnutrition is not detectable (111) or minimal (79). In our study, average decreases during routine episodes of peritonitis were 2% for body weight and 9% for serum albumin (79). Malnutrition can be severe, however, in complicated cases of CAPD peritonitis. We reported an average decrease of 7% in

body weight and 32% in serum albumin during persistent peritonitis (79).

Whether intravenous alimentation can prevent such profound malnutrition in severe peritonitis is not known. Metabolic acidosis frequently complicates peritonitis. In Gram-negative infections, the metabolic acidosis may be accompanied by respiratory acidosis (113) with direct adverse effects on nutrition. Thus, avoidance of malnutrition is an important reason to consider prompt catheter removal during persistent peritonitis (79).

Septic Sequelae and Delayed Mortality

Septic sequelae of CAPD peritonitis include fungal superinfection, intraperitoneal abscess formation, and, rarely, disseminated sepsis.

Abscesses develop in fewer than 1% of infections (114), with organisms recovered including *S. aureus* (115), *Pseudomonas* (114), and *Candida* (114); abscesses are diagnosed by abdominal ultrasound, computed tomography scans, and indium scans (114).

Toxic shock can follow *S. aureus* peritonitis. Shock with leukopenia and digital gangrene has also been observed in *Pseudomonas* peritonitis. The development of septic portal vein thrombosis is rare.

In addition to the direct mortality from sepsis, there is also an indirect but clear association between frequent episodes of PD peritonitis and mortality (116). Deaths tend to occur within 1 month of the onset of peritonitis, usually after removal of the peritoneal catheter and in the absence of clinical features of infection. Although the deaths are mainly cardiac in nature, this delayed mortality is statistically associated with persistent peritonitis, *P. aeruginosa* infection, severe malnutrition, and diabetes mellitus (78).

In addition to mortality, several other outcomes of PD-related peritonitis are far worse with infections caused by Gram-negative bacteria and *S. aureus* than those caused by other Gram-positive cocci (117,118).

Prevention

The most successful efforts aimed at preventing CAPD peritonitis have addressed the problem of accidental contamination. Patient and family education in aseptic technique is critical and cannot be overemphasized. Improvements to the PD apparatus, particularly the connecting devices, have significantly reduced the incidence of peritonitis.

The use of double-bag or Y-set transfer systems has reduced the incidence of PD peritonitis (119). This encouraging fact should be viewed in the proper perspective, however. The new disconnect systems have decreased the frequency of peritonitis caused by touch contamination, which usually involves skin flora such as coagulase-negative staphylococci and is less severe. Unfortunately, the incidence of peritonitis caused by more virulent pathogens, such as enteric Gram-negative bacilli and *S. aureus,* has not been reduced (120).

Other strategies employed to prevent peritonitis have not been as successful. They are discussed in the next section.

EXIT-SITE AND TUNNEL INFECTIONS

Infections of the peritoneal catheter exit site and tunnel are usually discussed together, because a clear distinction is not always possible. Although less common than CAPD peritonitis, these infections arouse great concern, because (a) they are persistent and often dictate catheter removal (121) and (b) in contrast to peritonitis, which has declined in frequency in recent years, their apparent incidence has remained stable at approximately 0.6 episodes per patient-year. This incidence may be misleading because acute episodes of exit-site and tunnel infection responding to treatment within 3 to 4 weeks are usually classified the same as chronic episodes requiring antibiotics for months (122). Occasionally, the delay between apparent cure of exit-site infection and onset of peritonitis with the same microorganism may be several months (123).

Diagnosis

The diagnosis of exit-site and tunnel infection presents difficulties not encountered with CAPD peritonitis. Table 41.15 presents Twardowski et al.'s (124) classification of the morphology of the exit site.

Gentle manipulation of the catheter allows expression of drainage and inspection of the catheter sinus (125). Certain manifestations such as erythema, pericatheter induration, and serosanguineous drainage from the exit site are signs of either exit-site infection or trauma, which predisposes patients to infection (126). Purulent discharge from the exit site is considered a clear sign of infection (127) and is a risk factor for catheter loss (123). Occasionally, exit-site infection presents as hypertrophic, friable tissue with purple discoloration, the so-called proud flesh.

Bacteriologic studies of the exit site can be difficult to interpret. Dry swabs of the exit site or cultures of serosanguineous exudate will usually reveal skin flora unrelated to the cause of infection. Even recovery of *S. aureus* in culture should be interpreted in the context of the clinical picture, because chronic dialysis patients are frequently staphylococcal carriers. Infection may develop several months after colonization of the exit site

with the same bacterial species. However, recovery of a single species of bacteria from a purulent exudate is a fairly reliable indicator of the cause of exit-site infection, generally *S. aureus*, *S. epidermidis*, or *Pseudomonas* species (128).

Tunnel infections can occasionally develop in the absence of exit-site infection (128). The diagnosis of deep tunnel infection requires special effort. In some cases, there are no clinical clues suggesting tunnel infection other than relapsing or persistent peritonitis (53). In other cases, dialysate cultures may remain positive after apparent cure of staphylococcal CAPD peritonitis (115). Ultrasonography is a sensitive and relatively inexpensive method of demonstrating a fluid collection in the tunnel (91,129,130). Indium scan and computed tomography may also be useful (53,115). Tunnel ultrasonography is indicated in patients with persistent or recurrent exit-site infection, those with simultaneous exit-site infection and peritonitis, those with relapsing peritonitis, and (for prognostic purposes) those treated for tunnel infection (131).

Management

The management of exit-site infection is shown in Fig. 41.3. Empiric antibiotic therapy should be started as soon as the diagnosis is made. Oral first-generation cephalosporins (cephradine, cephalexin) or penicillinase-resistant semisynthetic penicillins (dicloxacillin) can be used against sensitive staphylococci (132). Sulfamethoxazole-trimethoprim may also be used (133). Prolonged treatment courses, usually 4 weeks or longer, are required (132).

Quinolones reach therapeutic tissue levels and are commonly used against both Gram-positive and Gram-negative organisms, but their absorption may be reduced with concurrent ingestion of calcium salts, iron salts, zinc preparations, sucralfate, magnesium/aluminum antacids, and milk. Therefore, a period of 2 hours between the ingestion of ciprofloxacin, which should be taken first, and the other preparations is recommended (134). *Pseudomonas* exit-site infections require long treatment courses, and, if aminoglycosides are used, blood levels should be monitored.

TABLE 41.15. EXIT-SITE APPEARANCE

Classification	Clinical Characteristics
Acute infection	Pain, swelling, erythema ≥13 mm, purulent/bloody external drainage, sinus not entirely covered with epithelium, exuberant granulation tissue ("proud flesh") in exit-site/sinus, duration <4 weeks
Chronic infection	Purulent/bloody external discharge, sinus not entirely covered with epithelium, exuberant granulation tissue, duration >4 weeks; pain, swelling, erythema may be absent
External cuff infection without exit-site infection	Intermittent or chronic purulent/bloody "gluey" drainage after pressure on the cuff, intermittent or chronic maceration of epithelium in the sinus, proud flesh deep in the sinus, sinus covered with epithelium, tenderness/induration of tissues around the cuff, exit site looks normal
Equivocal exit	Purulent/bloody drainage expressed by pressure on the sinus, sinus not entirely covered with epithelium, slightly exuberant granulation tissue in exit/sinus, no pain, no swelling/redness >13 mm in diameter
Good exit	Epidermis covering part of sinus, epithelium covering the rest of sinus, thick drainage in sinus, specks of crust on dressing, no pain/swelling/redness/external drainage/exuberant granulation tissue
Perfect exit	Exit at least 6 months old, only epidermis in sinus, sinus track dry or with minute amount of clear or thick drainage, specks of crust on dressing, natural exit-site color, no pain/swelling/red or pink color around the exit/external drainage/granulation tissue
Exit trauma	Trauma, pain, bleeding, crusts, deterioration of exit appearance

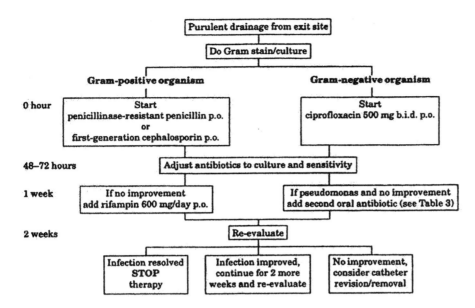

FIG. 41.3. Management of exit site infection. (Reprinted from Keane WF, et al. Adult peritoneal dialysis-related peritonitis treatment recommendations: 2000 update. *Perit Dial Int* 2000;20:396–411, with permission.)

Antibiotic sensitivities should guide the choice of agents used against unusual pathogens. Adjunctive therapy includes increased frequency of exit-site care (135) and application of compresses saturated with hypertonic saline (136). Local antibiotic preparations should not be used for the treatment of exit-site infections but may be indicated for the care of equivocal exit sites (123,137). Exit-site infection manifested as proud flesh can be managed by silver nitrate cauterization, repeated if necessary (127), with care taken to avoid touching healthy skin with the silver nitrate sticks.

Persistence of exit-site infection beyond 4 weeks of appropriate antibiotic treatment is considered an indication for surgical intervention. The usual procedure, especially for infections caused by *S. aureus,* is tunnel exploration and removal or "shaving" of the outer catheter cuff (127). If the infectious exudate encroaches on the inner cuff, the peritoneal catheter should be removed (138) and antibiotics continued for at least 7 to 10 days before implantation of a new catheter through a different route. The minimal waiting period before new catheter placement is extended to 3 to 4 weeks if peritonitis coexists (127).

For *Pseudomonas* tunnel infections, shaving of the outer cuff and draining of the tunnel abscess are unlikely to effect a cure. Many believe that persistence of *Pseudomonas* exit-site infection beyond 3 weeks of appropriate antibiotic coverage automatically mandates catheter removal (132). Deep tunnel infections without exit-site infections, in our experience, invariably lead to catheter loss (53,115).

Prevention

The prevention of exit-site and tunnel infection should involve efforts to minimize risk factors. The association between exit-site trauma and infection was discussed earlier. Careful anchoring of the catheter and avoidance of any potentially traumatic movements or procedures are of paramount importance. Nasal carriage with *S. aureus* is a risk factor for staphylococcal exit-site infection and staphylococcal peritonitis (139–142). Eradication of the nasal carriage led to a substantial reduction of the incidence of staphylococcal exit-site infection (143). Both oral rifampin and topical mupirocin are effective in reducing staphylococcal nasal carriage. Further studies are required to establish the effectiveness of mupirocin or rifampin in the prevention of tunnel infection or peritonitis (144).

Rifampin is taken in a dose of 300 mg twice a day for 5 days every 12 weeks, whereas mupirocin ointment is applied in the nares three times daily for 7 days for each positive nasal culture and then two times daily for 5 days each month. In addition, mupirocin is applied daily on the exit site during exit-site care. Mupirocin is well tolerated, but rifampin causes severe nausea and vomiting in a substantial number of patients and abnormal liver function tests in a smaller number of patients. However, emergence of staphylococcal strains resistant to mupirocin has been reported after long-term use of the agent in PD patients (145). Staphylococcal vaccines have proven ineffective. Prophylactic antibiotics before PD catheter placement and after breaks in PD technique are potentially useful (62).

Other risk factors for exit-site infection include the type and position of the peritoneal catheter exit (see later), wound hematoma, diabetes, and obesity (146,147). Preventive measures for exit-site and tunnel infections have been directed toward optimizing catheter design and implantation techniques. The Tenckhoff peritoneal catheter (148) is still widely used. The two-cuff Tenckhoff catheter configuration may offer some advantages of stability but has been associated with a higher rate of exit-site infections than the single-cuff Tenckhoff design in adults (149).

The swan-neck catheter (150) has a built-in bend allowing downward (caudal) direction of the exit-site sinus in the erect position, facilitating drainage of the exit site. Lower rates of exit-site infection were reported with the swan-neck than with the Tenckhoff catheters in some studies (150) but not in others (151). Low rates of exit-site infection were reported in high-risk patients with the placement of the exit site of a swan-neck catheter in the lateral wall of the chest parasternally, using a long tunnel instead of the abdominal wall (152).

The Moncrieff catheter (153) allows healing and growth of tissue into the cuffs, and the outer portion of the catheter rests in the subcutaneous tissue with the overlying skin intact. The skin is incised several weeks after catheter implantation. This method prevents contamination of the catheter with skin flora while the operative wound is fresh. Low rates of exit-site infection were initially reported with the Moncrieff catheter (154). However, a randomized study failed to reproduce this finding (155).

Impregnation of the catheter with antibiotics has not been proved effective (156). Silver rings around the catheter (157) and silver-impregnated catheters (158) have also not been established as effective preventive measures. Ultraviolet irradiation of the exit site was reported to reduce the rate of exit-site infections (159). The disconnect Y-set was reported to reduce not only the rate of peritonitis but also the rate of exit-site infections, probably because of less trauma to the catheter (160). Recent efforts to reduce adherence of *S. aureus* and, therefore, biofilm formation provided encouraging preliminary results (161).

Peritoneal catheters are implanted surgically in the operating room, blindly at the bedside, or peritoneoscopically. Good results have been claimed for all techniques. Meticulous aseptic technique during implantation; proper positioning of the cuffs; and avoidance of excessively long incisions, open spaces for fluid collection in the tunnel, and tissue damage are far more important than the insertion technique chosen. The operator's experience is much more important than the implantation technique in ensuring both good catheter function and lower infection rates. Short courses of antibiotics around catheter implantation, such as first-generation cephalosporins or gentamicin are recommended. Prophylactic antibiotics are also recommended during procedures prone to produce transient bacteremia, such as dental extraction or colonoscopy (132,162).

Exit-Site Care

Proper exit-site care is important for all CAPD patients, but particularly for those especially at high risk for infections and catheter loss such as diabetic women (163) and obese patients (164). Care should be delegated to specially trained staff.

Immediately after catheter implantation, the exit site and operative site are covered with sterile nonocclusive dressings, which should remain untouched for 7 days to allow for healing, unless excessive bleeding is noticed (127). Exit-site care involves aseptic technique with mask and gloves, avoidance of irritating or toxic solutions for cleansing, application of cleansing material only on the skin and not in the catheter sinus or the wound, use of absorbent dressings, immobilization of the catheter, and avoidance of moisture at the exit site (165).

After initial flushing of the peritoneal cavity to remove the blood, the catheter is capped and small volumes of dialysate (100 to 200 mL) containing 500 to 1,000 units of heparin are allowed to remain in the peritoneal cavity. The catheter may be flushed daily or every 2 days, but regular PD should not start for 10 to 14 days after catheter implantation to avoid early dialysate leaks, which increase the risk of tunnel infection.

For chronic exit-site care after healing, the patients are instructed to clean the exit site with a disinfectant, clear the excessive disinfectant from the skin with a sterile gauze, and cover the exit site with a dry nonocclusive dressing. Exit-site care is recommended daily to once every 5 days. Low rates of exit-site infections were reported with the use of antibacterial soap (135) or povidone iodine (166), whereas cleansing with hydrogen peroxide was associated with a high rate of exit-site infections (119). Tub baths should be avoided; showers should be taken with an occlusive dressing in place. Hand-washing before exit-site care and avoidance of force during removal of crust or scabs and during drying of the exit site are important.

REFERENCES

1. Conn HO, et al. Spontaneous bacterial peritonitis on cirrhosis: variations of a theme. *Medicine (Balt)* 1971;50:161–197.
2. Keane WF, et al. Peritonitis. In: Gokal R, et al., eds. *The textbook of peritoneal dialysis.* Dordrecht, the Netherlands: Kluwer Academic, 1994:473–501.
3. Vas SI. Microbiologic aspects of chronic ambulatory peritoneal dialysis. *Kidney Int* 1983;23:83–92.
4. Eisenberg ES, et al. Colonization of skin and development of peritonitis due to coagulase negative staphylococci in patients undergoing peritoneal dialysis. *J Infect Dis* 1987;156:478–482.
5. Sombolos K, et al. Propionibacteria isolates and asymptomatic infections of the peritoneal effluent in CAPD patients. *Nephrol Dial Transplant* 1986;1:175–178.
6. Williams PS, et al. Routine daily surveillance cultures in the management of CAPD patients. *Perit Dial Bull* 1987;7:183–186.
7. Singh MM, et al. Tuberculous peritonitis: an evaluation of pathogenic mechanisms, diagnostic procedures and therapeutic measures. *N Engl J Med* 1969;281:1091–1094.
8. Khanna R, et al. Fungal peritonitis in patients undergoing chronic intermittent or continuous peritoneal dialysis. *Proc EDTA* 1980;17:291–296.
9. Lindblad AS, et al., eds. *Continuous ambulatory peritoneal dialysis in the USA. Final Report of the National CAPD Registry 1981–1988.* Dordrecht, the Netherlands: Kluwer Academic, 1989:243–252.
10. Golper TA, et al. Risk factors for peritonitis in long-term peritoneal dialysis: Network 9 Peritonitis and Catheter Studies. *Am J Kidney Dis* 1996;28:428–436.
11. Juergensen PH, et al. Psychosocial factors and the incidence of peritonitis. *Adv Perit Dial* 1996;12:196–198.
12. Huang J-W, et al. Systemic lupus erythematosus and peritoneal dialysis: outcomes and infectious complications. *Perit Dial Int* 2001;21:143–147.
14. Spiegel DM, et al. Serum albumin: a marker for morbidity in peritoneal dialysis patients. *Am J Kidney Dis* 1993;21:26–30.
14. Furth JL, et al. Peritoneal dialysis catheter infections and peritonitis in children: a report from the North American Pediatric Renal Transplant Cooperative Group. *Pediatr Nephrol* 2000;15:179–182.
15. Lewis S, et al. Host defense mechanisms in the peritoneal cavity of continuous ambulatory peritoneal dialysis patients. First of two parts. *Perit Dial Int* 1991;11:14–21.
16. Holmes C, et al. Host defense mechanisms in the peritoneal cavity of continuous ambulatory peritoneal dialysis patients. 2: humoral defenses. *Perit Dial Int* 1991;11:112–117.
17. Coles GA, et al. Host defense and effects of solution on peritoneal cells. In: Gokal R, et al., eds. *The textbook of peritoneal dialysis.* Dordrecht, the Netherlands: Kluwer Academic, 1994:503–528.
18. Verbruch HA, et al. Peritoneal macrophages and opsonins: antibacterial defense in patients undergoing chronic peritoneal dialysis. *J Infect Dis* 1983;147:1018–1029.
19. Poyrazoglou HM, et al. Humoral immunity and frequency of peritonitis in chronic peritoneal dialysis patients. *Pediatr Nephrol* 2002;17:85–90.

20. Zarrinkalam KH, et al. Expression of defensin antimicrobial peptides in the peritoneal cavity of patients on peritoneal dialysis. *Perit Dial Int* 2001;21:501–508.

21. Goldstein CS, et al. Fibronectin and complement secretion by monocytes and peritoneal macrophages in vitro from patients undergoing continuous ambulatory peritoneal dialysis. *J Leuk Biol* 1986;39:457–464.

22. Davies SJ, et al. Activation of immunocompetent cells in the peritoneum of patients treated with CAPD. *Kidney Int* 1989;36:661–668.

23. Runyon BA. Low protein concentration ascitic fluid is predisposed to spontaneous bacterial peritonitis. *Gastroenterology* 1986;91:1343–1346.

24. Keane WF, et al. Opsonic deficiency of peritoneal dialysis effluent in continuous ambulatory peritoneal dialysis. *Kidney Int* 1984;25:539–543.

25. Coles GA, et al. Can the risk of peritonitis be predicted for new continuous ambulatory peritoneal dialysis (CAPD) patients? *Perit Dial Int* 1989;9:69–72.

26. Bennett-Jones DV, et al. Strain differences in the opsonization of *Staphylococcus epidermidis. Perit Dial Int* 1989;9:334–339.

27. Keane WF, et al. Opsonic deficiencies of peritoneal dialysis effluent in CAPD. *Kidney Int* 1984;25:539–543.

28. Davies SJ, et al. Peritoneal defense mechanisms and *Staphylococcus aureus* in patients treated with continuous ambulatory peritoneal dialysis (CAPD). *Perit Dial Int* 1990;10:135–140.

29. Holmes CJ, et al. Comparison of peritoneal white blood cell parameters from CAPD patients with a high or low incidence of peritonitis. *Am J Kidney Dis* 1990;15:258–264.

30. Peterson PK, et al. Antimicrobial activities of dialysate-eluted and resident human peritoneal macrophages. *Infect Immunol* 1985;49:212–218.

31. Lewis SL, et al. Phenotypic characterization of monocytes and macrophages from CAPD patients. *ASAIO Trans* 1990;36:M575–M577.

32. Carcano C, et al. Long-term, continuous ambulatory peritoneal dialysis reduces the expression of CD11B, CD14, CD16, and CD64 on peritoneal macrophages. *Perit Dial Int* 1996;16:582–589.

33. Giacchino F, et al. Lymphocyte subsets assayed by numerical tests in CAPD. *Int J Artif Organs* 1984;7:81–84.

34. Nagai T, et al. Oxidative metabolism of polymorphonuclear leukocytes in continuous ambulatory peritoneal dialysis. *Perit Dial Int* 1997;17:167–174.

35. Topley N, et al. The role of the peritoneal membrane in the control of inflammation in the peritoneal cavity. *Kidney Int* 1994;46:S71–S78.

36. Topley N. The cytokine network controlling peritoneal inflammation. *Perit Dial Int* 1995;15[Suppl]:S35–S39.

37. Duwe AK, et al. Effects of the composition of peritoneal dialysis fluid on chemiluminescence, phagocytosis, and bactericidal activity in vitro. *Infect Immunol* 1981;33:130–135.

38. Ing TS, et al. Lactate-containing peritoneal dialysis solutions. *Int J Artif Organs* 1993;16:688–693.

39. Jonasson P, et al. Heat-sterilized PD fluid blocks leucocyte adhesion and increases flow velocity in rat peritoneal vessels. *Perit Dial Int* 1996;[Suppl 2]:S137–S140.

40. Scambye HT, et al. Bicarbonate is not the ultimate answer to the bioincompatibility problems of CAPD solutions. *Adv Perit Dial* 1992;8:42–46.

41. Mahiout AM, et al. Pyruvate anions neutralize peritoneal dialysate cytotoxicity. *Nephrol Dial Transplant* 1995;10:391–394.

42. Peterson PK, et al. Current concepts in the management of peritonitis in continuous ambulatory peritoneal dialysis patients. *Rev Infect Dis* 1987;9:604–612.

43. Fried L, et al. Peritonitis. In: Gokal R, et al., eds. *Textbook of peritoneal dialysis,* 2nd ed. Dordrecht, the Netherlands: Kluwer Academic, 2000:545–564.

44. Korzets SZ, et al. CAPD peritonitis—initial presentation as an acute abdomen with clear peritoneal effluent. *Clin Nephrol* 1992;37:155–157.

45. Tranaeus A, et al. Peritonitis in continuous ambulatory peritoneal dialysis (CAPD): diagnostic findings, therapeutic outcome and complications. *Perit Dial Int* 1989;9:179–190.

46. Vas SI. The diagnosis of peritonitis in patients on continuous ambulatory peritoneal dialysis. *Semin Dial* 1995;8:232–237.

47. Beserra DA, et al. The diagnostic value of gram stain for clinical identification of the etiologic agents of peritonitis. *Perit Dial Int* 1997;17:269–272.

48. Everett ED. Peritonitis risk assessment and management. In: Twardowski ZJ, et al., eds. *Contemporary issues in nephrology: peritoneal dialysis.* New York: Churchill Livingstone, 1990:145–165.

49. Bunke M, et al. Culture negative CAPD peritonitis: the Network 9 study. *Adv Perit Dial* 1994;10:174–178.

50. Tuncer M, et al. Chemical peritonitis associated with high dialysate acetaldehyde concentrations. *Nephrol Dial Transplant* 2000;15:2037–2040.

51. Chan MK, et al. Peritoneal eosinophilia in patients on continuous ambulatory peritoneal dialysis: a prospective study. *Am J Kidney Dis* 1988;11:180–183.

52. Piraino B, et al. Chemical peritonitis due to intraperitoneal vancomycin (Vancoled). *Perit Dial Bull* 1987;7:156–159.

53. Murphy G, et al. Intraperitoneal thrombolytic agents in relapsing or persistent peritonitis in patients on continuous ambulatory peritoneal dialysis. *Int J Artif Organs* 1991;14:87–91.

54. Van der Reijden HJ, et al. Fecal peritonitis in patients on continuous ambulatory peritoneal dialysis; an end-point in CAPD? *Adv Perit Dial* 1988;4:198–203.

55. Tzamaloukas AH, et al. Peritonitis associated with intraabdominal pathology in continuous ambulatory peritoneal dialysis (CAPD) patients. *Perit Dial Int* 1993;13[Suppl 2]:S335–S337.

56. Chang JJ, et al. Pneumoperitoneum in peritoneal dialysis patients. *Am J Kidney Dis* 1995;25:296–301.

57. Wakeem MJ, et al. Viscus perforation in peritoneal dialysis patients: diagnosis and outcome. *Perit Dial Int* 1994;14:371–377.

58. Holley JL, et al. Polymicrobial peritonitis in patients on continuous peritoneal dialysis. *Am J Kidney Dis* 1992;19:162–166.

59. Kiernan L, et al. Outcome of polymicrobial peritonitis in continuous ambulatory peritoneal dialysis. *Am J Kidney Dis* 1995;25:261–264.

60. Kern EO, et al. Abdominal catastrophe revisited: the risk and outcome of enteric peritoneal contamination. *Perit Dial Int* 2002;22:323–334.

61. Wu G, et al. Is extensive diverticulosis of the colon a contraindication for CAPD? *Perit Dial Bull* 1983;3:180–183.

62. Keane WF, et al. Adult peritoneal dialysis-related peritonitis treatment recommendations: 2000 update. *Perit Dial Int* 2000;20:396–411.

63. Warady BA, et al. Consensus guidelines for the treatment of peritonitis in pediatric patients receiving peritoneal dialysis. *Perit Dial Int* 2000;20:610–624.

64. Troidle L, et al. Nine episodes of CPD-associated peritonitis with vancomycin-resistant enterococci. *Kidney Int* 1996;50:1368–1372.

65. Shemin D, et al. Effect of aminoglycoside use on residual renal function in peritoneal dialysis patients. *Am J Kidney Dis* 1999;34:14–20.

66. Singhal MK, et al. Rate of decline of residual renal function in patients on continuous peritoneal dialysis and factors affecting it. *Perit Dial Int* 2000;20:429–438.

67. Michel C, et al. Fungal peritonitis in patients on peritoneal dialysis. *Am J Nephrol* 1994;14:113–120.

68. Goldie SJ, et al. Fungal peritonitis in a large chronic peritoneal dialysis population: a report of 55 episodes. *Am J Kidney Dis* 1996;28:86–91.

69. Amici G, et al. Fungal peritonitis in peritoneal dialysis: critical review of six cases. *Adv Perit Dial* 1994;10:169–173.

70. Lo W-K, et al. Fungal peritonitis—current status 1998. *Perit Dial Int* 1998;19[Suppl 2]:S286–S290.

71. Lewis SL. Recurrent peritonitis: evidence for possible viral etiology. *Am J Kidney Dis* 1991;17:343–345.

72. Schloth T, et al. Peritonitis and the patient with human immunodeficiency virus (HIV). *Adv Perit Dial* 1992;8:250–252.

73. Lewis M, et al. Incidence and spectrum of organisms causing peritonitis in HIV positive patients. *Adv Perit Dial* 1990;6:136–138.

74. Breyer JA, et al. Isolation of human immunodeficiency virus from peritoneal dialysate. *Am J Kidney Dis* 1993;21:23–25.

75. Manley HJ, et al. Pharmacokinetics of intermittent intravenous cefazolin and tobramycin in patients treated with automated PD. *J Am Soc Nephrol* 2000;11:1310–1316.

76. Digenis GE, et al. Peritonitis-related deaths in continuous ambulatory peritoneal dialysis (CAPD) patients. *Perit Dial Int* 1990;10:45–47.

77. Krishnan M, et al. Prediction of outcome following bacterial peritonitis in peritoneal dialysis. *Perit Dial Int* 2002;22:575–581.

78. Tzamaloukas AH, et al. Peritoneal catheter loss and death in CAPD peritonitis. *Perit Dial Int* 1993;13[Suppl 2]:S339–S340.

79. Fox L, et al. Metabolic differences between persistent and routine peritonitis in continuous ambulatory peritoneal dialysis (CAPD). *Adv Perit Dial* 1992;8:346–350.

80. Murata GH, et al. Predicting the course of peritonitis in patients on continuous ambulatory peritoneal dialysis. *Arch Intern Med* 1993;153:2317–2321.

81. Bernardini J, et al. Analysis of continuous ambulatory peritoneal dialysis-related *Pseudomonas aeruginosa* infections. *Am J Med* 1987;83:829–832.

82. Chan MK, et al. *Pseudomonas* peritonitis in CAPD patients: characteristics and outcomes of treatment. *Nephrol Dial Transplant* 1989;4:814–817.

83. Bunke M, et al. *Pseudomonas* peritonitis in peritoneal dialysis patients: the Network 9 peritonitis study. *Am J Kidney Dis* 1995;25:769–774.

84. Craddock CF, et al. *Pseudomonas* peritonitis in continuous ambulatory peritoneal dialysis: laboratory prediction of treatment failure. *J Hosp Infect* 1987;10:179–186.

85. Krothapali R, et al. *Pseudomonas* peritonitis and continuous ambulatory peritoneal dialysis. *Arch Intern Med* 1982;142:1862–1863.

86. Al-Wali W, et al. Differing prognostic significance of reinfection and relapse in CAPD peritonitis. *Nephrol Dial Transplant* 1992;7:133–136.

87. Davies SJ, et al. Peritoneal defense mechanisms and *Staphylococcus aureus* in patients treated with continuous ambulatory peritoneal dialysis (CAPD). *Perit Dial Int* 1990;10:135–140.

88. Dasgupta MK, et al. Biofilms in peritoneal dialysis. *Perit Dial Int* 2001;21[Suppl 3]:S213–S217.

89. Finkelstein ES, et al. Patterns of infection in patients maintained on long-term peritoneal dialysis therapy with multiple episodes of peritonitis. *Am J Kidney Dis* 2002;39:1278–1286.

90. Glancey GR, et al. Peritoneal drainage: an important element in host defense against staphylococcal peritonitis in patients on CAPD. *Nephrol Dial Transplant* 1992;7:627–631.

91. Holley JL, et al. Ultrasound as a tool in the diagnosis and management of exit-site infections in patients undergoing continuous ambulatory peritoneal dialysis. *Am J Kidney Dis* 1989;14:211–216.

92. Williams AJ, et al. Tenckhoff catheter replacement or intraperitoneal urokinase: a randomized trial in the management of recurrent continuous ambulatory peritoneal dialysis (CAPD) peritonitis. *Perit Dial Int* 1989;9:65–67.

93. Posthuma N, et al. Simultaneous peritoneal dialysis catheter insertion and removal in catheter-related infections without interruption of peritoneal dialysis. *Nephrol Dial Transplant* 1998;13:700–703.

94. Innes A, et al. Treatment of resistant peritonitis in continuous peritoneal dialysis with intraperitoneal urokinase: a double-blind clinical study. *Nephrol Dial Transplant* 1994;9:797–799.

95. Buckman RF, et al. A unifying pathogenetic mechanism for the etiology of intraperitoneal adhesions. *J Surg Res* 1976;20:1–5.

96. Selgas R, et al. Tissue plasminogen activation (t-PA) and plasminogen activator inhibitor-I (PAI-I) levels in plasma and peritoneal effluent in patients on CAPD. *Adv Perit Dial* 1992;8:160–164.

97. Shusterman NH, et al. Management of refractory peritonitis to maintain the peritoneum for subsequent dialysis. *Perit Dial Int* 1992;12:211–213.

98. Dobbie JW. Pathogenesis of peritoneal fibrosing syndromes (sclerosing peritonitis) in peritoneal dialysis. *Perit Dial Int* 1992;12:14–27.

99. Slingeneyer A. Preliminary report on a cooperative international study on sclerosing encapsulating peritonitis. *Contr Nephrol* 1987;57:239–247.

100. Suzuki K, et al. Spontaneous peritonitis and peritoneal fibrosis in rats on peritoneal dialysis for nine weeks. *Adv Perit Dial* 1995;11:52–56.

101. Dobbie JW, et al. Role of imbalance of intracavity fibrin formation and removal in the pathogenesis of peritoneal lesions in CAPD. *Perit Dial Int* 1997;17:121–124.

102. Krediet RT, et al. Markers of peritoneal membrane status. *Perit Dial Int* 1996;16[Suppl 1]:S42–S49.

103. Mlambo NC, et al. Increased levels of transforming factor beta 1 and basic fibroblast growth factor in patients on CAPD: a study during non-infected steady state and peritonitis. *Inflammation* 1999;23:131–139.

104. Rampino T, et al. Hepatocyte growth factor/scatter factor released during peritonitis is active on mesothelial cells. *Am J Pathol* 2001;159:1275–1285.

105. Fukudome K, et al. Peritonitis increase MMP-9 activity of peritoneal effluent from CAPD patients. *Nephron* 2001;87:35–41.

106. Zemel D, et al. Analysis of the inflammatory predictors and peritoneal permeability for macromolecules starting before the onset of peritonitis in patients treated with CAPD. *Perit Dial Int* 1995;15:334–341.

107. Goel S, et al. The effect of peritonitis on the peritoneal membrane transport properties in patients on CAPD. *Adv Perit Dial* 1996;16:181–184.

108. Andreoli SP, et al. Adverse effects of peritonitis on peritoneal membrane function in children on dialysis. *Pediatr Nephrol* 1999;13:1–6.

109. Hendricks PMEM, et al. Peritoneal sclerosis in chronic peritoneal dialysis patients: analysis of clinical presentation, risk factors and peritoneal transport kinetics. *Perit Dial Int* 1997;17:136–143.

110. Blumenkrantz MJ, et al. Protein losses during peritoneal dialysis. *Kidney Int* 1981;19:593–602.

111. Dulaney JT, et al. Peritoneal dialysis and loss of proteins: a review. *Kidney Int* 1984;26:253–262.

112. Bannister DK, et al. Nutritional effects of peritonitis on continuous ambulatory peritoneal dialysis (CAPD) patients. *J Am Diet Assoc* 1987;87:53–56.

113. Sennesael JJ, et al. The impact of peritonitis on peritoneal and systemic acid-base status of patients on continuous ambulatory peritoneal dialysis. *Perit Dial Int* 1994;14:61–65.

114. Boroujerdi-Rad H, et al. Abdominal abscesses complicating peritonitis in continuous ambulatory peritoneal dialysis patients. *Am J Kidney Dis* 1994;23:717–721.

115. Tzamaloukas AH, et al. Persistence of positive dialysate cultures after apparent cure of CAPD peritonitis. *Adv Perit Dial* 1993;9:198–201.

116. Fried LF, et al. Peritonitis influences mortality in peritoneal dialysis patients. *J Am Soc Nephrol* 1996;7:2176–2182.

117. Bunke CM, et al. Outcomes of single organism peritonitis in peritoneal dialysis: gram negatives versus gram positives in the Network 9 peritonitis study. *Kidney Int* 1997;52:524–529.

118. Troidle L, et al. Differing outcomes of gram-positive and gram-negative peritonitis. *Am J Kidney Dis* 1998;32:623–628.

119. Daly C, et al. Double bag or y-set versus standard transfer systems for continuous ambulatory peritoneal dialysis in end-stage renal disease. *Cochrane Database Syst Rev* 2001(2):CD003078.

120. Churchill DN, et al. Peritonitis in continuous ambulatory peritoneal dialysis (CAPD): a multicentre randomized clinical trial comparing the Y-connector disinfectant system to standard systems. *Perit Dial Int* 1989;9:159–163.

121. Bernandini J, et al. An analysis of ten year trends in infections in adults on continuous ambulatory peritoneal dialysis (CAPD). *Clin Nephrol* 1991;36:29–34.

122. Nolph KD, et al. How to monitor and report exit/tunnel infections. *Perit Dial Int* 1996;16[Suppl 3]:S115–S117.

123. Kazmi HR, et al. *Pseudomonas* exit site infections in continuous ambulatory peritoneal dialysis patients. *J Am Soc Nephrol* 1992;2:1498–1501.

124. Twardowski ZJ, et al. Classification of normal and diseased exit sites. *Perit Dial Int* 1996;16[Suppl 3]:S31–S50.

125. Gonthier D, et al. Erythema: does it indicate infection in a peritoneal catheter exit site? *Adv Perit Dial* 1992;8:230–233.

126. Ferguson BJ, et al. Peritoneal dialysis exit site infections in CAPD patients wearing tight clothes. *ANNA J* 1988;15:180–181.

127. Oreopoulos DG, et al. Peritoneal catheter and exit-site practices: current recommendations. *Perit Dial Bull* 1987;7:130–138.

128. Piraino B. Management of catheter related infections. *Am J Kidney Dis* 1996;27:714–718.

129. Plum J, et al. Results of ultrasound-assisted diagnosis of tunnel infections in continuous ambulatory peritoneal dialysis. *Am J Kidney Dis* 1994;23:99–104.

130. Korzets Z, et al. Frequent involvement of the internal cuff segment in CAPD patients and exit-site infection—an ultrasound study. *Nephrol Dial Transplant* 1996;11:336–339.

131. Vychytil A, et al. Ultrasonography of the catheter tunnel in peritoneal dialysis patients: what are the indications? *Am J Kidney Dis* 1999;33: 722–727.

132. Gokal E, et al. Peritoneal catheters and exit-site practices: toward optimum peritoneal access. *Perit Dial Int* 1993;13:29–39.

133. Flanigan MJ, et al. Continuous ambulatory peritoneal dialysis catheter infections: diagnosis and management. *Perit Dial Int* 1994; 14:248–254.

134. Lomaestro BM, et al. Absorption interactions with fluoroquinolones: 1995 update. *Drug Safety* 1995;12:314–337.

135. Prowant BF, et al. Peritoneal catheter exit site care. *ANNA J* 1988; 15:219–222.

136. Strauss FG, et al. Hypertonic saline compresses: therapy for complicated exit-site infections. *Adv Perit Dial* 1993;9:248–250.

137. Khanna R, et al. Recommendations for treatment of exit-site pathology. *Perit Dial Int* 1996;16[Suppl 3]:S100–S104.

138. Gibel LJ, et al. Soft tissue complications of Tenckhoff catheters. *Adv Perit Dial* 1989;5:299–333.

139. Luzar MA, et al. *Staphylococcus aureus* nasal carriage and infection in patients on continuous ambulatory peritoneal dialysis. *N Engl J Med* 1990;322:505–509.

140. Kreft B, et al. Clinical and genetic analysis of *Staphylococcus aureus* nasal colonization and exit-site infection in patients undergoing peritoneal dialysis. *Eur J Clin Microbiol Infect Dis* 2001;20: 734–737.

141. Wanten GJA, et al. Nasal carriage and peritonitis by *Staphylococcus aureus* in patients on continuous ambulatory peritoneal dialysis: a prospective study. *Perit Dial Int* 1996;16:352–356.

142. Lye WC, et al. *Staphylococcus aureus* CAPD-related infections are associated with nasal carriage. *Adv Perit Dial* 1994;10:163–165.

143. Mupirocin Study Group. Nasal mupirocin prevents *Staphylococcus aureus* exit-site infection during peritoneal dialysis. *J Am Soc Nephrol* 1996;7:2403–2408.

144. Ritzau J, et al. Effects of preventing *Staphylococcus aureus* carriage on rates of peritoneal catheter-related staphylococcal infections. Literature synthesis. *Perit Dial Int* 2001;21:471–479.

145. Perez-Fontan M, et al. Mupirocin resistance after long-term use for *Staphylococcus aureus* colonization in patients undergoing chronic peritoneal dialysis. *Am J Kidney Dis* 2002;39:337–441.

146. Piraino B. Which catheter is the best buy? *Perit Dial Int* 1995;15: 303–304.

147. Lye WC, et al. A prospective randomized comparison of the Swan neck, coiled and straight Tenckhoff catheters in patients on CAPD. *Perit Dial Int* 1996;16[Suppl 1]:S333–S335.

148. Tenckhoff H, et al. A bacteriologically safe peritoneal access device. *Trams Am Soc Artif Intern Organs* 1968;14:181–186.

149. Oxton LL, et al. Risk factors for peritoneal dialysis-related infections. *Perit Dial Int* 1994;14:137–144.

150. Twardowski ZJ, et al. Six-year experience with Swan-neck catheters. *Perit Dial Int* 1992;12:284–289.

151. Eklund BH, et al. Peritoneal dialysis access: prospective randomized comparison of the Swan neck and Tenckhoff catheters. *Perit Dial Int* 1995;15:353–356.

152. Twardowski ZJ, et al. Four-year experience with Swan neck presternal peritoneal dialysis catheters. *Am J Kidney Dis* 1996;27:99–105.

153. Moncrief JW, et al. The Moncrief-Popovich catheter: a new peritoneal access technique for patients. *ASAIO J* 1993;39:62–65.

154. De Alvaro F, et al. Moncrieff's technique for peritoneal catheter placement: experience in a CAPD unit. *Adv Perit Dial* 1994;10:199–202.

155. Danielson A, et al. A prospective randomized study of the effect of a subcutaneously "buried" peritoneal dialysis catheter technique versus standard technique on the incidence of peritonitis and exit-site infection. *Perit Dial Int* 2002;22:211–219.

156. Trooskin SZ, et al. Failure of demonstrated clinical efficacy of antibiotic-bonded continuous ambulatory peritoneal dialysis (CAPD) catheters. *Perit Dial Int* 1990;10:57–59.

157. Pommer W, et al. Efficiency of a silver ring in preventing exit-site infection in adult PD patients: results of the SIPROCE study. *Adv Perit Dial* 1997;17:227–232.

158. Dasgupta MK. Silver-impregnated peritoneal catheters reduce bacterial colonization. *Adv Perit Dial* 1994;10:195–198.

159. Shimomura A, et al. The effect of ultraviolet rays on the prevention of exit-site infections. *Adv Perit Dial* 1995;11:152–156.

160. Burkart JM, et al. Comparison of exit-site infections in disconnect versus non-disconnect systems for peritoneal dialysis. *Perit Dial Int* 1992;12:317–320.

161. Balaban N, et al. Prevention of *Staphylococcus aureus* biofilm on dialysis catheters and adherence to human cells. *Kidney Int* 2003;63: 340–345.

162. Verrina E, et al. Prevention of peritonitis in children on peritoneal dialysis. *Perit Dial Int* 2000;20:625–630.

163. Holley JL, et al. Risk factors for tunnel infections in continuous peritoneal dialysis. *Am J Kidney Dis* 1991;18:344–348.

164. Piraino B, et al. The effect of body weight on CAPD related infections and catheter loss. *Perit Dial Int* 1991;11:64–68.

165. Prowant BF, et al. Recommendations for exit site care. *Perit Dial Int* 1996;16[Suppl 3]:S94–S99.

166. Luzar MA, et al. Exit-site care and exit-site infection in continuous ambulatory peritoneal dialysis (CAPD): results of a randomized clinical trial. *Perit Dial Int* 1990;10:25–29.

42

PREPARING DIALYSIS PATIENTS FOR RENAL TRANSPLANTATION

MATTHEW R. WEIR, CHARLES B. CANGRO, AND DAVID K. KLASSEN

CHOOSING THE APPROPRIATE TRANSPLANT PROCEDURE

Kidney transplantation procedures can be divided into several types based on the relationship between the recipient and the donor. These include cadaveric renal transplants, living-related renal transplants, and living nonrelated transplants. Living-related transplants may be further distinguished by the degree of relationship between the recipient and donor. These are commonly sibling to sibling transplants in which the genetic matching can range from a complete human leukocyte antigen (HLA) match to a complete HLA mismatch, or parent to child transplants in which a one haplotype or three HLA antigen match occurs. Cadaveric renal transplantation remains the most common transplant procedure with little change in the number of transplants done over the last decade. Living-donor transplantation, however, has been steadily increasing. In 2001 there were slightly more than 8,200 cadaveric transplantation procedures done. This compares with more than 5,100 living-donor transplants done during the same year (1). For dialysis patients, the choice of procedure has an important impact on patient survival, allograft organ survival, and time spent waiting for transplantation. Kidney transplantation is now regarded as the treatment of choice for end-stage renal disease (ESRD). A successful kidney transplant reduces the risk of dying for patients when compared with maintenance dialysis and improves the quality of life. Multiple studies comparing patients who have undergone transplantation with those who have not yet received a renal transplant and remain on the waiting list have clearly shown that renal transplantation is associated with better patient survival (2–6). This survival benefit was seen in all age groups including the elderly and among African-Americans and diabetics. Repeat renal transplantation after a failed initial transplant may also confer survival benefit.

The success of renal transplantation has resulted in an increase in the number of patients being listed for cadaveric transplantation. At the present there are more than 53,000 patients awaiting cadaveric transplantation (1). Unfortunately, the number of cadaveric donors has not kept pace with this increase. Over the past decade there have been only marginal increases in the number of donors. In 2001, there were 6,081 cadaveric donors. In that year for the first time the number of living donors exceeded the number of cadaveric donors with 6,499 individuals donating an organ (1). The ever-increasing number of patients seeking a transplant coupled with the relatively fixed number of cadaveric organs available has resulted in a substantial increase in the time spent on the cadaveric transplant waiting list. At present about 4% of patients per year die while waiting for a transplant (7). Patients who are fortunate enough to have a preemptive transplant (one done before the initiation of dialysis) or patients who spent less than 1 year on the waiting list have shown to have an improved survival following transplantation (8–10). The survival benefit of a shorter waiting time has also been documented in children. Patients who entered the transplant waiting list in 1990 had a mean waiting time of slightly more than 1 year. Patients who entered the waiting list in 1997 have waited an average of 3 years before receiving a transplant (11).

Because of the differences in outcome associated with cadaveric renal transplantation and living-donor renal transplantation, the dialysis patient able to choose between these procedures will have control over the profound differences in both graft survival and patient survival between these procedures. With cadaveric transplantation, 1-year allograft survival rates have gradually improved over the past decade and now have reached 89%. This is not dramatically different from the 95% 1-year graft survival for all living-donor transplants (11). The truly important differences between cadaveric renal transplantation and living-donor renal transplantation emerge with examination of the long-term graft survival rates. With cadaveric renal transplantation there is a substantial fall in graft survival over time. By 5 years, cadaveric allograft survival has decreased to 65%, whereas living-donor transplant graft survival remains at 78% (11). The half-life of cadaveric organs transplanted in the 1990s has averaged 8.6 years, whereas the half-life of living-donor transplants done at the same time has been 14.3 years (12) (Table 42.1). The results of renal transplantation using kidneys from living nonrelated donors such as spouses also compare favorably with the results obtained with cadaveric organs. The most recent data have shown that the half-life of these allografts ranges between 13 and 14 years (13). In both cadaveric and living-donor transplantation there is a significant effect of HLA matching on allograft survival,

TABLE 42.1. GRAFT SURVIVAL HALF-LIVES FOR RECIPIENTS OF CADAVER AND LIVING DONOR RENAL TRANSPLANTS 1988–2000

Transplant	Half-Life (Years)
All living	14.3
All cadaveric	8.6
HLA-identical living	22.2
Living unrelated	13.6

HLA, human leukocyte antigen.

particularly in long-term graft survival (Table 42.2). Five-year allograft survival of a zero mismatched HLA cadaveric organ is 72%, whereas a six-antigen mismatched cadaveric organ has a 5-year survival of 59% (11). This can be contrasted with a two haplotype matched or (zero antigen mismatch) living-donor transplant that has a 5-year survival of 87% and a projected half-life of 22 years (12). In addition to the benefits of living-donor renal transplantation on allograft survival there is a substantial benefit on patient survival as well. Patients who received cadaveric transplants in the decade of the 1990s have a projected 10-year survival of 63%. This is in contrast to a projected 80% 10-year patient survival for recipients of living-donor transplants (12).

Because of the demand for kidney transplantation and the ever-increasing waiting times, cadaveric kidneys have been used from donors who in the past might have been passed over. These "expanded criteria" organs have been obtained from donors older than 60 years old, donors with a history of high blood pressure, donors who have died with stroke, or donors whose kidney function was somewhat reduced. Patients receiving these expanded criteria organs have been shown to have improved survival compared with patients who remain on the transplant waiting list. These transplants do, however, have a shortened allograft survival compared with kidneys obtained from ideal donors. The United Network for Organ Sharing (UNOS), the federal contract agency that governs transplant policy and organ distribution, has developed a second waiting list to facilitate the distribution of expanded criteria organs to patients who are willing to accept these organs. The increase in live-donor kidney transplantation has resulted from the perceived need of the patients on the waiting list and the well-documented excellent outcome associated with these transplants. Newer surgical techniques such as laparoscopic donor nephrectomy have also been credited with an increase in individuals willing to undergo the donor procedure. The laparoscopic donor nephrectomy has

TABLE 42.2. FIVE-YEAR KIDNEY ALLOGRAFT SURVIVAL RELATED TO HLA MISMATCH

	Cadaveric % Survival	Live Donor % Survival
0 mm	72	87
1 mm	69	79
3 mm	65	76
6 mm	59	71

HLA, human leukocyte antigen.

been shown to have less morbidity and a more rapid return to usual activities than the traditional open donor nephrectomy. This procedure has been documented to result in increased rates of organ donation (14). The recipient outcomes have also been shown to be equivalent between traditional open nephrectomy and laparoscopically obtained organs (15).

The benefits of living-donor transplantation for dialysis patients can perhaps best be appreciated by noting that the outcome for both patient and allograft survival with any category of living-donor transplant is superior to even well-matched cadaveric transplantation. In addition, patients able to undergo living-donor transplantation can have this procedure scheduled on an elective basis and are able to avoid a prolonged period on the transplant waiting lists. Dialysis patients desiring to undergo transplantation who have a willing living donor should be encouraged to make use of this opportunity.

Combined kidney and pancreas transplantation for patients with ESRD and type 1 diabetes is now widely available. Dialysis patients who have previously received a cadaveric or living-donor kidney transplant are also potential candidates for a solitary pancreas transplant. The major benefits of kidney and pancreas transplantation are an improved quality of life, freedom from insulin therapy, the potential of avoiding additional secondary complications, and a normalization of fasting glucose with a decrease in the incidence of hypoglycemic episodes (16–18). The results of studies of secondary complications of diabetics undergoing pancreas transplantation are difficult to interpret in light of the fact that most of these patients have had diabetes for up to two decades. Successful pancreas transplantation is associated with normalization of serum insulin responses and a normalization of glycosylated hemoglobin. Glucose counter regulation associated with hypoglycemia improves after pancreas transplantation. The symptom recognition of hypoglycemia is restored, and dangerous episodes of hypoglycemia can be avoided. Diabetic neuropathy has been shown to be stabilized and in some instances autonomic and peripheral diabetic neuropathy improves (19). At the present there has been no clear benefit in halting the progression of the advanced diabetic retinopathy following pancreas transplantation. Recurrent diabetic nephropathy in the transplant kidney is prevented by pancreas transplantation and native kidney diabetic nephropathy may improve (20). In addition, some data suggest that combined kidney and pancreas transplantation may be associated with improved patient survival compared with diabetics who undergo kidney transplantation alone. Although the potential for significant improvement in outcome for diabetics with renal failure exists, the combined kidney pancreas transplantation procedure has an increased morbidity compared with kidney transplantation alone. Surgical complications are increased with a significant incidence of wound problems, intraabdominal infections, recurrent urinary tract infections, and primary technical failure of the pancreas allograft. In addition, successful kidney and pancreas transplantation requires a more aggressive antirejection immunosuppression strategy and results in the increased risk of infection associated with this procedure (21,22). The decision to undergo kidney and pancreas transplantation is perhaps best made by the patient in conjunction with the patient's nephrologist in consultation with a transplant center experienced in pancreas transplantation.

MEDICAL EVALUATION OF THE PATIENT WITH END-STAGE RENAL DISEASE

Organ transplantation improves the duration of life for the patient with ESRD (5). This result is in part due to the selection process of healthier individuals but is also related to other issues such as progression of atherosclerotic cardiovascular disease (5). However, in the perioperative period, the relative risk of death is greater in the transplant recipient compared with the same patient remaining on dialysis. Only at the point 3 to 4 months posttransplantation does the relative risk of death equalize between the patients remaining on dialysis versus those receiving a kidney transplant. It is for this reason that a very thorough medical evaluation of each patient must be performed pretransplant to ensure that the recipient is medically and nutritionally stable to undergo the rigors of an elective surgical procedure and be capable of tolerating not only the medications but also various treatments during the posttransplantation course (Table 42.3).

The leading causes of death posttransplantation are cardiovascular (23,24). Hence, management strategies for patients with incipient or existing cardiovascular disease remain most important. In addition, issues relating to lung disease, malignancy, preexisting viral infections, and risk for recurrent kidney disease also play an important role in stratifying the risk among candidates and may require specific therapy before transplantation and may influence the strategy for donor selection and even immunosuppression.

Cardiovascular Disease

Cardiovascular disease is the leading cause of death and graft loss after renal transplantation (23,24). Almost half of deaths with graft function that occur within 30 days of transplantation are due to cardiovascular disease, primarily myocardial infarction (24). Risk stratification before transplantation is critical to avoid perioperative mortality and minimize the risk for long-term morbidity and mortality. The presence or absence and the extent of cardiovascular disease may also play a role in the decision whether or not to undergo elective transplantation.

Although there is a large body of literature evaluating cardiovascular risk of nontransplant populations having elective surgery (25), there is limited study of transplant populations despite the fact that they have a substantial increased risk for cardiovascular disease (23,24). In nontransplant populations, mal-

TABLE 42.3. Contraindications to Transplantation

Active infection
Recent or current malignancy
Severe uncorrectable nonrenal disease
Active substance abuse
Severe psychiatric illness

nutrition, poorly controlled blood pressure, and diabetes are among those factors associated with the greatest risk for cardiovascular events during elective surgery (26–28). Myocardial infarction within 6 months, angina, recent history of pulmonary edema, atrial premature contractions (APCs) or ventricular premature contractions (VPCs), age greater than 70 years, and debilitated general medical status have also been noted as useful predictors for developing ischemic events in nontransplant populations undergoing elective noncardiac surgery (29).

Thus, those patients with ESRD with any of the previous risk factors should have noninvasive cardiac stress testing and those with a positive stress test should have coronary angiography (30). In addition, all patients with a prior history of myocardial infarction, congestive heart failure, or prior revascularization should probably undergo coronary angiography, if there is any evidence that a stress test is positive. Some have suggested that, because the prevalence of ischemic heart disease is so high in diabetic patients, they should all have angiography. However, investigators who have routinely performed coronary angiograms in consecutive diabetic patients have shown that only about 50% have angiographically significant coronary disease (31). Thus, noninvasive cardiac stress testing should be the initial focus followed by angiography, if there are any suspicions of active ischemic heart disease.

For asymptomatic patients who have risk factors for ischemic heart disease such as diabetes, male gender, age greater than 50 years, positive family history, cigarette smoking, hypertension, dyslipidemia, and so forth, noninvasive stress testing should be part of the evaluation (32). The use of a test with a high predictive value will prevent patients from being subjected to angiography unnecessarily, whereas a high negative predictive value will ensure that high-risk patients are not missed.

Most of the available data on the effectiveness of noninvasive screening techniques come from studies examining either dipyridamole, thallium or sestamibi scintigraphy (33,34), or dobutamine echocardiography (35,36). Although most of the available data with these screening techniques has been in patients without ESRD, some well-defined studies have looked at patients being screened for transplantation (33–36).

The advantage of the dobutamine echocardiography compared with thallium scintigraphy is its price. However, direct comparisons between these two screening modalities in ESRD patients are lacking. In the non-ESRD population, some investigators have suggested that dobutamine echocardiography was more specific for detecting coronary artery disease than dipyridamole sestamibi scanning, whereas the sensitivities of the two tests were very similar (37).

Thus, noninvasive cardiac testing plays an important role in assessing the ischemic heart disease risk in renal transplant candidates. However, these tests are less than perfect in predicting angiographically documented coronary disease or cardiovascular events. Dobutamine echocardiography may be an acceptable and more cost-effective alternative; however, less data is available than with thallium or sestamibi scintigraphy

Patients who appear to have critical lesions should undergo revascularization or angioplasty, stenting, and so forth before transplantation. One study demonstrated that patients randomized to revascularization before transplantation had fewer posttransplant cardiovascular disease events compared with patients managed medically (38). These findings suggest that in particular, diabetics and those with high risk for severe coronary artery disease should undergo elective revascularization before rather than after renal transplantation. However, this study was small and, thus, cannot be generally extrapolated to the whole ESRD population group in large part because morbidity and mortality are increased in dialysis patients who undergo coronary artery bypass surgery compared with non-ESRD patients (39).

Congestive heart failure is an important clinical consideration as part of the kidney transplant evaluation. Fifty percent of hemodialysis patients have a history of volume overload at some point during their clinical course during dialysis (40). As many as 20% may have decreased systolic function on echocardiogram (41). However, it is important to note that many patients have left ventricular hypertrophy and diastolic dysfunction with impaired lusitropy. This interferes with ventricular filling during diastole and can ultimately lead to output failure. The rationale for treatment is entirely different depending on ventricular function. Those with systolic heart failure will require preload and afterload reduction, whereas those with diastolic dysfunction will need antihypertensive agents, especially those that slow heart rate and facilitate ventricular relaxation (41). There are no overt contraindications to transplantation in patients with left ventricular hypertrophy or ventricular dysfunction unless the ejection fraction (EF) is less than 20%. There is much less information on the suitability of these types of patients for transplantation. Consequently, an echocardiogram is an important part of the evaluation. On a positive note, renal transplantation improves ventricular function in most patients with EFs in the 20% to 40% range (42,43).

Reversible causes of myocardial dysfunction should also be identified and treated. Problems related to alcohol abuse, anemia, and hypertension need to be considered. Reversible ischemia also may impair ventricular function.

Cerebral vascular disease is also an important consideration that must be considered as part of the pretransplant evaluation. The increasing age and prevalence of hypertension and diabetes as a cause of ESRD with the associated macrovascular disease increases the likelihood of cerebral vascular disease. This will likely increase. Patients with audible bruits or prior histories of transient ischemic attack (TIA) or stroke should have carotid artery Dopplers and consideration for carotid endarterectomy if significant disease is noted. Data from studies in the general population indicate that prophylactic surgery may be effective in selected patients, especially those with a surgical risk of less that 3% and a greater than 60% diameter reduction on ultrasound or those patients whose surgical risk is slightly higher but have more substantial stenoses in the presence of contralateral internal carotid artery stenosis of greater than 75% (44). In addition, whether patients with cerebral vascular disease are symptomatic or not, aspirin prophylaxis should be considered, although there are no data in transplant patients to support its use. In the presence of chronic atrial fibrillation, anticoagulation should be considered for guideline as in the general population (45).

Patients with polycystic kidney disease as a cause of ESRD with a family history of intracranial aneurysms or with a previous episode of intracranial bleeding should undergo computed tomography (CT) scan or magnetic resonance imaging (MRI) to evaluate the presence of intracranial aneurysm (46). Those aneurysms greater than 10 mm should be considered for prophylactic surgical removal to prevent bleeding (47).

Peripheral vascular disease is common in patients with ESRD (48). Its presence may help identify patients who need more careful evaluation of potential coronary artery disease or cerebral vascular disease. Because the renal transplant is connected to the iliac vessels, it is important to know the status of vasculature. Disruption of compromised iliac flow with a kidney transplant could render more distal vascular beds to impair blood supply. Some patients may require reconstructive surgery of aorto-iliac disease before or at the time of renal transplantation. Consequently, in high-risk patients lower extremity noninvasive testing should be considered followed by angiography if there is any question concerning the adequacy of the circulation.

In summary, atherosclerotic cardiovascular disease involving the heart, brain, and peripheral vasculature is one of the most important aspects of the pretransplant evaluation. Careful evaluation of all risk factors, adequacy of treatment, and provision of optimal medical management is necessary. In addition, preoperative evaluation of all possible areas of vascular compromise should be rigorously pursued and surgically corrected if indicated.

Cancer

Malignancies are responsible for 1% to 4% of all deaths in the dialysis population and 9% to 12% of deaths in the renal transplant population (49). Consequently, careful pretransplant screening is important to rule out transplantation occurring in a patient with a preexisting malignancy. What is not known is whether pretransplant screening may have a benefit in reducing the incidence of posttransplant malignancies.

Patients with prior episodes of cancer deserve a waiting period before transplantation because most forms of immunosuppression will likely inhibit surveillance mechanisms that would otherwise counteract the development of a malignancy (Table 42.4). The Cincinnati Transplant Tumor Registry indicates that 54% of recurrences occur in patients transplanted within 2 years of treatment, whereas 33% of recurrences

TABLE 42.4. RECOMMENDED TUMOR-FREE INTERVALS PRIOR TO TRANSPLANTATION

Malignancy	Time
Basal cell	None
In situ cervical	None
In situ bladder	None
Clark's level 1 melanoma	None
Duke's A colon	None
In situ lobular breast	None
Prostate	2 Years
Uterine	2 Years
Lymphoma	2 Years
Breast	2–5 Years
Invasive cervical	2–5 Years
Colorectal	2–5 Years

occurred in patients 2 to 5 years before transplantation (50). Only 13% of recurrences occurred in patients treated more than 5 years before transplantation. These statistics provide some general consideration in terms of the duration of wait between the time of treatment for cancer and transplantation.

Cutaneous malignancy is the most common form of cancer posttransplantation (50). There is a high recurrent rate of non-melanoma skin cancers that occurs over time after renal transplantation despite timely removal of lesions. However, this is rarely a cause of death.

The most important cancers to screen for are those that occur with greater frequency in the general population including cancers of the lung, prostate, breast, and cervix (50). In addition, renal cell cancer is more common in the ESRD population than in the general population, particularly in younger patients and those with ESRD from toxic, infectious, or obstructive uropathies (51). In addition, uroepithelial malignancies need to be screened for if there is any evidence of abnormalities in urinary sediment. High-risk patients may deserve an abdominal CT scan as part of their pretransplant workup.

For women, a pelvic examination with cervical evaluation and manual examination of the uterus should be part of every workup and should be continued on an annual basis while on the waiting list of a transplant.

Because of the increasing age of male renal transplant recipients, it is important to consider yearly evaluation of prostate specific antigen and digital rectal examination before transplantation, particularly for those older than 50 years (52). This may also be even more important in the African-American population in which there is a higher incidence of prostate cancer (53). If identified, it should be treated before transplantation. In the Cincinnati Transplant Tumor Registry, 40% of prostate cancer recurrences occurred within 2 years after treatment (54). Consequently, it may be best to wait at least 2 years after treatment before transplantation.

Lung cancer is an important malignancy not to miss before transplantation. It is the leading cause of cancer deaths (55). Screening chest x-ray film and a possible low-dose CT of the lung may be appropriate in high-risk patients with a family history who are smokers. Preferably, every patient who smokes should be made to stop before transplantation.

Cancer of the breast is the most common form of in situ cancer in female ESRD patients after nonmelanoma skin cancer and cancer of the uterine cervix (56). Interestingly, renal transplant recipients appear to have a lower relative risk of breast cancer than the general population. The explanation for this may be due to improved screening or previously unidentified effects of the immunosuppression (57). Factors associated with an increased risk of recurrence posttransplantation include prior nodal involvement, bilateral disease, inflammatory carcinoma, and prior bone metastases (50). Most clinicians would recommend a waiting period of 2 years after treatment and preferably longer (5 years) for most patients given the fact that the recurrence rate may be as high as 23% and mortality associated with it is substantial (50).

Manual breast examination and mammography should be performed annually for all women between the ages of 50 and 69 years being evaluated and waiting for a kidney transplant; screening should start earlier for those with a family history of breast cancer.

Although the incidence of colorectal cancer in dialysis patients is not increased compared with the general population, it remains a common cancer; therefore, fecal occult blood screening and sigmoidoscopy or colonoscopy should be considered in all patients older than 50 years as would be standard for the general population (56). Patients with previously treated colon cancer should wait at least 5 years before renal transplantation because the recurrence rate diminishes with time and mortality from recurrent colon cancer after renal transplantation is very high (50).

Lymphoproliferative disorders are more common in patients with ESRD than the general population (51) and may be substantially higher in renal transplant patients if they are exposed to the Epstein-Barr virus (EBV) de novo in the posttransplantation period (58). There is a question as to whether or not prophylactic treatment with acyclovir would be capable of suppressing EBV infection and the likelihood of EBV-associated posttransplantation lymphoproliferative disease (59,60).

In general, complete medical history and physical examination coupled with standard laboratory screening and judicious use of imaging techniques in higher risk patients should be considered as part of the standard workup. Individual determination of time to wait posttreatment of cancer before transplantation should be made on a case-by-case basis. In general waiting at least 5 years is preferred for most previously treated cancers.

Pulmonary Disease

Anticipating respiratory complications posttransplantation in the ESRD patient is no different than would be seen for non-ESRD patients facing elective surgery. The primary focus should be elimination of smoking and evaluation of pulmonary function if there is a history of chronic obstructive pulmonary disease or other forms of lung disease that interfere with oxygenation. All patients should be screened with a careful history and physical examination and a chest x-ray film. As mentioned previously, specific focus should be addressed on the smoker, because studies in the general population indicate that smokers were 5.5 times more likely to develop pulmonary complications postsurgery compared with those who did not smoke (61).

Endocrine Disease

The endocrine evaluation of a dialysis patient should primarily focus on issues surrounding diabetes, obesity, and ESRD-related bone disease.

Because diabetes is the leading cause of ESRD, the proportion of patients on dialysis awaiting a transplant with diabetes is substantial. Patients with diabetes, which is most commonly type 2, have advanced risk for atherosclerotic cardiovascular disease and death (62). Consequently, all diabetic patients need careful focus on evaluation of vascular beds pretransplantation. Retinopathy, neuropathy, autonomic dysfunction, and associated complications from diabetes persist and/or progress during dialytic therapy. Despite greater likelihood of progression of complications of the diabetes posttransplantation, survival is demonstrably improved for diabetics with renal transplantation compared with remaining on dialysis (5).

Pancreas transplantation may also be an appropriate strategy for a patient with type 1 diabetes who requires renal replacement therapy. With improving techniques and immunosuppression, pancreas transplantation has become an accepted therapy for patients with type 1 diabetes with patient survival rates exceeding 90% and rates of insulin independence of more than 80% at 1 year (63–65). Obesity is associated with increased morbidity and mortality posttransplantation (66). Although malnutrition increases mortality in the ESRD population and conversely higher body mass index (BMI) is associated with a reduced mortality among dialysis patients (67), obesity becomes an important risk factor for morbidity and mortality in the transplant patient. Obese patients have higher rates of delayed graft function, suffer from more surgical complications and wound infections, and will frequently require prolonged hospitalization (67,68). Posttransplant diabetes mellitus is more common in obese patients, and some transplant centers even suggest that increased risk of acute rejection and graft loss occurs in obese patients compared with nonobese patients (66,69). Most transplant centers suggest that BMI be less than 30 for renal transplantation candidates and that a recommendation should be made for weight loss therapy if this goal cannot be immediately achieved.

Pretransplant planning for the treatment of metabolic bone disease is important, because there is growing evidence that preemptive strategies may prevent the development of pathologic fractures. Patients with ESRD can suffer from high-turnover bone disease because of secondary hyperparathyroidism, low-turnover bone disease resulting from osteomalacia, or variance of both (70,71). Patients may also have dialysis-related amyloid bone disease. Renal transplantation is an effective treatment for most causes of low-turnover bone disease and for dialysis-related amyloid bone disease. However, persistence of hyperparathyroidism after successful renal transplantation is common (72). Therefore, parathyroid hormone (PTH) levels should be checked pretransplantation, and, if persistent, posttransplantation surgical removal of the parathyroid should be planned. Pretransplant parathyroidectomy should be considered for transplant candidates who have failed medical management and/or have severe persistent complications of hyperparathyroidism such as refractory hypercalcemia, markedly elevated calcium-phosphorus products, or progressive extraskeletal calcifications or calciphylaxis (70).

Gastrointestinal Disease

The primary gastrointestinal issues in the ESRD patient revolve around the presence or absence of diverticulosis or diverticulitis or other forms of colonic disease; peptic ulcer disease; or chronic liver disease, usually resulting from major hepatitis viruses or gallbladder disease.

Colon disease resulting from diverticulosis or diverticulitis is not uncommon in the ESRD patient, in many cases it is due to sedentary lifestyle and the medications predisposing to constipation (73). Although posttransplantation colonic perforation is a morbid and mortal consequence (74), it is unknown how to best diagnose and treat it preemptively. Patients with severe diverticulosis may require partial colectomy pretransplant. However, there is no accepted standard in terms of how to approach this problem. Patients with polycystic kidney disease have an even greater risk for colonic perforation posttransplantation as high as 5%, which is substantially more than the 0.5% to 2% that is seen in patients receiving renal transplantation with ESRD resulting from nonacquired polycystic kidney disease (non-APKD) disease (75).

Peptic ulcer disease can be a serious complication posttransplantation (76,77). The perioperative use of corticosteroids and infections such as herpes virus, cytomegalovirus (CMV), or *Candida* markedly increase the risk for gastritis and gastrointestinal hemorrhage. Prior history of peptic ulcer disease should prompt physicians to perform upper gastrointestinal endoscopy and fecal occult blood testing. During endoscopy, screening for *Helicobacter pylori* should be planned (78). With the advent of proton pump inhibitors, the risk of serious complications of gastrointestinal hemorrhage posttransplantation has markedly improved (79). Patients with a history of peptic ulcer disease have a threefold greater incidence of ulceration posttransplantation compared with those patients without a history of peptic ulcer disease (77). However, progressive screening and proton pump inhibitor use largely mitigates this risk.

Liver disease is a significant cause of late morbidity and mortality among renal transplant recipients (80). In fact, death from liver failure has been reported in anywhere from 8% to 28% of renal transplant recipients (81). Chronic posttransplant liver disease is usually related to viral hepatitis, primarily hepatitis B (HBV) and hepatitis C (HCV). Serum transaminases should be routinely followed pretransplantation, and if persistently abnormal a liver biopsy should be obtained. Renal transplant recipients should be routinely screened for HBV surface antigen and HCV. Patients who are HBV surface antigen positive will also have circulating HBV antigen or serologic evidence of acute viral replication [HBV deoxyribonucleic acid (DNA)] and are at increased risk of progressive liver disease posttransplantation (82). Although chronic dosing of lamivudine may help control viral replication in these patients, drug resistance likely limits the long-term effectiveness of this therapy (83,84). Consequently, there is some debate as to whether or not these patients should be transplanted because there are no data demonstrating whether the long-term survival advantage of renal transplantation is counterbalanced by the increased risk for progression of liver disease (5). A liver biopsy may be helpful to prognosticate, because patients with cirrhosis may have an unacceptable risk for progression to liver failure and should probably remain on dialysis. The primary use of the liver biopsy is to screen for cirrhosis or active hepatitis given the poor sensitivity of chronic serum transaminase elevations in predicting the type of histology one would observe on liver biopsy. All patients who are HBV surface antigen negative should receive the recombinant HBV vaccine.

HCV-related liver disease is a substantial problem for hemodialysis patients because of its frequency (85,86). Roughly 10% to 20% of hemodialysis patients are positive for HCV (see Chapter 22). Up to 50% of the cases of liver disease posttransplantation can be attributed to HCV infection (85,86). All transplant candidates should be screened for anti-HCV radioimmunoassay with confirmation testing by radioimmunoblot assay (RIBA). If positive, serum should be tested for HCV ribonucleic acid (RNA) to confirm current HCV infection. Because serum transaminases are poor indicators of degree of disease, liver biopsy should be strongly considered. Patients with cirrhosis on liver biopsy should, in most instances, remain on dialysis because of an unacceptable increased risk for progressive liver failure posttransplantation (87). Patients who are HCV RNA positive may benefit from a course of interferon-alpha before transplantation (88). Interestingly, HCV is also associated with an increased incidence of glomerulonephritis and diabetes posttransplantation (86,89). Without evidence of cirrhosis, the presence of HCV antibody per se should not be a contraindication to transplantation.

It has been routine over the past few years to give HCV-positive transplant candidates HCV-positive donor kidneys (90). Most reported experiences do not suggest that there is any increased risk of progressive liver disease to the recipient in the short term (91). However, long-term observation will ultimately be necessary to demonstrate the safety of this practice. It is important to note that waiting times on the transplantation list are reduced if HCV-positive kidneys are used in HCV-infected recipients (91).

Infections

An important part of the pretransplant evaluation in the dialysis patient is to eliminate infection that may persist posttransplantation and that may become more difficult to treat or possibly become life threatening. A careful history and physical examination are important to identify possible sites of infection such as at the site of hemodialysis or peritoneal dialysis access. Peritoneal fluid should be cultured. A serologic evaluation of past viral exposures is important and may help in the design of proper posttransplantation prophylaxis treatment, as well as guide decisions with regard to transplantation of a kidney from an infected donor. Transplant candidates should receive immunizations for known infections that are prevalent before transplantation, such as HBV and any childhood immunizations that may have been missed. Seroscreening for CMV, EBV, and all the hepatitis viruses is routinely recommended. However, it is not possible to exclude possible infection with other unusual pathogens such as syphilis, strongyloidiasis, toxoplasma, or herpes. In addition, newer viruses, which may be pathogenic and are being identified such as the polyoma virus (BK), cannot yet be screened for. Seroscreening for human immunodeficiency virus (HIV) and tuberculin testing should also be routine.

CMV infection, until the recent development of effective anti-CMV drugs, was a morbid and mortal event that could occur in the transplant recipient. The incidence of CMV disease is generally less than 5% for recipients who do not have antibodies to CMV and who receive kidneys from donors who are antibody negative (92,93). However, the incidence of primary CMV disease among antibody-negative recipients of CMV-positive kidneys is high, on the order of 50% to 75% without specific and effective prophylactic regimens (92,93). CMV disease in antibody-positive recipients receiving either positive or nega-

tive donor kidneys is about 25% to 40% (92,93). Thus, this illness is frequent in the posttransplant patient and will require careful assessment of the amount of immunosuppression because this directly influences the incidence and severity of CMV disease.

A recent metaanalysis of controlled clinical trials demonstrated that specific antiviral agents (acyclovir or ganciclovir) were effective in preventing CMV infection in solid organ transplant recipients (94). However, it is important to note that this regimen is associated with side effects and can be expensive. Therefore, judicious and appropriate screening pretransplantation can help identify those patients who will derive greatest benefit from the investment in prophylactic therapy. There is concern that (even with newer and more effective therapies such as valganciclovir) ganciclovir-resistant CMV strains can develop in patients receiving prophylaxis, which could undermine this therapeutic strategy (95).

Patients with ESRD are at greater risk for mycobacterial disease. This is frequently asymptomatic despite the fact that up to a third of ESRD patients may be anergic. Purified protein derivative (PPD) testing is recommended so that isoniazid prophylaxis can be used, and performance of a chest x-ray examination can be helpful to rule out the likelihood of active infection. There is no evidence that prophylaxis with isoniazid reduces the incidence of reactivation of tuberculosis after transplantation (96). Despite this, many centers require pretransplant and/or posttransplant isoniazid prophylaxis for patients with a positive PPD skin test.

Peritoneal dialysis patients must be carefully screened for occult tunnel track or peritoneal fluid infections. In particular, *Staphylococcus epidermidis* may cause an occult peritonitis that can flourish once immunosuppression is started posttransplantation. Clinical studies indicate that patients on peritoneal dialysis more frequently develop infections within the first month posttransplantation compared with patients on hemodialysis. More often than not, these sites are located in the abdominal cavity, the surgical wound, or in the peritoneal fluid. Peritoneal dialysis patients with active infections should have transplantation delayed, if at all possible, if they have a history of active or recent peritonitis to ensure that proper therapy can be employed. Documentation of clearing of the infection is appropriate.

Careful evaluation of the dentition is appropriate pretransplantation in all dialysis patients. Periodontal infections and active periodontitis could worsen posttransplantation because of the use of immunosuppressive agents, particularly cyclosporine because it induces gingival hyperplasia (97). Although there are no controlled clinical trials demonstrating that treatment of periodontal disease reduces the likelihood of recurrence posttransplantation, it is appropriate to consider strategies to care for active disease processes before using medications that will stimulate gingival growth and could cover up underlying infectious processes.

Pulmonary infections posttransplantation are an important concern. Some studies suggest that renal transplant recipients develop pneumococcal infections at a rate of about 1% per year (98). Pneumococcal immunization is currently recommended for all chronic dialysis patients (99). It is particularly important for those who have been previously splenectomized. Annual immunization with influenza vaccine is also currently recommended for all chronic dialysis patients (99). However, there are no good studies to indicate that influenza is more severe when it occurs in an immunosuppressed transplant patient compared with a dialysis patient. Most childhood vaccinations should be employed pretransplantation, if they have never been received.

Patients who are HIV positive and have a strong desire for transplantation may be evaluated for transplantation specifically at centers with protocols designed to examine the effects of immunosuppression on outcome in these high-risk individuals. At the current time, there is no recommended immunosuppression strategy. As such, protocol testing is required to understand more as to the optimal regimen in these patients.

Genitourinary Disease

The ESRD patient needs a careful examination of the genitourinary tract for a number of important reasons. First, there may be abnormalities in the drainage system that lead to the original renal dysfunction, such as bladder disease, stones, prostatic disease, or urethral strictures. These underlying abnormalities would need to be identified and corrected before the same urinary tract is used for drainage for the transplanted kidney. For this reason, a careful history and physical examination are needed. Routine recommendation for a voiding cystourethrogram (VCUG) should be considered in patients with a history of genitourinary abnormalities. Up to 25% of pretransplant VCUGs are abnormal in ESRD patients (100). Most of the time, the abnormalities are minor and do not require surgical correction. Among younger individuals, the likelihood of congenital abnormalities is greater, whereas in older individuals prostatic hypertrophy either from benign growth or malignancy are possibilities. In addition, bladder cancer is 1.4 to 4.8 times more common in dialysis patients than in the general population (51). Thus, any abnormalities on urinalysis should be carefully followed up with either a VCUG or cystoscopy. Urine cytology may also be helpful.

A neurogenic bladder is also an important problem that should be identified pretransplant. Although there are many causes, the most common are due to neurogenic issues usually related to diabetes. Patients may require intermittent catheterization or urinary diversion. In addition, patients with small bladders may need a bladder augmentation procedure or bladder stretching.

Patients with a history of urinary tract infections or stones need careful evaluation to ensure that there are no structural abnormalities that could predispose them to recurrence of these infections posttransplantation. Patients with bladder diverticula, large stones, or infected cysts, such as patients with polycystic kidney disease, may benefit from either unilateral or bilateral nephrectomy to reduce the likelihood of recurrent infection.

Other causes for a nephrectomy could include the identification of a renal cell carcinoma on ultrasound, oversized kidneys resulting from polycystic kidney disease that could impair placement of a new allograft, or possibly an inability to control blood pressure.

Recurrent Kidney Disease

It is important to identify the cause of ESRD in patients being evaluated for a kidney transplant. Almost all causes of kidney failure can recur in the kidney transplant with few exceptions such as polycystic kidney disease, Alport's syndrome, or toxic nephropathies resulting from drug ingestion. Although the risk of recurrence is small, in notable cases it can be substantial and possibly lead to graft loss. There is substantial variation in the risk for recurrence and its severity. For those patients who do have recurrent kidney disease, the risk of graft failure is 1.9 times higher than for patients without recurrent disease (101). In large part, the physician's assessment of the risk of recurrence is difficult because many patients progress to ESRD without proper identification of the cause. In addition, the incidence of recurrent disease may depend on the length of follow-up, and sometimes the ability to diagnose recurrent disease from chronic allograft nephropathy may be difficult.

Recurrent glomerulonephritis is most commonly seen with focal segmental glomerulosclerosis (FSGS), IgA nephropathy, and membranoproliferative glomerulonephritis (MPGN). Other glomerulonephritides such as membranous glomerulonephritis, Wegener's granulomatosis, and hemolytic uremic syndrome (HUS) can also recur (101) (Table 42.5).

TABLE 42.5. RECURRENCE OF GLOMERULONEPHRITIS AFTER RENAL TRANSPLANTATION

Disease	Histologic Recurrence %	Graft Loss with Recurrence %
Focal segmental glomerulosclerosis	20–40	40–50
IgA nephropathy	20–40	6–33
Membranoproliferative		
Type I	20–30	30–40
Type II	80–90	10–20
Membranous nephropathy	10–20	0–50
Anti-GBM nephritis	10–25	Rare
Henoch-Schönlein purpura	15–35	Rare
Hemolytic uremic syndrome	10–25	10–40
Lupus nephritis	Rare	Rare

GBM, glomerular basement membrane.

FSGS recurs in 20% to 40% of patients, and, of those that do recur, 40% to 50% will lose their grafts (102,103). Those patients with rapid progression to original ESRD with FSGS are at greatest risk. African-Americans and patients with younger age at onset of disease are more likely to have recurrence (104). The strongest predictor, however, is recurrence in a previous transplant. Unfortunately, there does not appear to be a serologic predictor for recurrence or an appropriate prophylactic therapy. Despite this, FSGS is not viewed as a contraindication to renal transplantation because it is a heterogenous disease process and it is impossible to predict who would not be an ideal candidate.

IgA nephropathy can also recur frequently (20% to 40%) (105). Although graft failure can occur in 6% to 33% of patients with recurrent disease (106), a shorter interval between onset and the development of ESRD with IgA nephropathy appears to correlate with the likelihood of recurrence (106). It is also more common to recur in recipients of living-related transplants. However, donor source has not affected graft survival in patients transplanted with ESRD resulting from IgA nephropathy. Graft loss because of recurrent IgA nephropathy is not a contraindication for retransplantation because good long-term graft survival is observed after repeat renal transplantation.

Henoch-Schönlein purpura recurs in 15% to 35% of patients but rarely causes graft failure (107). It usually recurs in individuals with disease that has been recently active. However, occasionally it can recur in patients who have had no evidence of disease for several years. Most data suggest that a shorter duration of original disease makes recurrence more likely (107). However, only 11% of graft failure can be attributed to recurrent disease despite the fact that histologic evidence of recurrence is common (107).

Patients with MPGN have recurrence rates of 20% to 30% (108). Graft loss may be seen in 40% of patients (108). In patients with type 2 MPGN, the risk of recurrence is nearly 80%; however, graft loss is less common than in type 1 MPGN occurring in about 10% to 20% of patients with recurrence (108). It is important to differentiate these idiopathic forms of MPGN from that which occurs secondary to HCV infection. It is also important to differentiate MPGN from chronic rejection by careful histologic evaluation, including immunofluorescence and electron microscopy.

Less common glomerulonephritides include membranous glomerulonephritis, which occurs in 10% to 20% of patients (109). Graft loss may be as high as 50% if patients are followed for greater than 10 years (109). There are no readily identifiable risk factors to determine the likelihood of recurrence.

HUS can recur in 10% to 25% of patients. However, it can be primary (without obvious cause) or secondary (related to the use of calcineurin inhibitors such as cyclosporine or tacrolimus) (110). It has even been reported with the use of antilymphocyte globulin and OKT3 monoclonal antibody (111,112). The older the age of onset of HUS, the shorter the interval for recurrent HUS posttransplantation and the shorter the interval between HUS onset and ESRD. The use of living donors should be contraindicated in these patients because it increases the risk for recurrence (109). The risk for graft failure is substantial. It may be as high as 50% (109). It is reported to be more than five times higher than for patients without posttransplant HUS. Strategies to provide necessary immunosuppression, particularly with the need for cadaveric donors in these patients, is important because most transplant centers would prefer not to use calcineurin inhibitors. Some centers have suggested that the use of prophylactic antiplatelet therapy may help reduce the chances of recurrence. However, there are no data to support this effort.

Antiglomerular basement membrane (anti-GBM) disease may recur in 10% to 25% of patients, although histologic recurrence may be seen in about 50% of patients. Anti-GBM antibodies should be documented as undetectable in the pretransplant workup to minimize the likelihood of recurrence.

Patients with ESRD resulting from Wegener's granulomatosis may also experience a recurrence rate as high as 15% to 50% (113). Data from small uncontrolled studies indicate that patients with recurrent disease can be successfully treated with cyclophosphamide (113). Most centers would recommend waiting until the disease is quiet before transplantation, although there are no data to indicate optimal timing of renal transplantation in patients with this disease process.

Patients with ESRD resulting from systemic lupus erythematosus (SLE) have a low risk of recurrence, perhaps less than 10% (114). It is generally recommended that patients not have any evidence of clinical disease before transplantation. It is preferable that the serologic parameters such as complements and antinuclear anti-DNA antibody be normal or at least stable before transplantation. Recurrence that results in graft failure is unusual, and there does not appear to be any effect of prior SLE on patient or graft survival (114).

Unusual causes of ESRD such as oxalosis, cystinosis, Fabry's disease, and sickle cell disease can recur. Oxalosis is the most important with regard to its recurrence rate, and preferably the patient should receive a simultaneous liver transplant at the time of the kidney transplant to reduce the likelihood that hyperoxalosis will destroy the transplanted graft.

Amyloidosis can recur in the kidney in about one third of patients posttransplantation (115). If patients have severe multiorgan involvement with amyloidosis, transplantation should be generally discouraged because their survival is low. However, with primary injury to the kidneys, transplantation should not be precluded. More often than not, the outcome of transplantation appears to be determined by the severity of systemic disease affecting survival rather than recurrence in the allograft leading to graft dysfunction.

Because diabetes is the most common cause of ESRD, it is important to note that both type 1 and type 2 diabetes can recur within the transplanted kidney. For type 1 patients, this explains the rationale behind simultaneous pancreas kidney transplantation. In the patients with type 2 diabetes, careful attention should be focused on blood pressure, cholesterol, and glycemic control. In addition, therapeutic strategies incorporating drugs that block the renin-angiotensin system should be used. Although no studies have indicated effects on graft survival using this approach, it has certainly been demonstrated to be effective in patients with type 2 diabetes and kidney disease without renal transplantation.

Coagulopathies

Patients with a history of recurrent graft clotting on dialysis or deep vein thrombosis should have special attention focused on their clotting studies. Limited studies have attempted to determine the prevalence of coagulation abnormalities among renal transplant candidates. Patients with SLE may have antiphospholipid antibodies, which may manifest as a lupus anticoagulant, and may have increased thrombotic risk (116). Other clotting abnormalities may also occur. Unfortunately, they may increase the risk for perioperative graft thrombosis. Consequently, a proactive approach is necessary to screen high-risk patients for coagulation abnormalities and to use prophylaxis to prevent clotting.

Psychosocial

A complete psychosocial evaluation should be performed on all prospective transplant recipients. The importance of this evaluation is to be sure that there are not psychosocial barriers to transplantation or potential problems with compliance or chemical dependency that could interfere with the complicated medical regimen posttransplantation. In addition, reversible medical causes of cognitive impairment could be identified with a dementia workup such as evaluating thyroid function and obtaining thiamin, vitamin B_{12}, and folate levels.

In particular, alcohol and drug abuse must be identified and dealt with. Underreporting of individuals with substance abuse is common and in many cases may lead to graft loss because of noncompliance (117,118).

Mental illness is common in patients with ESRD. The stress of a transplant and concern about the viability of the transplant could lead many patients into significant depression that could interfere with the maintenance of proper medical care. Consequently, susceptible individuals should be identified pretransplant so that careful support systems can be used during the transplantation course.

Well-managed schizophrenia is generally not considered a transplantation contraindication. Certainly those patients who are not well controlled deserve an opportunity for proper treatment before transplantation.

In summary, a careful examination of psychosocial issues is imperative before transplantation because noncompliance is the third leading cause of graft failure (119). Moreover, a poor home situation and financial or social problems could interfere with proper delivery of care and may lead to an adverse outcome posttransplantation.

MANAGEMENT OF PATIENTS ON THE CADAVERIC KIDNEY WAITING LIST

How should the health status of dialysis patients on the UNOS cadaver kidney waiting list be followed? Unfortunately, evidence-based guidelines describing the best mechanism to manage the health and psychosocial well being of patients on the cadaveric renal transplant waiting list have never been published. Knowledge about the correct management of patients on the waiting list for cadaveric kidney transplantation is in its infancy (120). Recognition of the significant death rate and the demonstration that the length of time on the waiting list is an independent determinant of long-term posttransplant prognosis has prompted intense interest in this subject (8,121).

The Clinical Practice Guidelines Committee of the American Society of Transplantation recently published the results of a survey, which polled transplant centers in the United States and asked how they managed patients on the cadaveric transplant waiting list (122). Sixty-seven percent (192 of 287) of centers polled responded to the survey. Despite a lack of evidence-based guidelines for the management of dialysis patients awaiting renal transplantation, certain important points merit discussion. During the months and years that a patient is maintained on hemodialysis awaiting a renal transplant, many things may change including demographics, psychosocial support, general medical condition, and cardiovascular status.

The transplant procedure has been described as an urgent surgery performed on an elective population. When a kidney becomes available, time is of the essence. The patient must be easily contacted, and a mechanism to transport the patient to the transplant center must be readily available. Patients undergoing maintenance hemodialysis must be continually reminded to update their telephone numbers and addresses with the transplant center. It should be pointed out to the patient that his or her diligence in this regard will benefit the patient greatly. Notifying the transplant center when going on a prolonged vacation, temporarily residing at an alternative location, or when changing residence will ensure that the patient can be promptly contacted when an organ becomes available. Delay in contacting a candidate or a lack of a means of expedited transport prolongs cold ischemia time, which increases the risk for delayed graft function, may increase the risk of early acute rejection, and negatively affects graft survival (123,124).

Many important psychosocial issues change for patients on maintenance hemodialysis. Unfortunately, these issues can be viewed as being of secondary importance compared with the general and more specifically cardiovascular health of potential recipients on the waiting list. Nevertheless, a patient's employment status, marital status, state of residence, insurance coverage, and psychologic support mechanisms can all change while on hemodialysis and on the waiting list. Although it is unlikely that any of these issues would directly prevent a patient from receiving a kidney transplant, these issues are important. For example, patients who stop working, graduate from school, relocate to a nearby state, or suffer the loss of spousal support as a result of death or divorce might find themselves nearly destitute in the posttransplant period as they face the financial cost of medications, repeat hospitalizations, and professional fees during the months and years following transplantation. Currently, maintenance medications for a renal transplant patient approach $15,000 per year. Few, if any, are able to cover these costs out-of-pocket. As a result, every patient should be reminded, while on the waiting list, to seek advice about how changes in psychosocial issues could alter benefits, insurance, and prescription coverage and thereby affect posttransplant life (11). Dialysis patients on the waiting list and transplant centers should maintain a routine dialogue about such issues. Patients should seek advice from social workers and financial counselors at their transplant center or dialysis unit when contemplating major life changes, such as changing jobs, seeking early retirement, seeking disability, and moving to another state. Ideally, individuals would have all the appropriate information to make the best decision before irreversible loss of coverage or benefits occur.

Ensuring that a patient, who might be on dialysis for several years before transplantation, is medically fit to undergo surgery is a daunting task for many transplant centers. At this time, given the lack of evidence-based data from studies of this population, the recommendation is to follow age-appropriate health maintenance and screening guidelines for colon, prostate, breast, and uterine malignancy (120,125).

Dialysis patients are catabolic; are at risk for malnutrition; suffer recurrent life-threatening infections; and most significantly of all, live with the atherogenic burden of chronic renal disease (126–129).

Strict medical guidelines for the initial listing of patients with renal insufficiency are standard at most transplant centers. Once a patient is listed, however, the frequency with which a patient on dialysis is reevaluated and the integrity of their cardiovascular reserve to permit a safe surgical procedure varies widely (130).

Given the importance of appropriate cardiovascular clearance and the often asymptomatic deterioration of cardiovascular function on dialysis, many centers surveyed responded that they closely followed patients on the waiting list. Most centers (79%) indicated that they screened patients on an annual basis. Of these, 40% employed nuclear perfusion scanning, 33% used exercise thallium scanning, 31% employed dobutamine echocardiography, and only 15% required coronary angiography (122). Unfortunately, these diagnostic studies are less reliable among patients with ESRD. Noninvasive testing for coronary artery disease among asymptomatic patients with ESRD is of limited value (131). Dobutamine stress echocardiography has been proposed as the best noninvasive method for long-term follow-up and repeated study of this population. Unfortunately, the frequency of follow-up assessments required and long-term studies comparing this with gold standard angiographic evidence are lacking. Dobutamine stress echocardiography has a sensitivity of 75% and a specificity of only 71%, compared with angiography when evaluating lesions of greater than 70% stenosis (14). Dipyridamole and thallium imaging has a sensitivity of only 37% and a specificity of only 73% in this population. It does not clearly predict cardiac prognosis among patients with ESRD (132). Efforts to facilitate communication and to educate patients, primary care physicians, local subspecialists (especially cardiologists), dialysis social workers, and dialysis center staff about the importance of updating the transplant center about changes in demographic, psychosocial, and health issues must be stressed. Most importantly, patients themselves, their nephrologists, and the pretransplant coordinators should work in concert and communicate frequently and freely to maximize preparedness at all times. It has been suggested that regular contact between the patient, nephrologist, and transplant centers, perhaps during site visits to dialysis centers by members of the transplant center team, could serve to educate patients, maintain motivation, diminish a sense of hopelessness, and offer time to reevaluate living-donor options.

REFERENCES

1. Transplant Statistics Organ Donation and Transplantation Trends. www.ustransplant.org/annual_reports/ar02/highlights/ar02_chapter _one.htm.
2. Schnuelle P, et al. Impact of renal cadaveric transplantation on survival in end-stage renal failure: evidence for reduced mortality risk compared with hemodialysis during long-term follow-up. *J Am Soc Nephrol* 1998;9:2135–2141.
3. Port FK, et al. Comparison of survival probabilities for dialysis patients vs. cadaveric renal transplant recipients. *JAMA* 1993;270: 1339–1343.
4. Ojo AO, et al. Comparative mortality risks of chronic dialysis and cadaveric transplantation in black end-stage renal disease patients. *Am J Kidney Dis* 1994;24:59–64.
5. Wolfe RA, et al. Comparison of mortality in all patients on dialysis, patients on dialysis awaiting transplantation, and recipients of a first cadaveric transplant. *N Engl J Med* 1999;341:1725–1730.
6. Meier-Kriesche HU, et al. Survival improvement among patients with end-stage renal disease: trends over time for transplant recipients and wait-listed patients. *J Am Soc Nephrol* 2001;12:1293–1296.
7. Harper AM, et al. The OPTN waiting list, 1988–2000.   In: Cecka JM, et al., eds. *Clinical transplants 2001.* Los Angeles: UCLA Immunogenetics Center, 2001:82.
8. Meier-Kriesche HU, et al. Effect of waiting time on renal transplant outcome. *Kidney Int* 2000;58:1311–1317.
9. Matas AJ, et al. 2,500 living donor kidney transplants: a single-center experience. *Ann Surg* 2001;234:149–164.
10. Vats AN, et al. Pretransplant dialysis status and outcome of renal transplantation in North American children: a NAPRTCS Study. North American Pediatric Renal Transplant Cooperative Study. *Transplantation* 2000;69:1414–1419.
11. 2002 Annual Report of the U.S. Organ Procurement and Transplantation Network and the Scientific Registry of Transplant Recipients: Transplant Data 1992–2001. Department of Health and Human Services, Health Resources and Services Administration, Office of Special Programs, Division of Transplantation, Rockville, MD; United Network for Organ Sharing, Richmond, VA; University Renal Research and Education Association, Ann Arbor, MI, 1–7.
12. Cecka JM. The UNOS renal transplant registry. In: Cecka JM, et al., eds. *Clinical transplants 2001.* Los Angeles: UCLA Immunogenetics Center, 2001:2–4.
13. Gjertson DW, et al. Living unrelated donor kidney transplantation. *Kidney Int* 2000;58:491–499.
14. Schweitzer EJ, et al. Increased rates of donation with laparoscopic donor nephrectomy. *Ann Surg* 2000;232:392–400.
15. Nogueira JM, et al. A comparison of recipient renal outcomes with laparoscopic versus open live donor nephrectomy. *Transplantation* 1999;67:722–728.
16. Osei K, et al. Physiological and pharmacological stimulation of pancreatic islet hormone secretion in type I diabetic pancreas allograft recipients. *Diabetes* 1990;39:1235–1242.
17. Robertson RP, et al. Time-related, cross-sectional and prospective follow-up of pancreatic endocrine function after pancreas allograft transplantation in type 1 (insulin-dependent) diabetic patients. *Diabetologia* 1991;34[Suppl 1]:S57–S60.
18. Katz H, et al. Effects of pancreas transplantation on postprandial glucose metabolism. *N Engl J Med* 1991;325:1278–1283.
19. Navarro X, et al. Long-term effects of pancreatic transplantation on diabetic neuropathy. *Ann Neurol* 1997;42:727–736.
20. Fioretto P, et al. Reversal of lesions of diabetic nephropathy after pancreas transplantation. *N Engl J Med* 1998;339:69–75.
21. Sollinger HW, et al. Experience with 500 simultaneous pancreas-kidney transplants. *Ann Surg* 1998;228:284–296.
22. Cheung AH, et al. Simultaneous pancreas-kidney transplant versus kidney transplant alone in diabetic patients. *Kidney Int* 1992;41: 924–929.
23. Kasiske BL, et al. Cardiovascular disease after renal transplantation. *J Am Soc Nephrol* 1996;7:158–165.

24. Ojo AO, et al. Long-term survival in renal transplant recipients with graft function. *Kidney Int* 2000;57:307–313.
25. Goldman L. Multifactorial index of cardiac risk in noncardiac surgery: ten-year status report. *J Cardiothorac Anesth* 1987;1: 237–244.
26. Hensle TW, et al. Metabolism and nutrition in the perioperative period. *J Urol* 1988;139:229–239.
27. Goldman L, et al. Risks of general anesthesia and elective operation in the hypertensive patient. *Anesthesiology* 1979;50:285–292.
28. Charlson ME, et al. Preoperative characteristics predicting intraoperative hypotension and hypertension among hypertensives and diabetics undergoing noncardiac surgery. *Ann Surg* 1990;212:66–81.
29. American College of Physicians. Guidelines for assessing and managing the perioperative risk from coronary artery disease associated with major noncardiac surgery. *Ann Intern Med* 1997;127:309–312.
30. Lewis MS, et al. Factors in cardiac risk stratification of candidates for renal transplant. *J Cardiovasc Risk* 1999;6:251–255.
31. Manske CL, et al. Atherosclerotic vascular complications in diabetic transplant candidates. *Am J Kidney Dis* 1997;29:601–607.
32. Kasiske BL, et al. The evaluation of renal transplant candidates: clinical practice guidelines. *Am J Transplant* 2001;1:1–95.
33. Dahan M, et al. Diagnostic accuracy and prognostic value of combined dipyridamole-exercise thallium imaging in hemodialysis patients. *Kidney Int* 1998;54:255–262.
34. Brown JH, et al. Value of thallium myocardial imaging in the prediction of future cardiovascular events in patients with end-stage renal failure. *Nephrol Dial Transplant* 1993;8:433–437.
35. Herzog CA, et al. Dobutamine stress echocardiography for the detection of significant coronary artery disease in renal transplant candidates. *Am J Kidney Dis* 1999;33:1080–1090.
36. Bates JR, et al. Evaluation using dobutamine stress echocardiography in patients with insulin-dependent diabetes mellitus before kidney and/or pancreas transplantation. *Am J Cardiol* 1996;77:175–179.
37. Smart SC, et al. Dobutamine-atropine stress echocardiography and dipyridamole sestamibi scintigraphy for the detection of coronary artery disease: limitations and concordance. *J Am Coll Cardiol* 2000; 36:1265–1273.
38. Manske CL, et al. Coronary revascularisation in insulin-dependent diabetic patients with chronic renal failure. *Lancet* 1992;340:998–1002.
39. Liu JY, et al. Risks of morbidity and mortality in dialysis patients undergoing coronary artery bypass surgery. Northern New England Cardiovascular Disease Study Group. *Circulation* 2000;102:2973–2977.
40. Longenecker JC, et al. Validation of comorbid conditions on the end-stage renal disease medical evidence report: the CHOICE study. Choices for Healthy Outcomes in Caring for ESRD. *J Am Soc Nephrol* 2000;11:520–529.
41. Parfrey PS, et al. Outcome and risk factors for left ventricular disorders in chronic uraemia. *Nephrol Dial Transplant* 1996;11:1277–1285.
42. Burt RK, et al. Reversal of left ventricular dysfunction after renal transplantation. *Ann Intern Med* 1989;111:635–640.
43. Foley RN, et al. Serial change in echocardiographic parameters and cardiac failure in end-stage renal disease. *J Am Soc Nephrol* 2000;11: 912–916.
44. Biller J, et al. Guidelines for carotid endarterectomy: a statement for healthcare professionals from a Special Writing Group of the Stroke Council, American Heart Association. *Circulation* 1998;97:501–509.
45. American College of Physicians. Guidelines for medical treatment for stroke prevention. American College of Physicians. *Ann Intern Med* 1994;121:54–55.
46. Chapman AB, et al. Intracranial aneurysms in autosomal dominant polycystic kidney disease. *N Engl J Med* 1992;327:916–920.
47. International Study of Unruptured Intracranial Aneurysms Investigators. Unruptured intracranial aneurysms—risk of rupture and risks of surgical intervention. *N Engl J Med* 1998;339:1724–1733.
48. Sung RS, et al. Peripheral vascular occlusive disease in renal transplant recipients: risk factors and impact on kidney allograft survival. *Transplantation* 2000;70:1049–1054.
49. US Renal Data System. Causes of death. USRDS 1999 Annual Report. Bethesda, MD: National Institutes of Health, National Institute of Diabetes, Digestive and Kidney Diseases, 1999:89–100.
50. Penn I. Evaluation of transplant candidates with pre-existing malignancies. *Ann Transplant* 1997;2:14–17.
51. Maisonneuve P, et al. Cancer in patients on dialysis for end-stage renal disease: an international collaborative study. *Lancet* 1999;354:93–99.
52. Konety BR, et al. Prostate cancer in the post-transplant population. Urologic Society for Transplantation and Vascular Surgery. *Urology* 1998;52:428–432.
53. Screening for prostate cancer. In: de Guiseppe C, et al., eds. *Screening for prostate cancer,* 2nd ed. 1996:119–134.
54. Penn I. The effect of immunosuppression on pre-existing cancers. *Transplantation* 1993;55:742–747.
55. Screening for lung cancer. In: de Guiseppe C, et al., eds. *Guide to clinical preventive services,* 2nd ed. Baltimore, 1996:135–139.
56. Brunner FP, et al. Malignancies after renal transplantation: the EDTA-ERA registry experience. European Dialysis and Transplantation Association-European Renal Association. *Nephrol Dial Transplant* 1995;10[Suppl 1]:74–80.
57. Stewart T, et al. Incidence of de-novo breast cancer in women chronically immunosuppressed after organ transplantation. *Lancet* 1995; 346:796–798.
58. Ellis D, et al. Epstein-Barr virus-related disorders in children undergoing renal transplantation with tacrolimus-based immunosuppression. *Transplantation* 1999;68:997–1003.
59. Birkeland SA, et al. Preventing acute rejection, Epstein-Barr virus infection, and posttransplant lymphoproliferative disorders after kidney transplantation: use of aciclovir and mycophenolate mofetil in a steroid-free immunosuppressive protocol. *Transplantation* 1999;67: 1209–1214.
60. Darenkov IA, et al. Reduced incidence of Epstein-Barr virus-associated posttransplant lymphoproliferative disorder using preemptive antiviral therapy. *Transplantation* 1997;64:848–852.
61. Bluman LG, et al. Preoperative smoking habits and postoperative pulmonary complications. *Chest* 1998;113:883–889.
62. Friedman EA. Management choices in diabetic end-stage renal disease. *Nephrol Dial Transplant* 1995;10[Suppl 7]:61–69.
63. Gruessner AC, et al. Analysis of United States (U.S.) and non-U.S. pancreas transplants as reported to the International Pancreas Transplant Registry (IPTR) and to the United Network for Organ Sharing UNOS. In: Cecka JM, et al., eds. *Clinical transplants 1998.* Los Angeles: Tissue Typing Laboratory, 1998:53–71.
64. Becker BN, et al. Simultaneous pancreas-kidney transplantation reduces excess mortality in type 1 diabetic patients with end-stage renal disease. *Kidney Int* 2000;57:2129–2135.
65. Ojo AO, et al. The impact of simultaneous pancreas-kidney transplantation on long-term patient survival. *Transplantation* 2001;71: 82–90.
66. Meier-Kriesche HU, et al. The effect of body mass index on long-term renal allograft survival. *Transplantation* 1999;68:1294–1297.
67. Leavey SF, et al. Simple nutritional indicators as independent predictors of mortality in hemodialysis patients. *Am J Kidney Dis* 1998; 31:997–1006.
68. Pirsch JD, et al. Obesity as a risk factor following renal transplantation. *Transplantation* 1995;59:631–633.
69. Modlin CS, et al. Should obese patients lose weight before receiving a kidney transplant? *Transplantation* 1997;64:599–604.
70. Sakhaee K, et al. Update on renal osteodystrophy: pathogenesis and clinical management. *Am J Med* 1997;52:1412–1421.
71. Massari PU. Disorders of bone and mineral metabolism after renal transplantation. *Kidney Int* 1997;52:1412–1421.
72. Tajima A, et al. Parathyroid function after kidney allografting. *Transplant Proc* 1996;28:1629–1630.
73. Pirenne J, et al. Colon perforation after renal transplantation: a single institution review. *Clin Sci* 1997;11:88–93.
74. Stelzner M, et al. Colonic perforations after renal transplantation. *J Am Coll Surg* 1997;184:63–69.
75. Lederman ED, et al. Complicated diverticulitis following renal transplantation. *Dis Colon Rectum* 1998;41:613–618.
76. Reese J, et al. Peptic ulcer disease following renal transplantation in the cyclosporine era. *Am J Surg* 1991;162:558–562.
77. Troppman C, et al. Incidence, complications, treatment, and outcome

of ulcers of the upper gastrointestinal tract after renal transplantation during the cyclosporine era. *J Am Coll Surg* 1995;180:433–443.

78. Teenan RP, et al. *Helicobacter pylori* in renal transplant recipients. *Transplantation* 1993;56:100–103.

79. Skala I, et al. Prophylaxis of acute gastroduodenal bleeding after renal transplantation. *Transplant Int* 1997;10:375–378.

80. Weir MR, et al. Liver disease in recipients of long-functioning renal allografts. *Kidney Int* 1985;28:839–844.

81. Pereira BJG, et al. Hepatitis C virus infection in dialysis and renal transplantation. *Kidney Int* 1997;51:981–999.

82. Fairley CK, et al. The increased risk of fatal liver disease in renal transplant patients who are hepatitis B antigen and/or HBV DNA positive. *Transplantation* 1991;52:497–500.

83. Jung YO, et al. Treatment of chronic hepatitis B with lamivudine in renal transplant recipients. *Transplantation* 1998;66:733–737.

84. Fontaine H, et al. HBV genotypic resistance to lamivudine in kidney recipients and hemodialyzed patients. *Transplantation* 2000;69:2090–2094.

85. Pereira BJG, et al. The impact of pre-transplantation hepatitis C virus infection on the outcome of renal transplantation. *Transplantation* 1995;60:799–805.

86. Cosio FG, et al. The high prevalence of severe early posttransplant renal allograft pathology in hepatitis C-positive recipients. *Transplantation* 1996;62:1054–1059.

87. Mathurin P, et al. Impact of hepatitis B and C virus on kidney transplantation outcome. *Hepatology* 1999;29:257–263.

88. Izopet J, et al. High rate of hepatitis C virus clearance in hemodialysis patients after interferon-alpha therapy. *J Infect Dis* 1997;176:1614–1617.

89. Bloom RD, et al. Association of hepatitis C with posttransplant diabetes in renal transplant patients on tacrolimus. *J Am Soc Nephrol* 2002;13:1374–1380.

90. Kiberd BA. Should hepatitis C-infected kidneys be transplanted in the United States? *Transplantation* 1994;57:1068–1072.

91. Mandal AK, et al. Shorter waiting times for hepatitis C virus seropositive recipients of cadaveric renal allografts from hepatitis C virus seropositive donors. *Clin Transplant* 2000;14:391–396.

92. Jassal SV, et al. Clinical practice guidelines: prevention of cytomegalovirus disease after renal transplantation. *J Am Soc Nephrol* 1998;9:1697–1708.

93. Sagedal S, et al. A prospective study of the natural course of cytomegalovirus infection and disease in renal allograft recipients. *Transplantation* 2000;70:1166–1174.

94. Couchoud C. Cytomegalovirus prophylaxis with antiviral agents for solid organ transplantation. *Cochrane Database Syst Revs* 2000;CD001320.

95. Limaye AP, et al. Emergence of ganciclovir-resistant cytomegalovirus disease among recipients of solid-organ transplants. *Lancet* 2000;356:645–649.

96. Apaydin S, et al. Mycobacterium tuberculosis infections after renal transplantation. *Scand J Infect Dis* 2000;32:501–505.

97. Margiotta V, et al. Cyclosporin- and nifedipine-induced gingival overgrowth in renal transplant patients: correlations with periodontal and pharmacological parameters, and HLA-antigens. *J Oral Pathol Med* 1996;25:128–134.

98. Linnemann CC Jr, et al. Risk of pneumococcal infections in renal transplant patients. *JAMA* 1979;241:2619–2621.

99. Rangel MC, et al. Vaccine recommendations for patients on chronic dialysis: the Advisory Committee on Immunization Practices and the American Academy of Pediatrics. *Semin Dial* 2000;13:101–107.

100. Kabler RL, et al. Pre-transplant urologic investigation and treatment of end-stage renal disease. *J Urol* 1983;129:475–478.

101. Hariharan S, et al. Recurrent and de novo glomerular disease after renal transplantation: a report from Renal Allograft Disease Registry (RADR). *Transplantation* 1999;68:635–641.

102. Artero M, et al. Recurrent focal glomerulosclerosis: natural history and response to therapy. *Am J Med* 1992;92:375–383.

103. Toth CM, et al. Recurrent collapsing glomerulopathy. *Transplantation* 1998;65:1009–1010.

104. Stephanian E, et al. Recurrence of disease in patients retransplanted for focal segmental glomerulosclerosis. *Transplantation* 1992;53:755–757.

105. Briggs JD, et al. Recurrence of glomerulonephritis following renal transplantation. Scientific Advisory Board of the ERA-EDTA Registry. European Renal Association-European Dialysis and Transplant Association. *Nephrol Dial Transplant* 1999;14:564–565.

106. Freese P, et al. Clinical risk factors for recurrence of IgA nephropathy. *Clin Sci* 1999;13:313–317.

107. Meulders Q, et al. Course of Henoch-Schönlein nephritis after renal transplantation: report on ten patients and review of the literature. *Transplantation* 1994;58:1179–1186.

108. Andresdottir MB, et al. Renal transplantation in patients with dense deposit disease: morphological characteristics of recurrent disease and clinical outcome. *Nephrol Dial Transplant* 1999;14:1723–1731.

109. Couchoud C, et al. Recurrence of membranous nephropathy after renal transplantation: incidence and risk factors in 1,614 patients. *Transplantation* 1995;59:1275–1279.

110. Ducloux D, et al. Recurrence of hemolytic-uremic syndrome in renal transplant recipients: a meta-analysis. *Transplantation* 1998;65:1405–1407.

111. Franz M, et al. Posttransplant hemolytic uremic syndrome in adult retransplanted kidney graft recipients: advantage of FK506 therapy? *Transplantation* 1998;66:1258–1262.

112. Hebert D, et al. Recurrence of hemolytic uremic syndrome in renal transplant recipients. *Kidney Int* 1986;[Suppl 19]:S51–S58.

113. Doutrelepont JM, et al. Early recurrence of hemolytic uremic syndrome in a renal transplant recipient during prophylactic OKT3 therapy. *Transplantation* 1992;53:1378–1379.

114. Nachman PH, et al. Recurrent ANCA-associated small vessel vasculitis after transplantation: a pooled analysis. *Kidney Int* 1999;56:1544–1550.

115. Ward MM. Outcomes of renal transplantation among patients with end-stage renal disease caused by lupus nephritis. *Kidney Int* 2000;57:2136–2143.

116. Heering P, et al. Renal transplantation in secondary systemic amyloidosis. *Clin Transplant* 1998;12:159–164.

117. Stone JH, et al. Antiphospholipid antibody syndrome in renal transplantation: occurrence of clinical events in 96 consecutive patients with systemic lupus erythematosus. *Am J Kidney Dis* 1999;34:1040–1047.

118. Rundell JR, et al. Psychiatric characteristics of consecutively evaluated outpatient renal transplant candidates and comparisons with consultation-liaison inpatients. *Psychosomatics* 1997;38:269–276.

119. Kimmel PL, et al. Psychologic functioning, quality of life, and behavioral compliance in patients beginning hemodialysis. *J Am Soc Nephrol* 1996;7:2152–2159.

120. Matas AJ, et al. Proposed guidelines for re-evaluation of patients on the waiting list for renal cadaver transplantation. *Transplantation* 2002;73:811–831.

121. Ojo AO, et al. Survival in recipients of marginal cadaveric donor kidneys, compared to other recipients and wait-listed transplant patients. *J Am Soc Nephrol* 2001;12:589–597.

122. Danovitch GM, et al. Management of the waiting list for cadaveric kidney transplants: report of a survey and recommendations by the Clinical Practice Guidelines Committee of the American Society of Transplantation. *J Am Soc Nephrol* 2002;13:528–535.

123. Tullius SG, et al. Contribution of donor age and ischemic injury in chronic renal allograft dysfunction. *Transplant Proc* 1999;31:1298–1299.

124. Cecka M, et al. Clinical impact of delayed graft function for kidney transplantation. *Transplant Rev* 2001;15:57–67.

125. Sox HC. Preventative health services in adults. *N Engl J Med* 1994;330:1589–1595.

126. Rostand SG. Coronary heart disease in chronic renal insufficiency: some management considerations. *J Am Soc Nephrol* 2000;11:1948–1956.

127. Danovitch GM. The epidemic of cardiovascular disease in chronic

renal disease: a challenge to the transplant physician. *Graft* 1999; 2[Suppl]:S108–S112.

128. Levey AS, et al. Controlling the epidemic of cardiovascular disease in chronic renal disease: what do we know? what do we need to know? where do we go from here? *Am J Kidney Dis* 1998;32: 853–906.

129. Braun WE, et al. Coronary artery disease in renal transplant recipients. *Cleve Clin J Med* 1994;61:370–385.

130. Middleton RJ, et al. Left ventricular hypertrophy in the renal patient. *J Am Soc Nephrol* 2001;12:1079–1084.

131. Schmidt A, et al. Informational contribution of noninvasive screening tests for coronary artery disease in patients on chronic renal replacement therapy. *Am J Kidney Dis* 2001;37:56–63.

132. Marwick TH, et al. Ineffectiveness of dipyridamole SPECT thallium imaging as a screening technique for coronary artery disease in patients with end-stage renal failure. *Transplantation* 1990;49:100–103.

CURRENT OUTCOMES FOR DIALYSIS PATIENTS

JEFFREY C. FINK

The diagnosis of end-stage renal disease (ESRD) carries potentially grave consequences for the patient who has been afflicted with this condition. Unfortunately, the onset of ESRD calls for exceptional care by a committed health care team to maintain an individual's productive and fulfilling life, given the challenges of the disease. In most cases, a patient with ESRD can expect a lifestyle disrupted by the necessity for several life-sustaining measures often not anticipated before the onset of the illness. With recognition of ensuing ESRD the patient and physician are faced with critical decisions regarding whether or not renal replacement therapy is a realistic option and, if so, what modality should be chosen and when to prepare for this inevitability.

The process of education and preparation for ESRD should begin long before its onset. Given the dismal prognosis of this disease and the importance of early intervention, it is essential that the nephrologist understand the implications of choosing any of the modalities for renal replacement at his or her disposal. Even with the institution of timely renal replacement therapy, the physician must continue to invest substantial effort to ensure the best quality of care with the purpose of improving the well being of the ESRD patient after starting on renal replacement therapy. An important rule for any clinician, and with particular resonance for the nephrologist, is that decisions regarding care and therapeutic choices must be made after review of clinical evidence with particular emphasis placed on outcomes. This chapter provides a review of the information available on the outcomes of patients with ESRD to provide an evidence-based approach for the physician caring for a patient with ESRD.

EPIDEMIOLOGIC AND DEMOGRAPHIC TRENDS IN END-STAGE RENAL DISEASE

Nephrologists and health care providers in this country and the rest of the world will face a growing population of ESRD patients as we enter the twenty-first century. The United States Renal Data System (USRDS) has tracked trends in the ESRD population including Medicare beneficiaries and, more recently, non-Medicare patients since 1988 and documented a dramatic growth in the number of people with this disease. The USRDS has shown that there has been a virtually constant increase in the incidence and prevalence of ESRD over the last several years.

The prevalence of ESRD reported by the USRDS increased from 179,000 in 1990 to 344,000 in 1999, and the population is projected to increase to more than 650,000 by the end of this decade (1,2). Fig. 43.1 demonstrates the increasing population of ESRD patients based on renal replacement modality over the last decade. The growth in the prevalent population of ESRD has been in part fueled by a simultaneous increase in the incidence of this disease. In 1990, there were 48,000 patients who developed ESRD, whereas 89,000 developed the disease in 1999 (1).

The rapidly increasing incidence of ESRD is almost certainly attributable to a burgeoning cohort with chronic kidney disease. It is difficult to accurately measure the number of Americans with chronic kidney disease in part because the essential elements of the early phase of this disease have not, as of yet, been well defined and there have been few national surveys to identify the portion of the population at highest risk for developing ESRD. Studies of the third National Health and Nutritional Examination Survey (NHANES III) have defined chronic kidney disease as a serum creatinine of 1.5 mg/dL or greater (hypercreatinemia). Using this definition, the population with chronic kidney disease has been estimated to be more than 6 million Americans (3). Other studies have used NHANES III data to estimate creatinine clearance using serum creatinine and other clinical parameters and reported that the prevalence of chronic kidney disease might be even higher depending on the threshold under which a diminished creatinine clearance represents kidney disease (4).

The prevalence of hypercreatinemia is higher in African-Americans relative to the remainder of the U.S. population. In NHANES III, African-American men had a mean serum creatinine of 1.25 mg/dL versus 1.16 mg/dL for all men in the United States. African-American women had a similar disparity with a mean creatinine of 1.01 mg/dL compared with 0.96 mg/dL for all women in the United States. (3).

The preponderance of hypercreatinemia among African-Americans is consistent with the finding that blacks are at increased risk for developing chronic kidney disease related to hypertension and diabetes. Among those patients with the diagnosis of either diabetes or hypertension, African-Americans are at a greater risk for chronic kidney disease than whites (5,6). It is still not clear, however, who among those with either hyper-

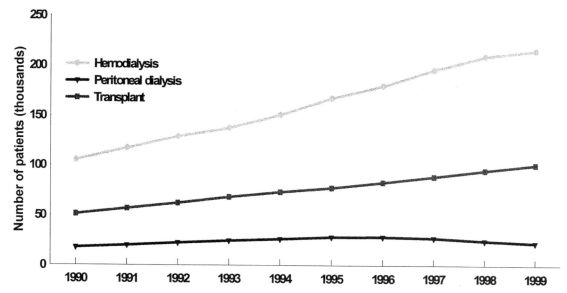

FIG. 43.1. The December 31 point prevalence counts of the end-stage renal disease patients by modality in the United States. (Reprinted from Annual data report of the USRDS, 2001.)

creatinemia or chronic kidney disease can expect to develop ESRD as opposed to remaining with stable renal function or succumbing to another illness like cardiovascular disease.

The growing population with ESRD has changed in its demographic characteristics over the last several years. Persons who are incident with ESRD are more likely than they might have been a decade ago to be older than 65 years, with diabetes, and of a racial or ethnic minority. Although a pathologic confirmation of the disease underlying ESRD is rarely made, diabetes is the most common diagnosis of renal failure submitted to the USRDS and accounts for an increasing number of ESRD cases each year. In the year 2000, 45% of new ESRD patients had diabetes designated as the cause of renal failure. The incidence of renal failure among diabetics has also dramatically increased throughout the 1990s as

shown in Fig. 43.2 (1). Hypertension ranks as the second most common cause of ESRD, although it remains unclear how often hypertension is a cause rather than a consequence of renal disease (7,8). African-Americans have become particularly prone to ESRD related to either diabetes or hypertension, as depicted in Fig. 43.2, with increased incidence rates of renal failure also observed among Hispanics, Asians, and Native Americans (1,9). Among those patients with diabetes, African-American race is a strong predictor for the development of diabetic nephropathy and progression to ESRD (10,11). Similarly, the higher risk of ESRD among African-Americans seems to be independent of the fact that blacks tend to be diagnosed with more severe hypertension, later in the disease course, and with more frequent concomitant presence of diabetes than whites (12).

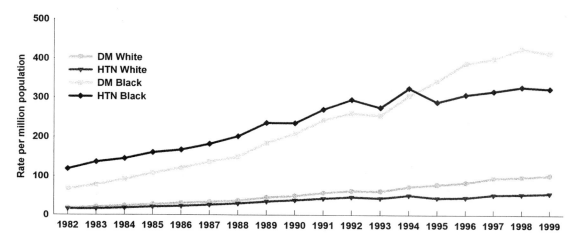

FIG. 43.2. Incidence rates of end-stage renal disease resulting from hypertension and diabetes by race. (Reprinted from the Annual data report of the USRDS, 2001.)

The ESRD population has become increasingly elderly over the years monitored by the USRDS. Incident rates of renal failure for people aged 65 or greater have virtually doubled through the 1990s. The prevalence of ESRD patients aged 65 or greater has increased from 30% to 34% of the total group from 1990 to 1999. In 1999, the median age of prevalent white dialysis patients was 67 years, whereas their African-American counterparts were just younger than 60 years. The aging trend among the ESRD population is expected to continue into the next decade (1).

The United States is not the only nation with a growing ESRD population. The incidence of ESRD has been reported to be increasing in several other nations including Japan, Canada, France, the Netherlands, Australia, and Poland to name a few that track such data, and Japan exceeds the United States in its prevalence rate of ESRD. Several countries also have a higher proportion of patients than the United States with diabetes as the cause of their renal failure. Chile stands out as one nation with an explosive increase over the last few years of the proportion of patients with diabetic nephropathy as the cause underlying their renal failure with the percentage increasing from approximately 25% in 1997 to more than 80% in 1999. Several nations can also claim to have even higher proportions of elderly ESRD patients than the United States. Germany ranks the highest with 58% of its ESRD patients aged 65 years or more (1).

The ESRD population has not only aged but also become increasingly ill at the initiation of renal replacement therapy. More patients developed ESRD with two or more comorbidities in 1999 relative to 1995. The preponderance of cardiovascular disease and congestive heart failure has increased among ESRD patients from 1995 to 1999. Furthermore, the proportion of patients with cerebral or peripheral vascular disease, cancer, or chronic obstructive pulmonary disease has risen over the same time period (1). There is also a large body of evidence demonstrating that patients who develop ESRD are not receiving adequate care before the need for renal replacement. Review of Health Care Financing Administration (HCFA) 2728 forms, which document demographic characteristics and several clinical parameters on new ESRD patients, show that more often than not patients who begin renal replacement therapy are anemic and undertreated for their anemia (13). These patients are frequently malnourished as indicated by low serum albumin levels (13). There is a high prevalence of left ventricular hypertrophy in this population, which is indicative of both poorly controlled hypertension and undertreated anemia (14). Furthermore, patients who begin dialysis are poorly educated about the dietary requirements of this illness (15). There continues to be a high preponderance of vascular catheters rather than arteriovenous accesses as the means by which dialysis is initiated, and very often the first consultation by a nephrologist is at the time of dialysis initiation (15,16). Several studies have documented that initiation of dialysis without appropriate and early referral to a nephrologist has deleterious effects on patients who develop ESRD (17,18).

The increasingly morbid, older, and poorly prepared ESRD population is also burdened by an unacceptably high mortality rate. It is commonly stated that the diagnosis of ESRD portends a prognosis that is worse than some types of cancer. Fig. 43.3 shows the life expectancy of a 49-year-old man diagnosed with ESRD relative to a similarly aged healthy man from the U.S. population and comparably aged men with one of three different cancers. The patient with ESRD only ranks better in life expectancy than the individual with lung cancer but can anticipate dying sooner than his counterparts diagnosed with either colon or prostate cancer (19). It is important to note that although mortality rates among ESRD patients continue to be unacceptably high, there have been improvements over the last few years as depicted in Fig. 43.4. First- and second-year mortality rates tracked by the USRDS over the last decade have significantly decreased by as much 13% and 15%, respectively. Despite this trend of improvement, however, the age, race, gender, and diagnosis-adjusted first-year mortality rates remained 275 deaths per 1,000 patient-years in 1998, which is the most recent year for which these data are available (1).

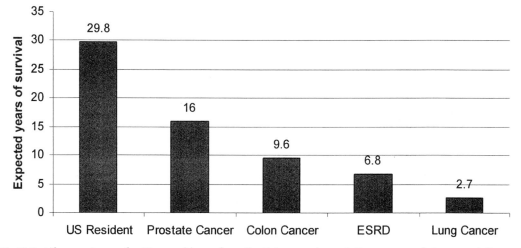

FIG. 43.3. Life expectancy of a 49-year-old man from the U.S. general population versus end-stage renal disease and various cancers. (Modified from Annual data report of the USRDS, 1994.)

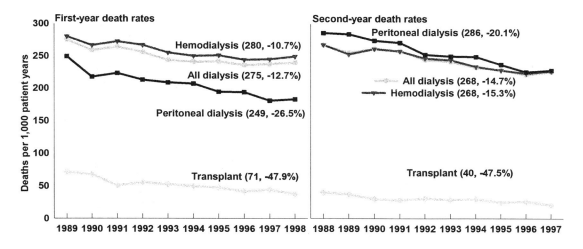

FIG. 43.4. First- and second-year death rates for incident end-stage renal disease patients by modality. The number of deaths per 1,000 patient-years in the first year are shown in parentheses with percentage change over all 10 years. (Reprinted from the Annual data report of the USRDS, 2001.)

The exceptional mortality rates observed in the ESRD population differs across races with African-Americans fairing better than whites. In one analysis from USRDS data it was found that, among hemodialysis patients, whites had a 29% higher risk of death than blacks (20). Similar results have been observed in Canada where the risk of death among whites on dialysis was significantly greater than their Asian and black counterparts on dialysis (21). Among those ESRD patients who are treated strictly with peritoneal dialysis, the disparity between races is the same, with African-Americans experiencing better survival rates than whites treated with peritoneal dialysis (22).

The most common cause of death in the ESRD population is cardiovascular disease (23) (see Chapter 18 for a detailed discussion). The risk of death from cardiovascular disease among dialysis patients of any age far exceeds that of similarly aged individuals in the general population. The higher risk of cardiovascular disease observed among ESRD patients is consistent with the growing preponderance of patients with diabetes and older age. Of note, white dialysis patients appear to have a higher risk of cardiovascular death than African-Americans (20). The occurrence of myocardial infarction among dialysis patients has particularly devastating consequences with grim survival prospects after the incident (24). Other manifestations of cardiovascular disease are also observed with high frequency in ESRD including cardiac arrest and congestive heart failure along with other manifestations of atherosclerotic vascular disease such as cerebrovascular and peripheral vascular disease (1).

MEDICARE END-STAGE RENAL DISEASE PROGRAM AND THE COST OF CARING FOR THIS POPULATION

One important reason behind the growth and demographic changes observed in the U.S. ESRD population is the nearly universal access to renal replacement therapy, which has offered renal failure patients with several options once they are faced with this diagnosis regardless of underlying health or financial status. The wide availability of renal replacement therapies in this country can be credited to the U.S. government and its establishment of the ESRD provision under Medicare. In 1972, the U.S. Congress passed bill HR 1, which designated ESRD as a disability to be covered by Medicare. Starting on July 1, 1973, more than 90% of ESRD patients became eligible for Medicare coverage of their renal replacement therapy including dialysis and renal transplantation. The Medicare provision for ESRD resulted in a dramatic increase in both the number of patients seeking dialysis and dialysis units serving them. Initially the ESRD population was comprised of insured, compliant patients who were cared for with high staff-to-patient ratios and dialysis sessions of 6 to 8 hour duration in dialysis units associated with hospitals but with common use of home hemodialysis. The federal government through the HCFA [now referred to as the Centers for Medicare and Medicaid Services (CMS)] has recognized the rising cost of the ESRD program. The total expenditures for this disease were approximately $18 billion in 1999, and the Medicare contribution to the total cost increased from slightly more than $5 billion in 1991 to almost $12 billion dollars in 1999 (1). As shown in Fig. 43.5, the increased cost of caring for the ESRD population has paralleled the growing number of patients with this disease, but the actual cost per capita rose slightly for dialysis patients from 1995 to 1999 while it decreased for transplant patients over the same time period. Hospitalizations increased over the same time period by 2.9% as might be expected for the increasingly morbid ESRD population (1). In concordance with the expected increase in the number of ESRD patients over the next decade, the projected Medicare and non-Medicare expenditures are expected to reach $28 billion (2). As a result of rising cost the Medicare ESRD program was a pioneer in the use of capitation as the method of reimbursement for dialysis. This method of reimbursement has led to a unique interaction between public policy and medical progress that has influenced the treatments and standards of care for ESRD patients in this country perhaps as it has for no other disease.

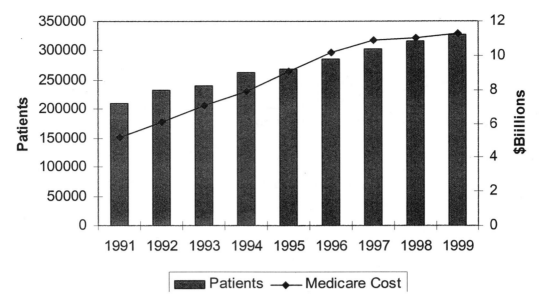

FIG. 43.5. The Medicare end-stage renal disease (ESRD) expenditures shown with the prevalence of ESRD in the United States from 1991 to 1998. (Modified from Annual data report of the USRDS, 1997, 2001.)

CHOICES FOR RENAL REPLACEMENT THERAPY

When a patient is faced with the diagnosis of ESRD, he or she has several choices to consider as a modality of renal replacement. The most common form of renal replacement in the United States continues to be hemodialysis with 64% of prevalent ESRD patients on this modality in 1999. Hemodialysis, along with transplantation, has grown in frequency as therapy selections over the years tracked by the USRDS while peritoneal dialysis has become less common. Hemodialysis is more common in ESRD patients who are older, of a racial minority, and with a cause of renal disease other than diabetes or hypertension;

hence, the increasing preponderance of this dialytic therapy at least in part relates to the demographic changes in the ESRD population (1). Although hemodialysis is the most common modality in patients who have survived with ESRD for up to 5 years, transplantation becomes equally common as a modality in patients who are living 6 to 7 years with ESRD and then surpasses hemodialysis as the most common form of renal replacement in patients who have survived more than 7 years with ESRD (1). Each renal replacement modality has substantially different costs. Fig. 43.6 shows the Part A Medicare payments per year of diabetic and nondiabetic patients maintained on hemodialysis, peritoneal dialysis, or transplantation. Cost for

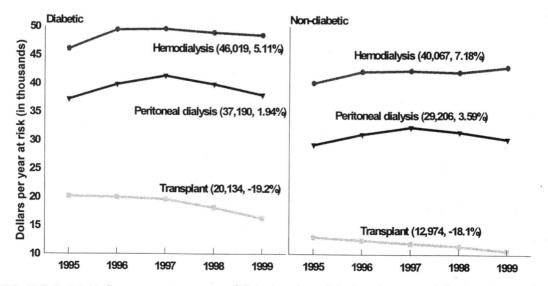

FIG. 43.6. Part A Medicare payments per year of diabetic and nondiabetic end-stage renal disease patients maintained on hemodialysis, peritoneal dialysis, or transplantation. (Reprinted from Annual data report of the USRDS, 2001.)

caring for an ESRD patient on hemodialysis is substantially greater than on peritoneal dialysis. The cost of both modalities has increased over the last 5 years with the rate of increase greater for hemodialysis than for peritoneal dialysis, which has demonstrated a trend toward decreased costs more recently. The cost of transplantation has significantly dropped over the same time period (1).

In devising a strategy of renal replacement therapy for a patient with impending ESRD therapy it is important to have a familiarity with the evidence, which compares the different modalities. Because most renal failure patients are treated with dialysis we must first consider the comparison of hemodialysis to peritoneal dialysis as a choice for renal replacement. The selection of dialysis modality must take into account the substantial differences in preparation and schedules required for both (see Chapter 8). The fundamental difference between hemodialysis and peritoneal dialysis relates to the schedule of treatment required of each. Peritoneal dialysis is essentially a home therapy, which offers the patient an opportunity to maintain a fair degree of autonomy and flexibility with the activities of daily living. This autonomy requires the patient to be relatively high functioning or with a dedicated caregiver to ensure competent and aseptic technique. Hemodialysis is predominantly a center-based therapy, although a small number of hemodialysis patients take dialysis at home. The decision to receive hemodialysis requires the patient to relinquish much of his or her autonomy and adhere to a structured schedule often requiring up to 20 hours a week dedicated to dialysis. It is possible that many patients, especially those previously uninsured, benefit from the increased interaction with the health care team that comes with center-based hemodialysis. Both therapies call for significant pre-ESRD education and preparation; however, hemodialysis is too often initiated urgently during a visit to the local emergency department with extreme azotemic symptoms or complications.

There have been several studies investigating the outcome of patients treated with hemodialysis versus peritoneal dialysis; however, the results of these reports have not provided a clear answer as to which is the superior modality. Table 43.1 summarizes the larger studies available and demonstrates the differences in populations studied and reported results. In 1995, Bloembergen et al. (25) studied a large group of prevalent USRDS patients comparing mortality rates of hemodialysis patients relative to peritoneal dialysis patients. The authors reported that hemodialysis was associated with a better survival than peritoneal dialysis. This study was followed by a report from Fenton et al. (26) that investigated an incident cohort of Canadian patients started on either hemodialysis or peritoneal dialysis and found a lower risk of mortality among those started on peritoneal dialysis; however, this survival benefit varied over time. Vonesh et al. (27) revisited USRDS data and studied several patient cohorts including those studied by Bloembergen et al. and composed of both incident and prevalent patients. The investigators evaluated differences in mortality rates between hemodialysis and peritoneal dialysis across the study cohorts. They concluded that there was little or no overall difference between hemodialysis and peritoneal dialysis in mortality rates when looking across several years tracked by the USRDS. Collins et al. (28) looked at a more contemporary cohort of incident USRDS population who initiated renal replacement between 1994 to 1996 and found peritoneal dialysis to confer a survival benefit relative to hemodialysis in the first few months after starting renal replacement; however, this survival benefit was not sustained over longer periods of follow-up. Most recently, Keshaviah et al. (29) combined data from the Regional Kidney Disease Program in Minnesota with the Canadian-USA prospective cohort of peritoneal dialysis patients to compare peritoneal dialysis and hemodialysis with regard to survival after adjusting for differences in dialysis clearance. The authors found that after adjusting the two groups for variations in delivered dialysis dose there was no difference in mortality rates between the two modalities (29). It is difficult to make definitive conclusions regarding the survival benefit of hemodialysis versus peritoneal dialysis; therefore, I believe that both modalities should be available and discussed after weighing the risks and benefits of each for individual patients.

In the evaluation of any patient who is approaching ESRD it is important to consider renal transplantation because this is the

TABLE 43.1. SUMMARY OF STUDIES COMPARING PERITONEAL DIALYSIS (PD) AND HEMODIALYSIS (HD)

Study	Patients	N	Years	Conclusions about Mortality
Bloembergen et al. (25)	USRDS: prevalent dialysis patients	170,700 patient-years	87 to 89	PD mortality >HD mortality
Fenton et al. (26)	Canadian Registry: incident dialysis patients	11,970 patients	90 to 94	PD mortality <HD mortality early after initiating therapy Differences were time dependent
Vonesh et al. (27)	USRDS: overlapping cohorts of incident and prevalent dialysis patients	1,256,745 patient-years	87 to 89 88 to 90 89 to 91 90 to 92 91 to 93	PD mortality ≅ HD mortality across all cohorts
Collins et al. (28)	USRDS: incident dialysis patients	117,158 patients	94 to 96	PD mortality <HD mortality early after initiating therapy and in several subgroups
Keshaviah et al. (29)	RKDP: incident HD patients CANUSA: incident PD patients	1,648 patients	87 to 95 90 to 92	PD mortality ≅ HD mortality after adjusting for adequacy of dialysis

Canadian Registry, Canadian Organ Replacement Registry; CANUSA, Canada-United States prospective trial database for continuous ambulatory peritoneal dialysis; RKDP, Regional Kidney Disease Program; USRDS, United States Renal Data System.

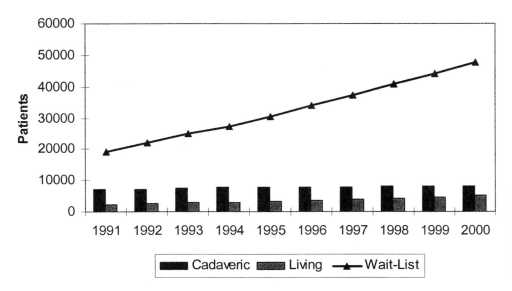

FIG. 43.7. The number of end-stage renal disease patients on wait-list for a kidney transplant with the number of living and cadaveric transplants performed over the same time period. (Modified from Organ Procurement and Transplant Network/Scientific Registry of Transplant Recipients as of August 2001.)

preferred option of renal replacement for many patients with renal failure. In conjunction with the growth of the ESRD population there has been an increasing demand for renal transplantation. Fig. 43.7 shows the growing number of wait-listed patients through 2000, despite a relatively stable number of renal transplants over the same years. Several studies have now demonstrated (among patients who are healthy enough to be on the transplant waiting list) that a renal allograft offers a significant survival advantage over dialysis (30–32). This survival advantage is not only realized in first-time renal transplant recipients but has also been reported for patients who receive a second transplant and among those who receive a so-called marginal kidney that does not have ideal function (31,32). Unfortunately, there have been several reports indicating that underreferral for transplant evaluation is common in the nephrology community (33,34).

CLINICAL PERFORMANCE MEASURES FOR DIALYSIS

The most commonly evaluated clinical parameter measured in the ESRD population is the delivered dose of dialysis as quantified by the urea reduction ratio (URR) and the parameter, *Kt/V*. Several studies have shown a strong relationship between dialysis adequacy as measured by URR or *Kt/V* and mortality (35–40). Although the relationship between dialysis adequacy and mortality is not completely linear, one can estimate that with each increment of *Kt/V* by 0.1% or 5% increment in URR there is a 7% and 11% reduction in mortality rates, respectively (40). Dialysis adequacy is also strongly associated with morbidity and cost of care of patients with ESRD. The National Cooperative Dialysis Study done in the early years of dialysis therapy showed that more intensive dialysis delivered over longer duration was associated with lower rates of treatment failure defined as hospitalization, study dropout, and mortality than that seen with patients treated with a lower dose of dialysis or a similar dose delivered over shorter duration (41). In a contemporary

group of hemodialysis patients it was also demonstrated that lower *Kt/V* values are associated with more days in the hospital and higher Medicare inpatient expenditures (42). A large prospective multicenter hemodialysis (HEMO) study evaluating both standard and high-dose hemodialysis prescriptions along with low- and high-flux hemodialysis membranes has recently been conducted (43). Preliminary results from this study have not shown a benefit to higher dose dialysis or high-flux filters beyond the minimum recommended dose of hemodialysis. More detailed analyses from this study are soon to come (see Chapter 10).

After evidence began to emerge showing the significant association between dialysis adequacy and ESRD outcomes there were several initiatives to improve the delivered dialysis around the country (44,45). The National Kidney Foundation established the Dialysis Outcome Quality Initiative (DOQI) in an effort to set up guidelines for quality care in the dialysis community. To ensure the quality of care provided to beneficiaries of the Medicare ESRD program, CMS established the Health Care Quality Improvement Program (HCQIP). The primary byproduct of HCQIP was the National/Network ESRD Core Indicators Project (CIP), which set out to maintain a database of key clinical indicators to provide insight into the quality of care delivered to dialysis patients. The CIP monitored these intermediate outcomes of dialysis patients from 1994 to 1999 at which time it was merged with the ESRD Clinical Performance Measures (CPM) Project, which was mandated by the U.S. Congress to ensure quality care in dialysis patients. The CPM project now measures several clinical performance measures in random samples of dialysis patients on an annual basis and evaluates the results in relation to established targets for each parameter (46).

The result of all these quality improvement initiatives has been some improvement in overall dialysis adequacy with the average Kt/V increasing by 9.7% from 1996 to 1999 and the URR increasing by 9.6% from 1994 to 1998 across the United States. (1). The target for adequacy established in the CPM project for in-center hemodialysis patients dialyzed for 6 months or longer at a frequency of three times per week was set at a *Kt/V* of 1.2 or greater when calculated using formal urea kinetic modeling or the Daugirdas II formula (47). Using this benchmark, the most recent CPM project report revealed that despite aggregate improvement in dialysis, 14% of hemodialysis patients sampled in October through December in 2000 continue to have *Kt/V* values below 1.2. Moreover, there was a substantial geographic variation in achieved dialysis adequacy and a wide disparity between the prescribed dose of dialysis and amount actually delivered to each patient (46).

The DOQI and CPM project have also established practice guidelines and targets for anemia management. Anemia is a strong indicator of outcome in dialysis patients. Hemodialysis patients who are anemic with hematocrit values less than 30% have 18% to 40% higher mortality rates than their counterparts with hematocrit values between 30% and 33%. Those hemodialysis patients with hematocrit values greater than 33% have as much as a 7% reduction in mortality risk relative to those patients with a hematocrit of 30% to 33% (48). Similar trends were shown for cost and hospitalization with the lowest Medicare expenditures and hospitalization rates for patients with hematocrit values greater than or equal to 36% (49). The CPM project set the target hemoglobin for in-center hemodialysis patients at 11 to 12 g/dL and early reports revealed that more than one fourth of prevalent hemodialysis patients sampled in December of 1996 had hematocrit values less than 30% (corresponding to a hemoglobin of 10 g/dL), and only half of the patients had hematocrit values greater than 33% (hemoglobin of 11 g/dL) (50). Anemia management has improved in the most recent CPM project report, which has shown a trend toward higher hemoglobin values since 1996; however, 26% of in-center hemodialysis patients sampled continued to have hemoglobin levels less than 11 g/dL in 2000.

The CPM project has also issued targets for iron management in conjunction with the established benchmarks for anemia management. For all anemic dialysis patients or those prescribed epoetin alfa therapy, iron parameters must be assessed at least once within a 3-month period, and there should be documentation of at least one ferritin concentration greater than or equal to 100 ng/mL and one transferrin saturation greater than or equal to 20%. In the most recent CPM project report 71% of in-center hemodialysis patients sampled had at least one transferrin saturation ≥20% and a ferritin ≥100 ng/mL, and, of those patients who had at least one transferrin saturation less than 20% or ferritin less than 100 ng/mL, 73% were prescribed intravenous iron (46) (see Chapter 32).

The serum albumin concentration has also been used as a clinical performance measure reflecting nutritional status in the ESRD patient with an inverse relationship between albumin concentration and risk for mortality in this population. Patients with a serum albumin less than 3.5 g/dL have an increased risk of death relative to those patients with higher albumin concentrations, and those patients with albumin concentrations of ≥4.0 g/dL have the lowest mortality (36,51). The CPM project has set an albumin ≥4.0 g/dL or ≥3.7 g/dL by the bromocresol green (BCG) and bromocresol purple (BCP) method, respectively, as the target albumin concentration for adult in-center dialysis patients. In the most recent report by the CPM, only

29% of hemodialysis patients had serum albumin concentrations of ≥4.0 g/dL or ≥3.7 g/dL, by BCG or BCP method, respectively, which is down from a peak of 37% greater than the same values in 1995 (46) (see Chapter 30).

DOQI states that hemodialysis patients should have a patent and competent vascular access placed with a priority on the establishment of a native arteriovenous fistula where and when possible. Based on these guidelines the CPM project has set the placement of a native arteriovenous fistula in 50% of new hemodialysis patients as a benchmark with the expectation that 40% of prevalent hemodialysis patients will have a native arteriovenous fistula as their primary access. In the most recent report from the CPM project, 27% of incident in-center hemodialysis patients sampled in 2000 had an established arteriovenous fistula and only 30% of all in-center hemodialysis patients sampled in 2000 had an arteriovenous fistula. Chronic venous catheters were used as vascular access for more than 90 days in 17% of the patients in the CPM project report (46). Data from the USRDS shows that, although frequency of fistula placements has increased in hemodialysis patients, the use of permanent catheters has also risen. This is in contrast to a drop in use of temporary catheters for chronic hemodialysis (1) (see Chapter 4).

In addition to the clinical performance measures for hemodialysis patients, the DOQI has also established guidelines for peritoneal dialysis adequacy. The target for a weekly dose of peritoneal dialysis in those patients on continuous ambulatory peritoneal dialysis (CAPD) is a *Kt/V*_urea of 2.0 and a total creatinine clearance of at least 60 L/week/1.73 m². These guidelines were based on observational studies of peritoneal dialysis patients in which a correlation was noted between achieved dialysis adequacy and subsequent survival. The most notable of these studies was the Canada-USA Peritoneal Dialysis (CANUSA) study that prospectively followed a cohort of 680 patients started on CAPD in the United States and Canada. The study showed that for each 0.1 unit per week decrement in *Kt/V* there was a 5% increase in the risk of death. Similarly, for each decrease in weekly creatinine clearance of 5 L/1.73 m², there was a 7% increase in the relative risk of mortality in the cohort (52). The CPM project sampled ESRD patients treated with peritoneal dialysis during the final quarter of 2000 and reported that only 69% of the sampled patients treated with CAPD reached the benchmark for adequacy set by DOQI. Only 62% of the patients sampled who were treated with continuous cycling peritoneal dialysis reached the target for adequacy set by DOQI, which was a weekly *Kt/V* of 2.1 or creatinine clearance of 63 L/week/1.73 m² (46).

The significance of peritoneal dialysis targets has been put into question by the results of some recently completed studies. A follow-up analysis of the CANUSA data revealed that the determinant of mortality risk was not differences in CAPD clearance but changes in residual renal function as the cohort was followed. In the recently completed Adequacy of Peritoneal Dialysis in Mexico (AMEDEX) trial, CAPD patients were randomly assigned to one of two adequacy regimens including a standard prescription and an intensive regimen. The baseline characteristics were the same in both groups including residual renal function. The patients were followed for an average of 18 months with significantly higher clearances in the intensive versus conventional group overall at all time points during the study (mean CrCl: 62.9 ±0.7 L/week/1.73 m^2 versus 54.1 ±1.0 L/week/1.73 m^2, respectively, p <0.001). The survival rates were no different in the two groups (53). Therefore, one must continue to question the importance of altering small-solute clearance versus preserving residual renal function in improving the survival of ESRD patients treated with peritoneal dialysis (see Chapter 14).

CHRONIC KIDNEY DISEASE CARE AND END-STAGE RENAL DISEASE OUTCOMES

Perhaps the greatest opportunity to improve the outcome of ESRD patients exists before the initiation of renal replacement therapy. Treating the complications of chronic renal disease as they evolve in association with the deterioration of renal function is critical to improving the well being of patients destined for ESRD (54,55). There is substantial evidence demonstrating that many of the ravages of kidney disease develop long before the onset of ESRD but only inflict damage after a patient requires renal replacement therapy. For instance, a large proportion of the ESRD population has diabetes as the primary cause of their renal disease and have poor glycemic control at the onset of renal replacement therapy (56). The complications of poorly controlled diabetes are a common cause of morbidity and mortality in ESRD patients. In addi-

tion, left ventricular hypertrophy is the result of the hypertension and anemia common with chronic kidney disease and is a major determinant of cardiac morbidity and mortality in patients after ESRD develops (57).

There is growing evidence that therapeutic interventions employed in patients before the need for renal replacement have demonstrable effect on survival after onset of ESRD. Glycemic control in patients with diabetes before they reach the dialysis unit has an enduring impact on survival after onset of ESRD (56). Pre-ESRD use of epoetin alfa has been shown to have an important benefit on survival after initiation of dialysis as shown in Fig. 43.8, which depicts the cumulative survival in a cohort of ESRD patients from the start of renal replacement and classified by their use of epoetin alfa before onset of ESRD. Interestingly, the survival benefit of epoetin alfa used before ESRD was realized within a year and a half of dialysis initiation but diminished in patients who continued on dialysis for a longer duration (58). This is plausible, because the beneficial effect of epoetin alfa enjoyed by a relatively small proportion of patients treated with the drug before onset of dialysis is equaled by use of epoetin alfa in virtually all patients after onset of ESRD. Indeed, those patients who are treated with epoetin alfa before onset of ESRD may have benefited from better predialysis care, and these results may reflect this quality of care rather than actual epoetin alfa administration. Nevertheless, either conclusion supports the notion that the interventions delivered before the onset of ESRD have a demonstrable effect on outcome after initiating renal replacement.

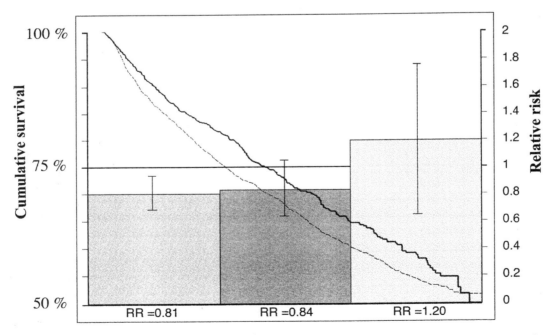

FIG. 43.8. Survival curve shows mortality rates of new end-stage renal disease (ESRD) patients in ESRD Network 5 treated with epoetin alfa before the initiation of dialysis *(solid line)* versus patients not treated *(dashed line)*. Histograms represent the adjusted relative risk of mortality associated with epoetin alfa use within three tertiles of follow-up after initiating dialysis: 0 to 19 months, 20 to 31 months, greater than 31 months. *y-axis* on the left represents the fraction of the cohort who survive at any given time; *y-axis* on the right represents relative risk; and *x-axis* represents time on dialysis. *p <0.05. (Reprinted from Fink JC, et al. Use of erythropoietin before the initiation of dialysis and its impact on mortality. *Am J Kidney Dis* 2001;37:348–355, with permission.)

CONCLUSION

In conclusion, the ESRD population is burdened by high morbidity and mortality rates. The number of persons with this disease is expected to grow rapidly over the next decade as the U.S. population, in general, ages and develops other diseases such as hypertension and diabetes, which are the primary causes of renal failure. The patient with impending ESRD has several choices for renal replacement therapy, and the nephrologists and other health care providers involved with his or her care should understand and present these choices in a timely fashion to the patient. There is no clear superior modality when comparing hemodialysis to peritoneal dialysis, and both options should be made available given the unique needs and preferences of each patient. Every patient should be offered the option of renal transplantation and undergo a timely evaluation to assess eligibility for placement on the transplant waiting list if a living donor is not available because there is compelling evidence that transplantation is the superior mode of renal replacement for many patients with ESRD. In most patients who are on dialysis it is important to follow their quality of care by tracking preestablished clinical performance measures. Although incremental improvements can be made in patients' quality of life while on dialysis, the most significant time point at which a provider can influence a patient's health and survival with ESRD is before he or she develops this condition. There is growing evidence that aggressive care and early intervention while a patient is afflicted with diminished but viable renal function has a beneficial effect on outcomes that endures after the onset of ESRD.

REFERENCES

1. U.S Renal Data System. USRDS 2001 annual data report: atlas of end-stage renal disease in the United States. Bethesda, MD: National Institute of Diabetes and Digestive and Kidney Diseases, 2001.
2. Xue JL, et al. Forecast of the number of patients with end-stage renal disease in the United States to the year 2010. *J Am Soc Nephrol* 2001; 12:2753–2758.
3. Jones CA, et al. Serum creatinine levels in the U.S. population: Third National Health and Nutrition Examination Survey. *Am J Kidney Dis* 1998;32:992–999.
4. Clase CM, et al. Prevalence of low glomerular filtration rate in nondiabetic Americans: Third National Health and Nutrition Examination Survey (NHANES III). *J Am Soc Nephrol* 2002;13:1338–1349.
5. Tierney WM, et al. Renal disease in hypertensive adults: effect of race and type II diabetes mellitus. *Am J Kidney Dis* 1996;13:485–493.
6. Tierney WM, et al. Effect of hypertension and type II diabetes on renal function in an urban population. *Am J Hypertens* 1990;3:69–75.
7. Klag MJ, et al. End-stage renal disease in African-American and white men: 16-year MRFIT findings. *JAMA* 1997;277:1293–1298.
8. Klag MJ, et al. Blood pressure and end-stage renal disease in men. *N Engl J Med* 1996;334:13–18.
9. Feldman HI, et al. End-stage renal disease in U.S. minority groups. *Am J Kidney Dis* 1992;19:397–410.
10. Brancati FL, et al. The excess incidence of diabetic end-stage renal disease among blacks: a population-based study of potential explanatory factors. *JAMA* 1992;268:3079–3084.
11. Smith SR, et al. Racial differences in the incidence and progression of renal diseases. *Kidney Int* 1991;40:815–822.
12. Whittle JC, et al. Does racial variation in risk factors explain black-white differences in the incidence of hypertensive end-stage renal disease? *Arch Intern Med* 1991;151:1359–1364.
13. Obrador GT, et al. Pre–end-stage renal disease care in the United States: a state of disrepair. *J Am Soc Nephrol* 2000;9:S44–S54.
14. Levin A, et al. Prevalent left ventricular hypertrophy in the predialysis population: identifying opportunities for intervention. *Am J Kidney Dis* 1996;27:347–354.
15. Stack AG. Determinants of modality selection among incident U.S. dialysis patients: results from a national study. *J Am Soc Nephrol* 2002; 13:1279–1287.
16. Stehman-Breen CO, et al. Determinants of type and timing of initial permanent hemodialysis access. *Kidney Int* 2000;57:639–645.
17. Bonomini V, et al. Benefits of early initiation of dialysis. *Kidney Int* 1985;28:S57–S59.
18. Ifudu O, et al. Excess morbidity in patients starting uremia therapy without prior care by a nephrologist. *Am J Kidney Dis* 1996;28: 841–845.
19. U.S. Renal Data System: USRDS 1994 annual data report. National Institutes of Health, National Institute of Diabetes and Digestive and Kidney Diseases. Bethesda, MD: National Institutes of Health, 1994.
20. Bloembergen WE, et al. Causes of death in dialysis patients: racial and gender differences. *J Am Soc Nephrol* 1994;5:1231–1242.
21. Pei YP, et al. Racial differences in survival of patients on dialysis. *Kidney Int* 2000;58:1293–1299.
22. Korbet SM, et al. Racial differences in survival in an urban peritoneal dialysis program. *Am J Kidney Dis* 1999;34:713–720.
23. Levey AS, et al. Controlling the epidemic of cardiovascular disease in chronic renal disease: what do we know? what do we need to learn? where do we go from here? *Am J Kidney Dis* 1998;32:853–908.
24. Collins AJ, et al. Cardiovascular disease in end-stage renal disease. *Am J Kidney Dis* 2001;38:S26–S29.
25. Bloembergen WE, et al. A comparison of mortality between patients treated with hemodialysis and peritoneal dialysis. *J Am Soc Nephrol* 1995;6:177–183.
26. Fenton SS, et al. Hemodialysis versus peritoneal dialysis: a comparison of adjusted mortality rates. *Am J Kidney Dis* 1997;30:334–342.
27. Vonesh EF, et al. Mortality in end-stage renal disease: a reassessment of differences between patients treated with hemodialysis and peritoneal dialysis. *J Am Soc Nephrol* 1999;10:354–362.
28. Collins AJ, et al. Mortality risks of peritoneal dialysis and hemodialysis. *Am J Kidney Dis* 1999;34:1065–1074.
29. Keshaviah P, et al. Survival comparison between hemodialysis and peritoneal dialysis based on matched doses of delivered therapy. *J Am Soc Nephrol* 2002;13:S48–S52.
30. Wolfe RA, et al. Comparison of mortality in all patients on dialysis, patients on dialysis awaiting transplantation, and recipients of a first cadaveric transplant. *N Engl J Med* 1999;341:1725–1730.
31. Ojo AO, et al. Survival in recipients of marginal cadaveric donor kidneys compared with other recipients and wait-listed transplant candidates. *J Am Soc Nephrol* 2001;12:589–597.
32. Ojo A, et al. Prognosis after primary renal transplant failure and the beneficial effects of repeat transplantation: multivariate analyses from the United States Renal Data System. *Transplantation* 1998;66: 1651–1659.
33. Garg PP, et al. Effect of the ownership of dialysis facilities on patients' survival and referral for transplantation. *N Engl J Med* 1999;341: 1653–1660.
34. Epstein AM, et al. Racial disparities in access to renal transplantation-clinically appropriate or due to underuse or overuse? *N Engl J Med* 2000;343:1537–1544.
35. Owens WF, et al. The urea reduction ratio and serum albumin concentration as predictors of mortality in patients undergoing hemodialysis. *N Engl J Med* 1993;29:1001–1006.
36. Collins AJ, et al. Urea index and other predictors of hemodialysis patient survival. *Am J Kidney Dis* 1994;23:272–282.
37. Parker TM, et al. Survival of hemodialysis patients in the United States is improved with a greater quantity of dialysis. *Am J Kidney Dis* 1994; 23:670–680.
38. Held PJ, et al. The dose of hemodialysis according to dialysis prescription in Europe and the United States. *Am J Kidney Dis* 1992;20: S16–S21.
39. Held PJ, et al. Five-year survival for end-stage renal disease patients in

the United States, Europe, and Japan, 1982 to 1987. *Am J Kidney Dis* 1990;15:451–457.

40. Held PJ, et al. The dose of hemodialysis and patient mortality. *Kidney Int* 1996;50:550–556.

41. Gotch FA, et al. A mechanistic analysis of the National Cooperative Dialysis Study (NCDS). *Kidney Int* 1985;28:526–531.

42. Sehgal AR, et al. Morbidity and cost implications of inadequate dialysis. *Am J Kidney Dis* 2001;37:1223–1231.

43. Greene T, et al. Design and statistical issues of the hemodialysis (HEMO) study. *Control Clin Trials* 2000;21:502–525.

44. Renal Physicians Association. *Clinical practice guidelines: adequacy of hemodialysis.* Washington, DC: Renal Physicians Association, 1993.

45. NKF-DOQI. NKF-DOQI clinical practice guidelines for hemodialysis adequacy. *Am J Kidney Dis* 1997;30[Suppl]:S15–S66.

46. Centers for Medicare & Medicaid Services. 2001 annual report: end-stage renal disease clinical performance measures project. *Am J Kidney Dis* 2002;39:S1–S98.

47. Daugirdas JT. Second generation logarithmic estimates of single-pool variable volume Kt/V: an analysis of error. *J Am Soc Nephrol* 1993;4:1205–1213.

48. Collins AJ, et al. Trends in anemia treatment with erythropoietin usage and patient outcomes. *Am J Kidney Dis* 1998;32:S133–S141.

49. Collins AJ, et al. Death, hospitalization, and economic associations among incident hemodialysis patients with hematocrit values between 36% to 39%. *J Am Soc Nephrol* 2001;12:2465–2473.

50. Frankenfield DL, et al. Racial/ethnic analysis of selected intermediate outcomes for hemodialysis patients: results from the 1997 ESRD Core Indicators Project. *Am J Kidney Dis* 1999;34:721–730.

51. Lowrie EG, et al. Death risk in hemodialysis patients: the predictive value of commonly measured variables and an evaluation of death rate differences between facilities. *Am J Kidney Dis* 1990;15:458–482.

52. Canada-USA Peritoneal Dialysis Study Group. Adequacy of dialysis and nutrition in continuous peritoneal dialysis: association with clinical outcomes. *J Am Soc Nephrol* 1996;7:198–207.

53. Paniaqua R, et al. Effects of increased peritoneal clearances on mortality rates in peritoneal dialysis: ADEMEX, a prospective, randomized, controlled trial. *J Am Soc Nephrol* 2002;13:1307–1320.

54. Obrador GT, et al. Early referral to the nephrologist and timely initiation of renal replacement therapy: a paradigm shift in the management of patients with chronic renal failure. *Am J Kidney Dis* 1998;31:398–417.

55. Levin A, et al. Multidisciplinary predialysis programs: quantifications and limitations of their impact on patient outcomes in two Canadian settings. *Am J Kidney Dis* 1997;29:533–540.

56. Wu MS, et al. Poor pre-dialysis glycaemic control is a predictor of mortality in type II diabetic patients on maintenance hemodialysis. *Nephrol Dial Transplant* 1997;12:2105–2110.

57. Foley RN, et al. The prognostic importance of left ventricular geometry in uremic cardiomyopathy. *J Am Soc Nephrol* 1995;5:2031.

58. Fink JC, et al. Use of erythropoietin before the initiation of dialysis and its impact on mortality. *Am J Kidney Dis* 2001;37:348–355.

SUBJECT INDEX

Page numbers in italics denote figures; those followed by *t* indicate tabular material.

A

Abdominal adhesions, 223, *223*
Access blood flow. *See also* Vascular access
    measurement, 57
    recirculation relationship, 65, 65*t*, 69
    thrombosis detection, 550
Access recirculation. *See* Recirculation
Access to treatment, 535
ACE inhibitors. *See* Angiotensin-
    converting enzyme inhibitors
Acebutolol, 240*t*, 242*t*
Acetaminophen poisoning, antidote, 570,
    571*t*, 575
Acetate buffer, 33–35, 396
    bicarbonate comparison, 33–35,
        396–397, 397*t*
    hemodynamic instability, 34, 34*t*,
        396–397
    high-efficiency, high-flux dialysis, 131
    and ventricular function, 34–35
Acetate-free biofiltration, 401
N-acetylcysteine
    in acetaminophen poisoning, 570,
        571*t*, 575
    in homocysteinemia poisoning, 270
N-acetyl procainamide poisoning, 576
N-acetyl-seryl-lysyl-proline levels, 469
Acid-base balance, 393–407
    and dialysate potassium, 31
    disorders in, 401–406
    general principles, 393
    in hemodialysis, 396–400, 397*t*, *398*
    in peritoneal dialysis, 393–396
Acidosis. *See* Metabolic acidosis
Acquired cystic kidney disease, 513–522
    clinical characteristics, 516–518
    complications, 517–518, 517*t*
    definition, 513
    demographics, 516, 517*t*
    and dialysis duration, 516, 517*t*
    differential diagnosis, 513
    pathogenesis, 515–516, *515*
    pathology, 513, *514–515*
    prevalence, 519*t*
    radiologic evaluation, 519–520

and renal cell carcinoma, 518–519
and renal transplantation, 519
screening, 521–522, 521*t*
ACTH, 370–372, 371*t*, 372*t*
ACTH stimulation test, 371, 371*t*
Activated charcoal, 570
    in hemoperfusion detoxification,
        573–574
    salicylate detoxification, 583
    theophylline detoxification, 586–587
Activated clotting time, 73
    appropriate level of, 74
    in children, 622, 624
Activities of daily living, and epoetin
    therapy, 473
Acute brain injury, 434
Acute hemodialysis. *See also* Acute renal
        failure
    children, 596–597, 596*t*, 620–623
    equipment-related complications, 108
Acute lymphoblastic leukemia, 431, 433
Acute on chronic hepatic failure, 431
Acute pancreatitis, 376–377
Acute renal failure, 160–180, 420–440
    and adult respiratory distress
        syndrome, 433
    children, 596–597, 596*t*, 620–623
    and congestive heart failure, 428–429
    continuous renal replacement
        therapies, 160–180, 420–440
        indications, 170, 421*t*
    definitions, 420
    dialysis dose and outcome, 421, *421*
    dialyzer membrane choice, 11
    extracorporeal blood purification,
        420–440
    and hepatic failure, 430–432
    intensive care units, 170–171,
        420–440
    mortality, 420
    and rhabdomyolysis, 427–428
    and sepsis, 425–427
Acute vascular access, 45–48, 528
Acyclovir, cytomegalovirus prevention,
    654

Adenosine, and intradialytic hypotension,
    285–286, *286*
Adequacy of hemodialysis. *See* Dialysis
    adequacy
Adhesions, peritoneal, 640
Adrenal hyperfunction, 371–372, 372*t*
Adrenal insufficiency, 370–371, 371*t*
Adrenomedullin, 234
Adult respiratory distress syndrome, 433
Advance directives, 536
Advanced glycosylation end-products
    and altered peritoneal function, 214
    atherosclerosis link, 271, 302
    β_2-microglobulin modification, 301
    inflammation role, 302, 313, *313*
    inhibitors, 303–304
    oxidative stress marker, 299, *300*, 301
    peritoneal membrane failure role,
        301–302
Advanced lipid peroxidation
    β_2-microglobulin modification, 301
    inhibitors, 303–304
    oxidative stress marker, 299, *300*, 301
Advanced oxidized protein products, 300,
    300, 301
Adynamic bone disease. *See* Aplastic
    adynamic bone disease
Aerobic work capacity, epoetin benefit,
    473
Affect Balance Scale, 559, 599*t*
African-Americans
    chronic kidney disease prevalence,
        662–663, *663*
    elderly dialysis patients, 526–527
    health-related quality of life, 565
    survival, 664–665
    underdialysis, 123
Age-adjusted estimation of creatinine
    clearance, 527, 527*t*
Age discrimination, dialysis access, 535
Age factors, quality of life, 564–565
Aging. *See* Geriatric dialysis patients
AIDS-associated nephropathy, survival,
    340
Air embolism, 47